ONCOLOGIC IMAGING

Pergamon Titles of Related Interest

Gross ONCOGENIC VIRUSES, Third Edition
Bentel TREATMENT PLANNING AND DOSE CALCULATION IN
RADIATION ONCOLOGY, Third Edition
Beall NMR DATA HANDBOOK FOR BIOMEDICAL APPLICATIONS
Foster MAGNETIC RESONANCE IN MEDICINE AND BIOLOGY

Related Journals*

INTERNATIONAL JOURNAL OF RADIATION
ONCOLOGY-BIOLOGY-PHYSICS
EUROPEAN JOURNAL OF CANCER AND CLINICAL ONCOLOGY
MEDICAL ONCOLOGY AND TUMOR PHARMACOTHERAPY
COMPUTERIZED RADIOLOGY
MAGNETIC RESONANCE IMAGING
ULTRASOUND IN MEDICINE AND BIOLOGY
INTERNATIONAL JOURNAL OF NUCLEAR MEDICINE & BIOLOGY
INTERNATIONAL JOURNAL OF APPLIED RADIATION
AND ISOTOPES

*Free specimen copies available upon request.

ONCOLOGIC IMAGING

Edited by

David G. Bragg, M.D.
University of Utah School of Medicine

Philip Rubin, M.D.
University of Rochester Cancer Center

James E. Youker, M.D.
Medical College of Wisconsin

PERGAMON PRESS
New York   Oxford   Toronto   Sydney   Frankfurt

Pergamon Press Offices:

U.S.A.	Pergamon Press Inc., Maxwell House, Fairview Park, Elmsford, New York 10523, U.S.A.
U.K.	Pergamon Press Ltd., Headington Hill Hall, Oxford OX3 0BW, England
CANADA	Pergamon Press Canada Ltd., Suite 104, 150 Consumers Road, Willowdale, Ontario M2J 1P9, Canada
AUSTRALIA	Pergamon Press (Aust.) Pty. Ltd., P.O. Box 544, Potts Point, NSW 2011, Australia
FEDERAL REPUBLIC OF GERMANY	Pergamon Press GmbH, Hammerweg 6, D-6242 Kronberg-Taunus, Federal Republic of Germany

Copyright © 1985 Pergamon Press Inc.

Library of Congress Cataloging in Publication Data
Main entry under title:

Oncologic imaging.

Includes index.
1. Cancer--Diseases--Diagnosis. 2. Diagnosis,
Radioscopic. 3. Imaging systems in medicine.
I. Bragg, David G. II. Rubin, Philip, 1927-
III. Youker, James E. [DNLM: 1. Neoplasms--radionuclide
imaging. 2. Neoplasms--radiography. QZ 241 O585]
RC270.O53   1984   616.99′40757   84-20578

ISBN 0-08-033653-1

Printed in Great Britain by A. Wheaton & Co. Ltd., Exeter

CONTENTS

1 THE STAGING AND CLASSIFICATION OF CANCERS

Philip Rubin
David G. Bragg

Once the histopathologic diagnosis of cancer is made, the most important decision in management is the first decision; the most important factor in the decision is the stage of the cancer or its anatomic extent.

Precise staging is one of the keys to cancer curability.[4] Rarely is there a second chance to salvage a cancer patient if the first decision regarding staging and treatment is ill-conceived. "For the purposes of classification of extent of cancer and of comparability of the results of treatment, a basic requirement is that the data be measurable, verifiable by others, and codifiable."[36]

The primary theme of this chapter is to place in perspective the process and purpose of tumor staging for both the oncologist and the radiologist. The foundation used for this discussion will be the *Manual for Staging of Cancer—1983*, published by the American Joint Committee for Cancer.[1] Because the specifics of staging and classification by body site will be the province of the chapters that follow, only a broad discussion of the principles and applications of this system will be covered here.

Clearly, the most important decision in the history of a cancer patient is the initial one, because it usually is the one that determines success or failure. A deliberate, well-designed program of tumor definition should be the hallmark of this initial decision, because it forms the basis of the staging process that follows. Consistent, well-designed imaging algorithms have not been widely accepted, therefore this process often appears to be more of an art than a science. To a large extent, the advantages and limitations of the various imaging procedures as well as their appropriate application to the demands of the staging process have not been defined in a deliberate, prospective manner.

The field of tumor imaging is no longer static; it is as dynamic as the rapidly evolving advances in imaging technology. As these imaging techniques become more refined, the microextensions of a neoplasm and its occult involvement of surrounding structures hopefully will be appreciated before the point at which therapeutic decisions are made.

DEFINITION AND TERMINOLOGY

Unfortunately, common usage has combined and confused the terms *staging* and *classification*. They refer to quite different but equally important aspects of tumor definition. In classifying a cancer, the clinician attempts to categorize all possible manifestations of the tumor. Classification is of necessity a multidimensional, multitemporal view of the disease and is a system for recording the facts observed by clinicians.

Staging may be defined as "a period or distinct phase in the course of a disease."[8] Staging is the process by which the anatomic extent of a tumor is defined at a certain point in time. Classification is therefore a means of recording facts, whereas staging implies an interpretation of these facts regarding prognosis.

The idea of the *stages* of a cancer does not imply a regular progression from stage I to stage IV; rather, these stages are arbitrary divisions, often related to prognosis and treatment. Final placement into a category depends on well-defined features. Diagnostic studies must be similarly applied in all cases. Factors that may prevent exact matching of patients in different series include such variables as age or associated medical diseases.

HISTORY OF STAGING AND CLASSIFICATION

The need for a universally acceptable scheme to classify cancers based on anatomic, histologic, and temporal variables became evident as soon as end results began to be reported. The literature reflected these differences in language, and cross comparisons of different patient series were impossible. The terms *early* and *late* and *operable* and *inoperable* had numerous individualized definitions and meanings.

In the 1920s, under the auspices of the League of Nations, gynecologists developed a system of classification and staging for cervical cancer. This scheme was used to characterize survival data from major cancer institutes worldwide. The concept of developing a consistent classification/staging system for all cancers remained largely dormant until after World War II. The Commission on Stage Grouping and Presentation of Results (ICPR) of the International Congress of Radiology (1953) and the International Union Against Cancer (UICC) subsequently did pioneering work in this field. The TNM (Tumor, Node, Metastasis) system was an outgrowth of these activities. Denoix,[25] working for the National Research Council Committee on Pathology, introduced the TNM language in an attempt to make the classification of cancer more consistent and accurate.

The American Joint Committee for Cancer Staging and End-Results Reporting was formally organized on January 9, 1959. The sponsoring organizations of the committee were the American Cancer Society, the American College of Pathologists, the American College of Physicians, the American College of Radiology, the American College of Surgeons, and the National Cancer Institute. The American College of Surgeons has served as the administrative sponsor of this committee since its inception. The charge of the committee was to develop a system of clinical staging of cancer by body site that was acceptable to the American medical community. Each of the sponsoring organizations has nominated members to serve on this committee. Development of the individual classification and staging systems was the product of various "task forces" appointed by the com-

mittee to consider cancers of respective anatomic sites. The scope of the American Joint Committee for Cancer Staging and End-Results Reporting gradually expanded to include the development of other staging systems (e.g., surgical evaluative staging, postsurgical treatment–pathologic staging), and the creation of checklists to allow more uniform characterization of each cancer site and thereby the promotion of the widespread use and appropriate application of classification/staging systems. In the interests of this expanded role, its name was changed in 1980 to the American Joint Committee on Cancer (AJC).

The older UICC, through its TNM Committee, adopted the TNM language for their classification system and began publication of their manual.[14] With the formation of the American Joint Committee for Cancer Staging and End-Results Reporting in 1959, a decision was made to adopt the TNM language in the development of their classification system. This was a landmark agreement in the history of the staging and classification of cancers. For the first time, the foundation for an international language and the potential for developing a unified staging classification system was at hand. Untold hours of effort on the part of the UICC and the AJC have continued to refine this system and promote its widespread acceptance. Both organizations have published pamphlets summarizing their systems of classification and staging. The first AJC manual for staging cancer was published in 1977 and the second edition was published in 1983.[1] Copies of this manual as well as booklets characterizing each anatomic site may be obtained free of charge through the offices of the American College of Surgeons.[1,14]

It is important to recognize that considerable controversy and differences in staging systems exist and that classification schemas continue to evolve. The use of the same letters (TNM) and Roman numerals (I–IV) have created a sense of uniformity in the literature. However, most systems have changed in the span of three decades that the UICC and AJC have been in existence. One needs only to scan the head and neck literature[2,3,32] as illustrated in Table 1-1 to recognize the degree of divergence as well as convergence among systems in different aspects. Diagnostic methods for Hodgkin's and non-Hodgkin's lymphomas have improved and increased in scope in recent years.[15] With the pragmatic adoption of the Ann Arbor system by the AJC and UICC, uniformity in reporting has eventuated. The histopathology is crucial to understanding non-Hodgkin's lymphomas[5,12,17,19,24] but classifications are constantly changing, whereas currently it is of less prognostic importance in Hodgkin's lymphoma. Occasionally a neoplastic disease undergoes a dynamic change and a new staging system emerges[16] as in Kaposi's sarcoma in AIDS patients. Some of the common cancer classifications respond to new imaging ap-

Table 1-1. Staging in Cancer of the Larynx

STAGE	UICC*	AJC†	NEILSON	LEDERMAN	TASKINEN AND HOLSTI	GARLAND	BRYCE ET AL.
I	$T_1N_0M_0$	$T_1N_0M_0$	$T_1N_0M_0$	$T_1N_0M_0$	$T_1N_0M_0$	$T_1N_0M_0$	$T_1N_0M_0$
II	$T_2N_0M_0$	$T_{2-4}N_0M_0$	$T_2N_0M_0^{\ddagger}$	$T_2T_3N_0M_0$§	$T_2N_0M_0$	$T_{2-3}N_0M_0$	$T_2N_0M_0$
	$T_1N_1M_0$				$T_1N_1M_0$		$T_1N_1M_0$
III	$T_{3-4}N_0M_0$	$T_{1-3}N_1M_0$	$T_2T_3N_0M_0$	$T_{2-4}N_0M_0$‖	$T_3N_0M_0$	$T_{1-3}N_1M_0$	$T_3N_0M_0$
	$T_{2-4}N_1M_0$			$T_1T_4N_1M_0$	$T_{2-3}N_1M_0$		$T_{2-3}N_1M_0$
	$T_{1-4}N_2M_0$				$T_{1-3}N_2M_0$		$T_{1-3}N_2M_0$
IV	$T_{1-4}N_3M_0$	$T_1N_1M_0$	$T_4N_0M_0$	$T_{1-4}N_{2-3}M_0$	$T_4N_{0-2}M_0$	$T_{1-4}N_2M_0$	$T_4N_0M_0$
	$T_{1-4}N_{0-3}M_1$	$T_{1-4}N_2M_0$	$T_{1-4}N_{1-3}M_0$	$T_{1-4}N_{0-3}M_1$	$T_{1-4}N_3M_0$	$T_{1-4}N_{0-3}M_1$	$T_{1-4}N_3M_0$
		$T_{1-4}N_{1-2}M_1$	$T_{1-4}N_{0-3}M_1$		$T_{1-4}N_{0-3}M_1$		$T_{1-4}N_{0-3}M_1$

*Unio Internationalis Contra Cancru (International Union Against Cancer).

†American Joint Committee on Cancer Staging and End Results Reporting.

‡Excluding cases with a fixed cord from Stage II even though the tumor may still be confined to the cords. Such cases are placed in Stage III.

§Mobility of larynx impaired but not lost or tumor extends beyond its tissue of origin.

‖Tumor with fixation of larynx or unilateral mobile cervical lymph node metastases or extralaryngeal infiltration.

Reprinted with permission from Vermund, H.: Role of radiotherapy in cancer of the larynx as related to the TNM system of staging. A review. *Cancer* 25:485–504, 1970.

proaches[27,33] and require refinement and alteration as in breast cancer[6,35] or because of different diagnostic or pathologic approaches as in colorectal cancer[7,22,28,39] or genitourinary cancers such as renal cancers,[13] bladder,[10,26] prostate[18,34,37] and testicular tumors.[21,23] Gynecologic cancer classification and staging systems have not changed considerably since their introduction in 1920, but they have been affected by new diagnostic operative procedures,[20] that is, laparotomy for staging of nodes to increase accuracy.[11] In these examples we have stressed the need for uniformity and agreement that recently evolved with the UICC and AJC systems. Furthermore, the "Unified and Symbolic Classification" approach advocated in this chapter is an attempt to have clinicians recognize the advantages of a simplified common cancer language to communicate their decisions and results.

PURPOSE AND OBJECTIVES OF CLASSIFICATION/STAGING SYSTEMS

As stated in the *Manual for Staging of Cancer—1983,* "proper classification and staging of cancer will allow the physician to determine treatment for the patient more appropriately, to evaluate results of management more reliably, and to compare statistics reported from various institutions more confidently."[1]

A classification scheme for cancers must encompass all the attributes of the tumor that define its life history. The AJC classification is based on the premise that cancers of similar histologic type or site of origin share similar patterns of growth and extension. Obviously, cancers exhibit a variety of different patterns of growth and ex-

tension based upon unique features of either the host or the tumor. A classification scheme must therefore encompass all potential manifestations of both the tumor and its host to be useful.

The complexities of cancer classification and staging are enormous, and it is a tribute to the efforts of the UICC and AJC to have developed a system that can be easily understood and applied in an unambiguous manner. It is only in this way that the information can be readily communicated to others, both to assist in institutional comparisons and to aid in the management of patients.

The objectives for a staging system can be briefly summarized:[14] (1) to aid the clinician in planning treatment; (2) to give some indication of prognosis; (3) to assist in the evaluation of end results; (4) to facilitate the exchange of information between treatment centers; and (5) to assist in the continuing investigation of cancer.

DEFINITION OF TERMINOLOGY—APPLICATION OF TNM SYSTEM

For the purposes of this book, the AJC classification system will be used, with notes commenting on other systems in broad use when appropriate. A proposed technique of description and classification applicable to all sites of cancer involves five basic steps:

1. Identification of the extent of disease by the use of the following symbols: T = extent of the primary tumor, N = condition of regional nodes, M = distant metastases—present or not evident.

2. Assignment of a series of subscripts to each of these three components, indicating ascending degrees of involvement (e.g., T_1, T_2, etc., and N_1, N_2, etc.).
3. Indication of the presence of metastatic disease by M_+ and absence by M_0. For certain sites, a number of specific M categories (M_1, M_2) may be desirable.
4. Grouping of the TNM assignments into a smaller number of clinical stages, usually four. This system makes it possible to regroup multiple categories (approximately 50) into similar staging systems.
5. Addition of supplementary information based upon the results of histologic examination by attaching the symbol (+), or symbols designating specific radiologic studies, such as lymphangiography (e.g., N_{1+}).

Histopathology is a vital attribute of any classification/staging system. The pattern of spread of a particular cancer often is a reflection of the specific cell type, its stage of differentiation, and the degree of anaplasia. The language for describing histopathology is now being standardized based on two major sources: the multiple volumes constituting the *Atlases of Tumor Pathology* published by the Armed Forces Institute of Pathology, and the World Health Organization efforts entitled *International Classification of Diseases for Oncology*.[25,38]

Temporal variables are defined in the TNM classification scheme to allow an update to occur after certain data have been obtained:

1. $_c$TNM clinical-diagnostic staging. This allows for the pretreatment characterization by the clinical examination and specific diagnostic studies to define the tumor and allow its comparison following treatment.
2. $_s$TNM surgical-evaluative staging. This terminology is applied following a major surgical exploration or biopsy.
3. $_t$TNM postsurgical treatment–pathologic staging. This term characterizes the extent of the cancer following thorough examination of the resected surgical specimen.
4. $_r$TNM retreatment staging. In instances in which the initial therapy has failed and additional treatment decisions are being considered, the disease is restaged under this terminology.
5. $_a$TNM autopsy staging. Final staging, after the postmortem study, is the terminology reserved for this designation.

There is no need to commit the various TNM systems to memory. The UICC and AJC manuals and, eventually, checklists serve this process elegantly. As Feinstein has indicated, the purpose of any classification is to affect the treatment decision and prognosis.[9]

Oncotaxonomy is the concept of one standard set of TNM definitions based on uniform criteria for all sites. The criteria are identified in Tables 1-2–1-4 and are based upon a linguistic analysis of the numerous TNM systems in which specific words defining extent of disease have been associated with certain categories.[30] The order of tumor progression is reflected in T_1, T_2, T_3, T_4, N_0, N_1, etc. A consistent cancer language allows for a uniform approach to tumor imaging and eventually to cancer staging and management decisions. Modifications will be required at individual sites, but the basic features will remain similar if not identical.

Tumor (T) Categories

The criteria for categorizing a primary tumor (T) is the apparent anatomic extent of the disease (Table 1-2) based on clinical, diagnostic imaging, surgical, or pathologic data. The extent commonly is dependent upon three features: depth of invasion, surface spread, and size. With the application of computed tomography, ultrasound, digital imaging techniques, and, in the near future, nuclear magnetic resonance imaging (NMR), these features should be more easily quantifiable.

Depth of invasion is a difficult yet a critical variable to be evaluated in defining any tumor. This is the main criterion used and primarily consists of the degree of invasion into adjacent or surrounding structures such as muscle, capsule, bone, cartilage, and other viscera. The loss of mobility or the fixation of the tumor to another structure is utilized in many schema.

Figure 1-1 illustrates, in a unified fashion, the variety of tissues that may be involved at different primary tumor sites in assessing tumor penetration. The fibrous capsule in solid organs, in contrast to the intrinsic muscle wall of hollow organs, is often the first tissue invaded by the cancer.

Surface spread is even more difficult to categorize, but may be related to the size of the tumor as well as the organ of origin. Whether the organ is solid or hollow also determines its description. In solid organs, the largest dimension of the measured tumor is the one most often used. In hollow organs, the size of the primary tumor is given in terms of the tumor's circumferential or longitudinal spread. Arbitrary divisions into regions can be used in some organs where a percentage of the surface area involved can be used in an attempt to quantify the extent of tumor spread (Table 1-2).

The size of a tumor is related to the number of cells present. This is more true "earlier" in the life of the tumor than later, when features such as hemorrhage or necrosis have intervened. Rate of tumor growth, cell removal or loss, and host resistance are obvious factors that will affect spread patterns. Even under the controlled conditions of the laboratory, the use of tumor volume as an estimate of rate of growth is fraught with error. As soon as the tumor becomes grossly palpable, changes in growth fraction, cell cycle, and cell loss occur. Nonethe-

Table 1-2. Specific Criteria Related to T Categories

	T_1	T_2	T_3	T_4
Depth of invasion				
Solid organs	Confined	Capsule muscle	Bone cartilage	Viscera
Hollow organs	Submucosa	Muscularis	Serosa	
Mobility	Mobile	Partial mobility	Fixed	Fixed and destructive
Neighboring structures	Not invaded	Adjacent (attached)	Surrounding (detached)	Viscera
Surface spread				
Regions (R)	$\frac{1}{2}$ or R_1	R_1	$R_1 + R_2$	$R_1 + R_2 + R_3$
Circumference	$< \frac{1}{3}$	$\frac{1}{3}$ to $\frac{1}{2}$	$> \frac{1}{2}$ to $\frac{2}{3}$	$> \frac{2}{3}$
Size (diameter)	< 2 cm	2 to 4–5 cm	> 4–5 cm	> 10 cm

less, these estimates are often provided as guidelines of tumor behavior and determine the stage.

Factors not used in categorizing primary tumors are location of the tumor within an organ, rate of tumor growth, multiplicity, and appearance of the tumor as either exophytic or endophytic. The reasons for this omission are the result of the difficulties involved in the relative weighting of each of these characteristics as well as their evaluation subsequent to treatment and in prognosis.

To understand the applications of this tumor classification, a *model system* is presented as an illustration. Two basic differences in application exist, depending upon whether the organ system in question is solid (Figure 1-1) or hollow (Figure 1-2) anatomically. The common example is as follows:

1. T_x—Tumor cannot be assessed.
2. T_0—No evidence of primary tumor, grossly or microscopically.
3. T_{is}—Carcinoma in situ.
4. T_1—A lesion confined to the organ of origin. The tumor is mobile, does not invade adjacent or surrounding structures or tissue, and is often superficial.
5. T_2—A localized lesion characterized by deep extension into adjacent structures or tissues. The invasion

CLASSIFICATION OF SOLID VISCERA

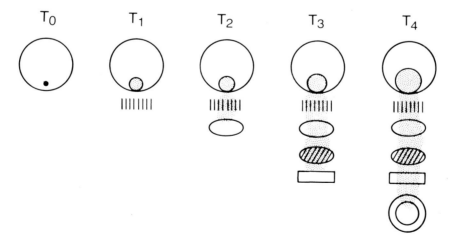

FIG. 1-1. Classification of solid viscera. This series of symbolic diagrams portrays the organ as a large circle and the dotted small circular areas as the cancer. The vertical lines are adjacent muscle, the clear oval is an adjacent attached structure, the lined oval is a surrounding—often detached—structure. The rectangle stands for bone or cartilage and the double circle, another viscera. The gravity of cancer spread or progress is identified in the sequential spread shown symbolically in most sites and is the basis of most classifications of T_1, T_2, T_3, and T_4. For a solid structure or site T_1 = confined to the organ of origin, usually 2.0 cm in its largest diameter, localized, mobile; T_2 = deeply invading, usually 2.0 cm to 4.0 or 5.0 cm in its largest diameter, localized, mobile, or partially mobile; T_3 = regionally confined, usually greater than 4.0 or 5.0 cm but less than 10 cm, fixed; T_4 = a massive lesion, greater than 10 cm in diameter, destructive, not confined to the region.

Reprinted with permission from Rubin, P.: A unified classification of tumors: An oncotaxonomy with symbols. *Cancer* **31**:963–982, 1973.

CLASSIFICATION OF HOLLOW VISCERA

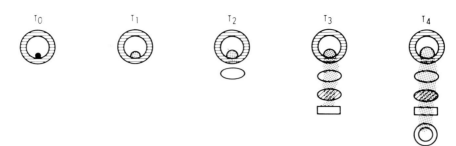

FIG. 1-2. Classification of hollow viscera. The model for classification of cancers of hollow viscera is illustrated by a linear arrangement of symbols for neighboring structures similar to the model for solid viscera. The major exception is the placement of muscle in the wall of the viscera compared with its juxtaposed relationship in numerous solid organs. The order of presentation of a hollow organ is T_1 = superficially invading, limited to mucosa or submucosa, less than one third of circumference, localized, occupying more than half of one region; T_2 = deeply invading, into muscularis, more than one third but less than one half of the lumen circumference, occupying more than half of the region, mobile; T_3 = invading all layers of the viceral wall, through serosa, into surrounding structures, fixed but not necessarily to bone, covering more than one half of a circumference, occupying more than one visceral region; T_4 = a massive, destructive lesion, causing a fistula or sinus, covering more than two thirds of the circumference, resulting in complete luminal obstruction, occupying more than two visceral regions.

Reprinted with permission from Rubin, P.: A unified classification of tumors: An oncotaxonomy with symbols. *Cancer* **31**:963–982, 1973.

is into the surrounding capsules, ligaments, intrinsic muscles, and adjacent, attached structures or similar tissues. There is some loss of tumor mobility, but it is not complete, therefore true fixation is not present.

6. T_3 — Advanced tumor that is confined to the region rather than the organ of origin, whether it is solid or hollow. The critical determinant is the presence of fixation, which indicates invasion into the adjacent, surrounding structures. These structures most often are bone or cartilage, but invasion of the extrinsic muscle walls, serosa, and skin should also be included. Invasion of surrounding detached structures of a different anatomy or function is in this category.

7. T_4 — A massive lesion extending into another hollow organ, causing a fistula, or into another solid organ, causing a sinus. Invasion of major nerves, arteries, and veins is also placed in this category. The destruction

of bone in addition to fixation is another advanced sign placing the tumor in this category.

Nodal (N) Categories

The establishment of lymph node categories is as critical in design as the T classification; however, the criteria currently used are more varied, vague in definition, and, occasionally, arbitrarily assigned. A unified code needs to be agreed upon more readily, and it is in this nodal category that more consistency needs to be achieved.

The criteria of node evaluation consist of size, firmness, capsular invasion, depth of invasion, mobility versus fixation, single versus multiple nodes, ipsilateral, contralateral, and bilateral distribution as well as distant nodal metastases (Table 1-3).

The *first station* is the cluster of lymph nodes receiv-

Table 1-3. Specific Criteria Related to N Categories

	N_1*	N_2	N_3	N_4
Station	First	First	First	Second
Drainage				
Unilateral	Ipsilateral	Ipsilateral	Ipsilateral	Contralateral
Bilateral	Ipsilateral	Contralateral or bilateral	Ipsilateral or contralateral	Distant
Number	Solitary	Multiple		
Size	<2 to 3 cm	>3 cm	>5 cm	>10 cm
Mobility	Mobile	Partial matted muscle invasion	Fixed to vessels, bone, skin	Fixed and destructive

*To distinguish N_0 from N_1 the specific criteria would include: Size—between 1–2 cm; Firmness—soft to hard; Roundness—½ cm to 1 cm. These are implied in most schemas and not spelled out.

ing direct drainage of a specific site or organ and is considered to be regional. The *second station* consists of those nodes that commonly receive lymph drainage from another lymph node rather than directly from the site or organ and is termed juxtaregional. The term that Rouvier introduced was that of a first and second station (echelon). When applied to lymph node anatomy, the first station is the first set of lymph nodes receiving the drainage of a specific organ but may not always be in the immediate anatomic region. This concept is a distinction with a meaningful clinical difference. It is important to note whether the drainage is unilateral or bilateral, since the assignment of contralateral nodes depends upon whether such contralateral nodes drain a site directly or indirectly, i.e., N_2 or N_4. There are many variations in nodal drainage, and in some sites there are multiple first stations.

Size is one of the most important criteria, in that a node must be palpable or detectable. When does a node reach a size to be considered significant, disregarding its firmness? Most place this size threshold at somewhat greater than 1.0 cm yet less than 3.0 cm. The use of size to categorize an ascending order of progression is not unlike the use of size in categorizing the primary tumor.

Firmness is another important criterion in differentiating the N_0 from the N_1.

Roundness refers to the measurement of nodal thickness and is implied in a hard "pea-sized" node. A discoid or flat node is usually a soft, ill-defined node. The rounder and firmer the node, the more likely it is to be involved by tumor.

The number of involved nodes is another variable in categorization. Solitary nodal involvement, as distinct from multiple nodal involvement, is commonly considered. The presence of multiple nodes is often associated with invasion of the capsule of the node, resulting in matting or clustering and eventually in a loss of mobility.

Mobility versus fixation is an important criterion in considering progression. The term *fixation* is used but rarely defined in classification schema. The loss of mobility of a lymph node is due to invasion of the nodal capsule. Matted nodes or invasion into the fascia of a muscle reduces lateral and vertical mobility. The node can no longer be rolled in all directions. Invasion into muscle can be determined by loss of mobility upon contraction of the muscle. Complete fixation refers to the direct invasion of bone, major blood vessels, or skin.

As in the primary (T) category above, a model classification for illustrating the application of a unified system to lymph node (N) involvement is presented. Figure 1-3 summarizes this model classification.

1. N_x — Regional nodes cannot be assessed clinically.
2. N_0 — Regional lymph nodes are not demonstrably abnormal. This category, quite surprisingly, represents

a significant point of conflict between the classifications used by the UICC and the AJC. The issue is the absence of palpable nodes versus the finding of palpable but not clinically significant adenopathy. In the latter situation, soft, ill-defined lymph nodes usually less than 1 cm in size are the clinical finding in question. These palpable, flat nodes of little significance are listed as N_0 in the AJC classification but N_{1a} in the UICC system. In the interest of reaching a common agreement, the AJC has adopted the UICC designations.

3. N_1 — A palpable, freely movable lymph node, 3 cm or less in diameter, limited to the first station of involvement. A distinction must again be made between an uninvolved node and an involved node. Metastases are suggested, but on lymph node firmness and roundness of the node rather than its size alone.
4. N_2 — Firm to hard lymph nodes, palpable yet partially movable, ranging in size from 3 cm to 5 cm. Such nodes may show microscopic evidence of capsular invasion, and clinically they may be matted together, demonstrating partial fixation to adjacent muscle. These nodes may be contralateral or bilateral if the primary tumor drains to both sides by virtue of its anatomy, but involvement is confined to the first station. The presence of multiple lymph nodes does not change this category provided the nodes are confined to the regional, primary station center and not matted together. Mobility is reduced and the nodes cannot be moved in all directions.
5. N_3 — Fixation is complete; the nodes have invasion beyond their capsule with complete fixation to adjacent bone, large blood vessels, skin (dermal lymphatic invasion), or to the nerves (perineural invasion).
6. N_4 — This category is reserved for lymph node involvement beyond the first station, in second or more distant stations. Extensive nodal necrosis, leading to destruction of bone and skin (fistula formation) or massive size (10 cm or greater) should also be placed in this category.

Metastases (M) Categories

Some debate exists over whether the metastatic category should be expanded to reflect solitary metastases as well as the number of metastatic lesions or anatomic sites involved. At the present time, the M category is dealt with simplistically as follows:

1. M_x — The presence of metastatic disease is not assessed.
2. M_0 — No evidence of metastatic disease.
3. M_1 — Distant metastases are present. The specific sites for metastatic disease should be individually noted.

The lack of a consistent and thorough attempt to categorize an anatomic extent of metastases is conspicuous

CLASSIFICATION OF LYMPH NODES

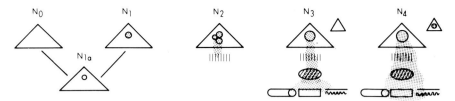

FIG. 1-3. Classification of lymph nodes. The triangle stands for a node-bearing region. The large triangle represents the first station node or regional node and the small triangle is the second station or juxtaregional node. The dotted small circular area(s) is the cancer. The vertical lines are muscle, the lined oval is a surrounding, separate structure(s), the rectangle is bone or cartilage, the cylinder represents blood vessels, and the horizontal double lines, skin. The order of progression of the cancer extends as shown with increasing involvement of surrounding structures in N_1, N_2, N_3, and in N_4 (see text).

Reprinted with permission from Rubin, P.: A unified classification of tumors: An oncotaxonomy with symbols. *Cancer* 31:963–982, 1973.

in current schema (Table 1-4). The important feature is the presence or absence of a metastasis, i.e., M_0 v M_1. The reason for this reflects the poor prognosis if metastases are present. Nevertheless, cure, although rare, is possible for some solitary metastases. As chemotherapy becomes more effective and results are assessed, there will be a need to categorize and subclassify this group of patients.

Our proposed classification,[30,31] of metastases is based upon the criteria of the number of metastases, the number of organ systems involved, and the degree of functional impairment present. The designation of M_x for no metastatic workup should only be used when the likelihood of metastatic disease is considered low, rather than merely using M_0. Subscripts for selected sites are shown.

The following classification schema is offered (Figure 1-4):

- M_0 — No evidence of metastases.
- M_{1a} — Solitary, isolated metastasis confined to one organ or anatomic site.
- M_{1b} — Multiple metastatic foci confined to one organ system or one anatomic site, i.e., lungs, skeleton, liver, etc., no function to minimal functional impairment.
- M_{1c} — Multiple organs involved anatomically, no or minimal to moderate functional impairment of involved organs.
- M_{1d} — Multiple organs involved anatomically, moderate to severe functional impairment of involved organs.
- M_x — No metastatic workup done.
- M modified to show viscera involved by letter subscript — pulmonary metastases (M_p), hepatic (M_h), osseous (M_o), skin (M_s), brain (M_b), etc.
- M_+ — Microscopic evidence of suspected metastases, confirmed by pathologic examination.
- NB — Visceral involvement by direct extension is not considered a metastasis.

Stage Grouping

The problem of having four categories for the primary tumor (T), and four categories for regional nodes (N), plus two categories for metastases (M) means that each patient can be placed in 32 different categories.

This number of stages is unmanageable for the clinician, and the reduction to four stage groupings has become clinical custom. The challenge in developing a unified stage grouping system thus is in determining which T and N categories to combine. The major clinical consideration is to determine which T and N categories have similar prognostic significance. Furthermore, the sum

Table 1-4. Specific Criteria Related to M Categories

	M_{1a}	M_{1b}	M_{1c}	M_{1d}
Number of metastases	1	>1	Multiple	Multiple
Number of organs	1	1	Multiple	Multiple
Impairments	0	Minimal	Minimal to moderate	Moderate to severe

M: Modified to show viscera involved by lettered subscript as: pulmonary (M_p), hepatic (M_h), osseous (M_o), skin (M_s), brain (M_b), etc.

M_+: Microscopic evidence of suspected metastases, confirmed by pathologic examination.

METASTATIC TAXONOMY

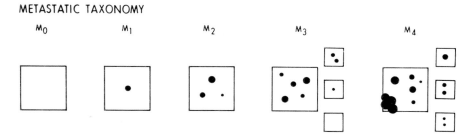

FIG. 1-4. Each box stands for a visceral organ(s) and the number of black dots for the number of metastatic lesions. The stages are explained in the text and the order of progression is M_{1a}, M_{1b}, M_{1c}, and M_{1d}. The number of organs and number of metastases increases (see text).

Reprinted with permission from Rubin, P.: A unified classification of tumors: An oncotaxonomy with symbols. *Cancer* 31:963–982, 1973.

total of both components may be greater than either of their parts, or the nodal category may outweigh considerations at the primary site. It is because of these varying circumstances that four possibilities with regard to stage of T lesion and to its N_1 equivalence are shown in a grid analysis, which has been employed as shown in four different cancers (Figure 1-5).

• $N_1 = T_1$ as in lung cancer.[1,9]
• $N_1 = T_2$ as in breast cancer.[1,9]

• $N_1 = T_3$ as in cervical cancer.[1,9]
• $N_1 = T_4$ as in larynx cancer.[9,25]

Is there a common characteristic or feature? Prognostic outcome is the most obvious consideration. Alternate considerations relate to (1) the resectability of the primary tumor and its node stations, and (2) the geographic extent of the primary tumor, which is equal to the distance of the lymph node station.

THE PROCESS OF CLASSIFICATION AND STAGING

There is a need to define both the minimum and optimum diagnostic workup that establishes the extent or stage of the cancer. It is here that the precision of the diagnostic oncologic imager must play a vital role. Differences exist here with respect to the UICC and AJC classification systems. The UICC system declares all diagnostic radiologic procedures and endoscopy used in the evaluation of the cancer to be acceptable but does not include the operative findings. Operative findings are allowed in some specific sites that are inaccessible, such as in ovarian tumor categories. The AJC allows inclusion of all types of examinations ordinarily available to the average specialist. Surgical and pathologic findings are not used in assigning a clinical stage, except in certain sites where specific procedures are necessary in the determination of the stage. One of the major sources for confusion is the use of different studies and criteria to arrive at the definition of extent of the cancer. Unless the criteria and examinations for definition are standardized, different groups of patients may be mistakenly placed in similar categories.

In brief, there are four steps in the definition of the extent of any given tumor:

1. Clinical staging: The evaluation of the apparent extent, based on physical examination, routine labora-

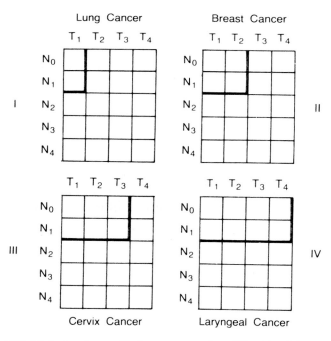

FIG. 1-5. In the above grid, the stage grouping of N_1 with a T lesion varies with different sites so that stage I disease in lung is T_1N_1. Stage II in breast is T_2N_1, stage III in cervix is T_3N_1, and stage IV in larynx is T_4N_1.

Reprinted with permission from Rubin, P.: A unified classification of tumors: An oncotaxonomy with symbols. *Cancer* 31:963–982, 1973.

tory studies, radiographic and endoscopic procedures.

2. Radiographic staging: The use of sophisticated radiographic procedures such as selective arteriography, computerized tomography, digital radiography, lymphangiography, etc., in tumor evaluation.

3. Surgical staging: Inclusion of the results of the exploratory procedure employed in the identification of the extent of a cancer, such a laparotomy in Hodgkin's disease or ovarian cancer.

4. Pathologic staging: The use of a biopsy procedure and histologic evaluation to determine the depth of invasion, histopathologic type, and presence or absence of nodal disease.

It is important to avoid interchanging clinical, surgical, or pathologic staging in reporting results unless it is specified and generally accepted. Categories for reporting these individual results are specified and summarized by the AJC system (see p. 6, *Manual for Staging of Cancer*[1]).

The inclusion of specific categories to modulate the classification system at different time periods using surgical, pathologic, and retreatment staging data is critical to the staging process. Often there is a tendency to supplant the clinical staging by surgical staging. This has been one of the missed opportunities in guiding clinical judgments because of the manner in which the data are recorded in the literature. If the clinical and radiologic assessments were made first, then restaging allocations into new categories based on surgical and pathological findings would improve the accuracy of both clinical and radiological evaluation. In fact, surgical exploration for staging rather than for resection is a redirection of surgical effort and is essential to multidisciplinary decision making. The criteria for each step in the staging sequence should be clearly indicated and the oncologist should not confuse these procedural steps and assignments. The transition from a clinical-diagnostic radiologic staging to a postsurgical pathologic staging, as an example, marks the transition from a unidisciplinary to a multidisciplinary cancer management strategy.

ONCOLOGIC ANATOMY AND STAGING FOR TUMOR DEFINITION

The normal anatomy of the site of origin of a neoplasm determines to a large degree its spread pattern and in turn its clinical manifestations. Although the tumor's spread pattern may appear to be random, it is largely predetermined by the surrounding anatomic structures, its lymphatics, and venous drainage. A cancer tends to follow the paths of least resistance and acts as a dissecting knife separating tissues along planes of cleavage. There are few tissues that can withstand its relentless

spread; with few exceptions, the outcome is ultimate invasion and destruction of virtually all tissues. Fascia, peritoneum, and the dura are tough, firm connective tissue barriers; regional lymph nodes may act as mechanical or immunologic barriers, and cartilage more than bone can halt its spread temporarily, containing the disease in a local or regional area.

If tissues are well vascularized or rich in lymphatics, the neoplasm will invade fine venules and lymphatic channels. Vocal cord cancers are poor in lymphatics and rarely involve lymph nodes, in contrast to supraglottic cancers and hypopharyngeal cancers, where lymph node spread is common, reflecting the richer lymphatic bed normally in these anatomic structures. The aggressiveness of the tumor is obviously a major factor determining tumor behavior, but the areolar planes and fat spaces present in most anatomic sites provide the receptive soil in which dissemination can occur (Figure 1-6).

The diagnostic imager needs to understand the exact location of regional lymph nodes. For lymph nodes, an ascending order of progression implies increasing lymph node involvement. As Rouvier advised,[29] the concept of regional node-bearing areas should be based upon sound anatomic and physiologic principles, since the lymph nodes in the anatomic region of the specific organ do not consistently receive all the lymph flow of that organ. Thus, the ovaries do not usually drain into the external iliac nodes, nor do the testes drain into inguinal nodes—each, in fact drains largely into the para-aortic lymph nodes.

Understanding normal anatomy is essential to oncologic diagnostic imaging. The anatomic structures should and can be visualized three-dimensionally. With the introduction of computerized transverse axial tomography and with nuclear magnetic resonance imaging on the horizon, reconstruction into other planes is providing a better window for cancer imaging. The primary purpose of this volume is to enable the oncologist, the radiologist, and the surgeon to become aware of the process of tumor staging after tumor diagnosis is made. It is essential to define as precisely as possible in three dimensions the neoplastic configuration wherever it is located. As stated initially, precise staging is the key to cancer curability.

CONCLUSION

The focus of this book is to fuse elements of the cancer, its anatomic site of origin, the classification staging process, and oncologic diagnostic procedural expertise. In each chapter, this theme will be developed and placed in the perspective of the imaging technology appropriate to that problem.

The use of decision trees accompanied by average procedural costs will be used as illustrations for each anatomic site. The choice of sequencing diagnostic imaging

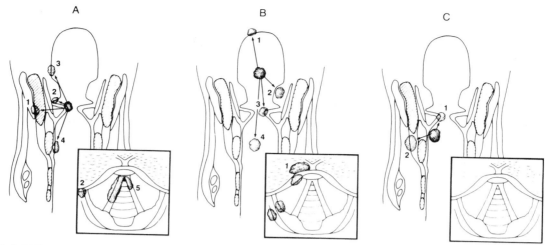

FIG. 1-6. The pattern of spread of laryngeal cancer is determined by the normal surrounding anatomy depending upon the location of the lesion. If it is in the true cord or glottis (A), it can spread into (1) the paralaryngeal space and thyroid cartilage: (2) the ventricle; (3) the supraglottic region; (4) the subglottic region; or (5) the opposite cord via the anterior commissure. If it is in the supraglottic area (B), it can spread into (1) the vallecula; (2) the pyriform sinus; as well as (3) the glottis, and (4) the subglottic region. If it is in the subglottic region (C), it can spread into (1) the true cord; and (2) the paralaryngeal and paratracheal space.

studies often is in a state of flux and is even controversial. Where data exist, comparative results will be used to guide the selection and sequencing of these studies. As mentioned earlier, the absence of well-controlled prospective trials of randomly designed imaging studies frustrates the evaluation of this process in the oncologic setting. Where appropriate, succinct illustrations will be used to persuade the reader of the correctness of the chosen imaging sequence. In the final analysis, however, each patient's imaging needs should be individualized depending upon his or her own unique tumor/host characteristics. The fusion of known pathologic patterns of tumor spread with different stages of advancement will also determine the aggressiveness of the staging workup. In summary, tumor imaging, precise staging, cancer curability, and multimodal management are interlocked and promise change and improvement in the future.

REFERENCES

1. American Joint Committee on Cancer: *Manual for Staging of Cancer*, 2nd ed. Philadelphia, J. P. Lippincott, 1983.
2. Baker, H. W.: Staging of head and neck cancer. *Int. Adv. Surg. Oncol.* 6:1–24, 1983.
3. Black, R. J., Gluckman, J. L.: Staging systems for cancer of the head and neck region—comparison between AJC and UICC. *Clin. Otolaryngol.* 8:305–312, 1983.
4. Carr, D. T.: Is staging of cancer of value? *Cancer* 51(Suppl.):2503–2505, 1983.
5. Castellino, R. A., Dunnick, N. R., Goffinet, D. R., Rosenberg, S. R., Kaplan, H. S.: Predictive value of lymphography for sites of subdiaphragmatic disease encountered at staging laparotomy in new-

ly diagnosed Hodgkin's disease and non-Hodgkin's lymphoma. *J. Clin. Oncol.* 1:532–536, 1983.
6. Cuschieri, A., Irving, A. D., Robertson, A. J., Clark, J., Wood, R. A.: Percentage malignant involvement: a new concept in staging of breast cancer. *Ann. R. Coll. Surg. Engl.* 65:11–13, 1983.
7. Davis, N. C., Newland, R. C.: Terminology and classification of colorectal adenocarcinoma: the Australian clinico-pathological staging system. *Aust. N.Z. J. Surg.* 53:211–221, 1983.
8. *Dorland's Illustrated Medical Dictionary*, 24th ed. Philadelphia, W. B. Saunders, 1965.
9. Feinstein, A. R.: *Clinical Judgement*. Huntington, NY, Robert E. Krieger Publishing Co., 1974.
10. Fryjordet, A., Skatun, J.: Staging of urinary bladder cancer by computerized tomography compared to clinical staging and postoperative pathologic staging. *J. Oslo. City Hosp.* 33:76–79, 1983.
11. Gerbie, M. V.: Malignant tumors of the vagina. Classification and approach to treatment. *Rostard Med.* 73:271–282, 1983.
12. Glimelius, B., Haeberg, H., Sundstrom, C.: Morphological classification of non-Hodgkin malignant lymphoma. II. Comparison between Rappaport's classification and the Kiel classification. *Scand. J. Haematol.* 30:13–24, 1983.
13. Hata, Y., Tada, S., Kato, Y., Onishi, T., Masuda, F., Machida, T.: Staging of renal cell carcinoma by computed topography. *J. Comput. Assist. Tomogr.* 7:828–832, 1983.
14. International Union Against Cancer: *TNM Atlas: Illustrated Guide to the Classification of Malignant Tumours*. Heidelberg, Springer-Verlag, 1982.
15. Joshua, D. E., Dalgleish, A., Kronenberg, H.: Is staging laparotomy necessary in patients with supradiaphragmatic stage I and IIA Hodgkin's disease? *Lancet* 1:847–848, 1984.
16. Krigel, R. L., Laubenstein, L. J., Muggia, F. M.: Kaposi's sarcoma: a new staging classification. *Cancer Treat. Rep.* 67:531–534, 1983.
17. Krueger, G. R., Medina, J. R., Klein, H. O., Knorads, A., Zach, J., Rister, M., Janik, G., Evers, K. G., Hirano, T., Kitamura, H., Bedoya, V. A.: A new working formulation of non-Hodgkin's lymphomas. A retrospective study of the new NCI classification proposal in comparison to the Rappaport and Kiel classifications. *Cancer* 52:833–840, 1983.

18. Lange, P. H., Narayan, P.: Understanding and undergrading of prostate cancer. Argument for postoperative radiation as adjuvant therapy. *Urology* **21**:113–118, 1983.

19. Leonard, R. C., Cuzick, J., MacLennan, I. C., Vanhegan, R. I., Mackie, P. H., McCormick, C. V.: Prognostic factors in non-Hodgkin's lymphoma: the importance of symptomatic stage as adjunct to the Kiel histopathological classification. *Br. J. Cancer* **47**:91–102, 1983.

20. Maggino, T., Bonetto, F., Catapano, P., Franco, F., Valente, S., Marchesoni, D.: Clinical staging versus operative staging in cervical cancer. *Clin. Exp. Obstet. Gynecol.* **10**:201–204, 1983.

21. Maricek, B., Brutschin, P., Triller, J., Fuchs, W. A.: Lymphography and computed tomography in staging nonseminomatous testicular cancer: limited detection of early stage metastatic disease. *Urol. Radiol.* **5**:243–246, 1983.

22. Mauro, M. A., Lee, J. K., Heiken, J. P., Balfe, D. M.: Radiologic staging of gastrointestinal neoplasms. *Surg. Clin. North Am.* **64**:67–84, 1984.

23. McCauley, R. L., Javadpour, N.: Supraclavicular node biopsy in staging of testicular carcinoma. *Cancer* **51**:359–361, 1983.

24. Moir, D. H.: War of the words: classification of non-Hodgkin's lymphomas. *Pathology* **15**:359–360, 1983.

25. National Research Council Committee on Pathology: *Atlas of Tumor Pathology*. Washington, Armed Forces Institute of Pathology, 1950–present.

26. Nelson, R. P.: New concepts in staging and follow-up of bladder carcinoma. *Urology* **21**:105–112, 1983.

27. Osborne, M. P., Meijer, W. S., Yeh, S. D., DeCosse, J. J.: Lymphoscintigraphy in the staging of solid tumors. *Surg. Gynecol. Obstet.* **156**:384–391, 1983.

28. Pheils, M. T.: Staging of large bowel cancer. *Med. J. Aust.* **1**:254–255, 1984.

29. Rouvier, H.: *Anatomie des Lymphatiques des l'Homme*. Paris, Masson, 1932.

30. Rubin, P.: A unified classification of tumors: An oncotaxonomy with symbols. *Cancer* **31**:963–982, 1973.

31. Rubin, P., Keys, H.: The staging and classification of cancer: A unified approach. In *Principles of Cancer Treatment*, Carter, S. K., Glatstein, E., Livingston, R. B. (Eds.). New York, McGraw-Hill, 1982, pp. 14–25.

32. Sakai, S., Ebihara, T., Ono, I., Taketa, C.: A comparison of AJC and JJC proposals on TNM classification of maxillary sinus carcinoma. *Arch. Otorhinolaryngol.* **237**:139–146, 1983.

33. Shibata, H. R.: Lymphoscintigraphy in the staging of breast cancer. *Can. J. Surg.* **26**:487–488, 1983.

34. Spirnak, J. P., Resnick, M. I.: Clinical staging of prostatic cancer: new modalities. *Urol. Clin. North Am.* **11**:221–235, 1984.

35. Stenkvist, B., Bengtsson, E., Eriksson, O., Jarkrans, T., Nordin, B., Westman-Naeser, S.: Histopathologic systems of breast cancer classification: reproducibility and clinical significance. *J. Clin. Pathol.* (Suppl.) (R. Coll. Pathol.) **36**:392–398, 1983.

36. Symposium: Obstacles to the control of Hodgkin's disease. *Cancer Res.* **26**:1047–1311, 1966.

37. Whitmore, W. E. Jr.: Natural history and staging of prostate cancer. *Urol. Clin. North Am.* **11**:205–220, 1984.

38. World Health Organization: *International Classification of Diseases for Oncology*, 1st ed. Geneva, WHO, 1976.

39. Zinkin, L. D.: A critical review of the classifications and staging of colorectal cancer. *Dis. Colon Rectum* **26**:37–43, 1983.

2 IMAGING STRATEGIES FOR ONCOLOGIC DIAGNOSIS AND STAGING

David G. Bragg

A well-designed imaging strategy is an implicit component of the approach to a patient with cancer. In the field of oncology, uncertainty augmented by unfamiliarity is often shared by both the clinician, with regard to the imaging technique, and the radiologist, with respect to the disease. The purpose of this chapter is to provide an introduction and an overview of the imaging process for the organ site chapters that follow. Specifically, the province of this section will be to create a template for setting the diagnostic process in motion as well as to provide a discussion of imaging techniques, including their current problems and opportunities in the near future.

Radiology plays a more dominant diagnostic role in most other disease settings than in oncology. The primary applications of imaging procedures in the patient with cancer are in tumor definition, staging and follow-up. There are notable exceptions to this statement (mammography and hollow organ GI examination). Nonetheless, experience has demonstrated that random screening, utilizing radiographic studies, cannot be justified in view of both yield and cost.

In taking stock of the advances that the field of oncology has enjoyed in the past few decades, most have involved improvements in treatment, with few in the area of cancer detection. Certainly diagnostic tools have become more sophisticated, accurate, and specific, but have these improved imaging techniques identified a population of smaller tumors that resulted in improved overall survival? In large measure, the answer is clearly no. The reasons are many, complex, and controversial, but they must be reviewed to place the problem in its proper perspective. Several factors will be considered, including such limitations as the imaging process, the disease, and treatment considerations that are relevant to the discussion.

TUMOR SIZE — IS THERE AN OPTIMAL DETECTION THRESHOLD?

Tumor size or volume (the T component of the American Joint Committee staging system) has an obvious, major impact on both the treatment decision process and patient outcome. Unfortunately, tumor size alone is only a part of the problem, since similarly sized cancers of varying location and histologic type may behave in vastly different manners. Nonetheless, there is evidence to suggest that the detection of a cancer at a smaller size or volume (hence "earlier age") that can be effectively treated should result in a more favorable outcome. It should therefore follow that those involved in oncologic imaging need to refine their diagnostic tools with a goal of detecting tumors at ever smaller sizes. Obvious relevant questions that should be asked are

1. What should this "threshold size" realistically be?
2. In what organ systems are the techniques most in need of improvement?
3. What data are available to validate the assumption that improved survival will result from cancer detection at an "earlier" stage or smaller volume?

4. What are the practical detection/resolution limitations of current and near term future imaging techniques?

Threshold tumor size is difficult to define. From an imaging standpoint, the limits of resolution of the various imaging systems in use today can be generally characterized. There are both objective and subjective limitations to these detection variables. In part, they are related to equipment (spatial and contrast resolution), patient and target organ considerations, and interobserver variations. Advances in equipment design, new techniques and systems, as well as the educational process have narrowed this gap, but, at present and probably for the foreseeable future, practical end points in lesion size resolution have been reached. Table 2-1 summarizes several common imaging techniques, broadly defines the advantages and limitations of each, and assigns an esti-

mate of the tumor detection threshold for each system by organ site. A number of assumptions are made to illustrate rough approximations of tumor size thresholds visible by each technique to serve the purposes of comparison.

Are current techniques adequate to meet this challenge? In most instances, the answer again is probably no. Experiments with a number of animal and human cancer models have shown that tumor growth is exponential (Figure 2-1) and proceeds along predictable lines until its volume reaches 3 or 4 mm^2. The nutrition of the cancer up to this time is derived from the extravascular compartment, probably by diffusion. Subsequent to this 3–4 mm^2 stage, the cluster of cancer cells develops an independent ability to induce its own vascular supply, possibly through the elaboration of a substance called tumor angiogenesis factor. From this time on, the tumor is able to stimulate new capillaries and ac-

Table 2-1. Imaging Detection Thresholds

IMAGING TECHNIQUE	THRESHOLD (CM) BRAIN	LUNG	LIVER	BONE	LYMPH NODE	PANCREAS	KIDNEY	COMMENTS
Plain films	N.A.	1.0	N.A.	2.0 +	N.A.	N.A.	N.A.	*Lung*—low-contrast objects with obscure margins amplify problem *Bone*—must be large in medullary cavity or involve cortex
Film tomography	N.A.	0.5	N.A.	0.5	N.A.	N.A.	N.A.	*Lung*—improves detection efficiency *Bone*—allows matrix of tumor and soft tissue component to be seen
Ultrasound	N.A.	N.A.	1.5–2.0	N.A.	2.0 +	1.5–2.0	1.0–2.5	Operator- and patient-dependent technology—"thresholds" variable and difficult to define
Computed tomography	1.0–1.5	0.2–0.5	1.0–1.5	0.5–1.0	1.0–2.0	1.5–2.0	1.0	Detection efficiency determined by anatomic location, size, and tumor type
Lymphography	N.A.	N.A.	N.A.	N.A.	0.5	N.A.	N.A.	Able to define intrinsic node defects. Fails to opacify many node groups visible by CT
Angiography	1.5–2.0	limited application	1.0–1.5	variable	N.A.	1.5–2.0	1.0–1.5	Detection efficiency based on tumor vascularity
Digital techniques	2.0–3.0	0.5–1.0	?	0.5–1.0	N.A.	N.A.	1.5–2.5	Used as angio substitute. Will have reduced detection efficiency in return for less cost and morbidity. Digital imaging will allow contrast enhancement
Magnetic resonance imaging	1.0–1.5	0.5	1.0–1.5	N.A.	1.0–2.0	1.5–2.0	1.0	Assumes similar spatial resolution with CT with improved detection efficiency in base of brain, head and neck. Unknown with body imaging
Conventional nuclear imaging	1.5–2.0	Variable (^{67}Ga)	2.0–2.5	0.5–1.0	variable (replaced nodes not visualized)	N.A.	N.A.	*Brain*—occasionally useful when CT not available or as adjunct *Liver*—cost-effective screen formats in appropriate setting *Bone*—Essential for screening
Monoclonal antibody imaging	?	?	?	?	?	?	?	Unknown impact—promises to define smaller tumor burdens in all body sites

N.A. = not applicable

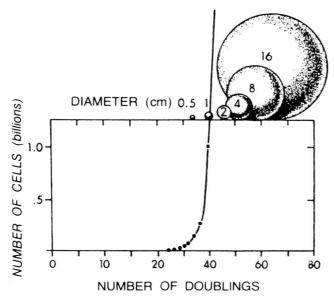

FIG. 2-1. Arithmetic depiction of the growth curve of a hypothetical tumor. Note the number of doublings necessary to reach a diameter of 1 cm and the relatively rapid increase thereafter. As the tumor grows, it assumes any of a number of forms that usually, but not always, correlate with biologic behavior. Benign tumors tend to have a spherical configuration corresponding to their symmetrical, controlled growth. This can be altered by their location and the confines of contiguous structures. These benign growths compress and push normal tissue. They also often demonstrate a capsule. In general, malignant neoplasms expand, invade, and destroy normal adjacent tissue. Their outline is usually irregular and poorly defined. When arising from an epithelial-lined surface, they often cause ulceration as they destroy and invade underlying tissue. In other instances, they grow as large fungating luminal masses. This growth pattern may have a bearing on prognosis, because the infiltrative, more destructive lesions are those most prone to dissemination. [Reprinted with permission from Collins, V. P., Loeffler, R. K., Tirey, H.: Observations on growth rates of human tumors. *Am. J. Roentgenol. Radium Ther. Nucl. Med.* 76:988–1000, 1956.]

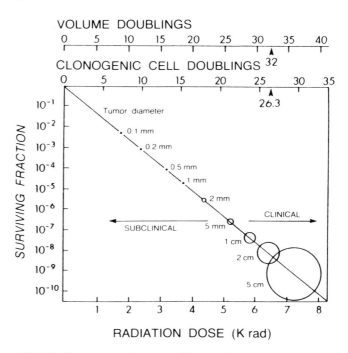

FIG. 2-2. Since a typical tumor cell has a volume of approximately 10^{-6} mm^3, a single mutant cell would have to undergo 32 volume doublings (ignoring stromal content of the tumor) to produce a tumor 2 cm in diameter. If the doubling time is constant, the spheres illustrate directly the increase in tumor size with time. Note that (1) even "early diagnosis" of, say, a 5-mm diameter tumor is not truly early in that 26 volume doublings have already occurred, and (2) the clinical illusion of accelerated terminal tumor growth can result from simple constant exponential growth; for example, the time to grow from 0.2 to 2 mm in diameter (a clinically undetectable change) is the same as that taken to increase from 5 mm to 5 cm (which is clinically most impressive). [Reprinted with permission from Withers, R. H., Peters, L. J.: Biological aspects of radiation therapy. In *Textbook of Radiotherapy*, 3rd ed., Fletcher, G. H. Philadelphia, Lea & Febiger, 1980, p. 143.]

quire nutrients by perfusion. Subsequent to this time, the cancer is also capable of metastasizing. It is presumed this same developmental process characterizes colonies of cancer cells, be they of primary or metastatic origin.[6,7] Extrapolating from this hypothesis, the challenge is to detect a cancer before it has reached a volume of 3 mm^2. Quite obviously, the resolution of a target of such size is uncommonly possible, even under the most optimal circumstances. With current imaging techniques, tumor nodules from 5 mm to 1.0 cm represent the minimal size of detection in most organ sites. Such tumor nodules, though small, are biologically advanced (Figure 2-2).

The age-adjusted cancer death rates by sex (Figures 2-3 and 2-4) fail to reflect the progress of diagnosis and treatment programs. The trends in survival by cancer site are summarized in Figures 2-5 and 2-6 illustrating the dramatic improvements between 1960 and 1980. The role that diagnostic oncologic imaging programs have

played in this process is difficult to document. Our improved and more sophisticated imaging techniques and procedures certainly have advanced the process of staging in all body sites. This ability to not only more accurately define, but in certain instances more specifically characterize, tumors has directed more aggressive treatment techniques to both the primary tumor and occasionally, its metastatic extensions. New techniques involving magnetic resonance and monoclonal antibodies promise future improvements in both diagnosis-staging and followup.

STATUS OF SCREENING PROGRAMS

The value of cancer screening has been questioned by many authors in recent years.[5] The only screening examination of unquestioned value is the Papanicolaou smear for cervical cancer. Random radiographic screening programs have neither resulted in an improved survival for

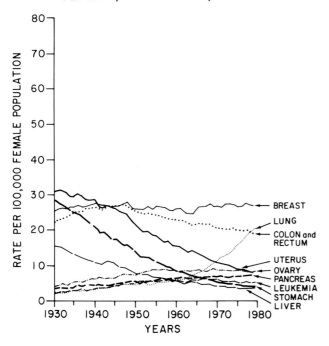

AGE ADJUSTED CANCER DEATH RATES FOR SELECTED SITES
FEMALES, UNITED STATES, 1930-1979

FIG. 2-3. The age-adjusted cancer death rate for females shows the striking increase in the lung cancer curve beginning in the early 1960s. Reprinted with permission from *CA – A Cancer Journal for Clinicians,* **34**:12, 1984.

the cancer in question nor been justified from the standpoint of cost effectiveness. The exception to this statement is the notable yield from mammographic screening, as illustrated by the results of the Breast Cancer Detection Demonstration Project (BCDDP).

These results[2] support a screening role for mammography in the detection of the more curable breast cancer in the asymptomatic patient. The impressive yield of noninfiltrating and minimal (under 1 cm) breast cancers detected during the BCDDP (59% and 52.6%, respectively), together with the improved detection efficiency in the 40-to-49 year age group in comparison with the earlier HIP study in the 1960s, has served to redefine the role of mammography.[2] Screening mammography should now be applied to patients over age 40 years, a recommendation adopted by the American Cancer Society in 1982. The controversy that emerged from the public discussions of the theoretical effect of radiation increasing the rate of occurrence of breast cancer, as extrapolated from three high radiation dose model studies, alarmed both the patient and physician communities regarding mammography. A concerted re-educational process must occur, in light of the impressive data reported from the BCDDP, to allow the intelligent and appropriate utilization of screening mammography to develop.

Preliminary results from the center trials evaluating diagnostic approaches for lung cancer have shown disappointing results. In brief, these three center programs differ to some degree in the structure and handling of their study groups, but all evaluate "high risk" male smokers over the age of 45 years, using chest X-ray studies and sputum cytologic examination at four-month intervals. To date, no difference in mortality has been apparent in comparing the study and control populations. Smaller and more peripheral tumors were detected by chest roentgenograms, and central lesions were usually detected by sputum examination. In addition, the vast majority of all cancers was detected by chest X-ray films rather than sputum cytologic examination. It is interesting to speculate that with additional experience, a mortality difference may yet emerge from these trials. Analysis of the data reveals that more advanced (stage III) lesions were detected in the control (70%) than in the study (35%) population. Also, there was a higher percentage of stage I lesions in the study (50%) compared with the control (20%) group.[1,10] Hopefully, these data indicate that the population of patients with advanced tumors will be selected out with time, and the continuing higher percentage of stage I lesions in the study

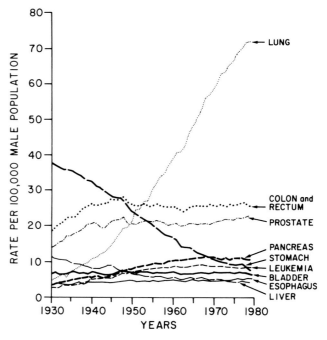

AGE ADJUSTED CANCER DEATH RATES FOR SELECTED SITES
MALES, UNITED STATES, 1930-1979

FIG. 2-4. The age-adjusted death rates for cancer sites in males shows the continuing slope of the curve representing lung cancer as well as the declining death rates for gastric cancer. Reprinted with permission from *CA – A Cancer Journal for Clinicians,* **34**:13, 1984.

TRENDS IN SURVIVAL BY SITE OF CANCER, BY RACE CASES DIAGNOSED IN 1960-63, IN 1970-73, AND IN 1973-80						
Site	1960-63[1] Relative 5-year Survival (Percent)		1970-73[1] Relative 5-year Survival (Percent)		1973-80[2] Relative 5-year Survival (Percent)	
	White	Black	White	Black	White	Black
Prostate	50	35	63	55	68	58
Kidney	37	38	46	44	50	52
Uterine Corpus	73	31	81	44	88	58
Bladder	53	24	61	36	73	48
Colon & Rectum	41	31	48	35	50	42
Uterine Cervix	58	47	64	61	68	62
Breast	63	46	68	51	74	62
Ovary	32	32	36	32	37	39
Brain and Central Nervous System	18	19	20	19	21	23
Lung and Bronchus	8	5	10	7	12	10
Stomach	11	8	13	13	14	14
Esophagus	4	1	4	4	5	3
Hodgkin's Disease	40	*	67	*	70	70
Lymphocytic Leukemia-Acute	4	*	28	*	43	*
Leukemia	14	*	22	*	32	27
Non-Hodgkin's Lymphomas	31	*	41	*	46	46
Larynx	53	*	62	*	67	57
Melanoma of Skin	60	*	68	*	79	*
Testis	63	*	72	*	82	67
Thyroid	83	*	86	*	92	89

[1] Rates are based on data from a series of hospital registries and one population-based registry.

[2] Rates are from the SEER Program and include patients diagnosed through 1980 and follow-up on all patients through 1981. They are based on data from population-based registries in Connecticut, New Mexico, Utah, Iowa, Hawaii, Atlanta, Detroit, Seattle-Puget Sound, and San Francisco-Oakland.

* Rates could not be calculated because of insufficient number of cases.

Source: Biometry Branch, National Cancer Institute.

FIG. 2-5. Trends in survival by cancer site 1960–63 and 1973–80, from *CA—A Cancer Journal for Clinicians*, 34:23 Jan.–Feb. 1984. With permission.

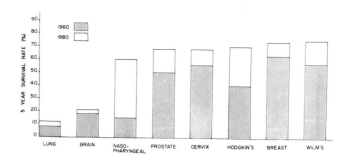

FIG. 2-6. Relative 5-year survival rates for selected sites 1960–1980 (NCI-SEER data, 1983). Survival rates have significantly improved between 1960 and 1980 in many sites, most notably nasopharynx and with Hodgkin's lymphoma. Little change in survival has occurred in the lung and brain during the same 20-year period.

technique and will remain so for the foreseeable future. Refinements in detection, perception-cognition, and resolution will improve chest radiographic accuracy; however, the returns, in terms of significantly advancing lung cancer detection efficiency, will probably be modest.[8,11] With lung cancers, as well as with most other primary tumor locations, the principal goal of imaging efforts should be tumor definition and staging, not random screening.

SPECIFIC ORGAN SITE DILEMMAS

Finally, with tumors such as pancreatic or esophageal cancers, screening of asymptomatic patients is obviously not feasible, since by the time symptoms are manifest, these cancers are not commonly curable. Again, refinements in imaging techniques are unlikely to improve upon this situation, placing the challenge of earlier detection into other arenas.

Hollow organ gastrointestinal tract examination has given radiologists a technique with which to detect cancer with acceptable sensitivity and specificity and cost. This is more applicable to large bowel cancer in North America and Europe but applies equally to gastric cancer, particularly where that disease is more prevalent, as in the Orient. Can the screening of asymptomatic individuals for gastrointestinal cancers with radiologic examination be justified based on questions of cost and yield? The answer at this time is also no. Undertaking such a random screening program would overwhelm examination resources and incur exorbitant costs. Symptoms, laboratory tests, and physical examination combined with endoscopy are all means with which to screen the population at risk and identify that patient group appropriate for radiologic study.

group will lead to a more favorable outcome in this population.

What, then, should be the focus of imaging efforts with lung cancer, both primary and metastatic? Again, it is not likely that significant improvement in lesion detection efficiency will occur in the near future. It is said that our diagnostic error rate with lung cancer varies from 20% to 50% and probably averages 30%. The recent (September 1983) update of the Mayo Clinic lung cancer study indicated that 90% of the peripheral lung cancers could be identified on earlier films in retrospect.[10] This report serves to illustrate the limitations of the chest radiograph in the detection setting, applied as a stereo PA and lateral technique and evaluated by multiple observers. In spite of these discouraging results, the chest X-ray is still the primary lung cancer detection

DECISION THEORY

The decision theory process in medicine has largely been an intuitive one in practice. The radiologist seldom has the privilege of analyzing the results of his or her examination just as the clinician infrequently applies the tools of decision theory analysis to the outcome of the imaging studies. These deficiencies add to the confusion that emerges when the data comparing imaging studies reported in the oncologic literature are analyzed.

A clear understanding of the decision theory process must accompany a knowledge of both the disease and imaging systems being applied to the clinical problem. The purpose of this section will be to place this concept in perspective, reviewing only a few of the aspects of the decision process and hopefully stimulating the reader to pursue the topic further through literature cited in the references.

Most oncologists are familiar with the common terms of sensitivity, specificity, true and false positivity, and predictive values of studies. Nonetheless, knowledge of these terms is usually superficial; this deficiency precludes an ability to apply them in everyday problem solving. The more widespread use of computers in medical environments will require oncologists to become more familiar with these terms, and the increasingly rigid demands of health care reimbursement policies will dictate the use of these terms in the prioritization of health care services.

Most, if not all, understand the definitions of the terms true and false, positive and negative; however, this simple illustration will serve as a review:

		Disease Present		No Disease
Exam Positive	* *	True Positive	* *	False Positive
Exam Negative	* *	False Negative	* *	True Negative

The sensitivity of a certain test or study is a function of the true-positive rate compared with the sum of the true positives and false negatives.

$$\text{Sensitivity} = \frac{\text{true positives}}{\text{true positives} + \text{false negatives}}$$

The specificity of a test is the relationship of the true-negative yield compared with the sum of the true-negative plus false-positive rate for the study.

$$\text{Specificity} = \frac{\text{true negatives}}{\text{true negatives} + \text{false positives}}$$

The predictive value of a study is a more important variable of its potential usefulness in a certain disease state. The predictive value of a positive examination is determined by the true-positive yield compared with the sum of the true-positive and false-positive rate.

$$\frac{\text{Predictive value of}}{\text{a positive test}} = \frac{\text{true positive}}{\text{true positive} + \text{false positive}}$$

$$\frac{\text{Predictive value of}}{\text{a negative test}} = \frac{\text{true negative}}{\text{true negative} + \text{false negative}}$$

This brief review of some of the more common and useful terms involved in the decision process should be enhanced by additional materials and applications cited in the references.[9,12]

SPECIFIC PROCEDURE LIMITATIONS AND APPLICATIONS

Table 2-2 lists the 10 common imaging procedures most often applied to oncologic problems. A number of assumptions have been made in an effort to illustrate common applications as well as limitations of each of these procedures.

Of all the studies listed, the film-screen system provides by far the greatest resolution, often more than can be used. The limiting problems with film radiography in tumor detection are primarily tissue discrimination and resolution of low contrast objects (e.g., lung nodules).

Signal-to-noise problems often limit the ability of radionuclide studies to resolve tumor masses. This has partially been the fault of focused scintillation cameras, and in part is a deficiency corrected by the tomographic scanning systems. Monoclonal antibody techniques may allow the identification of many tumors at a smaller size than currently is possible. Nonetheless, signal-to-noise problems, insufficient tumor tagging, and difficulty in developing tumor specific antibodies will be the major challenges of this new field.

In most body imaging areas, computed tomography (CT) has become the standard against which other tumor imaging systems are measured. The applications of CT to mass lesion detection in the brain and staging problems are now well established but inadequately utilized in the head and neck sites, as noted in the chapters about those areas. Computed tomography assumes a staging role in other body sites and has advantages for lesion definition in a number of specific organs. This has been inconsistently applied and unevenly reported in the staging of patients with lung cancer. This is, at least in part, a result of the differences in definition of abnormal lymph node size and operative proof of CT findings.

Table 2-2. Specific Imaging Procedure: Limitations and Applications

IMAGING PROCEDURE	RELATIVE COST	RELATIVE SENSITIVITY	RELATIVE SPECIFICITY	COMMENTS
Plain film radiography	low	varied	high	Plain films have excellent sensitivity and specificity in the soft tissues (mammography) and bones. In the chest, low-contrast tumor targets are a problem.
Xerography	low	high	moderate/high	Edge enhancement and wide exposure latitude allow soft tissue application (breast, neck, appendicular soft tissues, bone, and soft tissue tumor imaging).
Contrast GI studies	moderate	high	high	Cancer screening applications can be justified for high-risk groups (esophagus, stomach, and colon).
Radionuclide liver scan	moderate	moderate	low	Displaced by CT/US as screening liver imaging modality of choice. ? still initial screen of choice.
Radionuclide bone scan	moderate	high	low	Procedure of choice in skeletal scanning. Abnormal sites must be verified by film radiography.
Radionuclide brain scan	moderate	moderate	low	CT has replaced radionuclide brain scanning except where CT access is limited.
Ultrasound abdominal scanning	moderate	high	moderate	Lack of radiation exposure, cost, and availability lend ultrasound to abdominal screening. Technique is operator dependent.
Computed tomography Brain	high	high	moderate	Procedure of choice for screening mass lesion suspect using contrast enhancement only.
Lung	high	high	low	Highest sensitivity of all studies in detection of lung nodules. High false-positive rate.
Abdomen	high	high	moderate	
Angiography	high	high	moderate	Cost, invasiveness, and time limit applications.
Magnetic resonance (MRI)	high	high	high(?)	Resolution similar to CT. Elimination of bone artifacts makes CNS images better than CT. In chest, tumor and hilar node imaging improved over CT. Applications elsewhere—insufficient experience.

Magnetic resonance imaging (MRI) is emerging as a tumor imaging technique in a scenario quite similar to that of CT. Its role in CNS imaging is more easily understood and accepted than is its role in imaging other body sites. The prospect of tissue discrimination with MRI as well as in vivo spectroscopy must await the trial of new, higher field-strength magnets.

IMAGING STRATEGIES APPROPRIATE TO PATIENT CONDITION AND DISEASE STATUS

The challenge of oncologic imaging is complex and varies with each organ site and often, tumor type. In each of the organ-specific chapters that follow, we have attempted to develop an imaging template to be used in the definition of the tumor bulk (TNM of the American Joint Committee classification/staging system). The decision tree diagrams in each chapter follow a similar format when possible to aid the reader in understanding the concept of tumor staging. Obviously, the imaging process will often have to be tailored to suit the individual needs of the patient, the unique features of the tumor, and the characteristics of the disease.

Once the tumor is detected and a specific histologic diagnosis has been established, the definition of the T (tumor) component is performed as is illustrated in Table 2-3. Subsequently, imaging studies such as CT, ultrasound, or lymphography are used to define the N (node) compartments. Finally, a decision must be made about the need to explore the possibility of metastatic disease (M). This latter decision is often the most difficult and controversial of all. The decision must acknowledge the question, "Will the outcome of this study modify the therapeutic approach?" In addition, the specific tumor and its stage as well as the patient's status will affect the decision to evaluate the metastatic (M) compartment. In most instances, the imaging approach to the assessment of metastatic disease will be similar. The common organs targeted for the metastatic process are the lung, brain, liver, and skeletal system, making CT, radionuclide bone scans, and, to a lesser degree, sonographs, the most often employed imaging techniques in the detection of metastases.

The superior sensitivity of CT in the detection of

Table 2-3. Sequence of Imaging Process—Staging and Follow-up

PROCESS	PROBLEMS SPECIFIC TO PROCESS
Detection and diagnosis	Dictates staging workup
↓	
Staging workup (TNM)	Dictated by tumor type, patient status, organ site, and procedural limitations
↓	
Definition of tumor response to treatment	Imaging approach and sequence determined by therapeutic modality and tumor type
↓	
Follow-up	Imaging approach and sequence determined by therapeutic modality and tumor type
↓	
Detection of relapse	
↓	
Restage—before re-treatment	Abbreviated restaging tailored to the tumor, patient status, and retreatment modality considered

nodular lung disease must be considered in the perspective of questions about its lack of specificity and increased costs, both for the procedure and for validation of the positive examination. It may be appropriate to utilize film tomography to screen the chest for metastatic disease, either initially or on follow-up examination. Although the sensitivity of film tomography is lower than that of CT, the trade-off in cost may justify this

approach in the particular setting of the patient and type of tumor in question.

In some instances, the above sequence is best reversed. The initial exploration of the metastatic compartment occasionally may be more appropriate before assessing the node stations and tumor bulk. This situation would apply with clinically advanced primary tumors, patients presenting with a suspected metastatic disease, and in those particular cancers characterized by widespread disease at the time of initial presentation (e.g., small cell anaplastic lung cancer). Table 2-4 summarizes the sensitivity and specificity of imaging procedures.

Whenever possible, we have recommended a strategy for the posttreatment follow-up, with assumptions and guidelines similar to those developed for the staging workup before treatment. In no other instance is it more important for the radiologist to understand the treatment program than in the follow-up imaging process. Both the follow-up interval after treatment and the therapeutic approach will have a major influence on the selection and outcome of the imaging study. Once a relapse has been diagnosed, the staging process begins again, usually in an abbreviated form, tailored to both the patient and the tumor.

SUMMARY AND CONCLUSIONS

This review is intended to demonstrate that, with the exception of mammography and possibly chest radiography, imaging procedures for cancer detection cannot

Table 2-4. Imaging and the Detection of Metastases

MODALITY	SENSITIVITY/SPECIFICITY (1–4)*				
	LIVER	LUNG	BONE	BRAIN	LYMPH NODES
Isotope:					
^{99m}Tc-sulfur colloid	2/2				
^{99m}Tc-pyrophosphate			4/2†		
gallium 67					3/2
Ultrasound	3/4				2/3
Computed tomographic (CT) scan	3/4‡	4/3§		4/4	3/4‖
Plain x-ray		3/2	2/4		
Whole lung tomograms (WLT)		3/3			
Lymphangiogram (LAG)					3/4‖

*1 = Low; 4 = high.

†The bone scan may be positive up to 6 months prior to X-ray changes. Only 2–3% of bone lesions will be seen on x-ray with negative bone scan.

‡Denotes method of greatest overall accuracy.

§Most pulmonary metastases greater than 5 mm will be seen on plain x-rays. The other modalities (CT, WLT) should be reserved for critical decision making, i.e., when curative surgery is contemplated.

‖The choice of LAG vs. CT is both tumor and site dependent. Lymphomas are seen well with CT but solid visceral lymph node metastases (cervix, prostate, etc.) may be better demonstrated with LAG.

Reprinted with permission from Borg, S. A., Rubin, P., DeWys, W. D.: Metastases and disseminated diseases. In *Clinical Oncology for Medical Students and Physicians: A Multidisciplinary Approach*, 6th ed. Rubin, P. (Ed.). New York: American Cancer Society, 1983, p. 505.

be justified. This is a reality that will continue to be true in the foreseeable future. Only if some as yet unknown tumor-specific radionuclide procedure were developed that was capable of imaging tumors with volumes of 3 to 4 mm^2 or less, could the question of radiologic screening programs be readdressed.

The central theme of this book, as reviewed in each of the chapters that follow, is the application of imaging procedures in defining the tumor burden in both the primary site (T), the nodal stations (N), and the distant metastatic areas (M). To achieve this goal, not only must the applications and limitations of each of the imaging techniques be appreciated, but also the behavior of the cancer in question as well as the therapeutic options under consideration must be understood. The definition of the imaging strategy must also embrace the TNM staging requirements for the cancer, both initially and subsequent to treatment.

Specific imaging dilemmas have developed in almost every anatomic site. The more controversial of these are

1. Lung—which imaging procedure is most accurate in detecting the pulmonary nodule?
2. Liver—is mass lesion screening the province of CT, ultrasound, or radionuclide scanning?
3. Pancreas—should ultrasound or CT be the procedure of choice to detect pancreatic masses?
4. Kidney—how has the role of renal cancer detection and definition been modified with the introduction of ultrasound and CT?
5. Lymph nodes—what is the current position of lymphography and how has CT modified or replaced this examination?
6. Skeletal system—when should CT be applied; what is the role of angiography, radionuclide scanning, and film tomography?

All of these issues as well as many others are relevant to the process of oncologic imaging and are considered in the chapters that follow. Questions of detection efficiency must be placed in the context of how the information will be used or the manner in which the imaging results will modify the treatment program. If the returns of an invasive or expensive imaging procedure will not alter the therapeutic process, it should not be under-

taken. Also, concerns of sensitivity and specificity must be addressed for each examination considered. The final pathway selected should then be the result of the distillation of a review of the appropriateness of the imaging procedure and the needs of the specific oncologic process in question. We feel the decision tree will serve the needs for this dialogue between radiologists and oncologists and, in this spirit, have suggested such approaches in each of the anatomic sites. It should be understood that these decision trees are intended as guidelines and must be modified to meet the needs of the individual patient and the assets and liabilities of each imaging facility.

REFERENCES

1. American Cancer Society: *Report on the Cancer-Related Health Checkup.* New York, American Cancer Society, 1980.
2. Baker, L. F.: The Breast Cancer Detection Demonstration Projects: Five-Year Summary Report, *CA* **32**:194–225, 1982.
3. Borg, S. A., Rubin, P., DeWys, W.: Metastases and disseminated disease. In *Clinical Oncology for Medical Students and Physicians: A Multidisciplinary Approach*, 6th ed, Rubin, P. (Ed.). New York, American Cancer Society,1983.
4. Collins, V. P., Loeffler, R. K., Tivey, H.: Observations on growth rates of human tumors. *Am. J. Roentgenol. Radium Ther. Nucl. Med.* 76:988–1000, 1956.
5. Eddy, D.: *Screening for Cancer: Theory, Analysis, and Design.* Englewood Cliffs, NJ, Prentice-Hall, 1980.
6. Folkman, J.: Anti-angiogenesis: New concept for therapy of solid tumors. *Ann. Surg.* **175**:409–416, 1972.
7. Folkman, J., Merler, E., Abernathy, C., Williams, G.: Isolation of a tumor factor responsible for angiogenesis. *J. Exp. Med.* **133**:275–288, 1971.
8. Forrest, J. V., Friedman, P. J.: Radiologic error in patients with lung cancer. *Radiol. Clin. North Am.* 16:347–366, 1978.
9. McNeil, B. J., Keeler, E., Adelsten, S. J.: Primer on certain elements of medical decision making. *N. Engl. J. Med.* 293:211–215, 1975.
10. Muhm, J. R., Miller, W. E., Fontana, R. S., Sanderson, D. R., Uhlenhopp, M. A.: Lung cancer detected during a screening program using four-month chest radiography. *Radiology* **148**:609–615, 1983.
11. Stitik, F. P., Tockman, M. S.: Radiographic screening in early detection of lung cancer. *Radiol. Clin. North Am.* 16:347–366, 1978.
12. Weinstein, M. C., Fineberg, H. V.: *Clinical Decision Analysis.* Philadelphia, W. B. Saunders, 1980.
13. Withers, R. H., Peters, L. J.: Biological aspects of radiation therapy. In *Textbook of Radiotherapy*, 3rd ed, Fletcher, G. H. (Ed.). Philadelphia, Lea & Febiger, 1980, p. 143.

3 BRAIN AND SPINAL CORD NEOPLASMS

Robert E. Anderson
David G. Bragg
James E. Youker

Tumors of the central nervous system (CNS) constitute approximately 2% of all of the reported cancers in the United States, representing 12,000 new brain tumors and 4,000 spinal cord tumors annually and 10,000 deaths per year.[2] The incidence is higher for males than females (6.3 per 100,000 versus 4.4 per 100,000) and somewhat higher for whites versus blacks (5.6 per 100,000 versus 3.4 per 100,000).

Age plays a dominant role in both the incidence and behavior of brain tumors. The incidence of brain tumors rises gradually to a peak of 18.1 cases per 100,000 in the 65- to 69-year age group. It is also interesting that age affects behavior, in that astrocytomas occurring in individuals under the age of 40 to 45 tend to have a less aggressive course than those over the age of 45, the latter almost uniformly having a fatal outcome (personal communication from E. R. Laws, Jr., M.D., Mayo Clinic). Central nervous system tumors in children rank second in incidence to the leukemias and are responsible for 16,000 deaths annually.[34] The location of central nervous system tumors in children differs from that in adults, where they are more frequently located in an infratentorial area, usually in the cerebellum, brain stem, or medulla. In contrast, nearly 75% of all intracranial tumors in the adult population occur in a supratentorial location.

Primary tumors of the brain and spinal cord have unique characteristics not shared by cancers in other body organ sites. In spite of the rich blood supply, blood-borne metastases from brain tumors are extremely rarely reported. The absence of a lymphatic system in the brain precludes the possibility of lymph nodal metastases, except in rare instances, where presumably, seeding occurs following surgical intervention. Control of central nervous system tumors, therefore, depends almost entirely on the successful local management of the primary tumor. Local treatment is frequently frustrated by the critical location of brain tumors, limiting attempts at surgical excision and post-operative radiation therapy. In spite of the rarity of extracranial metastases from primary brain tumors, intracranial metastases from cancers in other body parts are frequent. The reason for this occurrence is unclear, other than to presume it is the result of the relatively high rate of blood flow to the brain compared with many other organs in the body. The most frequent extracranial primary tumor sites responsible for metastatic brain lesions are the lung, breast, extremities (sarcomas), and skin (melanoma).

Despite the application of a variety of multidisciplinary treatment protocols, long-term survival rates remain poor for many brain tumors.[31,38,52] Prognosis for brain tumors is correlated with both the histologic grade of the tumor and the age of the patient. Many brain tumors contain heterogeneous cell populations and in these instances, prognosis tends to be related to the highest grade of differentiation of the tumor.[92] The mortality for adults with central nervous system tumors has deteriorated in both white and black populations and both sexes. In 1950, mortality rates for blacks with central nervous system tumors were 3.5 per 100,000 population and increased to 4.6 per 100,000 in 1967. More recent data in the 1970s has shown this trend to continue.[27] Mortality figures for adolescents and young adults have remained constant during the same period of time.

Traditional means of detecting CNS neoplasms include plain film studies, isotope brain scans, angiography, pneumoencephalography, and myelography. Computed tomography (CT) scanning has replaced nearly all of these studies in both the initial detection and follow-up of brain tumors.[53]

Air studies (pneumoencephalography and ventriculography) have been virtually eliminated, except in certain unusual circumstances when two positions need to be checked, or hydrocephalus followed. The nuclear brain scan has a very limited role at present, being useful primarily for detecting skull or meningeal metastases. Myelography, however, remains a valuable imaging tool for the assessment of tumors of the spinal canal.

CT scanning has not only improved our ability to detect smaller brain tumors, but also CT-guided stereotactic biopsy techniques provide a safer means of obtaining tissue from these smaller lesions, regardless of location.[14,15] Surgical techniques, guided by CT stereotactic techniques, show promise as well, but the impact of these therapeutic techniques on survival statistics remains to be defined.[41,46,74]

CT has revolutionized the approach to the detection and diagnosis of space-occupying lesions in the brain. Tumors can be detected at a smaller site.[78,79] In addition, CT techniques provide important clinical data to aid therapeutic decisions including biopsy and post-treatment follow-up.[6,12,18] Despite the increased cost of CT, numerous studies have shown the cost-effective impact of these studies in patient management by their ability to eliminate expensive and invasive studies which are unnecessary with the new data provided by the CT images.[35] Magnetic resonance imaging (MRI) promises to provide additional information regarding the diagnosis and follow-up of central nervous system tumors.[11,56,67,89] The advantages of MRI include the absence of ionizing radiation; the ability to obtain three-dimensional images, as well as projections in axial, coronal, or sagittal planes; and the absence of bone artifacts in the skull base (Figure 3-1).[25] Most MRI images to date have been dependent upon proton imaging, with only experimental evidence to suggest applications utilizing other nuclei, especially phosphorous, fluorine, and sodium, in an effort to help differentiate normal and abnormal tissue in the central nervous system, as well as elsewhere in the body. These elements are in extremely low concentration relative to hydrogen, which will result in a weak biologic signal and, probably, limited spatial resolution. The future of magnetic resonance imaging in the brain appears promising now that improved spatial resolution has matched that of CT. The increased cost in comparison with CT will probably justify its use, particularly in areas near the skull

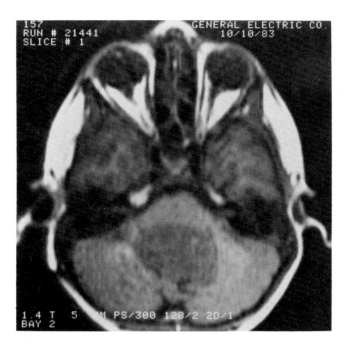

FIG. 3-1. Axial magnetic resonance image (MRI) through the skull base demonstrating an inferior vermian medulloblastoma. Note the absence of artifacts from bone.

base and posterior fossa, where CT images are compromised.

TUMOR BEHAVIOR AND PATHOLOGY

CNS tumors considered for staging by the American Joint Committee are the following:[3]

1. Astrocytoma
2. Oligodendroglioma
3. Ependymal and choroid plexus tumors
4. Glioblastomas
5. Medulloblastomas
6. Meningioma
7. Neurilemomas (neurinomas, schwannomas)
8. Hemangioblastomas
9. Neuronal tumors
10. Sarcomas
11. Reticulum cell sarcoma (microglioma)

Histopathology

A brief introduction to the pathology and behavior of these lesions follows, based largely on the opinions expressed by Russell and Rubinstein.[70]

Glioma and Glioblastoma. Astrocytoma and glioblastoma multiforme, originating from astrocytes or their primitive precursors, represent half of all intracranial tumors and three-fourths of all gliomas.[26,57,60,70] Although gliomas vary considerably in their aggressiveness, in general they behave unfavorably because of their unencapsulated growth within the brain.[60] Gliomas composed of mature elements which grow more slowly are considered to be relatively benign; those composed of immature elements which invade the brain rapidly are considered malignant.[60] Astrocytomas of the cerebellum, seen in the first decade of life, are usually well circumscribed and are rarely aggressive lesions. Astrocytomas have been classified by Kernohan as Grade I–IV, with Grade I being the least aggressive and Grade IV the most aggressive. (Grades III and IV are called glioblastoma multiforme.)[44] Rubinstein has classified these tumors as astrocytoma, malignant astrocytoma, and glioblastoma multiforme in order of their increasing malignancy.[69] Gliomas occur most often in the central white matter of the cerebrum in adults and the cerebellar hemispheres or brain stem in children and young adults.[60] Tumors with a lower grade of malignancy show calcification in as many as one-quarter of the cases while only a few percent of more malignant lesions calcify. Because of the high incidence of astrocytomas compared with other lesions that calcify, this tumor is the most common to show calcification on plain film examination. Spread of astrocytoma occurs by local extension. Deeper lesions may cross to the opposite cerebral hemisphere via the corpus callosum (Figure 3-2). The dura is rarely invaded. Cerebrospinal fluid (CSF) spread is also rarely observed. Glioblastoma multiforme is an anaplastic tumor occurring most frequently in the fourth and fifth decades of life, usually associated with survival times of less than 1 year. Despite the anaplastic histology of the lesion, spread via CSF is rarely observed.[17]

Oligodendroglioma. These slow-growing tumors represent approximately 5% of intracranial gliomas.[60,70,84] They originate from oligodendrocytes in the central white matter. Two typical features are location in the anterior half of the cerebrum and very large size at diagnosis.[60,84] Oligodendrogliomas exhibit calcification on roentgenograms in approximately half of the cases. Growth may be rapid in unusual cases, and the tumor may occasionally spread along ventricular or meningeal surfaces.

Ependymomas. These arise from the epithelial lining of the ventricular surfaces, along the spinal cord, and in the filum terminale. They are seen most frequently below the tentorium in children. Most ependymomas are histologically benign. There is a tendency for ependymomas to spread via CSF pathways.[40]

Choroid Plexus Neoplasms. Relatively rare tumors of epithelial origin, these are usually found in the first decade of life (Figures 3-3A, B). They comprise about 5% of brain tumors in children.[82] One-half of these tumors

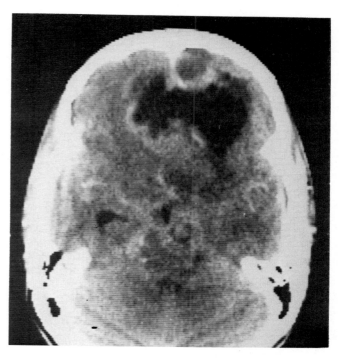

FIG. 3-2. Contrast-enhanced CT scan of a frontal lobe glioma, primarily cystic, with an irregular enhancing margin. Note that it crosses the midline in a "butterfly" configuration. This combination of findings is virtually diagnostic of a high-grade, primary neoplasm crossing the midline via the corpus callosum.

are found in the fourth ventricle. The tumors are commonly associated with hydrocephalus. Choroid plexus papillomas frequently metastasize via CSF pathways and produce secondary deposits in both the cranial cavity and spinal canal.

Medulloblastomas. These arise from the germinal cells of the medullary epithelium which normally differentiates into mature ganglion cells. Fifty percent occur in the first decade of life, with a smaller second age-incidence peak in the third decade of life. Medulloblastomas most commonly occur near the cerebellar midline and compress the fourth ventricle. The tumor is invasive and spreads readily via CSF upward into the third ventricle or downward along the spinal canal (Figure 3-4).

Meningiomas. Common, slow-growing, well encapsulated tumors, meningiomas often compress, but rarely infiltrate, the brain (Figures 3-5A, B, C). This tumor occurs most often during the middle decades of life, with a higher incidence in women. Sites of predilection include the parasellar regions, sphenoid wings, olfactory grooves, and parasagittal areas. Spread commonly occurs along the meninges near the primary mass, and the adjacent calvarium may become infiltrated with tumor cells. Multi-

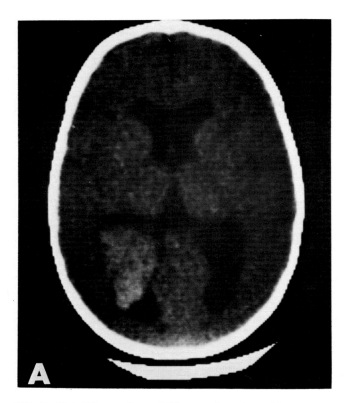 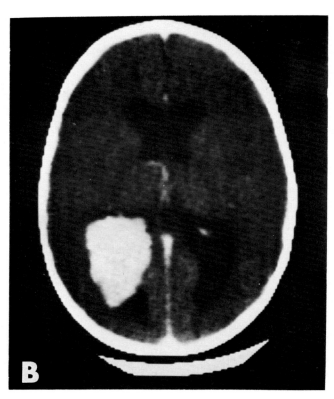

FIG. 3-3. Plain (A) and enhanced (B) scans of a patient with a mass within the ventricle. The position of the mass and uniform contrast enhancement limits the differential diagnosis to a very few lesions, in this case, choroid plexus papilloma.

ple meningiomas are found in the central type of Von Recklinghausen's neurofibromatosis. Multiple meningiomas also occur sporadically, either adjacent to one another or occasionally at remotely separate sites. Lesions usually appear clinically at different points in time. Histologically malignant meningiomas may invade the brain but distant spread is rare.

Neurilemomas (Neurinoma, Schwannoma). These are tumors originating in the connective tissue components of nerves. They are commonly seen in Von Recklinghausen's disease, affecting the peripheral nerves. Lesions involving intracranial nerve roots appear in the middle decades of life, affect women more than men, and are usually found along sensory, rather than motor, nerve roots. The most common intracranial site is the auditory nerve sheath (Figure 3-6). Single lesions along spinal nerve roots form the most common group of primary intrathecal neoplasms. Multiple and/or malignant examples are usually associated with Von Recklinghausen's neurofibromatosis.

Hemangioblastoma. A benign neoplasm of blood vessel origin, hemangioblastoma is usually located in the cerebellum in men, where a large cyst is frequently found associated with a smaller solid nodule (Figure 3-7). This tumor may also be found below the foramen magnum

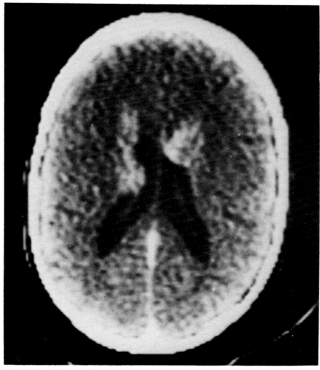

FIG. 3-4. CT scan of a young child 1 year after incomplete resection of a medulloblastoma from the cerebellum. A tumor has seeded in a retrograde fashion, and has become implanted along the margins of the lateral ventricles. (Case courtesy of G. DuBoulay, Radiology Department, Queens Square, London)

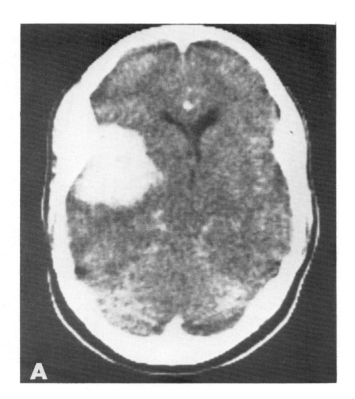

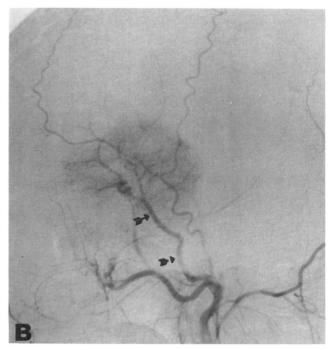

FIG. 3-5. (A) CT scan shows an enhancing mass in the middle fossa. The tumor could be either intra- or extra-axial in location. (B) External carotid angiogram, arterial phase, showing a hypertrophied middle meningeal artery (arrows) leading to the mass which already shows abnormal contrast enhancement.

in the spinal canal, but supratentorial examples are rare. The CNS mass may be associated with angiomatous lesions of the retina, cysts of the pancreas and kidneys, and renal, or suprarenal, tumors (Von Hipple-Lindau syndrome).

Neuronal Tumors. These include neuroblastomas, ganglioneuromas, and pheochromocytomas. These neoplasms derive from ganglion cells of the peripheral nervous system and their precursors, and therefore are usually found outside the brain or spinal canal. Neuroblastoma, usually arising in the adrenal gland in infants, may exhibit prominent metastases around the skull intracranially and extracranially (Figure 3-8). Less commonly, CNS spread may occur from a presacral mass infiltrating the spinal subarachnoid space. Ganglioneuroma is the name given to a more differentiated tumor of neuronal origin seen mainly in adults as a posterior mediastinal mass which may have an intraspinal component. These are benign lesions causing symptoms by local expansion.

Sarcomas. These may develop within the central nervous system, originating from meninges, or occasionally from the brain itself. Distant subarachnoid spread may occur. Sarcomatous degeneration has been reported years after radiotherapy for a tumor of another type or may be seen within a malignant glioma or initial biopsy.

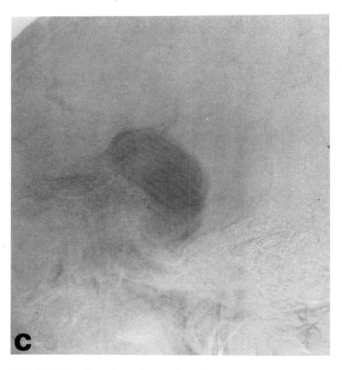

FIG. 3-5C. Capillary phase shows a dense, homogeneous tumor stain. In this instance, the angiogram not only helped define the tumor blood supply, but aided in the differential diagnosis. The angiographic pattern shown here is characteristic of meningioma.

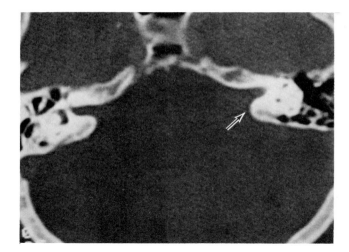

FIG. 3-6A. Thin section, high resolution bone technique CT scans now replace film tomography for the detection of erosion or expansion of the internal auditory canal in patients suspected of having an acoustic neuroma. Note the shortening and flaring of the medial end of the right internal auditory canal (arrow).

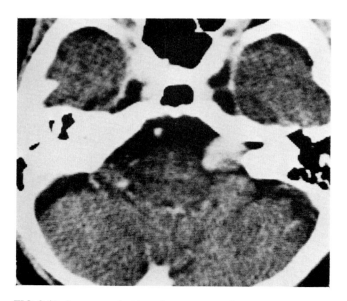

FIG. 3-6B. Same examination after contrast enhancement, using soft tissue image technique that reveals the contrast-enhanced acoustic neuroma protruding from the canal into the cerebello-pontine angle cistern.

Reticulum Cell Sarcomas. These usually involve the brain as part of a generalized malignant proliferation of primitive reticulum cells affecting lymph nodes, bone marrow, and other body structures. CNS involvement is most commonly meningeal, but parenchymal infiltration may occur. Infiltration along cranial and spinal nerve roots also occurs quite frequently. Some pathologists feel

that reticulum cell sarcomas may occur as isolated brain tumors. The same lesion is called microglioma by others, and in these cases is usually not associated with extracranial disease. Other varieties of lymphoma affect the brain and spinal cord, usually as part of systemic disease. Primary lymphoma of the brain does occur in rare instances, producing a CT appearance indistinguishable from other tumors.

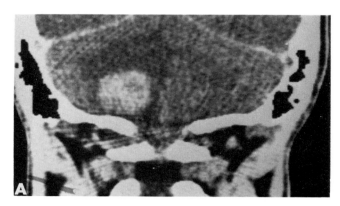

FIG. 3-7A. Coronal CT scan through the posterior fossa, following contrast infusion intravenously, shows a dense enhancing lesion surrounded by a sharply demarcated area of low density in a young adult with a vascular lesion in the retina.

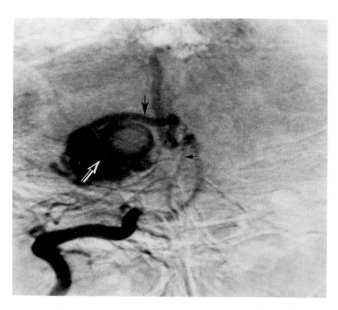

FIG. 3-7B. Single frame from a digitally subtracted intra-arterial angiogram, AP view, capillary phase. Note right–left deviation of an enlarged PICA artery (small arrow), and an enlarged single early draining vein (large arrow). Note also that the small cyst seen within the enhancing mass (white arrow) is not the cyst seen on the CT study: the two sets of information from the two tests are clearly complimentary in this instance.

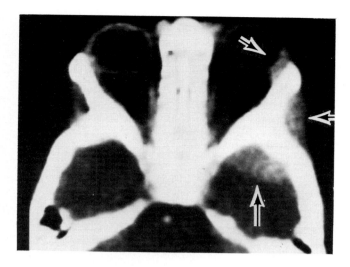

FIG. 3-8. Orbital, extracranial (temporal), and intracranial enhancing lesions typical for neuroblastoma (arrows).

Pineal Neoplasms. Although not included in the American Joint Committee staging list, pineal neoplasms will be briefly described since these lesions may spread via central nervous system pathways and pose unusual problems in staging and treatment (Figure 3-9). Tumors of the pineal gland area include teratomas, pinealomas, gliomas, and cysts. A variety of teratoma known as germinoma is the most common neoplasm at the site of the pineal gland. It appears clinically between ages 15 and 25 years, usually in men. Distant spread to the spinal canal has been reported. Tumors of the pineal gland itself sometimes are further divided into pineoblastoma or pineocytoma, and metastasize much more frequently. In one series of 21 cases, widespread cerebrospinal metastases developed in 10. Like germinomas, these tumors are usually found in the first decade of life.

Metastases. Metastases comprise nearly 40% of all intracranial tumors.[75] Twenty percent of patients dying of malignant tumors have intracranial metastases at the time of autopsy.[36,68] Malignant tumors which metastasize intracranially, in decreasing order of frequency, are from lung, breast, skin (melanoma), colon, rectum, and kidney.[19] Solitary intracerebral metastases, although less common than multiple, may be more difficult to recognize as metastases.

Patterns of Spread

Unlike neoplasms in most of the other parts of the body, distant spread via lymphatic channels or the bloodstream is a rare occurrence with virtually all CNS tumors. Local extension of the primary lesion is the usual cause of death. Most CNS tumors spread primarily by extension to contiguous tissue by local infiltration. As ependymal or pial surfaces are reached, these tissues may become involved at some distance from the primary mass. Considering how frequently tumors abut either a meningeal or ependymal surface, it is remarkable how seldom CSF-borne metastases occur. Medulloblastomas and ependymomas are known frequently to establish CSF-borne distant metastases. However, undifferentiated astrocytomas, pinealomas, and malignant tumors of the choroid plexus may also spread by these means.[16] Remote (extracranial) spread from a primary CNS neoplasm is rare.[8] Spread to local or regional lymph nodes may occur after surgery, presumably as a result of tumor seeding along the path of the incision. CSF shunt tubes have occasionally been implicated in tumor spread to the abdomen.[92]

Spread only rarely occurs via cerebral veins or dural sinuses to the lungs, bone, etc. Medulloblastomas may metastasize to bone, lymph nodes, and liver, whereas glioblastomas and ependymomas may go to lymph nodes, lung, and bone.[21,42,69] Skeletal metastases from meningiomas and gliomas have been recorded. Extracranial metastases most commonly involve the lungs and abdominal viscera.[62] Pineal germinomas may metastasize to lung, lymph nodes, and bone.[10]

CLASSIFICATION AND STAGING

The American Joint Committee for Cancer Staging and End Results Reporting has recommended the following staging classification.[3]

Evaluating the Primary Tumor (T)

A. *Supratentorial tumor:*

T_1 — Greatest diameter is 5 cm or less; confined to one side.

T_2 — Greatest diameter is more than 5 cm; confined to one side.

T_3 — Invades or encroaches upon the ventricular system; greatest diameter may be 5 cm or less.

T_4 — Crosses the midline, invades the opposite hemisphere, or extends infratentorially.

B. *Infratentorial tumor:*

T_1 — Greatest diameter is 3 cm or less; confined to one side.

T_2 — Greatest diameter is more than 3 cm; confined to one side.

T_3 — Invades or encroaches upon the ventricular system; greatest diameter may be 3 cm or less.

T_4 — Crosses the midline, invades the opposite hemisphere, or extends supratentorially.

Nodal Involvement (N) — This category does not apply to this site

Distant Metastases (M)

M_x — Not assessed

M_0 — No (known) distant metastasis

M_1 — Distant metastasis present.

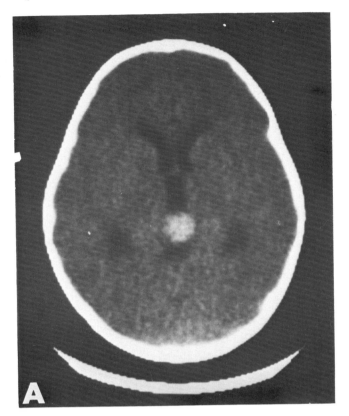
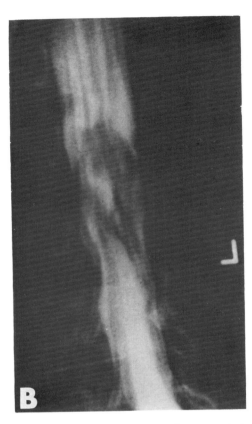

FIG. 3-9. (A) Youngster with headaches and lower extremity symptoms and signs. Contrast-enhanced CT brain scan shows mass lesion in the region of the pineal gland. (B) Myelogram reveals metastatic spread to the spinal subarachnoid space.

Schematic representation of tumors in the T categories are presented in Figures 3-10 and 3-11. Note that the difference between T_1 and T_2 is based upon tumor size. Larger masses are less likely to be curable. The diameters chosen to separate these two categories are arbitrary. The T_3 category is based upon the increased risk of spread via CSF pathways once the tumors come in contact with the ventricular surface. Further spread through the tentorial notch, or across to the opposite hemisphere, places the tumor in the T_4 category since this additional spread compromises both surgical and radiation therapy approaches.

Stage Grouping

Central nervous system tumors are placed into four stages based on histological differentiation of the tumor (see Table 3-1).[3] Grade I (G1) is well differentiated, whereas Grade IV (G4) is poorly differentiated, with frequent metastases, necrosis, and marked pleomorphism. Stages I through III are subdivided into A and B groups. The A groups include tumors whose size places them in the T_1 category and the B subgroup consists of tumors of the T_2 and T_3 size. Any metastasis, regardless of the size or position of the primary mass, puts the CNS tumor into Stage IV.

IMAGING PROCEDURES AND ASSESSMENT

Primary Brain Tumor

Imaging modalities for the detection and staging of CNS tumors include plain films; isotope brain scans, including positron emission tomography; pneumoencephalography; cerebral angiography; myelography; X-ray computed tomography (CT scan); and magnetic resonance imaging (MRI). The staging of most brain tumors involves a precise definition of the size of the primary tumor and the extent of involvement of vital structures within the brain. There is not often a need to detect nodal involvement or distant metastatic spread since it occurs so rarely. The detection and staging of most brain tumors is, at this time, most effectively demonstrated on high quality CT brain scans. Numerous articles have reported the value of CT head scanning in the detection and characterization of intracranial masses, including

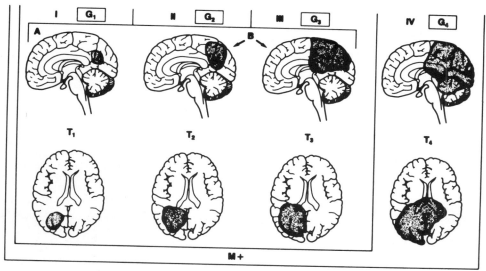

FIG. 3-10. Anatomic staging for supratentorial CNS tumors. *Tumor (T) categories: Size* is the critical factor and *extension* in a ventricle across the midline. For supratentorial lesions, <5 cm or >5 cm, and for infratentorial lesions, <3 cm or >3 cm. Extensions into ventricular region are T_3 and across midline, T_4. *Node (N) categories:* There are no N categories since the central nervous system has no regional lymph nodes. *Stage grouping:* The stage is primarily determined by grade. Appropriately, G_4, T_4, and M_1 are considered very uncommon and constitute stage IV. Modified from *AJC.*

their location, size, and effect on the ventricular system (Figures 3-9, 3-12, 3-13).[4,37,55,59,90] In summarizing the overall results of the National Cancer Institute Study of CT in the Diagnosis of Intracranial Neoplasms, Baker et al.[7] conclude that CT should be the first test employed in patients with suspected brain tumor. Butler et al.[19] conclude from a study of CT and radionuclide scans that contrast-enhanced CT scans are now the primary tool in the investigation of patients with possible brain tumors. Similar results have been found in brain neoplasms in infants and children.[45,73]

The detectability of a brain tumor depends on a number of factors, including its size, location (in relation to the ventricles or skull), the relative density before and after contrast infusion, the resolving power of the CT scanner, and the presence or absence of motion or other

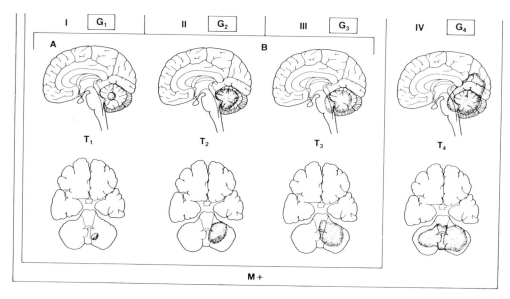

FIG. 3-11. Anatomic staging for infratentorial CNS tumors. See legend for Fig. 3-10.

Table 3-1. Stage Grouping for Central Nervous System Tumors

STAGE	GRADE	TUMOR	METASTASES
I:			
IA	G1	T_1	M_0
IB	G1	$T_{2,3}$	M_0
II:			
IIA	G2	T_1	M_0
IIB	G2	$T_{2,3}$	M_0
III:			
IIIA	G3	T_1	M_0
IIIB	G3	$T_{2,3}$	M_0
IV:			
	G4	$T_{1\text{-}4}$	M_0
	G1–3	T_4	M_0
	Any G	Any T	M_1

Reprinted from American Joint Committee on Cancer: *Manual for Staging of Cancer*, 2nd ed. Philadelphia, J. B. Lippincott, 1983, pp. 219–226.

artifacts in the image. For example, a fleck of calcium less than 1 mm may be easily seen, while an isodense tumor 1 cm in diameter may not be detected unless it deforms the ventricles or other anatomic features. Bone artifacts are still prevalent in the posterior fossa despite numerous improvements in scanner design. Intravenous contrast material should be given in every instance where a tumor is even remotely suspected, since a majority of tumors reveal abnormal post-infusion density changes. Butler[19] and Potts[66] found virtually no cases in which contrast-enhanced scans failed to show lesions seen on plain scans and concluded a single contrast-enhanced scan series is sufficient to detect both primary and metastatic tumors.[19,45,54]

Enhancement of a tumor is due to an abnormality of

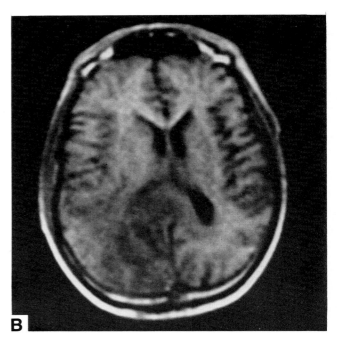

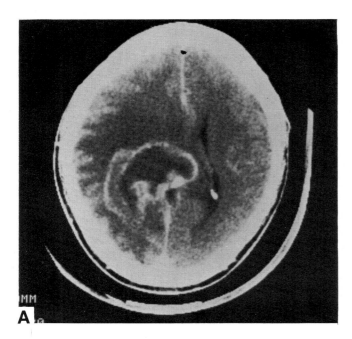

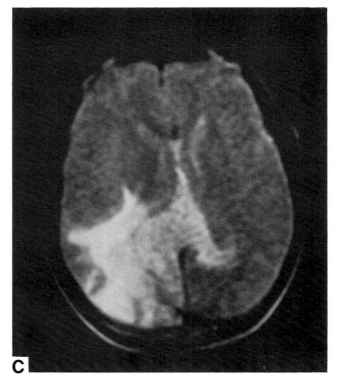

FIG. 3-12. Malignant astrocytoma (glioblastoma multiforme) in a contrast-enhanced CT image (A), T_1 weighted MRI image (B), and T_2 weighted MRI image (C). In the CT image, it has a rim of contrast enhancement, surrounding edema, and a necrotic center. In the T_1 weighted image (B), the tumor is poorly defined. In the T_2 weighted image (C), it appears as a region of bright signal, surrounded by edema which has an even brighter signal. The infiltration of the corpus callosum in the left hemisphere is best shown with MRI.

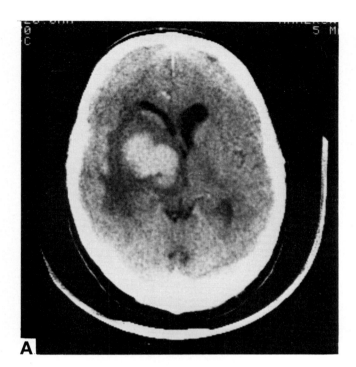

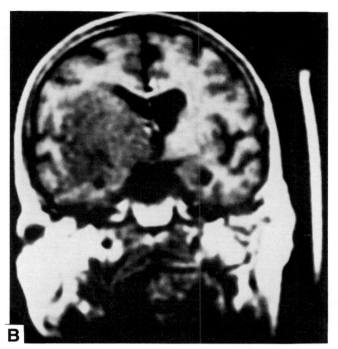

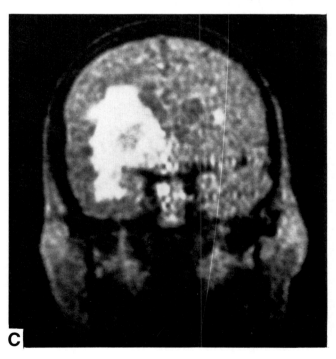

FIG. 3-13. Lymphoma involving the right cerebral hemisphere shown by CT (A) and coronal MRI images (B, C). In partial saturation images (B), the long T_1 of the tumor is demonstrated. In spin echo images (C), infiltration into the temporal lobe and the seeding in the opposite hemisphere are clearly shown.

the blood brain barrier within the lesion. An effective intravenous contrast administration protocol for adults is the rapid infusion of approximately 150 mL of 30% iodinated contrast agent prior to scanning and then the slower infusion of about 150 mL of contrast during scanning. With this protocol, the blood iodine concentration rises rapidly and is maintained at a high level during scanning. A higher volume of contrast material and delayed scanning are not recommended for routine use with modern CT equipment because of the possibility of impaired renal function. Patients with known cardiac disease should be limited to a total volume of 150 mL of 60% iodinated contrast agent. One milliliter of 60% iodinated contrast agent per pound of body weight is recommended in children, who are usually given a dose in an intravenous bolus for convenience.

Dynamic scanning is a rapid sequence of CT scans obtained during contrast injection which permits the visualization of arteries and has, in part, supplanted angiography. It has particular value in evaluating structures around the sella turcica. Aneurysms can be distinguished from tumor masses. For dynamic scanning, 1.5 mm-thick CT images are obtained at a single level. The first scan is obtained 5 seconds after initiation of the bolus injection of 50 mL of 60% iodinated contrast agent. Subse-

quently scans are obtained every 10–15 seconds for 90 seconds. Time density curves can be used to differentiate vascular and soft tissue structures.[24,65,91] Hypervascular tumors can be distinguished from aneurysms.

Although CT findings in brain tumors can never substitute for histopathology, a good deal of information can be gleaned about the tumor from the CT findings.[90] With gliomas, CT findings vary with tumor grade. A typical low-grade astrocytoma is characterized by slight hypodensity (with respect to brain), minimal mass, and no peritumoral edema or contrast enhancement. Tumor margins are frequently well defined, but may be indistinct if the density of the tumor in the adjacent brain is similar. Cysts and necrosis are uncommon in low-grade gliomas. Calcification, which is a frequent CT finding in these tumors, is usually central. An uncalcified low-grade astrocytoma may resemble an acute infarct on CT.

Intermediate-grade astrocytomas are usually characterized by inhomogeneous matrix, central hypodense cystic or necrotic zones, infrequent calcification, and moderate peritumoral edema. Cysts within the tumor are usually distinguished from necrosis by their sharply defined, rather than irregular and indistinct, margins on CT. Contrast enhancement in intermediate-grade gliomas varies from abundant to none. A subacute (1–6-week old) infarction may simulate a hypodense glioma; however, an infarct has a distinctive shape which corresponds to the distribution of a specific vessel or vessels, and has a characteristic pattern of peripheral, rarely central, enhancement. Cerebral abscess is characterized by a thin, uniform ring of enhancement; considerable reactive edema; and usually is associated with a strongly suggestive clinical picture. Glioblastoma multiforme or astrocytoma Grade III and IV appears in unenhanced CT images as a large inhomogeneous mass with irregular, poorly defined margins and central hypodense zones. Contrast enhancement is usually intense and inhomogeneous. The CT appearance of a typical glioblastoma multiforme may be mimicked by a large solitary necrotic metastasis. The most characteristic appearance of a parenchymal metastasis in the brain is a mass surrounded by edema. Contrast enhancement in metastases depends on the size and type of metastatic lesion. Following intravenous contrast infusion, small metastases appear as round, well-marginated, homogeneously enhancing nodules. Larger metastases often have a lucent center because of necrosis. Metastases from squamous cell carcinoma of the lung may demonstrate little contrast enhancement.[68] An oligodendroglioma typically appears on unenhanced CT scans as a large, irregular inhomogeneous mass containing calcium and hyperdense zones. Peritumoral edema is variable, as is contrast enhancement. Ganglioglioma and ganglioneuroma appear on unenhanced CT scans as small, well-defined hypodense or ill-defined isodense masses. Calcified and cystic areas are frequent, and homogeneous contrast enhancement is seen in three-quarters of these tumors.[93] Primary lymphoma appears typically on unenhanced CT scans as one or more isodense or slightly hyperdense basal ganglia, corpus callosum, or periventricular masses.[77] These tumors may be large masses or small nodules. Peritumoral edema is usually slight, and following intravenous contrast infusion, lym-

phomatous masses enhance homogeneously and often intensely. Primary cerebral neuroblastoma on unenhanced CT scans demonstrates a hypodense, isodense, or mixed density mass which is frequently large with well-defined margins. These tumors often contain coarse, dense calcification; central cystic or necrotic zones; and hemorrhage.[22,94] Contrast enhancement is typically inhomogeneous. The combination of intracerebral calcification and hemorrhage in a young patient should suggest primary neuroblastoma.

In tumors of the pineal region, radiologic detection is less difficult than differentiation. CT's role in patients with pineal region neoplasms is to localize the mass precisely, identify invasion of adjacent structures, detect metastases, and evaluate ventricular size.

Choroid plexus papillomas on unenhanced CT scans appear as a homogeneous isodense or hyperdense intraventricular mass having smooth, well-defined, frequently lobulated, margins. Focal calcification within the tumor is common, and occasionally a hypodense zone representing central necrosis is identified. Intense homogeneous enhancement following intravenous contrast infusion is the rule. The adjacent ventricle is almost always enlarged. Ependymomas are characterized by moderate contrast enhancement, with half of the tumors being homogeneous and half inhomogeneous with hypodense cystic areas or punctate calcification. A meningioma typically appears on unenhanced CT scans as a well-defined, smoothly marginated, isodense or hyperdense mass abutting a meningeal surface. The hyperdense matrix of a meningioma is the result of a diminished water-content tumor with hypervascularity and microscopic psammomatous calcification. Focal peripheral or central punctate or globular calcification is identified in up to 20% of intracranial meningiomas. Most meningiomas demonstrate intense homogeneous contrast enhancement.

Because of the exceptional ability of the CT scan to reveal relatively small lesions in the brain, problems in locating the lesion for biopsy have become more frequent. CT scanning fortunately can now be used to direct the biopsy procedure to an accuracy of 2–3 mL.[14] The system developed by Brown may be used with any wide aperture CT scanner with target computations made using a portable calculator.[14,15] A high degree of geometric accuracy, along with a low complication rate has been found with this system in clinical trials in several centers.

Angiography. Angiography is still requested before surgery in many cases when the surgeon wishes to visualize the vascular supply of the lesion detected by a CT scan as well as to localize major arteries and veins along the surgical path. Occasionally the angiographic pattern aids in differential diagnosis (Figure 3-5). Some tumors have a characteristic "blush" or "stain" as a result of their abnormal hypervascularity. This is particularly marked on meningiomas. Rapid sequence CT scanning, however, has substituted for angiography in many circumstances.

Digital Subtraction Angiography.

Digital subtraction angiography with injection of contrast intravenously has had its main utility in the demonstration of atherosclerotic disease in the extracranial arteries. Because of dilution of the contrast material by the intravenous injection, no fine vascular detail can be appreciated, although tumor stains can be visualized. Digital subtraction angiography with intra-arterial injection has been more widely used in CNS tumor evaluation. The ability of the computer to enhance the density of the contrast material in the arteries allows the radiologist to use small amounts of relatively dilute contrast material for intra-arterial studies. (For example, 5–6 mL of 40% contrast material in the common carotid artery, compared with 10–12 mL of 60% contrast material for standard film arteriography.) This low injection rate and low concentration of contrast material reduces the risk of embolization from the contrast jet, virtually eliminates the unpleasant burning sensation that accompanys standard angiographic methods, and allows the use of very small catheter sizes, which should further reduce the hazards of intra-arterial studies.[58] The ease of handling the multiple images from digital subtraction angiography has contributed to the increased popularity of the technique.

Plain Roentgenograms.

Plain roentgenograms of the skull may reveal abnormal calcifications and alterations caused by intracranial pressure. In children, separation of cranial sutures may be observed; prolonged pressure may result in exaggeration of the cranial imprint of the cerebral convolutions. In temporal tumors, the main changes are observed in the sella turcica,[20] where there may be loss of lamina dura, amputation of the posterior clinoids, undercutting of the anterior clinoids, and flattening of the sella. Craniopharyngiomas may have dense or flaky calcifications. Meningiomas may produce cloud-like or stippled calcification.

Radioisotope Scanning.

Radionuclides with short half-life, especially technetium 99m, may be used for detection and localization of intracranial lesions. Until the availability of computed tomography (CT), brain scans were carried out on all patients in whom there was a suspicion of an intracranial tumor. However, computerized tomography has largely supplanted radioisotope scanning of the brain.

Ventriculography and Pneumoencephalography.

Ventriculography and pneumoencephalography are invasive procedures with considerable risk and discomfort, and have been largely replaced by CT.

Spine.

Roentgenologic examination for tumors of the spinal cord is basically limited to plain roentgenograms and to myelography. The combination of myelography with dilute water soluble contrast and CT has proven to be particularly useful.

Magnetic Resonance Imaging (MRI).

MRI is a method of forming cross-sectional images of the body by use of magnetic fields and radiowaves. MRI utilizes the fact that certain nuclei will orient themselves in a magnetic field and absorb and emit radiowaves at their "resonant" frequency. Through complex calculations (performed by a computer), an image can be formed from the emitted radiowave.

In addition to forming images, MRI can give information about local physiological and biochemical abnormalities.

Magnetic resonance imaging of protons has recently been evaluated in oncology patients (Figures 3-12, 3-13). From the studies reported to date, MRI appears to equal CT in demonstrating cerebral neoplasia. It has a number of advantages over CT and a number of applications in which it clearly excels over CT. Numerous reports show that MRI detects small infiltrating malignancies more effectively than CT. In cases in which CT demonstrates no abnormality or only a subtle mass effect, MRI defines a region of abnormal signal intensity, affording a much better localization of the tumor. In brain stem pathology, MRI demonstrates the abnormality more consistently than CT because of the greater contrast sensitivity of the technique, and because CT studies of the posterior fossa are degraded by artifacts from the petrous bones, while MRI images are not, since little signal is produced by bone (Figures 3-14, 3-15). Also, MRI provides coronal (Figure 3-16) and sagittal projections which are difficult to achieve with CT. MRI effectively demonstrates infiltrating osseous neoplasms, since as neoplasm replaces bone, the faint signal is replaced by a relatively intense one. Almost every type of cerebral and cranial tumor has been studied with MRI although the objective comparisons of CT and MRI are still lacking (Figure 3-17). Benign tumors are more difficult to demonstrate effectively with MRI since the T1 and T2 characteristics of benign tumors do not differ substantially from normal intracranial structures. One problem with the MRI image of malignant tumors is that edema in tumors is difficult to differentiate, since each is associated with a prolonged T1 and T2 relaxation. With the combination of CT and MRI, tumor (the enhancing portion of the neoplasm) and the edema (the halo of low attenuation around the tumor) can be better differentiated. The sen-

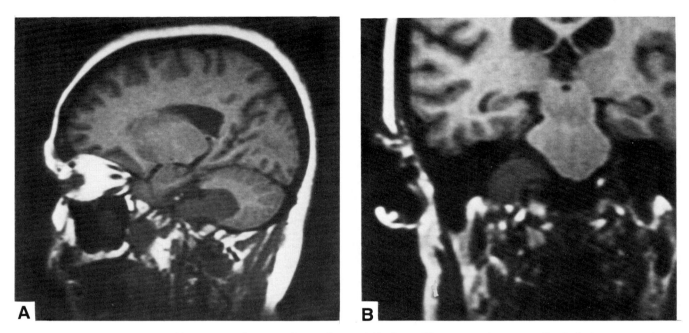

FIG. 3-14. Jugular foramen neurofibroma imaged in sagittal (A) and coronal (B) planes. These projections more effectively demonstrate the extent of tumor than did the axial CT images. The detection of the tumor is facilitated by the negligible signal from adjacent bone.

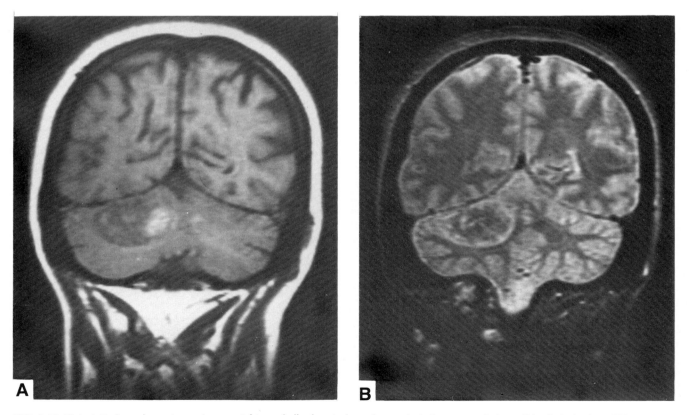

FIG. 3-15. Metastatic bronchogenic carcinoma, right cerebellar hemisphere demonstrated on coronal views. (A) relatively short TR sequence which reveals tissue of a short T_1, presumably blood. (B) a longer TR sequence which produces improved contrast between gray and white matter.

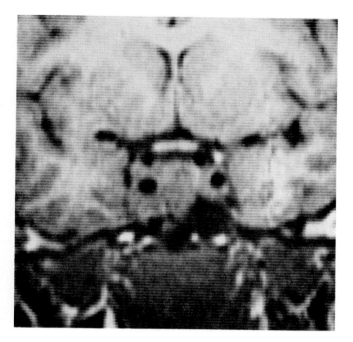

FIG. 3-16. Pituitary adenoma. Note that in the T_1 weighted image, the normally low-intensity signal from the cavernous sinuses has been replaced by the higher-intensity signal associated with the tumor. Cavernous sinus invasion is better evaluated by MRI than by CT.

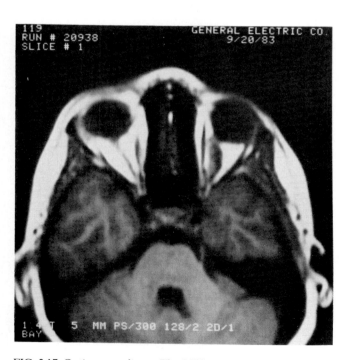

FIG. 3-17. Optic nerve glioma. The MRI appearance is not specific, but the extent of tumor is easily evaluated by MRI.

sitivity of MRI may increase, following greater experience in choosing the ideal pulse sequences. Applications of tissue characterization, spectroscopy, and surface coils have just begun. The role of MRI in the evaluation of tumors of the central nervous system is bound to increase.

Histopathologic Diagnosis. The importance of obtaining histologic diagnosis in managing deep brain lesions has been emphasized by the study of Broggi and Franzini who found that the histology in 10 of their series of 35 patients differed from their preoperative diagnosis based on clinical and radiologic studies. They feel, therefore, that they may have avoided inappropriate therapy in as many as 28% of the patients.[13]

The principal means of follow-up of brain neoplasms is also the X-ray CT scan at the present time. The study by Norman et al.[61] suggests that serial scans done at arbitrary intervals after treatment may be worthwhile, since CT scans revealed evidence of progression of a brain tumor an average of 2 months before clinical deterioration occurred in 9 of their 33 patients. Marks and Gado,[54] however, found that the CT findings correlated well with the clinical course in 93% of their patients, and conclude that the routine use of serial CT scans for follow-up was not justified. Recurrence rates as high as 47% may be found in follow-up scans in certain tumors such as medulloblastoma and ependymoma, either at the primary site or seeded throughout the ventricular system of subarachnoid spaces (Figure 3-4).[30]

Spinal Cord Seeding vs. Metastases. In most brain neoplasm cases, patient outcome depends upon the successful management of the primary lesion. However, certain tumors do seed to other parts of the craniospinal axis via CSF pathways. Since CT scanning has not proven effective in detecting intraspinal metastases, a decision must be made regarding the use of myelography in staging a number of CNS tumors. Bryan[16] collected 96 cases of CSF seeding by intracranial tumors, and found that 61.4% of these were malignant astrocytomas that had invaded ventricular surfaces. Since it was the primary mass that killed these patients, however, he concluded that myelography was not indicated in cases of astrocytoma.

Medulloblastoma is notorious for spread via CSF pathways, including extension antegrade to the third ventricle, lateral ventricles, basal cisterns, and spinal canal (Figure 3-4).[81] Deutsch and Reigel[28] found spinal metastases in 7 of 16 newly diagnosed medulloblastomas. None of the patients had spinal cord symptoms. CSF cytology was not accurate in detecting these metastases. They therefore recommend myelography in all cases for staging of medulloblastoma before treatment. Dorwart et al.[29] found spinal lesions in only one of nine patients with medulloblastoma at the time of initial diagnosis, but three of nine showed spinal metastases on myelograms at the time of the first signs of intracranial recurrence.

Ependymomas also seed relatively frequently to the spinal canal.[83] Spinal metastases were seen in 11 of 32 patients in a study by Kim and Fayos.[48] Of the 11 ependymomas producing metastases, 10 were infratentorial. Nine of these lesions were poorly differentiated histologically. They conclude that infratentorial, poorly differentiated ependymomas should therefore receive spinal axis irradiation as part of the initial therapy.

Pineal tumors may also seed the spinal axis (Figure 3-9), but in one study of 140 cases, only nine showed spinal metastases. A minority of these cases were biopsied, so the relation of CFS seeding to histology was not determined. The authors conclude that prophylactic irradiation to the spinal column is not justified as a routine procedure, in view of the morbidity associated with spinal radiotherapy in children.[88]

The decision to employ myelography in staging medulloblastomas, infratentorial, poorly differentiated ependymomas, and tumors of the pineal region should be made based on probabilities of spinal metastases indicated in the previous section, and also upon how a negative myelographic study will or will not affect treatment decisions at a given institution.

Metastatic Brain Tumors. Extracranial, remote metastases from intracranial primary tumors are rare occurrences, so that no imaging procedures are indicated for staging purposes when a lesion is known to represent a central nervous system primary tumor.[8,37] A special problem confronts the clinician, however, when a single lesion is found on CT scans without the assurance that it represents a brain neoplasm: Is it a primary brain tumor, metastasis from elsewhere in the body, or even a single brain abscess? There are no CT criteria that reliably distinguish between these possibilities (Figure 3-12). Primary brain malignancies may be less dense, isodense, or more dense than normal brain tissue on plain CT scan, and their enhancement is extremely variable. A single metastasis may be similar in appearance, but in the cooperative study summarized by Potts et al.,[66] 90% of the metastatic lesions in that study exhibited necrotic centers, and surrounding edema was moderate or marked. A single brain abscess is usually less dense than brain on the plain scan and shows a relatively thin wall-enhancing ring following intravenous contrast infusion. A thick or nodular wall is more characteristic of tumor than abscess.[76] The National Cancer Institute study revealed no distinct CT features that would permit the identification of the site of primary lesion in a series of 343 cases of brain metastases.[66] Voorhies et al.[85] studied 210 adult patients with single supratentorial lesions and found that in 23 cases the brain mass had produced the initial symp-

toms that brought the patient to medical attention. Ten of these 23 lesions were metastases from the lung, three were from kidney, and only one from a primary colon tumor. The primary site in the other nine cases remained unknown despite an extensive radiological workup. These authors conclude that a chest X-ray and IVP are sufficient prebiopsy screening studies in patients with a brain mass on CT scan but no evidence of an extracranial primary tumor site.

Both skull and meningeal metastases may be missed on CT scans, and are best detected by isotope studies.[5,47] Lymphomatous involvement of the meninges is more reliably detected by CSF cytology than by CT scan.[63] If meningeal disease is detected by CT scan, no clue to the type of tumor is generally seen, with the possible exception of neuroblastoma, in those instances when extracranial and orbital disease is also present (Figure 3-18).

Spinal Cord Neoplasms. Supratentorial lesions that seed via CSF to the spinal canal are discussed in earlier sections. Primary tumors of the spinal cord itself are uncommon, compared with brain neoplasms in all age groups. In a study of 488 central nervous system tumors in chil-

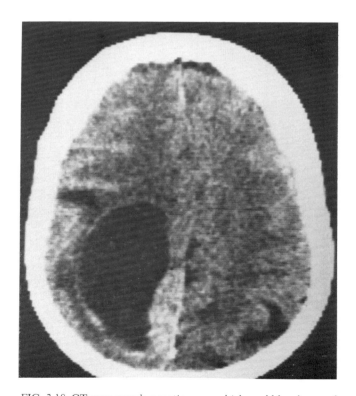

FIG. 3-18. CT scan reveals a cystic mass, which could be abscessed, primary, or secondary neoplasm. The thickening of the wall of the lesions medially favors neoplasm, but does not help in determining whether it is a primary brain tumor or metastasis. Biopsy revealed metastatic carcinoma.

dren, for example, only 21 were intraspinal.[34] Most primary malignancies of the cord are astrocytomas or ependymomas, and cause symptoms secondary to local growth.[32] Nerve sheath tumors such as neurilemomas and meningiomas also produce pain and other symptoms relative to the site of the primary mass only.

CT has shown promise in limited series as a method for detection of spinal cord mass lesions.[33,43] Cysts in the cord, and certain vascular tumors such as hemangioblastoma, can be demonstrated. Gliomas, however, may be isodense and may not enhance after AV contrast infusion.[51] Standard film myelography appears to remain the most practical means of screening a patient for a possible intraspinal mass. CT is particularly valuable in studying a short segment of the spinal canal thought to be abnormal clinically or by myelography (Figure 3-19). MRI is capable of demonstrating the spinal cord in both cross-sectional and longitudinal views. With refinements in this technology and widened availability of the equip-

ment, MRI may become the method of choice for spinal cord imaging.

IMAGING STRATEGIES AND DECISIONS

A flow diagram for the evaluation of a suspected brain tumor is presented (Figure 3-20). Assuming that a single lesion is found, the clinician must consider the possibility that the CT scan abnormality is a metastasis from an occult or silent primary tumor. This is even more true if multiple lesions appear suddenly. Chest X ray and IVP may be indicated before brain biopsy[85] to rule out two common sites: lung cancer and renal carcinoma. The intracranial vascular study is considered optional, based on the desire of the neurosurgeon to know the position of major vessels near the mass and general tumor vascularity before biopsy. A standard film angiogram may be done, or an intravenous digital study may suffice. A biopsy diagnosis of medulloblastoma, ependymoma, or pineal cytoma should be followed by myelography, if the presence or absence of spinal metastases will alter the therapy protocol. As a baseline study, follow-up scan series should be made after treatment. Additional CT scans are recommended only as indicated by the patient's clinical status.

A flow diagram for the evaluation of a suspected spinal

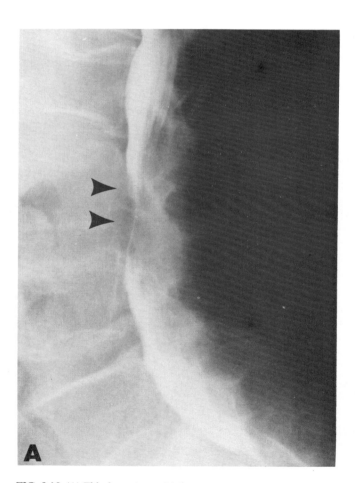

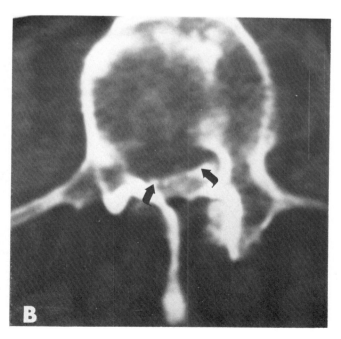

FIG. 3-19. (A) Elderly patient with known osteoblastic prostate metastases in the pelvis. Severe low back pain. Lateral view from myelogram series shows an extradural mass impinging upon the dye column, crossing a disc space but extending a considerable distance above it (arrows). The posterior cortical line adjacent to this extradural lesion is indistinct. (B) Single CT scan from a series of adjacent scan sections clearly demonstrates tumor involvement in the vertebrae with destruction of the posterior vertebral body margin, and extension of tumor into the canal (arrows). Nerve roots are crowded into the dorsal aspect of the spinal canal. Surgical biopsy revealed prostatic carcinoma.

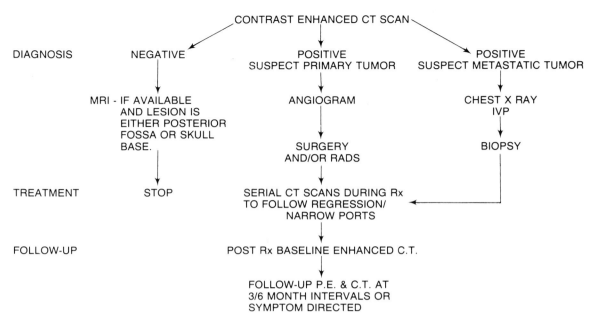

FIG. 3-20. Decision tree: suspected brain mass.

cord tumor is presented in Figure 3-21. Since most spinal masses prove to be metastases, routine X rays of the spine to define local bone involvement, together with a radionuclide bone scan to search for other skeletal lesions, are suggested. Myelography with water soluble contrast medium, both above and below the base of the obturator, is recommended to better define the subarachnoid space in relation to the lesion. Occasionally, multiple metastatic obstructing lesions can be found. CT scan imaging at the level of myelographic abnormality may be very useful in defining the extent of an extradural mass if lymphomas are suspected, particularly if bone films and scans are negative (Figure 3-13). Myelography or CT may be used in follow-up evaluation, based

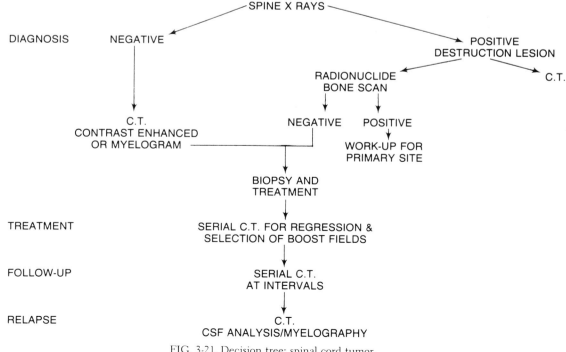

FIG. 3-21. Decision tree: spinal cord tumor.

upon the patient's symptoms. The cost-benefit ratio for these imaging modalities is shown in Table 3-2.

TREATMENT DECISIONS

The challenge, therapeutically, is to obtain local control and/or ablation, since this is synonymous with cure and long-term survival.[9,23,49,55,71] Although surgery is the first modality to be used, it is very limited in its ability to eradicate most truly invasive brain tumors because of the destruction of vital structures and the neurologic impairment that may result. Therefore, radiation therapy is commonly used, both in a definitive and adjuvant fashion, depending upon tumor residuum. A real improvement in survival has occurred with supervoltage techniques in common childhood brain tumors such as medulloblastoma, ependymomas, optic gliomas, craniopharyngiomas, and in both low and high grade gliomas. Chemotherapy, although frequently used in association with irradiation, is largely investigational in nature (Table 3-3).[9]

Supratentorial Tumors

For stage I, grade 1 tumors, the histopathology of a primary brain tumor determines the use of a modality, and its success, more than any other factor. For benign and low-grade tumors such as meningiomas, grade 1

astrocytomas, neurilemomas, pituitary adenomas, and craniopharyngiomas, complete resection is attempted, short of producing serious morbidity or running the risk of a mortality. Most often, postoperative irradiation is required as an adjuvant with a high degree of success in pituitary adenomas and craniopharyngiomas.[1,50] At the time of relapse, or if resection is incomplete, irradiation is used for low-grade astrocytomas and meningiomas. Meningiomas are best resected as completely as possible before undertaking radiation therapy.

For stage II, grade 2 gliomas, which include astrocytomas, ependymomas, oligodendrogliomas, or mixtures, surgical resection is always attempted, but however complete the resection, the risk of recurrence is high and postoperative adjuvant radiation therapy is advised. Rarely is chemotherapy used initially; it should be reserved for relapse.

For stage III, IV, and grade 3, 4 gliomas, particularly large tumors that cross the midline (T_4), resections are limited and are largely used for decompression of a rapidly expanding mass, rather than for a curative resection. All modalities are used since tumor control is difficult. Full-dose photon irradiation, even with doses as high as 7,000 to 8,000 cGy is rarely successful.[72] The addition of BCNU to irradiation is widely practiced but seldom adds more than 3 to 6 months to median survival.[86] Once relapse occurs, investigational combinations of

Table 3-2. Imaging Modalities for Evaluating Brain and Spinal Cord Tumors

MODALITY	STAGING CAPABILITY	COST BENEFIT RATIO	RECOMMEND AS ROUTINE STAGING PROCEDURE
A. Non-Invasive Plain X ray	Useful mainly in detecting osseous metastases from non-CNS neoplasms.	Low	Brain—No Spine—Yes
Nuclear medicine scan	Will detect most brain tumors. Best for detection of bone metastases from non-CNS neoplasms.	High	Brain—No Spine—Yes
Magnetic resonance scan	Unproven. Probably best in posterior fossa. Will play a role in spinal cord imaging.	?	?
B. Minimally Invasive Contrast-enhanced CT scan	Best test at present for detection, definition, and follow-up of brain tumors. Limited use in cord tumors.	High	Yes
C. Invasive Angiography	Aids in brain tumor characterization. Rarely used for either detection or follow-up.	Low	No
Myelography	Best test at present for spinal cord mass detection, whether I° or II°.	High	Yes
Biopsy	Required for most CNS tumors. May be done very accurately in the brain with CT guidance.	High	Yes

Table 3-3. Treatment Decisions for Central Nervous System Tumors

TUMOR	SURGERY		RADIATION THERAPY	CHEMOTHERAPY
Stage/Grade I, II	Complete resection, if possible		For residual and recurrent tumor: 5,000–6,000 cGy	NR
Stage/Grade III, IV	Partial resection Decompression		High doses are used: 6,000–8,000 cGy	BCNU simultaneously at start of RT
Medulloblastoma Ependymoblastoma	Complete resection, if feasible		Moderate doses are used: 4,500–5,500 cGy, depending on age	MAC is under investigation
Meningiomas	Complete resection, if possible	AND/OR	For residual and recurrent tumor: 6,000 cGy	NR
Pituitary Adenoma	Complete resection, if possible	AND/OR	As an adjuvant or definitive RT: 4,500–5,500 cGy	NR
Craniopharyngioma	Partial or complete resection		As an adjuvant or definitive RT: 5,500–6,000 cGy	NR
Pinealomas	No biopsy or attempt to resect		5,000 cGy	NR
Midbrain and brain stem	No biopsy or attempt to resect		5,000–6,000 cGy	NR

Key: NR = Not recommended
        RT = Radiation therapy
        MAC = Multiagent chemotherapy
        BCNU = 1,3 bis (2-chloroethyl)-1-nitrosourea

drugs are often used but rarely produce complete remissions. Agents such as BCNU, procarbazine, VM26, CCNU, vincristine, and methotrexate may be used alone or in combination.[23] Neutron beam therapy has produced a high degree of tumor sterilization, but unfortunately has also produced a large complication rate of white matter atrophy.[9] The Third Conference in Brain Tumor Therapy in 1979 updated the accomplishments of 5 years of intensive multimodal investigations. At best, all modes investigated—surgery, radiation therapy, and chemotherapy—were palliative only for adult malignant tumors.[80] This conclusion is still valid five years later.

Infratentorial Tumors

Most infratentorial tumors occur in childhood, and include medulloblastomas, ependymomas, cystic astrocytomas, and rarely, hemangioblastomas. Resection and decompression are the essential first steps in treatment. The tumors that have a high propensity to seed the subarachnoid space are medulloblastomas and ependymomas of intermediate and high grade; extended field radiation therapy is recommended to include the spinal axis. Pineal tumors such as pinealblastomas are also included in the group that tend to spread in this fashion. Posterior fossa tumors, such as medulloblastoma, or ependymomas in children, are particularly prone to seeding out in the subarachnoid space. Although the clinical incidence is 10% to 15%, the autopsy studies are as high as 30% (Table 3-4). Fortunately, these tumors are radiosensitive,

Table 3-4. Estimated Survival* for the More Common Brain Tumors

TUMOR	PERCENT SURVIVAL	
	5-YEAR	10-YEAR
Astrocytoma		
Grade I (cerebellar)	90–100	85–100
Grade I (all sites)	50–60	30–40
Grade II	16–46	8–15
Grade III	10–30	0–10
Grade IV	0–10	0–1
Medulloblastoma	40–50	20–30
Ependymoma	40–55	35–45
Oligodendroglioma	50–80	20–30
Brain stem**	20–30	0–10
Third ventricle and midbrain**	25–35	5–10
Pinealoma**	50–90	55–65
Pituitary adenoma	80–95	70–90
Craniopharyngioma	80–90	65–80
Optic	75–100	70–85
Meningioma†	70–80	50–60

*All figures are rounded and represent ranges of reported series in the literature. With the exception of grade I (cerebellar) astrocytomas, radiation therapy has been employed as an adjuvant to surgery.

**Radiation therapy alone is employed for the treatment of these tumors.

†Chemotherapy in adjuvant setting has not been established to add to 5- or 10-year survival.

Reprinted from Salazar, O. M.: *Moments of Decision in Primary Brain Tumors.* Chicago, American College of Radiology, 1977. With permission.

and the majority of patients (i.e., 50% or more) are able to survive, depending upon age and tumor grade, with modern techniques.[9]

Treatment Response Evaluation and Follow-up

CT scanning is the best method currently available for following the progress of treatment of brain tumors. A baseline CT scan is essential to establish how much of the tumor is left after surgery, and appearance prior to radiation therapy.[4,87] An early systematic study showed that serial CT scans were useful in following regression or growth, the development of brain necrosis and edema, changes in tumor density, and changes in the size of the ventricles, due either to loss of brain volume or ventricular obstruction.[64] As presented earlier, follow-up scans done at arbitrary intervals are probably of no more value than timing the scans related to some change in a patient's clinical status.[54] Postoperative baseline scans should be made in the first day or two following surgery to avoid mistaking early granulation tissue enhancement for residual tumor. Enhancing zones may appear after combined radiotherapy and chemotherapy because of damage to the blood-brain barrier by these treatment modalities.[87] Biopsy may be necessary to exclude residual tumors.

Myelography with water-soluble agents supplemented by CT scanning provides useful follow-up information after treatment for spinal tumors. Film myelography shows the longitudinal anatomy within the spinal canal best, while the axial CT scan is best for demonstrating paraspinal disease.

Treatment considerations have little effect on the choice of imaging follow-up studies in CNS tumors. CT scanning is the best method for defining the amount of residual tumor present, the effect of steroids on edema, the presence or absence of ventricular obstruction, etc. Myelography supplemented by CT provides follow-up information regarding cord tumors, regardless of the mode of therapy employed. Magnetic resonance imaging may eventually be the imaging method of choice for the post-treatment follow-up of spinal cord neoplasms, but at present this is speculation.

IMPACT OF NEW TECHNOLOGY

The proved tumor detection capability provided by CT scanning presents more of an opportunity for improved surgical cure rates for small brain tumors than was possible before CT. CT-guided stereotactic methods are now evolving, which should further improve both diagnostic and therapeutic results. Accurate biopsy of small, deep-seated tumors will improve histologic grading, and CT-guided stereotactic resection methods may improve cure rates by providing the neurosurgeon more

accurate spatial data than is presently obtainable under direct vision.[46,74] Coupling the CT-guided stereotactic neurosurgical apparatus to real-time, intraoperative ultrasonic B-scan monitoring should also improve the accuracy of small tumor resection.[41] Interstitial radiation implants placed using CT-guided stereotactic procedures also show promise, both in improving accuracy of dosimetry in the tumor volume, and also reducing the incidence of late CNS complications in long-term survivors due to high-dose whole brain radiation.[59]

The impact of magnetic resonance imaging on the diagnosis and management of CNS tumors awaits broader availability of new equipment and prospective studies. The absence of ionizing radiation, and the elimination of bone artifact on posterior fossa scans in particular, favor MRI over CT. The ease with which images from axial, coronal, and sagittal planes can be obtained also offers significant advantages to the study of both the brain and the spinal cord. A variety of dynamic processes may also be studied clinically at some point in the future. For example, blood flow studies comparing one area of the brain to another may be useful. The CT variables for tumor response to therapy may be supplanted by improved criteria using MRI methods. Since different tissue components respond differently to MRI excitation processes in vitro, MRI offers hope that certain chemical variables may be studied which could improve fundamental differential diagnostic information, such as differentiating inflammatory from neoplastic masses, and possibly even help distinguish between certain tumors to a degree not possible using CT techniques.

REFERENCES

1. Amacher, A. L.: Craniopharyngioma: The controversy regarding radiotherapy. *Child's Brain* 6:57–64, 1980.
2. American Cancer Society: *Cancer Facts and Figures.* New York, American Cancer Society, 1982.
3. American Joint Committee on Cancer: *AJC Manual for Staging of Cancer,* 2nd ed. Philadelphia, J. B. Lippincott, 1983, 219–226.
4. Andreou, J., George, A. E., Wise, A., deLeon, M., Kricheff, I. I., Ransohoff, J., Foo, S. H.: CT prognostic criteria of survival after malignant glioma surgery. *A.J.N.R.* 4:488–490, 1983.
5. Ascherl, G. F., Hilal, S. K., Brisman, R.: Computed tomography of disseminated meningeal and ependymal malignant neoplasms. *Neurology* 31:567–574, 1981.
6. Bahr, A. L., Hodges, F. J.: Efficacy of computed tomography of the head in changing patient care and health costs: A retrospective study. *A.J.R.* 131:45–49, 1978.
7. Baker, H. L., Houser, O. W., Campbell, J. K.: National Cancer Institute study: Evaluation of computed tomography in the diagnosis of intracranial neoplasms: 1. Overall results. *Radiology* 136:91–96, 1980.
8. Banna, M., Lassman, L. P., Pearce, G. W.: Radiological study of skeletal metastases from cerebellar medulloblastoma. *Br. J. Radiol.* 43:173–179, 1980.
9. Bloom, H. J. G.: Intracranial tumors response and persistence to therapeutic endeavors, 1970–1980. *Int. J. Radiat. Oncol. Biol. Phys.* 8:1083–1113, 1982.

10. Borden, S. IV, Weker, A. L., Toch, R., Wang, C. C.: Pineal germinoma. *Am. J. Dis. Child* 126:214–216, 1983.

11. Brant-Zawadski, M., Badami, J. P., Mills, C. M., Norman, D., Newton, T. H.: Primary intracranial tumor imaging: A comparison of magnetic resonance and CT. *Radiology* 150:435–440, 1984.

12. Brismar, J., Stromblad, L. G., Salford, L. G.: Impact of CT in the neurosurgical management of intracranial tumors. *Neuroradiol.* 16:506–509, 1978.

13. Broggi, G., Franzini, A.: Value of serial stereotactic biopsies and impedance monitoring in the treatment of deep brain tumors. *J. Neurol. Neurosurg. Psychiatry* 44:397–401, 1981.

14. Brown, R. A., Roberts, T. S., Osborn, A. G.: Stereotactic frame and computer software for CT-directed neurosurgical localization. *Invest. Radiol.* 15:308–312, 1980.

15. Brown, R. A., Roberts, T. S., Osborn, A. G.: Simplified CT guided stereotactic biopsy. *A.J.N.R.* 2:181–184, 1981.

16. Bryan, P.: CSF seeding of intracranial tumors: A study of 96 cases. *Clin. Radiol.* 25:355–360, 1974.

17. Burger, P. C.: Pathologic anatomy and CT correlations in the glioblastoma multiforme. *Appl. Neurophysiol.* 46:180–187, 1983.

18. Butler, A. R., Leo, J. S., Lin, J. P., Boyd, A. D., Kricheff, I. I.: The value of routine cranial computed tomography in neurologically intact patients with primary carcinoma of the lung. *Radiology* 131:399–401, 1979.

19. Butler, A. R., Passalagna, A. M., Bernestein, A., Kricheff, I.: Contrast-enhanced CT scans and radionuclide brain scan in supratentorial gliomas. *A.J.R.* 132:607–611, 1979.

20. Cala, L. A.: Correlation of papilledema and sella changes with site of tumor (excluding pituitary tumors). *Neuroradiology* 5:142–144, 1973.

21. Cappelaere, P., Clay, A., Adenis, L., Demaille, A., Laine, E.: Les metastases des tumeurs cerebrale primitives en dehors du nevraxe: a propos de trois observations. *Bull. Cancer* (Paris) 59:235–254, 1972.

22. Chambers, E. F., Turski, P. A., Sobel, D., Wara, M. W., Newton, T. H.: Radiologic characteristics of primary cerebral neuroblastomas. *Radiology* 139:101–104, 1981.

23. Chang, C. S. (Ed.): *Tumors of the Central Nervous System.* New York, Masson Publ., 1981.

24. Cohen, W. A., Pinto, R. S., Kricheff, I. I.: Dynamic CT scanning for visualization of the parasellar carotid arteries. *A.J.N.R.* 3:185–189, 1982.

25. Crooks, L., Arakawa, M., Hoehninger, M. J., Watts, J., McRee, R., Kaufman, L., Davis, P. L., Margulis, A. R., DeGroot, J.: Nuclear magnetic resonance whole body imager operating at 3.5 K gauss. *Radiology* 143:169–174, 1982.

26. Davis, D. O.: CT in the diagnosis of supratentorial tumors. *Semin. Roentgenol.* 12:97–108, 1977.

27. del Regato, J. A., Spjut, H. J., Cox, J. D. (Eds.): *Cancer Diagnosis, Treatment and Prognosis,* 6th ed. St. Louis, C. V. Mosby, 1985.

28. Deutsch, M., Reigel, D. H.: The value of myelography in the management of childhood medulloblastoma. *Cancer* 45:2194–2197, 1980.

29. Dorwart, R. H., Wara, W. M., Norman, D., Levin, V. A.: Complete myelographic evaluation of spinal metastases from medulloblastoma. *Radiology* 139:403–408, 1981.

30. Enzmann, D. R., Norman, D., Levin, V., Wilson, C., Newton, T. H.: Computed tomography in the follow-up of medulloblastomas and ependymomas. *Radiology* 128:57–63, 1978.

31. EORTC Brain Tumor Group: Effect of CCNU on survival rate of objective remission and duration of free interval in patients with malignant brain glioma—Final evaluation. *Eur. J. Cancer.* 14:1851–1856, 1978.

32. Epstein, B. S.: *The Spine: A Radiologic Text and Atlas,* 4th ed. Philadelphia, Lea & Febiger, 1976.

33. Ethier, R., King, D. G., Melancon, D., Belanger, G., Taylor, S., Thompson, C.: Development of high resolution computed tomography of the spinal cord. *J. Comput. Assist. Tomogr.* 3:433–438, 1979.

34. Farwell, J. R., Dohrmann, G. J., Flannery, J. T.: Central nervous system tumors in children. *Cancer* 40:3123–3132, 1977.

35. Fineberg, H. V., Bauman, R., Sosman, M.: Computerized cranial tomography. Effect on diagnostic and therapeutic plans. *J.A.M.A.* 238:224–227, July 18, 1977.

36. French, L. A., Ausman, J. I.: Metastatic neoplasms to the brain. *Clin. Neurosurg.* 24:41–46, 1976.

37. Glasauer, F., Yuan, R. H. P.: Intracranial tumors with extracranial metastases. Case report and review of the literature. *J. Neurosurg.* 20:474–493, 1963.

38. Gold, E. M., Gordis, L.: Determinants of survival in children with brain tumors. *Ann. Neurol.* 5:569–574, 1979.

39. Gutin, P., Phillips, T. I., Hosobuchi, Y., Wara, W. M., MacKay, A. R., Weaver, K. A., Lamb, S., Hurst, S.: Permanent and removable implants for brachtherapy of brain tumors. *Int. J. Radiat. Oncol. Biol. Phys.* 7:1371–1382, 1981.

40. Healy, J. F., Rosenkrantz, H.: Intraventricular metastases demonstrated by cranial computed tomography. *Radiology* 136:124, 1980.

41. Heilbrun, M. P., Roberts, T. S., Apuzzo, M. L. J., Wells, T. H., Sabishin, J. K.: Preliminary experience with BRW CT stereotaxic guidance system. *J. Neurosurg.* 59:217–222, 1983.

42. Henriquez, A. S., Robertson, D. M., Marshall, W. J. S.: Primary neuroblastoma of the central nervous system with spontaneous extracranial metastases. *J. Neurosurg.* 38:226–231, 1973.

43. Hilal, S. K.: CT of the spinal cord with the submillimeter fourth generation scanner (meeting abstract). *J. Comput. Assist. Tomogr.* 3:567, 1979.

44. Ho, K. C.: Tumors of the central nervous system. In *Medical College of Wisconsin Neuropathology Course Syllabus,* K. C. Ho (Ed.). 1979.

45. Kazner, E., Meese, W., Kretzschmar, K.: The role of computed tomography in the diagnosis of brain tumors in infants and children. *Neuroradiology* 16:10–12, 1978.

46. Kelly, P. J., Alker, G. J.: A method for stereotactic laser microsurgery in the treatment of deep-seated CNS neoplasms. *Appl. Neurophysiol.* 43:210–215, 1980.

47. Kido, D. K., Gould, R., Taati, F., Dunacan, A., Schnurs, S.: Comparative sensitivity of CT scans, radiographs, and radionuclide bone scans in detecting metastatic calvarial lesions. *Radiology* 128:371–375, 1978.

48. Kim, Y. H., Fayos, J. V.: Intracranial ependymomas. *Radiology* 124:805–808, 1977.

49. Kornblith, P. L., Walker, M. D., Cassady, R. J.: Neoplasms of the central nervous system. In *Cancer—Principles and Practice of Oncology,* DeVita, V. T. Jr., Hellman, S., Rosenberg, S. A. (Eds.). Philadelphia, J. B. Lippincott, 1982.

50. Kramer, S., McKissock, W., Concannon, J. P.: Craniopharyngioma: Treatment by combined surgery and radiation therapy. *J. Neurosurg.* 18:217–226, 1961.

51. Lee, B. E., Kazam, E., Newman, A. D.: Computed tomography of the spine and spinal cord. *Radiology* 128:95–102, 1978.

52. Levition, A., Fulchiero, A., Gilles, G. H., Winston, K.: Survival status of children with cerebellar gliomas. *J. Neurosurg.* 48:29–33, 1978.

53. Male, R. S., Bronskill, M. J., Rideout, D. F., Blend, R., Herman, S., Poon, P. Y.: Efficacy of computed tomography in the management of cancer patients. *Cancer* 52:1604–1608, 1983.

54. Marks, J. E., Gado, M.: Serial computed tomography of primary brain tumors following surgery, irradiation, and chemotherapy. *Radiology* 125:119–125, 1977.

55. McDonald, J. V., Salazar, O. M., Rubin, P., Lapham, L. W., Bakemeier, R. F.: Central nervous system tumors. In *Clinical Oncology for Medical Students and Physicians: A Multidisciplinary Approach,* 6th ed., P. Rubin (Ed.). New York, American Cancer Society, 1983, pp. 262–278.

56. McGinnis, B. D., Brady, T. J., New, P. F., Buonanno, F. S., Pykett, I. L., DeLaPaz, R. L., Kistler, J. P., Taveras, J. M.: Nuclear magnetic resonance (NMR) imaging of tumors in the posterior fossa. *J. Comput. Assist. Tomogr.* 7:11–17, 1983.

57. Merrit, H. H.: *A Textbook for Neurology*. Philadelphia, Lea & Febiger, 1979, pp. 214–215.

58. Miller, F. J., Mineau, D. E., Koehler, P. R., Nelson, J. A., Luers, P. D., Sherry, R. A., Lawrence, F. P., Anderson, R. E., Kruger, R. A.: Clinical intra-arterial digital subtraction imaging; Use of small volumes of iodated contrast material or carbon dioxide. *Radiology* 142:273–278, 1983.

59. Mundiger, F., Ostertag, C. G., Birg, W., Weigel, K.: Stereotactic treatment of brain lesions. *Appl. Neurophysiol.* 43:198–204, 1980.

60. Nelson, J. S.: The importance of brain tumor pathology. In *Therapy of CNS Tumors Syllabus*. Oak Brook, IL, The Radiological Society of North America, 1983.

61. Norman, D., Enzmann, D. R., Levin, V. A., Wilson, C. B., Newton, T. H.: Computed tomography in the evaluation of malignant glioma before and after therapy. *Radiology* 121:85–88, 1976.

62. O'Connell, D. J., Frank, P. H., Riddell, R. H.: The metastases of meningioma – radiologic and pathologic features. *Skeletal Radiol.* 3:30–35, 1978.

63. Pagani, J. J., Libshitz, H. I., Wallace, S., Hayman, L. A.: Central nervous system leukemia and lymphoma: Computed tomographic manifestations. *A.J.R.* 137:1195–1201, 1981.

64. Pay, N. T., Carella, R. J., Lin, J. P., Kricheff, I. I.: The usefulness of computed tomography during and after radiation therapy in patients with brain tumors. *Radiology* 121:79–83, 1976.

65. Pinto, R. S., Cohen, W. A., Kricheff, I. I., Redington, R. W., Berninger, W. H.: Giant intracranial aneurysms: Rapid sequential computed tomography. *A.J.N.R.* 3:495–499, 1982.

66. Potts, D. G., Abbott, F. G., von Sneidern, J. V.: National Cancer Institute study: Evaluation of computed tomography in the diagnosis of intracranial neoplasms. III: Metastatic tumors. *Radiology* 136:657–664, 1980.

67. Randell, C. P., Collins, A. G., Young, I. R., Haywood, R., Thomas, D. J., McDonnell, M. J., Orr, J. S., Bydder, G. M., Steiner, R. E.: Nuclear magnetic resonance imaging of posterior fossa tumors. *A.J.R.* 141:489–496, 1983.

68. Rao, K. C. V. G., Williams, J. P.: Intracranial tumors: Metastatic. In *Cranial Computed Tomography*. Lee, S. H., Rao, K. C. V. G. (Eds.), New York, McGraw-Hill Book Co., 1983, pp. 345–369.

69. Rubinstein, L. J.: Tumors of the central nervous system. In *Atlas of Tumor Pathology*, 2nd series, Fascicle 6. Washington, DC, Armed Forces Institute of Pathology, 1972, pp. 263–292.

70. Russell, D. S., Rubinstein, L. J.: *Pathology of Tumors of the Nervous System*, 4th ed. London, Edward Arnold Publ., 1977.

71. Salazar, O. M.: *Moments of Decision in Primary Brain Tumors*. Chicago, American College of Radiology, 1977.

72. Salazar, O. M., Rubin, P., Feldstein, M. L., Pizzutiello, R. S.: High-dose radiation therapy in the treatment of glioblastoma multiforme: A preliminary report. *Int. J. Radiat. Oncol. Biol. Phys.* 1733–1740, 1979.

73. Schott, L. H., Naidich, T. P., Gan, J.: Common pediatric brain tumors. Typical computed tomographic appearances. *Comput. Tomog.* 7:3–15, 1983.

74. Sheldon, C. H., McCann, G., Jacques, S., Lutes, H. R., Frazier, R. E., Katz, R., Kuk, R.: Development of a computerized microstereotaxic method for localization and removal of minute CNS lesions under direct 3D vision. *J. Neurosurg.* 52:21–27, 1980.

75. Solis, O. J., Davis, K. R., Adair, L. B., Roberson, G. R., Kleinman, G. M.: Intracerebral metastatic melanoma: CT evaluation. *Comput. Tomog.* 1:135–143, 1977.

76. Stevens, E. A., Norman, D., Kramer, R. A., Messina, A. B., Newton, T. H.: Computed tomographic brain scanning in intraparenchymal pyogenic abscesses. *A.J.R.* 130:111–114, 1978.

77. Tadmor, R., Davis, K. R., Roberson, G. H., Kleinman, G. M.: Computed tomography in primary malignant lymphoma of the brain. *J. Comput. Assist. Tomogr.* 2:135–140, 1978.

78. Tadmor, R., Harwood-Nash, D. C., Savoiardo, M., Scotti, G., Musgrave, M., Fitz, C. R., Chuang, S.: Brain tumors in the first two years of life: CT diagnosis. *A.J.N.R.* 1:411–417, 1980.

79. Tadmor, R., Harwood-Nash, D. C., Scotti, G., Savoiardo, M., Musgrave, M., Fitz, C. R., Chuang, S., Modan, M.: Intracranial neoplasms in children: The effect of computed tomography on age distribution. *Radiology* 145:371–373, 1982.

80. *Third Conference on Brain Tumor Therapy*, 1979, Cancer Treatment Reports Supp. 2, 1981.

81. Tsuchida, T., Tanaka, R., Fukuda, M., Tadeda, N., Ito, J., Honda, H.: CT findings of medulloblastoma. *Child Brain* 11:60–68, 1984.

82. Turcotte, J. F., Copty, M., Bedard, F., Michaud, J., Verret, S.: Lateral ventricle choroid plexus papilloma and communicating hydrocephalus. *Surg. Neurol.* 13:143–146, 1980.

83. Vaquero, J., Cabezudo, J. M., Nombela, L.: CT scan in subependymomas. *Br. J. Radiol.* 56:1, 1983.

84. Vonofakos, D., Marcu, H., Hacker, H.: Oligodendrogliomas: CT patterns with emphasis on features indicating malignancy. *J. Comput. Assist. Tomogr.* 3:783–788, 1979.

85. Voorhies, R. M., Sundaresan, N., Thaler, H. T.: The single supratentorial lesion. An evaluation of preoperative diagnostic tests. *J. Neurosurg.* 53:364–368, 1980.

86. Walker, M. D., Alexander, E., Jr., Hunt, W. E., MacCarty, C. S., Mahaley, M. S., Jr., Mealey, J., Jr., Norrell, H. A., Owens, G., Ransohoff, J., Wilson, C. B., Gehan, E. A., Strike, T. A.: Evaluation of BCNA and/or radiotherapy in the treatment of anaplastic gliomas. A cooperative clinical trial. *J. Neurosurg.* 49:333–343, 1978.

87. Wang, A. M., Skias, D. D., Rumbaugh, C. L., Schoene, W. C., Zamani, A.: Central nervous system changes after radiation therapy and/or chemotherapy: Correlation of CT and autopsy findings. *A.J.N.R.* 4:466–471, 1983.

88. Wara, W. M., Jenkin, R. D., Evans, A., Ertel, I., Hittle, R., Ortega, J., Wilson, C. B., Hammond, D.: Tumors of the pineal and suprasellar region: Children's cancer study group treatment results 1960–1975. *Cancer* 43:698–701, 1979.

89. Weinstein, M. A., Modic, M. T., Pavlicek, W., Keyser, C. K.: Nuclear magnetic resonance for the examination of brain tumors. *Semin. Roent.* 19:139–147, 1984.

90. Williams, A. L., Haughton, V. M.: *Cranial Computed Tomography: A Comprehensive Text*. St. Louis, C. V. Mosby, 1985.

91. Wing, S. D., Anderson, R. E., Osborn, A. G.: Dynamic CT scanning of the head. *A.J.N.R.* 1:135–139, 1980.

92. Wood, B. P., Haller, J. O., Berdon, W. E., Lin, S. R.: Shunt metastases of pineal tumors presenting as a pelvic mass. *Pediatr. Radiol.* 8:108–109, 1979.

93. Zimmerman, R. A., Bilaniuk, L. T.: Computed tomography of intracerebral gangliomas. *J. Comput. Tomogr.* 3:24–30, 1979.

94. Zimmerman, R. A., Bilaniuk, L. T.: CT of primary and secondary craniocerebral neuroblastoma. *A.J.R.* 135:1239–1242, 1980.

4 CERVICAL LYMPH NODE METASTASES

Anthony A. Mancuso

Cervical metastatic disease is an issue of paramount importance in the diagnosis and management of head and neck malignancies.[23] An overwhelming majority of head and neck neoplasms are squamous cell carcinomas and the incidence of nodal metastases is quite high. This chapter is intended, in part, as an introduction to the imaging approach to cervical metastatic disease. The treatment issues related to the presence and extent of cervical metastases will also be discussed in light of the ability of computed tomography to assist in staging tumors of the neck. The evaluation of the patient with cervical metastatic disease believed to be caused by an occult upper aerodigestive tract carcinoma will serve as a clinical model for the CT approach to the upper aerodigestive tract and neck. Last, we will consider the patterns of distant metastatic disease seen mainly in advanced primary tumors of the head and neck.

The frequency of cervical metastases from squamous cell carcinomas of the upper aerodigestive tract varies mainly with the site of the primary tumor. In general, the presence of histologically confirmed metastases halves the five-year survival for any given primary tumor.[23] More specific data according to the site of origin will be presented in the following chapters. Overall five-year survival rates for patient with positive nodes at the time of initial examination of upper aerodigestive tract lesions is less than 30%.[3] Less frequently, patients have cervical metastases of unknown origin. Most of these nodes are the result of "occult" upper aerodigestive tract carcinomas, and overall five-year survival in this group is about 15%.[6] Adenocarcinomas or undifferentiated carcinomas metastatic to the neck carry 5.0% and 9.4% five-year survival rates.[6]

With improvements in treatment and resultant prolonged survival, the incidence of distant metastases from head and neck cancer has risen. Specific data on incidence vary so much depending on origin, histologic type, and stage of the primary tumor that only general statements are appropriate in the context of this text. Patients with T_3, T_4, N_2, and N_3 category disease are fairly likely to have disseminated metastases at the time of death. Persistent disease or recurrence at the primary site, but especially in the neck, is strongly associated with distant metastases. Lymphatic extension is usually to the mediastinal nodes.[2] Hematogenous spread is most commonly to the lungs, bone, and, less frequently, the liver.[2] Visceral involvement beyond that is not significant enough to warrant routine imaging of patients at risk of having distant metastases.

TUMOR BEHAVIOR AND PATHOLOGY

Histopathology

Squamous cell carcinoma is by far the most common malignancy that produces cervical lymphadenopathy. Adenocarcinomas (from the thyroid and other sites), melanomas, and sarcomas will also occasionally involve these nodal groups. Lymphoma is the second most common

cause of malignant cervical adenopathy. Not infrequent-ly histologic study will reveal an anaplastic or undifferen-tiated tumor, in which case the search for a primary source or distinction from lymphoma may prove more difficult. Surface marker and electron microscopic study may be required to distinguish lymphoma, poorly differ-entiated carcinoma, and melanoma in some cases.

The following discussions will be based on the behav-ior of metastatic squamous cell carcinomas. Similar pat-terns of spread are seen in other carcinomas arising from the upper aerodigestive tract. The gross appearance of CT patterns does tend to differ for untreated carcinomas and lymphomas; this is discussed subsequently.

The location of a nodal mass in the neck is also a use-ful predictor of likely histologic type. Nodes in the upper deep cervical (jugulodigastric region) are almost uniform-ly the result of a primary squamous cell carcinoma in the upper aerodigestive tract. Those in the middle to lower neck will most likely be a result of an aerodigestive tract carcinoma but thyroid carcinoma or metastatic disease from primaries "below the clavicles" require stronger consideration (Figure 4-1). Posterior triangle nodes will be from either a nasopharyngeal carcinoma or a lym-phoma most of the time, although other aerodigestive tract carcinomas and metastases from outside the head and neck areas will also involve this group. Supraclavi-cular nodes are likely the result of an "infraclavicular" primary.

Patterns of Spread—
Normal Anatomy

The nodes of the neck are classically divided into several groups including the deep cervical, posterior tri-angle, supraclavicular, submental, submandibular, and periparotid groups (Figure 4-2).[23] The deep cervical lymph nodes are further subdivided into upper, middle, and lower groups. The single most important node of the deep cervical group is the jugulodigastric (subdigastric) node. This particular lymph node drains many portions of the upper aerodigestive tract and is therefore a first order node (first echelon according to Rouvier) in most of the neoplasms under discussion.[23] It is located deep to the origin of the sternocleidomastoid and just below the posterior belly of the digastric where that muscle crosses the jugular vein. On CT scans this usually trans-lates into a section taken slightly above the level of the hyoid bone and below the posterior belly of the digastric. The jugulodigastric node marks the junction between the superior and middle deep cervical nodes. Likewise, the jugulo-omohyoid node marks the junction between the middle and inferior groups of the deep cervical nodes. The jugulo-omohyoid node is located at the crossing of the omohyoid muscle and internal jugular vein.[23] On CT scans this usually correlates with the level taken ap-proximately through the top of the cricoid cartilage.

The deep cervical nodes can be identified on CT scans in many normal individuals as nonenhancing, round or elliptical densities usually 5 mm or less in size.[14,15,16] These are easily seen within the fat surrounding the jugular vein. Occasionally, normal deep cervical nodes can be 1 cm in size and even up to 1.5 cm in the jugulodigastric region.[23] This correlates with the clinical impression that the jugulodigastric node is often palpable although not necessarily involved by metastatic tumor (Figure 4-3).

The posterior triangle nodes (spinal accessory nodes according to Rouvier) are located far behind the jugular vein and are less than 5 mm in size when normal (Figure 4-3). When enlarged these nodes project posteriorly be-

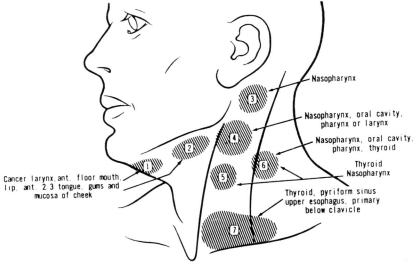

FIG. 4-1. The location of the lymph node involved by metastases can often suggest the site of a hidden primary. The common sites of head and neck cancers are indicated on this diagram in terms of the lymph node most commonly involved.

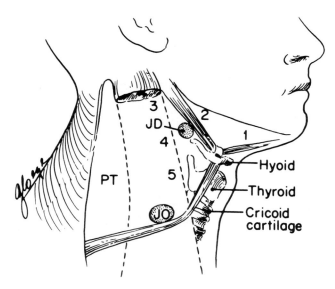

FIG. 4-2. The positions of the deep cervical nodes and other nodal groups within in the neck. 1 = Submental; 2 = Submandibular; 3, 4, 5 = upper, middle, and lower deep cervical; PT = posterior triangle nodes; JD = jugulodigastric node; JO = jugulo-omohyoid node. (This illustration is reprinted with permission of the *American Journal of Roentgenology* from Mancuso, A. A., Maceri, D., Rice, D., Hanafee, W. N.: CT of cervical lymph node cancer. *A.J.R.* 136:381–385, 1981.

tween the margin of the sternocleidomastoid and trapezius muscles.

The submandibular lymph nodes are located either just inferior and lateral to the gland or between the substance of the submandibular gland and the mandibular ramus (Figure 4-2).[10,23] Small nodes in this region, measuring 5 mm or less, are seen frequently and should be considered either normal variants or the result of prior inflammatory disease of the gland or anterior oral cavity.[15]

The submental lymph nodes are of the least clinical interest. Minimally enlarged nodes may be seen and are usually related to old dental or skin infections.[2] This nodal group is usually easily palpable when significantly enlarged.

The periparotid nodes are variable in number and position. The nodes may be located within the subcutaneous tissue surrounding the superficial portion of the gland. The nodes near the tail of the gland are located at the exit of the posterior facial vein.[10,23] In addition, intraparotid lymph nodes may be present within the substance of the gland along the course of the external carotid and posterior facial vein. Normally these nodes are not visible. Their major clinical significance is that their enlargement often leads to the mistaken clinical impression of a primary mass lesion of the parotid gland itself. The glandular substance of the parotid also normally contains some lymph follicles.[15,23]

An interesting and very important group of lymph nodes that were heretofore difficult or impossible to evaluate by physical examination or imaging techniques are the medial and lateral retropharyngeal nodes. The most well known of these is the node of Rouvier, which lies anterior to the longus colli muscle within the nasopharynx.[23] The lateral retropharyngeal nodes lie medial to the carotid sheath, basically between the carotid and its branches and the mucosal surface of the upper aerodigestive tract.[10,23]

Patterns of Spread—Pathologic Anatomy

A tumor usually reaches lymph nodes by emboli, which enter afferent lymphatic channels from the primary site or another node and lodge within the periphery of the node.[21] More rarely, a tumor may spread directly into the node if it is immediately adjacent to the primary site; this is more a phenomenon of local extension than it is a true expression of the natural history of cervical metastatic disease.

Once in the node, tumor emboli may grow to a size that completely replaces the lymphatic elements.[22] Continued enlargement may result in necrosis, a very frequent finding in nodes replaced by squamous cell carcinoma. Necrosis often occurs in nodes larger than 1.5 or 2 cm but may be seen earlier. It is common in nodes over 2.5 cm containing metastases (Figure 4-4).[4,15,18] Untreated lymphomatous nodes, on the other hand, are rarely grossly necrotic even when 3 to 4 cm in size (Figure 4-4).

Eventually the tumor invades the capsule of the node and spreads beyond it to the nearby soft tissues. Once extranodal spread has occurred, the tumor is free to invade surrounding muscle, vessels, and eventually bone (Figure 4-4).

Lymphatic spread tends to be along the pathways depending on the original primary site. Contiguous nodal group involvement is expected. "Skip areas" are unusual but do occur in previously untreated patients, probably because of anatomic variations.[23] Atypical patterns of nodal group involvement are more common in patients who have been treated by surgery or radiation, probably because of alteration of the normal paths of drainage.[9,15] Bilateral lymphatic spread is usually explained by a primary tumor arising in or crossing the midline (e.g., as is commonly seen in the nasopharynx and epiglottis) or by crossed lymphatic drainage (e.g., as is commonly seen in carcinoma of the tongue base).

The specific patterns of nodal involvement are highly dependent on the site of origin and extent of the primary tumor. These tendencies will be discussed in subsequent chapters.

The lymphatic channels ending at the base of the neck drain into the thoracic duct on the left and the right lymphatic duct. These both join with their respective bronchomediastinal trunks, providing a pathway to and from

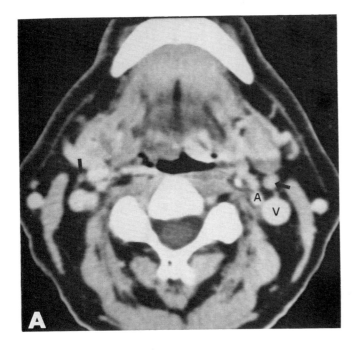

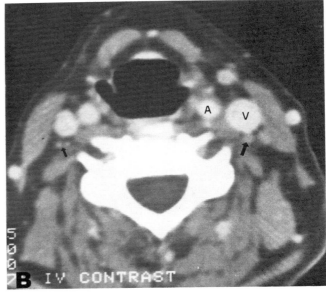

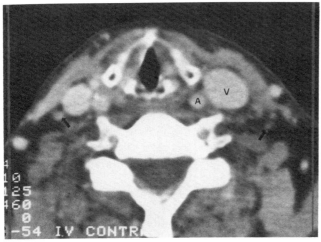

FIG. 4-3. Representative CT sections from the (A) upper, (B) middle, and (C) lower cervical regions. Normal lymph nodes are indicated by arrows. They are in large part located adjacent to the jugular vein (V). The carotid artery (A) lies medial to the jugular vein. Both of these vascular structures enhance on CT scans, while the nodes normally do not.

the neck that metastatic disease may follow. Both major collecting ducts communicate with the systemic venous system. This anatomy explains in part the hematogenous dissemination of tumors, the other mechanism being direct vascular invasion of the primary site or in cases of extensive extranodal spread of a nodal metastasis.

Metastases to bones will generally appear as lytic lesions. Depending upon the aggressiveness of the tumor, these may be discrete or show a permeative or "moth-eaten" pattern. Multiple discrete nodules are usually seen in the lung. Lymphangitic patterns in the lung would be distinctly unusual. Mediastinal adenopathy might also be seen.

CLASSIFICATION AND STAGING

Throughout the head and neck chapters of this book, the American Joint Committee (AJC) clinical-diagnostic staging system is used as a basis for discussion (Figure 4-5; Table 4-1). In some chapters, differences between the Union Internationale Contre Cancer (UICC) guidelines and those of the AJC will be presented when they emphasize important areas of controversy. The contrast between the two major staging systems is especially enlightening when it points to areas where CT imaging techniques might improve the clinical understanding of the extent of disease.

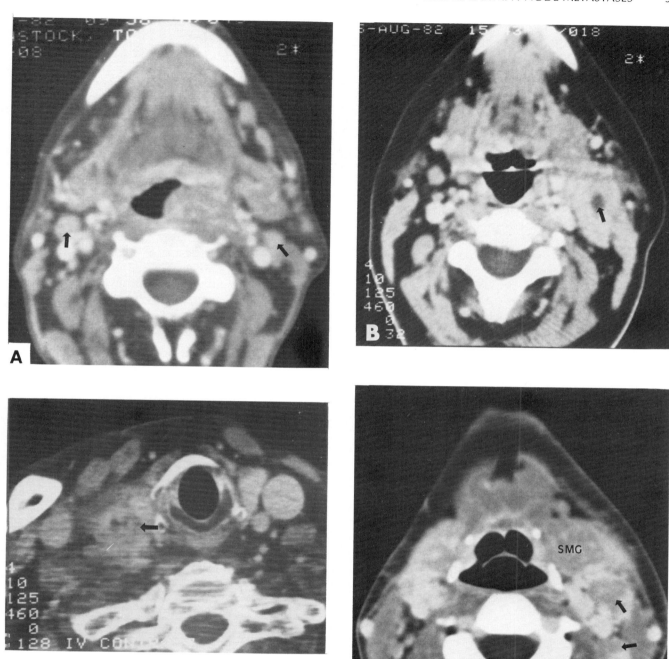

FIG. 4-4. Lymph nodes show differing morphologic structure depending on whether they are reactive or contain tumor. A through D show how this morphology may vary. (A) Reactive nodes (arrows) in the jugulodigastric regions in a patient with carcinoma of the oropharynx. (B) Cervical metastasis in a patient with supraglottic carcinoma shows a central area of necrosis (arrow). The nodal mass is well defined and shows fairly well-demarcated borders with surrounding muscles and vessels. This indicates that the tumor is likely still within the capsule of the nodal mass. (C) Metastatic carcinoma to the cervical nodes in a patient with a nasopharyngeal primary tumor. The tissue planes around the nodal mass (arrow) are obliterated and the carotid artery is not visible. The findings are characteristic of extracapsular extension. (D) Enlarged lymphomatous nodes (arrows) show no evidence of necrosis. The nodes have a morphology much the same as the reactive nodes seen in A; however, the intense peripheral enhancement is usually not seen in reactive nodes. It is difficult to differentiate the abnormally enlarged nodes from the normal submandibular gland (SMG).

A neck is considered to be N_0 when no clinically positive nodes are present. There are no specific size criteria attached to this classification. The separation of palpable nodes that are suspicious from those that are not suspicious is based on subjective criteria including approximate size (i.e., a 2.0-cm node might be more "suspicious" than a 1.0-cm node), firmness, and mobility.

A neck is considered to be N_1 when it contains a single, clinically positive homolateral node 3 cm or less in diameter. The measurement of nodal masses is again somewhat subjective because of the allowance that must be made for intervening soft tissues. Also, on occasion only the top of a nodal mass may be felt, especially when good bimanual examination is not possible. The UICC system requires that an N_1 neck contain evidence of moveable homolateral regional nodes; however, it gives no specific size criterion.

A neck that is considered to be N_2 will have a single homolateral nodal mass that is between 3 and 6 cm in size or multiple, clinically positive homolateral nodes, none of which is larger than 6 cm. It should be understood that any nodal mass larger than 3 cm is likely to be made up of more than one node. Multiple nodes may be adherent to one another or clearly separable: this is reflected in the two different criteria under the N_2 classification: N_{2a} and N_{2b}. The UICC system indicates that N_2 necks should contain moveable contralateral or bilateral regional nodes.

A neck staged N_3 may contain a homolateral nodal mass greater than 6 cm in diameter, contralateral nodes, or bilateral nodes. If bilateral neck disease is present, each side of the neck should be staged separately by the foregoing criteria. By UICC criteria any fixed nodal mass makes the neck N_3.

No clear-cut guidelines concerning evaluation of fixation are available in the AJC system. The UICC system does provide for this. Certainly additional comments such as "fixed," "mobile," and "decreased mobility" are often part of the clinical description of nodal mass. These are attempts to express the likelihood of capsular and extranodal extension. While this is reliable in advanced nodal disease, the subjectivity of these signs makes them less helpful in borderline cases. A more objective means of evaluating capsular and extranodal spread might prove useful in pretreatment clinical diagnostic staging.[4]

IMAGING PROCEDURES AND ASSESSMENT

Radiologists in the past have had little to do with staging cervical lymph node disease. Occasionally lateral soft tissue views have been used to assess possible retropha-

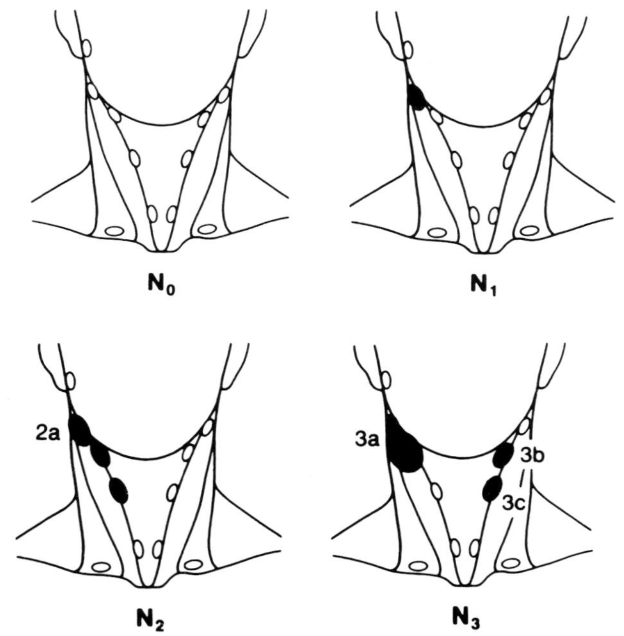

FIG. 4-5. Anatomic staging for cervical lymph node metastases. The size of the node and its mobility and the number and location are all factors in staging cervical nodes. The diameters, 2 cm, 3 to 5 cm, and 6 cm (N_1, N_2, N_3) were chosen because these are determined more objectively than fixation. Fixation implies adhesion to the carotid artery and, therefore, unresectability. Single and multiple nodes (N_1 v N_2), homolateral, and bilateral nodes (N_1, N_2, v N_3) are important factors.

Table 4-1. Nodal Involvement (N)

Cervical Node Classification. The following regional node classification is applicable to all squamous cell carcinoma of the upper aerodigestive tract. In clinical evaluation, the actual size of the nodal mass should be measured and allowance should be made for intervening soft tissues. It is recognized that most masses over 3 cm in diameter are not single nodes but are confluent nodes or tumor in soft tissues of the neck. There are three stages of clinically positive nodes: N1, N2, and N3. The use of subgroups a, b, and c is not required, but is recommended. Midline nodes are considered homolateral nodes.

NX   Minimum requirements to assess the regional node cannot be met.
N0   No clinically positive node
N1   Single clinically positive homolateral node 3 cm or less in diameter
N2   Single clinically positive homolateral node more than 3 cm but not more than 6 cm in diameter or multiple clinically positive homolateral nodes, none more than 6 cm in diameter
N2a Single clinically positive homolateral node more than 3 cm but not more than 6 cm in diameter
N2b Multiple clinically positive homolateral nodes, none more than 6 cm in diameter
N3   Massive homolateral node(s), bilateral nodes, or contralateral node(s)
N3a Clinically positive homolateral node(s), one more than 6 cm in diameter
N3b Bilateral clinically positive nodes (in this situation, each side of the neck should be staged separately; i.e., N3b: right, N2a; left, N1)
N3c Contralateral clinically positive node(s) only

Reprinted from *Manual for Staging of Cancer*, 2nd ed., O. H. Beahrs & M. H. Myers (Eds.), American Joint Committee on Cancer. Philadelphia, J. B. Lippincott, 1983, p. 39.

ryngeal metastases. Cervical lymphangiography is impractical and has never been done with any frequency.

Recommended Method of Study

Computed tomography is widely accepted as an imaging tool for staging lymph node disease in the abdomen and chest. The accessibility of the cervical nodes to physical examination has perhaps led to some delay in the widespread application of CT in staging cervical lymph node disease. We have been interested in the potential value of CT for this purpose since 1978.[16] Our early results have been so promising that further prospective studies have been undertaken that suggest that CT should be made the imaging tool of choice for staging cervical metastatic disease.[5,7,8,9,15,20,24,27] Moreover, our experience suggests that it would be very useful to require CT staging of most primary tumors and related regional metastatic disease.[9,15,20] Specific reasons for the superiority of CT to the clinical examination of the neck will be discussed in the following sections.

Technique of Examination

When evaluating the neck for regional lymphadenopathy related to primary tumors, whether of the lymph nodes themselves or of the upper aerodigestive tract, intravenous contrast should be used. The most convenient method is a rapid drip infusion. This is accomplished by placing a 19-gauge needle in a good-sized antecubital vein. The contrast bottle is then raised as high as possible on the IV pole. Since the aim is to scan while the contrast is at maximum levels in the intravascular compartment and within the primary tumor, we employ 60% meglumine iothalamate. One hundred-fifty milliliters usually is sufficient; however, an additional 75 ml of rapid drip infusion or bolus injections superimposed on the rapid drip infusion may be used. We prefer rapid drip infusion to bolus injections because the boluses occasionally create nausea and vomiting, which impedes scanning during the critical period of intravascular and tumor opacification.

The matter of section thickness and interval is fairly pragmatic. If a survey of the neck is required, then scans approximately 1-cm thick done at 2-cm increments may be done from the sternal notch to the skull base. Fill-in sections may be added as deemed appropriate. On the other hand, when studying a primary site in detail or searching for an occult primary tumor of the upper aerodigestive tract, contiguous sections of approximately 5 mm are indicated in the areas of critical interest. In searching for an unknown primary tumor, these critical areas include the nasopharynx, the oropharynx (including tonsillar fossae and tongue base), and the hypopharynx.

Contrast infusion is necessary for the following reasons:

1. Enhanced nodes are easier to detect with a bright rim and necrotic center and it is easier to distinguish the numerous branching vessels within the neck from the lymph nodes.
2. Contrast helps in determining whether capsular, limited extranodal, or marked extranodal extension with fixation of critical structures in the neck is present.
3. It is sometimes useful to distinguish the extent of the primary tumor and to differentiate it from related nodal masses.

The neck may be studied without contrast injection. If, for example, CT is being done for a limited glottic lesion, the likelihood of lymph node metastases is very low and contrast will add little if anything to the evaluation of the primary tumor. On the other hand, pyriform sinus lesions are better outlined with contrast injection and their extent along the pharyngeal wall may be better appreciated. In addition, these lesions are associated with lymph node metastases in a high percentage of cases, and the nodes should be evaluated in a definitive way.

In summary, contrast should never be injected in any CT examination of the body without clear rationale for its use. The use of intravenous contrast material is justified in nearly all instances of malignancies that involve the head and neck, although it is possible to evaluate both primary and regional nodal disease without contrast infusion if need be.

Limitations of CT

There are some limitations to imaging studies that most likely will never be overcome. This basically is due to the lack of specificity of morphologic findings. Computed tomography is not tissue specific. For example, tuberculous adenitis may result in nodal masses that appear identical to those secondary to metastatic disease. While MRI holds some promise for being more tissue specific, it will undoubtedly have its limitations. Even the pathologist is limited in his or her ability to examine a lymph node specimen. Error rates of up to 30% have been reported, depending mainly on how carefully the nodes are sectioned for microscopic examination.[28]

Nodes may not contain tumors, but may still be enlarged as a result of "reactive hyperplasia." This is very graphically illustrated in a study by McGavran et al.[18] in which the largest nodes in a positive neck specimen sometimes did not contain tumor tissue while smaller nodes in the same specimen were positive.[18] Reactive nodes clearly tend to be less than 1.5 cm in size; however, they may grow to 2.0 or 2.5 cm at times.[18] If a size criterion is then set for calling a node positive, a small percentage of false-positives will result.

Microscopic or macroscopic tumors may also be present in nodes that are completely within the size range seen in a normal population. Again, if size criteria are set, then false-negatives will result. This unfortunately is an unavoidable circumstance well known to those working in the field of oncology.

If a plane is visible between a nodal mass and the carotid artery or neck musculature, then one may be sure that the nodal mass is not fixed or adherent to these surrounding structures. If the mass is immediately adjacent to these structures, the difference between abutting, adherent, or fixed may be difficult to determine on a CT scan. The morphology of tumor margins (ill-defined, infiltrative vs. well encapsulated) may help make the differential[15] (Figure 4-4); (Table 4-1).

Interpretive Criteria for CT

The lymph node bearing areas of the head and neck as classically described by Rouvier have already been reviewed. Computed tomography shows each of these areas with great clarity and is free of the subjectivity involved with palpation of the neck[15,16] (Table 4-2). Computed tomography does, however, suffer from limitations imposed by the subjectivity of image interpretation. Nodal groups such as the retropharyngeal group have almost always been beyond evaluation; CT now demonstrates these node-bearing areas (Figure 4-6). Some of the deep cervical nodes lie immediately behind the jugular vein and deep to the sternocleidomastoid muscle, rendering them difficult to palpate.[15,16]

Normal nodes within the size ranges described by Rouvier are routinely identified by CT[15] (Table 4-2). The morphology of pathologically enlarged nodes can also be studied. Central necrosis or a thick (greater than 2 mm) rim of contrast enhancement is often visible in nodes involved with tumor. Edema or obliteration of soft tissue planes around nodal masses indicates extranodal spread.[15,16] The relationship of abnormal nodes to that of the carotid or surrounding musculature is demonstrated.[15,16] The size of solitary nodes and matted nodal masses may be precisely measured. All of these morphologic features which CT demonstrates can be used to lend objectivity to staging cervical metastases (Figure 4-4); (Table 4-1).

IMAGING STRATEGIES AND DECISIONS

Diagnostic Considerations

Patients with Neck Masses Caused by an Unknown Primary. Table 4-4 shows a suggested protocol for integrating CT, fine-needle aspiration biopsy, and triple endoscopy in patients with cervical adenopathy believed to be secondary to an occult carcinoma of the upper aerodigestive tract. It seems to be rational based on the clinical understanding of the problem as it has matured since Martin and Morfit's original article in 1944 and our own recent experience and that of others with CT scanning.[11,12,14,17,21,26]

Neck masses that subsequently prove to be malignant will most often be from regional lymph node metastases in a patient with carcinoma of the upper aerodigestive tract. In these patients clinical examination of the nasopharynx, oropharynx, hypopharynx, or larynx will most often reveal the site of the primary tumor. The task of the head and neck surgeon or radiation oncologist is then

Table 4-2. Size and Frequency of Visualization of Normal Cervical and Retropharyngeal Nodes

GROUP	SEEN IN NUMBER OF PATIENTS	SIZE RANGE	NUMBER OF PATIENTS WITH NODES AT UPPER LIMIT OF RANGE
Occipital	0/30	—	—
Mastoid	0/30	—	—
Facial	0/30	—	—
Lingual	0/30	—	—
Parotid	7/30	3–5	1/7
Retropharyngeal			
Median	0/30	—	—
Lateral	20/30	3–7	2/20
Submental-submandibular	28/30	3–10	3/28
Internal jugular			
Superior	30/30	3–10	6/30
Middle	30/30	3–10	2/30
Inferior	30/30	3–5	5/30
Anterior jugular	0/30	—	—
Juxtavisceral-scalene			
Spinal accessory	28/30	3–5	5/28

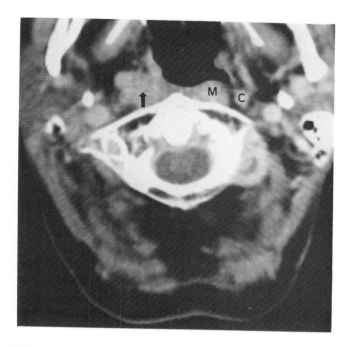

FIG. 4-6. This patient had recurrent Hodgkin's disease in the retro-pharyngeal nodes (arrow). Compare the abnormal with the normal side where the space between the prevertebral musculature (M) and carotid artery (C) is clear. The nodal mass disappeared completely with radiation therapy.

to stage the lesion as accurately as possible to arrive at the proper treatment plan. Occasionally the clinical examination of the aerodigestive tract will not reveal the site of the primary tumor. In this situation several possibilities exist to explain the source of the malignant node:

1. An occult primary tumor within the aerodigestive tract.
2. A metastasis from a primary tumor below the clavicles such as lung.
3. A primary tumor of lymph node origin (lymphoma). Under these circumstances the task of the head and neck surgeon or radiation oncologist becomes more difficult. Triple endoscopy and biopsy may turn up primary lesions of the aerodigestive tract that are not seen at routine clinical examination.

If triple endoscopy and biopsy are negative, then the situation becomes more complex. If the node is from a head and neck tumor, it is possible that:

1. The primary tumor is a very small one and therefore inapparent even at endoscopy.
2. The primary tumor metastasized to lymph nodes and then regressed.
3. The primary tumor is one that is growing primarily submucosally.[13,14]

It is in the last instance in which CT evaluation of the upper aerodigestive tract before triple endoscopy may

be of value (Table 4-4). We have shown that some tumors, especially those at the base of the tongue and in the nasopharynx, may grow primarily in the submucosal region and therefore escape clinical detection.[13,14] For this reason, we recommend CT scans of the nasopharynx, oropharynx, tongue base, and perhaps pyriform sinuses before triple endoscopy.[12] This may either turn up an obvious, deeply infiltrating mass or it may help direct biopsies during the triple endoscopy (Figure 4-7). If the primary site is suspected of being below the clavicles or if it might be a lymphoma, then the imaging approach is different. In order to make the choice between doing triple endoscopy and CT of the head and neck, or searching below the clavicles for the primary site, some preliminary workup is in order (see Table 4-4).

Some investigators have shown that an excisional biopsy of neck masses is detrimental to the patient if the mass turns out to be a nodal metastasis from a squamous cell head and neck primary tumor.[2,21] Because of this, head and neck surgeons are reluctant to do excisional biopsies unless definitive treatment of the neck is carried out at the same time. This might expose the patient to needless radical neck dissection. Recently, an alternative to excisional biopsy has been fine-needle aspiration biopsy (Table 4-4). With a well-trained cytopathologist this examination can be very accurate at determining the tissue type of the tumor. Fine-needle aspiration biopsy is not believed to be detrimental to the patient.[2,26] If the aspiration reveals squamous cell carcinoma and there is no apparent primary tumor from the routine clinical examination (indirect mirror, telescopic, or fiberoptic endoscopy), then we believe a CT examination of the upper aerodigestive tract is in order. Following this, triple endoscopy may be done and areas of abnormality on CT scans biopsied (Figure 4-8). If there are no abnormalities in the CT scan then triple endoscopy with or without random biopsies is indicated as in the past.

If the node is a squamous cell carcinoma and low in the neck, then a strong effort must be made to exclude the lung as the primary source. In female patients cervical carcinoma would be an additional consideration.

If the needle aspiration reveals probable lymphoma, then a larger excisional biopsy specimen may be obtained and appropriate staging workup carried out. The potential value of CT in the evaluation of lymphomas of the head and neck region will be discussed subsequently.

If the neck node is in the middle to lower neck and of another tissue type such as adenocarcinoma, then a search for a primary tumor below the clavicles is probably most appropriate if thyroid cancer is excluded. Strong considerations would have to be given to pancreatic and breast primaries. It would be even more appropriate to search the head and neck region if the node is in the jugulodigastric region or above.

If the needle aspiration is undifferentiated or indeter-

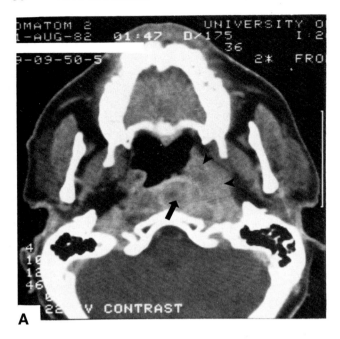

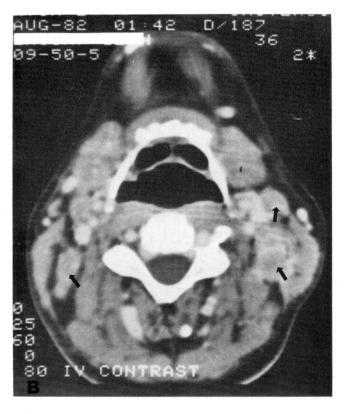

FIG. 4-7. This patient had bilateral cervical adenopathy; triple endoscopy under anesthesia revealed no evidence of a primary source. (A) A CT scan was done and showed the infiltrating mass of the nasopharynx (arrowheads). There was an associated retropharyngeal node (arrow). A repeat endoscopic examination under anesthesia again revealed entirely normal mucosa. Deep biopsies were obtained and returned carcinoma. (B) lower section illustrates the cervical lymph node involvement (arrow).

minate, then the search for the primary lesion should probably begin in the head and neck region or as the age and clinical situation of the patient dictate. Sometimes other neck masses will be in the lateral compartment of the neck and mimic lymph node metastases. Such lesions include neuromas of the carotid sheath, paragangliomas, laryngoceles, branchial cleft cysts, and, occasionally, nodes of infectious etiology. The clinical situation will usually sort out these cases; however, CT scans may be obtained and can prove definitive in confirming that the source of the neck mass is something other than a malignant nodal mass.

Symptomatic Patients Without Neck Mass. Sometimes patients have physical signs and symptoms that suggest involvement of the nerves that travel along the carotid sheath. Most often, this is seen in patients who have been treated for carcinomas of the upper aerodigestive tract or those who are at risk of developing metastases from more distant sites.[9] In such a group of patients CT is warranted in that tumor infiltration may be present even in the absence of a palpable mass. Sometimes the postradiotherapy and postsurgical changes in a neck make the findings of palpation less reliable. The decision of whether to do a myelogram or CT in this setting depends on the spectrum of the clinical findings.[9]

1. Involvement of the vagus nerve is usually heralded by vocal cord paresis and hoarseness. Other symptoms of glottic dysfunction such as aspiration may be present. Investigation of the course of the vagus nerve and recurrent laryngeal nerve should include CT of the neck and thoracic inlet continuing on to the aortopulmonary window if the symptoms are on the left.
2. Phrenic nerve paralysis resulting in an elevated ipsilateral hemidiaphragm may be seen with a tumor that has recurred in the neck or extended beyond the lymph nodes to involve the anterior scalene muscles. The phrenic nerve lies on these muscles.[10]
3. Unexplained hand, arm, and shoulder pain referable to the brachial plexus may also indicate involvement of the scalene group by extranodal extension of the tumor.
4. Horner's syndrome alone or combined with other symptoms should lead the search from the skull base to the thoracic inlet. Blood-borne direct metastases to these regions are also possible, but extranodal extension of lymphatic spread is most usual.
5. Neck pain may be related to direct invasion of the soft tissues or bones in the neck or perineural extension. Such symptoms in a patient with known tumor often go ignored if there are no clear-cut neurologic deficits and a negative physical examination.[9] Early study with CT can reveal very significant masses, which can be palliated without undue delay because of the lack

of physical findings. Various physical findings and neurologic complaints are possible in this setting. If the spectrum of findings indicates involvement of the middle to lower neck, then either a myelogram or a CT scan might be appropriate. A CT scan can definitely demonstrate epidural metastatic disease and may well show the source to be previously undiscovered nodal metastases in the retropharyngeal area.[7,9]

6. At times the neurologic syndromes are quite specific; this perhaps is best illustrated by the jugular fossa syndrome in patients with nasopharyngeal carcinoma and metastasis to the retropharyngeal nodes that surround the carotid sheath near the origin of the internal jugular vein. Cranial nerve deficits in the distributions of nerves IX through XII are possible. Incomplete syndromes are the rule.[26] Horner's syndrome is also possible because of the sympathetics that lie in this region.

A jugular fossa syndrome need not occur specifically in nasopharyngeal carcinoma in that metastases may occur from other regions of the aerodigestive tract to these nodes, and when clinical symptoms point to this region, a detailed CT study is indicated.[26] The cranial nerve syndromes related to involvement of the skull base and retropharyngeal lymph nodes will be discussed in more detail in subsequent chapters.

Staging Patients with Known Primary Stage Neck Nodes. There are two groups of patients of interest with known primary stage neck nodes; those with clinically positive and those with clinically negative necks. Another group of patients with suspicious but not definitely positive necks can also be identified. These are classified as either clinically positive or negative depending on the experience and bias of the examiner (see Table 4-5).

In patients with clinically positive necks, the aims of CT staging are as follows:

1. To determine the amount of involvement. A CT scan allows precise measurement. It also may show whether multiple matted nodes or a solitary node account for the palpable abnormalities. This might help to separate N_1 and N_2 categories more objectively.

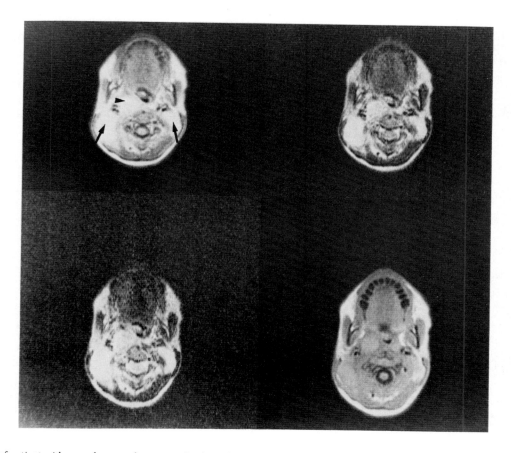

FIG. 4-8. MRI of patient with nasopharyngeal cancer and enlarged retropharyngeal and cervical nodes. Upper left—SE 2500/45 shows retropharyngeal node (arrowhead) and bilateral cervical nodes. Upper right and lower left—SE 2500/90 and 2500/135 images show nodes increase in relative signal intensity due to prolonged T_2. Lower right—SE 500/30 shows difference in tumor/muscle contrast on a relatively T_1 weighted image.

2. To assess the likelihood of capsular rupture and measure the amount of extranodal extension (i.e., carotid fixation or fixation to neck musculature).[15,16] This may lend more rationale to the designation of N_2 and N_3 nodes if criteria are modified to reflect CT staging variables.
3. To detect nodal disease not found on clinical examination such as occult contralateral spread or extension to retropharyngeal nodes.[15,16] This can upstage an N_1 or N_2 neck to N_3.
4. To help differentiate reactive nodes from tumor-positive nodes. This is difficult in many instances; however, central necrosis is virtually diagnostic of a tumor.

In the group of patients with clinically negative necks, CT serves mainly one of the two following purposes:

1. To detect nodes that are not felt at clinical examination. These usually lie deep to the sternocleidomastoid muscle or in the retropharyngeal region.[15,16] Prior radiotherapy or surgery may make the neck difficult to examine, in which case CT becomes even more useful for demonstrating clinically "occult" nodes. This may convert an N_0 to an N_1 neck.
2. To confirm the clinical impression of a negative neck and establish the size of the nodes that are present. This may have important implications in selecting the therapeutic approach to the neck. "Suspicious" necks that might be stage N_1 could be downstaged to N_0 (or vice versa) if appropriate CT criteria are established.

TREATMENT DECISIONS

Certainly information available from CT is very useful for prognostic purposes. One group of investigators has recently reinforced the importance of capsular rupture and extranodal spread in predicting the likelihood of survival.[4] Patients with carotid fixation will live no longer than one year. Fixation to other structures in the neck may have similar implications. It might be that patients with evidence of extranodal spread would be best handled by combined therapy; some authors argue that aggressive management is preferable in these patients if one is attempting cure.[2,4,19,25] Certainly patients with retropharyngeal nodal involvement usually have a dismal prognosis.[1]

The question of prophylactic (elective) treatment of the neck has been debated for many years by surgical and radiation oncologists. Numerous references on this are available in Batsakis's text.[2] N_0 necks may be equally well controlled by elective radiotherapy or surgery. It would seem appropriate to develop objective criteria for identifying (1) who should have prophylactic treatment of the cervical nodes, and (2) by what means they will be treated (radiation, surgery, or combined). Certainly

some of the factors that enter into these decisions are understood, such as the influence of the site and the extent of the primary tumor. Others are less clear, such as the effect of the host-tumor relationship. The limitation of the physical examination in staging cervical metastases has been documented by several groups. False-negative rates range from 15% to 65%.[2] False-positive rates are around 10% to 15%.[2] Enlarged reactive nodes and tumor foci in normal-sized nodes explain most of the errors; however, sometimes enlarged nodes are not felt because they lie in relatively inaccessible areas or because the patient's anatomy is unfavorable. Computed tomography does not suffer from the latter two circumstances; the former two will be a continued problem for any imaging study. Data available from CT might lead to a more objective basis for deciding on the indications and methods of prophylactic treatment of the neck.[15,16]

A brief summary of treatment guidelines follows but may be modified according to primary site.

1. N_0 nodes: The management of metastatic neck nodes is controversial; both surgery and radiation therapy are used in different circumstances (Table 4-3). Surgical treatment is used as an elective radical neck dissection (RND) when the neck is entered for resection of the primary tumor as in laryngeal/hypolaryngeal lesions. The one exception is oral cancers, which are controversial. Generally, elective neck radiation therapy is preferred for most primary sites and stages because

Table 4-3. Treatment Decisions: Cervical Lymph Nodes

STAGE	SURGICAL TREATMENT		RADIATION THERAPY
N_0	An elective radical neck dissection when the neck is entered for surgical resection of the primary as in laryngeal/hypopharyngeal lesions. Oral tongue is controversial.		Generally preferred for all stages T_2, T_3, T_4, and most sites of head and neck cancer.
N_1	Radical neck node dissection.	or	Definitive radiotherapy. Neck node is included with treatment field for primary tumor. Electron boost.
N_2	Radical neck node dissection.	and/or or	Postoperative radiotherapy. Definitive radiotherapy with interstitial implant, electron boost, or surgical shelling out of residuum after irradiation.
N_3	Unresectable, but nodes can be "excised" after irradiation.	and/or	Definitive radiotherapy ± chemotherapy, if partial response, then surgery.

it is extremely effective for subclinical disease. If radiation therapy is used to treat the primary tumor (T_2–T_4), the entire neck is treated with doses of 5,000 cGy with minimum morbidity and excellent control. With T_1 lesions that are well differentiated, such as in the oral cavity and oropharynx, large fields might not be used and only the jugulodigastric or jugulo-omohyoid neck nodes would be included with the primary lesion.

2. N_1 nodes: Radical neck dissection often with en bloc resection of the primary tumor is generally the preferred treatment, particularly if the cancers are moderately differentiated, even with unknown primaries. Alternately, definitive radiation therapy can be used, particularly when the primary tumor is treated by radiation therapy and fields include the involved node. An electron boost dose usually follows to the site of nodal involvement.

3. N_2 nodes: For N_2 nodes, a radical neck dissection is generally preferred if the nodes are mobile and there is no evidence of fixation. If the nodal capsule is invaded and there is some extension into the tissues of

the neck on CT scans at the time of surgery, postoperative radiation therapy should be given. In a similar fashion, if the preferred treatment to the primary tumor is external radiation that encompasses the nodes, then smaller fields can be employed with either an electron boost or an interstitial implant to involved nodes. Surgical shelling out of the residual nodal tissue is an alternative to boost doses and fields.

4. N_3 nodes: N_3 nodes are usually unresectable because of fixation to the carotid artery. Although this is difficult to determine clinically, CT can be very helpful. Definitive radiation therapy with or without chemotherapy is generally used, and if a good response occurs, then surgical removal of residual disease may be feasible.

5. Patients with extranodal spread with fixation of the carotid, scalene, or skull base or spread to retropharyngeal nodes (except for nasopharyngeal primaries) should be treated with palliative intent.

6. The position of nodes and likelihood of extranodal spread may be used to determine whether radical or

Table 4-4. Recommended Protocol for Evaluation of Unknown Primary Office Examination of Head and Neck Area Utilizing Indirect Mirror Exams or Scopes

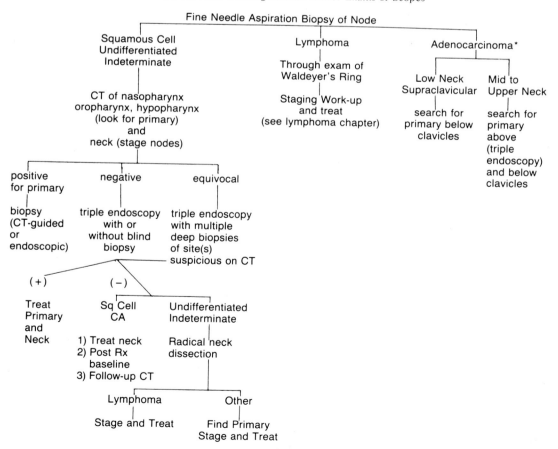

*Thyroid Carcinoma Excluded

Table 4-5. Computed Tomography to Stage Neck Nodes in Patients with Known Squamous Cell Carcinoma

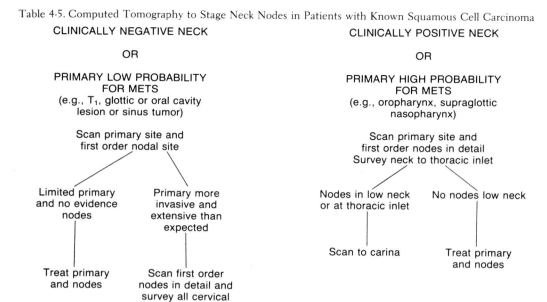

modified radical (preservation of spinal accessory nerve) neck dissection is the most appropriate operation.

In patients being followed for recurrent tumor, prior surgery or radiation often makes it difficult to evaluate the neck. Also, the incidence of retropharyngeal nodal involvement is higher. Computed tomography can be used to great advantage in these patients to detect recurrent nodal disease and perhaps institute salvage therapy sooner than if one were to wait for clinical signs of neck recurrence.[9]

IMPACT OF NEW TECHNOLOGY

Definitive data regarding new technology will be generated over the next five to ten years. Computed tomography must first be accepted as the oncologic imaging tool of choice for evaluating nearly all head and neck cancers. Its role in evaluating the neck must be studied prospectively by different investigators. From the foregoing discussions, it should be clear that CT has much to offer in staging and some role in the detection of head and neck malignancies. Its impact on survival and detection statistics will be difficult to assess, but some trends should emerge as this imaging tool is more widely applied and studied.

Magnetic resonance imaging promises to further enhance the role of imaging in the detection and staging of cervical lymph node disease. The benefits of studying the neck without ionizing radiation and without the small but definite risk of iodonated contrast infusion are attractive ones. More importantly, MRI holds the promise of increased sensitivity and specificity in diagnosis.

Hopefully, the signals from macroscopic tumor deposits in normal sized nodes will allow us to increase sensitivity. Perhaps the difference in signals between reactive and tumor-laden nodes will allow us to be more specific. These questions will be answered as this technology becomes more widely available.

REFERENCES

 1. Ballantyne, A. J.: Significance of retropharyngeal nodes in cancer of the head and neck. AM. J. Surg. 108:500, 1964.
 2. Batsakis, J. G.: Tumors of the Head and Neck. Clinical and Pathological Considerations, 2nd ed. Baltimore, Williams & Wilkins, 1979.
 3. Blady, J. V.: The present status of treatment to cervical metastases from carcinoma arising in the head and neck region. Am. J. Surg. 111:56, 1971.
 4. Cachin, Y., Sancho-Garnier, H., Micheau, C., Marandas, P.: Nodal metastasis from carcinoma of the oropharynx. Otolaryngol. Clin. North Am. 12:145–154, 1979.
 5. Chodosh, P. L., Silbey, R., Den, K. T.: Diagnostic use of ultrasound in disease of the head and neck. Laryngoscope 90:814–821, 1980.
 6. Didolkar, M. S., Fanous, N., Elias, E. G., Moore, R. H.: Metastatic carcinomas from occult primary tumors. A study of 254 patients. Ann. Surg. 186:625, 1977.
 7. Friedman, M., Shelton, V. K., Mafee, M., Bellity, P., Grybauskas, V., Skolnik, E.: Metastatic neck disease. Evaluation of computed tomography. Arch. Otolaryngol. 110:443–447, 1984.
 8. Gonsalves, C. G., Briant, T. D., Harmand, W. M.: Computed tomography of the paranasal sinuses, nasopharynx, and soft tissues of the neck. Comput. Tomogr. 2:271–278, 1978.
 9. Harnsberger, H. R., Mancuso, A. A., Muraki, A. S., Parkin, J. L.: The upper aerodigestive tract and neck: CT evaluation of recurrent tumors. Radiology 149:503–509, 1983.
10. Last, R. J.: Anatomy—Regional and Applied, 6th ed. New York, Churchill Livingston, 1978.
11. Leipsiz, B., Winter, M. L., Hokanson, J. A.: Cervical nodal metastases of unknown origin. Laryngoscope 91:593–598, 1981.

12. Muraki, A. S., Mancuso, A. A., Harnsberger, H. R.: Metastatic cervical adenopathy from tumors of unknown origin: The role of CT. *Radiology* 152:749–753, 1984.
13. Mancuso, A. A., Hanafee, W. N.: *Computed Tomography of the Head and Neck.* Baltimore, Williams & Wilkins, 1982.
14. Mancuso, A. A., Hanafee, W. N.: Elusive head and neck tumors beneath intact mucosa. *Laryngoscope* 93:133–139, 1983.
15. Mancuso, A. A., Harnsberger, H. R., Muraki, A. S., Stevens, M. H.: Computed tomography of cervical and retropharyngeal lymph nodes: Normal anatomy, variants of normal, and applications in staging head and neck cancer. Part I: Normal anatomy. *Radiology* 148:709–714, 1983.
16. Mancuso, A. A., Maceri, D., Rice, D., Hanafee, W. N.: CT of cervical lymph node cancer. *A.J.R.* 136:381–385, 1981.
17. Martin, H., Morfit, H. M.: Cervical lymph node metastases as the first symptom of cancer. *Surg. Gynecol. Obstet.* 78:133–159, 1944.
18. McGavran, M. H., Bauer, W. C., Ogura, J. H.: The incidence of cervical lymph node metastases from epidermoid carcinoma of the larynx and the relationship to certain characteristics of the primary tumor. *Cancer* 14:55–66, 1961.
19. Million, R. R., Cassisi, N. J., Wittes, R. E.: Cancer in the head and neck. In *Cancer: Principles and Practice of Oncology,* DeVita, V. T., Jr., Hellman, S., Rosenberg, S. A. (Eds.). Philadelphia, J. B. Lippincott, 1982, pp. 301–386.
20. Muraki, A., Mancuso, A. A., Harnsberger, H. R., Johnson, L. P., Meads, G. B.: CT of the oropharynx, tongue base and floor of the mouth: Normal anatomy and range of variations, and applications in staging carcinoma. *Radiology* 148:725–731, 1983.
21. Razack, M. S., Sako, K., Marchetta, F. C.: Influences of initial neck node biopsy on the incidence of recurrence in the neck and survival in patients who subsequently undergo curative resectional surgery. *J. Surg. Oncol.* 9:347, 1977.
22. Robbins, S. L.: *Pathology,* 3rd ed. Philadelphia, W. B. Saunders, 1967.
23. Rouvier, H.: *Anatomy of the Human Lymphatic System.* Ann Arbor, Edwards Bros. 1938.
24. Sagerman, R. H., Chung, C. T.: CT in the management of head and neck cancer. *CT* 5:229–235, 1981.
25. Strong, E. W.: Preoperative radiation and radical neck dissection. *Surg. Clin. North Am.* 49:271, 1969.
26. Templer, J., Perry, M. C., Davis, W. E.: Metastatic cervical adenocarcinoma from unknown primary tumor. *Arch. Otolaryngol.* 107:45–47, 1981.
27. Vibhakar, S. D., Eckhauser, C., Bellon, E. M.: Computed tomography of the nasopharynx and neck. *CT* 7:259–265, 1983.
28. Wilkinson, E. J., Hause, L.: Probability in lymph node sectioning. *Cancer* 33:1269, 1974.

5 THE NASOPHARYNX, THE PARANASAL SINUSES, AND NASAL CAVITY

Anthony A. Mancuso

In considering malignancies of the head and neck region, a number of sites mutually lend themselves to the presentation of diagnostic imaging and treatment. Some of these sites are the nasopharynx, the paranasal sinuses, and the nasal cavity, which are primarily concerned with the intake of air and are, in essence, the beginning of the respiratory tract. Because of its function, the tract is exposed to many environmental antigens and pollutants. For example, carcinoma of the nasopharynx is especially common among southern Chinese and seems to be related to environmental rather than genetic factors.[22,59,62] However, the Epstein-Barr virus is associated with nasopharyngeal carcinomas in all races.[8,21] The incidence of carcinomas of the nasal cavity and the paranasal sinuses has been found to be increased in furniture workers and appears to be related to wood dust inhalation.[15]

NASOPHARYNX

Malignancies of the nasopharynx are among the less common lesions affecting the upper aerodigestive tract in the non-Asian population. In whites these represent about 0.25% to 0.50% of all malignancies.[2,5] They are, however, some of the most tragic because of their devastating natural history and because early symptoms are often ignored or misinterpreted.[2,5,35] The incidence in southern Chinese people is very high, making it a very common neoplasm on a worldwide basis. The relatively poor survival statistics for these lesions are at least in part

related to this almost routine delay in diagnosis. If no consideration is given to the stage at initial examination or to degree of differentiation, the overall five-year survival for nasopharyngeal carcinoma is 39%. Eight percent of these patients will be alive with evidence of persistent disease.[5,67] When considered by stage, T_1 lesions show a 44% five-year survival with no evidence of disease (NED). T_2 and T_3 patients are about one-half as likely to survive disease-free for five years at rates of 24% and 17%, respectively.[5,67]

A variety of imaging tools have been used to study the extent of nasopharyngeal malignancies. Historically there has been a steady refinement in the techniques. Plain films, xeroradiography, nasopharyngography and pluridirectional tomography have been used to good advantage to show bone destruction and gross soft tissue limits of tumor. Computed tomography has supplanted all of these. Magnetic resonance imaging (MRI) may soon add new information.

The histopathology of nasopharyngeal malignancy is mainly that of epidermoid carcinoma in its various states of keratinization (Table 5-1). The unique features of other primary tumors such as adenoidcystic carcinoma and non-Hodgkin lymphoma will be outlined, although their morphologic patterns as seen on CT are indistinguishable from the ubiquitous squamous cell carcinomas.

With CT we now have a tool that looks beyond the mucosa and can identify deeply infiltrating lesions that are sometimes not apparent on clinical examination.[40,41] The ability of CT to demonstrate the anatomy of the

Table 5-1. Approximate Distribution of
Histology of Nasopharyngeal Cancer

HISTOLOGIC TYPE	PERCENTAGE
Carcinoma	99
Epidermoid	86
Adenocarcinoma	1.7
Unclassified	11
Sarcoma/Lymphoma	1

tissue planes deep to the mucosa, including node-bearing areas not accessible to physical examination, makes it the perfect compliment to the modern clinical examination of the nasopharynx. These two techniques of examination allow exquisite accuracy in establishing whether the nasopharynx contains a tumor and, if it does, the extent of the disease.[39]

In the following section we will show that CT has an impact on the diagnosis and management of nasopharyngeal malignancies in the following ways:

1. Detecting tumors that are not apparent on even good physical examination of the nasopharynx, sometimes in the face of repeated blind biopsies (Figures 5-1, 5-2).[39,40]
2. By earlier detection and diagnosis in selected patients with:
   (A) unilateral serous otitis media;
   (B) atypical facial pain;
   (C) various patterns of cranial nerve dysfunction.

3. Making clinical diagnostic staging more accurate by:
   (A) showing submucosal extension that alters T components;
   (B) showing otherwise undectable retropharyngeal nodal metastases;[40,42,43] and
   (C) demonstrating nonpalpable nodal metastases.[40,43,44]
4. By providing the most accurate means of follow-up available for determining response and recurrence.[17,61]

The impact of earlier detection and hence diagnosis on overall survival really depends on clinicians identifying the population at risk and referring them for study as early as possible (Table 5-2). Delays in diagnosis of six months to one year are not uncommon in nasopharyngeal carcinomas.[5,40] Certainly with CT we now have a tool capable of screening patients with "persistent unilateral serous otitis" or "facial numbness in the distribution of the fifth cranial nerve." The judicious and timely use of CT can only improve the situation.

Tumor Behavior and Pathology

Histopathology. Carcinoma is by far the most frequent primary malignancy of the nasopharynx, accounting for 98% to 99% of malignancies (Table 5-1).[5] The histopathologic diagnosis of squamous cell (epidermoid) carcinoma is made nearly 80% of the time, although it may hide within a confusing array of names seeking to describe the keratinizing and nonkeratinizing varieties of this common lesion.[5] The terms *transitional cell carcinoma* and *lymphoepithelioma* have been used to describe the nonkeratinizing type. Again, all are squamous cell carcinomas and their degree of biologic aggressiveness is a matter quite separate from their keratinizing versus nonkeratinizing properties, although the latter tend to be more common and less well differentiated.[5] It is difficult to predict the frequency of the other carcinomas that infrequently involve the nasopharynx.[5] Adenocystic carcinomas are particularly insidious in that some are be-

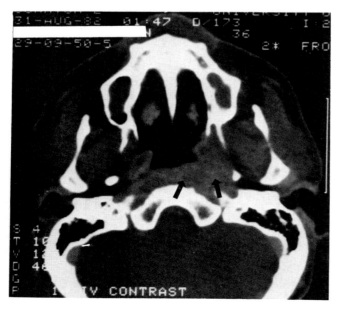

FIG. 5-1. Patient with cervical adenopathy of unknown origin. The CT scan revealed a deeply infiltrating mass in the nasopharynx (arrows). The mucosa was intact at triple endoscopy; however, a deep biopsy revealed squamous cell carcinoma.

Table 5-2. Common Symptoms and Syndromes and Nodes of Presentation in Patients with Nasopharyngeal Carcinoma

Otologic	Serous Otitis Media
	Otalgia
Neuralgic	Atypical Facial Pain
	Headache
	Sore Throat
Neuro-ophthalmologic	Cavernous Sinus Syndrome
	Jugular Fossa Syndrome
	Horner's Syndrome
	Proptosis
Nasal	Obstruction
	Discharge
	Bleeding
Cervical Adenopathy	

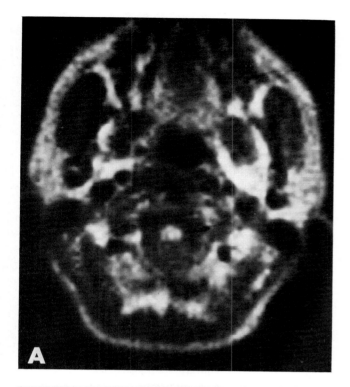

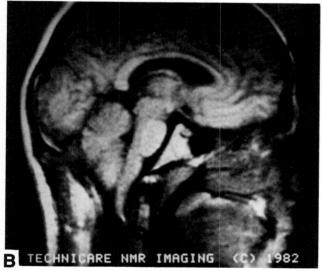

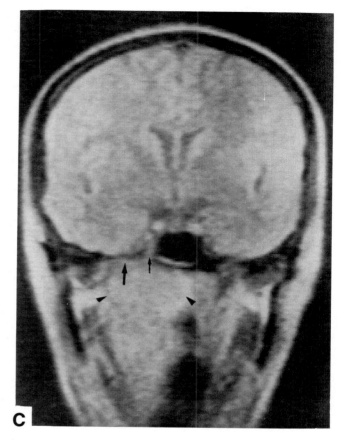

FIG. 5-2. (A) An early MRI image of the lower nasopharynx. The anatomic detail approximates that of CT (Courtesy of William Hanafee, M.D., UCLA Medical Center, Los Angeles). (B) Lateral view of the head and uppermost portion of the aerodigestive tract. Direct multiplanar imaging will be a distinct advantage of MRI (Image courtesy of Technicare Corporation). (C) Young patient with nasopharyngeal carcinoma. Coronal MR image SE 2000/30 shows primary tumor (arrowheads) eroding skull base (large arrow) and extending into cavernous sinus (small arrow).

lieved to arise in accessory salivary tissue within the parapharyngeal space and therefore may have a largely "submucosal" growth pattern. These may actually arise in the deep lobe of the parotid and appear as a nasopharyngeal lesion. The tumor is one of the few that spread primarily along nerves. The tumor is notorious for having spread beyond the grossly obvious primary site at the time of diagnosis and treatment via this nonencapsulated, infiltrating, and perineural pattern of spread. This tumor has a long natural history characterized by progressive local and perineural extension over periods of up to 15 to 20 years.

Lymphomas are probably the second most common histologic type found in the nasopharynx. These are mainly non-Hodgkin lymphomas, which may be associated with other areas of involvement in Waldeyer's ring or regional nodal or more remote disease.[5]

The relationship between nodal and extranodal lymphoma in the head and neck is difficult to sort out for a variety of reasons including: (1) the tendency for extranodal lymphoid tissue in the upper aerodigestive tract to undergo reactive hyperplasia, with the resulting atypia mimicking lymphoma;[5] (2) the inadequacy of biopsy material[5] (crushed or small samples are common); and (3) difficulties in being sure whether the head and neck disease is isolated or only part of a more generalized lymphoma.[5] In spite of these difficulties some general guidelines merit comment:

1. Extranodal involvement is common in non-Hodgkin lymphoma and rare in Hodgkin's lymphoma.[5]
2. If one portion of Waldeyer's ring is involved, it is likely that another will be.[5]
3. If extranodal disease is present in the head and neck, then systemic disease below the clavicles or diaphragm is a possibility. Historical data to document the frequency of systemic or nodal disease are difficult to define since few carefully controlled studies have been done.[5]

A variety of other malignant neoplasms round out the small percentage of "other" lesions that affect the nasopharynx. Rhabdomyosarcomas are common in children. Poorly differentiated tumors may be either lymphomas, carcinomas, or sarcomas. Rarely, primary tumors of the skull base such as chondrosarcomas, fibrosarcomas, or chondromas will appear as nasopharyngeal lesions. More rarely, metastases to the skull base or parapharyngeal space might appear as a primary nasopharyngeal mass; however, these patients usually have an established history of a tumor primary source.

Nasopharyngeal carcinoma does not seem to share the etiologic relationship with the use of alcohol and tobacco that carcinoma elsewhere in the upper aerodigestive tract does.[5] Other environmental factors have been indicted to explain the preponderance of this disease in the oriental population, although these are not clearly proven.[5]

Patterns of Spread. Lederman, in his excellent monograph on the nasopharynx, describes the natural history and spread of nasopharyngeal carcinoma.[35] With CT we now have an imaging tool that depicts these paths of local extension just as he and others[3,5] have described.

The course of tumor spread beyond the mucosal surfaces is vastly altered by the surrounding anatomic structures (Figures 5-3, 5-4). Some common pathways exist, including:

1. Spread along muscle bundles. Once there is invasion of a muscle, the tumor may spread from the muscle origin to its insertion and invade these osseous attachments (Figures 5-1, 5-5, 5-6).

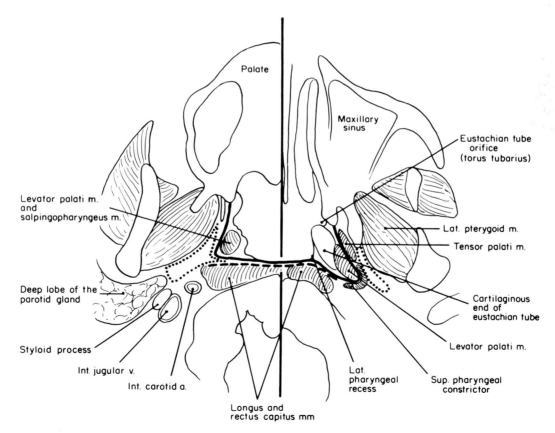

FIG. 5-3. The relationship of the pharyngobasilar fascia (solid black line) to the deep and superficial structures within the nasopharynx. The right-hand side of the diagram is more cephalad than the left. The limits of the parapharyngeal space are defined by black dots. The dashed line represents the prevertebral fascia.

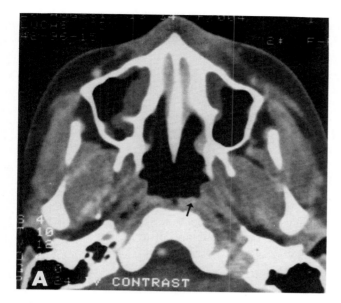

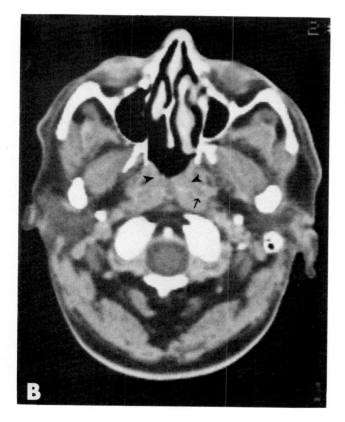

FIG. 5-4. Scans of normal patients done during contrast infusion. (A) The fine white line (arrow) is caused by capillary staining and is seen as a normal variant. Note that despite the fact that this patient has little fat in the deep tissue planes, these structures are still visible and symmetric. (B) Young patient with adenoidal tissue (arrowheads) lining the staining mucosal surfaces (arrow). Despite this mucosal "mass," the deep planes are normal and symmetric. Prominent adenoids are not uncommon up to 35 years of age and may be seen well beyond that age.

2. Spread within fibrofatty (areolar) tissue planes that surround the muscles (Figures 5-1, 5-5, 5-6).
3. Extension along neurovascular bundles to enter bones via the foramina created for the normal passage of these structures (Figure 5-6).
4. Spread along periosteal surfaces or expansion and spread within the marrow cavity of bones.

In general, tumors follow the "paths of least resistance" along existing anatomic structures. Cartilage is relatively resistant to invasion, probably because of its lack of vascularity.

In the nasopharynx, the patterns of spread differ little for individual histologic types, although some generalizations are possible. Adenocystic carcinomas may grow predominantly submucosally and tend to follow the nerves to and through the various basal foramina as well as peripherally. Rhabdomyosarcomas tend to ignore any particular boundary while spreading widely in the parapharyngeal and infratemporal spaces. Lymphomas probably present the widest spectrum of growth pattern. If a pattern "atypical" for carcinoma is present either clinically or on diagnostic studies, lymphoma should be placed higher on the differential list of possibilities.

Within the nasopharynx, deep extension of tumor follows the general pattern described above as modified by the pharyngobasilar fascia (Figure 5-3). This tough fascia is suspended from the skull base and surrounds the uppermost part of the aerodigestive tract. It is in itself a moderately resistant barrier to tumor growth, although aggressive malignancies are clearly capable of growing through it.[5,35] More importantly, it "channels" tumors along one of several mucosal and submucosal compartments.[5,35]

Growth of tumor on the airway side of the pharyngobasilar fascia carries it along the compartment that surrounds the levator palati.[35] The tumor can spread anywhere from the soft palate to the skull base (inferior petrous apex) within this tight tissue space (Figure 5-3). Such growth can result in tubal occlusive symptoms (unilateral serous otitis) by direct occlusion of the tube or interfering with the levator palati function. Spread in this space may also be in part submucosal and therefore inapparent on physical examination; this circumstance can lead to understaging.

Spread beyond the pharyngobasilar fascia may be direct or through the gap that exists between the upper margin of the fascia and the skull base. This brings the tumor into the parapharyngeal space. From the prestyloid portion of this space, the tumor may extend cephalad to contact the skull base at the foramen ovale and thus cause deficits in the third division of the fifth nerve.[35] The tumor may also extend to the poststyloid compartment, where it will reach the carotid artery first. Extension along the carotid canal brings the tumor into the

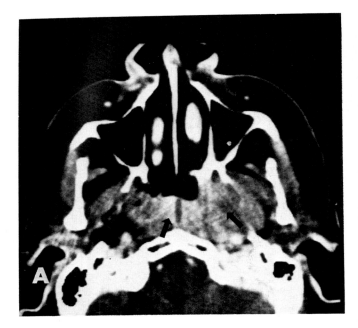

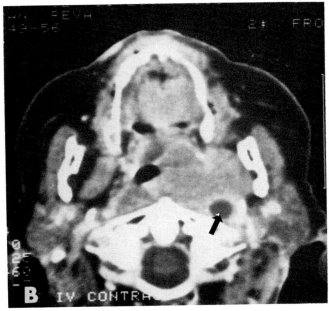

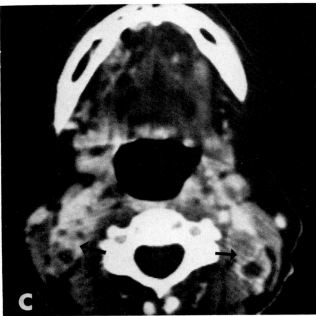

FIG. 5-5. Patient with typical nasopharyngeal carcinoma, with direct spread to the oropharynx and retropharyngeal and cervical nodal metastases. (A) An infiltrating mass extends across the midline (arrows). (B) A large mass involves the parapharyngeal space and soft palate. A necrotic retropharyngeal node is present (arrow). (C) A scan through the jugulodigastric region shows bilateral deep cervical and posterior triangle nodes (arrows), many of which are necrotic.

cavernous sinus where it may cause deficits in cranial nerves III, IV, V, and VI (Figure 5-2).[5,26,35] Direct extension to the carotid sheath may also result in partial or complete "jugular fossa syndrome," namely, deficits in cranial nerves IX through XII (Figures 5-5, 5-6).[5,35] Ero-

sion of the skull base accompanies all of these extensions; however, the region of the foramen lacerum may be spared because it is mainly composed of cartilage. Direct extension through the basisphenoid also carries the tumor intracranially. Such extension is more likely in tumors of the roof and fossa of Rosenmuller but also occurs in those areas along the lateral wall.[35] Destruction of the skull base and intracranial spread usually are characteristics of tumors that are advanced well beyond the stage of curability. Usually the spread is to the middle cranial fossa by the pathways described above. In very advanced lesions the basisphenoid and clivus may be extensively destroyed, with the tumor then gaining access to the posterior fossa.

Tumors may spread along the parapharyngeal musculature caudally to involve the tonsillar pillars, the base of the tongue, and even the floor of the mouth (Figure 5-3).[5,19] Later in the disease, extensive spread to the infratemporal fossa, pterygoid muscles, and mandible may result in trismus.

The patterns, incidence, and significance of nodal involvement will vary with the histopathology. Primary consideration in the following discussion is directed toward nodal disease associated with squamous cell carcinoma, since this represents the overwhelming majority of cases.

Nodal involvement in squamous cell carcinomas has important prognostic implications. The nasopharynx is rich in lymphatics, making cervical node involvement a common circumstance.[5,35,54] The retropharyngeal nodes (of Rouvier) lie between the carotid artery and the prevertebral muscles (Figure 5-3).[54] These are the first order nodes in nasopharyngeal carcinoma.[5,35,54] Involvement

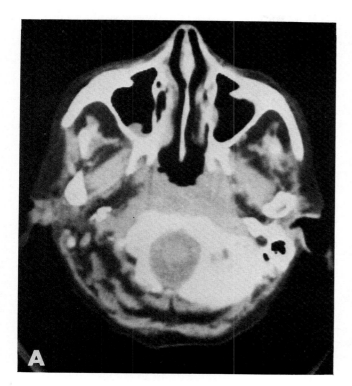
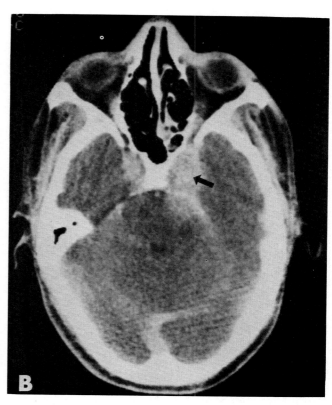

FIG. 5-6. Patient with nasopharyngeal carcinoma. (A) A circumferential deeply infiltrating mass extends across the midline. Spread to both carotid sheaths is present but is more prominent on the left. (B) The cavernous sinus is also involved with this end-stage tumor (arrow). (Photographs courtesy of Peter Som, M.D., Mount Sinai Hospital, New York).

of these nodes may result in compression or invasion of cranial nerves IX through XII and the upper cervical sympathetic trunk. This can lead to a partial or complete jugular fossa syndrome (Figure 5-5). Nodal disease is often bilateral because the disease commonly involves the midline and because the lymphatic drainage is crossed.[5,35,54] The frequency of cervical lymph node involvement at initial examination in 150 patients reviewed by Lederman[35] is as follows: Upper deep cervical, 70%; juguloomohyoid, 34%; spine accessory, 28%; inferior cervical, 20%. Other data support these trends.[31,58] Lymph node metastases are relatively unimportant modes of spread in adenoid cystic carcinomas, adenocarcinomas, and the other less common tumors that affect the nasopharynx. If involved nodes are found, they usually indicate a poor prognosis.[5]

Cervical lymph node metastases also account for one of the three most common presentations of nasopharyngeal carcinoma, the other two being tubal occlusive symptoms (most common) and neurological-ophthalmologic syndromes (least common). Nasal stuffiness, pain, or bleeding are uncommon complaints at initial examination and are usually indicative of a far advanced lesion.[5] Distant metastases involve bone (49%), the liver

(30%), and lungs (20%), most frequently occurring with an overall incidence of 28% in one series.[66] Metastases were more likely to occur with more advanced primary tumors and if cervical adenopathy was present. Assessment of metastatic disease should then include chest X-ray films, bone scans, and liver scan for patients with advanced tumors or with symptoms suggestive of metastatic disease.

Classification and Staging

Carcinoma of the nasopharynx is staged according to its superficial mucosal and deep extension by a combination of clinical and radiographic findings[1,5] (Figure 5-7; Tables 5-3, 5-4).

T_1 lesions are either mucosal and confined to one site (e.g., roof, one wall) or submucosal (i.e., positive biopsy and no visible tumor). The latter category raises important diagnostic and treatment implications relative to CT scanning which are discussed in subsequent sections.

T_2 lesions involve two sites (e.g., roof and lateral wall). T_3 lesions are those that have spread anteriorly to the nasal cavity or inferiorly to the oropharynx. The differentiation of T_2 and T_3 lesions is based on physical examination and biopsies. It must be emphasized that oc-

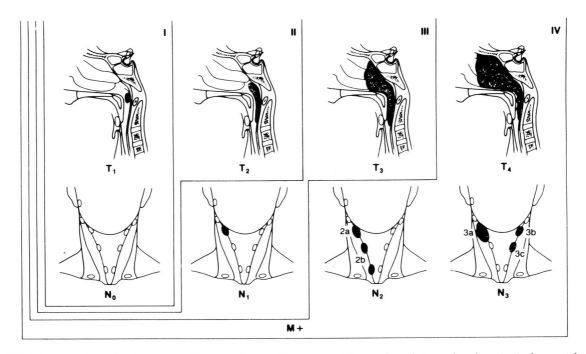

FIG. 5-7. Anatomic staging for cancer of the nasopharynx. T categories: The number of sites rather than size is the crucial factor. Sites are listed as vault (posterosuperior or roof) and lateral walls. The difference is between one site and two sites (T_1 v T_2) and anterior extension, which is T_3. Deep invasion into base of skull and nerves is T_4. Node (N) categories: The size of the node and its mobility and the number and locations are all factors in staging cervical nodes. The diameters ≤ 3 cm, 3 cm and 6 cm, and >6 cm were chosen because these are determined more objectively than fixation. Fixation implies adhesion to the carotid artery and therefore unresectability. Single and multiple nodes (N_1 v N_2), homolateral and bilateral nodes (N_1, N_2, N_3), are important factors. Stage grouping: The T category is the major determinant of stage. Note that N_1 nodes are equivalent to T_3 in advancement (stage III) and that N_2 and N_3 nodes and M_1, along with T_4 lesions, constitute stage IV. Modified from AJC[1].

cult (submucosal) extension may be present such that a T_1 lesion by clinical examination may in reality be a T_2 or T_3 lesion. The deep extensions resulting in such errors are along the pathways discussed in the *Patterns of Spread* section. The fallibility of blind biopsy in the nasopharynx has been well demonstrated, so that negative biopsies do not assuredly rule out the presence of tumor beneath intact mucosa (Figures 5-1, 5-8).[5,17,35,37,40,41,64,66]

T_4 tumors are those with clinical or radiographic evi-dence of skull base or cranial nerve involvement. These are obviously late phenomena characteristic of advanced tumors, most of which have a dismal prognosis (Figure 5-5). There are virtually no five-year survivors with T_4 lesions.[2,5,67] It should be apparent from prior discussion that deep extension may be present without invasion of the skull base or involvement of cranial nerves because most tumors must breach the pharyngobasilar fascia and extend along the deep tissue planes and neurovascular

Table 5-3. T Staging

T_x	Tumor cannot be assessed
T_0	No evidence of primary disease
T_{IS}	Carcinoma *in situ*
T_1	Tumor confined to one site
T_2	Involving more than one site in region of origin
T_3	Extension beyond region (nasopharynx to nose; larynx to pyriform sinus) or fixation of cord if laryngeal or hypopharyngeal
T_4	Massive tumor involving bone, cartilage, deep muscle or skin

Reprinted from American Joint Committee on Cancer: *Manual for Staging of Cancer*, 2nd ed. Philadelphia, J. B. Lippincott, 1983.

Table 5-4. Stage Grouping

Stage I	$T_1 N_0 M_0$
Stage II	$T_2 N_0 M_0$
Stage III	$T_3 N_0 M_0$
	T_1 or T_2 or T_3, N_1, M_0
Stage IV	$T_4 N_0 M_0$
	Any T, N_2 or N_3, M_0
	Any T, Any N, M_1

Reprinted from American Joint Committee on Cancer: *Manual for Staging of Cancer*, 2nd ed. Philadelphia, J. B. Lippincott, 1983.

bundles to produce such symptoms. It seems that there is room for improvement in the staging and quantitation of tumor within this portion of the upper aerodigestive tract.

Cervical metastases in nasopharyngeal carcinoma are staged according to the scheme established for cervical lymph node involvement in all primary head and neck malignancies.[1,5] These are presented in detail in the preceding chapter on the neck. The staging system does not directly take into account the likelihood of extranodal extension. This tendency increases directly with the size of the nodal mass.[7,46] Computed tomography is of help in evaluating extracapsular spread.

For nasopharyngeal carcinomas, there is an additional interesting omission in this classification, namely, the lack of accounting for retropharyngeal nodal metastases. Clearly, this has evolved because before the advent of CT these nodes were inaccessible to clinical or radiographic evaluation. Recall that the retropharyngeal nodes (of Rouvier) are the first-order drainage sites for carcinoma of the nasopharynx.[5,35,54] The status of these nodes would seem to be a worthwhile indication of stage of disease, likelihood of cervical metastases, and prognosis.[4,5]

Distant metastases are staged as M_0 (none known) or M_1 (present). If present they are usually pulmonary, osseous, or hepatic.[4,28]

T workup may include plain films and CT scans. N workup may be by CT scan. M workup should include chest X-ray films and, if clinically indicated, bone scans.

Imaging Procedures and Assessment

Numerous radiologic procedures have been used to aid in the evaluation of nasopharyngeal carcinoma (Table 5-5). Plain films (lateral and basal views) have been used for screening purposes and to define the extent of soft tissue as well as osseous involvement. These lack specificity and sensitivity and provide a definite answer only when gross destruction of the skull base is present.[10] Even in this regard they are inadequate because the extent of intracranial spread cannot be assessed. There is some role for plain films. This may include a lateral soft tissue view, which might aid in orienting those not familiar with the axial CT images to the extent of the lesion.

Contrast nasopharyngography has been used by several investigators who have refined the technique and produced exceptional images of the mucosal surfaces within the nasopharynx.[24,27] In this era of widespread expertise with flexible fiberoptic and rigid endoscopes, the status of the mucosa in the nasopharynx is rarely in question, and for this reason we feel this study is no longer indicated unless skilled endoscopic evaluation or CT is unavailable.

Conventional pleuridirectional tomography has been used with more precision than plain films for detecting subtle skull base invasion and the gross estimation of the soft tissue extension of lesions. This examination is less sensitive than CT for showing the extent of deep infiltration.[39] Conventional tomography is also less specific in that asymmetry of the soft tissues may often be attributed to malignancy when it is really caused by benign etiologies.[38] High-resolution CT of the skull base also provides images that are superior in quality and easier to interpret than pleuridirectional tomograms.[38,39,40] Pleuridirectional tomography in patients with known or suspected nasopharyngeal carcinoma should only be done if CT is not available.

Recommended Method of Study. Computed tomography is the imaging examination of choice for detecting and determining the extent of nasopharyngeal carcinomas. Computed tomography depicts the anatomy of the deep tissue planes surrounding the nasopharynx in a manner superior to all currently available imaging tools. Nuclear magnetic resonance imaging could replace CT in this regard, but the anatomic and clinical considerations will remain unchanged from those being presented (Figure 5-8). The CT image allows one to view the extensions of nasopharyngeal carcinoma along the pathways so aptly described by Lederman and others.[3,5,35,54,57,60,65] It explains clinical signs and symptoms by depicting correlative "disturbed" anatomy (e.g., a retropharyngeal no-

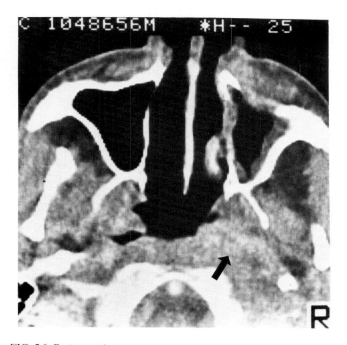

FIG. 5-8. Patient with recurrent tumor in the nasopharynx (arrow). Involvement was probably cephalad extension of an oropharyngeal primary. The mucosa was intact. Biopsy specimens were obtained on four different occasions because of the CT findings and persistent symptoms. Only the fourth deep biopsy was positive.

dal mass compressing cranial nerves IX to XIII in a jugular fossa syndrome).

Recommended uses of CT in helping to diagnose, stage, and follow up patients with nasopharyngeal cancer are presented in Figures 5-9, 5-10.

Technique of Examination. The technique of the CT examination will vary slightly with the scanner used. In general, scans are done with the patient supine with the Reid baseline perpendicular (or nearly so) to the table-top. The axial sections produced should be done "edge to edge" and at a thickness of 4 to 6 mm. Processing to obtain a reconstructed image "zoomed" to the region of interest provides excellent images. Also, processing that provides a better image of the bone at some expense to contrast resolution is desirable. This trade-off in density resolution is not significant on most units, since the inherent contrast—air, bone, soft tissues—in the area is high to begin with. Coronal sections may be necessary to confirm subtle findings on axial scans or to exclude pathologic entities near the roof of the nasopharynx or the skull base.

Contrast should be infused by the rapid drip infusion technique for the following indications:

1. Defining the extent of intracranial disease.
2. Evaluation of cervical and retropharyngeal lymph nodes.

3. Differentiation of tumor invading rather than obstructing paranasal sinuses.
4. Differential diagnosis of masses in the parapharyngeal space or those around the carotid sheath.

The first two of these are the indications usually operative for patients with known or suspected nasopharyngeal carcinomas.

The specific contributions of CT will be described under the individual headings that follow.

Limitations of CT. Certainly, data from CT are not tissue specific, and any critical management decision requires pathologic confirmation of CT findings. In general, the extent of deep infiltration as seen on CT scans correlates well with tumors seen elsewhere in the head and neck. This is probably best documented in studies of laryngeal and pyriform sinus carcinoma. Confirmation of the extent of malignancies elsewhere in the upper aerodigestive tract and especially in the nasopharynx is more difficult because of the limitations imposed on the surgeon by the surrounding anatomy. Multiple CT-directed biopsies are impractical and unnecessary for patient care. The spread of a nasopharyngeal carcinoma as seen on CT scans is in line with its natural history and correlates well with symptoms. Rarely, a deeply infiltrating mass will be a result of an inflammatory lesion, and, when present, it will be virtually indistinguishable from a malignant tumor. This is one of the circumstances that makes biopsy imperative. The other is the fact that the variety of tumors that appear in the nasopharynx are indistinguishable based on their morphologic structure; the histopathologic diagnosis of lymphoma would certainly have vastly different implications than that of carcinoma, which would differ from adenocystic carcinoma, etc.

There are no studies available to document the exact sensitivity, specificity, and accuracy of CT in evaluating nasopharyngeal carcinoma. It will probably prove to be both highly specific and sensitive when combined with the physical examination. Computed tomography may help avoid false-positive and false-negative interpretation of mucosal irregularities or "masses" seen on conventional roentgenograms (Figure 5-4). Moreover, it may help avoid clinical false-negatives caused primarily by submucosal tumors[2,5,41] (Figure 5-1). We are presently evaluating this in a prospective trial aimed at the detection of occult nasopharyngeal malignancies in patients with cranial nerve palsies, atypical facial pain, unilateral serous otitis media, and neck nodes. Preliminary results suggest that CT will be of benefit in this population at risk of developing nasopharyngeal cancer.[26]

The use of CT in evaluating cervical metastases in a methodical way was discussed in detail in that chapter.

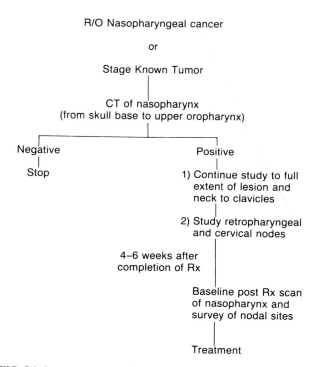

R/O Nasopharyngeal cancer

or

Stage Known Tumor

CT of nasopharynx
(from skull base to upper oropharynx)

Negative

Stop

Positive

1) Continue study to full extent of lesion and neck to clavicles

2) Study retropharyngeal and cervical nodes

4–6 weeks after completion of Rx

Baseline post Rx scan of nasopharynx and survey of nodal sites

Treatment

FIG. 5-9. Suggested protocol for initial CT evaluation of nasopharyngeal cancer.

Table 5-5. Imaging Modalities for Evaluating Nasopharyngeal Cancer

MODALITY	STAGING CAPABILITY	BENEFIT/ COST RATIO	RECOMMENDED ROUTINE STAGING PROCEDURE
Noninvasive			
Plain films nasopharynx (lateral soft tissue view) basal view skull	Gross screening: gross skull base destruction	Fair	Optional
Conventional tomography	Bone destruction skull base; suggest soft tissue extent of primary	Fair	No
Chest X-ray films	Look for metastases	High	Yes
Radionuclide studies; liver/spleen, bone scan	Look for metastases if suspected clinically	Fair	No
Nasopharyngography	Superficial extent	Low	No
MRI	Potentially primary site and regional nodes but no bone detail	?	?
Minimally Invasive			
CT	Primary site, nodes, skull base, intracranial spread	High	Yes

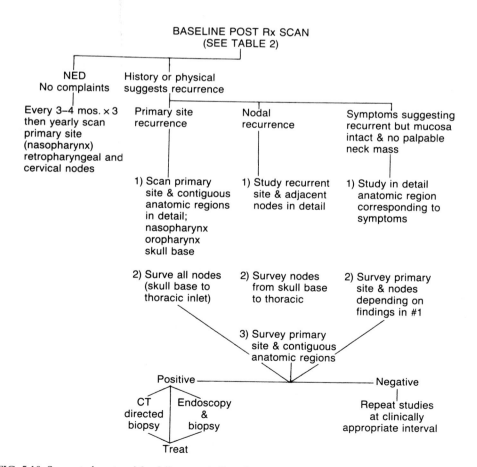

FIG. 5-10. Suggested protocol for follow-up studies of patients with known nasopharyngeal cancer.

Imaging Strategies and Decisions

Computed tomography has certainly refined our imaging approach to the nasopharynx. Nuclear magnetic resonance imaging may even improve it further (Figure 5-8). We now have an imaging tool that, when combined with physical examination of the nasopharynx, can render a diagnosis of normal or abnormal with a high degree of confidence. It is essential then to increase physician awareness of the impact of CT examination to the point where subpopulations of patients at risk of having nasopharyngeal carcinoma come to such definitive evaluation sooner. This would include an endoscopic examination by an experienced physician and a CT scan. The clinical settings in point have been enumerated in the prior discussion; they include patients with

1. Unilateral serous otitis media.
2. Deficits of cranial nerves that might be due to a nasopharyngeal lesion.
3. Atypical facial pain or numbness.
4. Cervical node of uncertain etiology.

If such a properly screened subpopulation receives CT scanning, then it can be expected that some tumors will be discovered with less delay and therefore at an earlier stage than usual. Theoretically this should improve survival statistics. This outcome remains to be proven.

Screening and Detection.

Delay in diagnosis occurs frequently in patients with nasopharyngeal malignancies. There are many reasons for such delay, and CT can solve some of them.[5,35] Any patient with persistent unilateral serous otitis media should have a CT scan of the nasopharynx even if the physical examination of the nasopharynx is normal. Patients with cranial nerve deficits or atypical facial pain (atypical for tic douloureux) that might be explained by a nasopharyngeal tumor should have a CT scan.[40,41] Patients with a neck node of uncertain cause may benefit from a CT scan of the nasopharynx (also the oropharynx and tongue base) before triple endoscopy and biopsy.[7,32,40,41] It cannot be overemphasized that in all of these settings, CT may show a tumor beneath intact mucosa (Figure 5-1). This phenomenon has been observed in negative blind biopsies;[38,40] moreover, even armed with the knowledge of where a tumor is according to the CT scan, circumstances of three negative biopsies before the fourth biopsy revealed a tumor may have been encountered[40] (Figure 5-2). A reasonable alternative is a percutaneous CT-directed biopsy through the mandibular notch.[14] This allows confirmation that the needle has been placed in the area of suspicion.

Diagnosis: Staging the Primary Tumor and Regional Nodes.

Tumors may spread along the mucosa, within the deep tissue planes, and by lymphatics.[3,5,35] Mucosal spread is evaluated by inspection, made more precise in recent years by the introduction of telescopic and flexible fiberoptic aids to physical diagnosis. Palpation of the neck is the accepted standard for detecting nodal metastases.

History, palpation, and roentgenographic examination, the latter looking mainly for bone destruction, have been the mainstay for diagnosing deep extension. However, deep extension may occur in the absence of significant history, beyond the palpating hand and certainly without gross evidence of bone destruction.[3,5,17,32,35,38,41,42,43,50,56]

While part of the primary tumor may be visible on the mucosa, a good deal of it may be spreading within the deep tissue planes surrounding the nasopharynx.[3,5,32] Ex-

Table 5-6. Treatment Decisions for the Nasopharynx[61]

STAGE	SURGERY	RADIATION THERAPY	CHEMOTHERAPY
I (T_1, N_0, M_0)	NR	Definitive RT, 6,500–7,000 cGy	NR
II (T_2, N_0, M_0)	NR	Definitive RT, 6,500–7,000 cGy	NR
III T_{1-3}, N_1, M_0) (T_3, N_0, M_0)	NR	Definitive RT, 7,000–7,500 cGy	Investigational chemotherapy
IV (T_4, N_2, N_3, M_0) (T_{any}, N_{any}, M_+)	NR	Definitive RT, 7,000–7,500 cGy	Investigational chemotherapy MAC
N_0	NR	Definitive RT, 5,000 cGy	NR
N_{1-3}	NR	Definitive RT, 6,000–7,000 cGy	Investigational chemotherapy
Relapse and recurrence	NR	Occasionally palliative RT	MAC

NR = Not Recommended
RT = Radiation Therapy
MAC = Multiagent Chemotherapy

tension along the levator palati and palatoglossus might take a lesion that is apparently confined to the lateral wall of the nasopharynx to the soft palate and oropharynx, respectively. A T_1 lesion thereby becomes T_3. Spread across the midline in the prevertebral spaces may not be appreciated on the physical examination; a T_1 lesion becomes T_2 (Figure 5-1). Spread into the infratemporal fossa from the parapharyngeal space may allow a tumor to spread along the pterygoid muscles and produce subtle erosion of the pterygoid plates; a T_1 or T_2 lesion becomes T_4. Computed tomography is obviously the best tool for detecting and determining the extent of intracranial spread.

Computed tomography has the proven capability to demonstrate tumor-involved nodes in patients who are normal on clinical examination;[40,42,43,44] this fact alone makes it a worthwhile study for many head and neck malignancies. When involved nodes are evident clinically, CT can quantitate the nodal involvement, may show otherwise undetectable contralateral nodes, and demonstrate the extent of extranodal spread (Figure 5-5).[40,42,43,44] In the nasopharynx the additional benefit of evaluating the retropharyngeal nodes now exists because of CT.[40,42,43,61]

Treatment Decisions[12,47,49,68]

Nasopharyngeal malignancies are treated almost exclusively with radiation therapy.[2,5,67] Surgery for cure is not possible. Limited local excision has been used as a palliative method when radiation is no longer feasible.[5] Both chemotherapy and immunotherapy have been used in attempts at salvage and palliation (Table 5-6).

Radical neck dissection is rarely used in an attempt to control cervical metastatic disease.[5] Its use is tempered by the fact that the first order nodes (retropharyngeal nodes) are beyond the limits of neck dissection and that the nodes occur in the posterior triangle. The latter circumstance requires sacrifice of the spinal accessory nerve and thus adds significantly to the morbidity of radical neck dissection.

CT data will do little to alter the basic treatment approach to known nasopharyngeal carcinoma because the mode of therapy is radiation and the incidence of nodal disease is so high that it requires elective treatment even in the absence of palpable disease.[2,5,67] However, it will show nodes in clinically negative necks or positive retropharyngeal nodes, which might suggest that a more radical approach to the neck be taken.

Pharyngeal cancers have always been the province of radiation therapists because of the inaccessibility of the nasopharynx and the proximity of the base of the skull and the cranial nerves. Large, generous fields are used with a shrinking-field technique for boosting the dose. Squamous cell carcinomas of varying degrees of differentiation usually require doses in the range of 6,500 to

7,500 cGy, depending upon their size and location (Table 5-6). Lymphoepitheliomas have responded to lower doses (6,000 to 6,500 cGy) with higher control rates than other tumors. Large neck nodes may require electron boost or interstitial techniques for boosting. If there is persistent nodal disease after irradiation, lymphadenectomy may be required if the primary is controlled and distant metastases remain absent.

Computed tomography may help in the management of the "unknown primary" appearing as a cervical metastasis.[40,41,42,43] If CT can depict the tumor in spite of a negative clinical examination or direct the endoscopists to the site most likely to yield a positive biopsy, then the field of treatment can be limited to the involved neck and biopsy-proven primary site.

Computed tomography also has the ability to detect a recurrent tumor in the absence of mucosal abnormality.[17,61] The patients usually complain of persistent pain or progressive symptoms suggestive of tumor but with a physical examination that shows only postradiotherapy changes. It is not unusual to "watch tumor grow" on CT scans in the absence of any mucosal expression of its presence[17] (Figure 5-2). This tendency has been documented in at least three studies as of this writing.[17,41,61] For this reason we and others[61] suggest that patients have a CT examination six to eight weeks following the completion of therapy and be followed at four to six month intervals for one year (Figures 5-5, 5-6). After that period, follow-up intervals should be individualized. It is essential not to delay rescanning patients who complain of pain or other symptoms of recurrent tumor even in the absence of confirmatory physical findings (Figure 5-2),[17] Such delay will only result in the needless postponement of salvage therapy in a significant number of patients.[17]

Impact of New Technology

Future developments should lead to a further refinement of exactly how CT and nuclear magnetic resonance imaging will be used to complement one another. More percutaneous CT-directed biopsies of suspicious lesions and possible sites of nodal involvement will probably be forthcoming.[14] The combination of the improved understanding of the clinical problems, refined imaging techniques, and more accurate treatment planning should lead to better patient management, reduction of morbidity, and, it is hoped, reduction of mortality.

THE PARANASAL SINUSES AND NASAL CAVITY

Malignancies of the paranasal sinuses and nasal cavity account for about 0.2% to 0.8% of all cancers and approximately 3% of cancers affecting the upper aerodigestive sinuses.[5] About 80% of cancers in this region begin in the maxillary sinuses.[5] Early diagnosis requires that both clinicians and radiologists maintain a high index of suspicion. Delay between onset of symptoms and final diagnosis averages six months.[5,13,18,19] This factor probably contributes to the poor overall survival statistics. A useful way of thinking of these lesions comes from Harrison,[19] who separates them into three groups: (1) Patients with early disease—small, localized lesions with 75% chance of five-year survival, which are uncommon; (2) Patients with late or advanced disease, whose chances of surviving five years are about 7%; and (3) an intermediate group, with overall five-year survival of about 50%.

The best hope for improving survival is to increase early detection rates. Another way is to be sure that the extent of the lesion is determined quickly and accurately, which allows precise treatment planning. Careful follow-up and early salvage of initial treatment failures may also improve survival statistics.

The following sections will discuss how CT may be useful in determining the extent of these malignancies and aid in the follow-up. Computed tomography is the imaging examination of choice for malignancies of this region because it defines the relationship of these tumors to the orbits, brain, intratemporal fossa, and nasopharynx in a manner so precise that it is unmatched by any other study.[39,40] Magnetic resonance imaging may improve on some aspects of CT; however, the studies should remain complementary because of superior depiction of bone detail by CT.

Tumor Behavior and Pathology

Histopathology. The histopathologic considerations of cancer in this region are primarily those of squamous cell carcinoma. Other lesions do occur here and are important to consider in the differential diagnosis related to the imaging workup and because the therapy and prognosis may differ vastly from that of squamous carcinoma. The reported incidence of squamous cell carcinoma in the nasal cavity and paranasal sinuses ranges from 80% to 90%.[13] About 80% of the cancers in this region arise from the maxillary antrum, and fully 80% of these will be squamous cell in origin. Primary carcinoma of the other sinuses is rare and, again, the dominant form is squamous cell.

Within the nasal and paranasal cavities other histologic types include melanoma, lymphoma, sarcoma, adenocarcinoma, and adenocystic carcinoma. These other lesions present no particular morphologic features on imaging studies that distinguish them from squamous cell carcinoma with the exception of a rare matrix-producing lesion such as chondrosarcoma. The histologic picture is usually a surprise to the clinician and diagnostic radiologist when it is something other than squamous cell.

Most of the adenocarcinomas of this region are felt to arise from surface epithelium or minor salivary gland tissue.[5] Adenoidcystic carcinoma originates in the latter and is particularly insidious because of its tendency to grow in a predominantly infiltrative pattern and perineurally. Adenocarcinoma comes from epithelial and minor salivary origins. The incidence of adenocarcinoma may be increased because of inhaled contact with wood shavings; cabinetmakers seem to be at increased risk of developing adenocarcinoma of the nasal cavity and ethmoids. These lesions tend to arise high in the nasal cavity and they are generally quite aggressive.[5] Mucoepidermoid is the third most common tissue type other than squamous cell in the sinonasal tract.[5] It ranks just behind adenoidcystic and adenocarcinoma in frequency. The clinical course of an aggressive mucoepidermoid carcinoma is similar to that of adenoidcystic or adenocarcinoma. Other carcinomas, including acinous cell, clear cell, and anaplastic, are much less common.

Malignant melanomas of the sinonasal tract account for 1% of all melanomas. Metastatic melanoma rarely involves these sites. The tumors arise mainly from melanocytes within the nasal mucosa over the turbinates and septum.[5] It is surprising that they tend not to arise from the olfactory epithelium, high in the nasal cavity, which is rich in melanin pigment.[5]

Lymphoma in the sinonasal tract is usually isolated, with no evidence of regional or distant nodal disease. Extramedullary plasmacystomas are unusual lesions. When they occur, about 80% are seen in the head and neck, with the sinonasal tract being a preferred site.[5]

Some further consideration should be given to differential diagnosis in this region, since other aggressive benign lesions may appear identical to malignancies on CT scans or other imaging studies. It is a sad fact that malignant tumors are frequently believed to be nasal polyps until they have proportions that make them incurable. Wegener's granulomatosis or the nonhealing midline granulomas may occasionally mimic malignancies. High in the nasal cavity one must always consider the rare possibility of esthesioneuroblastoma or inferior extension of a meningioma. An invasive pituitary adenoma may, on occasion, be mistaken for carcinoma of the sphenoid sinus; fortunately the latter lesion is very rare.

Patterns of Spread. Basic patterns of spread for malignancies of the upper aerodigestive tract were discussed in prior chapters. In the nasal cavity and paranasal sinuses, the anatomy is mainly that of an osseous framework covered with a mucoperiosteal lining. Superficial spread occurs along mucosal paths of least resistance; deep spread is primarily by bone destruction. Malignancies are usually beyond cure once they have spread to the point where they gain access to the muscle and fascial planes around this area. Spread to regional lymph

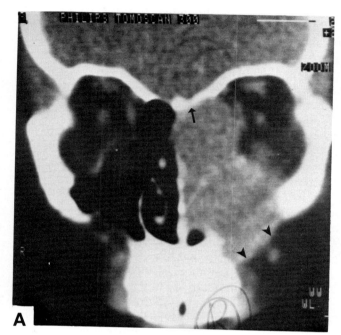

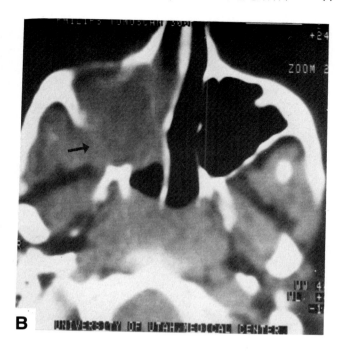

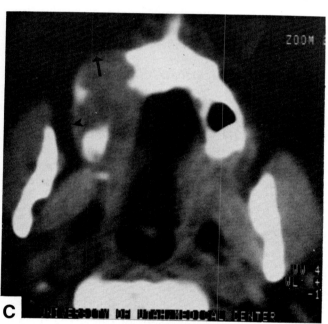

FIG. 5-11. Patient with squamous cell carcinoma of the maxillary antrum. (A) Coronal section shows the spread to the ethmoids stopping at the cribiform plate (arrow). The orbit is involved and spread to the cheek is likely (arrowheads). (B) Axial section, upper antrum. The tumor has eroded the posterior wall of the antrum and spread to the infratemporal fossa (arrow). (C) Axial section through the lower antrum and maxillary alveolar ridge. Spread to the cheek (arrow) and buccinator space (arrowheads) is demonstrated.

nodes in these malignancies is a late finding; again, it is in patients who are beyond the curative stage.

The importance of understanding where and how these lesions spread is best reflected in therapy planning issues. We will therefore consider how these tumors reach the posterior ethmoid and sphenoid region, the soft tissues of the deep face, orbit, skull base, brain, infratemporal fossa, and pterygomaxillary fossa, and the nasopharynx. Since maxillary sinus cancers represent the vast majority of sinonasal malignancies, it will be used as the prototype "typical" lesion.

Superior extension takes these tumors to the roof of the maxillary sinus and floor of the orbit (Figure 5-11). From the floor of the orbit they may grow directly into the muscle cone, and for a time the tumor will have breached the bony orbit leaving the periorbit intact. Direct spread into the orbit seems to be more common after the tumor has reached the antroethmoidal septum or has grown into the ethmoids (Figure 5-11). Tumors seem to penetrate the relatively thin lamina papryaceae more easily than the orbital floor.

While these aggressive tumors are perfectly capable of eroding directly through bone, they prefer paths of least resistance and will follow a neurovascular channel or natural ostium as a nidus for bone destruction. Extension to the roof and anterior wall of the antrum will produce point numbness below the orbit because of involvement of the infraorbital nerve. After destroying the anterior or lateral wall of the antrum, the tumors infiltrate the soft tissue of the face (Figures 5-11, 5-12). From here they have access to the dermal lymphatics that

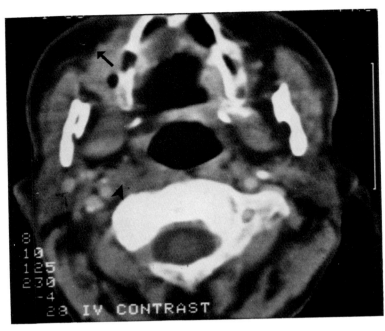

FIG. 5-12. Patient with squamous cell carcinoma of the hard palate and maxillary alveolar ridge. The primary mass has spread to the buccinator space (arrow). The mass had also spread through the hard palate to the floor of the nasal cavity, resulting in retropharyngeal nodal enlargement (arrowhead).

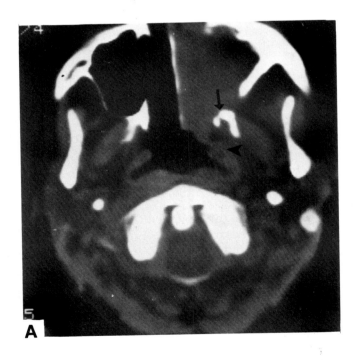

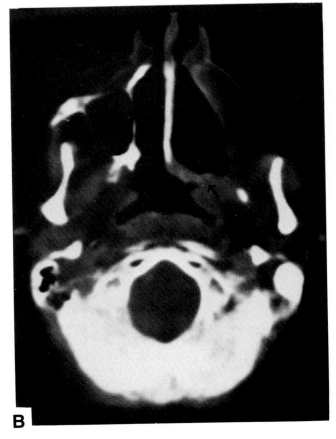

FIG. 5-13. Patient with antral carcinoma. (A) primary tumor has spread posteriorly to involve the pterygomaxillary fossa (arrow) and the wall of the nasopharynx (arrowhead). (B) Baseline study after radical maxillectomy and radiotherapy suggests residual disease (arrow). Several months later the patient developed a clinically obvious massive recurrence posteriorly in the maxillectomy cavity (no CT scan available).

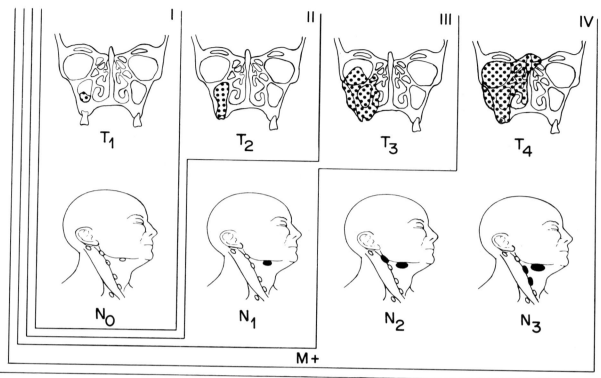

FIG. 5-14. Anatomic staging for cancer of the paranasal sinuses. T categories: The primary tumor is characterized by depth of penetration and extension to other contiguous structures in the region. Location in the sinus is an early factor. The presence or absence of bone destruction determines T_1 v T_2 and other categories. One extension to another site v multiple sites establishes whether it is T_3 or T_4. N categories and stage groupings: See legend for Figure 5-7. Modified from AJC[1].

drain to the submental, submandibular, and deep cervical groups; the submandibular nodes are mainly at risk.

Tumors spreading inferiorly erode into the maxillary alveolar ridge and may produce tooth loosening and pain patterns that suggest dental disease. Inferolateral spread takes lesions into the buccinator space, where again it has access to the deep facial and dermal lymphatics (Figures 5-9, 5-10). Inferomedial spread takes it to the hard palate, where it has all the implications discussed in the chapter on the oral cavity.

Medial spread is through the relatively thin medial antral wall. Once in the nasal cavity, the tumors may spread freely along all mucosal surfaces. Particularly disturbing patterns are posterior spread to involve the nasopharyngeal mucosa and invasion of the nasal septum with spread across the midline (Figure 5-13). Lymph drainage from the nasal cavity and nasopharynx is primarily to the retropharyngeal nodes.

Destruction of the posterior wall of the antrum brings the tumor to the infratemporal fossa (Figures 5-11, 5-13). This usually occurs medially and superiorly near areas of inherent weakness caused by the foramina for the terminal branches of the internal maxillary artery that supply the antrum and pterygomaxillary fossa. The tumors spread into the retroantral fat, infratemporal fossa, and pterygomaxillary fairly freely once they have spread beyond the posterior wall of the antrum (Figures 5-12, 5-13). Destruction of the pterygoid plates soon follows. Spread into the orbit via the inferior orbital fissure is also possible. Trismus is a late finding and is, in our experience, usually seen in fairly gross spread to the infratemporal fossa and pterygoid muscles.

Intracranial spread is most often at the cribiform plate. The tumors grow cephalad within the ethmoid sinus to reach this perforated bony margin. More cephalad extension brings invasion of the olfactory groove and bulb region and finally the frontal lobe. Rarely, tumors that have spread to the posterior ethmoids and sphenoid will reach the middle cranial fossa and cavernous sinus.

Intracranial perineural extension is uncommon in squamous cell carcinomas when they first appear. It is more usual in recurrent tumor.[9] Adenocystic tumors may spread primarily by the perineural route.

Some comments on nodal spread were made in passing during the preceding discussion. Nodal metastatic disease certainly is an important issue in sinonasal cancer; however, it is not as pivotal for management decisions as it is elsewhere in the head and neck. It occurs in about 25% of sinus cancer patients and is almost always to the submandibular node. For the most part, if nodal metastases are present, the patient has little or no chance of surviving. They are, then, mainly of prognostic significance.

It is estimated that 10% to 18% of patients with maxillary sinus carcinoma manifest nodes at initial examination.[32,45] Many nodes that become apparent clinically are probably related to the spread of lesions to the oral cavity, whereupon the characteristics of nodal drainage parallel primary lesions of that site.[33] During the period of observation about 25% to 35% of patients will manifest nodal disease clinically. This incidence is probably artificially low because the primary drainage to retropharyngeal nodes has been beyond routine clinical or imaging evaluation (Figure 5-12).

Classification and Staging

The proposed systems for staging carcinoma of the nasal cavity and paranasal sinuses have been modified by several authors, which is a testimony to the nuances of staging head and neck cancer in general and in this region in particular. Although it is probably most useful in individual patients to consider the exact location of the tumor, it seems that some staging systems will re-

main in place as a vehicle for end-results reporting. In this section we will adhere to the AJC guidelines (Figure 5-14; Table 5-3).

The staging system proposed in the AJC manual refers only to cancer of the maxillary atrum (see Table 5-4). The system is based on Ohngren's original observations, which indicated that tumors located anteroinferiorly (infrastructure) in the antrum tended to be more curable than those in the posterosuperior antrum (suprastructure).[51] Modernization of these original concepts produced the concept of separating the region into three compartments: (1) the suprastructure—demarcated by a horizontal line drawn along the inferior aspect of the orbits including the frontoethmoidal complex, the orbits, and the upper nasal cavity; (2) the mesostructure—demarcated by horizontal lines drawn through the floors of the orbits and the floors of the maxillary antra including the maxillary antra and midnasal fossa; and (3) the infrastructure—lying below the lines drawn through the floors of the antra and through the maxillary alveolar ridge. These are useful concepts in that they reflect the natural history of these tumors; however, the following staging scheme relies on Ohngren's line drawn from the medial canthus of the eye to the angle of the mandible. This line identifies an imaginary plane that divides the antrum into an anteroinferior portion (infrastructure) and a posterosuperior portion (suprastructure) (Figure 5-14).

Table 5-7. Imaging Modalities for Evaluating Sinus Cancer

MODALITY	STAGING CAPABILITY	BENEFIT/ COST RATIO	RECOMMENDED ROUTINE STAGING PROCEDURE
Noninvasive			
Conventional tomography	Good for detail of bone destruction; suggestive of extent of soft tissue invasion and likelihood of brain and orbital spread	Fair	No
Orthopantomography	Good for bone detail, hard palate, and maxillary alveolar ridge	Fair	No
Chest X-ray films	May detect metastases	High	Yes
Radionuclide studies; liver/ spleen, brain scan and bone scan	For detecting metastases only if clinically suspected	Low	No
MRI	Should be good for extent of primary tumor; will lack bone detail	?	?
Minimally Invasive			
CT	Invasive if contrast is infused; most useful tool for establishing extent of primary tumor	High	Yes
Invasive			
Angiography	Occasionally for diagnosis (e.g., juvenile angiofibroma); usually for adjunctive therapy (e.g., arterial infusion of chemotherapeutic agent)	Low	No

T_1 lesions are confined to the mucosa of the antral infrastructure with no evidence of bone destruction. T_2 lesions are confined to the suprastructure mucosa without evidence of bone destruction or to the infrastructure with bone destruction limited to the medial or inferior wall.

T_3 lesions are those that have spread beyond the confines of the antrum in one or more of the directions described in the previous section. Invasion of the skin of the cheek, the orbit, anterior ethmoids, or pterygoid muscles is indicative of these advanced lesions.

T_4 lesions are large, basically end-stage lesions that have invaded the cribiform plate, the posterior ethmoids, the sphenoid sinus, the nasopharynx, the pterygoid plates, or other parts of the skull base.

Cervical nodes are staged according to the criteria described in the chapter on the neck. No specific provision is made for retropharyngeal nodes since the criteria are at this point dependent on the physical examination.

Staging usually consists only of a T workup. Imaging procedures for this include plain films, conventional tomography, CT, and MRI. N workup, if necessary, may be accomplished with CT. M workup necessitates chest X-ray films and bone scans.

Imaging Procedures and Assessment

Plain films are usually the first examination done on patients suspected of having sinus disease. This still remains as the initial study for screening purposes, but plain films are never sufficient for staging known sinus or nasal cavity malignancies (Table 5-7).

Pluridirectional tomography was our most useful and precise imaging tool for staging these neoplasms before second, third, and fourth generation CT equipment became available. Even second generation CT has been shown to be more valuable for staging sinus cancer than pluridirectional tomography.[33,39]

Recommended Method of Study. Computed tomography is the recommended examination of choice for staging sinus malignancy and promised to be pivotal in staging cervical metastases as well.[20,25,29] The imaging approach to these patients is presented in Figure 5-15. Bone detail is so important in this process that CT will probably remain the first study of choice for initial evaluation of these tumors even if MRI lives up to its early promise. Plain films remain the initial screening procedure for patients with complaints referable to the paranasal sinuses. Conventional tomography or pantomography is reserved for those patients in whom information in the coronal plane is necessary and unavailable from CT studies.

Technique of Examination. The study should begin with axial sections usually from the cribiform plates to the maxillary alveolar ridge. Edge-to-edge 4- to 6-mm-thick sections usually provide sufficient detail. Images should be reviewed at window levels appropriate for both bone and soft tissue detail. Processing with a program emphasizing bone detail is desirable, but one should not

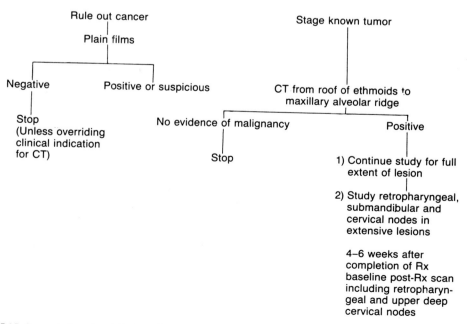

FIG. 5-15. Suggested protocol for initial CT evaluation of cancer of the paranasal sinuses and nasal cavity.

sacrifice too much soft tissue detail, since the normally processed images now usually provide adequate bone detail when viewed at wide window settings. Thin-section, high-resolution CT images processed for bone detail are unequivocally superior and easier to interpret than even the best pluridirectional tomographic images.

Coronal sections may be obtained if the relationship of the tumor to the orbital floor, cribiform plate, or hard palate is unclear on the axial scans. Reformations are sufficient for estimations of the extent of a lesion. Direct coronal sections are required if subtle detail of the orbital floor must be rendered. Anteroposterior pluridirectional tomograms may be substituted for direct coronal CT sections if the patient cannot cooperate for the latter study.

Contrast infusion may be used to distinguish tumor mass from obstructive sinus opacification. Contrast should always be injected if the tumor threatens the intracranial compartments. Coronal sections are required to detect subtle intracranial spread via the cribiform plate.[52]

If the tumor has spread so that it has access to the lymphatics of the nasal cavity, oral cavity, or dermis, then the cervical nodes should be staged. This requires rapid drip infusion of intravenous contrast. Scans in these instances should be carried caudally at about 1- to 1.5-cm intervals to at least the mid-neck. The area around the submandibular nodes should be studied with more detailed technique (i.e., 5-mm contiguous sections).

Imaging Strategies and Decisions

Screening and Detection. While plain films are usually the first study done in the search for sinus cancer, they are sometimes suggestive but not often definitive in this regard. A tomographic study is usually required to look for subtle evidence of bone destruction in an opacified sinus. If bone destruction is obvious on plain films, then tomography is necessary for definitive staging. Pluridirectional tomography may be used, but it is usually a needless step in the diagnostic process. The modern imaging approach to these lesions requires CT to establish the extent of the lesion. Moreover, it takes more training and experience to learn to interpret conventional sinus tomography than CT images. This is a critical issue when management decisions are being made on the basis of an image. For these reasons, we suggest that CT be used for studying patients suspected of harboring a malignancy as well as for those with known tumors.

Diagnosis — Staging. Clearly the problem of earlier diagnosis is not one that will be solved by CT. If a high index of suspicion for sinus malignancy is maintained in certain situations, some cases are likely to be confirmed at an earlier stage. Some of these circumstances of interest to the imaging physician include:

1. A middle-aged or older patient with persistent unilateral sinus opacification.
2. A patient with chronic sinus disease and excessive assymetric reactive bony changes.
3. Patients who have a history of nasal polyposis and long-standing sinus disease for whom plain films show diffuse pansinusitis, and the bony margins of the sinuses cannot be adequately evaluated on plain films.

The circumstances listed above will be related to benign sinus disease in the vast majority of instances. However, the imaging physician should be prepared to suggest a tomographic study despite the low yield situation. On the other hand, the head and neck surgeon who is maintaining a high index of suspicion should not hesitate to explore a sinus as these and other conditions suggest.

Computed tomography displays, in a manner far superior to any prior imaging tool, all of the anatomy of interest in staging sinonasal cancer. Magnetic resonance imaging will likely accomplish this also, with the exception of bone detail. A point-by-point anatomic summary is in order to correlate exactly how CT fits in with the staging issues discussed in prior sections.

Inferior Spread. Computed tomography shows the bone detail of the inferior sinus and defines the surrounding soft tissues with the nasal cavity, the buccinator space, or the oral cavity. This allows one to detect subtle infiltration into the cheek as well as the more gross finding of bone destruction (Figures 5-11, 5-12).

Anterior Spread. The relationship of the subcutaneous fat and dermis to the tumor mass is shown in all patients; even the most subtle breaches of the anterior antral wall and early soft tissue extensions are obvious (Figures 5-11, 5-12).

Medial Spread. The relationship of the tumor to the medial antral wall and nasal septum is clearly shown. Contrast infusion helps sort out obstructive versus invasive changes.

Superoposterior Spread. Axial and coronal sections display the floor of the orbit and structures of the muscle cone with great precision. The same projections define the limits of the antrum and ethmoids relative to each other and the orbit in such a manner that the relationship of tumor mass to the orbit, the anterior and posterior ethmoid, and the sphenoid sinuses is clearly shown (Figure 5-11).

Posterior Spread. Computed tomography clearly defines the relationship of tumor to the posterior wall of the an-

Table 5-8. Treatment Decisions for the Paranasal Sinuses

STAGE	SURGERY	RADIATION THERAPY (RT)	MULTIAGENT CHEMOTHERAPY (MAC)
I (T_1, N_0)	Complete resection of maxillary sinus sparing eye if possible	Optional postop RT	NR
II ($T_2 N_0$)	Surgical decompression before RT Complete resection of maxillary sinus except for exteneration of orbit	Preop and/or postop RT	NR
III ($T_3 N_1$)	Surgical decompression before RT Complete resection of maxillary sinus except for exteneration	Preop and/or postop RT	Investigational MAC
IV ($T_4 N_3$)	Unresectable	Definitive RT	Investigational MAC
Relapse after treatment	NR	NR	Investigational MAC
For N_0	NR	NR	NR
For $N_1 N_2$	Radical neck dissection if primary controlled	Postop RT	Investigational MAC

NR = Not Recommended

trum, retroantral fat, the pterygomaxillary fossa, and the infratemporal fossa (Figures 5-11, 5-12). It clearly defines whether a tumor involves just the soft tissues of the infratemporal fossa or has gone on to involve the pterygoid plates and other portions of the skull base. Spread to the nasopharynx via the infratemporal fossa (from its deep aspect) or via the mucosa through the posterior nares is usually easy to predict (Figure 5-13).

Nodal Disease. The major group of interest in nodal disease is the retropharyngeal nodes (Figure 5-12). A CT scan can detect enlarged nodes in this area more consistently than physical examination.

From the above listing it should be clear that CT is the imaging study of choice for staging sinus and nasal cavity malignancies. It provides all of the necessary data demanded by the staging system presented in the previous sections. It adds to this an ability to determine precise tumor volume, a way of evaluating retropharyngeal nodes, and, in many instances, a means of distinguishing obstructive and invasive changes in this area. A precise clinical-diagnostic stage for every neoplasm affecting this area is relatively simple to obtain using a CT as described in previous sections; this is true even for those who see very few of these lesions. Beyond this "labeling" process, the diagnostic imager is providing radiation, surgical, and medical oncologists with an accurate accounting of the extent of the lesion. This can only lead to more precise and rational treatment planning.

Treatment Decisions[11,23,36,48,53,68]

Initial treatment of many lesions is usually by a combination of radiation and surgery (Table 5-8). Chemotherapy and immunotherapy are usually reserved for salvage; however, the combination of intra-arterial infusion of chemotherapeutic agents followed by radiation has shown some promise as a primary mode of therapy.[11,23,36,48,55,68]

The use of combined surgery and radiation in most cases is a reflection of the advanced state of many lesions when they appear. Less than 10% of patients have T_1 or T_2 lesions, and the limited nature of the lesion is easily confirmed on CT scans. The main aim of imaging should be to identify an intermediate group of patients who do not have advanced lesions and in whom attempts to "treat for cure" have a reasonable chance of success. The intermediate group benefits most from imaging because it is here that careful planning of radical treatment is necessary to avoid recurrence in a potentially curable lesion. On the other hand, patients who are clearly beyond curative stages should be spared the extreme morbidity entailed in radical therapy. From the poor overall survival statistics (only one patient in four survives for five years), it should be clear that some attempts to treat for cure are in reality palliative from the outset.

It is useful to separate nasal cavity and antral carcinomas when considering therapy because most series show a 20% to 50% better survival in nasal cavity tumors.[5] The range is 38% to 63% five-year survivals compared with about 25% for sinus primaries. Radiotherapy may be used alone but it is often combined with surgery.[6]

Limited carcinoma of the antrum can be treated primarily by radical surgery. This presupposes that the encumbent mutilation can be tolerated and that adequate margins will be obtained. Absolute contraindications to a curvative surgical approach include destruction of the skull base, invasion of the pterygoid process, infiltration of the nasopharyngeal mucosa, and inoperable nodal metastases (retropharyngeal nodes). A borderline contraindication might be invasion of the infratemporal fossa without fixation to the pterygoid process. The usual surgical approach is radical maxillectomy sometimes combined with orbital exenteration.

The combined radiation-surgical approach is most often used because of the advanced nature of the lesions at initial examination. Preoperative radiation is usually followed by surgery if the lesion is considered operable. Radiation alone may be used as a palliative measure but will yield five-year survival rates of only 12% to 19%.[16,33] Nodes are treated with en bloc dissection with or without radiation.[30,34,63]

Recurrent tumor may be picked up earlier with CT than by physical examination.[61] Patients should have postoperative baseline studies and be followed at appropriate intervals. This has been discussed in detail in prior chapters (Figure 5-11).

The treatment decisions according to stage are:

1. For earliest stage I, T_1, N_0, M_0, surgical resection of maxillary bone and sinus is adequate if the margins are clear and the cancer is limited to the antrum without bone destruction of a wall.
2. For intermediate stage II and III, surgical resection of the maxillary sinus alone is often inadequate, and sparing the eye is not possible once the orbital floor is eroded. Preoperative or postoperative radiation therapy or both are used, most often with high-energy photons/electrons through a wedge pair arrangement. Surgical decompression, creating an opening in the palate through a Caldwell-Luck incision or a wider opening in the floor of the sinus is recommended to allow for adequate drainage. Selected CT scans are essential for treatment planning, tumor volume definition, and isodose selection. Postoperatively, a mold can be used and differentially loaded with radioactive sources depending upon residual disease or margins in operative specimens as determined by microscopic study.
3. For advanced stage IV nonresectable disease, radical radiation treatment combined with multiagent chemotherapy is often used. For nodal involvement, which is usually in the submandibular area, radical neck dissection should be done because radiation fields seldom extend to this level, since they would require incidental irradiation of large portions of a normal oral cavity and add considerably to morbidity. When positive nodes are found, particularly if they are advanced, radiation therapy should follow surgical resection.
4. For metastatic disease and relapse, multiagent chemotherapy or investigational phase II agents are advocated for palliation. Table 5-6 and Figure 5-14 present the treatment decisions and anatomic staging for paranasal cancer.

Impact of New Technology

Evaluation of tumors with CT may have an impact upon survival by making choices of therapy more precise; however, significant improvement in survival would be expected to come mainly from earlier diagnosis. Unfortunately this involves a set of patient and physician factors that are largely beyond the sphere of influence of the diagnostic radiologist. Computed tomography does have the ability to limit the substantial morbidity sometimes inflicted in an attempt to treat a patient for cure when only palliative measures are indicated; this is due to its ability to define tumor limits more precisely than any other imaging study. MRI will be the important new modality to evaluate since it may provide better imaging of tumor spread and infiltration.

Magnetic resonance imaging will be used to evaluate tumors of the nasal cavity and paranasal sinuses. It may become the imaging examination of choice, although the lack of bone detail with MRI might make the studies complimentary in some instances. An MRI study can potentially be more specific in that signals from a tumor and the contents of an obstructed sinus may differ enough to allow their distinction from one another. Multiplanar imaging will be easier with MRI, and interference from dental fillings may prove less bothersome than with CT. Computed tomography is a superb imaging tool for cancer in this region and care must be exercised to avoid making CT or MRI cost-additive without additional diagnostic benefit. Clinical studies comparing these imaging methods should determine which is the preferred method and in what instances both should be done.

REFERENCES

1. American Joint Committee on Cancer: *Manual for Staging of Cancer*, 2nd ed. O. H. Beahrs, M. H. Myers (Eds.). Philadelphia, J. B. Lippincott, 1983.
2. Bailar, J. C.: *Nasopharyngeal cancer in white populations — A world wide survey.* UICC Monograph series 1:18, 1967.
3. Ballantyne, A. J.: Routes of spread. In *Radiation Therapy in the Management of Cancers of the Oral Cavity and Oropharynx.* Fletcher, G. H., Maccomb, W. S. (Eds.) Springfield, IL, Charles C Thomas, 1962, pp. 91–116.
4. Ballantyne, A. J.: Significance of retropharyngeal nodes in cancer of the head and neck. *Am. J. Surg.* 108:500, 1964.
5. Batsakis, J. G.: *Tumors of the Head and Neck. Clinical and Patho-*

logical Considerations. Baltimore, Williams & Wilkins, 1979.

6. Bosch, A., Vallecillo, L., Frias, Z.: Cancer of the nasal cavity. *Cancer* 37:1458, 12976.

7. Cachin, Y., Sancho-Garnier, H., Micheau, C., Marandas, P.: Nodal metastases from carcinoma of the oropharynx. *Otolaryngol. Clin. North Am.* 12:145–154, 1979.

8. Coates, H. L., Pearson, G. R., Neel, H. B., Weiland, L. H.: Epstein-Barr virus-associated antigens in nasopharyngeal carcinoma. *Arch. Otolaryngol.* 104:427–430, 1978.

9. Dodd, G. D., Dolan, P. A., Ballantyne, A. J., Banez, M. L., Chau, P.: The dissemination of tumors and inflammatory disease as evaluated by CT and pluridirectional tomography. *Neuroradiology* 16:449–453, 1978.

10. Eller, J. L., Roberts, J. F., Ziter, F. M. H., Jr.: The normal nasopharyngeal soft tissues for adults. A statistical study. *A.J.R.* 112:537–541, 1971.

11. Fletcher, G. M., Goepfeit, H., Jesse, R. H., Jr.: Nasal and paranasal sinus carcinoma. In *Textbook of Radiotherapy*, 3rd ed. Fletcher, G. H. (Ed.). Philadelphia, Lea & Febiger, 1980, pp. 408–425.

12. Fletcher, G. H., Million, R. R.: Nasopharynx. In *Textbook of Radiotherapy*, 3rd ed. Fletcher, G. H. (Ed.). Philadelphia, Lea & Febiger, 1980, pp. 364–384.

13. Frazell, E. L., Lewis, J. S.: Cancer of the nasal cavity and accessory sinuses: A report of the management of 416 patients. *Cancer* 16:1293, 1963.

14. Galenby, R. A., Mulhern, C. B., Strawitz, J.: CT guided percutaneous biopsies of head and neck masses. *Radiology* 146:717–719, 1983.

15. Hadfield, E. H., Macbeth, R. G.: Adenocarcinoma of the ethmoids in furniture workers. *Ann. Otol. Rhinol. Laryngol.* 80:699–703, 1971.

16. Hamberger, C. A., Martensson, G., Sjogren, H. A.: Treatment of malignant tumors of the paranasal sinuses. In *Cancer of the Head and Neck*. Conley, J. (Ed.). Washington, DC, Butterworths, 1967, pp. 224–229.

17. Harnsberger, H. R., Mancuso, A. A., Muraki, A.: The upper aerodigestive tract and neck. CT evaluation of recurrent tumors. *Radiology* 149:503–509, 1983.

18. Harrison, D. F.: The management of malignant tumors of the nasal sinuses. *Otolaryngol. Clin. North Am.* 4:159, 1971.

19. Harrison, D. F. N.: Problems in surgical management of neoplasms arising in the paranasal sinuses. *J. Laryngol.* 90:69, 1976.

20. Hasso, A. N.: CT of tumors and tumor-like conditions of the paranasal sinuses. *Radiol. Clin. North Am.* 22:119–130, 1984.

21. Henderson, B. E., Louie, E., Jing, J. S. H., Buell, P., Gardner, M. B.: Risk factors associated with nasopharynx carcinomas. *N. Engl. J. Med.* 295:1101–1106, 1976.

22. Ho, J. H.: An epidemiologic and clinical study of nasopharyngeal carcinoma. *Int. J. Radiat. Oncol. Biol. Phys.* 4:183–198, 1978.

23. Jesse, R. H.: Preoperative vs postoperative radiation in treatment of squamous cell carcinoma of the paranasal sinuses. *Am. J. Surg.* 110:552–557, 1965.

24. Jing, B. S., McGraw, J. P.: Contrast nasopharyngography in diagnosis of tumors. *Arch. Otolaryngol.* 81:365–371, 1965.

25. Johnson, L. N., Krohel, G. B., Yeon, E. B., Parnes, S. M.: Sinus tumors invading the orbit. *Ophthalmology* 91:209–217, 1984.

26. Kalividouris, A., Mancuso, A. A., Dillon, W. P.: A CT-clinical approach to patients with symptoms related to the V, VII, IX–XII cranial nerves and cervical sympathetics. *Radiology* 151:671–676, 1984.

27. Kaseff, L. G.: Early x-ray diagnosis of occult infiltrating nasopharyngeal carcinoma. *Ann. Otol. Rhinol. Laryngol.* 86:864–870, 1977.

28. Khor, T. H., Tan, B. C., Chua, E. G., Chia, K. B.: Distant metastases in nasopharyngeal carcinoma. *Clin. Radiol.* 29:27, 1978.

29. Kondo, M. Horiuchi, M. Inuyama, Y., Dokiya, T., Tsutsui, T., Iwata, Y., Endo, M., Hashimoto, T., Kunieda, E., Hashimoto, S.: Value of computed tomography for radiation therapy of tumors of the nasal cavity and paranasal sinuses. *Acta. Radiol. (Oncol.)* 22:3–7, 1983.

30. Kurchara, S. S., Webster, J. G., Ellix, F., Fitzgerald, J. P., Shedd, D. P., Badib, A. O.: Role of radiation therapy and of surgery in the management of localized epidermoid carcinoma of the maxillary sinus. *A.J.R.* 114:35, 1971.

31. Laing, D.: Nasopharyngeal carcinoma. *Otolaryngol. Clin. North Am.* 2:703, 1969.

32. Larsson, L. G., Mancuso, A. A., Hanafee, W. N.: Computed tomography of the tongue and floor of the mouth. *Radiology* 143:493–500, 1982.

33. Larsson, L. G., Martensson, G.: Carcinoma of the paranasal sinuses and the nasal cavities. *Acta Radiol.* 42:149, 1954.

34. Larsson, L. G., Martensson, G. L.: Maxillary antral cancers. *J.A.M.A.* 219:342, 1972.

35. Lederman, M.: *Cancer of the Nasopharynx: Its Natural History and Treatment.* Springfield, IL, Charles C Thomas, 1961.

36. Lederman, M.: Cancer of the upper jaw and nasal chambers. *Proc. R. Soc. Med.* 62:65–72, 1969.

37. Loke, Y. W.: Lymphoepitheliomas of the cervical lymph nodes. *Br. J. Cancer.* 19:482, 1965.

38. Mancuso, A. A., Bohman, L. G., Hanafee, W. N., Maxwell, D.: Computed tomography of the nasopharynx. Normal and variants of normal. *Radiology* 137:113–121, 1980.

39. Mancuso, A. A., Hanafee, W. N., Winter, J., Ward, P.: Extentions of paranasal sinus tumors and inflammatory disease as evaluated by CT and pluridirectional tomography. *Neuroradiology* 16:449–453, 1978.

40. Mancuso, A. A., Hanafee, W. N.: *Computed Tomography of the Head and Neck.* Baltimore, Williams & Wilkins, 1982.

41. Mancuso, A. A., Hanafee, W. N.: Elusive head and neck tumors beneath intact mucosa. *Laryngoscope* 93:133–139, 1983.

42. Mancuso, A. A., Harnsberger, H. R., Muraki, A., Stevens, M. H.: Computed tomography of cervical and retropharyngeal lymph nodes. Normal anatomy, variants of normal, and applications in staging head and neck cancer. Part I: Normal anatomy. *Radiology* 148:709–714, 1983.

43. Mancuso, A. A., Harnsberger, H. R., Muraki, A., Stevens, M. H.: Computed tomography of cervical and retropharyngeal lymph nodes. Normal anatomy, variants of normal, and applications in staging head and neck cancer. Part II: Pathology. *Radiology* 715–723, 1983.

44. Mancuso, A. A., Maceri, D., Rice, D., Hanafee, W. N.: CT of cervical lymph node cancer. *A.J.R.* 136:381–385, 1981.

45. Marchetta, F. C., Sako, K., Mattick, W. L., Stinziano, G. D.: Squamous cell carcinoma of the maxillary antrum. *Am. J. Surg.* 118:805, 1969.

46. McGavran, M. H., Bauer, W. C., Ogura, J. H.: The incidence of cervical lymph node metastases from epidermoid carcinoma of the larynx and the relationship to certain characteristics of the primary tumor. *Cancer* 14:55–66, 1961.

47. Messic, J. B., Fletcher, G. H., Goepfert, H.: Megavoltage irradiation of epithelial tumors of the nasopharynx. *Int. J. Radiat. Oncol. Biol. Phys.* 7:447–453, 1981.

48. Million, R. R., Cassisi, N. J., Wittes, R. E.: Cancer in the head and neck. In *Cancer: Principles and Practice of Oncology*, DeVita, V. T., Jr., Hellman, S., Rosenberg, S. A. (Eds.) Philadelphia, J. B. Lippincott, 1982, pp. 301–395.

49. Million, R. R., Cassisi, N. J., Wittes, R. E.: Nasopharynx. In *Cancer: Principles and Practice of Oncolgoy.* DeVita, V. T., Jr., Hellman, S., Rosenberg, S. A. (Eds.). Philadelphia, J. B. Lippincott, 1982, pp. 365–369.

50. Muraki, A. S., Mancuso, A. A., Harnsberger, H. R., Johnson, L. P., Meads, G. B.: CT of the oropharynx, tongue base, and floor of the

mouth. Normal anatomy and range of variations, and applications in staging carcinoma. *Radiology* **148**:725–731, 1983.

51. Ohngren, L. G.: Malignant tumors of the maxillo-ethmoidal region; a clinical study with special reference to the treatment with electrosurgery and irradiation. *Acta Otolaryngol. (Suppl)* **19**:1, 1933.

52. Pagani, J., Thompson, J., Mancuso, A. A., Hanafee, W. N.: Lateral wall of the olfactory fossa in determining intracranial extension of sinus carcinomas. *A.J.R.* **133**:497–501, 1979.

53. Pearlman, A. W., Abadir, R.: Carcinoma of the maxillary antrum. The role of preoperative irradiation. *Laryngoscope* **84**:400–409, 1974.

54. Rouvier, H.: *Anatomy of the Human Lymphatic System*. Ann Arbor, Edwards Brothers, 1938.

55. Sakai, S., Fuchihata, H., Hamasaki, Y.: Treatment policy for maxillary sinus carcinoma. *Arch Otolaryngol.* **82**:172, 1976.

56. Sako, K., Pradier, R. N., Marchetta, F. C., Pickren, J. W.: Fallibility of palpation in the diagnosis of metastasis to cervical lymph nodes. *Surg. Gynecol. Obstet.* **118**:989, 1964.

57. Schaefer, S. D., Merkel, M., Burns, D. K., Close, L. G.: Computed tomography of upper aerodigestive tract squamous cell carcinoma. Assessment following induction chemotherapy. *Arch. Otolaryngol.* **110**:236–240, 1984.

58. Schnohr, P.: Survival rates of nasopharyngeal carcinoma in California: A review of 516 cases from 1942 through 1965. *Cancer* **25**:1009, 1970.

59. Shu-Chen, H.: Nasopharyngeal cancer: A review of 1,605 patients treated radially with Cobalt-60. *Int. J. Radiat. Oncol. Biol. Phys.* **6**:401–407, 1980.

60. Silver, A. J., Mawad, M. E., Hilal, S. K., Sane, P., Ganti, S. R.: Computed tomography of the nasopharynx and related spaces. Part II: Pathology. *Radiology* **147**:737–738, 1983.

61. Som, P., Shugar, J., Biller, H.: The early detection of antral malignancy in the postmaxillectomy patient. *Radiology* **143**:509–512, 1982.

62. Suen, J. Y., Myers, E. N. *Cancer of the Head and Neck*. New York, Churchill Livingstone, 1981.

63. Tabb, H. G., Barranco, S. J.: Cancer of the maxillary sinus. *Laryngoscope* **81**:818, 1971.

64. Tuick, D., Cutler, M.: Transitional cell epidermoid carcinoma: radiosensitive type of intraoral tumor. *Surg. Gynecol. Obstet.* **45**:320, 1927.

65. Vibhakar, S. D., Eckhauser, C., Bellon, E. M.: Computed tomography of the nasopharynx and neck. *CT* **7**:259–265, 1983.

66. Vilar, P.: Nasopharyngeal carcinoma: A report on 24 patients seen over six years. *Scott Med. J.* **11**:315, 1966.

67. Wang, C. C., Meyer, J. E.: Radiotherapeutic management of carcinoma of the nasopharynx. *Cancer* **28**:566, 1971.

68. Zagars, G., Norante, J. D.: Head and neck tumors. In *Clinical Oncology for Medical Students and Physicians: A Multidisciplinary Approach*, 6th ed. Rubin, P. (Ed.) New York, American Cancer Society, 1983, pp. 230–261.

6 ORAL CAVITY AND OROPHARYNX, INCLUDING THE TONGUE AND FLOOR OF THE MOUTH

Anthony A. Mancuso

Cancers of the oral cavity and oropharynx account for approximately 5% of all malignant tumors in the United States.[4,27] One would expect that tumors in an area so readily accessible to inspection and palpation would be diagnosed and treated early with a high likelihood for cure; however, this is not always the case. It seems clear that definitive treatment of T_1 or T_2 lesions of the anterior tongue or other anterior, superficial regions of the oropharynx is very likely to be successful.[13] Tumors of the tongue base or those elsewhere in the oropharynx prove much more difficult to cure, especially when positive nodes are present. To put this problem in some perspective relative to survival statistics and cure rates, one must split the region into several anatomic categories:

1. Carcinomas of the lower lip account for 25% to 30% of oral region cancer. Five-year survival rates are in the 80% to 90% range overall.[4] These lesions are rarely of interest to the diagnostic imager and therefore will not be discussed any further.
2. Tumors of the buccal mucosa may prove more aggressive than those of the lip. These may arise anywhere from the mucosa lining the cheek to the point where it joins the gingivobuccal sulcus (over the alveolar ridges) or in the retromolar trigone. The overall five-year survival rate for patients with buccal carcinoma is 30%.[4] However, this improves to 60% to 75% for verrucous carcinomas. The influence of location, therapy, and histology will be discussed in more detail subsequently.

3. Carcinomas of the gums (gingiva), gingival buccal sulcus, and alveolar ridge account for 10% of malignancies of the oral region. Cure rates measured by five-year survival average 40% to 70% in different series and decrease to 7% in the presence of cervical metastases.[1,27]
4. Carcinoma of the floor of the mouth carries an overall five-year survival rate of 65%. T_1 and T_2N_0 rates hover around 70% to 80%. The appearance of nodes before or after therapy roughly halves the probability of survival.[14]
5. Carcinomas of the oral portion, i.e., the anterior two thirds of the tongue have a good prognosis in the T_1 to T_2N_0 stages with 85% and 61% five-year survival rates, respectively.[27] Again, the presence of nodes more than halves the survival rate.[4,14,27]
6. Some authors (including myself) prefer to lump carcinomas of the oropharyngeal structures into one group. The region then encompasses the tonsillar pillars, the tongue base, and lingual tonsils. The soft palate is probably best considered separately. This can be conveniently referred to as the oropharynx. For simplicity the subsequent discussion on mode of spread and imaging evaluation will be split into two groups; specifically, lesions of the anterior oral cavity and the more posterior oropharynx. The rationale for this will become clear in later descriptions.

Survival statistics on carcinomas of the oropharynx are difficult to interpret in a specific way because of the variety of lesions included and the difficulty in determining the exact site of origin. In general, these lesions are more advanced when discovered and tend to have nodal metastases more frequently than those of the anterior oral cavity. Overall five-year survival figures range from 15% to 50%.[4]

Imaging has played only a minor role in the evaluation of patients with malignancies of the oral cavity and oropharynx in the past. Plain films, panoramic views of the mandible, and xeroradiography provided a gross assessment of bone invasion. Pluridirectional tomography was often of value in assessing invasion of the hard palate, the maxillary alveolar ridge, and the pterygoid processes. For the most part, however, the mainstay of clinical-pathologic staging has been the physical examination, the prevailing attitude among head and neck surgeons being that this area is relatively easy to examine by inspection and palpation. However, careful review of head and neck oncology literature reveals authors who have pointed out the limitations of physical examination not only of the oropharynx and tongue base but also of the neck.[1,3,4,14,17,20,21,27,33,34,36,39]

Computed tomography takes us a step beyond these present limitations. Magnetic resonance imaging may take us another. The information available from CT is complementary to that of the clinical examination. Computed tomography is relatively imprecise at showing the mucosal extent of the lesion, whereas it shows the deep extensions very well. The patterns of spread known to occur along the muscle bundles and fascial planes surrounding the oropharynx[3,20] can now be documented preoperatively (Figure 6-1). Lymph-node-bearing areas heretofore clinically silent (e.g., retropharyngeal nodes) until end-stage disease was present can now be evaluated more critically. Computed tomography may even prove more accurate than the clinical examination for staging deep cervical metastases.[23,24,25]

How does all of this translate into data that is useful to the surgical, radiation, or medical oncologist? Computed tomography can have an impact on early detection and diagnosis because it has the potential to show tumor growing beneath intact mucosa.[22,23] For instance, patients with complaints of ear pain and a "fullness in the throat" have had negative endoscopic examinations and CT scans showing large primary deeply infiltrating lesions at the tongue base (Figures 6-2, 6-3, 6-4). This phenomenon has been demonstrated throughout the upper aerodigestive tract.

The most significant impact of CT should be to enhance the accuracy of pretreatment clinical-diagnostic staging. Hopefully this will apply to both the primary site and regional nodal disease. Moreover, CT used properly can detect or confirm posttreatment recurrence more quickly than in the past, perhaps leading to improved salvage rates. The impact of this new imaging tool on overall survival is only speculative at present. Computed

tomography and, in the future, MRI, promise to provide a more precise approach to those planning the treatment of oropharyngeal carcinoma. This should at least reduce therapeutic morbidity, and it might improve survival.

TUMOR BEHAVIOR AND PATHOLOGY

Histopathology

A discussion of the histopathology of oral cavity and oropharyngeal cancer is basically that of squamous cell carcinoma. This cell type accounts for 90% of the malignancies in this region.[4] There seems to be a tendency for the histologic grade to increase as the point of origin of the tumor moves anteriorly to posteriorly in the oral cavity and oropharynx.[4] While histologic grade certainly has a bearing on therapy and prognosis, the status of the regional lymph nodes and the size of the primary are of far greater significance in this regard.[4] Lack of control may be manifest by local or nodal recurrence and generally carries a grave prognosis, so that early definitive management is usually the aim of therapy.

Verrucous carcinoma, which is a "low-grade" squamous cell carcinoma, is a particularly interesting lesion because cure rates are usually much higher than those of other more invasive squamous cell lesions. These lesions account for about 5%[8] of oral carcinomas. Unfortunately, they do invade deeply, and their "benign" surface appearance often hides this growth characteristic from the unwary. The warty tumors arise mainly along the gingivobuccal sulcus and along the alveolar mucosa of the mandible (not infrequently in the retromolar trigone). These may at times be confused with benign neoplasms of squamous cell origin.

Malignancies other than squamous cell carcinoma are very unusual in the oral cavity and oropharynx. Adenoid-cystic carcinoma arising from minor salivary glands or accessory salivary tissue is notorious for its infiltrative and perineural growth pattern. Local recurrences and a protracted clinical course are also common expressions of this tumor's natural history. While these lesions may move quickly and disseminate widely, survival statistics are usually measured in terms of 10 to 15 years rather than the "standard" five years. Adenocarcinoma, lymphoma (of oropharyngeal portion of Waldeyer's ring), and melanoma may also affect this anatomic region. Sarcomas arising from the mandible and tumors of odontogenic origin round out the group of less frequently encountered malignancies in the oropharynx and oral cavity.

Patterns of Spread

This discussion will be limited to the natural history of squamous cell carcinoma as described by earlier investigators,[3,20] whose work has been confirmed in vivo by

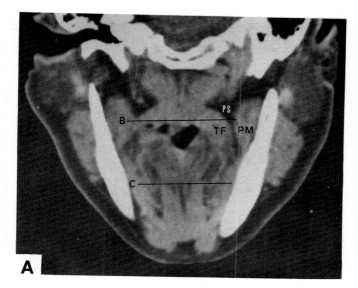

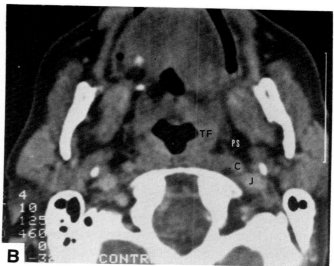

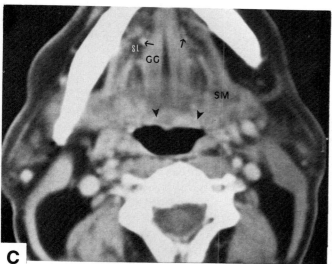

FIG. 6-1. Normal CT scans of the oropharynx, the tongue base, and the floor of the mouth. (A) Coronal scan with lines indicating the levels of the axial scans shown in B and C. TF = tonsillar fossa, PS = parapharyngeal space, PM = pterygoid muscles. (B) Axial section through upper oropharynx. TF = tonsillar fossa, PS = parapharyngeal space, C = carotid, J = jugular. (C) Axial section through tongue base and the floor of the mouth. Lingual vessels (arrows) course through the low-density sublingual space (SL). Lingual tonsil (arrowheads), submandibular gland = SM, genioglossus = GG.

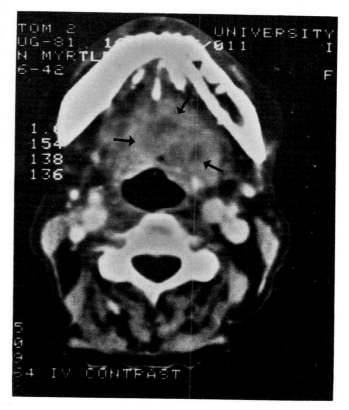

FIG. 6-2. A patient with a 12-to-18-month history of ear pain and dysphagia. Endoscopy under anesthesia showed normal mucosa and a vague mass.   Infiltrating carcinoma invades most of the tongue base and the floor of the mouth (arrows).

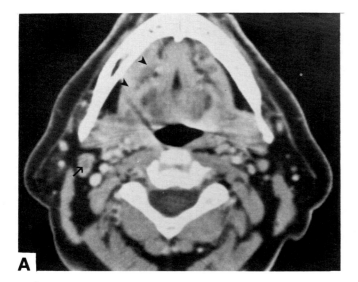

A

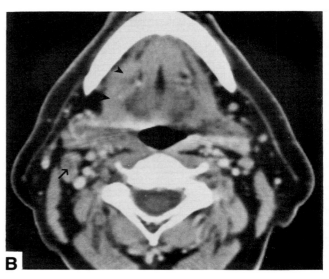

B

FIG. 6-3. A patient with a two-year history of ear pain. Over that two-year period, three blind biopsies of the tongue base were negative; a fourth blind biopsy several weeks before CT was positive. Examination of the neck was normal. (A) Infiltrating mass (arrowheads) thickens the mylohyoid and obliterates portions of the sublingual space. An

8-to-10-mm necrotic node (arrow) is also present. (B) More caudally, an infiltrating mass (arrowheads) is more obvious and a second 10-to-12-mm necrotic node is present. Clinically, this tumor was stage $T_x N_0$. According to CT criteria it is $T_2 N_2$.

our experience with CT scanning over the last several years.[3,12,18,20,21,23,30] Certainly the basic pathways of spread observed for squamous carcinoma are observed in the other histologic types.

Squamous cell carcinoma may grow by either super-

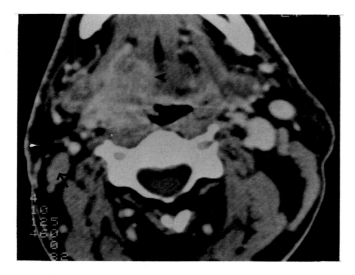

FIG. 6-4. This patient had prior radical neck dissection for cervical metastases because of a squamous cell carcinoma of unknown origin. He had new cervical adenopathy several years later (arrow). The primary tumor extends to the midline (arrowhead). Hemiglossectomy was deemed possible because the CT scan showed that the contralateral lingual vessels and hypoglossal nerve could be preserved. Surgery confirmed the CT findings and an extended hemiglossectomy was performed with adequate margins.

ficial (mucosal) or deep pathways. Ballantyne[3] and Lederman[20] suggest that the deep spread occurs along preexisting anatomic pathways of least resistance. This tendency has been confirmed elsewhere in the head and neck by exquisite whole-organ sections in the larynx and hypopharynx.[15,30,37] More recently, CT has supported these observations in the nasopharynx and oropharynx.[2,7,14,18,23,30] It is of course more difficult to get precise anatomic correlation in these more cephalad portions of the upper aerodigestive tract, but a combination of CT, surgical, and clinical data does agree with the natural history as presented by the earlier investigators.

Deep extension occurs along one of the following pathways:

1. Muscle bundle and surrounding fascial planes. Tumors that penetrate the mucosa and submucosa generally reach the muscles by growing across the parapharyngeal space. Upon reaching the various muscle groups within this loose fibrofatty space, growth seems to be directed along the muscles from their origin to insertion (Figures 6-3, 6-4, 6-5, 6-6, 6-7, 6-8). This is probably the single most important pathway to recognize since much of such spread goes on beyond the physician's ability to detect it even with modern endoscopic techniques and good palpation. For example, a tumor within the tonsillar fossa may penetrate the mucosa, the superior constrictor, and its fascia and spread to the soft palate and nasopharynx along the the palatoglossus or palatopharyngeus and the levator palati, respectively. All of this may occur beneath intact mucosa.[12,22,23]

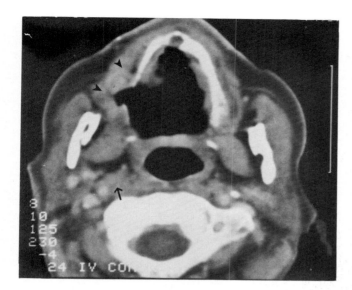

FIG. 6-5. This patient had carcinoma of the maxillary alveolar ridge–gingivobuccal sulcus. Tumor invades the alveolar ridge and buccinator space (arrowheads). Unsuspected retropharyngeal adenopathy (arrow) was the result of extension to the hard palate and inferior nasal cavity.

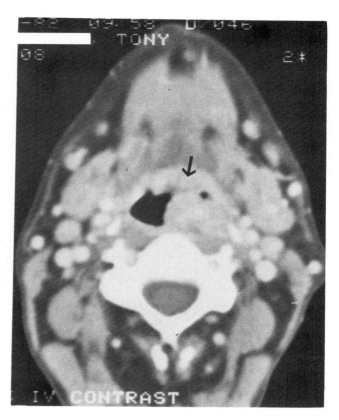

FIG. 6-6. This patient had throat pain and dysphagia. Endoscopy revealed an exophytic carcinoma of the lower oropharynx; there was some question whether it involved the tongue base. A CT scan showed the mass was confined to the posterior lateral wall of the lower oropharynx. The normal lingual tonsil (arrow) should not be mistaken for tumor. Surgery confirmed the CT findings.

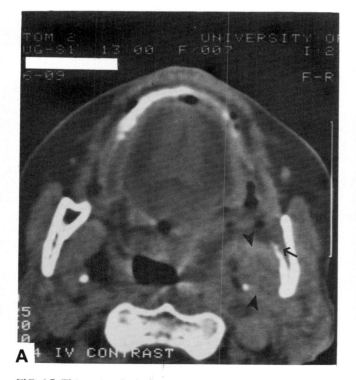

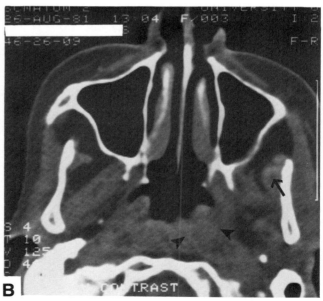

FIG. 6-7. This patient had recurrent carcinoma of the retromolar triangle after radiation therapy. (A) A mass (arrowheads) obliterates all deep tissue planes and has spread to the mandible (arrow). (B) Cephalad spread has occurred along the mandible and pterygoids to the infratemporal fossa (arrow) and along the tonsillar pillar to the lateral wall of the nasopharynx (arrowheads). All findings were confirmed at surgery.

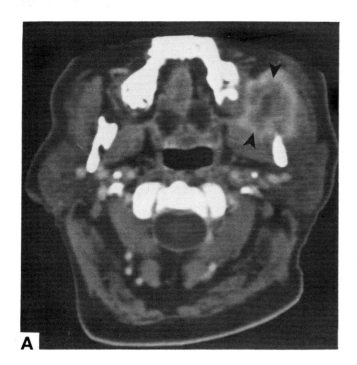

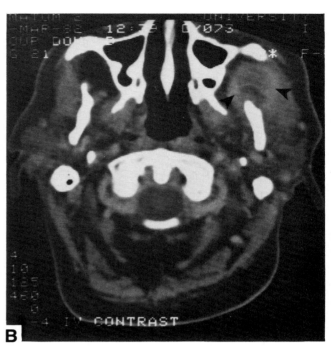

FIG. 6-8. This patient had persistent pain after radiotherapy and surgery for carcinoma of the oral cavity. The mucosa was normal on physical examination. (A) Recurrent tumor mass infiltrates the buccinator space and muscles of mastication (arrowheads). (B) The tumor spread cephalad to the infratemporal fossa. The mode of spread is along the mandibular periosteum and attachments of pterygoid and masseter muscles (arrowheads).

Just as likely is caudal extension of such a lesion, carrying it down the glossopalatine sulcus to the tongue base. From the tongue base, spread along the intrinsic tongue musculature can take a lesion anteriorly to the floor of the mouth (Figures 6-3, 6-4). Spread into the intrinsic tongue musculature and caudally takes the lesion into the pre-epiglottic space (Figure 6-3). It must be apparent from this single example that the deep tissue spaces surrounding the oropharynx are all interconnected by the muscles involved in deglutition. In fact, this may explain part of the frustration in trying to determine the site of origin of a large oropharyngeal lesion. As was mentioned previously, some authors have taken to "lumping" the lesions of the oropharynx (tonsillar pillars, posterior one third of the tongue), citing the fact that this seems to behave as a tumor "field." It does in fact, if one considers the anatomy of tumor spread in this region.

Tumors of the oral cavity may, of course, spread along these same pathways once they have grown large enough to invade the tonsillar pillars or floor of the mouth.

In advanced or recurrent lesions, tumors may reach the pterygoid or masseter muscles (Figures 6-8, 6-9, Tables 6-1, 6-2). Such extension often occurs long before trismus is evident clinically. Spread from the origin to the insertion of the muscles of mastication can then carry the tumor to the mandible or the pterygoid plates (and hence the skull base).

2. Spread along periosteal surfaces. Eventually, tumors spreading along muscle and fascial planes will reach the osseous attachments of the muscles and fascia. Growth continues along this surface until bony invasion occurs. This spread is especially important in carcinomas of the gingivobuccal sulcus and other lesions arising close to the maxillary and mandibular alveolar ridges where bone invasion may occur relatively early (Figure 6-6). Bone invasion in other, more posterior oral cavity lesions usually occurs with large, advanced lesions (e.g., invasion of the skull base, pterygoid plates, and mandible).

3. Spread within the marrow space. Once the periosteum has been breached, tumor may spread within the marrow cavity of the bone. In the head and neck region this pattern is best recognized following invasion of the mandible. Some authors have shown that tumors most likely penetrate the periosteum by first extending along the natural ostia formed by penetrating neurovascular bundles.[15] Another point of entry seems to be via dental sockets, where the periosteum may not be intact because of coexisting peridontal disease or missing teeth.[4]

4. Perineural spread. In addition to following neurovascular bundles, a tumor may grow in the perineural

Table 6-1. T Staging

T_X	Tumor cannot be assessed
T_0	No evidence of primary disease
T_S	Carcinoma in situ
T_1	Greatest dimension ≤ 2 cm
T_2	Greatest dimension > 2 cm and ≤ 4 cm
T_3	Greatest dimension > 4 cm
T_4	Massive tumor > 4 cm with deep invasion of muscle (root of tongue, pterygoid, neck) or invasion of bone, cartilage or skin

Reprinted from American Joint Committee on Cancer: *Manual for Staging of Cancer*, 2nd ed. Philadelphia, J. B. Lippincott, 1983.

Table 6-2. Stage Grouping

Stage I	$T_1 N_0 M_0$
Stage II	$T_2 N_0 M_0$
Stage III	$T_3 N_0 M_0$
	T_1 or T_2 or T_3, N_1, M_0
Stage IV	$T_4 N_0 M_0$
	Any T, N_2 or N_3, M_0
	Any T, Any N, M_1

Reprinted from American Joint Committee on Cancer: *Manual for Staging of Cancer*, 2nd ed. Philadelphia, J. B. Lippincott, 1983.

space. This growth characteristic is not usually seen in the first presentation of squamous cell carcinoma, although it is not infrequent in the setting of recurrent disease.[35] Adenoidcystic carcinoma, however, commonly spreads perineurally, and this tendency contributes to the great difficulty in effective long-term management of these malignancies.

A clinician treating malignancies in this part of the upper aerodigestive tract must be aware of the fore-going paths of local extension as well as the clinical expression of such spread. Equally important in most of these lesions is the status of the cervical lymph nodes. The presence of nodal metastases in squamous cell carcinoma of the oral cavity and oropharynx may vastly alter the therapeutic plan and probably halves the patient's chances of survival.[4] These tendencies seem to hold regardless of the stage or histologic grade of the primary lesion. Since the site and incidence

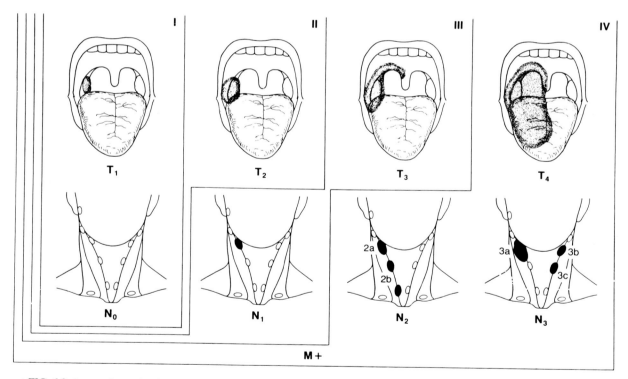

FIG. 6-9. Anatomic staging for cancer of the oropharynx and oral cavity. Tumor (T) categories: The primary tumor is largely characterized by size and then by extension to other sites. The diameters are ≤ 2 cm, > 2 cm, ≤ 4 cm, and > 4 cm for T_1, T_2, and T_3 lesions. As tumors become massive and expand to contiguous sites, they become T_4. Node (N) categories: The size of the node and its mobility and the number and location are all factors in staging cervical nodes. The diameters ≤ 3 cm, 3 cm and 6 cm, and > 6 cm were chosen because these are determined more objectively than fixation. Fixation implies adhesion to the carotid artery and, therefore, unresectability. Single and multiple nodes (N_1 v N_2), homolateral and bilateral nodes (N_1, N_2 v N_3) are important factors. Stage grouping: The T category is the major determinant of stage. Note that N_1 nodes are equivalent to T_3 in advancement (stage III) and that N_2 and N_3 nodes and M_1, along with T_4 lesions, constitute stage IV.

of nodal disease varies with the point of origin of the primary tumor, the following discussion will be divided according to anatomic categories that best reflect tumor behavior. In addition, specific local pathways of extension and related clinical signs or symptoms will be considered.

Oral Cavity

Buccal mucosa. Spread of tumor along the buccal mucosa occurs as tumors extend to the gingivae or retromolar trigone. Deep spread is usually direct along the buccinator muscle, which attaches to the maxilla, the mandible, and the pterygomandibular raphe. Most commonly, deep spread is limited to the cheek (buccal fat pad region); however, advanced lesions may spread around the mandible and go on to the submaxillary space.[19,23,38] The submandibular nodes are the earliest to be involved, and the jugulodigastric group is also considered a primary drainage site. About 36% to 50% of patients with exophytic or ulceroinfiltrative carcinoma will have nodal metastases on initial examination;[4,37] nodal metastases are unusual in the verrucous lesions.

Gingiva and alveolar mucosa. The bone of the alveolar ridges is less resistant to tumor spread because the mucosa invaginates into the tooth sockets.[3,4] Mucosal spread of lower (mandibular) gingival lesions takes them to the gingivolabial sulcus, the anterior floor of the mouth, the tongue, and the mandible. On the upper (maxillary) gingivae the lesions have access to the gingivolabial sulcus, the cheek, the hard palate, the inferior nasal cavity, and the nasal septum. Deep spread of a lower gingival lesion occurs along the buccinator and the muscles of the floor of the mouth as they attach along the myloid line. Spread along the medial pterygoid, the masseter, and the lingual nerve occurs with lesions at the molar level. Once the mandible is involved, perineural alveolar nerve involvement may carry the tumor to the skull base. The upper gingival lesions spread posterosuperiorly along the masseter and pterygoid groups. Superior extension takes them into the maxillary antrum.

The submandibular and jugulodigastric nodes again are first-order drainage sites. These nodes are involved about 30% to 35% of the time at first examination.[4,35] Lesions of the mandibular gingiva have a slightly greater tendency to produce nodal metastases than do those of the maxillar alveolar ridge.

Anterior two thirds (oral portion) tongue. There are no real anatomic boundaries to tumor spread in the tongue, and infiltration occurs freely along its intrinsic and extrinsic musculature. Such growth may carry lesions to the hyoid bone, the myloid line of the mandible, the mentum, the styloid process, and the palate, since all these sites are sites of origin of tongue muscle. Submucosal growth usually carries the lesion to the floor of the mouth, the mandible, the anterior tonsillar wall, and the pharyngeal wall.

Lymph drainage is primarily via the submandibular and digastric groups. About 30% to 40% of patients with T_1 or T_2 carcinomas of the oral tongue will have positive nodes at initial examination.[16,35,40] This increases to 72% for T_2 lesions. Bilateral nodal metastases and early nodal involvement are important features of tongue carcinoma.

Floor of the mouth. Spread here is primarily within the areolar tissue separating the intrinsic and extrinsic tongue musculature (Figures 6-3, 6-4, 6-5). The mass tends to grow centrifugally and along the submandibular duct, the lingual nerve, and the lingual artery as they course through these fibrofatty spaces.[3] Deeper spread takes the tumor along the mylohyoid line and mandibular periosteum; in this case, there need not be frank bone invasion. Continued growth brings the tumors to the submandibular and submental triangles or along the genioglossus muscle to the tongue base.

Submandibular and jugulodigastric nodes are the primary drainage sites; submental nodes are rarely involved. About 50% of patients with T_1 lesions will have clinically positive necks at the time of initial examination,[35] but there is a high incidence (30%) of patients who have no microscopic confirmation of nodal metastasis.[9] T_2 and T_3 tumors have a 65% and 71% rate of histologically confirmed nodal metastases.[16,40]

Oropharynx

Tonsillar fossa and pillars. A squamous cell carcinoma arising in or about the tonsillar fossa commonly spreads superiorly to the palate and inferiorly to the tongue base by both superficial and deep routes. Exophytic lesions tend to remain superficial, and ulceroinfiltrative lesions may have considerable deep spread with relatively little visible mucosal change. Deep spread takes the tumor immediately through the superior constrictor and its fascia to the parapharyngeal space. Cephalad extension may then occur to the soft palate (along the palatoglossus) or the nasopharynx (via the levator palati).[3,20] Anterior tonsillar pillar lesions spread upward by the same routes. Caudal extension takes these lesions to the retromolar trigone. Posterior and caudal extension take these lesions down the palatine arch (glossopalatine sulcus) to the tongue base and posterior pharyngeal wall.

Primary lymph node drainage is to the jugulodigastric and superior deep cervical groups. The retropharyngeal nodes are also considered first-order nodes for some of the tumors.[32] About 50% to 70% of patients will have nodal metastases at initial examination.[5,6,9] This area is relatively silent clinically and a majority of the lesions are graded T_2 or T_3N_1 or N_2 when they are discovered. Bilateral and subclinical nodal disease is not uncommon.

Tongue base (posterior third or oropharyngeal portion of the tongue). Lesions of the tongue base arise from the squamous epithelium within the numerous crypts lying caudal to the circumvallate papillae. They are often ulceroinfiltrative in character, sometimes making identification of a primary tumor difficult (Figures 6-3, 6-4).

The tumors arising within the valleculae spread to the epiglottis and pre-epiglottic space by both deep and superficial routes. As in the anterior two thirds of the tongue, there are really no barriers to deep spread. Growth along the intrinsic and extrinsic muscles and accompanying neurovascular bundles (hypoglossal nerve, lingual nerve and artery) goes on unrestricted. The more laterally placed tumors arising in the glossopalatine sulcus tend to group both cephalad and caudally along the lateral pharyngeal wall.

Ear pain is a symptom that should not be ignored or misinterpreted as caused by "ear problems" in a patient at risk of having oropharyngeal cancer. This is a common complaint related to glossopharyngeal nerve irritation with referral to the tympanic branch of this nerve (Figures 6-3, 6-4). The pain is perceived as being deep in the ear. Dysphagia and a sore throat or fullness in the upper throat are other common presenting complaints. Palpation is an essential part of the examination because these lesions often grow deeply, leaving little mucosal evidence of their presence.

An enlarged lymph node is often the initial complaint of patients with carcinoma of the tongue base. About 50% to 70% of patients will have metastatic nodes at initial examination;[5,35] 20% will have bilateral nodes.[11] The jugulodigastric group is most commonly involved.

The soft palate and palatine arch. Lesions of the soft palate and palatine arch tend to be better differentiated and easier to control than those of the more posterior oropharynx. They do, however, have a tendency to spread submucosally and more deeply. Spread along the numerous deep pathways described in prior sections can carry these lesions anteriorly to the hard palate and buccal mucosa, superiorly to the nasopharynx, and inferiorly along the lateral pharyngeal wall and tongue base.

Because the palate is a midline structure, nodal involvement may be bilateral. Primary drainage is to the upper deep cervical, the jugulodigastric, and the retropharyngeal nodes. About 35% to 50% of patients will have positive nodes at initial examination.[5,35]

Distant metastases are, in general, uncommon except in the terminal phases of carcinomas of the oral cavity and oropharynx. It is quite unusual to have clinical or imaging evidence of metastases at the initial examina-

tion. When seen, metastases usually involve the lungs, bone, or liver. The tendency for distant metastasis seems to parallel the biologic aggressiveness of the lesion.

In a practical sense, the occurrence of multiple primary tumors in the upper aerodigestive tract is a more important issue than distant metastases. A most convincing study is one from the Mayo Clinic[29] wherein 732 patients with squamous cell carcinoma of the oral cavity were studied: 8.7% had a second discrete oral primary tumor, 75% had leukoplakia, and 55 patients had a second primary tumor elsewhere in the aerodigestive tract. The trend is supported by studies on patients with laryngeal cancer and various autopsy series.[4] The overall rate of this phenomenon is probably in the range of 10% to 15%.

CLASSIFICATION AND STAGING

The clinical-diagnostic staging of carcinomas arising in the oral cavity and oropharynx is virtually the same. The staging of the primary tumor and nodes is by a combination of the clinical examination and imaging studies. Workup of distant metastases beyond chest X-ray films and routine blood work is dictated by the clinical situation.

The primary tumor is basically staged by size criteria (Figure 6-9).[41] This evokes thoughts that the system is somewhat arbitrary, i.e., some attempt has been made to relate size to the deep extent of a lesion, its likelihood of metastasizing to regional nodes and its prognosis. This is a rational approach, but not an infallible one. Computed tomography also has its liabilities; however, in the next section (Imaging Procedures and Assessment), we will indicate its potential to be more precise than the current clinical-diagnostic staging system.

The T_0 classification (no evidence of a primary tumor) is an interesting one in that it reflects the fact that tumors may be present within this region in the absence of abnormal mucosa, i.e., a palpable mass or tumor is demonstrated by blind biopsy. This phenomenon is well known in the palatine and lingual tonsillar areas, where primarily ulceroinfiltrative growth beginning deep in a tonsillar crypt may carry a lesion toward the deep (musculofascial plane) rather than superficial (mucosal) plane. Computed tomography may prove very valuable in studying patients with such lesions (Figures 6-3, 6-4).

T_1 lesions are 2 cm or less in greatest dimension; T_2 lesions are between 2 and 4 cm, and T_3 lesions are greater than 4 cm. T_4 lesions within the oral cavity are greater than 4 cm in diameter and demonstrate deep invasion to the maxillary antrum, the pterygoid muscles, the base of the tongue, or the skin of the neck. In the oropharynx, this T^4 category requires invasion of bone, the soft tissues of the neck, or the deep tongue musculature.

It is obvious that deep invasion is an important prognostic sign. The only place it is specifically mentioned is in the T_4 category; five-year survival rates in these lesions are 15% at very best if nodes are not present. Obviously, deep extension is going to be present in some lesions that measure 1, 2, 3, or 4 cm or it can be present in lesions that are not visible (Figure 6-3). This "occult" deep extension probably leads to some cases of failure to control the primary site. More accurate staging and therapy planning might be possible if the deep extent could be defined more precisely.

The cervical nodes from carcinoma are staged by the same criteria as discussed in the chapter on the neck. Again, the retropharyngeal nodes, which form an exceedingly important group (at least from a prognostic point of view), are omitted from the presently accepted staging scheme.

Distant metastases are staged as M_0 (none known) or M_1 (present). The lungs, liver, and bone are the most likely sites.

IMAGING PROCEDURES AND ASSESSMENT

Radiologic imaging procedures, while important, have played an adjunctive role in staging malignancies of the oral cavity and oropharynx. Plain films, panoramic views, and pluridirectional tomography have been used to good advantage for diagnosing bone invasion; this is most frequent along the alveolar ridges (Table 6-3). More advanced lesions may invade the maxillary antrum, the hard palate, and the skull base (usually the pterygoid plates). Xeroradiography has been used similarly. Contrast studies of the upper aerodigestive tract are of limited value; they are used mainly to determine the status of the larynx, the hypopharynx, or the cervical esophagus when necessary. Angiography now is rarely used for diagnostic purposes. Occasionally it is performed as an adjunct to local chemotherapy by intra-arterial infusion (Table 6-3).

Computed tomography, with recent improvements developed mainly from 1976 to 1981, has emerged as a primary oncologic imaging tool. It has the potential to provide very precise information about the extent of malignancies in this region, including the status of the cervical lymph nodes.[12,18,23-25,29] Magnetic resonance (MRI) imaging is now being studied and promises to take us another quantum jump in oncologic imaging.

Recommended Method of Study

Computed tomography is the imaging examination of choice for determining the deep extent of lesions of the oral cavity and oropharynx; however, plain films and pluridirectional tomography are still useful in some instances (Figures 6-10, 6-11).[3] Erosion of bone along the maxillary and mandibular alveolar ridges is probably studied more conveniently and cost effectively with panoramic (Panorex) views or plain films. Sometimes dental amalgams make portions of a CT study of the oral

Table 6-3. Imaging Modalities for Evaluating Carcinoma of the Oral Cavity and Oropharynx

MODALITY	STAGING CAPABILITY	BENEFIT/ COST RATIO	RECOMMENDED ROUTINE STAGING PROCEDURE
Noninvasive			
Chest X-ray films	Lung metastases, second primary detection	High	Yes
Plain films (mandible, soft tissue views)	Gross bone invasion	Fair	No
Orthopantomography	Mandibular, hard palate invasion	High	No
Pluridirectional tomography	Hard palate, maxillary antral spread	High	No
MRI	Potentially primary site and nodes— bone detail	?	?
Radionuclide bone scan, liver/spleen scan, and brain scan	Only in advanced lesions or symptomatic patients. CT or MRI better for brain metastases	Low	No
Minimally invasive			
CT	Primary site, nodes, brain metastases (in symptomatic patients)	High	Yes*
Invasive			
Angiography	Not used for diagnosis but sometimes as adjunct to therapy	N/A	No

*Not for superficial oral cavity lesions. Should be used for lesions T_2 or larger or if clinical suspicion of deep spread.

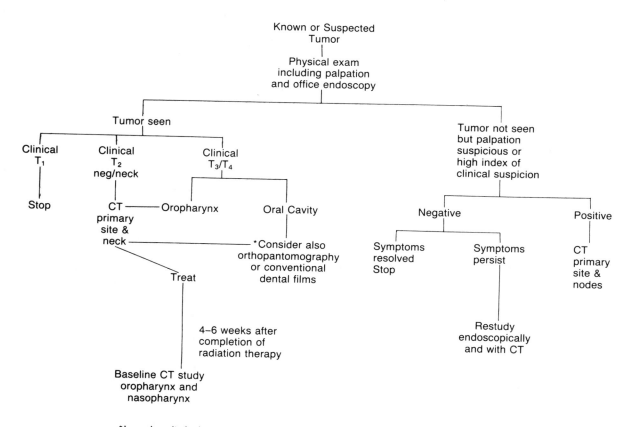

FIG. 6-10. General clinical imaging approach to cancer of the oral cavity and oropharynx.

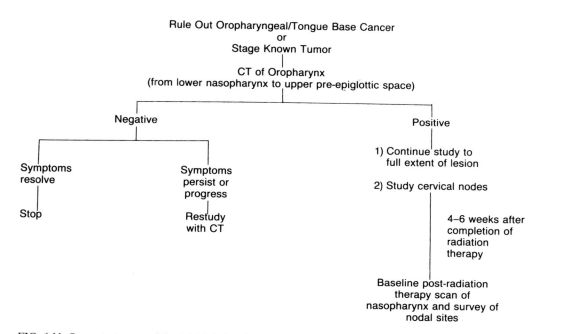

FIG. 6-11. Suggested protocol for initial CT evaluation of cancer of the oropharynx and base of the tongue.

cavity unsuitable for diagnostic purposes. For instance, erosion of the hard palate or the floor of the antrum might go undetected because of the artifacts produced by the dental fillings. Anteroposterior pluridirectional tomography provides superb images of these structures under such conditions. Magnetic resonance imaging might replace CT as the oncologic imaging tool of choice in this region. It is more likely that the studies will prove complementary. In any case, the anatomic data and treatment implications will remain basically unchanged from those being presented here.

Technique of Examination

The basic technique is unchanged from that presented in the chapter on the nasopharynx. Some variation is sometimes necessary to avoid the often devastating artifacts caused by dental devices and amalgams. First, all bridgework and similar items that can be removed should be removed. It is also wise to remove dentures because some of them contain metal that is hidden from view. If a significant amount of metal remains in the oral cavity, then several simple procedures can be used to produce diagnostic quality images of the oropharynx and floor of the mouth; the hard palate and alveolar ridges will have to be studied by other techniques.

Since the floor of the mouth is below the mandibular alveolar ridge, it can be studied in axial section. The patient's neck is then hyperextended to its maximum comfortable position. The gantry is angled $-20°$ (toward the feet). This will usually produce an angled off-axis section that roughly parallels the mandibular condyle. Sections begun at or slightly anterior to the angle of the mandible will then be at the anterior limit of the oropharynx and free of artifacts. Of course, localizing digital radiographs and more precise angle selection are possible on modern scanners, but this only prolongs the study.

The indications for contrast enhancement were outlined in the chapter on the nasopharynx along with suggested section thickness and increments.

The specific contributions of CT will be discussed in the following sections.

Limitations of CT

Computed tomography, of course, is not tissue specific, and "reactive changes" or superimposed infection may cause tumors to appear more extensive than they really are. In the oral cavity, dental fillings may produce artifacts that render a study nondiagnostic. This may be avoided in the oropharynx by methods described under Techniques.

In the detection of lymph node metastases CT is limited by two factors: (1) microscopic disease occurring in normal-sized nodes, and (2) reactive nodes that are enlarged but contain no tumor. These problems will re-main for the foreseeable future, although MRI has some promise for being more tissue specific.

Definite comments on the sensitivity and specificity of CT as a screening test will need to await more widespread application in this regard. Preliminary data suggest that it will be highly specific but not very sensitive for detecting occult carcinomas of the upper aerodigestive tract.[26] These variables must also be investigated relative to the ability of CT to stage cervical metastases compared with the physical examination. Early reports suggest a promising role for CT in this regard.[22,23,25]

IMAGING STRATEGIES AND DECISIONS

Detection

Although this portion of the upper aerodigestive tract is quite accessible to physical examination, there is a tendency for some lesions to grow mainly out of sight and beyond the limits of palpation even in the most cooperative patients. This usually occurs in the crypts of the facial and lingual tonsils (Figures 6-2, 6-3). Some patients may have an enlarged lymph node of unknown cause. Others may complain of vague pain or fullness in the throat or ear pain. In light of sufficient risk factors and clinical suspicion, such patients may benefit from a "screening" CT scan encompassing the oropharynx, even in the absence of abnormality on physical examination. A CT scan is capable of showing otherwise undetectable lesions under these circumstances.[22,23]

Diagnosis and Staging

Despite the accessibility of this area to physical examination and therefore theoretically to early detection, many authors emphasize relatively poor overall cure rates for oropharyngeal and oral cavity carcinoma. The best rates of cure are for early lesions located anteriorly in the oral cavity. The explanation for this is undoubtedly multifaceted; CT has begun to help us understand some of them. Lack of control of local disease is in part caused by deep extension that may not be evident on physical examination. The American Joint Committee (AJC) criteria (T category) have been arranged to account for this on the basis of size. The immediate fallibility of this somewhat arbitrary system is apparent when one considers that some tumors grow predominantly exophytically and others predominantly in an ulceroinfiltrative fashion. The Union International Centre Cancer (UICC) criteria try to be more specific; however, the "deep invasion regardless of size" is determined solely by subjective criteria. It seems that an imaging system such as CT can lend more objectivity to clinical-diagnostic staging. With continued improvements, CT should be able to provide very precise tumor volumes and a highly accurate appraisal of deep extension. Evidence is already accumulating to support these views.[12,16,19,20]

The incredibly rich lymphatic network draining the oropharynx and oral cavity is also, in part, responsible for lack of control in cancer of this region. Physical examination of the neck is good but suffers definite limitations for the purpose of staging nodal metastases. The incidence of microscopically positive nodes in clinically negative necks ranges from 25% to 60%.[17,21,33,34,36,39] It seems that there is room for improvement. Computed tomography can image all of the lymph-node-bearing areas related to these primary tumors, including those normally beyond the limits of physical examination (retropharyngeal, highest jugular).[23,24,25] While CT obviously cannot assess microscopic disease, it can very precisely show the size and staining (following IV contrast injection) characteristics of normal and abnormal masses.[23,24,25] Again, this should add a great deal more objectivity to the assessment of these nodal groups than the present N category in both the AJC and UICC schemes. This last fact needs to be confirmed by more investigators, but the following factors seem clear from limited studies of the capabilities of CT:

1. It can demonstrate retropharyngeal metastases.
2. It has shown nodal metastases in clinically N_0 necks.
3. It can provide data indicative of extranodal extension in the absence of physical findings suggesting such spread.
4. It can detect "occult" contralateral metastases.
5. It can predict fixation to structures within the neck (with limitations).

These factors certainly warrant further study because they are critical issues in management decisions.

In summary, studies available for the evaluation of the T components include CT, MRI, plain films, orthopantomography, and pluridirectional tomography (Table 6-3, Figures 6-10, 6-11), and perhaps MRI will be the mainstay of diagnostic imaging in the foreseeable future. The N component may be studied by CT or MRI. The M workup may include chest X-ray films, bone scans, and liver/spleen scans depending upon the extent of the primary and regional lymphatic disease.

The overall approach to the initial evaluation and follow-up of these patients is presented in Figures 6-10, 6-11, 6-12.

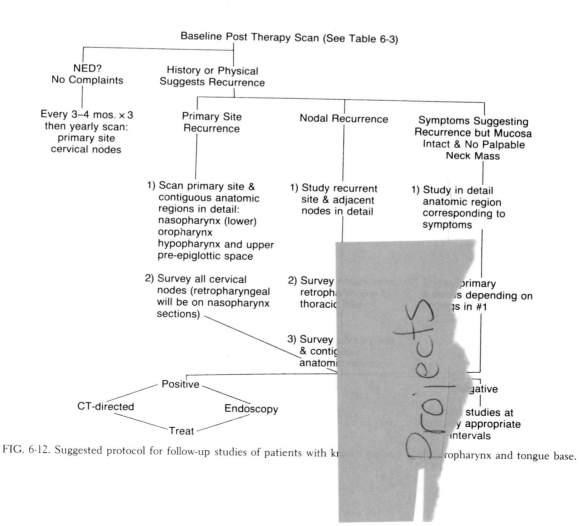

FIG. 6-12. Suggested protocol for follow-up studies of patients with k... ...ropharynx and tongue base.

TREATMENT DECISIONS

The oral cavity and oropharynx are notoriously controversial when one considers how to treat carcinomas of this region. The matter of primary and nodal control has been debated by radiation and surgical oncologists for many years.[10,28,31] The options are so varied, based on site of origin, stage, histology, and lymph node disease, that a comprehensive discussion is impossible within the scope of this text, this notwithstanding the patient's condition and desires or institutional bias.

The choice, seemingly, should be straightforward: radiation, surgery, or combined therapy. But heterogeneity in both staging and treatment approaches has made comparison of survival statistics difficult. The attendant morbidity of any therapy makes the "risk v benefit" issue extremely important in this region so that it is very important to look at management critically. It is hoped that CT (and perhaps MRI) will usher in a new era of understanding in patients with these lesions. Armed with a more precise idea of the deep extent of a lesion and the status of regional lymph nodes provided by CT, radiation, surgical, and medical oncologists may be able to decide on an appropriate course of therapy in a more rational way.

Tumor imaging defines the stage and tumor extent and allows for a multidisciplinary strategy to determine the choice of treatment. Decisions that are made are most often based on staging (Table 6-4).

For early localized stage I and II lesions, the choice usually rests between surgery or radiation therapy. Generally, radiation therapy is preferred for posterior lesions in the oral cavity, particularly those in the oropharynx or extending into this region. The dividing line between the resectable and nonresectable lesions usually rests between T_1 and T_2 v T_3 and T_4 primaries. Favorable neck nodes for surgery are usually considered to be N_1 (N_2 is intermediate), whereas N_3 fixed nodes are considered unresectable by definition, i.e., fixed usually to the carotid artery. N_0 necks are usually irradiated electively. Generally, stage I and II lesions when managed by definitive radiation therapy include a combination of techniques such as external supervoltage beam irradiation, interstitial implantation, or high energy electrons.

For stage III oral cavity cancers of borderline resectability, a combined modality approach is often used. Adjuvant radiation therapy or chemotherapy, preoperatively or postoperatively, is administered. Surgical resection or definitive radiation therapy alone with or without chemotherapy is considered, if surgery is not appropriate, which is more likely for oropharyngeal lesions.

For stage IV nonresectable cancers, radiation therapy is widely used with investigational agents such as a radiosensitizer or multiagent chemotherapy.

For recurrent local/regional lesions, salvage is usually attempted by an alternate mode such as radiation therapy salvage for surgical failures and surgical salvage for radiation therapy failures. When combined modalities have been used, particularly surgery and radiation and then chemotherapy, this is a viable alternative.

Metastatic disease is best palliated by multiagent chemotherapy, which provides good response rates but

Table 6-4. Treatment Decisions: Cancer of the Oral Cavity/Oropharynx

STAGE	SURGERY		RADIATION THERAPY (RT)	CHEMOTHERAPY
I (T_1,N_0,M_0)	Radical resection	or	Definitive RT 6,000–6,500 cGy*	NR
II (T_2,N_0,M_0)	Radical en bloc resection	or	Definitive RT 6,500–7,000 cGy*	NR
III (T_3,N_0,M_0) ($T_{any} N_1,M_0$)	Radical en bloc resection	and	Radiotherapy Preop v postop 5,000–6,000 cGy	Preop or postop RT
IV ($T_4,N_{2,3},M_0$)	Unresectable		Definitive RT 5,000 v 7,000 cGy*	Preop or postop RT plus investigational MAC
Local Regional	RT for surgery relapse		Surgery for RT relapse	Investigational MAC
Metastatic	NR		NR	Investigational MAC

NR = not recommended
MAC = multiagent chemotherapy
*Utilization of interstitial implant is combined with external irradiation for lesions whenever possible. The total dose can be increased by 500–1000 cGy.

is usually of short duration and as yet has not proved to be curative.

In summary, for early stage lesions, radiation therapy or surgery can be successful, but generally the treatment of choice for most oropharyngeal carcinomas is irradiation, whereas surgery is used for the oral cavity, particularly if deformity is minimal. Excellent control with radiation therapy exists for T_1 and T_2 lesions, which require doses of approximately 6,500 to 7,000 cGy. Elective node irradiation is recommended for all but the smallest primaries, and 5,000 cGy is effective to eradicate subclinical neck nodes (N_0).

In the multimodal approach to advanced disease (T_3, T_4, N_2, N_3), surgical techniques are radical and usually require en bloc resection of the primary tumor, neck nodes, and hemimandibulectomy with reconstruction. (With extensive oropharyngeal lesions, laryngectomy may be required to prevent aspiration.) As mentioned, radiation and chemotherapy are important to management.

Computed tomography has an important role to play in the follow-up of these patients (Figure 6-12). Theoretically, if one course of therapy (surgery or radiation) is planned with the thought of retaining the other for salvage, then careful follow-up with CT may allow one to establish the diagnosis of recurrence earlier than on clinical grounds or before obvious mucosal disease is apparent (Figures 6-8, 6-9). This is very important in that it seems that recurrent disease at or adjacent to the primary site not infrequently goes "underground" because its superficial pathways are so altered by surgery or radiation. Computed tomography also has the potential to detect persistent or recurrent nodal disease. All patients studied for recurrence should have a scan of the node-bearing areas of the neck. The effects of prior radiation or surgery make physical examination of the neck less reliable than the pretreatment examination. Patients who have primary tumors of the head and neck and complain of pain or develop neurologic deficits suggesting recurrent tumor should be studied immediately with CT.[13] Careful history and physical examination will often direct the study to a small anatomic region capable of explaining the symptoms or signs.

IMPACT OF NEW TECHNOLOGY

Computed tomography has not been widely applied to tumors in the oropharynx and oral cavity. It certainly has not been studied prospectively in a large number of patients to determine whether it can have an impact on survival. Our continuing experience in this region suggests that the use of CT will lead to more accurate staging. Theoretically, this should provide a more rational basis for selecting therapy; however, this will require a wide acceptance of CT and concomitant training of persons to interpret these studies in a manner useful for on-

cologists. When this occurs perhaps there will be a reduction in treatment morbidity. Improved survival seems to be more of a problem of early detection and preventive medicine. Computed tomography may have a small role to play in early detection and perhaps in this way could help improve overall survival.

Magnetic resonance imaging will certainly be used to study oropharyngeal and oral cavity carcinoma. It has the potential to be more specific and sensitive than CT in evaluating primary and nodal disease. Several years of investigation will be required before we fully understand the relationship between CT and MRI in this regard.

REFERENCES

1. Backstrom, A., Jakobsson, P. A., Nathanson, A., Wersall, J.: Prognosis of squamous cell carcinoma of the gums with cytologically verified cervical lymph node metastases. *J. Laryngol.* 89:391, 1975.
2. Bailar, J. C.: *Nasopharyngeal cancer in white populations—A world wide survey.* UIC Monograph series 1:18, 1967.
3. Ballantyne, A. J.: Routes of spread. In *Radiation Therapy in the Management of Cancers of the Oral Cavity and Oropharynx.* Fletcher, G. H., Macomb, W. S. (Eds.), Springfield, IL, Charles C Thomas, 1962.
4. Batsakis, J. G.: *Tumors of the Head and Neck. Clinical and Pathological Considerations.* Baltimore, Williams & Wilkins, 1979.
5. Blady, J. V.: The present status of treatment of cervical metastases from carcinoma arising in the head and neck region. *Am. J. Surg.* 111:56, 1971.
6. Conley, J.: *Concepts in Head and Neck Surgery.* Stuttgart, Georg Thieme Verlag, 1970.
7. Dodd, G. D., Dolan, P. A., Ballantyne, A. J., Ibanez, M. L., Chau, P.: The dissemination of tumors of the head and neck via the cranial nerves. *Rad. Clin. of N.A.* 8:445–462, 1961.
8. Duckworth, R.: Verrucous carcinoma presenting as mandibular osteomyelitis. *Br. J. Surg.* 49:332, 1961.
9. Erich, J. B., Kragh, L. V.: Treatment of squamous cell carcinoma of the floor of the mouth. *Arch. Surg.* 79:94, 1959.
10. Fletcher, G. H.: Oral cavity and oropharynx. In *Textbook of Radiotherapy* 3rd ed. Fletcher, G. H. (Ed.). Philadelphia, Lea & Febiger, 1980, pp. 286–329.
11. Frazell, E. L., Lucas, J. C.: Cancer of the tongue: Report of the management of 1,554 patients. *Cancer* 15:1085, 1962.
12. Harnsberger, H. R., Mancuso, A. A., Muraki, A., Parkin, J. L.: The upper aerodigestive tract and neck: CT evaluation of recurrent tumors. *Radiology* 149:503–509, 1983.
13. Harrison, D. F.: The management of malignant tumors of the nasal sinuses. *Otolaryngol. Clin. North Am.* 4:159, 1971.
14. Harrold, C. C. Jr.: Management of cancer of the floor of the mouth. *Am. J. Surg.* 122:487, 1971.
15. Kirchner, J. A.: Two hundred laryngeal cancers: Patterns of growth and spread as seen in serial section. *Laryngoscope* 87:474–482, 1971.
16. Krause, C. J., Lee, J. G., McCabe, B. F.: Carcinoma of the oral cavity. *Arch. Otolaryngol.* 97:354, 1973.
17. Kremen, A. J.: The case for elective (prophylactic) neck dissection. In *Cancer of the Head and Neck.* Conley, J. (Ed.). Washington, Butterworths, 1967, pp. 183–185.
18. Larsson, L. G., Mancuso, A. A., Hanafee, W. N.: Computed tomography of the tongue and the floor of the mouth. *Radiology* 143:493–500, 1982.
19. Lederman, M.: *Cancer of the Nasopharynx: Its Natural History and*

Treatment. Springfield, IL, Charles C Thomas, 1961.

20. Lederman, M.: Cancer of the pharynx. *J. Laryngol.* **81**:151, 1967.

21. Lyall, D., Shetlin, C. F.: Cancer of the tongue. *Ann. Surg.* **135**:489, 1952.

22. Mancuso, A. A., Hanafee, W. N.: *Computed Tomography of the Head and Neck.* Baltimore, Williams & Wilkins, 1982.

23. Mancuso, A. A., Hanafee, W. N.: Elusive head and neck tumors beneath intact mucosa. *Laryngoscope* **93**:133–139, 1983.

24. Mancuso, A. A., Harnsberger, H. R., Muraki, A., Stevens, M. H.: Computed tomography of cervical and retropharyngeal lymph nodes: Normal anatomy, variants of normal, and applications in staging head and neck cancer. *Radiology* **148**:709–714 and **148**:715–723, 1983.

25. Mancuso, A. A., Maceri, D., Rice, D., Hanafee, W. N.: CT of cervical lymph node cancer. *A.J.R.* **136**:381–385, 1981.

26. Mancuso, A. A., Muraki, A., Harnsberger, H. R., Parkin, J.: Metastatic cervical adenopathy from tumors of unknown origin: The role of CT. Submitted to *Radiology.*

27. Mendelson, B. C., Hodgkinson, D. J., Woods, J. E.: Cancer of the oral cavity. *Surg. Clin. North Am.* **57**:585, 1977.

28. Million, R. R., Cassisi, N. J., Wittes, R. E.: Cancer in the head and neck. In *Cancer: Principles and Practice of Oncology.* DeVita, V. T., Jr., Hellman, S., Rosenberg, S. A. (Eds.). Philadelphia, J. B. Lippincott, 1982, pp. 301–395.

29. Moertel, C. G., Dockerty, M. B., Baggenstoss, A. H.: Multiple primary malignant neoplasms. I, II, and III. *Cancer* **14**:221–230; 231–237; 238–245, 1961.

30. Muraki, A., Mancuso, A. A., Harnsberger, H. R., Johnson, L. P., Meads, G. B.: CT of the oropharynx, tongue base, and floor of the mouth: Normal anatomy and range of variations, and applications in staging carcinoma. *Radiology* **148**:725–731, 1983.

31. Olofsson, J., van Nostrand, A. W. P.: Growth and spread of laryngeal and hypolaryngeal carcinoma with reflections of effective preoperative radiation. 139 cases studied by whole organ serial sectioning. *Acta Otolaryngol.* (suppl. 308):1–84, 1973.

32. Rouvier, H.: *Anatomy of the Human Lymphatic System.* Ann Arbor, Edwards Brothers, Inc., 1938.

33. Sako, K., Pradier, R. N., Marchetta, F. C., Pickren, J. W.: Fallibility of palpation in the diagnosis of metastasis to cervical lymph nodes. *Surg. Gynecol. Obstet.* **118**:989, 1964.

34. Spiro, R. H., Alfonso, A. E., Farr, H. W., Strong, E. W.: Cervical node metastasis from epidermoid carcinoma of the oral cavity and oropharynx. A critical assessment of current staging. *Am. J. Surg.* **128**:562, 1974.

35. Spiro, R. H., Strong, E. W.: Mouth cancer, a surgical perspective. *Clin. Bull.* **6**:3, 1976.

36. Southwick, H. W., Slaughter, D. P., Trevino, E. T.: Elective neck dissection for intraoral cancer. *Arch. Surg.* **80**:905, 1960.

37. Tucker, G. F.: The anatomy of laryngeal cancer. *Can. J. Otolaryngol.* **3**:417–431, 1974.

38. Wang, C. C., Meyer, J. E.: Radiotherapeutic management of carcinoma of the nasopharynx. *Cancer* **28**:566, 1971.

39. Ward, G. E., Edgerton, M. T., Chambers, R. G., McKee, D. M.: Cancer of the oral cavity and pharynx and results of treatment by means of the composite operation (in continuity with radical neck dissection). *Ann. Surg.* **150**:202, 1959.

40. Wurman, L. H., Adams, G. L., Meyerhoff, W. L.: Carcinoma of the lip. *Am. J. Surg.* **130**:470, 1975.

41. Zagars, G., Norante, J. D.: Head and neck tumors. In *Clinical Oncology for Medical Students and Physicians: A Multidisciplinary Approach,* 6th ed. Rubin, P. (Ed.). New York, American Cancer Society, 1983, pp. 230–261.

7 LARYNX AND HYPOPHARYNX

Anthony A. Mancuso

Malignancies affecting the hypopharynx may be logically discussed along with those of the larynx or oropharynx. In this chapter, the larynx and hypopharynx will be considered as an anatomic unit, since the pathways of tumor spread from either of the two sources overlap in so many cases. It will, however, become immediately apparent that treatment and prognosis vary greatly depending upon which subdivision of this anatomic region is the primary site.

As with the oral cavity and oropharynx, it is necessary to split this small anatomic region into subdivisions so that natural history, treatment, and prognosis can be discussed in an orderly fashion. These subdivisions include:

1. The glottis. The true vocal cords are the most common site of origin for endolaryngeal carcinomas. Five-year survival rates of about 90% can be obtained with either surgery or radiation therapy in early lesions.[9] Once deep invasion has occurred, which is manifested mainly by a reduction in vocal cord mobility, this rate is nearly halved to 50%.[9]
2. The supraglottic larynx. This region includes tumors arising from the arytenoid cartilage, the laryngeal surface of the epiglottis, the aryepiglottic folds, the false cords, and the ventricle. It is probably best to separate tumors in this group into marginal (aryepiglottic folds) and anterior (mainly epiglottic origin) categories. This is based mainly on the data of Ogura et al.[46] which indicated survival rates of 53% for marginal lesions and 82% for other supraglottic lesions. This further

subdivision facilitates selection of patients for conservative surgery.
3. The infraglottic larynx. The exact limits of the infraglottis vary according to whether the undersurface of the true cords is included in this region. The undersurface is not included customarily in the infraglottic region, which extends from 5 mm to 1 cm below the true cords to the lower border of the cricoid cartilage. These arbitrary definitions have little value to the imaging physician, and, as will be emphasized in a subsequent section, the major issue of interest in this region is the relationship of tumor to the cricoid cartilage.

Infraglottic carcinomas are rare, accounting for perhaps 4% to 6% of all laryngeal tumors. Five-year survival rates are in the 40% range.[24,61] Infraglottic extention of glottic carcinoma is a much more common circumstance. Where such infraglottic spread takes place, the very favorable five-year survival rate of 90% for glottic carcinoma is more than halved to between 36% and 41%,[40,41] figures that are nearly identical to those for primary infraglottic tumors.
4. The hypopharynx. This region begins at the pharyngoepiglottic folds and includes the pyriform sinuses (fossae). Its medial boundary is the lateral surface of the aryepiglottic fold. The posterolateral wall of the pharynx and the postcricoid area are also included in this region of the upper aerodigestive tract.

Carcinomas in this area arise predominantly in the pyriform sinus. Three-year and five-year survival rates for surgery or combined therapy are in the 40% to 50% range.[9,17,42] Radiation alone yields low (6% to

8%) five-year cure rates except in small lesions without cervical metastatic disease.

Carcinomas of the postcricoid area have at best an overall salvage rate of 20% to 25%.[44,57] A similar, dismal cure rate of about 20% is quoted for carcinomas of the posterior pharyngeal wall. Note that the survival rates in these regions are similar to those for lesions of the tongue base and overall represent the poorest survival rates for lesions of the upper aerodigestive tract except for the cervical esophagus (5% gross five-year cure rate).[16]

Cervical lymph node metastases are uncommon with glottic lesions and very common with the remainder of the lesions affecting the larynx and hypopharynx. The status of these lymph nodes often has a dramatic impact on the likelihood of survival and the approach to therapy. These issues depend very much on the specific site of origin of the primary lesion and therefore will be discussed in detail in the appropriate sections.

Diagnostic imaging has always played a useful role in the evaluation of the larynx and hypopharynx. Plain films for soft tissue and cartilage detail were of great use to Baclesse.[8] Since then, laryngography, barium swallow, and conventional tomography have been used to define areas of critical interest in management decisions. Computed tomography (CT) with its unparalleled display of the deep tissue planes within and surrounding the larynx has replaced these older modalities under nearly all circumstances. Computed tomography proves to be complementary to clinical examination in that it demonstrates the patterns of deep infiltration and the status of the lymph nodes, while endoscopic examination defines the mucosal extent of disease and vocal cord mobility. Magnetic resonance imaging may improve on CT in some ways; however, with modern, fast scanners and detailed techniques there seems to be little acute need for advancement in this area of oncologic imaging. The surgical approach to laryngeal carcinomas requires especially accurate definition of the tumor margins if failures are to be avoided and laryngeal function preserved. A good deal of the following discussion will be directed toward how imaging with CT can make this "precision surgery"[50] even more precise.

TUMOR BEHAVIOR AND PATHOLOGY

Histopathology

Squamous cell carcinoma is by far the predominant histologic form affecting the larynx and hypopharynx. These tumors are usually moderately well differentiated and represent over 90% of the epithelial malignancies in the region.[18] The glottis is by far the most frequent site of primary origin. There is a tendency for the tumors to be more biologically aggressive proceeding from the glottis to the supraglottic region and then posteriorly to the hypopharynx.

The degree of biologic aggressiveness as well as the host–tumor relationship seems to be, at least in part, related to the growth pattern of the lesion. Growth of these carcinomas may range from primarily exophytic to ulceroinfiltrative. Verrucous carcinoma is at the more benign end of the spectrum. These warty, exophytic growths are highly curable if diagnosed and treated properly. Unfortunately, verrucous carcinomas account for only 1% to 2% of laryngeal lesions.[10,19] Ulceroinfiltrative lesions present quite a different problem because of their tendency for deep spread and fixation to critical structures and their greater tendency to metastasize.

The histologic evaluation of the deep and superficial margins of laryngeal carcinomas has been corrected with differentiation and host–tumor relationships.[28,30] While it is true that size and location are the more important criteria for staging, the pattern of growth might also prove valuable in treatment decisions and prognosis. The tumors with more well-defined, pushing margins seem to have a better prognosis than those with ill-defined infiltrative borders.[13,31,50]

Lymph node metastases are of paramount importance in the prognosis and management of laryngeal carcinomas. There are relatively high error rates in detecting whether metastases are present by clinical examination. These false-positive and false-negative results are attributable to the limitations and subjectivity of palpation, the presence of microscopic tumors in normal-sized nodes, and the presence of enlarged, "reactive nodes" that contain no tumor. The nodal response may also be used to judge the host–tumor relationship. Extranodal extension seems to be a very useful prognostic indicator in this regard.[9,14]

Other histologic types of carcinoma may involve the larynx. Carcinosarcomas are rare tumors with both epithelial and mesenchymal elements. Many of these lesions may in fact be anaplastic carcinomas or carcinomas with pseudosarcomatous reaction. Pleomorphic carcinomas differ somewhat in that they are strictly epithelial and do not contain a true sarcomatous component. Both of these lesions are highly aggressive. Adenoid cystic lesions, adenocarcinomas, acinous carcinomas, and others rarely involve the larynx.

Malignancies may also arise from the supportive tissues of the larynx. All are rare. Fibrosarcomas (about 32 reported cases) and those arising from cartilage (between 125 and 136 reported cases) make up the bulk of these tumors.[9] Rhabdomyosarcomas, paragangliomas, neuromas, lipomas, and lymphomas have been reported. All are extremely rare and are of little practical significance except to make one aware that exact diagnosis always requires histologic confirmation.

Patterns of Spread

Laryngeal carcinomas spread along the mucosa, deep to the mucosa, and via lymphatics. Deep extension patterns are all-important in staging. Such spread is "channeled" by the arrangement of the deep tissue planes in the larynx depending upon the relative resistance of the anatomic structures that surround the growing tumor (Figure 7-1). These patterns of deep spread must be considered in relatively limited increments because the pertinent anatomy changes dramatically at different levels within the larynx and hypopharynx. These will be divided in the following, fairly widely accepted, manner.

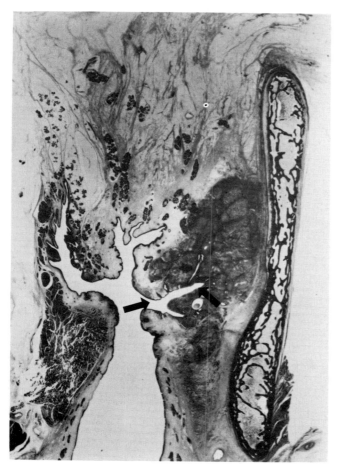

FIG. 7-1. Section through the mid-coronal plane of the larynx. This transglottic tumor probably arose in the laryngeal ventricle (arrows), but it spread freely in the fibroadipose tissue of the paralaryngeal space. (Courtesy of John Kirchner, M.D., Department of Otolaryngology, Yale University.)

The Glottis. The true vocal cords are of great importance in the larynx because they must be preserved or reconstructed in some form in order to provide adequate glottic function after therapy. As a result, a vast amount of data has been compiled relating to the critical anatomy necessary for glottic reconstruction. A detailed accounting of this is not possible since there are so many variations; however, a discussion of the pathways of tumor spread in this region will bring to light most of these considerations in a general way.

Fortunately, most glottic carcinomas are limited lesions that spread along the intrinsic laryngeal musculature; this in itself may lead to a fixed vocal cord. Probably the next most frequent occurrence is spread to the anterior commissure (Figure 7-2). This all important region in glottic cancer is formed by the joining of the vocal ligaments at the central tendon where the cords insert on the inner surface of the thyroid laminae. From here the tumors may extend to the contralateral true vocal cord or directly invade the thyroid cartilage. Superior extension takes them to the false vocal cords and the low pre-epiglottic space. Direct inferior spread carries them along the cricothyroid membrane, where they have access to the relatively rich infraglottic lymphatics and eventually the anterior cricoid ring.

Superior extension from a more lateral point of origin will take the lesions into the false vocal. This spread may be mucosal or within the paralaryngeal space and deep to the ventricle (Figure 7-2). Caudal spread carries the lesion to the aryepiglottic fold.

Some of the most clinically significant and most difficult to diagnose deep extensions occur posterolaterally in true cord tumors. Involvement of the cricoarytenoid joint may result in fixation of the cord or cartilage invasion (Figure 7-1). Spread to the interarytenoid region and on inferiorly is usually a superficial pattern of extension. Once the tumor has invaded the lower aspects of the paralaryngeal space it may spread to the space between the cricoid and thyroid cartilage.

Infraglottic spread was described in the prior section. One should recall that such inferior spread reaches the cricoid cartilage more readily as one proceeds posteriorly along the true cords. This is because the cricoid arches slope inferiorly from posterior to anterior. Moreover, the cords are 1 to 2 mm thick at the anterior commissure and progressively widen to a maximum of 4 to 5 mm in their middle portions.

Lymph node involvement is unusual in limited glottic lesions. Deep spread or extension beyond the true cord mucosa provides access to the richer lymphatic fields, and the likelihood of nodal metastasis increases. Specific patterns of nodal disease related to these more advanced lesions are discussed in the sections on the infraglottis and supraglottis.

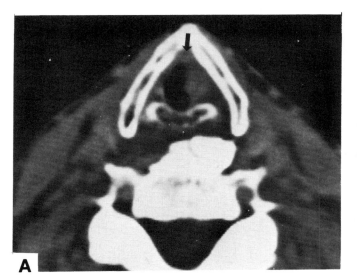

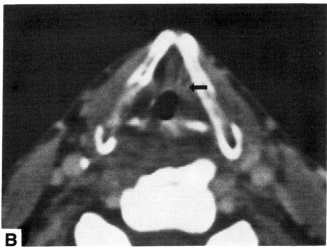

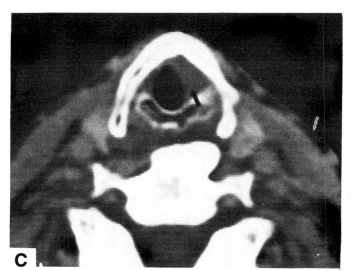

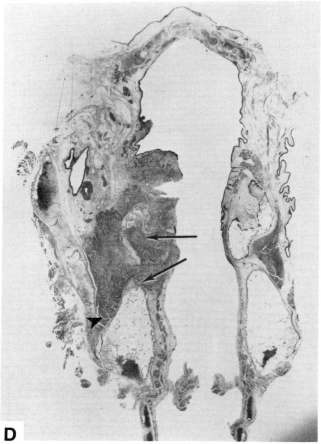

FIG. 7-2. Patient with transglottic carcinoma. (A) The undersurface of a true cord level section shows a thickened cord and involvement of the anterior commissure (arrow). (B) At the false cord level the normal fat density of the paralaryngeal space has been replaced by tumor (arrow). (C) Tumor adjacent to the cricoid (arrow) indicates that infraglottic spread is beyond the limits of conservation surgery (vertical hemilaryngectomy). (D) A coronal whole organ section through the cricoarytenoid joints. The tumor has eroded both cartilages (arrows). Spread into the cricothyroid space via the paralaryngeal space is present (arrowhead). (Courtesy of John Kirchner, M.D., Department of Otolaryngology, Yale University.)

The Supraglottis. The supraglottic region is of great interest in that it demonstrates very clearly how anatomic considerations limit and direct tumor growth and how these circumstances are used as a rational basis for choosing therapy. The growth patterns of supraglottic carcinomas occur in two basic forms: (1) predominantly anteriorly, on the laryngeal surface of the epiglottis and above the false cord, and (2) posterolaterally, involving the aryepiglottic fold (so-called marginal supraglottic lesions).[46] These are useful subdivisions because these lesions behave differently and because the surgical approach differs somewhat (supraglottic laryngectomy versus partial laryngopharyngectomy).

Anterior supraglottic carcinomas arise at or above the junction of the epiglottis and false cords.[9,13,31,46,57] These may be plaquelike exophytic lesions or they may be ulceroinfiltrative. Both tend to spread circumferentially along the laryngeal surface of the epiglottis. The ulceroinfiltrative lesions also tend to extend through the epiglottic cartilage and into the pre-epiglottic space (Figures 7-3, 7-4). This fibrofatty tissue space is in continuity with the paralaryngeal space, so that once the tumors have entered these deep planes they may extend both circumferentially and in a cephalocaudal direction. Since these deep spaces provide little resistance to tumor growth and obviously lie beneath the mucosa, the exact extent of the lesion may not be apparent from the amount of mucosal disruption. The junction of the false cords and the epiglottis provides both a physical and lymphatic barrier to tumor spread[50] (Figure 7-4B). The anatomic junction of the ventricular bands, the petiole, the thyroepiglottic ligament, and anterior commissure seems to resist invasion except by the more aggressive supraglottic lesions.[13,28,42,45,57] Thyroid cartilage invasion is unusual except in ulceroinfiltrative lesions that have crossed the anterior commissure. In these instances the tumor usually enters the cartilage along the central tendon of the anterior commissure. Advanced lesions may also spread back along or within the aryepiglottic folds (Figure 7-4). Supraglottic lesions very rarely extend beyond the confines of the larynx in any direction. The tumors also spread superiorly within the pre-epiglottic space to involve the tongue base.

Marginal supraglottic lesions arise on the aryepiglottic fold. Technically, the lateral surface of the aryepiglottic fold is considered to lie within the pyriform sinus; this is obviously an area of overlap. Deep infiltration immediately places the tumors in the posterolateral portion of the paralaryngeal space (Figure 7-5). Anteromedial growth takes the lesion to the pre-epiglottic space, and occasionally this circumferential pattern of spread continues across midline (Figure 7-4A). As with anterior supraglottic tumors, a good deal of this growth may occur beneath intact mucosa. The base of the aryepiglottic fold in the arytenoid region is a common site of involvement. From here the tumors may go on to the true vocal cord or the cricoarytenoid joint, but more commonly they end at or near the arytenoid. Spread to or across the true cord is uncommon; this would make these transglottic tumors. Cartilage invasion is unusual in true marginal supraglottic tumors.

The Infraglottis. In the scheme presented here, the undersurface of the true cords will be excluded from the

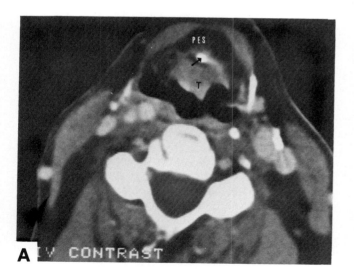
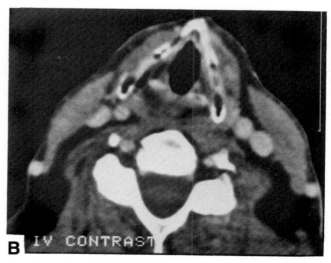

FIG. 7-3. Patient with exophytic epiglottic carcinoma. (A) Note that the tumor mass (T) lies to the airway side of the partially calcified epiglottis (arrow). The pre-epiglottic space (PES) is spared. (B) A section through the false cord level shows no tumor, indicating a margin at the anterior commissure should be adequate for supraglottic laryngectomy.

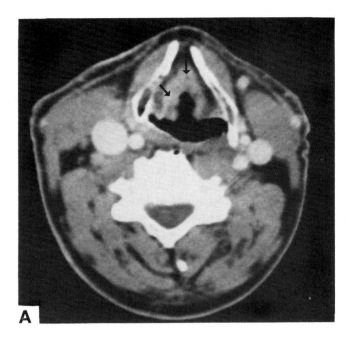

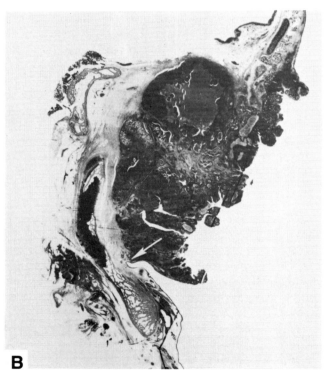

FIG. 7-4. (A) A circumferential supraglottic mass infiltrates the para-laryngeal and pre-epiglottic spaces (arrows). (B) A sagittal whole organ section shows an epiglottic tumor with "pushing" margins invading the pre-epiglottic space. The inferior margin of the tumor is at the false cord just above the anterior commissure (arrow). (Courtesy of John Kirchner, M.D., Department of Otolaryngology, Yale University.)

infraglottic region. The conus elasticus is resistant to tumor growth relative to the mucosa, submucosa, muscles, and fibrofatty tissue that lie within and around the cricoid cartilage.[13,31,48,60] This fibroelastic membrane extends from the vocal ligaments to the upper surface of the cricoid. This tough membrane obviously may be destroyed by tumor; however, there is a tendency for lesions originating on its mucosal aspect to remain more superficial and spread circumferentially within the confines of the cricoid cartilage and cricothyroid membrane. Tumors on its lateral (deep) surface tend to grow within the lower aspects of the paralaryngeal (paraepiglottic) space and into the soft tissues of the neck via the gap between the cricoid and thyroid cartilages[13,31,48,59] (Figure 7-2). Growth along the intrinsic and extrinsic laryngeal musculature, which is intimately related to the cricoid cartilage at this level, also occurs. Perineural spread may follow the course of the recurrent laryngeal nerve between the lateral aspect of the cricoid and the inferior cornu of the thyroid cartilage. In general, a tumor may reach and invade the cricoid cartilage by spreading along the conus elasticus. The inferior margins and cornua of the thyroid cartilage may also be destroyed in very advanced lesions.

The lymphatic drainage of the larynx changes fairly abruptly at the junction of the undersurface of the true cords and the infraglottis. A fairly rich lymphatic plexus begins at this junction and splits into three groups: one goes anteriorly through the cricothyroid membrane and on to the lower deep cervical groups; the other two groups go posterolaterally where they pierce the cricotracheal membrane and drain to the paratracheal nodes.[13,50,52]

The Hypopharynx. Tumors arising in the hypopharyngeal region are, of course, not endolaryngeal. These lesions do threaten glottic function and partial laryngeal resection is almost always included in surgical management. A good understanding of their growth patterns is necessary to differentiate them from marginal supraglottic lesions and to plan accurate therapy.

Mucosally, the lesions tend to grow in a circumferential manner, enveloping all surfaces of the pyriform sinus (Figure 7-6). The tumors may spread to the posterior pharyngeal wall. Very advanced lesions may grow up to and along the pharyngoepiglottic fold to involve the lower glossopalatine sulcus and the base of the tongue. Larger tumors may also "spill over" onto the medial aspect of the aryepiglottic fold.

The deep extensions of these lesions are particularly sinister. Anteriorly and medially they have access to the paralaryngeal space. Circumferential (in the horizontal plane) growth takes the tumor deep to the aryepiglottic fold and the laryngeal surface of the epiglottis, sometimes across midline within the latter. Vertical growth within the paralaryngeal space takes the tumor to the up-

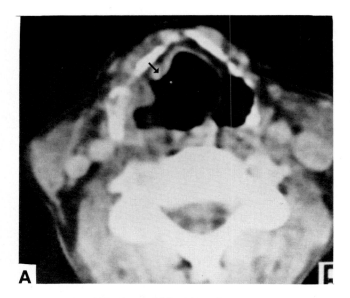

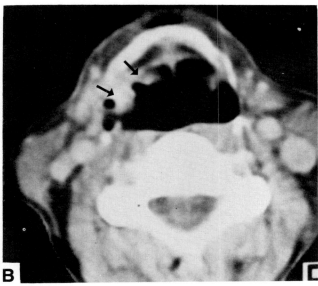

FIG. 7-5. Patient with a marginal supraglottic carcinoma. (A) A section through the lower supraglottic larynx shows thickening of the aryepiglottic fold (compare with opposite side) and anterolateral spread in the paralaryngeal space (arrow). (B) The tumor extends cephalad to involve the pharyngoepiglottic fold and lateral pharyngeal wall (arrows).

per limits of the endolarynx and on caudally to the cricothyroid space (Figure 7-6). The inferior spread is important because from the cricothyroid space the tumors may grow into the postcricoid region or into the soft tissues of the neck. Laterally, the tumors may grow directly through the thyroid cartilage and into the exolaryngeal soft tissue (Figure 7-6).

Thyroid cartilage invasion commonly occurs in pyriform sinus tumors. The inferior margin of the thyroid ala is a frequent site of invasion as the tumor spreads from the cricothyroid space to the soft tissues of the

neck. Areas of erosion in the mid portion of the thyroid lamina may be seen adjacent to a tumor growing within the paralaryngeal space (Figure 7-6). Occasionally tumors with "pushing" margins will grow superiorly within the paralaryngeal space and "dumbbell" into the exolaryngeal soft tissues through the thyrohyoid membrane, all of this occurring without destruction of the thyroid lamina.[13,48,60]

The lymphatic drainage network of the supraglottis and hypopharynx differs vastly from that of the other regions of the larynx. The supraglottis develops from buccopharyngeal anlage, and the glottis and infraglottis from the tracheobronchial anlage.[9,50] The glottis with its sparse submucosal lymphatic network can be logically considered a barrier to vertical lymphatic drainage.[50] The supraglottic region is relatively rich in lymphatics and the incidence of nodal metastasis is quite high, probably in the range of 30% overall. The frequency of nodal metastasis increases the more posterior the lesions;[8,9] the lowest incidence is noted in epiglottic lesions with progressively higher numbers for lesions of the aryepiglottic folds and pyriform sinuses.

Distant metastases from carcinomas of the larynx often occur late in the natural history of the disease. Lack of control of local or regional disease is the primary cause of death in most patients. The lungs, liver, and bone are the most usual sites of distant metastatic involvement.

It is of interest that histologic differentiation does not influence the ability of a tumor to disseminate widely.[1] Moreover, if the primary tumor is controlled initially by radiation or surgery, the exact method of therapy does not seem to influence the likelihood of the patient's developing metastases.[2]

CLASSIFICATION AND STAGING

The clinical-diagnostic staging of carcinomas of the larynx and hypopharynx is separated according to the anatomic regions described in previous sections. In the oral cavity and oropharynx, the primary site is staged mainly by the size criteria of the American Joint Committee (AJC) format with no real accounting of deep spread.[3] The International Union Against Cancer (UICC) format provides some leeway for upstaging because of deep invasion. In the larynx and hypopharynx, the primary tumor is staged mainly by three criteria: (1) the number of regions of the larynx involved; (2) in special instances, the presence of spread to or across critical adjacent sites (e.g., anterior commissure and pre-epiglottic space); and (3) evidence of deep infiltration, manifested mainly by fixation of the vocal cord or hemilarynx. Gross evidence of cartilage destruction on plain films has also been used to diagnose very advanced lesions. It is important to keep these three generalizations in mind to avoid becoming lost in what seems to be a confusing array of stages and substages in the clinical diagnostic scheme

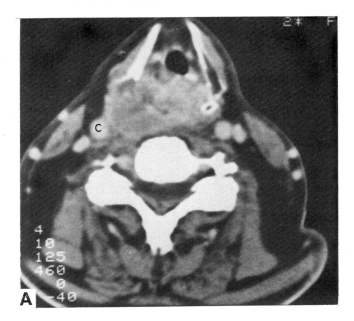

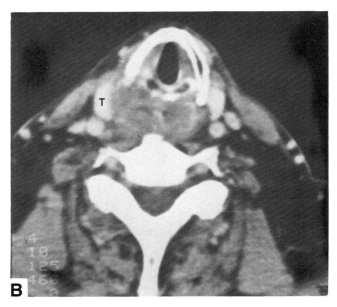

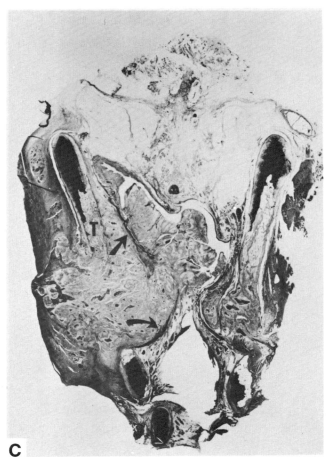

FIG. 7-6. Patient with a T_4 pyriform sinus carcinoma. (A) A section through the middle to lower supraglottic level. The mass has destroyed the posterior aspect of the thyroid lamina and extends to the exolaryngeal soft tissues. The mass is likely adherent to the medial aspect of the carotid **C**, but is not fixed. Spread within the paralaryngeal space and across the midline via the posterior pharyngeal wall is also evident. (B) Postcricoid and exolaryngeal spread eventually go on to involve the thyroid gland **T** and cervical esophagus. (C) A somewhat posterior coronal whole organ section shows typical pyriform sinus carcinoma. The tumor has destroyed the thyroid ala and has spread to exolaryngeal soft tissues. The conus elasticus is resisting tumor spread (curved arrow). Cephalad spread in the paralaryngeal space is sometimes limited by the quadrangular membrane (straight arrow). (Courtesy of John Kirchner, M.D., Department of Otolaryngology, Yale University.)

(see Figures 7-7, 7-8, 7-9, and 7-10). The major treatment issues are centered around whether deep invasion is present and the presence and likelihood of nodal metastases. Both of these factors should be foremost in the mind of a diagnostic radiologist being consulted in the management of patients with laryngeal carcinoma.[6,7]

The Glottis

T_1 lesions are confined to the vocal cord, which retains its normal mobility. These are of little interest for diagnostic radiologists in that they are limited lesions that can be handled well by surgical or radiation techniques. Diagnostic imaging may be necessary to determine the status of the anterior commissure in some cases.

T_2 lesions are those lesions which have spread to one adjacent region (supraglottis or infraglottis), and the vocal cords have either impaired or normal mobility. This is a very important category for the diagnostic imaging physician as well as the physicians treating the patient, since some of these lesions will have deep extension, which is difficult to confirm clinically but is highly significant in management decisions. A CT scan should help greatly in studying such patients.

T_3 lesions are those lesions which are confined to the larynx and have caused fixation of the vocal cord. There are several reasons for fixations of the vocal cord. These range from simple ones, such as infiltration of the cord musculature, to those ominous ones, such as thyroid cartilage invasion.

T_4 lesions are usually large tumors that destroy the thyroid (or rarely the cricoid) cartilages or extend beyond the confines of the larynx. Although these tumors are usually quite extensive (often massive), primarily ulceroinfiltrative lesions can reach the thyroid cartilage and extend to the cricothyroid space and begin an exolaryngeal course without reaching "massive" proportions. More subtle evidence of cartilage invasion is present on scans from current generation scanners than on lateral xeroradiograms and "soft tissue" views of the cartilages.[5] This may revise somewhat the equation of "cartilage invasion equals massive tumor."

Anatomic staging for cancer of the glottis is presented in Figure 7-7.

The Supraglottis

T_1 lesions are confined to the site of origin with normal vocal cord mobility. T_2 lesions are those lesions which have spread to an adjacent supraglottic site or sites or to the true cord level, but, again, the vocal cord is not fixed.

The designation T_3 differs in the supraglottis from that in the glottis and infraglottis, where it is based strictly on the presence of vocal cord fixation. T_3 supraglottic lesions may cause fixation; however, involvement of the medial wall of the pyriform sinus, the postcricoid region or the pre-epiglottic space also warrants this classification. A CT scan is of great value in identifying deep spread that is not apparent clinically and would cause lesions to be upstaged from T_2 to T_3.

T_4 lesions are usually massive tumors that have extended cephalad to involve the tongue base or other portions of the oropharynx. Exolaryngeal spread to the soft tissues of the neck or cartilage destruction are other signs indicative of this advanced stage.

Anatomic staging for cancer of the supraglottis is presented in Figure 7-8 and Table 7-1.

The Infraglottis

T_1 tumors are confined to the infraglottis. T_2 lesions involve the vocal cords but normal cord mobility is retained. T_3 lesions demonstrate cord fixation. T_4 lesions are large tumors that destroy cartilage or extend beyond the confines of the larynx.

The Hypopharynx

The staging of tumors in the hypopharynx is more logically considered with the larynx than the oropharynx, since the staging system and treatment plan relies heavily on fixation of endolaryngeal structures. T_1 lesions are confined to the site of origin, be it the pyriform sinus, the posterior pharyngeal wall, or the postcricoid region. T_2 lesions are those lesions which have spread to an adjacent region or site without fixation of the ipsilateral hemilarynx. T_3 lesions fix the hemilarynx. T_4 lesions invade the exolaryngeal soft tissues or bone. The tendency for these tumors to destroy the thyroid cartilage and extend into the soft tissues of the neck is high and may not be apparent clinically. A CT scan is especially valuable in this region if errors in therapy planning are to be avoided.

Anatomic staging for cancer of the hypopharynx is presented in Figure 7-9.

Lymph Nodes

The cervical nodes for carcinoma of the larynx and hypopharynx are staged by the same criteria as discussed before in the chapter on cervical lymph nodes. The retropharyngeal nodes may be involved in very advanced or recurrent lesions. The paratracheal, paraesophageal, and pretracheal groups are important in addition to the usual considerations of the deep cervical groups when infraglottic spread has occurred.[13,50,52] The paratracheal and paraesophageal groups are usually difficult to evaluate by palpation.

Distant metastases are staged M_0 (none known) or M_1 (present). The lungs, liver, and bone are likely sites.

IMAGING PROCEDURES AND ASSESSMENT

Radiologic imaging procedures have traditionally played an important role in staging malignancies of the larynx and hypopharynx. Baclesse has classically emphasized the importance of mineralization of the thyroid cartilage on plain film.[8] Barium studies, conventional pluridirectional and linear tomography, laryngography, and xeroradiography have been used to help stage these tumors. All have been somewhat limited in their ability to show the deep extent of lesions except in the most advanced cases. Computed tomography has refined these capabilities and magnetic resonance imaging (MRI) may even make further improvements.

Plain films and xeroradiographs, excluding port films, really play no constant role in the evaluation of malignancies in this region. Conventional tomography lacks the density resolution of CT, although some would still consider it part of the radiologic evaluation of laryngeal carcinomas.[22] In our experience, it is usually an addi-

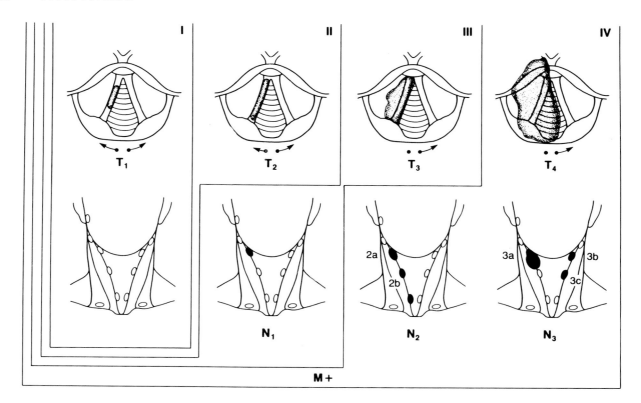

FIG. 7-7. Anatomic staging for cancer of the glottis. T categories: The essential factors are mobility and fixation and site of origin, not size. Normal mobility is T_1, compound mobility is T_2, and fixation is T_3. Massive lesions destroy cartilage and extend beyond the larynx into the soft tissue of the neck. N categories: The size of the node and its mobility and the number and location are all factors in staging cervical lymph nodes. The diameters ≤ 3 cm, 3 cm and 6 cm, and >6 cm were chosen because these are determined more objectively than fixation. Fixation implies adhesion to the carotid artery and therefore unresectability. Single and multiple nodes (N_1 v N_2), homolateral, and bilateral nodes (N_1, N_2 v N_3) are important factors. Stage grouping: The T category is the major determinant of stage. Note that N_1 nodes are equivalent to T_3 in advancement (stage III) and that N_2 and N_3 nodes and M_1, along with T_4 lesions, constitute stage IV. (Reprinted from Zagars, G., Norante, J. D.: Head and neck tumors. In *Clinical Oncology for Medical Students and Physicians: A Multidisciplinary Approach*, 6th ed. Rubin, P. (Ed.). New York, American Cancer Society, 1983, pp. 230–261. With permission.)

tive study and is not necessary if a good CT scan is available. Laryngography studies mainly the mucosa and function, therefore adding little to the endoscopic examination. Laryngograms do provide a good view of the infraglottis and anterior commissure as well as the pyriform sinuses and laryngeal ventricles; however, they have been shown to be less informative that CT in two correlative studies.[4,34] Barium swallow can be used to good advantage to study patients suspected of having lesions in the hypopharynx, the postcricoid region, or the cervical esophagus. Staging of known lesions in this area is best carried out with a combination of CT and endoscopy.

Recommended Method of Study

A CT scan is the examination of choice for evaluating malignancies of the larynx and hypopharynx if an imaging examination is deemed necessary[4,20,31] (Figure 7-10). There is little reason to do other studies for staging known malignant tumors. Positive contrast barium swallow may still be used in selected instances for screening patients with suspected pyriform sinus or postcricoid lesions. Rarely, positive contrast laryngography may be done to study the function and mucosal surfaces of the larynx in a patient who cannot be examined by endoscopy

Table 7-1. Stage Grouping—Glottis, Supraglottis, Hypopharynx

Stage I	T_1, N_0, M_0
Stage II	T_2, N_0, M_0
Stage III	T_3, N_0, M_0
	T_1, T_2 or T_3, N_1, M_0
Stage IV	T_4, N_0 or N_1, M_0
	Any T, N_2 or N_3, M_1

From American Joint Committee on Cancer: *Manual for Staging of Cancer*, 2nd ed. Philadelphia, J. B. Lippincott, 1983.

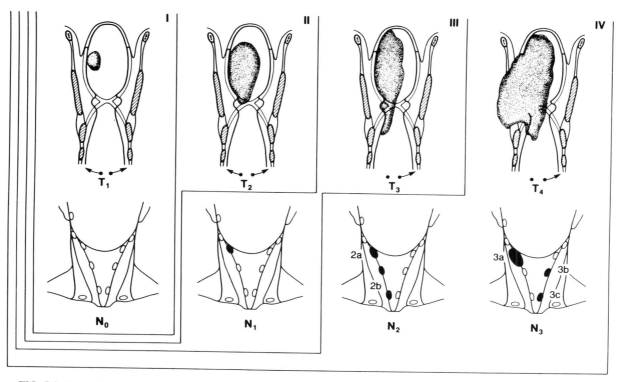

FIG. 7-8. Anatomic staging for cancer of the supraglottis. T categories: see legend for Figure 7-7. N categories: see legend for Figure 7-7. Stage grouping: see legend for Figure 7-7.

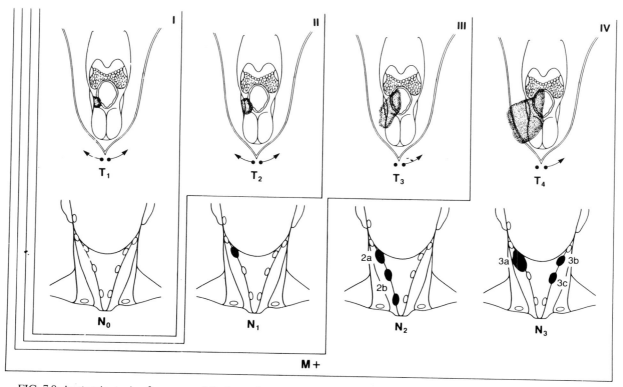

FIG. 7-9. Anatomic staging for cancer of the hypopharynx. T categories: The number of sites rather than size is the critical factor. Sites are listed as vault (posterosuperior or roof) and lateral walls. The difference is between one site and extension to involve another site (T_1 v T_2) and anterior extension or with cord fixation, which is T_3. Deep invasion into the base of the skull and nerves is T_4. N categories: See legend for Figure 7-7. Stage grouping: see legend for Figure 7-7.

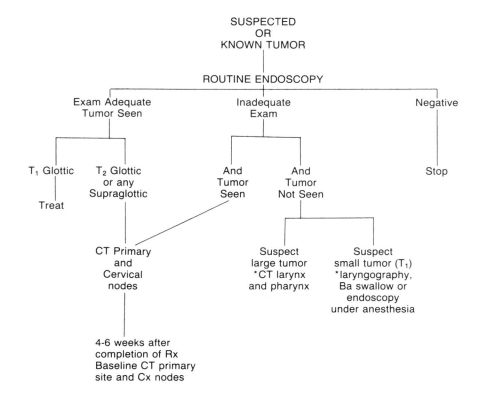

SUSPECTED
OR
KNOWN TUMOR

ROUTINE ENDOSCOPY

Exam Adequate
Tumor Seen

Inadequate
Exam

Negative

T₁ Glottic

T₂ Glottic
or any
Supraglottic

And
Tumor
Seen

And
Tumor
Not Seen

Stop

Treat

CT Primary
and
Cervical
nodes

Suspect
large tumor
*CT larynx
and pharynx

Suspect
small tumor (T₁)
*laryngography,
Ba swallow or
endoscopy
under anesthesia

4-6 weeks after
completion of Rx
Baseline CT primary
site and Cx nodes

*Such "screening" imaging only necessary in patients medically unable to undergo endoscopy under anesthesia. Should use CT if possible since these patients are usually poor candidates for laryngography.

FIG. 7-10. General clinical imaging approach to laryngeal and hypopharyngeal cancer.

without general anesthesia. Magnetic resonance imaging could play a role in this area in the near future but to date no experience in this anatomic region has been reported.

Technique of Examination

The patient should be placed supine in the scanner. With the neck slightly hyperextended, the central axis of the larynx will usually be oriented parallel to the table top. Lateral digital radiographs may be used to determine the limits of the examination. A scan of the larynx should normally begin at the inferior margin of the cricoid cartilage and extend to the tongue base (one or two sections above the hyoid bone). The study may certainly be limited to a lesser area in small lesions and if lymph node metastases are unlikely.

Sections should be no more than 5 mm thick and in general done edge to edge. Slightly thinner (3 or 4 mm) sections may prove useful at the glottic level for more precise delineation of tumor margins relative to the anterior commissure and cricoarytenoid joint regions. Overlapping of sections is necessary for high quality reformation. In general, reformatted images provide little

information that is necessary and not available from the axial scans.

Scans are routinely done with the patient in quiet respiration. If significant degradation occurs at 10-second scan times, we do a series through any critical area of interest with the patient in suspended inspiration. The patient should hold his or her breath as a routine on sections through the infraglottis and supraglottis to improve the image quality. At the glottic level, this may make scans difficult to interpret, since the true cords will be apposed in the midline because most patients perform a Valsalva's maneuver during breathholding. Phonation scans are not used because scan times of more than 1 or 2 seconds make phonating an "E" impractical. A modified Valsalva's maneuver (blowing the cheeks out) is a useful tool for distending the pyriform sinuses. This maneuver will also allow the base of the aryepiglottic folds to be visualized.

In cases of an advanced (T_3 or T_4) carcinoma of the glottis and any stage supraglottic or hypopharyngeal primary tumor, the lymph node areas of the neck should be studied. This requires rapid drip infusion of contrast. The contrast infusion also is of value in more precisely defining the limits of the primary tumor.

Limitations of CT

The most important fact to remember is that CT is not tissue specific. Pathologic confirmation is required, regardless of CT findings, before any course of treatment is considered.[55] Laryngeal tuberculosis can look exactly like laryngeal carcinoma.

Cartilage destruction is an important aspect of staging laryngeal carcinomas. Computed tomography is the best tool available to date for demonstrating such extension. Subtle cartilage invasion still remains difficult to diagnose because of normal variations in thyroid cartilage mineralization.

An inexperienced radiologist sometimes feels uncomfortable when trying to determine the demarcation of the true and false cord levels on axial sections. Re-formations may be used to overcome this insecurity until sufficient experience is gained to allay such anxieties. A "fallback" to conventional AP tomography may also suffice.

Extranodal extension with or without carotid fixation is an important prognostic sign in cervical metastatic disease. Unfortunately, it is sometimes difficult to decide whether nodal masses are abutting, adherent to, or fixing the carotid. Most of the time this seems to be predictable.

The staging of cervical nodes will always be somewhat in error when size and criteria are employed. Enlarged nodes will sometimes be purely "reactive hyperplasia," and normal-sized nodes will sometimes contain microscopic or macroscopic deposits of tumor. Magnetic resonance imaging may offer some improvement, but this will continue to be a problem for the forseeable future.

In summary, diagnostic imaging studies available for the T work-up include plain soft tissue views, xeroradiographs, conventional tomograms, laryngograms, CT scans, and MRI. For the N component, CT and perhaps MRI may be used. The M work-up should include a chest X-ray film, and may include a radionuclide bone scan or a liver/spleen scan. The interrelationship of suggested protocols for these lesions are outlined in Table 7-2 and Figure 7-10.

IMAGING STRATEGIES AND DECISIONS

Detection

There is little role for CT as a screening test for carcinoma of the larynx and hypopharynx. Occasionally, CT might turn up an "occult primary" in the hypopharynx that is responsible for otherwise unexplained cervical lymphadenopathy. It might also have some role in studying patients who are unable to cooperate for adequate endoscopic examinations for either emotional or physical reasons.

Diagnosis and Staging of Primary Tumor and Regional Nodal Disease

Despite the excellent visualization of the larynx and hypopharynx obtained by head and neck surgeons with flexible fiberoptic and telescopic devices, CT has much to offer in the clinical-diagnostic staging of cancers in the

Table 7-2. Imaging Modalities for Evaluating Carcinomas of the Larynx and Hypopharynx

MODALITY	STAGING CAPABILITY	BENEFIT/ COST RATIO	RECOMMENDED ROUTINE STAGING PROCEDURE
Noninvasive			
Chest X-ray films	Look for metastases, second primary	High	Yes
Xeroradiographs and lateral soft tissue views	Survey primary site. Look for gross cartilage destruction	Fair	No
Barium swallow	Detect, stage hypopharyngeal carcinomas	Fair	No
Laryngography	Stage primary laryngeal hypopharyngeal tumor	Fair	No
Conventional tomography	Stage primary laryngeal and hypopharyngeal tumor	Fair	No
Radionuclide scans: Bone, liver/ spleen, brain	To detect metastases in advanced tumors or symptomatic patients	Low	No
MRI	Stage primary site and regional nodes	?	?
Minimally Invasive			
CT	Stage primary and regional nodes	High	Yes*

*In T_2 or larger glottic carcinomas, all supraglottic and hypopharyngeal primaries.

larynx and hypopharynx. The clinical examination shows the physiology and mucosal surfaces, while a CT scan shows the deep extent. A CT scan also augments the clinical examination of the neck, usually confirming the clinical impression, sometimes showing it to be in error, and other times suffering the same limitations.[33,51] Computed tomography is the imaging tool that comes closest to being the perfect complement to the endoscopic and physical examinations.[27,54]

A CT scan is most useful in cases where it is difficult to decide on clinical grounds between radical (total laryngectomy) or conservative (partial laryngectomy) surgery. A CT scan is equally well applied when used to decide whether surgery or radiotherapy would be a more appropriate mode of therapy. These considerations are best understood by splitting the larynx and hypopharynx into its several subdivisions as in the prior sections:

The Glottis. There is little value in the study of T_1 glottic carcinomas, since these are limited lesions that are highly amenable to cure by radiation or surgery. It is only when glottic lesions spread beyond the limits of vertical hemilaryngectomy or to the point where the chance for cure by radiation diminishes that they become interesting to the diagnostic imager. Of course, any lesion may be studied to increase the confidence level of the surgical or radiation oncologist in his or her choice of therapy for the patient. The status of the anterior commissure may be in question even after a good endoscopic examination, and CT may be used to evaluate this point. Sometimes a CT scan will show invasion of the thyroid cartilage at the anterior commissure through a subtle asymmetry in mineralization, which must not be overinterpreted.

T_2 glottic lesions are very interesting from an imaging point of view. A CT scan may show deep extension, which accounts for the limited mobility of the vocal cord observed in many of these lesions. Computed tomography shows, in a very precise manner, the degree of infraglottic extension relative to the cricoid cartilage (Figure 7-2). It also shows cephalad extension via the paralaryngeal space to the false cords.

In T_3 glottic lesions, there are several potential reasons for fixation of the vocal cord, including (1) invasion of vocal cord muscles; (2) the bulk of the tumor interferes with mobility; (3) invasion of or fixation to the thyroid cartilage; (4) cricoarytenoid joint involvement; and (5) infraglottic extension with or without fixation to the cricoid. More than one of the factors listed above often will be present in a patient. Most often, invasion of the intrinsic laryngeal musculature is the primary reason for fixation.[31,39,48,60]

A CT scan is useful for demonstrating causes other than muscle invasion. Even with current scanners, exquisite images, and rapid drip infusion of contrast, it is difficult to be certain whether a bulky cord is attributable primarily to an exophytic or an infiltrative lesion. This may improve with further refinements in equipment. Even lacking this, CT can show one or more of the other factors that may account for cord fixation.

In T_4 lesions, CT can document cartilage invasion, show exolaryngeal spread, and depict the "transglottic" nature of these large tumors. The T_4 category is usually obvious from the clinical examination; however, lesions felt to be more limited on endoscopic evaluation occasionally are upstaged after a CT scan.

The Supraglottis. T_1 supraglottic lesions may be primarily exophytic or ulceroinfiltrative. If the status of the pre-epiglottic space is in question, then a CT scan should be done, because potentially T_1 lesions can be upgraded to T_3 if the pre-epiglottic space is involved (Figures 7-3, 7-4).

In large exophytic lesions, CT can be used to define the limits of the tumor relative to the anterior commissure when the bulk of the tumor makes this difficult by clinical means.

In marginal supraglottic lesions, CT can be used to define the status of the midline, the pre-epiglottic space, and the medial wall of the pyriform sinus. Sometimes marginal supraglottic lesions will be upstaged because of otherwise occult spread into the pre-epiglottic space.

Both anterior and marginal supraglottic lesions will spread superiorly into the tongue base. This is an ominous event that may be clinically silent. Palpation of the tongue base may be negative despite such cephalad extension of the tumor via the pre-epiglottic space. A CT scan can show such spread before symptoms or physical findings suggest that it is present.[37]

The Infraglottis. A CT scan shows the relationship of the primary tumor to the cricoid cartilage. Reasons for true cord fixation are described previously and operate here as well. In advanced lesions, CT may clearly show escape of the tumor past the lower margin of the cricoid. This means that the tumor has access to the tracheal lymphatics, and spread to the mediastinal nodes is likely. Stomal recurrences are also very frequent in such instances.

Cartilage invasion (other than of the epiglottic cartilage) is unusual in supraglottic tumors.[31,48,60] Very aggressive carcinomas of the supraglottis may follow the petiole and thyroepiglottic ligament to the anterior commissure and upper infraglottis. These lesions are really transglottic, and erosion of the thyroid cartilage at the anterior commissure may occur. A CT scan shows such spread to best advantage and confirms the clinical impression of a very advanced lesion.

The Hypopharynx. Pyriform sinus carcinomas are very often quite advanced by the time they are diagnosed and therefore come to imaging. These lesions have a very high incidence of exolaryngeal spread and thyroid cartilage invasion. Since a good deal of spread occurs deep to the mucosa in this type of lesion, CT can potentially differentiate T_1 from T_2 lesions very accurately. Unfortunately, relatively few true T_1 and T_2 lesions are encountered.

Causes for fixation of the hemilarynx again may be multifactorial, and CT offers the best chance for deciding just what factors are operative. The greatest strength of CT in studying these lesions is its ability to show exolaryngeal spread via the cricothyroid space or directly through or over the thyroid cartilage and postcricoid spread via the cricothyroid space; both of which may not be detectable clinically (Figure 7-6). All of these deep extensions are indicative of T_4 lesions.

Primary carcinomas of the posterior pharyngeal wall and postcricoid region are uncommon relative to the other areas of the larynx and hypopharynx. Their extent is also best depicted by CT.

Cervical Lymphadenopathy

A simple listing of the staging issues relative to CT of cervical lymph node disease should suffice for this section. A detailed discussion of these factors is presented in the chapter on the neck. Some have been raised in the other chapters on the upper aerodigestive tract.

1. A CT scan can very accurately depict the size of nodes, both normal and abnormal, in every lymph-node-bearing region of the neck of interest to those treating carcinomas of this region.
2. A CT scan can show 1.5 to 2.5 cm nodes in clinically negative necks after therapy and occasionally shows nonpalpable positive nodes in untreated necks.
3. The morphology of lymph node masses as seen on a CT scan can be used to predict extranodal extension

and the probability of fixation of critical anatomic structures of the neck within certain limitations.

From these three factors it should be evident that CT can lend a great deal of objectivity to the staging of necks in patients with carcinoma of the larynx and hypopharynx. Some of the clinical implications of this will be discussed subsequently.

TREATMENT DECISIONS[20,25,26,43,61,62]

Primary Tumor

It is impossible to discuss all of the nuances of treatment and remain within the scope of this text. The following general discussion should provide the insight necessary to develop an imaging approach to the larynx and hypopharynx using CT. If MRI replaces CT in this regard, the treatment issues and anatomy will remain unchanged; only the way of depicting the altered anatomy will be modified. A tabulation or decision tree based upon TNM staging and tumor imaging should be viewed with the following text (Table 7-3).

The Glottis. T_1 lesions require no diagnostic imaging unless the clinician wishes to increase his or her level of confidence that the clinical assessment of the lesion is accurate. These tumors may be managed with radiation or vertical hemilaryngectomy. Generally, radiation therapy is preferred, with very high cure rates of better than 90%. The voice quality is superior after radiation therapy of the vocal cord, and motion returns to normal. When relapse occurs, particularly in individuals who continue to smoke after radiation treatment, surgical salvage is used. T_1 lesions may spread to the anterior

Table 7-3. Treatment Decisions: Larynx

STAGE	SURGERY		RADIATION THERAPY (RT)	CHEMOTHERAPY
I (T_1,N_0,M_0)	Laryngofissure		Definitive RT preferred 6000–6500 cGy	NR
II (T_2,N_0,M_0)	Hemilaryngectomy or total laryngectomy		Definitive RT preferred 6500–7000 cGy	NR
III (T_3,N_1,M_0)	Radical laryngectomy and radical neck dissection		Definitive RT or post-op RT 6500–7000 cGy	NR
IV (T_4,N_1,M_0)	Radical laryngectomy and radical neck dissection	and	Definitive RT or post-op RT 6500–7500 cGy	Investigational MAC
Relapse	Salvage RT		Salvage surgery	Investigational MAC
Metastatic (M_1)	NR		Possibly	Investigational MAC

NR = Not Recommended
MAC = Multiagent Chemotherapy

commissure, where, again, surgery or radiation may be used. At this point one must determine whether more than 30% of the contralateral true cord is involved and whether thyroid cartilage invasion is present. Thyroid cartilage invasion requires a surgical approach to the lesion. Greater than 30% involvement of the contralateral true cord obviates vertical hemilaryngectomy in some institutions, although "extended" conservation surgery is possible in experienced hands.

T_2 lesions may spread infraglottically to a point that threatens the cricoid cartilage. Since the cricoid serves as the foundation for all reconstructive surgery, this is a critical management issue. Previous authors and investigators have justifiably placed much emphasis on relating the amount of infraglottic extension to choices of therapy.[11,12,29,49,58] This was based mainly on measuring the subglottic extent in millimeters as it was depicted on tomograms, laryngograms, or plain films. While such guidelines are useful, it must be remembered that the major issue is the status of the cricoid cartilage. It is certainly true that 10 mm of inferior extension in the anterior infraglottic space does not threaten the cricoid; however, this same amount of spread downward in the midcoronal plane or more posteriorly puts the tumor onto the cricoid cartilage. A CT scan images tumor bulk relative to the cricoid cartilage. This is done in the axial plane, which seems to be the optimal one for defining these changes. Under these circumstances the surgeon can be forewarned of the most subtle caudal extension that might limit the success of vertical hemilaryngectomy.

Cephalad extension of T_2 glottic lesions may occur within the paralaryngeal space. Some of this spread may be beneath intact mucosa. A CT scan can certainly show the extent of a lesion relative to the false cord and ventricle, although the uninitiated are sometimes insecure at making this determination from axial sections. Coronal reformations may be used to increase confidence levels or one may revert to conventional studies until sufficient experience with CT is acquired to be confident in this regard. Generally, radiation therapy is preferred, with cure rates of better than 80%, and the option of surgical salvage always remains. Surgery is used when relapse occurs after radiation therapy, and radiation is given after relapse when surgery is the treatment of choice for early lesions.

T_3 glottic tumors may be localized lesions that have invaded the intrinsic laryngeal musculature. They may also be lesions that have spread deeply beyond the limits of any voice conservation surgery. Computed tomography is usually followed by total laryngectomy, followed by full-dose radiation therapy. If N_1 nodes are present, a radical neck dissection would be done as part of the total laryngectomy. A sampling of ipsilateral nodes is done otherwise, and if nodes are found positive, a radical neck dissection follows.

T_4 lesions are massive tumors treated by total laryngectomy combined with radiation. Computed tomography is interesting only to confirm that the lesion is T_4 and to aid in the decision over how the neck should be treated. Neck nodes are often involved and radical neck node dissection en bloc with a primary tumor is often done.

Infraglottic carcinomas. These unusual lesions have a poor prognosis. The infraglottis clinically is relatively silent, difficult to examine, and tumors are usually advanced when the diagnosis is confirmed. Recurrences are frequent, mainly because of lymphatic spread. Computed tomography may be used effectively in that it can show the precise infraglottic extent of the lesion. Spread outside of the larynx through the cricothyroid membrane or spread along the mucosa beyond the inferior margins of the cricoid are both particularly bad prognostically. Treatment for the primary tumor is total laryngectomy combined with radiation.

Supraglottic tumors (Table 7-4). T_1 and T_2 lesions of the suprahyoid (free margin) or infrahyoid (fixed portion) epiglottis may be managed successfully by radiation or surgery.[46,56] A most important issue in lesions of the epiglottis is the status of the pre-epiglottic space. Infiltration of this space almost precludes successful management by radiation therapy. Spread to the pre-epiglottic space is nearly always silent clinically and cannot be accurately shown on other diagnostic imaging examinations unless it is massive.[4,32,34,53] Computed tomography is the examination of choice for determining whether involvement of the pre-epiglottic space is present. Supraglottic laryngectomy should be highly successful in managing patients with such spread but with otherwise limited tumors.

A 3-to-5-mm tumor-free margin relative to the anterior commissure is required for supraglottic laryngectomy.[15,47,56] It is usually not difficult to identify an adequate margin at endoscopy; however, CT may help establish whether one is present in cases that are unclear because of bulky tumors or other unfavorable clinical circumstances. Marginal supraglottic lesions may be managed by partial laryngopharyngectomy, but this is "precision surgery" and requires careful selection of patients.[46] A CT scan can help in the selection of patients for partial laryngopharyngectomy. For example, deep spread across the midline within the paralaryngeal and pre-epiglottic space would require total laryngopharyngectomy. Computed tomography has the potential to refine the selection criteria for the surgical approach to marginal supraglottic carcinomas but has yet to be widely applied and tested in a prospective study.

Carcinomas of both the anterior and marginal supraglottic groups may spread superiorly within the pre-epiglottic space to involve the tongue base. Surgery done

Table 7-4. Treatment Decisions: Supraglottic Larynx

STAGE	SURGERY		RADIATION THERAPY (RT)		CHEMOTHERAPY
I (T_1,N_0,M_0)	Supraglottic partial laryngectomy Spare vocal cord	or	Definitive RT 6000–6500 cGy		NR
II (T_2,N_0,M_0)	Supraglottic laryngectomy and radical neck dissection	and	DefinitiveRT 6500–7000 cGy		NR
III (T_3,N_1,M_0)	Radical laryngectomy	and/or	Definitive RT 6500–7000 cGy		NR
IV (T_4,N_2,N_3,M_0)	Radical laryngectomy plus radical pharyngectomy with reconstructive surgery if possible	and	Post-op RT 6500–7500 cGy		Investigational MAC
Local relapse	RT for surgical relapse		Surgery for RT relapse	and	Investigational MAC
Metastatic (M_1)	NR		Occasionally		Investigational MAC

NR = Not Recommended
MAC = Multiagent Chemotherapy

with curative intent would then need to be total glossectomy and laryngectomy, a difficult operation for most patients to tolerate both emotionally and physically.

When cartilage is invaded, treatment for the primary tumor is a total laryngectomy since it is very difficult to salvage these patients if radiation therapy fails. Radiation therapy, however, is an essential part of the treatment because of the high incidence of stomal recurrences that develop with subglottic extensions; these can be prevented by radiation treatment that includes the tracheal stoma. The surgical specimen needs to be carefully evaluated, particularly when subtotal laryngectomies are done, to determine whether there is residuum or adequate margins and whether radiation therapy is indicated.

T_3 supraglottic tumors depend on whether cartilage invasion is present. Supraglottic tumors are usually not difficult to stage clinically. Computed tomography can confirm the clinical impression of cartilage-involved invasion if necessary, particularly with extensions into the pre-epiglottic space and paralaryngeal spaces. Therapy is usually total laryngectomy combined with radiation therapy, which can be given either preoperatively or postoperatively. If there is any compromise of the airway, a tracheotomy is performed; postoperative irradiation then is given, particularly if one is attempting to avoid laryngectomy.

T_4 supraglottic tumors are usually not difficult to stage clinically. A CT scan can easily confirm the clinical impression if necessary. Therapy is total laryngectomy combined with radiation therapy. The staging of neck nodes in patients with such advanced lesions is probably the most important factor, rather than the extent of the primary tumor. The prognostic and therapeutic implications of cervical nodes were discussed in the chapter on the neck.

Hypopharyngeal carcinoma. The tendency for hypopharyngeal carcinomas to invade deeply and metastasize to lymph nodes frequently has been emphasized in the prior sections. Treatment for cure is usually by radical surgery, at times combined with postoperative irradiation. Radiation treatment is potentially curative only in the most limited lesions. Partial pharyngectomy or laryngopharyngectomy may be attempted in limited lesions. Spread across the midline, into the cricothyroid space or to the postcricoid region would obviate limited surgical approaches. Such spread is well demonstrated on CT scans. A CT scan may demonstrate exolaryngeal spread and cartilage invasion in tumors staged T_2 clinically; such upstaging (T_2 to T_4) might help to avoid treatment failures and needless patient morbidity.

A combined modality approach is generally used for advanced lesions; radiation therapy is used either preoperatively or postoperatively. Chemotherapy is also used for extensive lesions, particularly in investigational protocols. Radiosensitizers have been used in randomized studies with some promise of improved survival.

In summary, CT may be useful in the following situations relative to staging primary tumors in the larynx and hypopharynx:

1. To confirm that the tumor is limited and increase the confidence of the radiation or surgical oncologist that the choice of therapy is likely to be for cure.

2. To help determine whether limited "borderline" lesions would be best suited to radiation or surgical management.
3. To help decide whether radical surgery is more appropriate than conservation surgery or radiation in more advanced but still "borderline" lesions.
4. To help upstage tumors and in doing so perhaps avoid treatment failures, since CT shows deep extension of tumors that is unsuspected from their mucosal presentation.

Regional Nodal Disease

The staging of cervical nodes is an exceedingly important issue in treatment planning prognosis. The accurate staging of necks is certainly desired by most physicians who treat head and neck cancer. It seems that CT has the potential to help in management decisions. These were discussed in detail in the chapter on the neck.

Recurrent Tumor

In the preceding section, the discussion centered on how imaging by CT might help prevent treatment failures. Failures will occur despite the best efforts at diagnosis and management. Some patients are also treated with one mode of therapy (surgery or radiation) in the hope that a recurrence can be salvaged by the other. It then is important that the diagnostic radiologist develop his or her technique to the point where recurrent tumor is noted as early as possible.

Surgery will most often dramatically alter the anatomy at the operative site; however, it is surprising how often the deep tissue planes return to a relatively normal appearance after healing. In general, postoperative scarring does not produce masses or a diffusely infiltrative look in the remaining anatomy. Likewise, radiation, where curative, leaves little trace of "postradiation fibrosis." Certainly some slight thickening of the skin and platysma is often visible, but the tumor bed will most often return to a near normal appearance. Despite this we strongly urge that baseline scans be obtained six to eight weeks after the completion of surgery or radiation treatment. Progressive focal mass lesions are almost uniformly a result of recurrent tumor.[23,36,38] These may occur in the absence of a mucosal lesion; however, the patients are usually symptomatic.[23] Persistent or new pain is a symptom that should not be ignored in a patient at risk of developing a recurrence[23] (Figure 7-11). Investigation by endoscopy and CT is always indicated in these patients, unless there are mitigating clinical considerations.

The follow-up scans should be done about every three to four months at first. The interval may be widened as indicated clinically. These studies always include the primary and nodal sites. If patients have specific complaints, then a careful history will allow one to study the anatomic region that might explain the symptomatology in addition to the regions that are normally included.

With laryngeal carcinomas, persistent edema (beyond three to six months) suggests persistent or recurrent tumor. It may also be due to radiation-induced perichondritis or chondronecrosis. The latter condition can be aggravated by repeated biopsies seeking to sort out this diagnostic dilemma. A CT scan can help in this clinical situation by identifying patterns typical for chondronecrosis or by directing biopsy attempts to focal mass lesions.[36,38]

Failures may also occur in the cervical nodes. These are usually picked up clinically; however, CT has the ability to show them earlier than clinical examination. Moreover, the "woody" texture of the neck after radiotherapy or the scarring after surgery often make the clinical evaluation of the neck in these patients less than satisfactory (Figure 7-12).[56]

Radiotherapy, surgery, chemotherapy, and immunotherapy are used to salvage patients with recurrent tumor. The choices are based on the form of previous therapy used, extent of recurrent tumor, prognosis, and the general health and wishes of the patient. The permutations and combinations are therefore myriad; however, some specific comments are in order.

1. Computed tomography can indicate at times that "treatment for cure" is inadvisable and only palliative measures should be undertaken. For instance, involvement of the retropharyngeal nodes or recurrence of neck disease with evidence of carotid fixation is unlikely to be cured by any means. In primary tumor, recurrences that spread to the tongue base and postcricoid region or lower may indicate noncurability (Figures 7-10, 7-11).
2. If extensive bone or cartilage invasion has occurred, it is unlikely that radiation alone will be curative.
3. In the setting of chondronecrosis versus recurrent tumor, CT may indicate that the status of the laryngeal skeleton is so bad that laryngectomy is indicated whether or not tumor is present.[21,35,38]

IMPACT OF NEW TECHNOLOGY

There is little role for CT as a screening test for carcinomas of the larynx and hypopharynx. On occasion it will discover an otherwise inapparent lesion that is responsible for an "occult" cervical metastasis. It can, therefore, be used in searching for unknown primaries with the hope of earlier diagnosis of such lesions.

Computed tomography is more often used to stage known primary tumors. On most occasions it confirms the clinical impression of the extent of the tumor; on others it upstages the primary. In this regard it has the potential to reduce treatment failures resulting from the

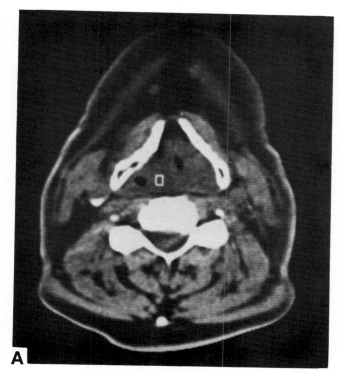

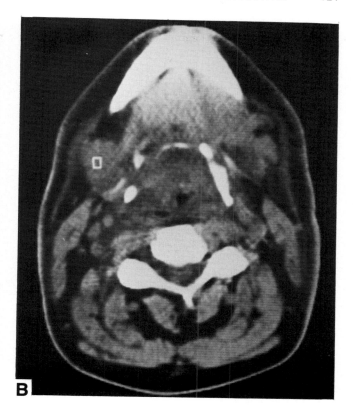

FIG. 7-11. Patient after radiation therapy for marginal supraglottic carcinoma and related bilateral cervical adenopathy. (A) Section through the low supraglottic larynx shows diffuse, mainly posterior, soft tissue swelling, most suggestive of edema. (B) A diffuse increased density obliterates the normal fatty density of the upper pre-epiglottic space. In the absence of frank chondronecrosis, such widespread abnormality suggests recurrent tumor. (C) A recurrent tumor mass extensively involves the tongue base and the floor of the mouth (arrowheads). Note that on all scans the fairly prominent pretherapy adenopathy has completely regressed, leaving the carotid sheath region relatively normal. Also note the thickening of the subcutaneous tissues and platysma, a normal finding after radiotherapy.

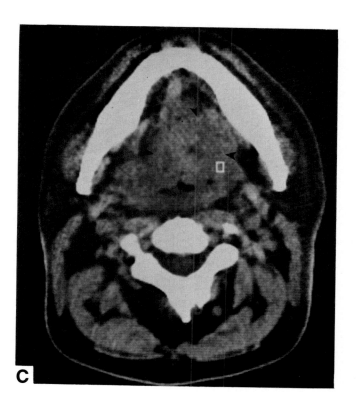

discovery of unsuspected deep spread. The impact of this on survival and morbidity statistics has not been studied to date.

Computed tomography can prove very valuable in staging cervical adenopathy. It can be no worse than the physical examination and promises to be better. Computed tomography should lend an objectivity to the staging of cervical metastatic disease that is not available with physical examination; this can only help provide a more rational basis for therapy. Again, the impact on survival statistics and the potential for reducing morbidity must be studied in a systematic way. Our preliminary experience is very encouraging in this regard (see neck chapter).

Magnetic resonance imaging can only improve on what CT has done. The studies may be complementary, or MRI may replace CT as the oncologic imaging tool

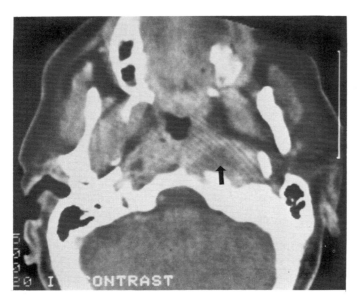

FIG. 7-12. Patient with history of prior radiation therapy and laryngopharyngectomy for pyriform sinus carcinoma. The chief complaint was upper neck pain for about six months; physical examination was negative for evidence of recurrence. The CT scan shows a necrotic retropharyngeal nodal metastasis.

of choice. Things can only improve with the coming of this exciting new imaging tool, since it promises to offer simple multiplanar imaging and perhaps higher sensitivity to altered normal tissue. Most exciting, and most speculative, is the possibility of MRI offering greater specificity than CT because of its potential to characterize tissue by signals other than that from the hydrogen nucleus. T1 and T2 values for hydrogen nuclei are unlikely to prove specific for tumor; however, this question will be answered in the next several years.

REFERENCES

1. Abramson, A. L., Parisier, S. C., Zamansky, M. J.: Distant metastases from carcinoma of the larynx. *Laryngoscope* **81**:1503, 1971.
2. Alonson, J. M.: Metastasis of laryngeal and hypopharyngeal carcinoma. *Acta Orolaryngol.* **64**:353, 1967.
3. American Joint Committee on Cancer: *Manual for Staging of Cancer.* 2nd ed. Beahrs, O. H., and Myers, M. H. (Eds.). Philadelphia, J. B. Lippincott, 1983, pp. 31–42.
4. Archer, C. R., Sagel, S. S., Yeager, V. L., Martin, S., Friedman, W. H.: Staging of carcinoma of the larynx. Comparative accuracy of CT and laryngology. *A.J.R.* **136**:571–575, 1981.
5. Archer, C. R., Yeager, V. L., Herbold, D. R.: Computed tomography vs. histology of laryngeal cancer: Their value in predicting laryngeal cartilage invasion. *Laryngoscope* **93**:140–147, 1983.
6. Archer, C. R., Yeager, V. L., Herbold, D. R.: Improved diagnostic accuracy in the TNM staging of laryngeal cancer using a new definition of regions based on computed tomography. *J. Comput. Assist. Tomogr.* **7**:610–617, 1983.
7. Archer, C. R., Yeager, V. L., Herbold, D. R.: Improved diagnostic accuracy in laryngeal cancer using a new classification based on computed tomography. *Cancer* **53**:44–47, 1984.
8. Baclesse, F.: Carcinoma of the larynx. *Br. J. Radiol.* (Suppl.) **3**:1, 1949.
9. Batsakis, J. G.: *Tumors of the Head and Neck: Clinical and Pathological Considerations.* 2nd ed. Baltimore, Williams & Wilkins, 1982.
10. Bauer, W. C.: Varieties of squamous carcinoma—biologic behavior. *Radiat. Ther. Oncol.* **9**:164, 1974.
11. Biller, J. J., Barnhill, F. R. Jr., Ogura, H. H., Perez, C. A.: Hemilaryngectomy following radiation failure for carcinoma of the vocal cord. *Laryngoscope* **80**:249, 1970.
12. Biller, H. J., Ogura, J. H., Pratt, L. L.: Hemilaryngectomy for T$_2$ glottic cancers. *Arch. Otolaryngol.* **93**:238, 1971.
13. Bryce, P. D.: The laryngeal subglottis. *J. Laryngol. Otol.* **89**:667–685, 1975.
14. Cachin, Y., Sancho-Garnier, H., Micheau, C., Marandas, P.: Nodal metastases from carcinoma of the oropharynx. *Otolaryngol. Clin. North Am.* **12**:145–154, 1979.
15. Calcaterra, T. C.: Supraglottic laryngectomy with preservation of laryngeal function. *Am. J. Surg.* **37**:393, 1970.
16. Cunningham, M. P., Catlin, D.: Cancer of the pharyngeal wall. *Cancer* **20**:1859, 1967.
17. Eisbeck, K. J., Krause, C. J.: Carcinoma of the pyriform sinus. A comparison of treatment modalities. *Laryngoscope* **87**:1904, 1977.
18. Ferlito, A.: Histological classification of larynx and hypopharynx cancers and their clinical implications. Pathologic aspects of 2052 malignant neoplasms diagnosed at the ORL Department of Padua University from 1966 to 1976. *Acta. Otolaryngol.* (Suppl. 342), 1976.
19. Ferlito, A., Antonutto, G., Silvestri, F.: Histological appearance and nuclear DNA content of verrucous carcinoma of the larynx. *ORL* **38**:65, 1976.
20. Fletcher, G. H., Goepfert, H.: Larynx and pyriform sinus. In *Textbook of Radiotherapy*, 3rd ed. Fletcher, G. H. (Ed.). Philadelphia, Lea & Febiger, 1980.
21. Gamsu, G., Webb, W. R., Shallit, J. B., Moss, A. A.: Computed tomography in carcinoma of the larynx and pyriform sinus—the value of phonation CT. *A.J.R.* **136**:577–584, 1981.
22. Gregor, R. T., Lloyd, G. A. S., Michaels, L.: Computed tomography of the larynx: A clinical and pathologic study. *Head Neck Surg.* **3**:284–296, 1981.
23. Harnsberger, H. R., Mancuso, A. A., Muraki, A.: Computed tomography evaluation of recurrent and residual tumors of the upper aerodigestive tract and neck. *Radiology* **149**:503–509, 1983.
24. Harrison, D. F. N.: The pathology and management of subglottic cancer. *Ann. Otol. Rhinol. Laryngol.* **80**:6, 1971.
25. Harwood, A. R., Hawkins, N. V., Rider, W. D., Bryce, D. P.: Radiotherapy of early glottic cancer. I. *Int. J. Radiat. Oncol. Biol. Phys.* **5**:473–476, 1975.
26. Hawkins, N. V.: VIII. The treatment of glottic carcinoma: An analysis of 800 cases. *Laryngoscope* **85**:1485–1493, 1975.
27. Horowitz, B. L., Woodson, G. E., Bryan, R. N.: CT of laryngeal tumors. *Radiol. Clin. North Am.* **22**:265–279, 1984.
28. Jakobsson, P. A.: Histologic grading of malignancy and prognosis in glottic carcinoma of the larynx. *Can. J. Otolaryngol.* **4**:885, 1975.
29. Jesse, R. H., Lindberg, R. D., Horiot, J-C.: Vocal cord cancer with anterior commissure extension: Choice of treatment. *Am. J. Surg.* **122**:437, 1971.
30. Kashima, H. K.: The characteristics of laryngeal cancer correlating with cervical lymph node metastasis. *Can. J. Otolaryngol.* **4**:893, 1975.
31. Kirchner, J. A.: One hundred laryngeal cancers studied by serial section. *Ann. Otol. Rhinol. Laryngol.* **78**:689, 1969.
32. Larsson, S., Mancuso, A. A., Hoover, L., Hanafee, W. N.: Differentiation of pyriform sinus cancer from supraglottic laryngeal cancer by computed tomography. *Radiology* **141**:427–432, 1981.
33. Mafee, M. F., Schild, J. A., Valvassori, G. E., Capek, V.: Computed tomography of the larynx: Correlation with anatomic and pathologic

studies in cases of laryngeal carcinoma. *Radiology* 147:123–128, 1983.

34. Mancuso, A. A., Hanafee, W. N.: A comparative evaluation of computed tomography and laryngography. *Radiology* 133:131–138, 1979.
35. Mancuso, A. A., Hanafee, W. N.: *Computed Tomography of the Head and Neck.* Baltimore, Williams & Wilkins, 1982.
36. Mancuso, A. A., Hanafee, W. N.: Computed tomography of the injured larynx. *Radiology* 133:139–144, 1979.
37. Mancuso, A. A., Hanafee, W. N.: Elusive head and neck tumors beneath intact mucosa. *Laryngoscope* 93:133–139, 1983.
38. Mancuso, A. A., Harnsberger, H. R., Hanafee, W. N.: The post radiation larynx and neck. In preparation.
39. Mancuso, A. A., Tamakawa, Y., Hanafee, W. N.: CT of the fixed vocal cord. *A.J.R.* 135:529–534, 1980.
40. Martensson, B.: Aspects on treatment of cancer of the larynx. *Ann. Otol. Rhinol. Laryngol.* 76:313, 1967.
41. Martensson, B.: Transconioscopy in cancer of the larynx. *Acta Otolaryngol.* (suppl) 224:476, 1967.
42. McGavran, M. H., Bauer, W. C., Spjut, H. J., Ogura, J. H.: Carcinoma of the pyriform sinus: The results of radical surgery. *Arch. Otolaryngol.* 78:826, 1963.
43. Million, R. R., Cassisi, N. J., Wittes, R. E.: Cancer in the head and neck. In *Cancer—Principles and Practice of Oncology.* DeVita, V. T., Jr., Hellman, S., Rosenberg, S. A. (Eds.). Philadelphia, J. B. Lippincott, 1982, pp. 301–395.
44. Ogura, J. H.: Cancer of the hypopharynx and larynx. *Am. J. Med. Sci.* 244:501, 1962.
45. Ogura, J. H., Biller, J. H.: Conservative surgery in carcinomas of the head and neck. *Otolaryngol. Clin. North Am.* 1:641, 1969.
46. Ogura, J. H., Sessions, D. G., Spector, G. J.: Conservation surgery for epidermoid carcinoma of the supraglottic larynx. *Laryngoscope* 85:1808, 1975.
47. Ogura, J. H., Spector, G. J., Sessions, D. G.: Conservation surgery for epidermoid carcinoma of the marginal area (aryepiglottic fold extension). *Laryngoscope* 85:1801, 1975.
48. Olofsson, J., van Nostrand, A. W. P.: Growth and spread of laryngeal and hypopharyngeal carcinoma with reflections on effective preoperative radiation. 139 cases studied by whole organ serial sectioning. *Acta Otolaryngol.* (suppl. 308):1–84, 1973.
49. Olofsson, J., Williams, G. T., Rider, W. D., Bryce, D. P.: Anterior commissure carcinoma: Primary treatment with radiotherapy in 57 patients. *Arch. Otolaryngol.* 95:230, 1972.
50. Pressman, J., Simon, M., Morell, C.: Anatomic studies related to the dissemination of cancers of the larynx. *Am. Acad. Opthalmol. Otolaryngol. Trans.* 64:628–638, 1960.
51. Reid, M. H.: Laryngeal carcinoma: High-resolution computed tomography and thick anatomic sections. *Radiology* 151:689–696, 1984.
52. Rouvier, H.: *Anatomy of the Human Lymphatic System.* Ann Arbor, Edward Brothers, 1938.
53. Sagel, S. S., Aufderheide, J. F., Aronberg, D. J.: High resolution computed tomography in the staging of carcinoma of the larynx. *Laryngoscope* 90:292–300, 1981.
54. Schaefer, S. D., Merkel, M., Burns, D. K., Close, L. G.: Computed tomography of upper aerodigestive tract squamous cell carcinoma. Assessment following induction chemotherapy. *Arch. Otolaryngol.* 110:236–240, 1984.
55. Silverman, P. M., Bossen, E. H., Fisher, S. R., Cole, T. B., Korobkin, M., Halvorsen, R. A.: Carcinoma of the larynx and hypopharynx: Computed tomographic-histopathologic correlations. *Radiology* 151:697–702, 1984.
56. Som, M. L.: Conservative surgery for carcinoma of the supraglottis. *J. Laryngol. Otol.* 84:655, 1970.
57. Som, M. L., Nussbaum, M.: Surgical therapy of carcinoma of the hypopharynx and cervical esophagus. *Otolaryngol. Clin. North Am.* 2:631, 1969.
58. Som, M. L., Silver, C. E.: The anterior commissure technique of partial laryngectomy. *Arch. Otolaryngol.* 87:138, 1968.
59. Spiro, R. H., Alfonso, A. E., Farr, H. W., Strong, E. W.: Cervical nodal metastasis from epidermoid carcinoma of the oral cavity and oropharynx. A critical assessment of current staging. *Am. J. Surg.* 128:562, 1974.
60. Tucker, G. F.: The anatomy of laryngeal cancer. *Can. J. Otolaryngol.* 3:417–431, 1974.
61. Vermund, H.: Role of radiotherapy in cancer of the larynx as related to the TNM system of staging. A review. *Cancer* 25:485, 1970.
62. Zagars, G., Norante, J. D.: Head and neck tumors. In *Clinical Oncology for Medical Students and Physicians: A Multidisciplinary Approach,* 6th ed. Rubin, P. (Ed.). New York, American Cancer Society, 1983, pp. 230–261.

8 MAJOR SALIVARY GLANDS

Anthony A. Mancuso

Salivary gland tumors account for less than 3% of all head and neck neoplasms.[1,18] About 75% to 85% of these affect the parotid gland. Fortunately, the majority of tumors of the parotid gland are benign. Depending upon the series, anywhere from approximately 35% to 70% of parotid tumors will be benign.[1] Most studies report an incidence of benign histologic diagnoses for parotid masses of well over 50%.[1] The submandibular gland, on the other hand, has an approximately equal incidence of benign and malignant neoplasms.[1] Submandibular gland tumors account for approximately 10% of all salivary gland neoplasms.[1] Consideration of survival statistics adds little to the general discussion of salivary gland neoplasms. Cure rates are highly variable depending upon the histologic type of the tumors. Recurrences notoriously occur beyond five-year follow-up. There is at least a 27% overall recurrence rate in patients with carcinomas involving the parotid gland.[10] This tendency to recur is increased to 60% in patients with advanced lesions. The tendency for local recurrence is even higher in submandibular gland malignancies. Overall, these tumors seem to behave in a biologically more aggressive manner than do the parotid lesions of similar histologic type.

Throughout this chapter we will deal with two important features of treatment of malignant tumors of the parotid and submandibular gland: (1) the lack of a satisfactory means of staging these lesions, and (2) the all-important treatment considerations relative to the facial nerve in parotid gland malignancies.[12] The imaging physician and the clinician should also consider that many suspected parotid mass lesions turn out to arise from structures extrinsic to the gland. We will discuss in detail the sources of such mass lesions as well as how CT can be used to differentiate these from intrinsic lesions in the parotid and submandibular glands (Figure 8-1).

Computed tomography and, perhaps in the near future, magnetic resonance imaging (MRI) will provide us with a means to diagnose these tumors earlier. This is especially true when studies are used in situations such as unexplained peripheral seventh nerve paralysis or in the early screening of patients with parotid or periparotid masses. Unfortunately, it is usually patient delay that leads to late diagnosis of palpable mass lesions in this region, and there is little that any imaging study can do to reduce this factor.

TUMOR BEHAVIOR AND PATHOLOGY

Unlike the other regions of the head and neck, where the cell type is squamous cell in about 80% to 90% of the cases, the histopathologic types of malignancies affecting the parotid gland are varied. There are several possible tissues of origin for these malignancies including acinar cells, which give rise to acinous cell carcinomas; the striated duct cells, which give rise to the oncocytic tumors; the excretory duct cells, which give rise to squamous cell carcinomas and mucoepidermoid carcinomas, with the remaining adenomas and adenocarcinomas

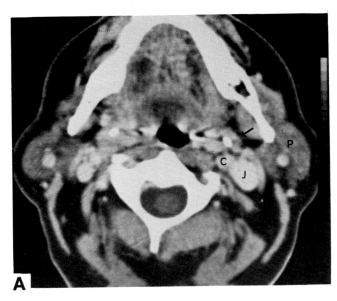

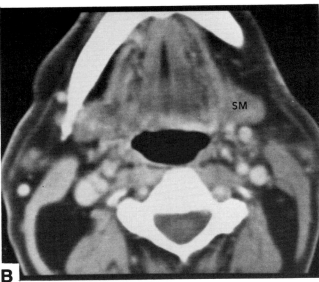

FIG. 8-1. Normal major salivary glands. (A) The mixed fatty tissue density of the parotid (P) differs from surrounding muscle planes and enhanced vascular structures. Masses in the parotid region may arise from the gland itself, the parapharyngeal space (arrow), the carotid sheath (C = carotid, J = jugular), the mandible, surrounding lymph nodes, or rarely, the cervical spine. (B) The normal submandibular gland (SM) is of a homogeneous density that is approximately the same as that of surrounding muscles. Masses in the submandibular region almost always arise from the gland or surrounding lymph nodes. Branchial cleft cysts and other masses are unusual.

duct reserve cells and the intercalated duct reserve cells.[1] This so-called "bicellular theory of origin" is supported by both light microscopic and electron microscopic studies.[14,23] Regardless of the theories concerning specific cells of origin, one must consider the different histologic types, since they occur in different age groups and manifest somewhat different growth characteristics. In a slight departure from the format of the other head and neck chapters, both the patterns of spread and histopathologic considerations will be discussed under individual tumor type.

Mixed Tumors

Histopathologically, two types of cells are generally found in mixed tumors: those of epithelial origin and those of myoepithelial origin. The relative content of these types of cells varies along a broad spectrum. Two types of malignant mixed tumors exist. Carcinoma ex pleomorphic adenomas are carcinomas that arise in mixed tumors. These are predominantly epithelial malignancies that are capable of assuming any epithelial subtype, usually a ductal carcinoma.[1] If metastases occur, only the carcinoma is expressed.[1] This is the most common variety of "malignant mixed tumor." A truly malignant mixed tumor is uncommon. This situation is characterized by unexplainable metastases that occur from a histologically benign mixed tumor. The other circumstance may be where the epithelial and supportive elements are frankly malignant and metastasize together. In the latter instance the neoplasm should be considered a carcinosarcoma.[1] It should be emphasized that these are very rare lesions and are mentioned only to distinguish them from the more common circumstance of the carcinoma arising in an otherwise benign-appearing mixed tumor.

In patients with carcinoma ex pleomorphic adenomas, the malignancy most often arises in a lesion that has been present for 10 to 15 years.[1] The patient may or may not have had recurrent tumor. Typically there will be a history of recent rapid enlargement. If the patient complains of pain or facial nerve paralysis, the tumor is almost certainly malignant. Perineural invasion is common in such circumstances.[19] In the appropriate clinical setting, the diagnosis of a malignant tumor might be suspected clinically but it requires histologic confirmation. The risk of "malignant transformation" seems to only be directly correlated with the amount of time that the tumor is present.[1,19]

In the past many mixed tumors were considered to be malignant because of their tendency to recur. Subsequently this was found to be mainly the result of incomplete excision of a benign mixed tumor. The occasional occurrence of a rapidly disseminating malignancy following years of quiescence seems to confirm malignant behavior. However, from the prior discussion it should be

arising from the intercalated duct cells.[1] An alternative scheme proposed by Batsakis simplifies the theories of cell origin for these neoplasms. He suggests that we consider two basic groups of cells, the stem groups from which all of the more differentiated cell types found in the salivary glands arise. These include the excretory

clear that both types of "malignant mixed tumors" are unusual circumstances occurring in the clinical setting outlined above.

While the absolute diagnosis of malignancy requires careful histologic examination, some of the growth characteristics of this tumor in its malignant form can lead to increased suspicion of a malignancy as observed on imaging studies (Figure 8-2). It is not unusual to observe an encapsulated malignant tumor, but disruption or abnormally prominent bulges in the capsule suggest more aggressive behavior. Areas of necrosis or hemorrhage within the tumor bed should also be interpreted as suspicious of malignancy. Any imaging study is only a gross estimation of these behavioral characteristics, and a lack of these findings should not lead to a false sense of security if malignancy is suspected on clinical grounds.

It is exceedingly important to recognize this entity mainly because of its high rates of recurrence and metastasis. One study reports an incidence of cervical metastases of 25% and of distant metastases of at least 32%.[29] The lungs, brain, and bone are the most likely sites of distant metastases. It is interesting that the distant metastatic spread occurs at a higher rate than regional lymph node metastases. This indicates that persistent tumors of the major salivary glands favor the hematogenous rather than the lymphogenous route of metastasis. Overall, a patient with a carcinoma arising in a pleomorphic adenoma has a very poor prognosis compared with patients with the other malignancies that affect the salivary glands. Five-year cure rates are in the range of 40% to 50%.[16,28]

Adenoid Cystic Carcinomas

Adenoid cystic carcinomas are malignant epithelial tumors that account for approximately 2% to 5% of all tumors in the parotid gland.[1] In the submandibular gland adenoid cystic carcinomas are the most common malignancy.[1]

While this tumor appears to be grossly well delimited, it is not encapsulated. The growth pattern of this tumor is basically infiltrative. Perineural growth and extension is a very common mode of spread in this tumor; this tendency and its infiltrative growth pattern make attempts at cure very frustrating, and recurrences are very common (Figure 8-3). In general, clinicians treating this lesion are quite aware of these growth tendencies; however, the tumor persists in eluding adequate resection because of its somewhat peculiar mode of spread.

In the short term the prognosis is quite good. In the parotid gland, nearly 75% of patients will be alive five years after diagnosis and initial treatment.[2] One must consider 10-year and 15-year survival rates in order to more fully understand the devastating nature of this particular tumor. Ten-year cure rates will be approximately 29% and 20-year cure rates 13%.[2,26] Overall, it is likely that a patient who develops adenoid cystic carcinoma will die of that disease at 15 years from the initial verification of its presence. Long-term survival prospects are even more pessimistic for submandibular and minor salivary gland origins.

Extension by lymphatic spread is unusual in this lesion and is more likely the result of direct invasion of a node rather than spread along the lymph channels. About 40% of patients will eventually manifest regional or distant metastatic disease.[1] These most often occur in the lungs.

Mucoepidermoid Carcinomas

Mucoepidermoid tumors account for approximately 3% to 9% of all salivary gland tumors.[1] They most commonly arise in the parotid gland; however, the relative incidence of this tumor is higher in the minor salivary glands. Overall, this is the most frequent malignant tumor arising in the salivary tissue.

These tumors demonstrate a very wide range of behavior, from a very nonaggressive, almost benign course, to a very aggressive and rapidly progressive one. In gross morphologic terms, evidence of an ill-defined or infiltrating margin or necrosis would suggest the tumor is of a more aggressive nature. This tumor is characteristically nonencapsulated (Figure 8-4).

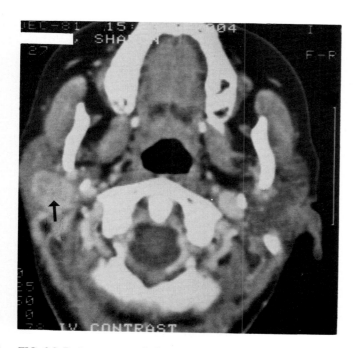

FIG. 8-2. Patient suspected clinically of having a parapharyngeal or deep lobe parotid mass. Fairly homogeneous, well-circumscribed mass (arrow) in the deep portion of the superficial lobe (i.e., in the plane of the facial nerve) is typical of a benign mixed tumor. Tumors in this location typically displace the facial nerve caudally and medially. Surgery confirmed the presence of a benign mixed tumor with downward and medial displacement of the facial nerve.

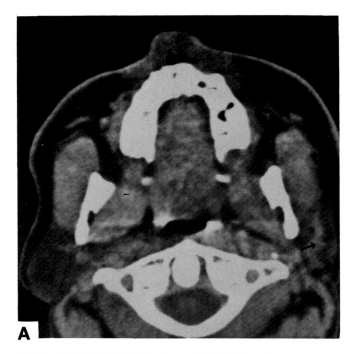

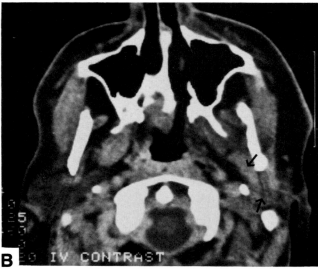

FIG. 8-3. Patient with a 1½-year history of facial weakness first, then pain in the second and third division distributions of the trigeminal nerve. (A) An irregular infiltrating mass (arrow) follows the course of the facial nerve. Compare with the normal side. (B) The entire parotid bed, including the deep lobe is replaced by tumor (arrows). The tumor reached the fifth nerve by this spread deep to the mandible and into the infratemporal fossa.

Unfortunately, even though malignant, these tumors may grow without any clinical signs or symptoms other than a persistent swelling or "lump" in the parotid tissue. With invasion of surrounding soft tissues, fixation to these tissues may occur. Eventually, perineural invasion causes facial pain or weakness. The latter symptoms are ominous and are most often indicative of malignancy

within the parotid gland. Recurrences usually occur within the first postoperative year, and their reported frequency varies. A reasonable figure is probably 30%.[1]

Both regional nodal and distant metastases are fairly frequent. The likelihood of metastasis increases directly with the grade of the primary tumor. High-grade malignancies are said to have a regional nodal metastatic rate of 66%; the rate of distant metastases is 33%.[15,16] These rates are markedly reduced for the low grade malignancies.

Overall survival rates are highly dependent upon the grade of the malignancy. High-grade lesions show a five-year survival of about 40%.[31] The cure rates in the intermediate and high-grade lesions are somewhat stage-dependent in that they are 100%, 65%, and 10% in stages I, II, and III, respectively.[27]

Acinous Cell Carcinomas

Acinous cell carcinomas account for approximately 2.5% to 4% of all tumors of the parotid gland.[1] They are usually not found in other salivary tissue and characteristically are found in patients in their 40s or 50s.

Acinous cell tumors tend to have well-delineated margins and may possess a capsule. Lobulated patterns are more characteristic of recurrent tumors. These have an approximately 3% incidence of bilaterality within the parotid glands.[1]

Some ambiguity over the relationship of the histologic appearance of the lesion and the relationship of the tumor to the host exists. This has caused some confusion over exactly how these tumors should be treated and in predicting outcome.[1] Recurrence rates are quite high if subtotal parotidectomy is chosen for the primary therapy. The range seems to be from 67% to 85%.[1,9] Approximately 10% of these will manifest cervical metastases.[1] Invasion of the facial nerve is not an early finding with these lesions.

As in the other parotid malignancies, survival rates must be considered in longer terms than five years. Overall, five-year survival is 90% and declines to approximately 56% at 20 years.[12] The clinical extent of the lesion is probably the thing that correlates best with ultimate survival rates. In conjunction with such data, determinant "cure" rates of 76%, 63%, and 55% have been reported, respectively.[26]

Adenocarcinomas

Adenocarcinoma represents a group of tumors that cannot be classified under one of the prior glandular cell categories. Some of these are probably carcinomas arising in mixed tumors while others are most likely elements arising in conjunction with adenoid cystic carcinomas. True adenocarcinomas do arise on their own in salivary tissue. The incidence of these in the parotid glands is unclear.[1] The age range at diagnosis is broad, being

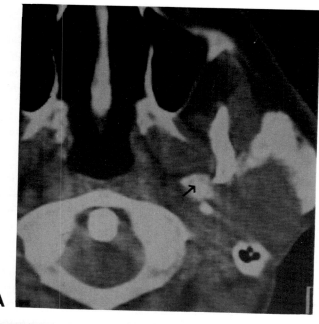

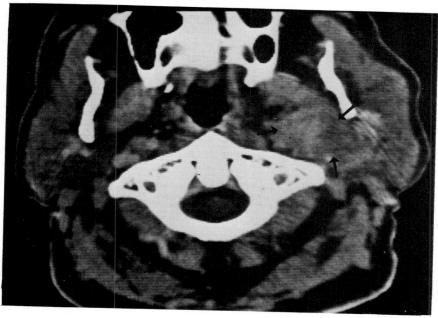

FIG. 8-4. Two patients with mucoepidermoid carcinoma of the parotid. (A) Tumor in the deeper portion of the superficial lobe demonstrated by the older technique of CT sialography. The deep lobe is normal (arrow). (B) On newer scanners CT sialography is almost never required. A deep lobe tumor (arrow) invades the carotid sheath, unmistakable evidence of its aggressive nature. A needle aspiration biopsy confirmed the presence of a mucoepidermoid carcinoma.

anywhere from 20 to 70 years.[1] As with other lesions, the time of appearance of the mass to histologic confirmation of adenocarcinoma is approximately four years. This is probably mainly due to a lack of symptoms associated with early growth.

These tumors have a locally infiltrative growth pattern, and the more invasive tumors tend to have high rates of metastases to regional nodes as well as hematog-

enous spread to bone and lungs. Patients with regional or distant metastases are very likely to die of their disease.[1]

Undifferentiated Carcinomas

Undifferentiated carcinomas are unusual and highly malignant lesions. Some investigators feel that they should not be separated from the more generic classification of adenocarcinoma. These tumors account for from 1% to 4% of all parotid malignancies.[3] They are most frequent in the elderly, but may appear at almost any age. One third of the cases may actually have arisen in patients with longstanding mixed tumors.[13,21] Overall, these tumors have a very aggressive clinical course and poor prognosis.

Primary Squamous Cell Carcinoma of the Parotid Gland

Primary squamous cell carcinoma is so unusual in the parotid gland that one should first consider that the tissue represents metastases to periparotid lymph nodes from a lesion at some other site in the upper aerodigestive tract.[1] The true incidence of these tumors in the parotid gland is difficult to ascertain and reported incidences range from 0% to 3.4%.[1]

Local recurrence and regional lymph node metastases are the usual natural history in these patients. Survival seems to be best correlated with initial clinical stage of the disease. Distant metastases are usually not a significant part of the clinical picture.[1]

Lymphoma of the Parotid Gland

Primary lymphoma of the parotid gland is an exceedingly unusual entity. Of course the most usual picture of head and neck lymphoma is that of cervical lymph node enlargement. Extranodal lymphoma alone accounts for a small percentage of primary head and neck tumors. Accepted criteria for diagnosing a primary lymphoma of the salivary gland include: (1) No known lymphoma in extrasalivary tissue; (2) histologic proof that the lymphoma is parenchymal and not restricted to the periparotid and intraparotid lymph nodes; and (3) histologic confirmation that the lesion is truly malignant and not a reactive phenomenon.[1]

Intraglandular lymphoid tissue is present within the parotid glands but is not found in the adult submandibular and sublingual glands.[1] It is most likely that lymphomas within the parotid arise from this intraglandular lymphoid tissue. There is an increased incidence of lymphoproliferative disease in patients with Sjogren's syndrome.[1]

If multiple masses are seen within and around the parotid gland, strong consideration should be given to the fact that this represents multiple enlarged lymph nodes from extraglandular lymphoma. This may be present in the absence of clinical disease elsewhere in the neck.

Many of the masses that develop in the parotid region are not in fact of parotid origin. Metastases to the peri- and intraparotid lymph nodes are not uncommon. These nodes drain the skin of the face and scalp, the lacrimal glands, the sinonasal tract, the nasopharynx, and the oro-pharynx. Lesions, usually squamous cell carcinomas, in any of these locations can produce enlargement of the nodes that must be differentiated from primary tumors in the gland. Metastases from melanomas or nodal enlargement caused by lymphoma are probably the other most frequent causes of metastatic enlargement of these nodal groups.

The paraparotid and intraglandular nodes can also enlarge in response to inflammatory disease within the various sites of drainage. These must be differentiated from enlarged nodes caused by other sources and primary parotid tumors. This is usually done on the basis of the clinical circumstances and imaging studies.

The parotid gland is intimately related to the parapharyngeal space and carotid sheath. Lesions growing in these spaces can therefore displace the gland from its deep aspect, mimicking a parotid mass lesion. Such tumors may arise from the parapharyngeal space, although these are unusual. Other tumors may arise in conjunction with the carotid sheath; these would most likely be neuromas of the cranial nerves or paragangliomas. It is important to differentiate these lesions from those arising in the deep lobe of the parotid glands (Figures 8-1, 8-2).

The parotid gland is also intimately related to the mandible, so that rarely lesions arising from the mandible or masseter hypertrophy will mimic parotid mass lesions.

Similar difficulties are encountered in the submandibular gland, although the range of diagnostic possibilities is more limited than in the parotid. Masses in this region usually are enlarged lymph nodes or submandibular gland masses (Figure 8-5). The differentiation is simply made by imaging studies, although it is often not clear from the physical examination. Occasionally, mass lesions arising from the mandible or other structures of the neck such as branchial cleft cysts are mistakenly diagnosed as being of submandibular gland origin.

CLASSIFICATION AND STAGING

Most authors agree that the staging system used for the salivary gland and parotid lesions in particular is not entirely satisfactory.[1] From the prior section it should be clear how difficult it is to predict the behavior of these tumors and the likelihood of survival even when the histologic type is known. When considering these tumors, therefore, it is of practical importance to study the relationship of the lesion to the facial nerve, its histologic type, and its degree of invasiveness in each patient. The system of classification and staging, even if improved in coming AJC revisions, will probably not be satisfactory.

T_1 lesions are 2 cm or less in diameter (Figure 8-6). They are solitary, freely mobile, and, if the lesion is of the parotid gland, facial nerve function must be intact. A very small percentage of parotid or submandibular gland malignancies appear at this point.

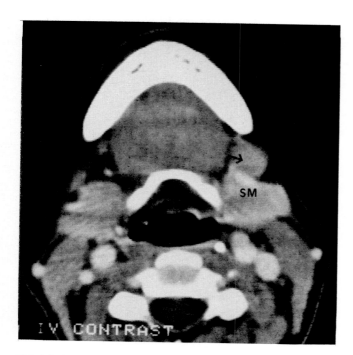

FIG. 8-5. Patient with a submandibular mass: clinical diagnosis of nodal origin versus submandibular gland origin. The CT scan clearly shows a mass (arrow) extrinsic to the gland (SM). The patient therefore was followed closely on antibiotic therapy and the node regressed.

T_2 tumors are between 2 and 4 cm in diameter. They may demonstrate some limited mobility or fixation to the skin. Again, if in the parotid gland the facial nerve must be intact. These must be solitary lesions.

T_3 tumors are between 4 and 6 cm in diameter. Multiple masses may be palpable. This could be due to either associated nodal disease or lobulation of the mass. These may demonstrate evidence of deep fixation or skin ulceration. In parotid lesions, facial nerve dysfunction distinguishes T_2 from T_3 lesions as well as the other criteria described above.

T_4 tumors are massive lesions, more than 6 cm in diameter. They invade the mandible or other adjacent bony structures.

The staging of cervical metastases is the same as that used elsewhere in the head and neck region. This is discussed in detail in the chapter on the neck.

The above staging system reflects the basic patterns of growth as described in the prior section. Tumors grow for a long period of time within the parotid gland except for very high grade tumors, which tend to progress more rapidly. The tumors spread mainly by direct extension. Fixation to adjacent tissues usually first occurs in the subcutaneous fat. Deeper spread takes the lesion to the mandible, the infratemporal fossa and parapharyngeal space (Figures 8-3, 8-4). Fixation to bony structures is not common with these lesions and indicates a far advanced

tumor with little or no hope of long-term survival. This is reflected in the T_4 category.

One of the most important classifications in parotid lesions is the T_2 versus T_3 distinction based on facial nerve dysfunction. All of the malignancies within the parotid gland have a tendency to invade and spread along the course of the nerve. This is an ominous prognostic sign.

Spread of these tumors to the cervical lymph nodes is mainly to the paraparotid and then the deep cervical chain so that the standard classifications of cervical metastases are appropriate; however, it would seem appropriate that some provision be made for distinguishing paraparotid nodal enlargement from that in the deep cervical nodes. Spread to the retropharyngeal nodes is not seen in these malignancies. The nodal disease is, in general, a less important feature of the malignancies of the salivary glands than it is elsewhere in the head and neck. Distant metastases are more usual than nodal spread in most lesions; therefore, in advanced tumors careful staging relative to this issue is indicated.

IMAGING PROCEDURES AND ASSESSMENT

Certainly the imaging study that has been used most often and with the greatest success in evaluating parotid neoplasms has been sialography (Table 8-1). This study is done simply by cannulating the parotid or submandibular ducts and injecting either water soluble or oily contrast medium. Filming may be accomplished either during fluoroscopy or with plain film techniques. Other studies used for evaluating parotid neoplasms include plain films of the mandible and facial structures to exclude bone invasion. For some patients with facial nerve dysfunction, pleuridirectional tomography has been used to assess the integrity of the bony facial canal. In advanced lesions, tomography of the temporal bone has also been used to assess the degree of invasion of the mastoid portion of the temporal bone.

More recently, CT techniques have been applied to the evaluation of parotid and submandibular gland masses. This began in approximately 1977 and 1978, with several investigators nearly simultaneously reporting the possibility that CT-assisted parotid sialography offered more definitive evaluation of the extent of mass lesions than did conventional sialography.[6,24,25,30] Experience between these first reports and in 1982 indicated that CT-assisted sialography was certainly the examination of choice over conventional sialography for almost all parotid mass lesions.[11,32] With the coming of thin section and high resolution techniques, it appears that CT without injection of the parotid or submandibular ducts will be sufficient for studying most parotid mass lesions.[5] This study must be done during the intravenous injection of contrast

Table 8-1. Imaging Modalities for Evaluating Major Salivary Gland Malignancies

MODALITY	STAGING CAPABILITY	BENEFIT/ COST RATIO	RECOMMENDED ROUTINE SCREENING PROCEDURE
Noninvasive			
Chest films	Detect metastases	High	Yes
Plain films of face, mandible	Show bone involvement or other etiology for mass	Low	No
Sialography	Mass intrinsic, extrinsic; Some suggestion of benign v malignant	Low	No
Pleuridirectional tomography	Invasion of facial canal or temporal bone	Fair	No
MRI	Extent of tumor, related adenopathy	?	?
Minimally Invasive CT	Intrinsic v extrinsic to gland. Extent of primary including spread to facial canal or temporal bone, related nodal disease	High	Yes

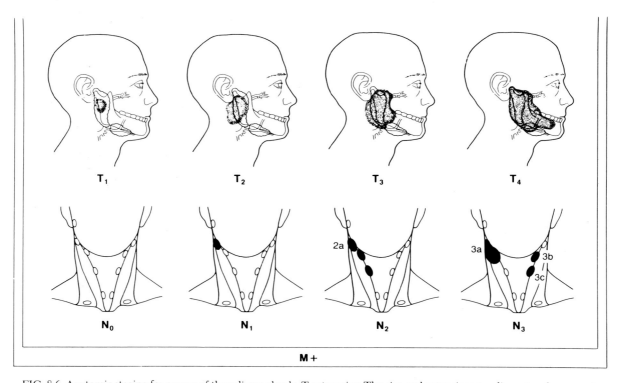

FIG. 8-6. Anatomic staging for cancer of the salivary glands. T categories: The size and extensions to adjuvant and surrounding structures are the key determinants to progression. The size is the same as oral cavity lesions, <2 cm, 2–4 cm, >4 cm, for T_1, T_2, and T_3. Invasion of the facial nerve is T_3, and invasion into mandible, T_4. N categories: The size of the node, its mobility, and the number and location are all factors in staging cervical nodes. The diameters ≤3 cm, 3 cm and 6 cm, and >6 cm were chosen because these are determined more objectively than fixation. Fixation implies adhesion to the carotid artery, and therefore, unresectability. Single and multiple nodes (N_1 v N_2), homolateral and bilateral nodes (N_1, N_2 v N_3) are important factors. Stage grouping: none; one is proposed.

and meticulous attention to optimizing the CT technique. Magnetic resonance imaging may replace CT as the imaging examination of choice for salivary gland masses.

Recommended Method of Study

It is safe to say that CT has replaced conventional sialography as the examination of choice for parotid and submandibular gland lesions (Figure 8-7).[22] The choice of whether the study is done is at present an individual one and based on the available CT technology and experience of the radiologist. From personal experience and that of others in doing CT without injection of the parotid or submandibular ducts, it seems that this technique will be sufficient in most instances.[5] A CT-assisted sialogram is likely to then become a "fall-back study." With modern CT technology the full extent of the lesion and its relationship to the temporal bone and mandible can be shown without the necessity of resorting to plain film or conventional tomography. As in other regions of the head and neck, an assessment of the regional lymph nodes is also possible, although less important in this disease because of its natural history as described in the prior section.

Technique of Examination

A CT-assisted sialogram is performed by injecting the parotid or submandibular duct with water-soluble contrast. Oily contrast medium may also be used. The use of oily contrast has the advantage of allowing delayed scanning; the medium may be injected into the ducts outside of the CT room and the patient brought in and scanned at a later time.

Sections should be approximately 5-mm thick and made at 5-mm increments. The patient should be positioned with the head tilted back and the gantry angled so that the entire parotid bed is studied without interference from dental fillings. This may be accomplished routinely by extending the patient's head approximately 30° and angling the gantry to 20°. If more precise localization is required or if the anatomic landmarks are unfamiliar, then localizing digital radiographs may be used for planning the angle of the sections. It is usually not necessary to go so far as to position the patient for direct coronal sections. Scans begun at approximately the anterior edge of the temporomandibular joint and carried posteriorly will adequately cover the entire parotid bed without interference from metallic artifacts. This off-axis scanning plane also has the advantage of depicting the relationship of the parotid gland to the posterior belly of the digastric muscle. The plane of the digastric muscle is a useful landmark for identifying the plane of the facial nerve. Additionally, this oblique plane identifies the stylomastoid foramen and clearly shows the relationship of tumor mass to the distal most aspect of the

descending facial canal. This scanning plane suffers the disadvantage of being less familiar to most radiologists. Moreover, it is probably less favorable than axial sections for characterizing cervical metastatic disease.

If the study is to be done without injection of the parotid or submandibular ducts then rapid drip infusion of contrast is used. The remainder of the scanning technique remains as described above. It seems unnecessary to do preinfusion scans; however, this point bears further investigation. The exact sensitivity and specificity of a CT study of the salivary glands without simultaneous sialography requires further investigation.

Limitations of CT

Unfortunately, gross morphology does not always correlate with histologic findings, and lesions with a very aggressive appearance on CT scans may turn out to be benign. Well-circumscribed lesions may also prove malignant. Histologic confirmation is necessary in all cases and may be obtained preoperatively by fine needle aspiration to facilitate treatment planning and patient awareness (Figure 8-4B).

Evaluation of facial nerve invasion is difficult. The relationship of the mass to the plane of the facial nerve is a relatively easy thing to show; actual invasion is a matter best left to clinical signs and symptoms and pathologic confirmation. One must also be aware that an intact bony facial canal does not necessarily exclude perineural extension into the portion of the nerve traveling within the temporal bone.

As in other areas, enlarged nodes may be purely "reactive" and normal-sized nodes may contain microscopic tumor; however, CT promises to lend a more rational basis to the evaluation of regional metastases in spite of these limitations. This has been discussed in detail elsewhere. Sometimes a nodal mass may be adherent to the primary tumor, making it as difficult to distinguish the two as it sometimes is on physical examination.

IMAGING STRATEGIES AND DECISIONS

Computed tomography has become the imaging procedure of choice in parotid and submandibular lesions for several reasons. In known tumors it is a method superior to conventional sialography for showing the exact position and extent of the primary mass. It can define the relationship of the mass to the expected position of the facial nerve. In known malignancies, high-resolution and edge-enhancement techniques can be applied to define the limits relative to the temporal bone and descending facial canal at the same time that the mass lesion is studied; this makes a second pleuridirectional tomographic study unnecessary. Again, in known malignancies computed tomography can be used to stage lymph node involvement, in this case the paraparotid and deep cervical lymph node groups.

Early in their course, many malignant lesions produce no significant clinical signs or symptoms that differentiate them from benign mass lesions within the parotid gland. The only reliable signs of malignancy are facial pain or weakness. Fixation of the mass to the surrounding facial structures and the presence of lymph node metastases are strongly suggestive of an aggressive lesion.

Detection

Computed tomography is of great value in screening parotid mass lesions for reasons discussed above. In almost all cases it will be very clear from the study whether a parotid region mass is truly an intrinsic parotid lesion or arises from some other site. A similar screening function is available in the submandibular region, where the differential is usually between enlarged nodes and an intrinsic submandibular mass. To date there are no large series evaluating the use of CT in submandibular gland tumors. My personal experience is limited, but it suggests that CT will be just as useful as it is in the parotid region in this regard.

Patients with peripheral seventh nerve dysfunction often present difficult management and diagnostic dilemmas (Figure 8-3). Surely most of these patients will turn out to have idiopathic seventh nerve palsies. If the cases are atypical for Bell's palsy in any way, then a CT scan might prove valuable to exclude a structural lesion of the parotid or temporal bone that might explain clinical findings. On recent generation scanners these studies may be done at the same sitting.

Staging

The staging of salivary gland lesions is essentially based on three factors: size, degree of fixation, and, in parotid lesions, status of the facial nerve. The probability of nodal metastasis and distant metastases is also an important variable. The AJC has an admittedly preliminary method of classification that was presented in an earlier section of this chapter.

Computed tomography can lend an objectivity to any staging system that is otherwise unavailable. The precise size of the lesion is the simplest data available. This becomes most significant when a tumor is growing in a "dumbbell" fashion through the stylomandibular notch. Only the "tip of the iceberg" may be palpable. Fortunately this occurs in a minority of lesions that arise in the deep lobe or the deep portion of the superficial lobe. If coronal as well as axial sections are obtained, precise tumor volumes may be calculated.

Computed tomography can show the relationship of the tumor to the plane of the facial nerve; however, clinical symptoms are probably a more reliable indicator of perineural extension (Figures 8-2, 8-3, 8-4). A CT scan can also be used to help decide if the tumor has grown in a retrograde manner along the facial nerve to enter the descending facial canal.

The morphology of a mass as seen on a CT scan may provide gross clues concerning its degree of invasiveness. Shaggy irregular margins or central necrosis are sugges-

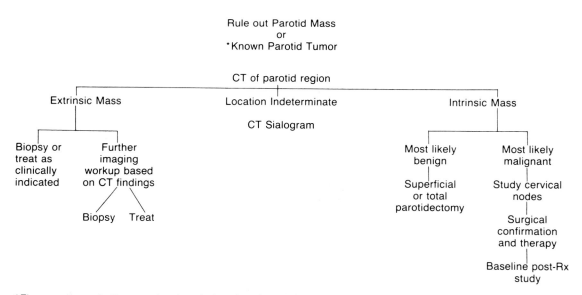

*Fine needle aspiration may be done before imaging evaluation or following CT localization.

FIG. 8-7. Suggested protocol for initial imaging evaluation of known or suspected parotid masses.

tive of an aggressive demeanor (Figures 8-3, 8-4); well-circumscribed margins usually indicate a benign lesion or less aggressive malignancy (Figure 8-2). Lobulated contours may be seen in either benign or malignant lesions.

Computed tomography allows an analysis of the relationship of the tumor margins to the surrounding anatomy. Invasion of the subcutaneous fat may be visible. Spread into surrounding muscles and bony structures can also be demonstrated (Figures 8-3, 8-4). Ultrasound has not been widely used but has been useful for some parotid pathologic entities.[4]

Nodes may be staged according to the criteria discussed in the chapter on the cervical lymph nodes. In the parotid we can add the ability to evaluate the paraparotid group. In both the parotid and submandibular gland regions, CT can help distinguish local (paraparotid and submandibular) nodes from the primary tumor; this is a distinction that is sometimes difficult to make by palpation.

TREATMENT DECISIONS

Most parotid lesions are treated primarily by surgery. This may range anywhere from simple parotidectomy to complete parotidectomy, sacrifice of the facial nerve, or radical temporal bone resection. The surgical plan is based on histopathologic considerations and the extent of the lesion. Radiation is often used in combination with surgery or as the primary treatment for tumors beyond the limits of resection. Chemotherapy may be used as an adjuvant in advanced lesions (Table 8-2). The choice of therapy really does not influence the CT imaging approach to the lesion, whereas the spread of the malignancy as seen on a CT (or MRI) greatly influence the choice of therapy.

The progress of therapy is best evaluated by obtaining a baseline scan six to eight weeks after the completion of treatment. The patient may then be followed at appropriate intervals. Most treatment failures are local;

however, contiguous nodal groups should be studied as deemed appropriate considering the natural history of the specific tumor in question.

The role of radiation therapy is becoming more widely accepted for aggressive cancers of the salivary gland and for recurrent salivary gland tumors that were initially managed surgically.[20] When conservative surgery is used in an attempt to preserve the facial nerve, particularly with tumor morcellation, residual disease is likely. Radiation therapy has proved to be very effective with photon radiation (supervoltage).[17] Unresectable and recurrent salivary gland cancers are very successfully treated with neutron beam therapy; this has been demonstrated particularly well by Catterall in London.[7,8] An RTOG clinical trial has been designed to determine the superiority of neutron compared with photon irradiation.[8] Adenoid cystic carcinomas tend to invade in a perineural fashion and require a very extended field, particularly in tracing the seventh and fifth nerves to their origins intracranially to avoid recurrence intracranially.[33] This failure pathway is very distressing, and patients are difficult to salvage. Multiagent chemotherapy is of limited value and remains largely investigational.

It is also important to note that metastatic lung disease is not hopeless, particularly for the cylindromas of adenoid cystic carcinomas where foci in lung are very slow moving and do not call for chemotherapy. Whole lung irradiation has produced some dramatic results and is worth trying with conservative doses.

IMPACT OF NEW TECHNOLOGY

From prior discussions it should be clear that CT will do little to alter detection rates and survival in patients with parotid and submandibular tumors. Its most useful contribution in this field is the determination of whether a periparotid or submandibular mass is intrinsic or extrinsic to the parotid or submandibular gland, respectively. In these cases, CT can limit unnecessary surgical explo-

Table 8-2. Treatment Decisions: Parotid Gland

STAGE	SURGERY	RADIATION THERAPY	CHEMOTHERAPY
T_1, N_0	Excisional biopsy including either, or both, superficial and deep lobes	Deferred unless relapse	NR
T_2, N_0	Excisional biopsy including either, or both, superficial and deep lobes	Intermediate and high grade 60–65 cGy Unilateral neck nodes 50 cGy	NR
T_3, N_1	Radical resection of parotid Radical resection of neck nodes, unless fixed	65–70 cGy wedge fields or mix of photons and electrons Unilateral neck nodes 50–60 cGy	Investigational MAC
T_4, N_2, N_3	Radical resection of parotid Radical resection of neck nodes, unless fixed	For perineural invasion extend fields to cover nerve paths to base of skull Boost fields to residuum 70 cGy	Investigational MAC
Relapse	Radical resection, if possible If nodes palpable, radical neck dissection	RT 65–70 cGy as for Stage IV disease	Investigational MAC

ration and direct the diagnostic or therapeutic evaluation along the most appropriate line.

Some role in screening and early diagnosis does exist in that "occult" tumors in patients with unexplained facial palsies may be discovered. Computed tomography may also be able to detect recurrences before they are obvious clinically, thereby leading to earlier "salvage" therapy.

Magnetic resonance imaging clearly offers the potential to study major salivary gland tumors in multiple planes and without the small inconvenience caused by dental fillings and the need for intravenous contrast injection. It is doubtful that it will add any more specificity to diagnosis, since the histopathologist is often unable to predict how aggressive a particular tumor will be in a given patient. The relative sensitivity of CT and MRI is a point of lesser interest, since almost all patients have a mass. Magnetic resonance imaging may prove more sensitive for detecting tumors in patients with chronic, progressive facial palsy and no palpable mass demonstrating perineural invasion.

REFERENCES

1. Batsakis, J. G.: *Tumors of the Head and Neck: Clinical and Pathological Considerations.* 2nd ed. Baltimore, Williams & Wilkins, 1982.
2. Blanck, C., Eneroth, C.-M., Jakobsson, P. A.: Adenoid cystic carcinoma of the parotid gland. *Acta Radiol. Scand.* 6:177, 1967.
3. Blanck, C., Eneroth, C.-M., Jakobsson, F., Jakobsson, P. A.: Poorly differentiated solid parotid carcinoma. *Acta Radiol. Scand.* 13:17, 1974.
4. Bruneton, J. N., Sicart, M., Roux, P., Pastaud, P., Nicolau, A., Delorme, G.: Indications for ultrasonography in parotid pathologies. *ROFO* 138:22–24, 1983.
5. Bryan, R. N., Miller, R. H., Ferreyo, R. I.: Computed tomography of the major salivary glands. *A.J.R.* 139:547, 1982.
6. Carter, B., Karmody, C. S.: Computed tomography of the face and neck. *Semin. Roentgenol.* 13:257–266, 1978.
7. Catterall, M.: Fast neutron therapy—Losing sight of the forest by counting the trees. *Int. J. Radiat. Oncol. Biol. Phys.* 7:287–289, 1981.
8. Catterall, M.: The treatment of malignant salivary gland tumors with fast neutrons. *Int. J. Radiat. Oncol. Biol. Phys.* 7:1737–1738, 1981.
9. Chong, G. C., Beahrs, O. H., Woolner, L. B.: Surgical management of acinic cell carcinoma of the parotid gland. *Surg. Gynecol. Obstet.* 138:65, 1974.
10. Conley, J., Hamaker, R. C.: Prognosis of malignant tumors of the parotid gland with facial paralysis. *Arch. Otolaryngol.* 101:39, 1975.
11. Conn, I. G., Wiesenfeld, D., Ferguson, M. M.: The anatomy of the facial nerve in relation to CT/sialography of the parotid gland. *Br. J. Radiol.* 56:901–905, 1983.
12. Eneroth, C.-M., Jakobsson, P. A., Blanck, C.: Acinic cell carcinoma of the parotid gland. *Cancer* 19:1761, 1966.
13. Evans, R. W., Cruickshank, A. H.: *Epithelial Tumors of the Salivary Glands.* Philadelphia, W. B. Saunders, 1970.
14. Eversole, L. R.: Histogenic classification of salivary tumors. *Arch. Pathol.* 92:433, 1971.
15. Foote, F. W. Jr., Frazell, E. L.: Tumors of the major salivary glands. *Cancer* 6:1065, 1953.
16. Frazell, E. L.: Clinical aspects of tumors of the major salivary glands. *Cancer* 7:637, 1954.
17. Guillamnondegui, O., Byers, R. M., duV. Tapely, N.: Malignant tumors of salivary glands. In *Textbook of Radiotherapy*, 3rd ed. Fletcher, G. H. (Ed.). Philadelphia, Lea & Febiger, 1980, pp. 426–443.
18. Leegaard, T., Lindeman, H.: Salivary gland tumors: Clinical picture and treatment. *Acta Otolaryngol.* 263:155, 1970.
19. LiVolsi, V. A., Perzin, K. H.: Malignant mixed tumors arising in salivary glands. I. Carcinomas arising in benign mixed tumors: A clinicopathologic study. *Cancer* 39:2209–2230, 1977.
20. Million, R. R., Cassisi, N. J., Wittes, R. E.: Cancer in the head and neck. In *Cancer—Principles and Practice of Oncology.* DeVita, V. T., Jr., Hellman, S., Rosenberg, S. A. (Eds.). Philadelphia, J. B. Lippincott, 1982.
21. Patey, D. H., Thackray, A. C., Keeling, D. H.: Malignant disease of the parotid. *Br. J. Cancer* 19:712, 1965.
22. Rabinov, K., Kell, T., Jr., Gordon, P. H.: CT of the salivary glands. *Radiol. Clin. North Am.* 22:145–159, 1984.
23. Regezi, J. A., Batsakis, J. G.: Histogenesis of salivary gland neoplasms. *Otolaryngol. Clin. North Am.* 10:297, 1977.
24. Som, P. H., Biller, H. F.: The combined CT-sialogram. A technique to differentiate parotid tumors from extraparotid pharyngomaxillary space tumors. *Ann. Otol. Rhinol. Laryngol.* 85:590–595, 1979.
25. Som, P. H., Biller, H. F.: The combined CT sialogram. *Radiology* 135:387–390, 1980.
26. Spiro, R. H., Huvos, A. G., Strong, E. W.: Adenoid cystic carcinoma of salivary origin. A clinicopathologic study of 242 cases. *Am. J. Surg.* 128:512, 1974.
27. Spiro, R. H., Huvos, A. G., Strong, E. W.: Cancer of the parotid gland. A clinicopathologic study of 288 primary cases. *Am. J. Surg.* 130:452, 1975.
28. Spiro, R. H., Huvos, A. G., Strong, E. W.: Malignant mixed tumor of salivary origin. A clinicopathologic study of 146 cases. *Cancer* 39: 388–396, 1977.
29. Spiro, R. H., Huvos, A. G., Strong, E. W.: Acinic cell carcinoma of salivary origin. A clinicopathologic study of 67 cases. *Cancer* 41: 924, 1978.
30. Stone, D., Mancuso, A. A., Rice, D., Hanafee, W. N.: CT parotid sialography. *Radiology* 138:393–397, 1981.
31. Thorvaldsson, S. E., Beahrs, O. H., Wooner, L. B., Simons, J. N.: Mucoepidermoid tumors of the major salivary glands. *Am. J. Surg.* 120:432, 1970.
32. Wiesenfeld, D., Ferguson, M. M., McMillan, N. C.: Simultaneous computed tomography and sialography of the parotid and submandibular glands. *Br. J. Oral Surg.* 21:268–276, 1983.
33. Zagars, F., Norante, J. D.: Head and neck tumors. In *Clinical Oncology for Medical Students and Physicians: A Multidisciplinary Approach*, 6th ed. Rubin, P. (Ed.). American Cancer Society, 1983, pp. 230–261.

9 THYROID CANCER

Anthony A. Mancuso

The management and prognosis for thyroid carcinomas is very much related to the histologic type of the lesion and its extent when discovered. Papillary and follicular malignancies have long-term survival rates approaching that of an age-matched population when tumors are "occult" or intrathyroidal.[5,11] The mortality rate for intrathyroidal tumors without capsular invasion is probably 2% to 3%.[2,5,6,11] Extrathyroidal spread raises mortality rates to the range of 38% to 50%. Lymph node involvement does not appear to alter survival rates where they are noted and treated at the initial diagnosis.[1] Patients older than 40 years of age at diagnosis are two to three times more likely to die of their disease than those under 40.[6]

Anaplastic carcinoma is a relatively uncommon lesion and has an exceptionally poor prognosis; about 60% of patients will be dead in six months.[2,5,6,11] Medullary carcinoma is again much less common than papillary or follicular carcinoma. The tumor shows a wide variation in growth rate and 20-to-30-year survivals with delayed recurrences are not uncommon.[2,5,6,11] Primary thyroid lymphoma is also variable in its natural history, depending mainly on the histologic type.

Several imaging techniques have been used to evaluate patients with known or suspected thyroid malignancies. Ultrasonography is used mainly for screening purposes; radionuclide imaging is useful for both detecting and staging malignancies; while computed tomography is used infrequently to show the extent of a tumor that is likely to have extended beyond the capsule to involve the trachea or esophagus. The interrelationships of these diagnostic imaging tools vary with the clinical circumstances; these differences will serve as the focus for later discussions.

TUMOR BEHAVIOR AND PATHOLOGY

Histopathology

Pathologic considerations weigh heavily in the prognosis and management of thyroid malignancies. Follicular cells are the most numerous type of the epithelial cells in the thyroid gland. These are probably the cells of origin for 90% of thyroid carcinomas. This cell type gives rise to two differentiated forms of thyroid carcinoma, papillary and follicular.[5] Papillary carcinomas account for 30% to 70% of thyroid carcinomas. These lesions tend to be multifocal and nonencapsulated, and typically invade lymphatics and metastasize to regional lymph nodes. The tumors tend to behave more aggressively in older patients (mean age at diagnosis is 42 years).[9] Extracapsular spread worsens the prognosis.[5] Microscopic papillary carcinoma is not an unusual autopsy finding. Radiation is an important etiologic factor in thyroid cancer, primarily of the papillary variety. The increased incidence of this malignancy in children treated with radiation for thymic and adenoid hyperplasia is a case in point.[4]

Follicular carcinomas account for 10% to 40% of thyroid carcinomas.[5,11] This tumor is typically solitary and encapsulated. It tends to invade veins and metastasize to bone and other distant sites. Prognosis is again worse in older patients. The tumors tend to be more frequent in iodine-deficient areas ("goitrous" areas) and perhaps related to the "drive" of the elevated thyroid stimulating hormone (TSH) levels. Radiation is a definite but less important etiologic factor in this cell type.

The C cell (parafollicular cell) is the other basic epithelial cell of the thyroid. These cells are difficult to identify in humans because they account for less than 1% of the epithelial components.[5] Tumors of these cells probably account for about 10% of thyroid malignancies.[5,6] Medullary carcinomas take their origin from these cells and account for 3% to 10% of thyroid carcinomas in various series. They appear in a very wide age range, with growth rates showing equally wide variation. Although prolonged survivals (20 to 30 years) are not uncommon, the patients usually die of the tumor. Genetic factors appear to be important in the etiology, with up to 20% of cases being genetically mediated.[5] The tumors may be associated with pheochromocytomas or multiple endocrinopathy syndromes.

Undifferentiated carcinomas are usually classified morphologically. Some of the small cell carcinomas appear to, in reality, be malignant lymphomas.[5] Anaplastic carcinomas make up about 5% to 30% of thyroid carcinomas in most series. The disease is rare in patients below 40 years of age and does not occur in children. It is extremely aggressive, and most patients are dead within six months. The tumors seem to be caused by a change in behavior of a pre-existing differentiated carcinoma; it must be emphasized that only a very small percentage of differentiated carcinomas will progress in this way.[5]

Malignant lymphomas account for up to 12% of thyroid malignancies. These are mainly tumors of the elderly, the mean age at diagnosis being 65. Chronic thyroiditis may be an etiologic factor leading to an increased incidence of this tumor.

Patterns of Spread

It should be clear from the prior discussion that the patterns of spread are related to the histologic cell type; however, there are common pathways that are of interest to the physician planning a logical imaging approach to these tumors.

Lesions may be encapsulated or not and contained within the capsule of the thyroid gland. Papillary carcinomas can be multifocal. Tumors may not be palpable; however, most patients have a palpable mass. The primary lesions may extend locally beyond the capsule of the gland, thereby directly invading the trachea, the esophagus, and various other soft structures of the neck surrounding the visceral compartment. Related symptoms include dyspnea, dysphagia, and pain. Posterior and medial spread may involve the recurrent laryngeal nerve, causing a vocal cord paresis.

Lymphatic spread begins in local nodes. The low-er deep cervical nodes are frequently a site of such spread and are accessible to physical examination. Deeper groups surrounding the trachea and esophagus are less amenable to evaluation by palpation. The mediastinal nodes are the next to be involved. Patients with thyroid cancer account for a significant number of cases of cervical metastases of "unknown" origin.

Distant spread is usually to the lungs, skeleton, and brain. Patients, on occasion, have symptoms referable to these sites.

The specific tendencies for individual tumors to demonstrate these patterns of spread were discussed under the histopathology section. In summary, papillary carcinomas tend to progress more slowly than the other types; they grow locally and spread first to the local nodes. Follicular carcinomas are less predictable in time course and tend to disseminate via the bloodstream. Anaplastic carcinomas grow wildly locally with widespread invasion of surrounding structures; nodes may or may not be involved. Medullary carcinomas show local lymphatic spread first and later distant metastases.[5]

CLASSIFICATION AND STAGING

The American Joint Committee on Cancer (AJC) classification and staging of thyroid cancer has been completely revised in the 1983 edition of their *Manual for Staging of Cancer* (Figure 9-1) (Table 9-1). There are major differences between the AJC and International Union Against Cancer (UICC) TN categories and stage groupings. For TNM staging, histopathologic type of lesion and the age of the patient are extremely important determinants for prognosis. Refer to the AJC and UICC manuals for detailed descriptions of the two staging systems.

IMAGING PROCEDURES AND ASSESSMENT

The imaging approach to the thyroid gland varies considerably depending upon the mode of presentation, the extent of the primary lesion, and the likelihood of metastasis. Several radiologic techniques have been used and are currently being used to screen patients for thyroid

---

Table 9-1. Tumor (T) Node (N) Classification* — Thyroid Cancer

T_1	Primary tumor ≤ 3 cm
T_2	Primary tumor > 3 cm
T_3	Multiple, intraglandular
T_4	Fixed/invasion through capsule
N_0	No clinical or histologic evidence of node metastasis
N_1	Clinically or histologically positive nodes

*Post-surgical
From American Joint Committee on Cancer: *Manual for Staging of Cancer*, 2nd ed. Philadelphia, J. B. Lippincott, 1983.

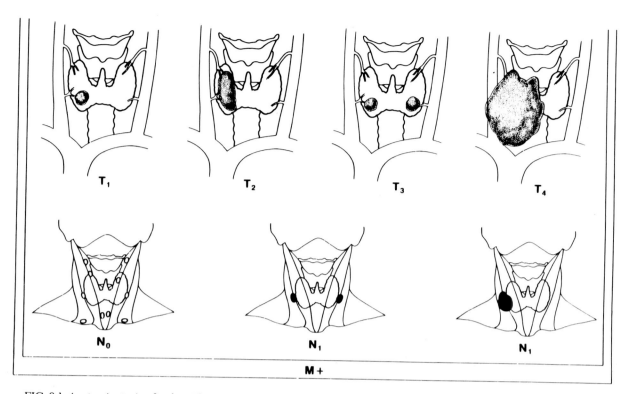

FIG. 9-1. Anatomic staging for thyroid cancer. Tumor (T) classifications: The size (less than or greater than 3 cm) determines T_1 and T_2; multiple nodules are T_3 and fixation is T_4. Node (N) categories: Nodes are either N_0, no clinically or histologically positive nodes, or N_1, clinically or histologically positive nodes. Fixed nodes are not staged differently in the AJC but are N_3 in the UICC system. AJC v UICC classification: The UICC classification is entirely different and has four categories. It is based on single v multiple nodules (T_1 v T_2), homolateral v bilateral (T_2 v T_3), mobility v fixation (T_3 v T_4), and extension beyond capsule. Pathologic (Presurgical) stage (p) TNM is totally different and is based on similar features, but nodules less than 1 cm in size are a critical distinction between pT_1 and pT_2. Modified from AJC.[12]

Table 9-2. Imaging Modalities for Evaluating Carcinoma of the Thyroid

MODALITY	STAGING CAPABILITY	BENEFIT/ COST RATIO	RECOMMENDED ROUTINE STAGING PROCEDURE
Noninvasive			
Chest films	Detect metastases	High	Yes
Bone films	Confirm metastases	Low	No
Ultrasonography	Detect primary, help determine nature of margins and extent	High	No
Radionuclide thyroid scan	Functioning v nonfunctioning solitary thyroid nodule	Fair	No
Radionuclide "total body" ^{131}I scan	For detecting functioning metastases after thyroid ablation	Fair	No
Radionuclide brain, bone, liver scan	For detecting metastases in symptomatic patients or advanced lesions	Low	No
MRI	Extent of primary and regional nodal disease	?	?
Minimally Invasive			
CT	Extent of primary and regional nodal disease	Fair-High*	No

*Depending on histologic type and clincal or surgical estimate of extent of lesion.

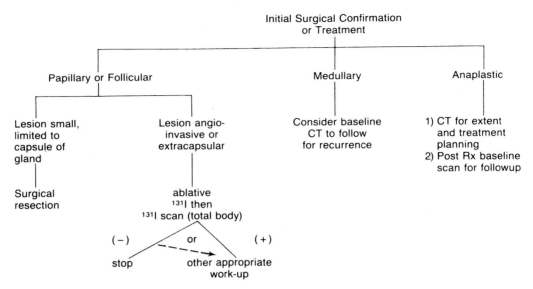

FIG. 9-2. General imaging approach to known thyroid carcinomas.

malignancy and to determine the extent of known malignancies (Table 9-2, Figure 9-2).

Plain films and xeroradiograms of the neck are of limited, if any, value and are probably an unnecessary expenditure of time and money. Thermography has been used for screening, but its lack of specificity makes it, again, an unnecessary additive test. Sometimes a barium swallow study may be used to determine esophageal involvement; however, modern imaging tools (CT) combined with fiberoptic endoscopy are probably more useful in this regard. The assessment of metastatic disease is accomplished with plain films, radionuclide imaging, and CT.

Recommended Methods and Limitations of Study (and Technique)

Radionuclide Imaging. Radionuclide scans have been a mainstay of diagnosis for many years. Imaging may be accomplished with technetium ^{Tc}99m pertechnetate, ^{131}I, or ^{123}I. Current techniques usually employ a gamma camera with a pinhole collimator. In the evaluation of solitary nodules, oblique views and localization and palpation with marking of nodules are routine techniques. This examination will usually show nodules down to 8 mm in size.[9]

In follow-up studies a patient must be off replacement therapy. One to 15 mCi of ^{131}I is administered and scanning is done 72 hours later. A rectilinear scanner or gamma camera may be used. Sometimes adjunctive TSH stimulation is necessary for patients who for some reason do not generate adequate levels of endogenous TSH.

Ultrasonography. Gray scale ultrasonography is of great value in assessing thyroid masses. Static B-mode images are most useful for determining whether solitary masses are solid or cystic (Figure 9-3). With the coming of high resolution real-time ultrasonography, the sensitivity of ultrasonography for identifying nonpalpable lesions has also increased dramatically. One recent study has revealed a 16% incidence of nonpalpable, solid nodules in patients being examined for carotid occlusive disease.[3] The implication is that this technique can be used to screen patients at risk of having thyroid carcinomas.

Adequate examination of the thyroid is easily accomplished using static B-mode equipment, although high resolution real-time ultrasound will likely become the preferred technique. Five-megahertz or 7-MHz transducers are used to scan the thyroid region in the transverse and longitudinal planes. Additional sector scans made in the groove between the sternocleidomastoid and the trachea are useful in selected "suspicious" areas or over palpable masses; these will show the character of the glandular tissue and lesion to best advantage.

Computed Tomography. Computed tomography is not used routinely for evaluating thyroid masses. It is most valuable when looking for the extent of extracapsular spread or fixation of surrounding neck structures by a known malignancy (Figure 9-4). It may also prove a valuable adjunct to staging local and mediastinal lymph node spread.

Computed tomography should be done with contiguous 5-mm sections through the thyroid bed. Contrast should be given by rapid drip infusion. The examination may be carried cephalad or caudally to evaluate neck and mediastinal adenopathy if indicated.

IMAGING STRATEGIES AND DECISIONS

Solitary Thyroid Nodule

A solitary nodule is the most common form of thyroid cancer. Patients with a solitary nodule usually have a radionuclide study; if the nodule is "cold," ultrasound examination may be done to determine whether it is solid or cystic. If the nodule is cystic, aspiration may suffice for pathologic confirmation of benignancy. If solid, ex-

cisional biopsy is usually the preferred method for management. Ultrasound or radionuclide studies may show that more than one nodule is present, in which case the management technique may switch to that for a multinodular goiter.

Patients at Risk of Having Thyroid Malignancy

Ultrasonography may be used to screen populations at risk of having thyroid malignancies. The most obvious of these is that group of patients who received radiation

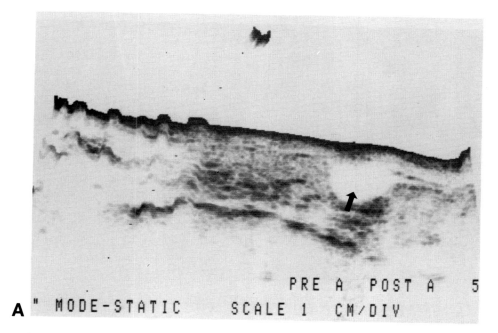

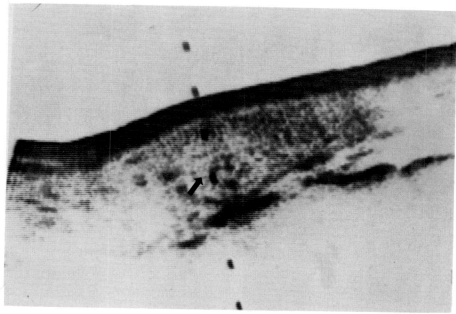

FIG. 9-3. (A) Longitudinal scan through the thyroid bed. The sonolucent area represents a simple thyroid cyst (arrow). (B) Longitudinal scan through the thyroid. A typical solid nodule is seen (arrow). This was a benign adenoma.

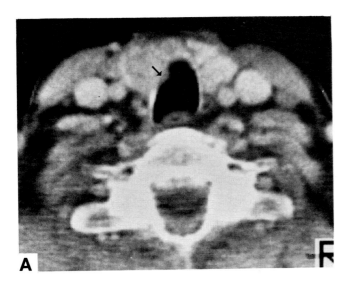

A

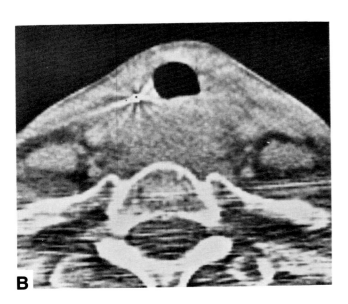

B

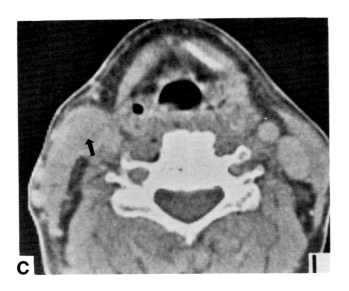

C

to the thyroid region for the treatment of hyperplastic adenoids or thymus glands. High resolution real-time or static B-mode techniques are adequate to survey patients for nonpalpable thyroid nodules. If a nonpalpable nodule is present, needle aspiration may be carried out under ultrasonic guidance.

Patients with Known Thyroid Carcinomas

If the physical examination suggests extracapsular spread, then a CT scan of the thyroid should be done. The extent of the primary relative to the trachea and esophagus can be determined. If nodes are present or strongly suspected, then the CT scan may be extended to include the mediastinal node-bearing areas. The middle to upper neck may also be studied in an effort to demonstrate occult cervical adenopathy.

A chest film should be obtained to search for pulmonary metastases. This may be augmented by conventional or computed tomography. Radionuclide bone scans and skeletal metastatic bone scans can be done to detect osseous metastases. Radionuclide scanning and ultrasonography are used to evaluate patients suspected of harboring liver metastases.

Differentiated thyroid carcinomas may also be studied by ^{131}I scanning. Follow-up of treated patients with differentiated tumors has two basic aims: (1) to determine if the initial surgery or radionuclide therapy has succeeded in ablating the tumor, and (2) to determine if any residual tumor has enough radioiodine uptake to justify further radioiodine therapy. If the normal thyroid tissue has been ablated one may expect that residual local tumor or metastases will pick up the tracer. This has three distinct advantages over other imaging techniques: (1) It is very specific for the diagnosis of recurrence; (2) it can localize metastases anywhere in the body; and (3) it can assess the potential value of radioiodine treatment.

TREATMENT DECISIONS[8,10,12]

Differentiated tumors of the thyroid are treated primarily by surgery. In papillary carcinoma, this will usually be by thyroidectomy or subtotal thyroidectomy.[2,5,6,11] Supportive medical treatment may be aimed at TSH suppression as well as thyroid replacement. Radioiodine irradiation may be used as an ancillary therapeutic measure. Imaging is important in these patients to assess the extent of disease before and after surgery.[131]I scanning in particular may be used to determine if radioiodine therapy is necessary and likely to be successful. If symp-

FIG. 9-4. (A) Early invasion of the trachea (arrow) is present in a patient with a thyroid carcinoma. (B, C) A patient with an anaplastic carcinoma of the thyroid gland has a large retrotracheal mass. Higher in the neck a cervical lymph node is present (arrow). (Reprinted with permission of Williams & Wilkins from *Computed Tomography of the Head and Neck* by Mancuso, A. A., and Hanafee, W. N., 1982, Baltimore.)

tomatology, the extent of the primary, or radioiodine scanning indicate a more extensive tumor is present than was thought to be the case preoperatively, then the metastatic work up must be more aggressive. One should, however, recall that the overwhelming majority of the lesions are localized and highly curable, especially under the age of 40 years.

Limited follicular carcinomas are also treated primarily by surgery.[2,5,6,11] Subtotal thyroidectomy may be used with or without postoperative ablative therapy. Where a follicular carcinoma is angioinvasive, total thyroidectomy and ablative radioiodine therapy are usually the choice of therapy.[4] Ablative therapy is necessary if di-

agnosis and treatment of metastases or remaining local disease with radioiodine is contemplated. If the resection of tumor has been subtotal, then external beam radiation is used as adjunctive treatment along with radioiodine (if tumor is shown to be a functioning one). External beam irradiation is also used for patients who have inoperable lesions or who have local recurrence.[5] Computed tomography may be useful in demonstrating extracapsular spread preoperatively and should probably be used for patients with evidence of partial or complete fixation. A CT scan can also show clinically occult recurrence (Figure 9-5).

A medullary carcinoma of the thyroid is treated by sur-

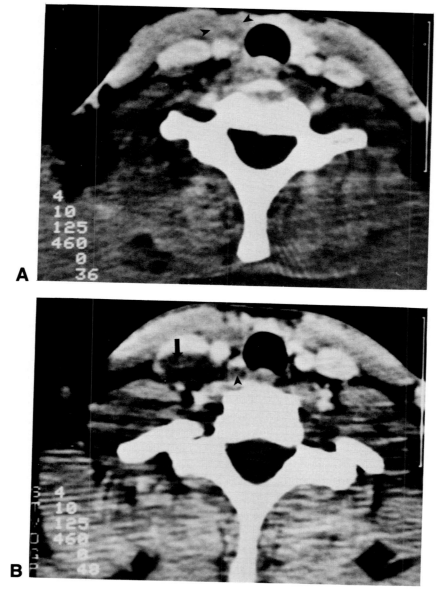

FIG. 9-5. This 23-year-old woman had a history of prior surgical removal of a papillary carcinoma of the thyroid. She had a six- to eight-month history of a feeling of fullness in the neck. No masses were palpable. (A) A CT scan showed a tissue density in the resected thyroid bed (arrowheads). (B) A section slightly lower showed nodal metastases in the scalene group of nodes (arrow) and in a juxtavisceral node in the tracheoesophageal groove (arrowhead).

gery. These tumors may also respond to external beam radiation.[5] Computed tomography may be used in therapy planning or to follow these patients.

Anaplastic carcinomas are treated primarily by irradiation. These tumors are usually inoperable at the time of diagnosis. A CT scan is useful to determine their extent. It can help in the decision whether surgery can be attempted for cure or whether it should be done as an adjunctive "debulking" procedure. A CT scan may also be useful in port planning and follow-up. Lymphomas of the thyroid gland are treated primarily by radiation; chemotherapy may also be used.

IMPACT OF NEW TECHNOLOGY

The most promising area for the newer imaging techniques is in screening. High resolution real-time or static B-mode ultrasonography can prove very useful in identifying nonpalpable nodules in patients at risk of having thyroid carcinoma. These patients can be followed closely without risk by this simple, noninvasive technique. The trade-off for this early detection will probably be the morbidity associated with the removal of a number of benign adenomas. The benefit will be detection of carcinomas at a highly curable stage of the disease.

Computed tomography promises to be of some value in evaluating the local and regional extent of disease in patients with known carcinomas. This may have some useful impact in therapy planning. Computed tomography could help in improving survival by detecting recurrent disease before it is evident clinically; however, this requires further study (Figure 9-5).

Magnetic resonance imaging may replace CT with regard to thyroid cancer; however, it is unlikely to be any more specific or sensitive than ultrasonography as a screening examination.

REFERENCES

1. American Joint Committee on Cancer: *Manual for Staging of Cancer*, 2nd ed. Philadelphia, J. B. Lippincott, 1983.
2. Cady, B., Sedgwick, C. E., Meissner, W. A. Bookwalker, J. R., Romagosa, V., Werber, J.: Changing clinical, pathologic, therapeutic, and survival patterns in patients with papillary carcinoma of the thyroid. *Ann. Surg.* 5:541, 1976.
3. Carroll, B. A.: Asymptomatic thyroid nodules—incidental sonographic detection. *A.J.R.* **138**:499, 1982.
4. Duffy, B. F., Fitzgerald, P. J.: Cancer of the thyroid in children, a report of 28 cases. *J. Clin. Endocrinol. Metab.* 10:1296–1308, 1950.
5. Duncan, W.: *Recent Results in Cancer Research—Thyroid Cancer.* New York, Springer-Verlag, 1980.
6. Greenfield, L. D.: *Thyroid Cancer.* West Palm Beach, FL, CRC Press, 1978.
7. International Union Against Cancer: *TNM Atlas.* Berlin, Springer-Verlag, 1982.
8. Lindberg, R. D.: External beam irradiation in thyroid cancers. In *Textbook of Radiotherapy*, 3rd ed. Fletcher, G. H. (Ed.). Philadelphia, Lea & Febiger, 1980, pp. 384–388.
9. Maisey, M. N., Moses, D. C., Hurley, P. J., Wagner, H. N.: Improved methods for thyroid scanning. *J.A.M.A.* **223**:761–763, 1963.
10. Million, R. R., Cassisi, N. J., Wittes, R. E.: Cancer in the head and neck. In *Cancer—Principles and Practice of Oncology.* DeVita, V. T. Jr., Hellman, S., Rosenberg, S. A. (Eds.). Philadelphia, J. B. Lippincott, 1982.
11. Woolner, L. B., Beahrs, O. H., Black, B. M., McConafey, W. M., Keating, F. R.: Classification and prognosis of thyroid carcinoma. *Am. J. Surg.* 102:354–387, 1961.
12. Zagars, G., Norante, J. D.: Head and neck tumors. In *Clinical Oncology for Medical Students and Physicians: A Multidisciplinary Approach*, 6th ed. Rubin, P. (Ed.). New York, American Cancer Society, 1983, pp. 230–261.

10 THORACIC NEOPLASMS: IMAGING REQUIREMENTS FOR DIAGNOSIS AND STAGING

John D. Armstrong, II
David G. Bragg

Neoplasms of the thorax constitute one of the most frustrating yet important challenges facing the oncologist. The incidence of primary lung cancer continues to rise, particularly in women, yet no significant improvement in survival has resulted from more vigorous efforts toward early detection through screening. The much less common primary neoplasms of the pleural surfaces also appear to be increasing in frequency, again with no measurable improvement in survival. The complex group of mediastinal primary neoplasms is now more easily detected and staged with computed tomography (CT), yet again, gains in survival statistics have not resulted from this technological advance. Each type of intrathoracic tumor will be covered separately here, with a major emphasis on the primary tumors of the lungs and the mediastinal and pleural compartments.

Treatment decisions for patients with lung cancer are dependent upon accurate detection and histologic and staging information. The goal of this chapter is to place the imaging requirements in the perspective of the histologic and behavioral features of the major intrathoracic cancers. A brief discussion of specific problems related to chest metastatic disease also is included; however, most of this information can be found in the chapters covering the respective organ sites.

PRIMARY LUNG CANCER

Introduction

Primary lung cancer is the most frequently occurring neoplasm in men and the second most frequently occur-ring neoplasm in women. Improved diagnostic, staging, and treatment techniques have indeed yielded improved survival in several specific tumor settings, but little substantive improvement in lung cancer mortality has occurred in the 50 years since Graham's first pneumonectomy for lung cancer. The same frustration has persisted in most reported lung cancer series, where only 25% to 40% of tumors are resectable at the time of discovery.[54] The challenge to individuals concerned with early detection of lung cancer must be the discovery of this neoplasm at a time when the tumor is still localized. This probably will not be possible in the undifferentiated and small cell cancers, but it is conceivable with the other primary lung tumors.

Survival Statistics of Primary Lung Cancers. Analysis of the statistical aspects of primary lung cancer reveals little cause for optimism. Table 10-1 lists the estimated numbers of new cancer cases for 1985 including newly diagnosed cases of lung cancer and mortality.[12] Figures 10-1 and 10-2 show that the lung cancer death rate continues to climb in men, although less steeply than in the recent past. Particularly alarming is the same curve for women. A striking increase in newly diagnosed cases and mortality has been reported in the past 10 to 15 years. If this trend continues, it is anticipated that the lung cancer death rate in women will exceed that for breast cancer by 1990. The overall five-year survival for lung cancer is less than 10%. If the present death rate continues, about 2 million people in the United States will have died of lung cancer by the year 2000.[12]

Table 10-1. Lung Cancer Statistics

Estimated New Cancer Cases Diagnosed—1985

All sites	910,000
male	455,000
female	455,000

Lung Cancer Cases Diagnosed

Total	144,000
male	98,000
female	46,000

Estimated Cancer Deaths—1981

All sites	462,000
male	249,000
female	213,000

Lung Cancer Deaths

Total	125,600
male	87,000
female	38,600

Reprinted from Cancer Statistics, 1985. CA 35:26–27, 1985. With permission.

The criteria for resectability differ between surgical centers. Most thoracic surgeons would concur that for a tumor to be considered resectable, the patient must be physiologically able to tolerate the procedure (operable), and the primary tumor must be technically resectable, with lymph nodes limited to the ipsilateral tracheobronchial angle or subcarinal node group or both. Unfortunately, approximately 50% of patients will have distant metastases at the time of diagnosis.[54]

These depressing features of primary lung cancer suggest that the disease is being diagnosed at a time late in its natural history and that improved survival cannot be anticipated unless a strategy for earlier diagnosis can be developed.

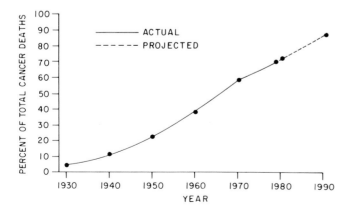

FIG. 10-1. Age adjusted lung cancer death rates for males, 1930–1990. (Modified from Cancer Statistics, 1981. CA 31:13–21, 1981.)

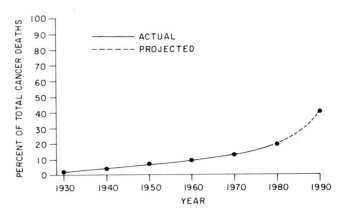

FIG. 10-2. Age adjusted lung cancer death rates for females, 1930–1990. (Modified from Cancer Statistics, 1981. CA 31:13–21, 1981.)

Tumor Behavior and Pathology

Four major types of lung primary parenchymal cancers characterize both the World Health Organization (WHO) and the Working Party for the Therapy of Lung Cancer (WP-L) nomenclature and classification schemes.[45] Over 90% of lung cancers belong to one of these categories. Each of these four primary cancers has unique histologic and behavioral characteristics as well as commonly observed radiographic features (Table 10-2).[12]

Squamous (Epidermoid) Carcinoma. Squamous (epidermoid) carcinomas are histologically characterized by the presence of keratin, squamous pearls, and intercellular bridges. They are divided by degree of differentiation into well-differentiated, moderately differentiated, and poorly differentiated types. About 60% of these tumors arise centrally within the mainstem, lobar, segmental, or subsegmental bronchial mucosa, the latter two being the most common sites. When central lesions are confined to the bronchial wall, pulmonary function is not impaired and the lesion is radiographically occult. In fact, central squamous cancers account for almost all occult lung cancers. Sputum cytologic examination is often positive for malignant cells in early central lesions. As the lesion invades the bronchial wall and surrounding lung tissue and lymph nodes, radiographic abnormalities become evident. A central ill-defined infiltrate is characteristic, and hilar and mediastinal lymph node enlargement is observed in about 40% of patients. Progressive submucosal growth may occlude the bronchus, producing volume loss (Table 10-2) or obstructive pneumonia (Figure 10-3).[11,45] Grossly, these tumors tend to be bulky, large, yellow-white masses with central caseous necrosis, and the site of origin may be difficult to determine. Approximately 10% of squamous carcinomas cavitate. These

Table 10-2. Pathologic Characteristics and Radiologic Features of Lung Cancer

HISTOLOGY	APPROXIMATE FREQUENCY (%)	PARENCHYMAL ABNORMALITY	FEATURES	FIVE-YEAR SURVIVAL* (%)
Squamous	35–50	Central, ill-defined mass, infiltrate or lobar collapse	Grows by direct invasion Obstructive pneumonia and collapse Cavitation Late metastasis	37
Small cell	20–30	Hilar mass	Grows by submucosal lymphatic extension Early hematogenous metastases Obstructive pneumonia and collapse	1
Adenocarcinoma	20–35	Peripheral, ill-defined nodule, mass or infiltrate	Early hematogenous metastases Rare cavitation Scar carcinoma	27
Large cell	5–15	Peripheral large ill-defined mass	Very rapid growth Early lymphatic and hematogenous metastases Infrequent cavitation	27

*Adapted from Cancer Statistics, 1981. CA **31**:13–21, 1981.

excavated lesions usually have thick irregular walls and eccentrically placed air or air–fluid levels. A spectrum of thick-to-thin-walled cavitary squamous carcinomas have been observed; thus no specific appearance of a cavitary lung mass is characteristic of a primary lung cancer.

Approximately 40% of squamous lesions are peripheral in origin and, like cancers of other cell types, show radiographic evidence of poorly defined infiltrative or lobulated lesions. Squamous carcinomas are also the most frequently encountered cell type in Pancoast's tumors; however, any cell type may be observed. These so-called

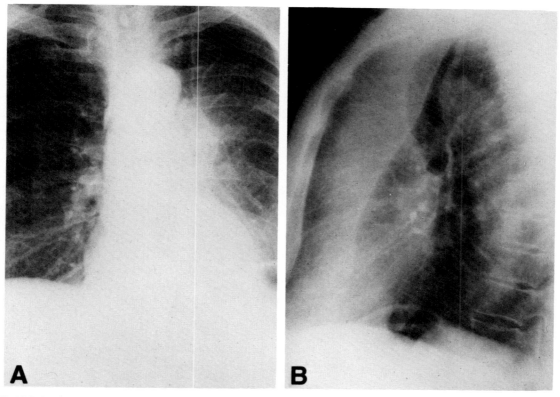

FIG. 10-3. Squamous carcinoma. (A) posteroanterior and (B) lateral chest roentgenograms illustrating left upper lobe collapse in a 63-year-old male smoker with squamous carcinoma obstructing the left upper lobe bronchus confirmed bronchoscopically.

superior sulcus tumors arise in the thoracic apex and were first observed radiographically by Pancoast.[61] Tumors at this location may invade the ribs (varying involvement of the first three) and vertebrae, producing local pain; they may involve the brachial plexus, producing sensory and motor disturbances in the upper extremity and atrophy of the hand; and they may involve the sympathetic nerve chain, producing an ipsilateral Horner's syndrome. Pancoast reported seven cases of this "peculiar neoplastic entity" of epithelial histopathology in 1932 and advised careful radiologic examination of the lung apex in patients complaining of shoulder and neck pain because it may escape detection.

Squamous carcinoma is characterized by slow growth and has the most favorable prognosis of the four major cell types. It tends to remain localized longer than other cancers and is usually associated with late extrathoracic metastases.

Small Cell Carcinoma. Small cell carcinomas have been subdivided into small (oat cell or lymphocyte-like) cell and an intermediate form that includes somewhat larger and more fusiform, spindle, oval, or polygonal-shaped nuclei. Either type is characterized by cells that have little or no cytoplasm. The classic "oat cell" has a round or oval small dark nucleus approximately twice the size of the lymphocyte. Characteristic histologic features are the abundance of small naked cells with a "cord and ribboning" pattern. Electron microscopy (EM) may confirm small cell carcinoma with the identification of neurosecretory-like granules in these cells. The tumor tends to rapidly invade lymphohematogenous channels and metastasize widely before pulmonary symptoms have been provoked.[45] Small cell carcinomas have the poorest prognosis of the four major cell types. They account for about 20% to 30% of primary lung tumors, and 70% to 80% arise centrally near the hilum.[55] Rapid submucosal growth in this region accounts for the common radiographic finding of an ill-defined hilar or perihilar mass. Bronchial obstruction with volume loss or obstructive pneumonia may also occur. The radiographic features of these tumors merge closely with those of squamous cell origin (Figure 10-4).

The metastatic potential of small cell carcinoma is high. Hilar and mediastinal lymph nodes are involved in 80% as shown by radiography at initial examination and 100% at necropsy.[79] Bone marrow spread has been reported in 50% of cases at the time of initial staging.[28] Approximately 10% to 15% of patients with small cell cancer have evidence of brain metastases at initial examination.[58,71] Nearly one half of patients will eventually develop brain involvement during the course of their illness, which has become evident as survival increases[82] (Table 10-2).

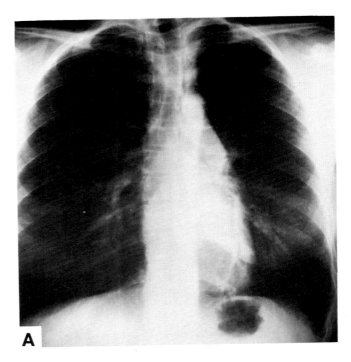

A

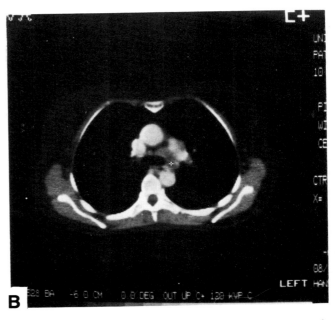

B

FIG. 10-4. Small cell carcinoma (A) PA chest roentgenogram made 8/15/80 of a 43-year-old woman, a heavy smoker with low back pain, that shows a left anterior mediastinal mass in the aortopulmonary window. (B) Enhanced CT scan made three days later at the level of the carina shows aortopulmonary, left tracheobronchial, and paraesophageal lymphadenopathy. Left anterior mediastinal biopsy produced a specimen of a small cell carcinoma. Positive bone scan. (C) PA chest roentgenogram made 9/25/80 shows disappearance of the adenopathy after chemotherapy. (D) PA film made 2/12/81 shows complete collapse of the left lower lobe caused by recurrent small cell carcinoma obstructing the left lower lobe bronchus; this was confirmed by CT and bronchoscopic biopsy.

and occasional peripheral infiltrates, lobar collapse, pleural effusions, and nodules (always associated with hilar disease). Of the 17 patients who became symptomatic during the interval between annual examinations, an average of 8.6 months elapsed between the last yearly chest roentgenogram read as normal and the roentgenogram on which the cancer was diagnosed. The authors conclude that the extremely short asymptomatic phase of oat cell carcinoma precludes early detection by present techniques.[30]

Small cell cancer accounts for 75% of the clinical syndromes related to secretion of ectopic hormones. The most frequently observed syndrome is ectopic secretion of adrenocorticotropic hormone and is usually associated with clinical or laboratory signs of Cushing's syndrome. Inappropriate secretion of antidiuretic hormone is diagnosed by finding hyponatremia with decreased serum osmolality and urinary sodium levels. The Eaton-Lambert syndrome is a myasthenia-like disorder that is frequently associated with small cell cancer and includes the clinical features of easy fatigability of the proximal muscles, weak or absent muscle-stretch reflexes, and a suboptimal response to neostigmine.[70]

Adenocarcinoma. In well-differentiated adenocarcinomas, cells are arranged in distinct glandular or acinar patterns, and mucin may be identified within cells or acinar lumina. In moderately differentiated tumors, cells tend to be arranged in nests, cords, or isolated cell pattern, forming acinar or glandular structures. In poorly differentiated tumors, the predominant cell is anaplastic, although distinct foci of acinar or glandular formation, with or without mucin, may be present.[45]

Adenocarcinomas account for 20% to 35% of all lung cancers and 60% to 70% appear as a peripheral mass alone or in combination with other lesions. These slowly growing peripheral lesions are usually 4 cm or less in diameter and often show ill-defined spreading or infiltrative margins, which are often related to desmoplasia at the edges of the tumor (Figure 10-5).[11,45] The metastatic potential of adenocarcinoma is similar to large cell tumors and generally intermediate between the high frequency of small cell metastases and the lower frequency of squamous carcinomas, as shown in Table 10-3.

Squamous carcinoma has historically been the most common type of lung cancer. Recent studies indicate that adenocarcinoma has emerged as the most common.[13,86,89] It is curious to note that most of this increase in the incidence of adenocarcinoma is reported in the male population. Further work is required to clarify the explanation and significance of this finding.

Adenocarcinoma, including the bronchioloalveolar variety, may arise in a focus of granulomatous scar or pulmonary fibrosis; hence, the designation of "scar cancer."

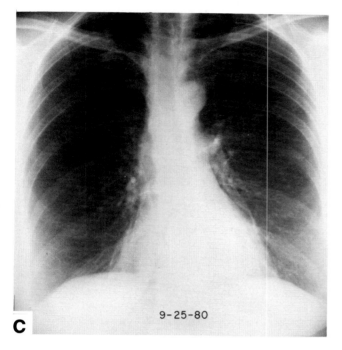

9-25-80

C

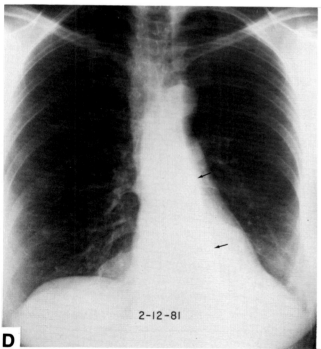

2-12-81

D

The behavior of this tumor is illustrated in the 27 cases of small cell cancer detected in the National Lung Program at Memorial Sloan-Kettering Cancer Center in New York. Twenty-four of the 26 patients had advanced (stage III) disease. These 24 patients had bulky, usually hilar, involvement with extension to the mediastinum

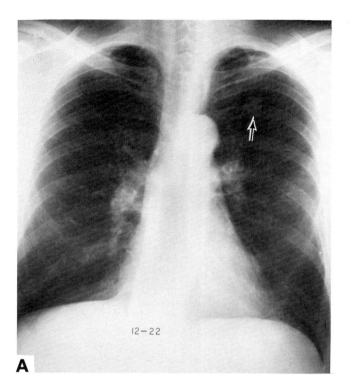

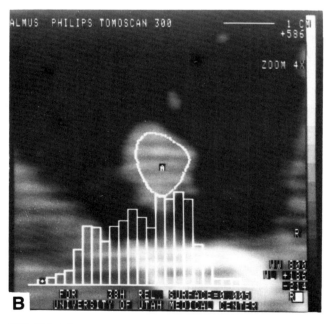

FIG. 10-5. Adenocarcinoma (A) PA chest roentgenogram of a 59-year-old man with a "stroke" shows an ill-defined, 1.5-cm nodule in the left upper node overlying the left posterior sixth rib. Percutaneous needle aspiration biopsy produced evidence of adenocarcinoma. A CT scan of the patient's head showed a brain metastasis. (B) A CT scan through the equator of the nodule shows ill-defined margins. The histogram shows the distribution of CT numbers in a region of interest within the nodule, the mean is 104 Hounsfield units (HU). Siegelman et al. have shown that CT numbers below 164 HU in solitary pulmonary nodules are most often malignant.[76]

Fibrosis, however, may actually develop within adenocarcinomas during their growth and result in apparent stability of the lesion during radiographic observation. With certain adenocarcinomas, extensive collagen formation within a region of central fibrosis is correlated with pleural involvement, lymph node metastases, vascular invasion, and a prognosis that is poor compared with tumors that show little or no collagenation.[75]

Bronchioloalveolar tumors are composed of proliferating cuboidal or tall columnar epithelial cells with uniform to pleomorphic nuclei and abundant pink or vacuolated cytoplasm. Abundant mucin may be produced. In some of these tumors—the so-called alveolar cell carcinomas—the neoplastic cells proliferate to produce permanent intra-alveolar papillary structures using pre-existing alveolar walls almost entirely as a framework for their growth. Distinction between primary and metastatic adenocarcinomas cannot always be made and much reliance is placed on coexistent chronic pulmonary disease and associated bronchioloalveolar epithelial hyperplasia and atypia in zones away from the neoplasm. Electron microscopy is useful but may not be able to differentiate primary from metastatic neoplasm, especially pancreatic carcinoma. Radiographically, the local form of bronchiolar carcinoma consists of a solitary nodule or a poorly defined parenchymal infiltrate. The diffuse form may appear as a lobar or segmental alveolar opacity simulating pneumonia, multiple bilateral pulmonary nodules, or patchy opacities simulating infection or metastatic disease to the lung.[31]

Large Cell Carcinoma. Large cell carcinomas show no evidence of maturation or differentiation, and diagnosis is largely based on exclusion of other cell types. Individual cells tend to be large and pleomorphic, with irregular enlarged vesicular or hyperchromatic nuclei and prominent nucleoli. The formation of nests and sheets gives a number of these tumors an epidermoid appearance, although similar patterns may be reproduced by poorly differentiated adenocarcinomas. Grossly, anaplastic tumors tend to be fairly massive, bulky, hemorrhagic, and necrotic gray-white masses frequently located in the peripheral portions of the lungs. These tumors invade locally and may disseminate widely.[45]

Large cell undifferentiated cancer is estimated to account for 5% to 15% of lung cancers. The most common radiographic abnormality is a rapidly growing peripheral mass. In one review, over 60% of 97 patients had a peripheral mass alone or in combination with other abnormalities, and in 65% of 59 patients it was the only lesion described. Approximately 70% of 39 single peripheral masses were larger than 4 cm in diameter, and most had poorly defined margins. Cavitation in these lesions occurs but is infrequent.[11] Table 10-3 shows the

Table 10-3. Correlation between Histologic Type of Lung Cancer and Site of Spread

| | CELL TYPE (%) | | | |
SITE	SQUAMOUS	SMALL CELL	ADENO-CARCINOMA	LARGE CELL
Scalene lymph node biopsy	23	32	48	46
Mediastinal lymph node				
Mediastinoscopy biopsy	27	73	50	52
Bone; routine marrow	3	24	17	17
autopsy	24	37	40	29
Brain; clinical	14	30	25	21
autopsy	22	40	34	24

correlation between large cell carcinoma and frequency of metastases by site.

Bronchial Adenoma. Bronchial adenomas are considered malignant pulmonary neoplasms that by virtue of their location, rate of growth, and low level of malignancy differ from other primary lung carcinomas. It is typically a slowly growing, circumscribed tumor, which may be polypoid or sessile, situated in the submucosal tissues of proximal bronchi. Bronchial adenomas have been categorized as carcinoids, cylindromas, and mucoepidermoid tumors. Carcinoids constitute 80% to 90% of this group and those that are "malignant" show invasion of surrounding structures and metastasize to hilar and mediastinal lymph nodes. These lesions are typically highly vascular and hemoptysis is a prominent clinical feature. Cylindromas and mucoepidermoid tumors arise from bronchial glands.[16,40]

Bronchial adenomas account for 1% to 3% of all malignant lung tumors. There is a slight predominance of female patients. The age incidence is 30 to 50 years and delay in the correct diagnosis is typical because of slow tumor growth. There is no characteristic radiographic appearance. Some cases show no abnormalities because the lesion is endobronchial and nonobstructing. Occasionally occurring as a solitary nodule, bronchial adenoma is often associated with postobstructive pneumonia or atelectasis (Figure 10-6). With long-standing bronchial obstruction, extensive chronic suppuration, abscess, bronchiectasis, or fibrosis may occur. A hilar mass alone or in combination with parenchymal infiltration is a situation that should suggest an obstructing bronchial adenoma.[16,40] Adenomas may metastasize, usually to the liver, adrenal glands, brain, and bone. Radiographically, bone metastases are often osteoblastic. About 50% of patients survive 10 years.[40]

Classification and Staging

The American Joint Committee for Cancer Staging and End Results Reporting (AJC) was organized in 1959 to develop systems of staging by primary site that were acceptable to the American medical profession. The task force on lung with AJC approval first published the system for staging lung cancer in 1973, and the following section was updated in 1979. The TNM system can be applied to most patients with lung cancer with certainty and the proper stage designated with consistency.[3,56]

In this system, the letter T represents the primary tumor; N, regional node involvement; and M, distant metastases. Numerical suffixes are added to each letter to define the extent of disease (Table 10-4). For example, a tumor 3 cm in diameter that is surrounded by normal lung has no associated atelectasis or obstructive pneumonitis, and does not extend proximal to a lobar bronchus (e.g., a typical solitary pulmonary node) is designated T_1. Spread of the tumor to the ipsilateral hilar lymph nodes is designated N_1, and if there is no evidence of distant metastasis, the designation is M_0. Certain TNM groups have been combined into specific stages, as in Table 10-5 and Figure 10-7. A work sheet provided in the publication is helpful in characterizing T, N, and M as well as patient performance status and histologic cell type.[3] Clinical diagnostic and surgical-evaluative staging tend to underestimate the extent of T and N and all staging tends to underestimate the M portion. There is no reliable method of detecting the microscopic foci that occur frequently in lung cancer.[3]

Imaging Procedures and Assessment

Detection. In recognition of lung cancer survival statistics, a three-center cooperative trial was begun at the

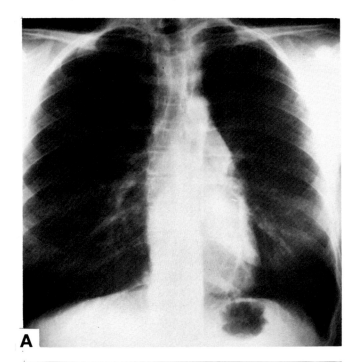

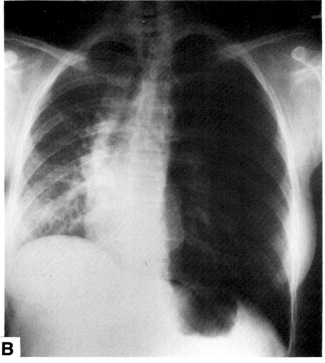

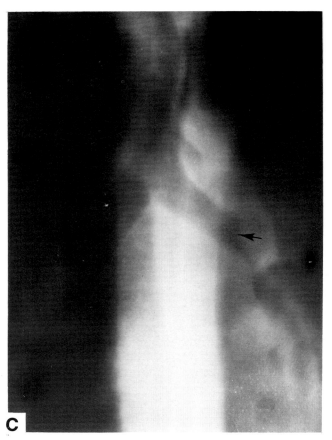

FIG. 10-6. Carcinoid adenoma. (A) PA chest roentgenogram of a 27-year-old woman with a two-year history of intermittent left-sided wheezing. (B) PA chest roentgenogram obtained in expiration showing left lung hyperinflation and mediastinal shift toward the normal right side. (C) AP conventional tomogram shows endobronchial lesion at the left upper lobe orifice obstructing the left main bronchus (arrow) originally detected on the plain films. Endoscopic biopsy showed bronchial carcinoid. A left upper lobectomy with sleeve resection of the main bronchus was performed, confirming the diagnosis.

Memorial Sloan-Kettering center, the Mayo Clinic, and the Johns Hopkins center to study a group of patients at an earlier stage of their disease.[43,47,83,92] This study addressed a high-risk group of patients over the age of 45 years who smoked 20 or more cigarettes a day. A study group was matched with a control population. The study group differed between the centers in some ways but were analyzed periodically with pooled sputum cytologic examination, chest roentgenograms, and physical examination. It was hoped that improved early detection would yield better survival, as had been noted in earlier trials.[23] To date, the initial reports of these trials suggest that screening can detect more lung cancers, more resectable cancers, and more early stage cancer. Lung cancers that have been detected by chest roentgenograms include those lesions in the periphery of the lung and central tumors of the small cell type. Sputum cytologic examination serves a complementary diagnostic role and is the best detector of occult central squamous carcinomas. The five-year survival rate for those who developed lung cancer is higher in the screened group than in the control group; however, the mortality rates in both the study and control groups are virtually identical (26% and 27% at two years), and this is the crucial issue. More advanced

Table 10-4. TNM Classification

Primary Tumor (T)

T_X — Tumor proven by the presence of malignant cells in bronchopulmonary secretions but not visualized roentgenographically or bronchoscopically, or any tumor that cannot be assessed as in a retreatment staging.

T_0 — No evidence of primary tumor.

T_{IS} — Carcinoma in situ.

T_1 — A tumor that is 3.0 cm or less in greatest diameter, surrounded by lung or visceral pleura, and without evidence of invasion proximal to a lobar bronchus at bronchoscopy.

T_2 — A tumor more than 3.0 cm in greatest diameter, or a tumor of any size that either invades the visceral pleura or has associated atelectasis or obstructive pneumonitis extending to the hilar region. At bronchoscopy, the proximal extent of demonstrable tumor must be within a lobar bronchus or at least 2.0 cm distal to the carina. Any associated atelectasis or obstructive pneumonitis must involve less than an entire lung, and there must be no pleural effusion.

T_3 — A tumor of any size with direct extension into an adjacent structure such as the parietal pleura or chest wall, the diaphragm, or the mediastinum and its contents; or a tumor demonstrable bronchoscopically to involve a main bronchus less than 2.0 cm distal to the carina; or any tumor associated with atelectasis or obstructive pneumonitis of an entire lung or pleural effusion.

Nodal Involvement (N)

N_0 — No demonstrable metastasis to regional lymph nodes.

N_1 — Metastasis to lymph nodes in the peribronchial or the ipsilateral hilar region, or both, including direct extension.

N_2 — Metastasis to lymph nodes in the mediastinum.

Distant Metastasis (M)

M_X — Not assessed.

M_0 — No (known) distant metastasis.

M_1 — Distant metastasis present.
  Specify _____.

  Specify sites according to the following notations:

Contralateral Pulmonary — PUL
Osseous — OSS
Hepatic — HEP
Brain — BRA
Lymph Nodes — LYM
Bone Marrow — MAR
Pleura — PLE
Skin — SKI
Eye — EYE
Other — OTH

Reprinted from American Joint Committee on Cancer: *Manual for Staging of Cancer*, 2nd ed. Philadelphia, J. B. Lippincott, 1983, pp. 99–105. With permission.

(stage III) lesions were found in the control (70%) than in the study group (35%) and significantly more stage I lesions were found in the study group (50%) compared with the control group (20%). These data suggest that further experience with these cooperative lung cancer trials will demonstrate an improved survival in the screened study groups. In general, screening is promising for squamous carcinoma and adenocarcinoma but not for small cell or large cell carcinoma. The results to date do not yet provide a basis for recommending large scale screening programs for early lung cancer detection by sputum cytologic examination and chest radiography. These clinical trials are still in progress and final results will not be available for several years. Meanwhile, the American Cancer Society has shifted its emphasis from early detection programs to prevention of smoking.

Diagnostic Assessment by Intrathoracic Location. *Lung:* Detection and localization of a lung cancer demands careful evaluation of high-quality chest roentgenograms. High kilovoltage (about 140-kilovolt [peak]) exposures in posteroanterior (PA) and lateral projections produce an image of optimum latitude such that the lung can be "seen through" overlying structures such as the ribs, heart, mediastinum, and diaphragm. Tumors that arise in the bronchial wall centrally near the hilum often shed

Table 10-5. Stage Grouping

Occult Carcinoma

$T_X N_0 M_0$

An occult carcinoma with bronchopulmonary secretions containing malignant cells but without other evidence of the primary tumor or evidence of metastasis to the regional lymph nodes or distant metastasis.

Stage I

$T_{IS} N_0 M_0$
Carcinoma in situ

$T_1 N_0 M_0$
$T_1 N_1 M_0$
$T_2 N_0 M_0$

A tumor that can be classified T_1 without any metastasis or with metastasis to the lymph nodes in the peribronchial or ipsilateral hilar region only, or a tumor that can be classified T_2 without any metastasis to nodes or distant metastasis.

Note: $T_X N_1 M_0$ and $T_0 N_1 M_0$ are also theoretically possible, but it would be difficult if not impossible to make such a clinical diagnosis. If such a diagnosis is made, it would be included in Stage I.

Stage II

$T_2 N_1 M_0$

A tumor classified as T_2 with metastasis to the lymph nodes in the peribronchial or ipsilateral hilar region only.

Stage III

T_3 with any N or M
N_2 with any T or M
M_1 with any T or N

Any tumor more extensive than T_2, or any tumor with metastasis to the lymph nodes in the mediastinum, or any tumor with distant metastasis.

Reprinted from American Joint Committee on Cancer: *Manual for Staging of Cancer*, 2nd ed. Philadelphia, J. B. Lippincott, 1983, pp. 99–105. With permission.

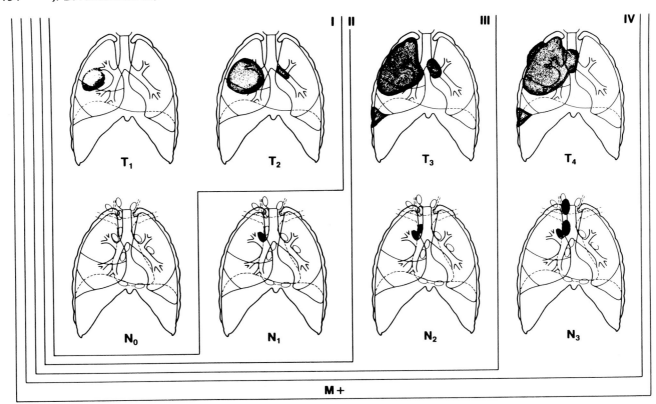

FIG. 10-7. Anatomic staging for lung cancer. Tumor (T) categories: Size and confinement to lung are the major considerations in the progression of non-oat cell cancers: squamous cell carcinoma and adenocarcinoma. T_1 v T_2 depends on the mass being less or more than 3 cm. The depth of invasion is reflected by extension through the pleura, which is akin to an organ capsule (T_3). Further advancement into mediastinum or chest wall has been designated as T_4, although this is not part of the American Joint Committee (AJC) or International Union Against Cancer (UICC) criteria. Node (N) categories: Location within the lung hilar (N_1) or mediastinal (N_2) indicates the common progression. Supraclavicular nodes are considered metastatic, although an N_3 notation would be reasonable. Stage grouping emphasizes the early resectable stages confined to a lobe or lung (T_1 and T_2) with and without hilar disease (N_1) as I and II respectively. Advanced disease (T_3), pleural invasion, and mediastinal nodes are stage III, with metastases reflecting stage IV. Special T_x and N_3 categories are not officially used by the AJC/UICC. Tumor (T) and node (N) equivalents are: $T_2 = N_1$, $T_3 = N_2$, $T_4 = N_3$. AJC[3] v UICC classifications: T_4 is not an official designation. Oat cell cancers are usually metastatic or premetastatic and are categorized as intrathoracic or extrathoracic. (Adapted from Van Houtte, P., Salazar, O. M., Phillips, C. E., Asbury, R. F.: Lung cancer. In *Clinical Oncology for Medical Students and Physicians: A Multidisciplinary Approach*, 6th ed. Rubin, P. (Ed.). New York: American Cancer Society, 1983, pp. 142–153.)

cells recovered in the sputum but remain radiographically occult until the invasive lesion attains threshold size or is associated with hilar or mediastinal lymph node enlargement.

The visibility of the roentgenographic shadow of a lung nodule is related to several variables. Lesion size is an important factor affecting visibility because (1) as the size increases, the nodule becomes more distinguishable from background structures in the surrounding lung, and (2) as nodule thickness increases, the contrast of the image increases, becoming more visually apparent and therefore detectable. The presence of calcification within a nodule also affects visibility, such that nodule image contrast increases with greater calcium content. Another factor affecting detection is margin sharpness. For a given size, density, and location, a sharply marginated nodule may be more readily detected than a nodule with less well-defined edges. These principles apply to all lung nodules, including primary cancers and metastatic lesions.

Under ideal circumstances, a nodule in the periphery with few overlying structures may be detectable when as small as 4 mm in diameter; however, a central lesion may be virtually invisible up to sizes of several centimeters in diameter. Lesions in the central regions of the chest often escape detection because (1) these areas are not searched as carefully as peripheral areas, and (2) there is decreased image contrast in the poorly penetrated areas such as the hila, mediastinum, retrocardiac region, and subdiaphragmatic region. Finally, larger complex background structures are present in the central lung compared with the periphery, making discrimination between a lung nodule and normal structures more difficult.

The search–detection–recognition process by which an observer finds a nodule on chest roentgenograms is complex. It is well known, however, that a single reader (radiologist) looking at a single film will not detect 30% to 50% of lung nodules present.[4,23] Multiple readers improve detection accuracy and multiple films with single or multiple readers further improve detection.[78,81] Comparison with previous chest roentgenograms is often very helpful. If the nodule was present and remains unchanged in size for two years or more, the lesion is almost certainly benign. If the lesion is new, enlarging, or of indeterminate age, further study is indicated to exclude cancer. Often, a lesion was present on earlier roentgenograms but was not detected or recognized as a significant abnormality.[68]

Conventional linear tomography may be helpful in the evaluation of lung lesions for the demonstration of calcification, margin or border characteristics, and cavitation. These features, however, are not pathognomonic, and unexplained lung lesions require tissue diagnosis when the index of suspicion for cancer is high.

Calcification within a pulmonary nodule is typical of benign or inflammatory lesions. It is often obvious on routine films and may be confirmed with low-kilovolt (peak) (e.g., 80) films, fluoroscopy with spot filming, or conventional linear tomography. Cancers rarely contain sufficient calcification to be detected on conventional films except when an adenocarcinoma arises within a granulomatous scar and the obvious calcified focus is eccentric within the nodule.

Recently, Siegelman et al.[76] described their experience with computed tomography (CT) in the study of solitary pulmonary nodules. In 91 apparently uncalcified lung nodules, no lesion with CT numbers of 148 Hounsfield units (HU) or greater proved to be malignant. They recommend using 164 HU as the lower threshold for benign pulmonary lesions (Figure 10-5B). It was their assumption that diffuse calcification or dense fibrous tissue explained the high CT numbers found in benign lesions.[76] Unfortunately, this technique is equipment-limited, and further study is required to evaluate its diagnostic role. Other centers have had difficulty in finding benign lesions, not visibly calcified on plain films, with CT numbers of 164 HU or greater. Changing surgical practice by such techniques represents yet an additional challenge.

Computed tomography is the most sensitive technique available for detection of additional or multiple pulmonary nodules, especially in the peripheral subpleural regions where metastatic nodules are frequent and otherwise difficult to detect. In one study, CT detected 48% more nodules than conventional tomography and 78% of all lesions over 3 cm found at surgery (in contrast to 59% with conventional tomography.[74] Computed to-

mography lacks specificity, however, and 25% to 50% of the additional nodules detected by CT proved to be nonneoplastic. Computed tomography provides additional information but this usually does not influence patient treatment.[51]

Lymph node involvement in patients with lung cancer is reason for concern that a tumor has escaped the confines of the lung. In fact, in practice very few T_1, N_1, M_0 and T_2, N_1, M_0 tumors are encountered.[22] The bronchopulmonary hilar lymph nodes are contiguous with the tracheobronchial and paratracheal nodes. The former are N_1, the latter constitute N_2 nodes (Figure 10-8). When

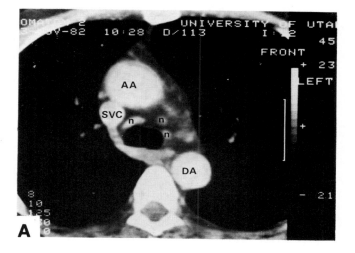

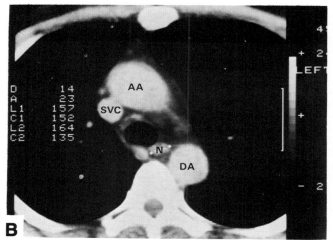

FIG. 10-8. Mediastinal CT. (A) Axial enhanced CT image above the carina clearly shows the azygous arch entering the superior vena cava (SVC), ascending aorta (AA), descending aorta (DA), and normal lymph nodes (n). (B) Axial enhanced CT image above A, also below the aortic arch, shows the structures seen in A; however, the left lower paratracheal/paraesophageal node (N) measures approximately 1.4 cm and was called "indeterminate." The patient underwent left thorocotomy following a normal ^{67}Ga scan. The lymph nodes (n and N) were sampled, found to be "reactive" and contained no tumor, and a lobectomy was performed for a T_2N_1 lesion of the left lower lobe.

sufficiently enlarged, these nodes may be detectable on plain roentgenograms, conventional tomograms, 55° oblique hilar tomograms (OHT), or CT.[51] A study of CT detection of hilar lymph node involvement showed (1) hilar lymph node enlargement could be identified on CT scans in 9 of 16 patients (56% sensitivity) proved to have metastatic tumor involvement; scans were indeterminate in three and falsely negative in four, and (2) CT scans were normal in 39 of 41 patients who had no evidence of hilar lymph node metastases and indeterminate in two.[6]

Overall accuracy of hilar evaluation was similar for plain roentgenograms, OHT, and CT in another recent study. Hilar lymph node enlargement could be identified on plain films in 9 of 17 patients (53%) proved to have metastatic tumor involvement; OHT detected 12 of 17 (70%), and CT detected 11 of 17 (65%). Plain films were normal (negative) in 21 of 25 patients (85%) who had no evidence of hilar lymph node metastases; OHT was normal in 20 of 25 (80%), and CT was normal in 22 of 25 (88%). When the 17 patients with malignant involvement of hilar nodes are considered alone, the proportion of false-positive results is striking: 47% for plain films, 29% for OHT, and 35% for CT.[60]

Mediastinum: To properly select patients who have surgically resectable disease, staging must include assessment of mediastinal (N_2) lymph node involvement. A variety of imaging techniques have been used to detect mediastinal involvement with inconsistent success, lacking either sensitivity or specificity. Chest roentgenograms detect an abnormality in mediastinal contour in, at most, 50% of patients with lymph node metastases. Conventional tomography adds little additional information compared with a well-penetrated, carefully evaluated PA chest film. A barium esophagram may demonstrate abnormal left paratracheal and subcarinal nodes. Table 10-6 shows a summary of seven recent attempts to evaluate the role of CT staging in mediastinal metastases.[14,19,21,52,60,67,85] Note the striking variation in sensitivity from 0.28 to 0.95 and specificity from 0.46 to 1.0. Despite the stated advantages of CT, the wide scatter in data obtained in these 261 patients is undoubtedly a reflection of the variation in scan quality, interpretive expertise, and, especially, the criteria for lymph node size and mediastinal invasion. No agreement exists between authors on the "normal" size of lymph nodes in the hilum and mediastinum. Some authors regard all visible lymph nodes as abnormal.[67] Others suggest that nodes that are solid, round, or oval and larger than most nodes seen in patients without lung cancer (5–6 mm) should be interpreted as abnormal.[52] Others regard 1 cm as the threshold for abnormal;[19] yet neither sensitivity nor specificity data (Table 10-6) support this conclusion.

A recent paper evaluated CT staging in 98 lung cancer patients with the criteria that (1) invasion was diagnosed when the tumor interdigitated with mediastinal fat, (2) surrounded mediastinal vessels or main stem bronchi, and (3) mediastinal lymph nodes were greater than 1.5 cm in diameter.[6] Computed tomography correctly staged 33 of the 35 patients (94%) found to have resectable disease and 41 of the 45 patients (91%) found not to have resectable disease. In the remaining 18 patients (25%), determination of resectability by CT was called indeterminate. These cases had mediastinal lymph node enlargement of 1.0 to 1.5 cm or mediastinal tumor invasion was not certain, as illustrated in Figure 10-8. Ultimately, in one half of the indeterminate cases the tumors were resectable and in one half they were unresectable; however, designation of an indeterminate group is an important step in identifying a smaller set of patients who require invasive confirmation of tumor involvement. By combining the use of CT and mediastinoscopy (otomy) when appropriate during the study period, the resectability rate for patients undergoing thoracotomy for cure at Barnes Hospital was 92.5%.[6] Thus, with CT demonstration of direct mediastinal invasion (34 of 34 cases), thoracotomy can be avoided. Indeterminate or definitely enlarged mediastinal lymph nodes demonstrated on CT allow appropriate use of biopsy procedures to sample suspected metastatic disease. The major limitations of CT are that contiguity of a neoplasm with the mediastinum is not equivalent to definite invasion and that CT cannot detect neoplastic involvement in normal-sized lymph nodes.[6]

Forty-two patients with T_2 lung cancers investigated in another study underwent plain roentgenography, conventional tomography, and CT for mediastinal evaluation.[52] Plain films detected mediastinal lymph node involvement in 1 of 18 patients (5% true positive) proved to have metastatic tumor involvement; conventional tomography detected 9 of 18 (50%), and CT detected 17 of 18 (94%) patients. Plain films were normal (negative) in 24 of 24 patients (100% true negative) who were shown to have no evidence of mediastinal lymph node metastases; conventional tomography was normal in 23 of 24 (95%), and CT was normal in 15 of 24 (62%).[52] Thus, CT of the mediastinum was more sensitive but not more specific than the other two modalities in this study. Clearly, lymph node enlargement does not always signify tumor involvement and nodes infiltrated with tumor are not always enlarged.[6,14,19,51,52,60,67,85] These limitations are particularly evident in plain roentgenography, which is grossly insensitive to nodal involvement with a high false-negative rate. Conversely, plain roentgenography is specific (1.0), whereas the predictive value of a negative (normal plain film) is only 0.62. Nonetheless, plain films are the most useful first imaging tool overall in evaluation of patients with lung cancer.

Table 10-6. N$_2$ Staging of Lung Cancer (Mediastinum): CT Data from 261 Patients

AUTHORS	YEAR	NUMBER OF CASES	SCAN TIME (SEC)	TRUE POSITIVE (+ +)	FALSE NEGATIVE (− +)	FALSE POSITIVE (+ −)	TRUE NEGATIVE (− −)	SENSITIVITY (%)	SPECIFICITY (%)	ACCURACY (%)
Crowe et al.[14]	1978	44	18	21	1	0	22	95	100	98
Underwood et all.[85]	1979	18	18	4	5	1	8	44	89	67
Ekholm et al.[19]	1980	35	4.2	2	5	15	13	28	46	43
Rea et al.[67]	1981	22	2	4	1	4	13	80	76	77
Faling et al.[21]	1981	49 (51)*	2	(15)	(2)	(2)	(32)	88	94	87
Moak et al.[52]	1982	51 (68)*	18	(25)	(26)	(1)	(16)	48	59	60
Osborne et al.[60]	1982	42	5	17	1	9	15	94	62	76

*Number of observation and result is given in parentheses.

The data shown in Table 10-6 represent small series and the results show considerable variability. An excellent diagnostic imaging procedure would ideally yield 95% sensitivity and 95% specificity; to date, none meets these criteria. The gold standard has traditionally been surgical exploration of the thorax. Computed tomographic staging can be expected to improve significantly for several reasons. Equipment improvements occur rapidly, and recent changes include shorter scan times (<2 seconds), smaller image elements, which improve resolution, and improved "software" reconstruction techniques. Second, criteria for lymph node enlargement and tumor invasion will become better established, based upon observation and experience, and interpretive decisions will become more accurate. As illustrated by the more recent experience of Barnes Hospital,[6] patients with negative CT scans are candidates for resection (high true negative), those with positive CT scans are not (with some exceptions), and patients with indeterminate scans are candidates for tissue sampling procedures (mediastinal surgical exploration or needle aspiration/biopsy).

Table 10-7 shows a summary of 213 patients evaluated for mediastinal tumor involvement using gallium.[2,17,24,37,39] Concentration of ⁶⁷Ga in a lung lesion scanned 48 to 72 hours after administration is very suggestive of cancer. While 85% to 95% of primary lung cancers concentrate ⁶⁷Ga, as few as 65% of adenocarcinomas are ⁶⁷Ga avid. If the tumor is peripheral and concentrates ⁶⁷Ga, radionuclide deposition in the hilum/mediastinum (N$_1$, N$_2$) and distant organs (M) is evaluated to determine "tumor involvement." Ideally, absence of ⁶⁷Ga deposition in the mediastinum would allow the patient to proceed directly to thoracotomy without mediastinoscopy. Sensitivity varies in these five studies from 0.65 to 0.92 and specificity from 0.67 to 0.90. One study is notable for the absence of false negatives.[2] However, in six cases (all adenocarcinomas) ⁶⁷Ga failed to concentrate, precluding the test from contributing to staging in these patients; thus, they are included in Table 10-7 as false negatives.

The data shown in Table 10-7, like those in Table 10-6, are disappointing and represent early experience with an imaging modality used to stage lung cancer. As with CT, radionuclide imaging technology continues to improve. Gallium scanning may prove useful in selected patients in routine staging, particularly peripheral non-adenocarcinomas.

Finally, a brief discussion of surgical mediastinal exploration is appropriate. Mediastinoscopy is performed via a small transverse suprasternal incision and allows inspection and biopsy along the anterior trachea, right and left paratracheal regions, the carina and subcarinal space, the right upper lobe bronchus, and 1 to 3 cm of each main bronchus.[27] Mediastinotomy is performed with a vertical parasternal incision extended into the anterior second, third, or fourth intercostal space. It is usually

Table 10-7. N$_2$ staging of lung cancer: ⁶⁷Ga data from 213 patients

AUTHORS	YEAR	NUMBER OF PATIENTS	TRUE POSITIVE (+ +)	FALSE NEGATIVE (− +)	FALSE POSITIVE (+ −)	TRUE NEGATIVE (− −)	SENSITIVITY (%)	SPECIFICITY (%)	ACCURACY (%)
DeMeester et al.[17]	1976	47	18	6	4	19	75	83	79
Alazraki et al.[2]	1978	31	11	6	4	10	65	71	71
Lesk et al.[37]	1978	34	17	2	5	10	89	67	79
Fosburg et al.[24]	1979	26	14	2	1	9	88	90	88
Lunia et al.[39]	1981	76	48	4	7	16	92	70	85

performed on the left side, which permits examination of anterior mediastinal, aortopulmonary, left bronchopulmonary and tracheobronchial nodes.[46] Contraindications to pulmonary resection include (1) small cell carcinoma, (2) contralateral paratracheal node involvement, (3) ipsilateral paratracheal node involvement (except for squamous carcinoma involving the tracheobronchial nodes), and (4) direct mediastinal invasion.[42,57] A 5% to 36% false-negative rate is found when the results of mediastinoscopy are evaluated at thoracotomy. Thoracotomy staging produces an approximate 10% false-positive staging rate.

A committee of the American Thoracic Society was charged with developing a map of regional lymph nodes that would receive wide acceptance and develop multifactorial criteria for the extent, degree, and type of nodal involvement in primary lung cancer. The proposed ATS schema revises the AJC classification shown in Figure 10-9, introduces a map of regional pulmonary nodes with anatomic definitions, and should become the standard for staging by radiologists, surgeons, and pathologists.[84]

Chest wall, pleura: Plain roentgenography may demonstrate pleural effusion or rib destruction. Computed tomography allows diagnosis of chest wall invasion when the tumor obliterates fat planes between the pleura and chest wall muscles or invasion of the rib or sternum. However, the CT appearance of both benign and malignant focal pleural and pericardial thickening appears identical. Computed tomography is an invaluable imaging technique and should be used to detect and define chest wall involvement.[6,32]

Extrathoracic extension: All clinical staging tends to underestimate M extension.[3] In recent years, radionuclide or CT scanning for brain, liver, and bone metastases have become standard procedures in the search for asymptomatic disease. All three are recommended in small cell cancer because approximately 50% of these patients have disseminated disease at the time of initial examination. With non-small cell lung cancer, without signs or symptoms to suggest extrathoracic metastatic disease, the role of radiologic staging is less clearly defined.

In the brain, contrast enhanced CT scans are the most accurate studies in detecting space-occupying mass lesions. Butler et al.[10] found 3 of 55 (5%) neurologically intact lung cancer patients with clinically unsuspected cerebral metastases on CT scans. Despite the low yield, they believe the cost of CT could be justified in patients with primary lung cancer, before definitive treatment, in preventing unnecessary surgery.[10] Martini and Posner[44] made similar recommendations for preoperative brain CT scans in all patients who are candidates for curative resection. They found that two thirds of brain metastases appear within three months of initial treatment unrelated to the stage of the tumor. Also, they found the incidence of brain metastases was twice as frequent with adenocarcinoma than with squamous cell cancer.[44] In general, CT brain scanning is not a routine examination in non-small cell cancers; rather, the decision is based upon the index of suspicion (e.g., cell type), symptoms, and clinical signs.

Extracranial screening for metastatic disease is less easily justified. Mintz et al.[50] analyzed the impact of initial staging (physical examination, laboratory studies and chest X-ray films), clinical staging (radionuclide liver and bone scans, CT brain scans, and total-body gallium 67 citrate scans) with final pathologic staging. In 38 of 115 patients, clinical staging led to advancement of disease stage, with the gallium scan being the most useful study. In addition, their clinical stage correlated well with the final stage as determined by subsequent histologic analysis.[50] In contrast, Ramsdell et al.[65] prospectively analyzed the impact of multiorgan radionuclide scans in a series of 52 operable patients with primary lung cancer. They found that 16 of 17 positive radionuclide liver scans were false positive with but one true-positive study. No brain scan abnormality was detected that was not clinically suspected. Of 13 positive radionuclide bone scans, only one was a true positive. Their data do not

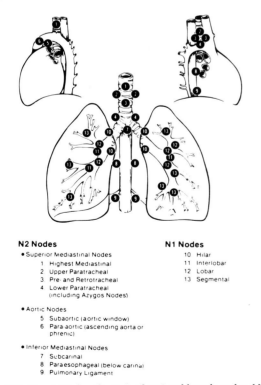

N2 Nodes
- Superior Mediastinal Nodes
  1. Highest Mediastinal
  2. Upper Paratracheal
  3. Pre- and Retrotracheal
  4. Lower Paratracheal (including Azygos Nodes)

- Aortic Nodes
  5. Subaortic (aortic window)
  6. Para-aortic (ascending aorta or phrenic)

- Inferior Mediastinal Nodes
  7. Subcarinal
  8. Paraesophageal (below carina)
  9. Pulmonary Ligament

N1 Nodes
10. Hilar
11. Interlobar
12. Lobar
13. Segmental

FIG. 10-9. The AJC classification of regional lymph nodes. Note that all single digit nodes are mediastinal (N2) and all hilar, peribronchial, and intrapulmonary nodes (N1) are assigned double digits. (Modified from American Joint Committee on Cancer: *Manual for Staging of Cancer,* 2nd ed. Philadelphia, J. B. Lippincott, 1983, p. 105.)

support the routine use of multiorgan radionuclide scans in patients with resectable primary lung cancer.[65]

In the non-small cell lung cancer patient, there may be a role for preoperative contrast-enhanced brain CT scans. Until these studies become more sensitive and specific, it would seem prudent to rely primarily upon the patient's symptoms and physical and laboratory findings to direct further imaging and biopsy procedures.

Biopsy Techniques. Cytologic examination of sputum has become an extremely helpful technique in the diagnosis of lung cancer. Centrally located cancers that involve major bronchi will yield the highest proportion of positive tests, especially squamous carcinomas, including in situ and minimally invasive occult lesions. The lowest yield will be in those patients with small peripheral primary cancers.[72]

Fiberoptic bronchoscopy is indicated in most patients with suspected primary lung cancer.[41] Diagnostic yield will be greatest when a visible endobronchial lesion is brushed and biopsied. Fluoroscopically guided bronchoscopic biopsy of lesions that are not endoscopically visible may also be successful, with experience, when the lesion is sufficiently large to be fluoroscopically visible. Posterior and apical upper lobe lesions are somewhat more difficult to visualize because of the bend required of the scope. A newly devised retractable needle at the end of a flexible core, passed through the biopsy channel, may extend the potential for bronchoscopic tissue retrieval because tissue penetration with blunt biopsy forceps is often difficult to achieve.

Percutaneous transthoracic needle aspiration biopsy (PTNAB) is a well described and widely used technique.[29] A small gauge needle (Figure 10-10) is passed into a lung lesion under single or biplane fluoroscopic or CT control with local anesthesia. Larger bore biopsy needles yield larger tissue specimens; however, greater complication rates and occasional deaths have forced large bore needles to be abandoned. Cells and often grossly visible tissue specimens are coaxed into the needle lumen by applying suction with a syringe connected to the aspirating needle and manipulating the needle in vertical and rotational directions within the lung lesion. A single pleural puncture minimizes the complication of pneumothorax and may be accomplished in two ways; the pleura may be punctured once with the aspiration needle and then withdrawn and the needle contents expressed onto a glass slide or into iced normal saline. If multiple punctures are desired, a larger or sheathed needle may be used to puncture the pleura, and multiple passes are then made through the lumen of the larger needle or sheath with a smaller needle. Complications of PTNAB include hemoptysis, which occurs in less than 10% of patients and is usually mild and self-limited. Apparent enlargement or change in the margins of a lung lesion on chest

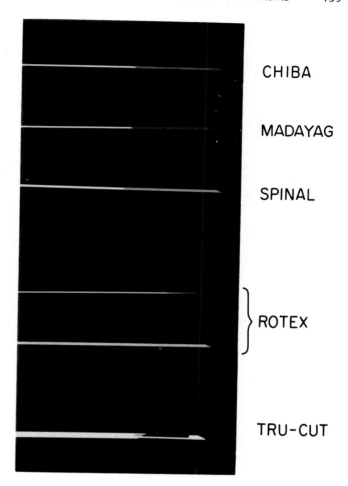

FIG. 10-10. Percutaneous biopsy needles. Roentgenogram of representative thin-walled needles used for percutaneous thansthoracic biopsy. The Chiba or 22-gauge spinal needle, Madayag needle with pointed stylet, and 21-gauge spinal needle are each shown with their stylets partially withdrawn; aspiration is used to draw specimen into lumen. The Rotex needle, approximately 20 gauge, with spiral screw withdrawn and 18-gauge Tru-cut needle are cutting needles.

roentgenograms suggest hemorrhage at the biopsy site. Pneumothorax may occur in up to 50% of patients but is usually small and asymptomatic, and only 10% to 15% of patients require thoracostomy tube drainage. The incidence of pneumothorax increases with smoking, chronic lung disease (chronic bronchitis and emphysema), increasing age, apical lesions, large biopsy needles, and multiple punctures. Pneumothorax is minimized by operator experience, small needle, fewer punctures, breathing oxygen-enriched air (5 L/min by nasal cannula before and approximately four to eight hours after the procedure), and by placing the patient in a position such that the pleural site of puncture is dependent (e.g., supine following a posterior biopsy) immediately after the biopsy. A pneumothorax can be easily managed with an angiographic 7F catheter with multiple side holes introduced percutaneously over a trocar. The catheter is connected to a Heimlich valve with a connecting tube across a stopcock. During expiration, air on the pneumothorax side leaves the catheter from the pleural space through the compliant rubber valve. Upon inspiration, when the pressure gradient is reversed, the valve collapses (closes), preventing air from moving into the pleural space. This simple apparatus may be taped to the chest wall and the patient sent to the hospital ward or home. If after 48 to 72 hours the pneumothorax has resolved and does not recur when the catheter is clamped, the catheter may be withdrawn. The technique of PTNAB and complication management can be readily learned by physicians who perform interventional studies.

Virtually any chest wall or lung parenchymal lesion is amenable to PTNAB if it can be visualized on a fluoroscope or CT scan, including small or central lesions. Diagnostic accuracy exceeds 90% in malignant lesions but is less reliable in confirming benignancy. Adequate tissue obtained from three passes into a suspicious lesion that fails to show evidence of neoplastic cells is generally considered sufficient evidence for a decision, together with the patient's age, sex, smoking history, symptoms, clinical signs, and geographic living and travel history. Careful follow-up or thoracotomy are the options in doubtful cases. When a lesion is approached vigorously or with a screw-obturator needle, the absence of neoplastic cells is more likely to suggest a benign diagnosis. PTNAB is particularly helpful in evaluating (1) indeterminate lesions despite thorough evaluation including bronchoscopy, (2) patients deemed inoperable by virtue of underlying disease, and (3) patients with evidence of disseminated disease, which precludes thoracotomy for resection (e.g., N_2, M_1).

Imaging Strategies and Decisions

Imaging recommendations in lung cancer are debatable because no streamlined, cost-effective, ideal imaging sequence has yet been established. The reasons for this circumstance are several: (1) imaging technology continues to advance rapidly, but change; (2) well-controlled prospective imaging trials are lacking; and (3) the "gold standard" for evaluating lymph node involvement remains surgery and is definitive only at pathologic examination following resection. We propose a diagnostic approach in Figures 10-11, 10-12, and 10-13 based upon the TNM classification. Each schema strives to be conservative and cost-effective and relies upon state-of-the-art imaging technology and interpretive expertise; moreover, the ideal result in lung cancer is to perform curative resection in patients with local disease and to avoid major surgery in patients with disseminated disease. The sputum-positive, roentgenographically negative lesion (T_x) is not included in Figure 10-11. The localization of in situ or minimally invasive tumors in the central bronchial tree ultimately depends upon meticulous endoscopy and biopsy. These lesions may become roentgenographically visible, in which case staging would proceed according to these proposed schemata for T, N, and M.

The T decision tree (Figure 10-11) begins with the common roentgenographic presentations of lung cancer: peripheral nodule/mass, central mass/infiltrate, and chest wall lesion. The goal is to completely characterize T as

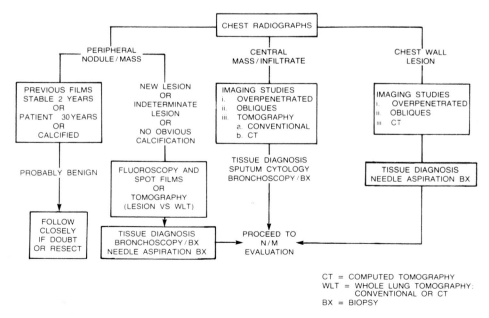

FIG. 10-11. Diagnostic and staging steps in evaluating patients with primary lung cancer based on the T system. The pathway strives to be conservative and cost-effective and relies upon state-of-the-art imaging technology and interpretive expertise.

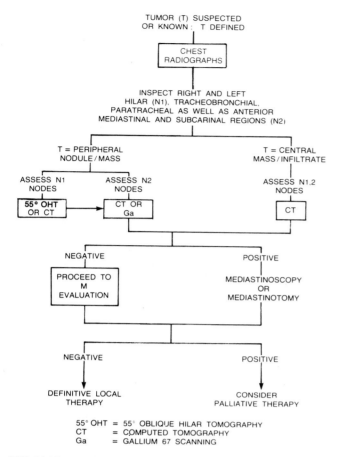

FIG. 10-12. N (node) evaluation. Diagnostic and staging steps in evaluating patients with primary lung cancer based on the TNM system. The pathway strives to be conservative and cost-effective and relies upon state-of-the-art imaging technology and interpretive expertise.

T_1, T_2, or T_3 in any of its manifestations. Cost-effective imaging and tissue diagnosis are the essence of this table.

The N decision tree (Figure 10-12) begins with a careful inspection of lymph-node-bearing regions on the chest roentgenogram followed by tomography or ^{67}Ga scanning. One imaging study, such as CT, may fulfill requirements for T and N imaging in a given patient; for example, CT would allow examination of the chest wall, tumor location/invasion, and hilar and mediastinal lymph nodes. On the other hand, 55° OHT may be best suited for N_1 nodes.[51] Gallium scanning is useful when the primary tumor concentrates the radionuclide and is not central in location. Under these conditions, the absence of activity in the hilum/mediastinum or distant sites militates against tumor spread. Overall, CT will probably prove to be the most valuable method for evaluating N extension, especially when a separate indeterminate group is added to results such that true positives and true negatives are significantly increased. The small group of indeterminate tumors (25% of patients) can be further evaluated with mediastinal exploration and biopsy (med-

iastinoscopy traditionally used in right-sided tumors, mediastinotomy most frequently used for left-sided lesions, especially left upper lobe), while patients with CT-positive tumors are treated nonsurgically and patients with CT-negative tumors undergo thoracotomy for cure.[6]

The M diagnostic tree (Figure 10-13) separates small cell from non-small cell tumors because the former are so frequently disseminated and treatment planning requires differentiation between limited and widespread disease. Non-small cell cancers, on the other hand, have differing probabilities for metastases, and M evaluation is based upon the index of suspicion, the presence of symptoms or signs, and abnormal serum chemistry values. If a thoracotomy is planned, confirmation of the absence of metastases by organ scans of the brain, liver, and bone is a desirable step. Confirmation of a positive bone or liver scan largely depends upon how a positive scan affects the treatment plan (e.g., an isolated positive scan in a patient with otherwise limited disease would require confirmation) and whether an alternative explanation exists for a "positive" scan (such as healing fracture, arthritis, benign lesion, and so forth). Table 10-8 shows imaging modalities for evaluating carcinoma of the lung and gives estimates of cost/benefit ratio and usefulness of each modality. Table 10-9 summarizes guidelines for the efficient evaluation of patients with suspected lung cancer.[35]

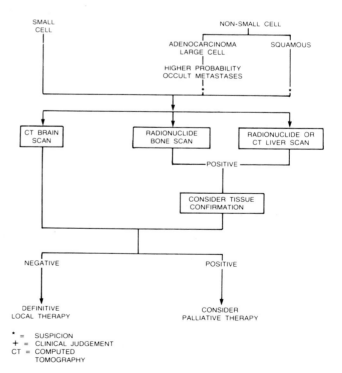

FIG. 10-13. M (metastatic) evaluation. Diagnostic and staging steps in evaluating patients with primary lung cancer based on the TNM system. The pathway strives to be conservative and cost-effective and relies on state-of-the-art imaging technology and interpretive expertise.

Table 10-8. Imaging Modalities for Evaluating Carcinoma of the Lung

MODALITY	STAGING CAPABILITY	BENEFIT/ COST RATIO	RECOMMENDED ROUTINE STAGING PROCEDURE
A. Noninvasive			
1. Chest Films			
a. Posteroanterior and Lateral	Baseline high resolution image to assess T, less reliable for N and M	High	Yes
b. Previous	May establish change in T, N_1/N_2, or M	High	Yes
c. Follow-up	Useful to evaluate change; growth, recurrence, new or other disease	High	Yes
d. Overpenetrated	Useful to show bone, mediastinum, retrocardiac, and subdiaphragmatic lung	High	No
e. Oblique	15° or 45° useful to show lung, hilum and mediastinum in different projection	High	No
2. Fluoroscopy Spot Films	Permits evaluation of the patient, lung function, density and location of the lesion, biopsy site(s); may obviate tomography	High	No
3. Tomography			
a. Lesion	Defined size, borders, calcification, relationship to adjacent structures	Fair	No
b. 55° Oblique Hilar	Sensitive to node (N_1) enlargement, useful to define anatomy	High	No
c. Whole Lung	May show unsuspected lung, hilar or mediastinal lesion(s)	Low	No
4. Bone Films	Useful only to confirm metastases	Low	No
5. Radionuclide (RN) Bone, Brain Liver Scans	Useful in evaluation of clinically suspected metastases. CT better than RN for liver and brain	Low	No
Gallium 67	Fairly useful for metastases, variable sensitivity and specificity	Fair	Maybe
6. Magnetic Resonance Imaging	Easily distinguishes hilar masses and lymphadenopathy from blood vessels and fat for evaluation of T and N	?	?
B. Minimally Invasive			
1. CT	Invasive if intravenous contrast material given. Most useful of all modalities for determining characteristics of T and N in the thorax and M in the brain and liver	High	Yes
C. Invasive			
1. Percutaneous Needle Biopsy	Guided by fluoroscopy or CT, accurate in establishing cytologic diagnosis from T (particularly peripheral lung lesions); M (especially liver or bone); less experience with N	High	Yes
2. Angiography	Pulmonary angiography, azygous venography, superior venacavography reserved for special cases	Low	No

Treatment Decisions in Lung Cancer

At present, surgery and radiotherapy represent the only hope for cure for non-oat cell lung cancer patients. Chemotherapy has found its greatest success in small cell cancer patients, where significant improvements in survival have been reported in recent years. Radiation therapy is reserved for the patients who are considered to be inoperable or who have incompletely resected disease or metastatic disease.[5,49,69,88]

The trend in the past 30 to 40 years of lung cancer surgery has been toward the use of less extensive procedures. At the Massachusetts General Hospital during the decade from 1931 to 1940, 73% of lung cancer patients were treated primarily by pneumonectomy. From 1961 to 1970, only 32% of patients had a pneumonectomy for treatment of their primary lung cancer.[90] In reviews justifying the less extensive surgery, patient survival, regardless of cell type, was found to be 26% in the pneumonectomy group (9.1% hospital mortality), 35.2% in the lobectomy group (7.5% mortality), and 44.5% in the segmenectomy population (0% mortality).[90]

In non-oat cell carcinomas, mediastinal lymph node disease and malignant pleural effusions significantly af-

Table 10-9. Guidelines for Efficient Evaluation in the Patient with Suspected Lung Cancer: Simultaneous Determinations

DIAGNOSIS	STAGING T,N & M	OPERATIVE STATUS
establish histologic diagnosis	determine extent of disease	operability and attitude
i. squamous (40%)	i. biopsy palpable node	i. functional status
ii. small cell (20%)	ii. most patients are inoperable	a. assess with history and arterial blood gasses
iii. adeno (20%)	iii. metastatic evaluation is time consuming and expensive	b. decreased survival poor functional status
iv. large cell (15%)	iv. routine radionuclide scans not indicated in asymptomatic pts.	ii. cardiopulmonary reserve
v. other, mixed (5%)	v. inoperable signs—effusion, hoarseness, Horner's, SVC syndrome (N_2)	iii. attitude toward operation—a substantial percent refuse, obviating extensive work-up

Reprinted from Koh, H. K., Prout, M. N.: The efficient work-up of suspected lung cancer. *Arch. Intern. Med.* 142:966–968, 1982. With permission.

fect survival. In the series of Mountain et al.,[57] survival fell to nearly 0% at five years if an effusion was present. Also in their series, overall five-year survival of patients with resected disease without lymph node involvement was 48%. This figure dropped to 35% if hilar nodal disease was present and 8% if mediastinal nodes were involved. Survival was even lower for patients with adenocarcinoma in whom mediastinal node involvement was found; only 2% of that group survived five years. Therefore, adenocarcinoma patients with mediastinal metastases are not candidates for surgery.

Certain T_3 lesions are amenable to surgical resection: (1) peripheral cancers exhibiting direct invasion of the parietal pleura, intercostal muscles, or ribs, (2) Pancoast's tumors, and (3) cancers closer than 3 cm to the carina amenable to resection and reconstruction.[57]

Radiation therapy has remained controversial as a treatment of non-small cell carcinoma, but it is widely used in both definitive and palliative fashions. Based on Radiation Therapy Oncology Group studies that have been completed randomizing patients to three different dose levels, optimum doses are considered in the range of 5,000–6,000 cGy delivered in 5 to 6 weeks through a shrinking-field technique.[63,64] With the introduction of CT scans, a more precisely defined volume can be treated, allowing the radiation oncologist to be more accurate in modern treatment planning by locating and avoiding vital intrathoracic structures, such as the spinal cord, in a changing body contour. Radiation therapy has also been combined with surgery in preoperative[7,34] and postoperative[33,62,87] radiation programs with limited success. Table 10-10 summarizes the various combinations of treatment that have been or may be used for the treatment of bronchogenic carcinoma.[88]

With small cell carcinoma, prolongation of life rather than "cure" has been the major objective of treatment

Table 10-10. Bronchogenic Carcinoma, Squamous Cell, and Adenocarcinoma

STAGE	SURGERY	RADIATION THERAPY		CHEMOTHERAPY
I T_1,T_2,N_0,M_0	Lobectomy Pneumonectomy Plus hilar node resection	NR		NR
II T_1,T_2,N_1,M_0	Lobectomy Pneumonectomy Plus hilar node resection	Postoperative RT optional 5,000 cGy/5–6 weeks		NR
III T_3,N_0,M_0	Lobectomy or Pneumonectomy And hilar node resection if possible	Definitive RT if unresectable 5,000–6,000 cGy/5–6 weeks		Investigational MAC
T_{any}, N_2M_0	Usually no resection attempted	Definitive RT if unresectable 5,000–6,000 cGy/5–6 weeks		Investigational MAC
IV T_4,N_3,M_0	NR	Palliative RT	and/or	MAC
T_{any},N_{any}, M_+	NR	Palliative RT	and/or	MAC

RT = radiation therapy.
NR = not recommended.
MAC = multiagent chemotherapy.

programs to date (Table 10-11). Bone marrow and CNS invasion are the principal sites of metastases with these aggressive lesions. At the time of diagnosis, marrow involvement can be found in approximately 50% of patients and CNS lesions in 10% to 13% of patients. During the course of their disease, CNS involvement will develop in approximately 50% of patients. Prophylactic treatment of the brain with drugs (nitrosoureas) or radiation has not dramatically changed either the incidence of subsequent relapse or survival.[71]

Multiple drug chemotherapy is the cornerstone of treatment for small cell tumors of the lung. The role of radiation therapy is primarily to consolidate the tumor regression in connection with chemotherapy or to palliate symptomatic metastatic sites in caval obstruction or in CNS prophylaxis. It is not effective as an independent primary treatment modality.

The role of consolidation radiation therapy is full-dose treatment to 4,500 to 5,000 cGy with a shrinking-field technique being combined with chemotherapy, since there is a high incidence of local regional relapses with chemotherapy alone in trials of a variety of cooperative group studies.[73] Again, the use of CT imaging is valuable for boosting fields to higher doses.

Although small cell tumors are not considered in the province of surgery, peripheral small cell lesions have been cured by surgical resection. Routine surgical approaches for this type of tumor are not recommended at present. With current chemotherapy regimens, response rates of 60% to 90% can be expected, although these are not long lasting. Long-term survival in a limited number of patients can now be anticipated and five-year survivals are now being reported.[28,38]

Impact of New Technology

The past decade of progress in medical imaging has been as dramatic as any since Roentgen's initial discovery in 1895. In spite of these exciting improvements no parallel changes in survival have resulted. It is hoped that screening of high-risk patients will afford improved survival with time, but this is still an unrealized goal.

Applications of CT have certainly yielded valuable staging and treatment planning data. The learning and application phases of this "new technique" will continue to provide rewards, but these will be limited in terms of survival gains.

Magnetic resonance imaging (MRI) is the exciting new technology for the 1980s.[8] Its status, to date, parallels that of CT in the 1970s.[9] Early acceptance of CT imaging in the brain was followed by a gradual understanding and acceptance of CT body imaging. In 1983, MRI was in a similar position. To date, the gains of MRI in oncologic imaging have been small and principally in improved sensitivity rather than tumor specificity. Possibly later, with the larger superconductive magnets undergoing initial trials, some new data may emerge from clinical changes in carbon and phosphorus compounds in cancers or other metabolic signatures.[9]

Experimental applications of MRI techniques have shown, in vivo, the potential specificity of the technique in discriminating normal from cancerous tissue. These observations are based on differences in tumor cell water content and changes in MRI imaging characteristics (T_1 and T_2 relaxation times).[19] Theoretical and experimental applications of MRI in animal tumor models have recently been reviewed.[8,15]

Nuclear magnetic resonance imaging of the human thorax has been very limited. Ten normal adults and 12 patients, nine with advanced lung cancer, were studied at the University of California with spin-echo images using a 0.35 Tesla superconducting magnet. Mediastinal and hilar structures were seen equally well in MRI images and CT scans (Figure 10-14). Spin-echo images showed several features of tumor behavior, including mediastinal invasion, vascular and bronchial compression and invasion, and hilar and mediastinal adenopathy. Tumor could be separated from mediastinal and hilar fat on these images because of its larger T_1 relaxation time. Lung le-

Table 10-11. Small Cell Carcinoma

STAGE	SURGERY	RADIATION THERAPY		CHEMOTHERAPY
I Limited intrathoracic disease T_1, T_2, N_0	Complete resections, if possible	Definitive RT 4,500–5,000 cGy to primary nodes Elective brain RT	and	Pre- and postoperative RT MAC
II Limited intrathoracic disease T_1, T_2, N_0	Investigative resections	Definitive RT 4,500–5,000 cGy to primary nodes Elective brain RT	and	MAC
III Limited intrathoracic disease T_3 or N_2, M_0	Unresectable	Definitive RT 4,500–5,000 cGy to primary nodes Elective brain RT	and	MAC
IV Metastatic	Unresectable	Palliative RT		MAC

RT = radiation therapy.
MAC = multiagent chemotherapy.

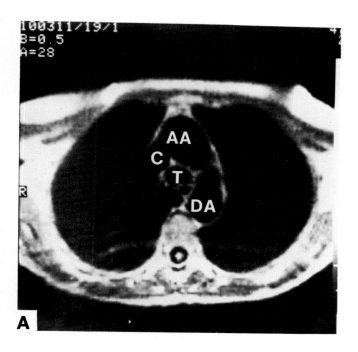

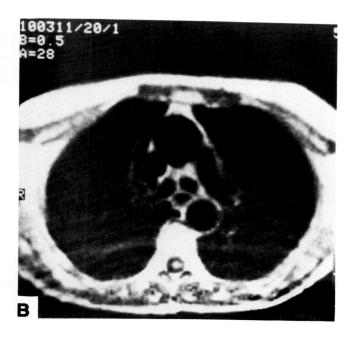

FIG. 10-14. (A) Normal MRI spin-echo image through the aortic arch of a 45-year-old man. The ascending aorta (AA), descending aorta (DA), trachea (T), and superior vena cava (C) are clearly shown. (B) Normal MRI spin-echo image through the main pulmonary artery of the same man. The main pulmonary artery (MPA) and left pulmonary artery (LPA) are clearly seen. The trachea has divided into right and left main bronchi (MB). Only the walls of vessels are demonstrated. No signal is seen within the great vessels, pulmonary arteries, or veins. The spin-echo delays and pulse sequence intervals used in this study precluded obtaining any signal from the lungs.[26] (MRI images provided by Dr. Gordon Gamsu, University of California, San Francisco.)

sions as small as 1.5 cm could be seen on spin-echo images. Further evaluation of MRI in lung cancer staging is required to determine the sensitivity and specificity of this technique.[26]

A prototype digital apparatus dedicated to chest imaging received an initial clinical trial at the University of Alabama during 1982. From approximately 400 patients who were examined with the device, 50 were selected for observer studies comparing digital images with conventional roentgenograms. Visualization of seven mediastinal structures was significantly improved on digital images because of increased exposure latitude. Pathologic states were seen equally well with both systems.[25] The role of digital imaging in tumor diagnosis and staging is yet unknown.

Radionuclide diagnostic and staging procedures are, at present, either nonspecific or quantum limited in chest tumor imaging. Advances in the development of radiopharmaceuticals or tagged monoclonal antibodies possibly may extend the current role of nuclear imaging in diagnosis and staging.

PLEURAL NEOPLASMS

The group of primary pleural mesotheliomas have an interesting, rather well understood profile in spite of being a distinct clinicopathologic entity for such a brief period of time. Prior to 1931, mesotheliomas were described but rarely reported, probably most often being confused with metastatic pleural disease. It is estimated at present that some 500 deaths annually result from mesothelioma in the United States.[36] With both pleural and peritoneal mesotheliomas, a clear etiologic link to asbestos exposure has been established. All types of asbestos fibers have been responsible for mesotheliomas; however, the crocidolite fiber is believed to be both the most ubiquitous and potent in this regard. Asbestos exposure increases the risk of developing a mesothelioma by 300 times, with a long latent period averaging 29 years from initial exposure to death. Since approximately 1 million workers are now at risk, and a 5% to 7% incidence of mesotheliomas has been estimated, the increasing frequency of this tumor can be appreciated.[1]

There are two gross types of mesothelioma, the localized and the diffuse forms (25% v 75% of cases, respectively). The diffuse type is always malignant and is linked to asbestos exposure, whereas no definite association has been shown with the solitary form. The localized lesion is believed to be a benign tumor; however, eight malignant neoplasms were encountered in a recent review of 60 cases from the Mayo Clinic.[59]

The three histologic types of mesothelioma are epithelial (most often the one confused with metastases), mesenchymal (also called sarcomatous or fibrosarcomatous type), and mixed forms.

These tumors arise from either the visceral or parietal

pleural surface (Figure 10-15). The malignant, diffuse mesothelioma is an inexorably progressive, locally aggressive tumor that encases the pleural surface, invading the adjacent structures of the mediastinum and chest wall. Effusions are common and usually apparent on presentation. Symptoms are almost universally present with the diffuse lesion and include chest pain, dyspnea, weight loss, and fever. Metastases outside the thorax have been described but are uncommon, since the tumor usually limits itself to the chest and contiguous intrathoracic structures.

The diagnosis of primary or metastatic pleural tumors may be difficult and requires a high index of suspicion in a patient with an obscure pleural effusion, chest pain, or a pleural mass. Open thoracotomy and biopsy are essential to assess the extent of disease and to obtain adequate tissue for histologic diagnosis. Thoracoscopy and biopsy may obviate thoracotomy. Cytologic analysis of sputum samples or pleural fluid is seldom diagnostic.[20] Percutaneous needle biopsy usually yields insufficient and occasionally even misleading histologic material for diagnosis.

Mesothelioma survival figures have been disappointing, with surgery being the only effective curative option. The median survival without treatment in the diffuse lesion is 2 months, increasing to 11 months with surgery. A number of alternative approaches to treatment have been tried (chemotherapy, topical radionuclides, and external radiation therapy) with only a temporary, palliative influence on the tumor.[1]

Metastatic involvement of the pleural space is most frequently found to be caused by adenocarcinomas. This is, in part, because of the primary tumors that predilect the pleural space (breast, upper GI tract, lung, and ovary). Pleural effusions are the universal finding but seldom can mass lesions be identified (as noted with mesotheliomas), since the tumor implants are usually small.

Plain roentgenograms may reveal extent of disease in malignant mesotheliomas but a large pleural effusion may obscure much of the tumor. Thoracentesis and diagnostic pneumothorax with decubitus roentgenograms in various body positions may be very helpful in assessing pleural tumor. Computed tomography, however, is the single most valuable imaging procedure.[32] Transverse section imaging encompasses the mediastinum, lung, and chest wall in a single image; eliminates overlying structures; and allows precise demonstration of size, contour, and extent of tumor. Invasion of the mediastinum and chest wall may be diagnosed when a tumor obliterates fat planes between the pleura and chest wall muscles or when tumor invades bone.

MEDIASTINAL NEOPLASMS

Several generalities help to illustrate the problems posed by mediastinal neoplasms: age and anatomic com-

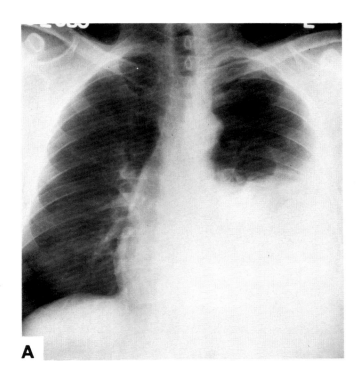

A

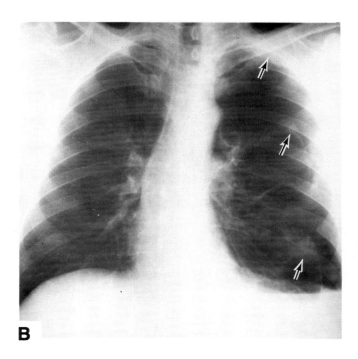

B

FIG. 10-15. Malignant mesothelioma. (A) PA chest roentgenogram of a 64-year-old man with 40-year history of asbestos exposure. Exudative left pleural effusion was nondiagnostic. (B) PA chest roentgenogram following thoracentesis and diagnostic pneumothorax shows multiple masses of various sizes on the visceral and parietal pleural surfaces, including a large lobulated apical mass obscured by the large effusion. Surgical exploration and histologic examination confirmed epithelial type malignant mesothelioma.

partment of origin are major diagnostic determinants, symptoms tend to closely correlate with tumor behavior, and therapy of this tumor subset is largely within the province of surgery.

Although mediastinal primary and metastatic tumors occur at any age, the reported incidence of malignant mediastinal masses is greater in children than in adults (40% to 45% v 20% to 25%). This discrepancy is best illustrated by the differences in types of posterior mediastinal tumors in children and adults. Far more malignant neural tumors are found in the posterior mediastinum in children compared with adults. In balance, thymomas are rare childhood tumors, with almost all instances reported in adults over the age of 20 years.[77]

Table 10-12 summarizes the anatomic compartment most commonly associated with the respective mediastinal neoplasms. These anatomic compartments are arbitrarily defined as superior mediastinum (thoracic inlet to the plane inferiorly defined by T-4 to the sternomanubrial junction), anterior (sternum to the pericardium anteriorly), middle (anterior pericardium to the anterior margin of the thoracic vertebrae), and posterior (anterior vertebral bodies to the posterior pleural margin). Arbitrary locational assignments have been made with the lymphomas as well as in some instances with mesenchymal tumors and the ill-defined, rare primary carcinomas. The incidence figures are derived from a total of 1,906 solid tumors in children and adults summarized by Ravitch and Sabiston.[66] The most frequently observed neoplasms are those of a neurogenic origin: thymomas, lymphomas, and germ cell tumors.

Symptoms are usually attributable to either local invasion or compression. They consist of pain, cough, and dysphagia. Relating tumor behavior to symptomatology, some 50% of symptomatic mediastinal masses prove to be malignant, whereas 90% of benign lesions are asymptomatic.

Thymomas are the most common anterior mediastinal primary neoplasm, accounting for nearly 20% of all tumors summarized in Table 10-12. Virtually all thymomas

occur in adults. Blalock originally drew attention to the association of myasthenia gravis and thymoma in 1939. Estimates over the association of myasthenia and thymoma vary from 10% to as high as 50%. Present figures suggest that thymectomy will relieve the myesthenic symptoms in approximately 25% of patients and help control the disease in another 50%.[22] It is estimated that nearly 70% of patients with solid thymic tumors have an associated systemic syndrome (red cell aplasia, hypogammaglobulinemia, malignancy, collagen vascular disease, etc.). The pathologist is usually unable to distinguish benign from malignant thymomas on histologic criteria. Their gross appearance is most important in predicting tumor behavior, with the noninvasive, encapsulated lesions usually being benign. Invasive thymomas tend to be locally aggressive lesions with rare distant metastases. Survival following surgical resection averages 10% to 13% for these invasive neoplasms.

A discussion of the mediastinal lymphomas will be found in the chapter on lymphomas.

The germ cell neoplasms account for some 13% of mediastinal solid tumors. Their location in the anterior mediastinum must have a congenital basis because the tumors resemble those of a gonadal origin. Teratomas are the most frequent subtype, of which some 80% are benign. The malignant types have a carcinomatous morphology rather than being sarcomatous. As with the solid thymomas, preoperative differentiation of the malignant and benign lesions is not possible; hence, surgery is the only effective diagnostic and treatment approach available at present.[66] Seminomas, choricocarcinomas, and embryonal tumors also occur. The latter two neoplasms are highly aggressive, widely metastatic lesions that occur in young males and have a uniformly fatal outcome. Seminomas, on the other hand, are radioresponsive, curable lesions that also are limited to the young adult male population, particularly if the mediastinal mass is truly primary, not metastatic.

The mesenchymal mediastinal tumors constitute a broad group of uncommon neoplasms of fat, muscle, vessel, or connective tissue origin. They include lipomas, liposarcomas, fibromas and their sarcomatous subtypes, as well as hemangiomas and lymphangiomas.

Of all mediastinal solid tumors, the neurogenic category is the most common (Table 10-12). Some 50% of these tumors in children are malignant, whereas the vast majority in adults are benign.[66] The spectrum of these tumors ranges from the most common benign neurilemmoma to neurofibroma and its malignant counterpart, the neurosarcoma. The incidence of the sarcomatous form increases with age and in the presence of neurofibromatosis.[66] Sympathetic ganglia tumors include the benign ganglioneuroblastomas and neuroblastomas. The latter tumors are usually limited to young children and frequently are widely metastatic at the time of diagnosis, challenging the radiologist to localize all distant sites of

Table 10-12. Mediastinal Neoplasms:
Compartmental Location and Incidence

MEDIASTINAL COMPARTMENT	TYPE OF TUMOR	INCIDENCE* (%)
Superior Mediastinum	Endocrine tumors (thyroid, parathyroid, carcinoid)	5
Anterior Mediastinum	Thymoma	19
	Lymphoma	17
	Germ Cell Tumors	13
	Mesenchymal Tumors	9
	Primary Carcinomas	4
Posterior Mediastinum	Neurogenic Tumors	31

*Adapted from Heitzman, E. R.: Computed tomography of the thorax: Current perspectives. A.J.R. 136:2–12, 1981.

disease in the osseous system, liver, brain, and lymph nodes.

Computed tomography cannot establish the histologic diagnosis in mediastinal tumors; however, after plain roentgenograms, CT may (1) precisely demonstrate size, contour, and extent of tumor; (2) detect direct invasion of the mediastinal contents and chest wall; (3) allow separation of vascular structures using intravenous contrast; (4) characterize tissue attenuation, thus differentiating fat, tissue, and calcification; (5) determine the best site for tissue source to establish histologic diagnosis; and, finally, (6) provide a baseline for measurable tumor and follow-up.

PULMONARY METASTATIC DISEASE

The lung is the most common site for metastases regardless of the primary tumor site.[91] The chest roentgenogram is usually the first indicator of tumor extension. The initial manifestation of non-lung cancer as metastatic pulmonary disease is uncommon and a search for the primary tumor site is often fruitless. Radiographic patterns of metastatic disease to the lung may be useful in searching for the primary site or in differentiating metastatic disease from nonneoplastic processes. Multiple pulmonary nodules are the most common radiographic and pathologic form of metastatic disease to the lung. The so-called lymphangitic pattern is most often associated with metastatic adenocarcinoma from breast or gastrointestinal primaries. A lymphangitic tumor is almost always accompanied by pulmonary symptoms and may be confused with the diagnosis of left ventricular failure and pulmonary edema. Tumor overwhelms the pulmonary lymphatic system, producing lymph vessel engorgement, increased interstitial lung water with bronchial and vascular cuffing, and visible septal lines mimicking the radiographic changes of heart failure.

Nodular metastatic disease presents an imaging challenge analogous to primary lung cancer detection as discussed earlier. The margins of metastatic pulmonary nodules tend to be sharp and well-defined from bone and soft tissue sarcomas as well as renal and testicular carcinomas. In contrast, metastatic epidermoid carcinomas tend to have ill-defined margins that are more difficult to recognize radiographically until nodule size exceeds 1 to 1.5 cm because of the inherent low contrast of these lesions. Cavitary nodular lesions occur most often with tumors of epidermoid origin. Examples of these cavitary lesions are most frequently found with primaries of the head and neck and cervix; however, virtually any type of tumor may excavate.

Nodular pulmonary metastases, most often of a sarcomatous origin, occasionally seed the pulmonary vascular bed in a subpleural location. Necrosis within these

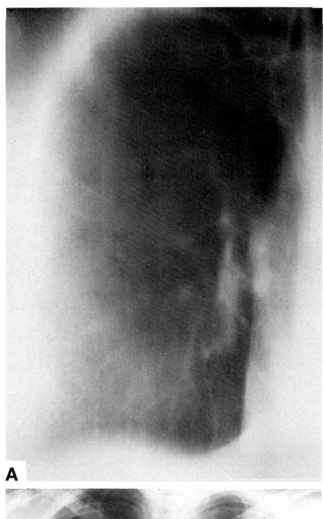

A

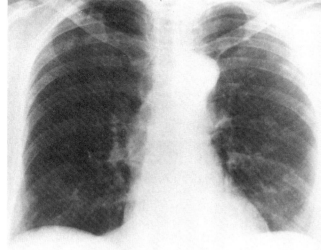

B

FIG. 10-16. Metastatic adenocarcinoma—colon primary. (A) A standard PA chest roentgenogram shows the ill-defined nodular lesions distributed throughout both lung fields. The ill-defined margins and low contrast densities emphasize the difficulty of detecting these nodules. (B) Tomograms show the nodules at one focal plane in the right lung. (C) CT scan at the same level, with variations in the window settings, shows variations in the displayed size of the nodules.

tumors can cause a bronchopleural fistula, resulting in pneumothorax. Pneumothorax associated with metastatic sarcomas is most frequently noted in young patients.[93]

A miliary pattern of metastatic disease is uncommon and presumably results from hematogenous embolization of tumor cells. It is described in tumors of epithelial origin, especially carcinoma of the cervix, following surgery and is usually associated with a dismal prognosis. The differential diagnostic considerations in this pattern include silicosis and inflammatory or drug-induced disease as well as metastatic tumor.

When a patient has plain film evidence suggesting pulmonary metastatic disease without a clinically obvious primary site, only a limited search for the primary location should be undertaken. Initially a complete history and physical examination, appropriate laboratory studies, and review of previous roentgenograms are necessary. A tissue diagnosis is then established without delay, based upon biopsy of a clinically detected site or lung lesion using excisional, endoscopic, or needle techniques. If the histologic examination reveals adenocarcinoma, a breast primary is usually obvious on careful clinical examination; if not, mammograms rarely identify a clinically occult lesion. If the patient is a middle-aged or older man with nodular metastatic adenocarcinoma, the primary site will most often be discovered in the lower gastrointestinal tract (Figure 10-16). In contrast, multiple nodules of epidermoid carcinoma in a middle-aged or older man are most often metastates from a head and neck primary site (Table 10-13).

Steckel and Kagan[80] reviewed 255 patients with metastases from an unknown primary site. Of 34 patients with autopsy information, no primary tumor site could be found in 20. In the 14 in whom a primary site was identified, it was concluded that this information would not have influenced patient outcome or treatment. Based on these and other data, the authors urged restraint in searching for the primary site in this situation.[80]

Patients with primary tumors capable of spreading to the lung are appropriately followed with chest roentgenograms to detect metastatic disease and correlate change in measurable lesions (e.g., lung nodules) with therapy. Other cost effective screening imaging studies, including "unsharp masking" with improved antiscatter grids and digital chest imaging, may improve the detection accuracy of metastatic disease.[4] However, routine use of expensive, highly sensitive imaging techniques such as computerized tomographic chest imaging should be avoided and reserved for selected patient groups. Improved sensitivity of CT must be balanced against cost, time, and nonspecificity. Sophisticated imaging studies may be superfluous when the possibility of lung metastasis is remote or when the detection of metastases has no influence on therapy.

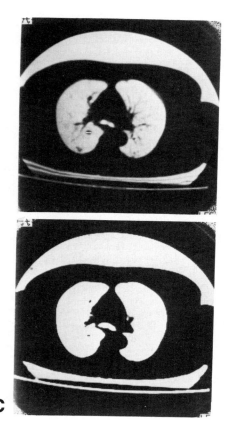

C

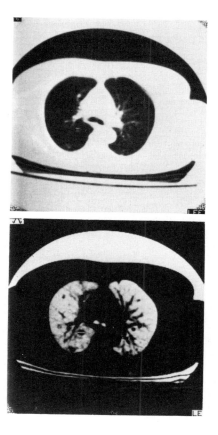

Table 10-13. Pulmonary Metastatic Disease: Patterns and Probable Primary Sites

NODULAR PATTERN			LYMPHANGITIC PATTERN
SARCOMAS	EPIDERMOID	ADENOCARCINOMA	
	head and neck	colon	"Always"
		prostate	adenocarcinoma (may be
	lung cancer	lung	sarcomatous or epithelial)
	head and neck	kidney	

			Male Patient	*Female Patient*
	cervix	colon	lung primary	breast
		prostate	(unilateral	ovary
		lung	pattern)	
		kidney	pancreas/	
		breast	stomach	
		uterus	prostate	

In conclusion, the radiographic appearance of metastatic disease is nonspecific and can be mimicked by a variety of diseases. Tissue confirmation will be required in most circumstances to establish the diagnosis. An organized and conservative imaging search should be considered for patients who initially have pulmonary metastatic disease with an occult primary site.[48,53]

REFERENCES

1. Aisner, J., Wiernick, P. H.: Malignant mesothelioma. Current status and future prospects. *Chest* 74:438–444, 1978.
2. Alazraki, N. P., Ramsdell, J. W., Taylor, A. T., Friedman, P. J., Peters, R. M., Tisi, G. M.: The reliability of gallium scan chest radiography compared to mediastinoscopy for evaluating mediastinal spread in lung cancer. *Am. Rev. Respir. Dis.* 117:415–420, 1978.
3. American Joint Committee on Cancer: *Manual for Staging of Cancer*, 2nd ed. Philadelphia, J. B. Lippincott, 1983, pp. 99–105.
4. Armstrong, J. D., Sorenson, J. A., Nelson, J. A., Tocino, I., Lester, P. D., Janes, J. O., Niklason, L. T., Stanish, W.: Clinical evaluation of unsharp masking and slit scanning techniques in chest radiography. *Radiology* 147:351–356, 1983.
5. Barkley, H. T., Jr., Bloedorn, F. G., Hussey, D. H.: Thorax. In *Textbook of Radiotherapy*, 3rd ed. Fletcher, G. H. (Ed.). Philadelphia, Lea & Febiger, 1980, pp. 662–703.
6. Baron R. L., Levitt, R. G., Sagel, S. S., White, M. J., Roper, C. L., Marberger, J. P.: Computed tomography in the preoperative evaluation of bronchogenic carcinoma. *Radiology* 145:727–737, 1982.
7. Bloedorn, F. G.: Rationale and benefit of preoperative irradiation in lung cancer. *J.A.M.A.* 196:340–341, 1966.
8. Brady, T. J., Burt, C. T., Goldman, M. R., Pykett, I. L., Buonnanno, F. S., Kistler, J. P., Newhouse, J. H., Hinshaw, W. S., Pohost, G. M.: Tumor characterization using ^{31}P NMR spectroscopy. In *NMR Imaging — Proceedings of an International Symposium on NMR Imaging*. Winston-Salem, NC, Bowman-Gray School of Medicine, 1982.
9. Budinger, T. F.: Medical application of nuclear magnetic resonance scanning: Some perspectives in relation to other techniques. In *NMR Imaging — Proceedings of an International Symposium on NMR Imaging*. Winston-Salem, NC, Bowman-Gray School of Medicine, 1982.
10. Butler, A. R., Leo, J. S., Lin, J. P., Boyd, A. D., Kricheff, I. I.: The value of routine cranial computed tomography in neurologically intact patients with primary carcinoma of the lung. *Radiology* 131:399–401, 1979.
11. Byrd, R. B., Carr, D. T., Miller, W. E., Payne, W. S., Woolner, L. B.: Radiographic abnormalities in carcinoma of the lung as related to histologic type. *Thorax* 24:573–575, 1969.
12. Cancer Statistics, 1985. *CA* 35:26–27, 1985.
13. Cox, J. L. D., Yesner, R. A.: Adenocarcinoma of the lung: Recent results from the Veterans Administration lung group. *Am. Rev. Respir. Dis.* 120:1025–1029, 1979.
14. Crowe, J. K., Brown, L. R., Muhm, J. R.: Computed tomography of the mediastinum. *Radiology* 128:75–87, 1978.
15. Davis, P. L., Sheldon, P., Kaufman, L., Crooks, L., Margulis, A. R., Miller, T., Watts, J., Nakawa, M., Hoenninger, J.: Nuclear magnetic resonance imaging of mammary adenocarcinomas in the rat. *Cancer* 51:433–499, 1983.
16. deLima, R.: Bronchial adenoma. *Chest* 77:81–84, 1980.
17. DeMeester, T. R., Bekerman, C., Joseph, J. G., Toscano, M. S., Golomb, H., Bitran, J., Gross, N. J., Skinner, D. B.: Gallium-67 scanning for carcinoma of the lung. *J. Thorac. Cardiovasc. Surg.* 72:699–708, 1976.
18. Eggleston, J., Saryan, L., Hollis, D.: Nuclear magnetic resonance investigations of human neoplastic and abnormal non-neoplastic tissues. *Cancer Res.* 35:1326–1332, 1975.
19. Ekholm, S., Albrechtsson, U., Kugelberg, J., Tylen, U.: Computed tomography in preoperative staging of bronchogenic carcinoma. *J. Comput. Assist. Tomogr.* 4:763–765, 1980.
20. Ellis, K., Wolff, M.: Mesotheliomas and secondary tumors of the pleura. *Semin. Roentgenol.* 12:303–311, 1977.
21. Faling, L. J., Pugatch, R. D., Jung-Legg, Y., Daly, B. D. T., Hong, W. K., Robbins, A. H., Snider, G. L.: Computed tomographic scanning of the mediastinum in the staging of bronchogenic carcinoma. *Ann. Rev. Respir. Dis.* 124:690–695, 1981.
22. Fontana, R. S.: *Lung Cancer and Asbestos Related Pulmonary Disease*. A national correspondence course sponsored by the National Cancer Society and American College of Chest Physicians, 1981.
23. Forrest, J. V., Friedman, P. J.: Radiologic errors in patients with lung cancer. *West. J. Med.* 134:485–490, 1981.
24. Fosburg, R. G., Hopkins, G. M., Kan, M. K.: Evaluation of the mediastinum by gallium 67 scintigraphy in lung cancer. *J. Thorac. Cardiovasc. Surg.* 77:76–82, 1979.
25. Fraser, R. G., Breatnach, E., Barnes, G.: Digital radiography of the chest: Clinical experience with a prototype model. Presented at the Radiologic Society of North America, 68th Scientific Assembly and Annual Meeting, Chicago, Ill., 1982.
26. Gamsu, G., Webb, W. R., Sheldon, P., Kaufman, L., Crooks, L. E., Birnberg, F. A., Goodman, P., Hinchcliffe, W. A., Hedgecock, M.:

Nuclear magnetic resonance imaging of the thorax. *Radiology* 147: 473–480, 1983.

27. Goldberg, E. M., Shapiro, C. M., Glicksman, A. S.: Mediastinoscopy for assessing mediastinal spread in clinical staging of lung carcinoma. *Semin. Oncol.* 1:205–215, 1974.

28. Hansen, M., Hansen, H. H., Dombernowsky, P.: Long term survival in small cell carcinoma of the lung. *J.A.M.A.* 244:247–250, 1980.

29. Heaston, D. K., Mills, S. R., Moore, A. V., Johnston, W. W.: Percutaneous thoracic needle biopsy. In *Pulmonary Diagnosis, Imaging and Other Techniques.* Putman, C. E. (Ed). New York, Appleton-Century-Crofts, 1981, pp. 289–305.

30. Heelan, R. T., Melamed, M. R., Zaman, M. B., Martini, N., Flehinger, B. J.: Radiologic diagnosis of oat cell cancer in a high-risk screened population. *Radiology* 136:593–601, 1980.

31. Heitzman, E. R.: *The Lung Radiologic Pathologic Correlations.* St. Louis, C. V. Mosby Co., 1973.

32. Heitzman, E. R.: Computed tomography of the thorax: Current perspectives. *A.J.R.* 136:2–12, 1981.

33. Isreal, L., Bonadonna, G., Sylvester, R., and Members of the EORTC Lung Cancer Group.: Controlled study with adjuvant radiotherapy, chemotherapy, immunotherapy, and chemoimmunotherapy in operable squamous carcinoma of the lung. In *Lung Cancer: Progress in Therapeutic Research.* Muggia, F., Rozencweig, M. (Eds.). New York, Raven Press, 1979, pp. 443–452.

34. Kent, C. H., Schwade, J. G.: Preoperative radiation therapy in carcinoma of the lung. In *Lung Cancer: Progress in Therapeutic Research.* Muggia, F., Rozencweig, M. (Eds.). New York, Raven Press, 1979, pp. 289–293.

35. Koh, H. K., Prout, M. N.: The efficient work-up of suspected lung cancer. *Arch. Intern. Med.* 142:966–968, 1982.

36. Legha, S. S., Muggia, F. M.: Pleural mesothelioma: Clinical features and therapeutic implications. *Ann. Intern. Med.* 897:613–621, 1977.

37. Lesk, D. M., Wood, T. E., Carroll, S. E., Reese, L.: The application of 67Ga scanning in determining the operability of bronchogenic carcinoma. *Radiology* 128:707–709, 1978.

38. Livingston, R. B.: Small cell carcinoma of the lung. *Blood* 56: 575–584, 1980.

39. Lunia, S. L., Ruckdeschel, J. C., McKneally, M. F., Killam, D., Baxter, D., Kellar, S., Ray, P., McIlduff, J., Lininger, L., Chodos, R., Horton, J.: Noninvasive evaluation of mediastinal metastases in bronchogenic carcinoma. *Cancer* 47:672–679, 1981.

40. Marks, C., Marks, M.: Bronchial adenoma. A clinicopathologic study. *Chest* 71:376–380, 1977.

41. Marsh, B. R., Frost, J. K., Erozan, Y. S., Carter, D.: Fiberbronchoscopy. In *Lung Cancer. Clinical Diagnosis and Treatment.* Straus, M. J. (Ed.). New York, Grune & Stratton, 1977, pp. 107–112.

42. Martini, N., Flekinger, B. J., Zaman, M. B., Beattie, E. J.: Prospective study of 445 lung carcinomas with mediastinal lymph node metastases. *J. Thorac. Cardiovasc. Surg.* 80:390–399, 1980.

43. Martini, N., Melamed, M. R.: Occult carcinoma of the lung. *Ann. Thorac. Surg.* 30:215–223, 1980.

44. Martini, N., Posner, J.: Brain metastases in resected non-oat cell lung cancer. *Proc. Am. Assoc. Cancer Res.* 20:421, 1979.

45. Mathews, M. J.: Morphology of lung cancer. *Semin. Oncol.* 1: 175–182, 1974.

46. McNeill, T. M., Chamberlain, J. M.: Diagnostic anterior mediastinotomy. *Ann. Thorac. Surg.* 2:532–539, 1966.

47. Melamed, M. R., Flehinger, B. J., Zaman, M. B., Heelan, R. T., Hallerman, E. T., Martini, N.: Detection of true pathologic Stage I lung cancer in the screening program and the effect on survival. *Cancer* 47(suppl):1182–1187, 1981.

48. Milne, E. N. C.: Pulmonary metastases: Vascular supply and diagnosis. *Int. J. Radiat. Oncol. Biol. Phys.* 1:739–742, 1976.

49. Minna, J. D., Higgins, G. A., Glatstein, E. J.: Cancer of the lung. In *Cancer: Principles and Practice of Oncology.* DeVita, D. V. T.,

Hellman, S., Rosenberg, S. A. (Eds.). Philadelphia, J. B. Lippincott Co., 1982, pp. 396–474.

50. Mintz, U., DeMeester, T. R., Golomb, H. M., Cimochowski, G., Rezai, K., MacMahon, H., Sovik, C., Bitran, J. D.: Sequential staging in bronchogenic carcinoma. *Chest* 76:653–657, 1979.

51. Mintzer, R. A., Malave, L. S. R., Neiman, H. L., Michaelis, L. L., Vanecko, R. M., Sanders, J. H.: Computed vs conventional tomography in evaluation of primary and secondary pulmonary neoplasms. *Radiology* 132:653–659, 1979.

52. Moak, G. D., Cockerill, E. M., Farber, M. O., Yaw, P. B., Manfredi, E.: Computed tomography vs standard radiology in the evaluation of medastinal adenopathy. *Chest* 82:69–75, 1982.

53. Mountain, C. F.: Pulmonary metastatic disease—Progress in a neglected area. *Int. J. Radiat. Oncol. Biol. Phys.* 1:755–757, 1976.

54. Mountain, C. F.: Assessment of the role of surgery for the control of lung cancer. *Ann. Thorac. Surg.* 24:365–373, 1977.

55. Mountain, C. F.: Clinical biology of small cell carcinoma. Relationship to surgical therapy. *Semin. Oncol.* 5:272–279, 1978.

56. Mountain, C. F., Carr, D. T., Anderson, W. A. D.: A system for the clinical staging of lung cancer, *A.J.R.* 120:130–138, 1974.

57. Mountain, C. F., McMurtrey, M. J., Frazier, O. H.: Regional extension of lung cancer. *Int. J. Radiat. Oncol. Biol. Phys.* 6:1013–1020, 1980.

58. Newman, S. J., Hansen, H. H.: Proceedings: frequency, diagnosis and treatment of brain metastases in 247 consecutive patients with bronchogenic carcinoma. *Cancer* 33:492–496, 1974.

59. Okike, N., Bernatz, P. E., Woolner, L. B.: Localized mesothelioma of the pleura. Benign and malignant variants. *J. Thorac. Cardiovasc. Surg.* 75:363–372, 1978.

60. Osborne, D. R., Korobkin, M., Ravin, C. E., Putman, C. E., Wolfe, W. G., Sealy, W. C., Young, G. W., Breiman, R., Heaston, D., Ram, P., Halber, M.: Comparison of plain radiography, conventional tomography and computed tomography in detecting intrathoracic lymph node metastases from lung carcinoma. *Radiology* 142:157–161, 1982.

61. Pancoast, H. K.: Superior pulmonary sulcus tumor. *J.A.M.A.* 99:1391–1396, 1932.

62. Paterson, R., Russell, M. H.: Clinical trails in malignant disease: Part IV—lung cancer. Value of postoperative radiotherapy. *Clin. Radiol.* 13:141–144, 1962.

63. Perez, C. A., Stanley, K., Rubin, P., Kramer, S., Brady, L. W., Marks, J. E., Perez-Tamayo, R., Brown, G. S., Concannon, J. P., Rotman, M.: Patterns of tumor recurrence after definitive irradiation for inoperable non-oat cell carcinoma of the lung. *Int. J. Radiat. Oncol. Biol. Phys.* 6:987–994, 1980.

64. Perez, C. A., Stanley, K., Rubin, P., Kramer, S., Brady, L. W., Marks, J. F., Perez-Tamayo, R., Brown, G. S., Concannon, J. P., Rotman, M. Prospective randomized study of various irradiation doses and fractionation schedules in the treatment of inoperable non-oat cell carcinoma of the lung. Preliminary report of the Radiation Therapy Oncology Group. *Cancer* 45:2744–2753, 1980.

65. Ramsdell, J. W., Peters, R. M., Taylor, A. T., Alazraki, N. P., Tisi, G. M.: Multiorgan scans for staging lung cancer. Correlation with clinical evaluation. *J. Thorac. Cardiovasc. Surg.* 73:653–659, 1977.

66. Ravitch, M. M., Sabiston, D. C.: Mediastinal infections, cysts and tumors. In *Pediatric Surgery*, 3rd ed. Ravitch, M. M., Welch, K. J., Benson, C. D., Aberdeen, E., Randolf, J. G. (Eds.). Chicago, Year Book Medical Publishers, 1979, pp. 492–512.

67. Rea, H. H., Shevland, J. E., House, A. J. S.: Accuracy of computed tomographic scanning in assessment of the mediastinum in bronchial carcinoma. *J. Cardiovasc. Thorac. Surg.* 81:825–829, 1981.

68. Rigler, L. G.: An overview of cancer of the lung. *Semin. Roentgenol.* 12:161–164, 1977.

69. Rosenberg, J. C.: Neoplasms of the mediastinum. In *Cancer: Principles and Practice of Oncology.* DeVita, V. T., Jr., Hellman, S.,

Rosenberg, S. A. (Eds.). Philadelphia, J. B. Lippincott Co., 1982. pp. 475-498.

70. Rosenow, E. C., Carr, D. T.: Bronchogenic carcinoma. CA 29: 233-245, 1979.

71. Ruckdeschel, J. C., Caradonna, B., Paladine, W. J., Hillinger, S. M., Horton, J.: Small cell anaplastic carcinoma of the lung: Changing concepts and emerging problems. CA 29:233-245, 1979.

72. Saccomanno, G.: Diagnostic Pulmonary Cytology. Chicago Education Products Division, American Society of Clinical Pathologists, 1978.

73. Salazar, O. M., Creech, R. H.: "The State of the Art:" Toward defining the role of radiation therapy in the management of small cell bronchogenic carcinoma. Int. J. Radiat. Oncol. Biol. Phys. 6:1103-1117, 1980.

74. Schaner, E. G., Chang, A. E., Doppman, J. L., Conkle, D. M., Flye, M. W., Rosenberg, S. A.: Comparison of computed and conventional whole lung tomography in detecting pulmonary nodules: A prospective radiologic-pathologic study. A.J.R. 131:51-54, 1978.

75. Shimosata, Y., Hashimoto, T., Kodama, T.: Prognostic implications of fibrotic focus (scar) in small peripheral lung cancers. Am. J. Surg. Pathol. 4:365-373, 1980.

76. Siegelman, S. S., Zerhouni, E. A., Leo, F. P., Khouri, N. F., Stitik, F. P.: CT of the solitary pulmonary nodule. A.J.R. 135:1-13, 1980.

77. Silverman, N. A., Sabiston, D. C., Jr.: Mediastinal masses. Surg. Clin. North Am. 60:757-776, 1980.

78. Sorenson, J. A., Armstrong, J. D., Nelson, J. A.: Value of multiple films and multiple readers for detection of lung nodules in chest radiography. Presented at 67th Scientific Assembly and Annual Meeting, Radiological Society of North America-American Association of Physicists in Medicine, Chicago, November 15-20, 1981.

79. Spencer, H.: Pathology of the Lung, 4th ed. Elmsford, NY, Pergamon Press, 1985.

80. Steckel, R. J., Kagan, A. R.: Diagnostic persistence in working up metastatic cancer with an unknown primary site. Radiology 134: 367-369, 1980.

81. Stitik, F. P., Tockman, M. S.: Radiographic screening in the early detection of lung cancer. Radiol. Clin. North Am. 16:347-366, 1978.

82. Takita, H., Brugarolas, A., Marabella, P., Vincent, R. G.: Small cell carcinoma of the lung. Clinicopathological studies. J. Thorac. Surg. 66:472-477, 1973.

83. Taylor, W. F., Fontana, R. S., Uhlenhopp, M. A., Davis, C. S.: Some results of screening for early lung cancer. Cancer 47:1114-1120, 1981.

84. Tisi, G. M., Friedman, P. J., Peters, R. M., Pearson, G., Carr, D., Lee, R. E., Selawry, O.: Clinical staging of primary lung cancer. Am. Rev. Respir. Dis. 127:659-664, 1983.

85. Underwood, G. H., Hooper, R. G., Axelbaum, S. P., Goodwin, D. W.: Computed tomographic scanning of the thorax in the staging of bronchogenic carcinoma. N. Engl. J. Med. 300:777-778, 1979.

86. Valaitis, J., Warren, S., Gamble, D.: Increasing incidence of adenocarcinoma of the lung. Cancer 47:1042-1046, 1981.

87. Van Houtte. P., Rocmans, P., Smets, P., Goffin, J., Lustman-Maréchal, J., Vanderhoeft, P., Henry, J.: Postoperative radiation therapy in lung cancer: A controlled trial after resection of curative design. Int. J. Radiat. Oncol. Biol. Phys. 6:983-986, 1980.

88. Van Houtte, P., Salazar, O. M., Phillips, C. E., Asbury, R. F.: Lung cancer. In Clinical Oncology for Medical Students and Physicians: A Multidisciplinary Approach, 6th ed., Rubin, P. (Ed.). New York, American Cancer Society, 1983, pp. 142-153.

89. Vincent, R. G., Pickren, J. W., Lane, W. W., Bross, I., Takita, H., Houten, L., Gutierrez, A. C., Rzepka, T.: The changing histopathology of lung cancer: A review of 1682 cases. Cancer 39:1647-1655, 1977.

90. Wilkins, E. W., Scannell, G., Craver, J. B.: Four decades of experience with resections for bronchogenic carcinoma at the Massachusetts General Hospital. J. Thorac. Cardiovasc. Surg. 76:364-368, 1978.

91. Willis, R. A.: The Spread of Tumors in the Human Body, 3rd ed. London, Butterworths. 1973.

92. Woolner, L. B., Fontana, R. S., Sanderson, D. R., Miller, W. E., Muhm, J. R., Taylor, W. F., Uhlenhopp, M. A.: Mayo lung project. Evaluation of lung cancer screening through December 1979. Mayo Clin. Proc. 56:544-555, 1981.

93. Wright, F. W.: Spontaneous pneumothorax and pulmonary malignant disease—a syndrome associated with cavitating tumors. Clin. Radiol. 27:211-222, 1976.

11 BREAST CANCER

John R. Milbrath
David G. Bragg
James E. Youker

Breast cancer is a disease of awesome proportions that afflicts one in every eleven American women and is still the leading cause of cancer mortality in women.[2,3] In recent years, public attention has been focused on breast cancer as a result of the medical debate regarding screening, detection and treatment. This chapter will review the major elements of this controversy, summarize the different pathologic forms of breast cancer, describe the imaging process from the vantage point of both screening and detection as well as staging, and, finally, discuss some of the treatment controversies.

The American Cancer Society estimates that 115,900 new cases of breast cancer occurred in 1984 with 38,000 deaths, representing 26% of the total number of cancers diagnosed in women and 18% of the female cancer deaths.[3] Breast cancer is uncommon in men, with an estimated 900 new cases detected and 300 deaths in 1984. Environment plays a role, since the frequency of the disease in countries with a high fat diet is much greater than that found in countries with a low fat, high fiber diet.[4] In the continental United States, the incidence of breast cancer is highest in northern urban cities, particularly those bordering the Great Lakes.

Survival rates have improved little during the past 50 years in spite of dramatic changes in both diagnosis and treatment. As an example, the five-year survival rate for all stages of breast cancer was 53% in the 1940s and 65% in the 1970s.[2] The importance of early diagnosis is emphasized by the five-year survival of 97% for minimal cancer and 85% if the tumor is localized to the breast. Once spread occurs to the regional lymph nodes, how-

ever, the survival drops to 56%. It is a general assumption that once systemic metastatic disease occurs, the opportunity for "cure" approaches zero.[52,53]

The cause of breast cancer is unknown, yet risk factors have drawn the attention of the medical and lay public.[66] Risk factors are defined as those features, factors, or conditions that increase the incidence of breast cancer in a given person or group from the level of the base population. Space precludes an in-depth discussion of the multiple different risk factors that fall into general groups of:

1. Genetic. A person with a first-degree relative with breast cancer carries a two-fold to three-fold greater risk than the general population; it also appears that certain families are at greater risk than the general population; it also appears that certain families are at greater risk for onset of breast cancer at an early age, which is often bilateral.

2. Hormonal. Women with early menarche or late natural menopause have an increased risk; castration decreases the chance of developing breast cancer;[97,100] women whose first full-term birth occurred under age 18 years have one third the risk of breast cancer as those whose first child was born after they were 30 years of age.

3. Nutrition/geographic/environmental. The above-mentioned differences in the incidence of reast cancer must be based on lifestyle and nutritional variables, since they do not appear racially stratified.

4. Radiation. Radiation, delivered at high doses, has been

173

shown to increase the spontaneous rate of development of breast cancer.

5. Proliferative disease of the breast. Many authors believe there is an increased risk of breast cancer developing in women with a previous history of benign, proliferative disease.[75]

An American woman has an 8.2% chance of acquiring breast cancer before age 75 years. A woman with no special risk factors, as summarized above, still has a 5.9% chance of developing breast cancer.[11] Unfortunately, no combination of risk factors can identify a group of women at a significantly higher risk, hence any screening/detection program *must* be focused upon the population at large.[33,55]

The therapy of breast cancer in recent years has moved toward less radical surgical procedures. Today most patients are treated with either a modified radical mastectomy or with a "lumpectomy" along with axillary sampling and primary radiation therapy. Regional radiation therapy appears to improve local control but probably does not affect survival. A number of clinical trials are now underway comparing different treatment modalities. To date, there appears to be no statistically significant difference in the number of recurrences or the survival rate between radical mastectomy and more modest surgical procedures such as "lumpectomy" combined with radiation therapy.[54, 55]

The real impact of medical imaging in the management of malignant disease of the breast has been the detection by mammography of minimal breast cancer in asymptomatic women. The mortality rate of breast cancer has been shown to be reduced by the combination of mammography and physical examination. This landmark study, the Health Insurance Plan of New York (HIP), began in 1963 and compared 31,000 women who were offered mammography and physical examination with a control group of the same size.[89] The screened population in this program experienced a reduced breast cancer mortality of around 40%. This decrease in mortality was initially observed only in women over the age of 50 years, but recent studies indicate a mortality reduction even in women under age 50.[77]

Encouraged by the results of the HIP study, the National Cancer Institute (NCI) and the American Cancer Society (ACS) in 1973 created the Breast Cancer Detection Demonstration Project (BCDDP).[7] Over 280,000 asymptomatic women aged 35 to 74 years were examined at 29 centers nationwide with a combination of clinical history, physical examination, mammography, and thermography. Because of poor results with thermography, this technique was dropped from the screening armamentarium. Routine mammography screening under the age of 50 years was discontinued during the course of the program except for women with a personal history

of breast cancer or a strong family history. The results of the BCDDP screening program have been most impressive. The overall cancer detection rate for the first annual BCDDP screen (prevalent screen) was 5.54 per 1,000. The detection rate increased from 1.5 per 1,000 at ages 35 to 39 to 11.28 per 1,000 at ages 65 to 74. The second annual screen (incidence screen) quite naturally had detection rates that were lower; 1.9 per 1,000 for all ages, 0.57 for ages 35 to 39, and 2.78 for ages 65 to 74.

Great strides in the technique of mammography and its ability to detect very small cancers were made in the interval between the HIP study of 1963 and the BCDDP study of 1973. The impact of improved mammography technique in the early detection of breast cancer was described in the Five Year Summary Report of the Breast Cancer Detection Demonstration Project[7] (see Tables 11-13, 11-14). Mammography was the only reason for biopsy in 41.6% of the cancers discovered in the BCDDP compared with 33.3% in the earlier HIP study.[7,89] Approximately one third (32.4%) of the BCDDP cancers were either nonfiltrating or less than 1 cm in size. Mammography alone was the means by which 57.1% of these very early cancers were discovered.

The great improvement rates by mammography occurred in the 40-to-49-year-old age group where mammography was the sole reason for biopsy in 19.4% of the HIP women and 35.4% of the BCDDP women. Moskowitz makes a plea for aggressive screening for women under the age of 50 years.[77] No breast cancer deaths were encountered at the end of five years of study in 4,000 Cincinnati women aged 40 to 49 who had participated in an aggressive mammography screening program. The authors believe that this reduced rate is almost exclusively the result of the emphasis placed on the detection of minimal breast cancer by mammography.

There are inherent problems with any screening program. If the screening procedure has a low sensitivity and picks up only a small portion of the asymptomatic patients with the disease, then patients may be given false assurance and delay seeking medical advice when the disease becomes symptomatic. Also, there may be far too many biopsies if the procedure has a low specificity. The evaluation of screening programs is made difficult because of two potential biases, a lead-time bias and a length-time bias sampling.[52,53] The lead-time bias refers to the fact that early detection may increase the time between the discovery of the disease and death but not actually change the patient's survival. Length-bias sampling occurs because a slowly growing tumor is more likely to be detected in an initial screening examination and the more rapidly growing tumors are more apt to appear in the interval between examinations. Thus, the patient whose tumor is discovered by screening may have a less virulent tumor because of this bias.

Because of the great number of small cancers detected in the BCDDP by mammography in women under age 50, the American Cancer Society recently adopted new guidelines for the appropriate use of mammography. They recommend (1) monthly breast self-examination starting at age 20; (2) physical examination of the breast by a physician every three years from age 20 to 40 and every year thereafter; (3) a baseline mammogram from age 35 followed by annual or biennial mammograms from age 40 through 49, and (4) annual mammograms from age 50 on. The American College of Radiology adopted similar guidelines in September, 1982.

The early success of the BCDDP screening program became clouded by public concern over the radiation risk of mammography that bordered on hysteria. This media-induced concern resulted in an unfortunate situation where many symptomatic patients avoided mammography, often at the suggestion of their personal physician. This misunderstanding arose from the concern of patients and physicians over the possible risk of radiation-induced breast cancer. These concerns developed because of the documented increased rate of breast cancer that was described in three different population groups who had been previously exposed to large doses of radiation, far in excess of those encountered during mammography.[101] These patient groups included (1) young American and Canadian women treated with radiation therapy for postpartum mastitis; (2) young women subjected to multiple fluoroscopic chest examinations to follow the course of their artificial pneumothorax, which was used in the treatment of pulmonary tuberculosis in the 1940s; and (3) Japanese women who had survived exposure to atomic bomb radiation during the Hiroshima/Nagasaki detonations. In this latter group, it was shown that the younger the age at exposure, particularly in those women under the age of 20, the greater the risk of subsequent breast cancer. Exposures to women over the age of 30 did not appear to materially affect subsequent breast cancer incidence rates. As a result of these studies, there clearly appears to be an increased risk with increasing dose and, possibly, younger age at exposure. However, the danger of radiation-induced breast cancer from screening mammography is largely theoretical and speculative. A review panel convened by the National Cancer Institute concluded that there was an estimated theoretical risk of six cases of breast cancer per million woman per year per rad of radiation per year at risk, following a 10-to-15 year latency period. For an individual woman at the age of 35 years exposed once to one rad of radiation, the estimated increased lifetime risk of breast cancer would be less than 1%. In an older patient, the risk should be much less. The development of new imaging techniques has permitted a steady reduction in the amount of radiation needed for mammographic diagnosis. According to Hempelmann, the mid-breast doses for a typical BCDDP mammography averaged 0.37 rad for xeromammography and 0.04 rad for film-screen techniques.[10,51]

TUMOR PATHOLOGY AND BEHAVIOR

Carcinoma of the breast is a term used to characterize the malignant neoplasms that arise from the epithelium lining the ducts and lobules of the breast. Malignant neoplasms arising from other cells in the breast (i.e., sarcoma) are rare. The causes of breast cancer are as yet unknown. Although an increased risk of cancer occurs with a variety of interrelated genetic, environmental, sociobiologic, and physiologic factors, no single factor or combination of variables is sufficient to explain the cause of the disease.

Although inconclusive, recent studies have indicated a relationship between atypical epithelial hyperplasia and carcinoma.[14,40,56,59] These studies have suggested that this is a morphologic continuum from normal through varying degrees of hyperplasia to carcinoma in situ and eventually to invasive carcinoma.

Malignant Tumors of the Breast

The classification of breast cancer according to McDivitt and Stewart is useful (Table 11-1).[69,70] The vast majority of malignant tumors of the breast are carcinomas (95% or more) (Table 11-2).[1] Minor modifications for the purpose of simplicity have been suggested by many authors. Carcinoma of the breast may be divided into those tumors arising from the major ducts and those originating from the smaller ducts, lobules, and acini.

Table 11-1. Classification of Histologic Types

Paget's disease of the nipple
Carcinoma of mammary ducts
  Noninfiltrating
    1. Papillary carcinoma
    2. Comedocarcinoma
  Infiltrating
    1. Papillary carcinoma
    2. Comedocarcinoma
    3. Carcinoma with fibrosis (scirrhous carcinoma)
    4. Medullary carcinoma with lymphoid infiltration
    5. Colloid carcinoma
Carcinoma of lobules
  Noninfiltrating
  Infiltrating
Relatively rare carcinomas
  So-called "sweat gland carcinoma"
  Intracystic carcinoma
  Adenoid cystic carcinoma
  Squamous cell carcinoma
  Spindle cell carcinoma
  Carcinoma with osseous and cartilaginous metaplasia

Reprinted from Stewart, F. W.: Tumors of the breast. In *Atlas of Tumor Pathology*. Armed Forces Institute of Pathology, 1950, p. 12. With permission.

Table 11-2. Incidence of Histologic Types of Invasive
Breast Cancer (1,000 Cases)

	NUMBER	PERCENT
Pure tumor groups		
Infiltrating duct NOS		
(not otherwise specified)	526	52.6
Medullary	62	6.2
Lobular invasive	49	4.9
Mucinous	24	2.4
Tubular	12	1.2
Adenocystic	4	0.4
Papillary	3	0.3
Carcinosarcoma	1	0.1
Paget's disease	23	2.3
With intraductal carcinoma	2	0.2
Infiltrating duct NOS	16	1.6
Infiltrating duct NOS + tubular	4	0.4
Infiltrating duct NOS + mucinous	1	0.1
Combinations with infiltrating duct NOS	280	28.0
Infiltrating duct NOS:		
+ Tubular	165	16.5
+ Lobular invasive	33	3.3
+ Mucinous	16	1.6
+ Lobular invasive + tubular	16	1.6
+ Papillary	12	1.2
+ Adenocystic	10	1.0
+ Tubular + adenocystic	8	0.8
+ Tubular + papillary	8	0.8
+ Mucinous + papillary	4	0.4
+ Adenocystic + mucinous	2	0.2
+ Lobular invasive + adenocystic	1	0.1
+ Lobular invasive + mucinous	1	0.1
+ Lobular invasive + papillary	1	0.1
+ Tubular + mucinous	1	0.1
+ Adenocystic + papillary	1	0.1
+ Lobular invasive + tubular + adenocystic + mucinous	1	0.1
Other combinations of tumor types exclusive of NOS	16	1.6
Tubular + papillary	5	0.5
Lobular invasive + tubular	4	0.4
Tubular + mucinous	2	0.2
Lobular invasive + mucinous	1	0.1
Tubular + adenocystic	1	0.1
Adenocystic + mucinous	1	0.1
Mucinous + papillary	1	0.1
Lobular invasive + tubular + adenocystic + papillary	1	0.1
Total	1,000	100.0

Reprinted from National Surgical Adjuvant Breast Project. *Cancer* 36:8, 1975. With permission.

Invasive Ductal Carcinoma. Invasive ductal carcinoma, which represents approximately 75% of all invasive types, is the most common of all mammary carcinomas. Grossly, it is a poorly defined mass that cuts with a resistant gritty sensation, like cutting through an unripe pear. The degree of hardness depends on the amount of connective tissue present. The tumor is usually grayish-yellow with radiating fibrous trabeculae running toward the periphery of the tumor. The size of the tumor varies from nonpalpable nodules detectable only by mammography and careful microscopic inspection to enormous tumors that infiltrate the entire breast, including the skin and pectoralis muscle.

Intraductal Carcinoma. Intraductal carcinoma refers to a carcinoma that grows predominantly within the mammary ducts. It is multifocal in about one third of the cases. On gross examination, the breast parenchyma may appear normal or the mammary ducts may be dilated. When the characteristic "comedo" appearance is present, wormlike masses of necrotic tumor can be expressed from the ducts. Microscopically, the tumor cells are similar to those of the usual breast carcinoma. The malignant cells filling the ducts may be arranged in various patterns—solid, papillary, or cribriform. Calcification within the tumor is frequent and can be identified by mammography. Diffuse or scattered microcalcifications on the mammogram suggest the diagnosis of intraductal carcinoma.

Not all intraductal carcinomas are small and clinically occult. One third of the intraductal carcinomas recently reported were between 2 and 5 cm in diameter, while another 20% were greater than 5 cm in diameter.[1,57] Intraductal carcinomas may be accompanied by areas of stromal invasion. There is no correlation between the overall size of the tumor and the degree of infiltration. The incidence of axillary metastases correlates better with the size of the infiltrating component than with the overall size of the tumor.[95] Even in those cases in which a breast biopsy shows tumor confined entirely to the ducts and there is no definite mass palpable in the breast, metastatic spread to the low axillary lymph nodes has been reported.[13]

Medullary Carcinomas. Medullary carcinoma often appears in patients under 50 years of age and constitutes between 5% and 7% of all mammary carcinomas. The tumor is very well circumscribed with a soft, fleshy cut surface that bulges rather than retracts. The tumor tissue usually has a homogenous gray color and contains small yellow and red focal areas of necrosis and hemorrhage. Microscopically, the cells of medullary carcinomas are large and anaplastic, with prominent nucleoli and numerous metastatic figures. An important histologic feature of the entity is the presence of a prominent lymphoid infiltrate, which occasionally is so striking that it may be confused with malignant lymphoma. The prognosis of medullary carcinoma is more favorable than for the ordinary invasive ductal carcinoma, particularly in tumors smaller than 3 cm.[1]

Mucinous (Colloid) Carcinoma. Mucinous carcinoma represents approximately 3% of all breast carcinomas. It tends to occur in elderly patients and to have a slow growth of long duration. Generally, it is well delineated with a soft bulging translucent cut surface divided by fibrous septae. Microscopically, the tumor demonstrates nests and strands of epithelial cells floating in a sea of mucin. The prognosis tends to be good.

Papillary Carcinomas. Papillary carcinomas are rare, representing 1% or less of all mammary carcinomas. The tumors tend to be well circumscribed and are either solid or cystic. The cystic lesions may be either single or multilobular. The cavity of the cyst contains necrotic tissue or hemorrhagic fluid. Microscopically, the cells in these tumors demonstrate a papillary arrangement. Papillary carcinoma rarely invades the surrounding stroma and the five-year survival rate is better than with the usual duct carcinoma. Complete excision of papillary carcinomas is important, since recurrence may appear after a relatively long interval.

Lobular Carcinoma. Lobular carcinoma, a tumor that arises from the small end ducts of the breasts has generated considerable interest in recent years. Lobular carcinoma-in-situ, the noninvasive variety, is characterized by clusters of anaplastic small cells lying within the lobules of the breast.[6,44,48,63,85,106] This lesion may extend beyond the boundary of the lobular terminal duct from which it arises, in which case it is known as invasive lobular carcinoma, and it may be indistinguishable from the standard infiltrating duct carcinoma. Lobular carcinoma-in-situ usually is a non-palpable incidental finding in 1% to 2% of all breast biopsy specimens. It frequently is serendipitously detected on a mammogram. Finely stippled calcification is observed on the mammogram. Microscopically, the calcification may be in the surrounding normal breast lobules rather than in the cancer itself. Lobular carcinoma-in-situ is frequently multicentric and bilateral. Thirty percent to 40% of women with biopsy-proven lobular carcinoma-in-situ will develop infiltrating carcinoma within the ensuing 20 years. Subsequent infiltrating carcinoma may develop as frequently in the contralateral breast as in the ipsilateral breast. The infiltrating carcinomas are usually of the ductal type and do not resemble the original in situ lesions.

Tubular or Well-Differentiated Adenocarcinoma. Tubular carcinomas are well-differentiated infiltrating ductal carcinomas in which the neoplastic cells form small structures that resemble tubules, lined with a single layer of cells. These tumors are usually small. Patients with tubular carcinoma have a lower incidence of axillary metastases and a better survival rate than patients with ordinary ductal carcinoma.[19,20]

Rare Types of Invasive Carcinoma. There is a group of rarely encountered, histologic types of mammary carcinoma that are so few in number that no meaningful association with prognosis is available.

Epidermoid carcinoma is a tumor of elderly women in which the mammary carcinoma histologically is virtually all epidermoid carcinoma.

Adenoid cystic carcinoma is a rare form of infiltrating ductal carcinoma that is identical morphologically to the adenoid cystic carcinoma of the salivary gland. The neoplastic cells, surrounded by hyalinized stroma, are so well differentiated that they frequently form a basal lamina. Patients with this form of carcinoma have an extremely low incidence of axillary metastases.

Sweat gland carcinoma has no unique gross features to distinguish it from ordinary infiltrating ductal carcinoma. Some authors feel that there is no need to separate these apocrine carcinomas, since there appear to be no differences in their natural history.[1] The tumor consists of large cells with eosinophilic cytoplasm and resembles, but does not arise from, the cutaneous apocrine sweat glands.

Carcinoma with osseous or cartilaginous metaplasia, carcinosarcomas, pure squamous cell carcinomas, basal cell carcinomas, and the so-called lipid-rich carcinomas have been observed.

Special Manifestations of Breast Cancer. *Paget's disease*: Paget's disease, which occurs in 1% to 4% of all patients with breast cancer, is manifested clinically as an eczematoid lesion of the nipple associated with itching, burning, oozing, or bleeding. The nipple changes are always associated with an underlying carcinoma of the breast that can be palpated in about two thirds of the patients. This underlying tumor may be either intraductal or of the invasive ductal type. Microscopically, the tumor consists of nests of large, malignant cells with clear cytoplasms situated among the normal cells of the epidermis. Currently, the Paget's cell is felt to be an extension of the underlying malignant tumor to the epidermis of the nipple. The prognosis for patients with Paget's disease depends on the histologic type of the associated tumor.

Inflammatory carcinoma: The term "inflammatory carcinoma" was originally used to describe a type of breast cancer in which the entire breast was red and warm with widespread edema of the skin, thus simulating the appearance of mastitis. Biopsy specimens of the edematous areas as well as the adjacent normal-appearing skin demonstrate undifferentiated cancer cells in the subdermal lymphatics producing an obstructing lymphangitis. However, patients may have the clinical picture of inflammatory carcinoma in the absence of dermal invasion and, conversely, there may be widespread permeation of dermal lymphatics in the absence of the clinical features of inflammatory carcinoma (so-called occult inflammatory carcinoma).[86] The entity of inflammatory carcinoma is associated with an extremely poor prognosis. Most patients have advanced cancer, including palpable axillary nodes, supraclavicular nodes, and distant metastases at the time of diagnosis. Surgery is contraindicated and a combination of chemotherapy and radiation therapy is the recommended treatment.

Stromal or Nonepithelial Neoplasms of the Breast. A number of stromal or nonepithelial neoplasms of the breast have been described. Most of these are sarcomas and include fibrosarcomas, leiomyosarcomas, rhabdomyosarcomas, and angiosarcomas. These extremely rare tumors have an ominous prognosis and usually result in a rapid death from widespread dissemination. Liposarcomas of the breast, which are also rare, may have a more favorable prognosis. Malignant lymphoma can appear as a primary mammary neoplasm or can involve the breast as part of a generalized process.[1] The prognosis is poor. Cystosarcoma phylloides is an uncommon tumor that has both epithelial and nonepithelial elements. The majority of cystosarcoma phylloides are benign, and they may be derived from fibroadenomas. They may become very large and infrequently demonstrate some invasion of adjacent breast tissue. There have been distant metastases with a fatal outcome. It is difficult to determine which tumors will have a malignant behavior and metastasize based on the clinical and histologic appearance. Axillary metastases are extremely unusual and so there is little if any justification for routine axillary dissection in patients suspected of having cystosarcoma phylloides.

Histologic Type and Prognosis

It is possible for the pathologist to identify certain histologic types of carcinoma that are associated with a better prognosis than others. Tumors with a favorable prognosis are recognizable on the basis of their gross and microscopic features. A convenient classification system has been developed by Ackerman and Rosai, who classified the carcinomas of the breast into four categories.[1]

Type 1. Includes all in situ neoplasms, whether arising from ductal or lobular epithelium.
Intraductal carcinoma (with or without Paget's disease)
Intraductal papillary carcinoma
Lobular carcinoma in situ
Type 2. Invasive with well-delineated margins
Pure mucinous carcinoma
Well-differentiated (tubular) carcinoma
Invasive papillary carcinoma
Medullary carcinoma
Adenoid cystic carcinoma
Type 3. Invasive (most numerous and includes all carcinomas not definitely classified as type 1, 2, or 4).
Invasive ductal carcinoma not otherwise specified
Intraductal carcinoma with invasion
Invasive lobular carcinoma
Epidermoid carcinoma

Type 4. Invasive, undifferentiated carcinomas
Undifferentiated carcinomas composed of cells without ductal or lobular arrangement and tumors clearly invading blood vessels, regardless of type.

The incidence of the various histologic types of breast cancer was documented in a recent review of 1,000 cases by Fisher and his colleagues[35] (Table 11-2).

More than half of the tumors (52.6%) were pure infiltrating duct lesions. A combination of infiltrating ductal carcinoma was found with other tumor types in 28% of the tumors.

Histologic Differentiation and Nuclear Grade

A relationship between the degree of anaplasia of the tumor and the patient's clinical course has long been postulated.[16,103] Mammary carcinomas have been divided into three histologic grades of malignancy depending upon the degree of tubule formation, the size of cells, the size of nuclei, and degree of hyperchromatism and the number of mitoses. Grade I represents the lowest grade of malignancy and grade III the most malignant. Overall, patients with low grade tumors have better prognosis than do those with high grade tumors.

The nuclei of tumor cells also have been characterized into three distinct nuclear grades according to their differentiation. In this system grade I is the most malignant and grade III the least malignant.[15] Black and associates report a relationship between patient survival, nuclear grade of the tumor, and sinus histocytosis of the axillary lymph nodes.

Characteristics of Primary Tumor

Primary tumor size correlates well with the incidence of lymph node metastases and with five-year survival rates.[34]

Gallager and Martin propose the term "minimal breast carcinoma" to describe all in situ carcinomas and those invasive carcinomas with the invasive component no larger than 0.5 cm in diameter.[41] Other authors have extended the definition of minimal breast cancer to include lesions measuring less than 1 cm in diameter. A very favorable cure rate (greater than 90% ten-year survival) is possible with these minimal breast cancers.[65]

Cancer of the breast is frequently a multifocal process. A woman treated for cancer of one breast is five times more likely to develop a second breast cancer.[84] Donegan and Spratt in their experience at Ellis Fischel State Cancer Hospital found that 2% or 52 of 2,620 women with cancer of the breast initially had bilateral mammary cancers.[26] From the same institution, a review of 704 women with no previous cancers who were treated with a radical mastectomy for an initial unilateral mammary cancer and observed for five to 18 years revealed that 14 women

(2%) developed a second clinical primary tumor in the remaining breast within seven years. It appears that the number of clinically detected second primaries is a function of the period of observation. The longer a group of patients are followed, the greater will be the incidence of additional cancers. The use of modern mammography as a diagnostic tool has also increased the detection of otherwise occult second cancers. Using mammography, Egan reported the discovery of new contralateral cancers in 6% of 1,112 women examined at Emory University between 1963 and 1973.[29] A careful pathologic examination of the entire breast leads to the discovery of far more cancers than ever become clinically apparent.[40] Utilizing serial whole organ histologic preparations in 47 breasts removed because of invasive cancer, Gallager and Martin found two or more and usually many independent foci of cancer in 47% of the breasts examined.

The identification of estrogen and progesterone receptors in breast cancer has important prognostic and therapeutic implications. Estrogen receptors are cytoplasmic proteins responsible for the uptake of estrogen into target cells. Estrogen receptor is found in about two thirds of human breast cancer specimens. Since estrogen receptors are necessary for estrogen activity, their presence correlates well with the response of advanced breast cancer to endocrine therapy.[87] Only 8% of tumors lacking estrogen receptors regress with endocrine therapy, whereas about 60% of those containing estrogen receptors respond. The assay also has prognostic value, since a number of studies have confirmed that estrogen receptor-negative tumors are often poorly differentiated and have a poorer prognosis than estrogen receptor-positive tumors. This relationship between the presence of estrogen receptors and prognosis is independent of other variables.

Progesterone receptor is an end product of estrogen action and therefore its presence implies an intact estrogen response mechanism. Tumors lacking both receptors are usually endocrine independent and rarely regress with endocrine therapy. The highest response rate occurs in those tumors containing both estrogen receptor and progesterone receptor, suggesting that, indeed, progesterone receptor may be a good marker for endocrine independence. Estrogen receptor-negative and progesterone receptor-positive tumors are rare, but responses to endocrine therapy have been observed.

The time required for a tumor to double in volume may provide information on its biologic behavior.[26] Gershon-Cohen measured primary tumor volume changes by means of mammography in patients who did not have surgery until two or more mammograms had been performed. The tumor volume doubling time varied from 23 to 209 days. Breast cancer doubling times vary considerably, and the method has had very little clinical importance to date. Meyer and Kopans reported a small group of breast cancers that showed no change in size on mammography during a follow-up period of 2 to 4.5 years.[74] A lack of interval change on serial mammograms does not exclude the possibility of malignancy.

Patterns of Spread of Breast Cancer

According to Haagensen, breast cancer spreads through the breast: (1) by direct infiltration into the breast parenchyma, (2) along mammary ducts, and (3) via breast lymphatics.[47]

The typical stellate appearance of breast cancer seen either on gross examination or on the mammogram is the result of tentacles of tumors that extend out from the central tumor. Involvement of the overlying skin and infiltration of the deep pectoral fascia occurs if the breast is not treated. Tumor spread is frequently observed along the ducts with resultant involvement of large areas of the breast.

Donegan and Spratt,[26] in their series of 2,045 cases, found 37% of primary tumors to be located in the upper outer quadrant, 12% in the upper inner quadrant, 18% in the lower outer quadrant and 6% in the lower inner quadrant, with 15% in the central region, defined as within 1 cm of the areola, and an additional 20% being described as diffuse because of multifocal origin or massive involvement of the entire breast. Cancers were located in the left breast in 52% of the cases in the Donegan and Spratt series, 47% in the right breast and 1% were bilateral. The greater amount of breast tissue in the upper outer quadrant of the breast is thought to be responsible for the increased incidence of cancer in that area. A large series from the National Surgical Adjuvant Breast Project demonstrates no significant differences in prognosis as a result of primary location of the breast tumor[35] (Table 11-3).

The most common regional spread of breast cancer is to the axillary, internal mammary, and supraclavicular lymph node regions. Axillary lymph node involvement is most common. Approximately 40% to 50% of patients with breast cancer have involvement of the axillary lymph nodes. The frequency of axillary lymph node involvement is in part related to the size of the primary tumor (Table 11-4). Location of the primary tumor within the breast is of much less importance in determining the likelihood of axillary lymph node involvement. The presence or absence of histologic involvement of axillary lymph nodes is probably the single most important factor in predicting survival. Patients with histologically negative axillary nodes have markedly improved survival statistics compared with patients with positive axillary nodes. Furthermore, patients with one to three positive nodes have improved survival compared with patients having four or more positive nodes (Tables 11-4, 11-5).

The axilla is commonly divided into three levels for the purpose of categorizing the extent of lymph node involvement.

Table 11-3. Five-Year Relapse Rate According to the Location
of the Primary and Nodal Status

LOCATION	NEGATIVE NODES (%)	POSITIVE NODES (%)
Upper, outer quadrant	17 (208)*	63 (239)
Upper, inner quadrant	25 (75)	59 (37)
Lower, inner quadrant	22 (23)	55 (22)
Lower, outer quadrant	26 (46)	70 (44)

*Numbers in parentheses indicate the number of patients in each subgroup.
Reprinted from DeVita, V. T., Jr., Hellman, S., Rosenberg, S. A. (Eds.). *Cancer: Principles and Practice of Oncology*. Philadelphia, J. B. Lippincott, 1982, p. 918. With permission.

Table 11-4. Five-Year Relapse Rate According to the Size or Primary and Axillary Node Involvement

	SIZE OF PRIMARY (%)		
	<2 cm	2–5 cm	>5 cm
Axillary nodes negative			
Fisher et al.	12	24	27
Nemoto et al.	13	19	25
Valgussa et al.	8	24	19
Axillary nodes positive			
Fisher et al.	50	60	79
Nemoto et al.	39	50	65
Valagussa et al.	37	64	74

Reprinted from DeVita, V. T., Jr., Hellman, S., Rosenberg, S. A. (Eds.). *Cancer: Principles and Practice of Oncology*. Philadelphia, J. B. Lippincott, 1982, p. 921. With permission.

I. Proximal—tissue inferior to the lower border of the pectoralis minor muscle.
II. Middle—tissue directly beneath the pectoralis minor.
III. Distal—tissue superior to the pectoralis minor.

Histologic involvement of the nodes in the upper axilla carries a worse prognosis than involvement of the proximal level nodes alone. In the series of Berg and Robbins,[12] the 20-year survival rate with negative axillary lymph nodes was 60%. When the nodes low in the axilla at level I were involved, the 20-year survival rate was 38%, at level II it was 30%, and when level III nodes high in the axilla were involved, the rate was only 12% (Tables 11-5, 11-6).

The size of the primary tumor and axillary node involvement have both been shown to be important variables in predicting prognosis. The data of Valagussa and colleagues demonstrated a five-year relapse rate of 37% for patients with positive nodes and small (0–2 cm) primaries and 79% for patients with positive nodes and large (greater than 5 cm) primaries.[102]

The internal mammary lymph node chain is the second major drainage area for carcinoma of the breast. Because this lymph node group is intrathoracic in location, it is unusual for its involvement to appear clinically. Handley,[49] reporting on internal mammary lymph node biopsies in 1,000 patients, observed that internal mammary lymph node involvement is more common when the primary is in the inner quadrant than when it is in the outer quadrant of the breast (Table 11-7). However, even in those patients with inner or central

Table 11-5. Prognosis Related to Histologic Involvement of Axillary Lymph Nodes for Patients Treated by Radical Mastectomy

	VALAGUSSA (10-YEAR DISEASE-FREE SURVIVAL) (%)	HAAGENSEN (10-YEAR SURVIVAL) (%)	SCHOTTENFELD* (10-YEAR SURVIVAL) (%)	FISHER (10-YEAR DISEASE-FREE SURVIVAL) (%)	SPRATT AND DONEGAN (10-YEAR SURVIVAL) (%)	PAYNE* (10-YEAR ACTUAL SURVIVAL) (%)
Histologically negative	72	76	72	76	68	76
Histologically positive	25	48	43	24	27	35
1–3 Nodes positive	34	63	—	36	—	—
≥4 Nodes positive	16	27	—	14	—	—

*Significant number of patients received postoperative irradiation.
Reprinted from DeVita V. T., Jr., Hellman, S., Rosenberg, S. A. (Eds.). *Cancer: Principles and Practice of Oncology*. Philadelphia, J. B. Lippincott, 1982, p. 920. With permission.

Table 11-6. Ten-Year Survival Related to Primary Size
and Level of Axillary Involvement

AXILLARY STATUS	<2 cm (%)	2–5 cm (%)	>5 cm (%)	TOTAL (%)
Negative	82	65	44	72
Positive, proximal only	73	74	39	65
Positive, middle or distal	*	28	37	31
Positive all	68	51	37	

*Insufficient data.
Reprinted from Schottenfeld, D., Nash, A. G., Robbins, G. F., Beattie Jr., E. J., Ten-year results of the treatment of primary operable breast carcinoma. *Cancer* 38:1005, 1976. With permission.

primary tumors, axillary lymph node involvement is more common than internal mammary node involvement (42% v 28%). In those patients in which the axillary lymph nodes are uninvolved, internal mammary node involvement is very uncommon, occurring in only 8% of the patients. The size of the primary is important in relation to internal mammary node involvement. Only 19% of internal mammary nodes are involved when the primary is less than 5 cm compared with 37% when the primary is greater than 5 cm.

The spread of tumor to the supraclavicular lymph node chain is through the axillary lymph node chain. Dahl-Iverson[25] observed supraclavicular lymph node involvement in 18% of 125 patients with involvement of the axillary nodes and in none of 149 patients who did not have involvement of the axillary nodes. It is evident that supraclavicular lymph node spread represents a late stage of axillary node involvement and carries an ominous prognosis. Although the regional intercostal lymph nodes are a site of potential lymph node involvement, the incidence of spread to this area has not been established. It would appear to be uncommon except in advanced or recurrent cases.

Widespread metastases from carcinoma of the breast are commonly encountered. The most frequent sites for

metastatic involvement other than the breast itself and its draining lymph nodes are the liver, bone, pleura, and adrenals (Table 11-8).

CLASSIFICATION AND STAGING

A staging system is a grouping of patients by the extent of their disease. The extent of their disease may be described before treatment (clinical staging) or after surgical intervention (surgical-pathologic staging). Clinical staging is based on physical examination as well as laboratory and radiologic evaluation. Staging is important in the selection of the most appropriate treatment regimen, in predicting prognosis, and as a means of comparing patient outcomes from various institutions. A variety of methods of staging carcinoma of the breast have developed over the years. The most widely used clinical staging system is that developed by the American Joint Committee on Cancer and by the International Union Against Cancer.[5] Although there have been minor differences in the past in the systems of these two organizations, they are now consistent. They are based on the TNM system, with the T standing for primary tumor extent, the N for regional node involvement, and the M for metastases (Table 11-9). Accurate clinical staging requires careful inspection of the skin and palpation of the breast and regional nodes. Mammography is recommended as part of the staging process (Figure 11-1).

Imaging Procedures and Assessment

The most important methods used in detecting carcinoma of the breast are physical examination and mammography. Thermography, ultrasound, computed tomography, magnetic resonance imaging, diaphanography, and heavy ion imaging have, at present, less defined roles (Table 11-10).

Table 11-7. Internal Mammary Node Involvement Related to Location of Primary and Axillary Node Involvement

AMOUNT OF INTERNAL MAMMARY NODE INVOLVEMENT	UPPER, INNER QUADRANT (%)	LOWER, INNER QUADRANT (%)	CENTRAL (%)	UPPER, OUTER QUADRANT (%)	LOWER, OUTER QUADRANT (%)
Total	27 (67/248)	33 (20/61)	32 (70/216)	14 (54/382)	13 (12/93)
Axilla Not Involved	14 (20/143)	6 (2/36)	7 (5/76)	4 (7/170)	5 (2/40)
Axilla Involved	45 (47/105)	72 (18/25)	46 (65/140)	22 (47/212)	19 (10/53)

Reprinted from Handley, R. S.: Carcinoma of the breast. *Ann. R. Coll. Surg.* 57:65, 1975. With permission.

Table 11-8. Sites of Metastases from Breast Cancer in
Three Collected Series

SITE	160 CASES (%)	43 CASES (%)	100 CASES (%)
Organ	59	65	69
Liver	58	56	65
Bone	44	—	71
Pleura	37	23	51
Adrenals	31	41	49
Kidneys	Not recorded	14	17
Spleen	14	23	17
Pancreas	—	11	17
Ovaries	9	16	20
Brain	—	9	22
Thyroid	—	—	24
Heart	—	—	11
Diaphragm	—	—	11
Pericardium	5	21	19
Intestine	—	—	18
Peritoneum	12	9	13
Uterus	—	—	15
Lymph Nodes	72	—	76
Skin	34	7	30

Reprinted from DeVita, V. T., Jr., Hellman, S., Rosenberg, S. A. (Eds.). *Cancer: Principles and Practice of Oncology.* Philadelphia, J. B. Lippincott, 1982, p. 922. With permission.

Physical Examination. Palpation of the breast has long been the mainstay in the detection of breast cancer. Breast self-examination (BSE) is one of the main thrusts of the American Cancer Society's patient education program. Over 90% of women still detect their cancer themselves, although not necessarily during periodic examination.[1] Examination of the breast is considered an integral part of a general physical or gynecologic examination, even if the patient has no breast complaints. In this setting, however, physical examination is being used as a screening test and, unfortunately, there are no data confirming the value of physical examination in this role.

In the HIP study, mammography and physical examination contributed independently to the reduction in mortality, but the magnitude of the contribution of each could not be measured from this study. There is no controlled study that shows a reduction in breast cancer mortality can be affected by BSE. In a study correlating BSE and routine physical examination by physicians and the stage of cancer discovered, there was no statistically significant difference in stage between tumors detected by BSE and those found by routine physician examina-

Table 11-9. TNM Classification

Primary Tumor (T)

T_x Minimum requirements to assess primary tumor cannot be met.
T_0 No evidence of primary tumor.
T_{is} In situ cancer (in situ lobular, pure intraductal and Paget's disease of the nipple without palpable tumor).
T_1 Tumor 2 cm or less in greatest dimension
  T_{1a} No fixation to underlying pectoral fascia or muscle
  T_{1b} Fixation to underlying pectoral fascia or muscle
    i   tumor ≤ 0.5 cm
    ii tumor 0.5–1.0 cm
    iii tumor 1.0–2.0 cm
T_2 Tumor more than 2 cm but not more than 5 cm in its greatest dimension.
  T_{2a} No fixation to underlying pectoral fascia or muscle.
  T_{2b} Fixation to underlying pectoral fascia or muscle.
T_3 Tumor more than 5 cm in its greatest dimension.
  T_{3a} No fixation to underlying pectoral fascia or muscle.
  T_{3b} Fixation to underlying pectoral fascia or muscle.
T_4 Tumor of any size with direct extension to chest wall or skin. (Chest wall includes ribs, intercostal muscles, and serratus anterior muscle, but not pectoral muscle.)
  T_{4a} Fixation to chest wall.
  T_{4b} Edema (including peau d'orange), ulceration of the skin of the breast, or satellite skin nodules confined to the same breast.
  T_{4c} Both of the above.
  Dimpling of the skin, nipple retraction, or any other skin changes except those in T_{4b} may occur in T_1, T_2, or T_3 without changing the classification.

Nodal Involvement (N)

Definitions for Clinical-Diagnostic Stage

N_x Regional lymph nodes cannot be assessed clinically.
N_0 Homolateral axillary lymph nodes not considered to contain growth.
N_1 Movable homolateral axillary nodes considered to contain growth.
N_2 Homolateral axillary nodes considered to contain growth and fixed to one another or to other structures.
N_3 Homolateral supraclavicular or infraclavicular nodes considered to contain growth or edema of the arm. (Edema of the arm may be caused by lymphatic obstruction and lymph nodes may not then be palpable.)

Definitions for Surgical-Evaluation and Postsurgical Resection—Pathologic Stage.

N_x Regional lymph nodes cannot be assessed (not removed for study or previously removed).
N_0 No evidence of homolateral axillary lymph node metastasis.
N_1 Metastasis to movable homolateral axillary nodes not fixed to one another or to other structure.

(continued)

Table 11-9. (*continued*)

N_{1a} Micrometastasis <0.2 cm in lymph node(s).
N_{1b} Gross metastasis in lymph node(s).
     I   Metastasis more than 0.2 cm but less than 2.0 cm in one to three lymph nodes.
     II   Metastasis more than 0.2 cm but less than 2.0 cm in four or more lymph nodes.
     III   Extension of metastasis beyond the lymph node capsule (less than 2.0 cm in dimension).
     IV   Metastasis in lymph node 2.0 cm or more in dimension.
N_2 Metastasis to homolateral axillary lymph nodes that are fixed to one another or to other structures.
N_3 Metastasis to homolateral supraclavicular or infraclavicular lymph node(s).

Distant Metastasis (M)

M_X Minimum requirements to assess the presence of distant metastasis cannot be met.
M_0 No (known) distant metastasis.
M_1 Distant metastasis present.

Stage Grouping

Stage T_{is}	In situ	Stage IIIA	T_0, N_2, M_0
Stage X	Cannot stage		T_{1a} or T_{1b}, N_2, M_0
Stage 1	T_{1ai}, N_0, M_0		T_{2a} or T_{2b}, N_2, M_0
	T_{1aii}, N_0, M_0		T_{3a} or T_{3b}, N_0, M_0
	T_{1aiii}, N_0, M_0		T_{3a} or T_{3b}, N_1, M_0
Stage 1	T_{1bi}, N_0, M_0		T_{3a} or T_{3b}, N_2, M_0
	T_{1bii}, N_0, M_0	Stage IIIB	Any T, N_3, M_0
	T_{1biii}, N_0, M_0		Any T_4, any N, M_0
Stage II	T_0, N_{1a} or N_{1b}, M_0	Stage IV	Any T, any N, M_1
	T_{1a} or T_{1b}, N_{1a} or N_{1b}, M_0		
	T_{2a} or T_{2b}, N_0, M_0		
	T_{2a} or T_{2b}, N_{1a} or N_{1b}, M_0		

Reprinted from the American Joint Committee on Cancer. *Manual for Staging of Cancer*, 2nd ed. Philadelphia, J. B. Lippincott, 1983, p. 130. With permission.

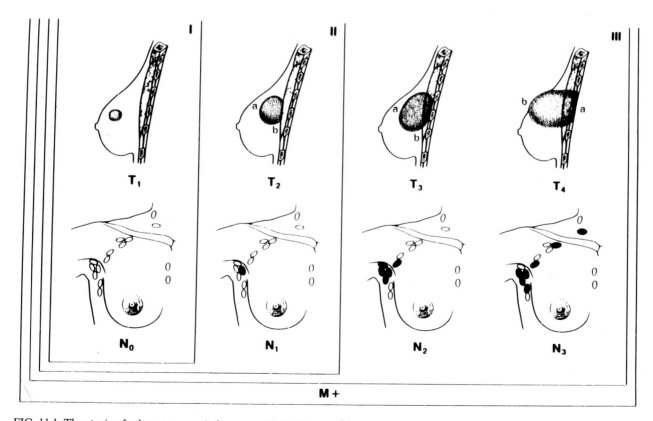

FIG. 11-1. The staging for breast cancer is diagrammatically illustrated in this illustration by the tumor size and node status. The line brackets convert the T and N designations to their respective stages, indicated by roman numerals.

Table 11-10. Imaging Modalities for Evaluation of Breast Cancer

MODALITY FOR TUMOR (T)	STAGING CAPABILITY	COST/BENEFIT RATIO*	SCREENING POTENTIAL	COMMENTS
Mammography	Visualizes approximately 90% of breast cancers	High	Yes	Film/screen and xeromammography have similar diagnostic accuracy
Ultrasound:				
Dedicated	Limited to identification of cystic lesions and evaluation of dense breast	Low	No	Dedicated units are expensive and not suitable for stand-alone screening
Small part		High	No	
Diaphanography	Unproven	Unproven	Unproven	Experimental evaluation studies pending
Computed Tomography	Limited to evaluation of chest wall and internal mammary node involvement	Low	No	Dedicated CT breast imaging system has been abandoned
Thermography	Not effective	Low	No	Biological basis unproven
Magnetic resonance imaging	Unproven	Low	Unproven	Experimental studies pending

*A high cost/benefit ratio refers to a favorable situation for use of the study.

tion.[46] A five-year mortality reduction of only 8% to 9% was estimated for women with cancers discovered either during routine BSE or routine physical examination by physicians. This is a significant decrease from the 40% reduction in mortality demonstrated in the HIP study utilizing routine mammography in addition to a physical examination.

Mammography. Mammography was probably performed soon after the discovery of X rays, but it was not until 1930 that Warren first reported its usefulness in the diagnosis of breast disease.[105] In 1960, Egan reported the use of fine-grain industrial film mammography in 1,000 cases.[27,28,31] This report was a milestone in the radiographic evaluation of the breast. Training programs were developed to instruct large numbers of radiologists in the technique and interpretation of mammography. The most widely utilized mammography techniques at present are xeromammography and screen-film mammography.

A series of technical improvements on the original Egan technique has resulted in improved image quality of mammograms and a very significant reduction in radiation dose.[10] Gros and Franz, in the mid 1960s, substituted a molybdenum target for tungsten in the anode of the X-ray tube. The greater photoelectric effect of the molybdenum X rays at 26 to 28 kV(p) increased the contrast between low-density structures, resulting in better visualization of tumors and calcifications. Compression of the breast with the resultant elimination of motion artifacts and the separation of mammary structures was another improvement introduced by Gros. X-ray units specifically dedicated to the examination of the breast resulted in further improvement.

Wolfe's development of xeromammography in 1972 was a major advance.[107] Xeromammography employs a photoconductive plate of selenium-coated aluminum instead of X-ray film as an image receptor. The charged plate is placed underneath the breast and then exposed to X rays. The exposure results in a latent electrostatic image on the plate corresponding to differing densities within the breast. Processing results in the transfer of the latent image onto a permanent blue and white paper. An edge enhancement phenomenon accentuates borders of structures such as masses and calcifications. The radiation exposure to the midbreast is in the range of 250–400 mrad. Xeromammography functions best with a tungsten tube operating at 45 to 55 kV(p).

In the 1970s, the Dupont Company began marketing a system combining an intensifying screen with a single emulsion X-ray film.[82] The intimate contact required between the film and the screen was accomplished by enclosing the system in a sealed air-evacuated envelope. The system permitted short exposures with significantly reduced radiation. Variations of this system have been widely adopted and are now produced by several manufacturers.

There is no difference in diagnostic accuracy between the two techniques. Xeromammograms are easier to interpret, which is important when viewing large numbers of studies. The screen-film technique has the advantage of requiring less radiation.

Our routine views for xeromammography are the craniocaudal and mediolateral (to include the chest wall). In the craniocaudal projection, the patient is usually sitting with the height of the cassette adjusted so that the breast is flat on top of the cassette with no gap between the breast and the cassette. Compression is applied either with the Xerox paddle or with balloon compression from the cone. The average technique for the craniocaudal projection is 300 mA and 50 kV(p). For the mediolateral projection, the patient lies on the side to be examined with the cassette underneath her. The opposite breast is retracted out of the way and compression applied. A 2 kV(p) increase over that used for the craniocaudal view is usually necessary. Supplemental views with a change in the direction of the X-ray beam are important when an abnormality is observed on one view and not the other.

Low-dose film mammography requires a dedicated unit. Routine views are a craniocaudal view and an oblique view. The craniocaudal view is done with the patient either standing or sitting. Rigorous compression is very important. In order to obtain patient cooperation, the technique should be explained to the patient in considerable detail. The oblique view, which is a modification of the lateral view, is obtained with the unit angled at approximately 45°.[9] If a nonpalpable lesion is discovered, then a true lateral view is necessary so that the lesion can be accurately located. Although some authors have advocated a single oblique-view mammogram, most authors feel that two views of each breast (oblique and craniocaudal) are essential.[79] Modern, dedicated film-screen units utilize phototiming and a grid. The operator selects a kV(p) setting usually in the range of 25 to 28 kV(p) with a slight increase with the oblique view. Our average mid-breast radiation dose from two views is 0.750 cGy with xeromammography and 0.075 cGy with film-screen mammography.

Mammographic techniques that enhance the image contrast are helpful in visualizing small calcifications and slight differences in tissue density. Egan et al. and other authors propose the use of scatter-absorbing grids in mammography in order to increase contrast and object visibility.[30] A typical 5-to-1 ratio grid designed for mammography and used in conjunction with a molybdenum anode X-ray tube at 30 kV(p) will produce primary X-ray beam penetration of approximately 70%.[30,39] The use of grids in mammography is particularly important in the search for calcification in the larger breasts. Although the use of a grid does produce an increase in breast surface exposure, this can be partially offset by using more sensitive film and a slightly increased peak kilovoltage.

Another approach that has been used in an effort to obtain finer mammographic detail is direct radiographic magnification. This technique, in which the distance between the breast and the X-ray film is increased, requires a microfocal spot X-ray tube with an anode that is no greater than 0.3 mm in diameter. Sickles and his colleagues, who have utilized magnification mammography extensively, believe that the optimum degree of magnification is approximately 1.5 times life size.[91,92] In a comparative study of 750 patients by conventional mammography v conventional mammography plus magnification mammography, the authors detected nine proven malig-

nant tumors by the magnification technique that were not seen by conventional technique. Sickles thinks that the use of magnification mammography in equivocal cases will permit the surgeon to defer biopsy in favor of clinical observation. The current major use of magnification mammography is in the equivocal or difficult-to-examine patient. Magnification requires approximately double the radiation dose of standard mammography.

The mammographic features of cancer have been divided into "primary" and "secondary" signs of malignancy (Table 11-11). Primary signs include a mass of a relatively high density with an ill-defined spiculated border and numerous tiny calcifications (Figures 11-2, 11-3). The mass usually appears larger by palpation than by mammography. Secondary signs of breast cancer include retraction of the nipple, thickening of the skin, venous engorgement on the side of the tumor, fibrous tissue proliferation and axillary node enlargement. These secondary signs almost invariably represent an advanced cancer of the breast.

Benign lesions of the breast tend to be well circumscribed and are often surrounded by a lucent line thought to represent a "mach effect" of the eye. Fibroadenomas are often lobulated (Figure 11-4). Cysts are usually round to oval and are frequently multiple (Figure 11-5). Medullary and colloid carcinomas may be quite well circumscribed and may be confused with benign lesions. However, there usually is some irregularity along the margin of the tumor (Figure 11-6). Sclerosing adenomas, breast abscesses, and fat necroses all result in irregular appearing lesions on mammograms that resemble a carcinoma (Figure 11-7).

The emphasis today is on the detection by mammography of early cancers that are asymptomatic and too small to be palpable.[10] Gold has described the following mammographic signs associated with such small cancers: (1) a circumscribed cluster of microcalcifications (Figure 11-8), (2) a segmental prominence of one or more ducts, or (3) a localized distortion of breast architecture.

Table 11-11. Mammographic Signs

I. Malignant
  A. Primary signs
    1. Mass with ill-defined spiculated borders
    2. Innumerable tiny calcifications
  B. Secondary signs
    1. Retraction of nipple
    2. Skin thickening
    3. Venous enlargement
    4. Fibrous tissue proliferation
    5. Axillary node enlargement
II. Benign
  A. Well circumscribed mass often surrounded by lucent line
  B. Large coarse calcifications

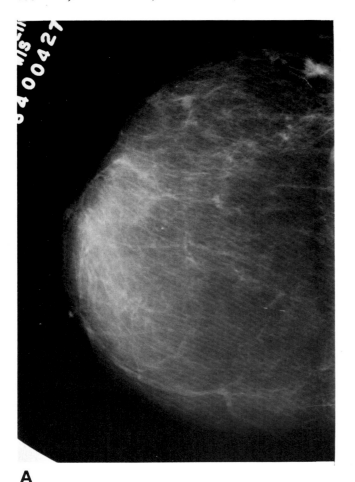

A

Calcifications seen on the mammograms, which are typical for cancer (Figure 11-8), tend to be so numerous as to be difficult to count, and may be tiny, clustered, polymorphic, finely stippled, angular, irregularly shaped, and sometimes branching. On the other hand, benign calcifications (see Figure 11-3) tend to be large, round, few in number, and less varied in size. Frequently, however, benign and malignant calcifications can not be differentiated, making biopsy imperative. Scattered, large ring-shaped or coarse linear calcifications are typical of benign secretory disease (Figure 11-9). Approximately half of the cancers demonstrate calcifications on a mammogram. The benign conditions of sclerosing adenosis, fat necrosis, and apocrine metaplasia may manifest microcalcifications similar to those seen in malignancy. Fibroadenomas are characterized by very large and amorphous calcifications (Figure 11-10).

Moskowitz has evaluated the predictive value of certain mammographic signs in patients with both negative and positive clinical examination of the breast.[76]

When the clinical examination was negative, 11.5% of the microcalcifications seen on mammography proved to be cancer at biopsy. Seventy-one percent of these cancers were minimal. However, when the clinical examination was positive, only 5.16% of the microcalcifications were proved malignant by biopsy and, of these, 38% were minimal. Masses felt to be definitely malignant on mammography proved to be malignant on biopsy in 100% of the cases with a positive physical examination

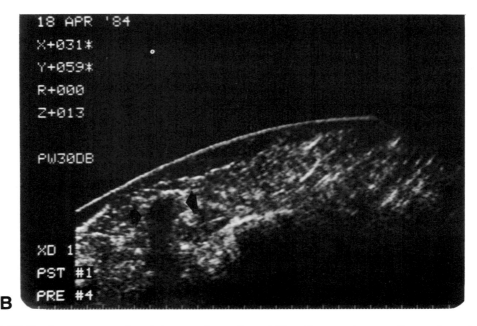

B

FIG. 11-2. (A) Classic appearance of a scirrhous carcinoma (arrow). Note the tentacles extending out from the tumor. (B) Ultrasonogram of same patient showing poorly defined solid mass (arrow) with posterior shadowing.

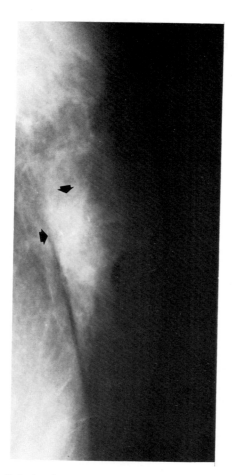

FIG. 11-3. Spiculated carcinoma (arrows) containing typical calcifications.

and in 73.68% of the cases with a negative clinical examination. The probability of a positive biopsy in a radiographically benign dominant mass over 1 cm in size, palpable or not, was 2%. Half of these tumors were minimal.

In 1967, Wolfe proposed that it was possible to predict which women were more likely to develop breast cancer based on their "parenchymal patterns" on mammography.[108] Wolfe divides the breast into four distinct patterns in order of increasing risk: (1) N_1, at lowest risk in which the parenchyma is composed almost entirely of fat and with no visible ducts; (2)P_1, low risk, in which the parenchyma is primarily fat but with prominent ducts in the anterior portion of the breast occupying up to one fourth of the breast volume; (3) P_2, at high risk, with severe duct prominence occupying more than one fourth the breast volume; (4) DY, at high risk with severe dysplasia, which, in its most severe form, appears homogeneous. N_1 and P_2 were considered by Wolfe as low-risk patterns whereas P_2 and DY were considered as high-risk patterns. Wolfe, in a follow-up study published in 1982, again stated that mammographic parenchymal pat-

terns were an indicator of breast cancer risk.[109] Of the prevalent breast cancers, 63% were found in P_2 breasts, 25% in DY breasts, 9.6% in P_1 breasts and 2.4% in N_1. If Wolfe's contentions are correct, it should be possible to identify, based on the mammographic appearance of the breast, a group of patients at higher risk of developing breast cancer than the general population. This relative high-risk group could then be subjected to more vigorous screening techniques. In Wolfe's population, 93% of the breast cancers could be found in 57% of the population. Although several authors have presented data that tend to agree with Wolfe's thesis, most recent papers dispute the theory.[31,99]

Thermography. Thermography in breast cancer screening has been a controversial subject throughout its 20-year history. Lawson first made the observation that breast cancers were associated with the elevation of the temperature of the skin over the lesion.[64] Electronic scanners, previously used in the military, were modified for use in evaluating skin temperatures.

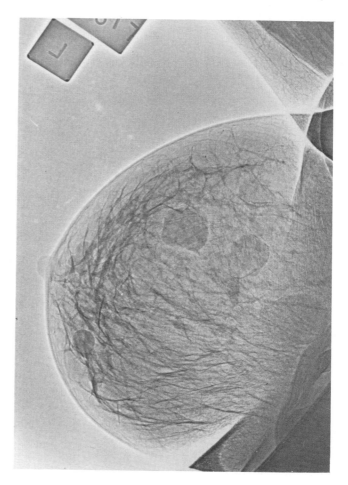

FIG. 11-4. Xeromammogram showing multiple fibroadenomas in a young patient. Note the well-defined lobulated borders.

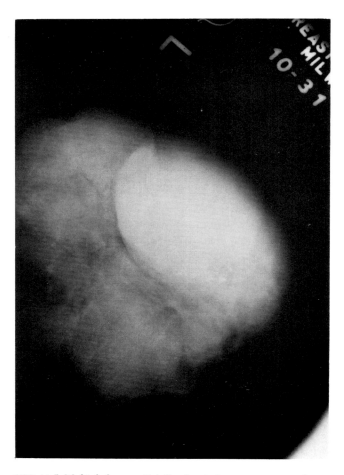

FIG. 11-5. Multiple large well-defined cysts in a premenopausal woman who had numerous cyst aspirations in the past.

An initial wave of enthusiastic reports followed.[58,104] Unfortunately most of these were either anecdotal or nonobjective. Thermography, however, was included in the 29 BCDDP's even though many of the radiologists in the study had little or no previous thermographic experience. Continued poor results, even from many centers where radiologists had experience with thermography, caused the National Cancer Institute to discontinue thermography as a routine screening test. In 1976, the American College of Radiology and the American Thermographic Society jointly declared that thermography was "not an adequate screening method for the detection of breast cancer or other breast disease when used *alone* or with only a physical examination."[88] This statement, coupled with several reports disputing the value of thermography, particularly in identifying small cancers, has caused many to be disillusioned with the technique.[78]

Breast thermography is usually performed by one of three methods: telethermography, contact thermography, or computerized thermography. In telethermography,

infrared radiation emitted from the body is focused by an optical mirror on a thermistor that converts infrared energy to an electrical signal, which is then displayed on a cathode-ray tube. The image may then be photographed for permanent record (Figure 11-11B).

In contact liquid-crystal thermography (LCT), a sheet of thin plastic containing heat-sensitive encapsulated liquid cholesterol esters is placed on the breast. Infrared radiation causes the black cholesteric crystals to change colors, which vary with the infrared energy being emitted from the breast surface. The color image on the plate is photographed while the plate is in contact with the breast.

In computerized thermography, multiple thermistors are used to detect infrared radiation. The electronic signals are fed to a computer, which uses various algorithms to calculate whether the measurements are normal or abnormal. An image of the breast is not usually obtained.

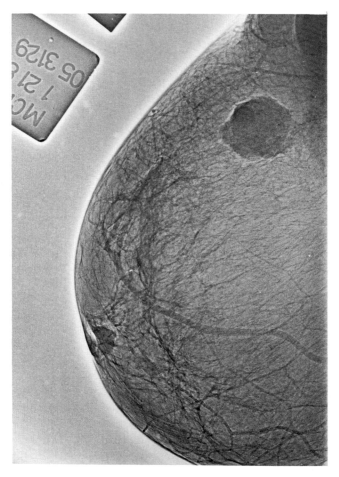

FIG. 11-6. Xeromammogram showing a typical medullary carcinoma that is fairly well circumscribed but tends to have somewhat nodular borders. Differentiation from a benign lesion is frequently difficult.

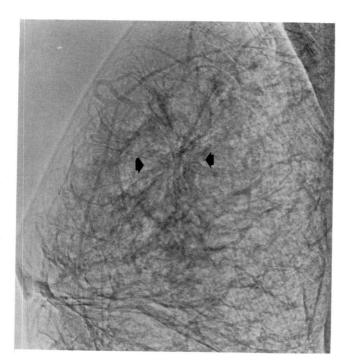

FIG. 11-7. Xeromammogram demonstrating nonpalpable spiculated mass (arrows) thought to be highly suspicious for carcinoma. A biopsy showed fat necrosis.

In a recent objective analysis of telethermography in detecting small breast cancers, recognized experts could not distinguish women with minimal breast cancer from women without cancer.[78] While thermography has been alternately proposed as an indicator of risk for future development of breast cancer, there are presently no objective data to support this contention.[17,55]

The American College of Radiology recently stated that thermography is not useful in screening for breast cancer because it misses so many of the small cancers that are the most curable types.

Ultrasound. Ultrasonography has recently become a useful method of imaging of the breast. High-frequency sound waves are produced by the vibrations of an electronically stimulated crystal transducer and pass into the breast, where they reflect from tissue interfaces back to the transducer. The signals are then transmitted electronically to a cathode-ray tube, where they are displayed as a cross-sectional image. Diagnostic ultrasound, which uses no radiation, has not been shown to be hazardous to human health. A specific area of the breast can be evaluated with a hand-held, high-resolution, real-time transducer or the entire breast can be evaluated with automatic water-bath units capable of imaging multiple thin sections of the breast.

The major role of breast sonography is its ability to dis-

tinguish cystic from solid masses[62] (Figures 11-12, 11-13). It is more accurate than either mammography or physical examination in this role.[36]

Ultrasonography is especially useful in evaluating masses that are nonpalpable and cannot be readily aspirated. In women with multiple masses, ultrasound is useful for the detection of a suspicious lesion requiring biopsy. However, ultrasound can rarely demonstrate cancers under 1.0 cm in size or microcalcifications.

Cancer detection rates for ultrasonography are considerably higher in women with radiographically dense breasts than in those women whose breasts are mostly fatty. Also, cancers that are detected by mammography and not by ultrasound are frequently small and nonpalpable, whereas carcinomas detected by ultrasound and not by mammography are almost always detected by physical examination. Therefore, at the present time, ultrasonography for breast cancer detection should be limited to women with dense breasts and then only as a supplemental technique to mammography.[94]

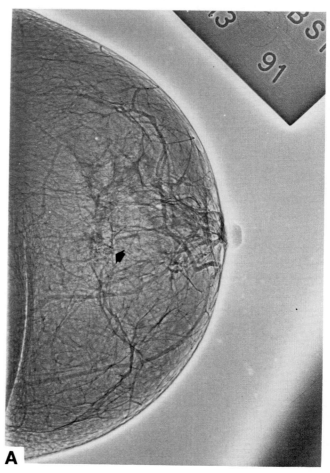

FIG. 11-8. (A) Cluster of calcifications (arrow) on xeromammogram.

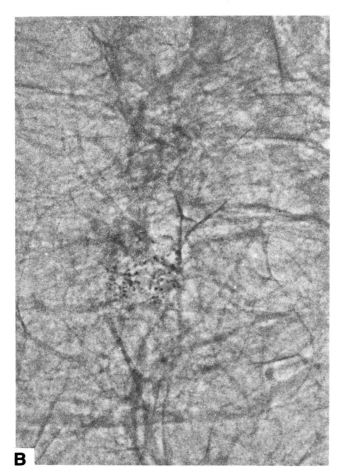

B

FIG. 11-8, continued. (B) Close-up view demonstrates numerous calcifications of varying size and shape. Histologic examination showed intraductal carcinoma.

Computed Tomography. A dedicated breast CT scanner has undergone extensive clinical trials and produced some interesting results. Contrast-enhanced scans have resulted in the detection of small cancers even in dense breast tissue, suggesting the possibility of an abnormal iodine-blood barrier.[21,22,24] Unfortunately, the cumbersome, dedicated equipment required for these studies precludes its widespread application. In addition, other reports failed to validate the detection efficiency for breast cancers.[45,71] Conventional CT scanners also have been reported to be able to detect small cancers on scans after contrast enhancement. In a practical clinical setting, this technique is not useful in terms of cost, radiation dose, and lesion specificity.

Computed tomographic scanning may be useful in pretreatment staging, particularly for the deep tumor, near the chest wall (Figure 11-14E,F). When chest wall invasion or internal mammary lymph node enlargement is suspected, CT is the examination of choice in evaluating these sites.

Diaphanography. Transillumination of the breasts with real-time viewing of the breast by a dark adapted examiner was described by Cutler in 1929.[24] However, the technique lapsed into relative obscurity until the 1950s because of lack of resolution and specificity.

Gros refined the technique with an improved design of the transilluminating light source and the recording of hard-copy images. More recently, in the United States, Carlsen has constructed a diaphanoscopy-diaphanography system using an infrared light source with the images recorded on an infrared-sensitive television camera and viewed on a standard television monitor. This technique allows real-time viewing of the images. There have been very enthusiastic reports, suggesting that the technique of diaphanography has an accuracy comparable with that of xeromammography. With diaphanography, the increased vascularity around the tumor may cause a reduction in light transmission either because blood is a strong absorber in the red and near infrared part of the

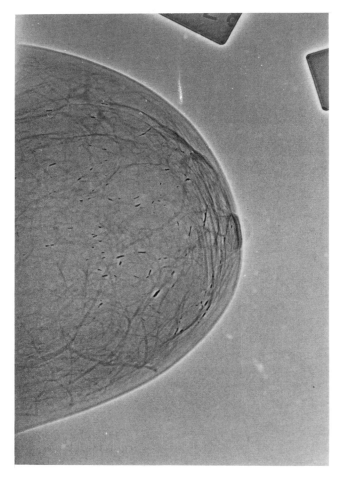

FIG. 11-9. Xeromammogram showing diffuse rodlike calcifications typical of secretory disease.

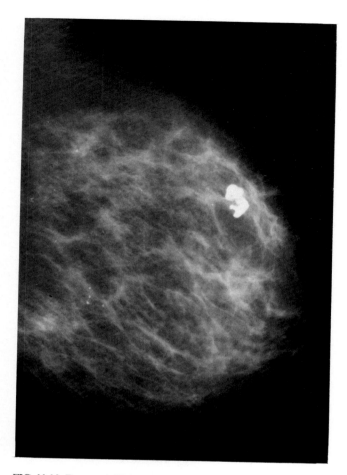

FIG. 11-10. Dense calcifications typical of a degenerating fibroadenoma.

spectrum or because the nitrogen-rich compounds found in growing tumors preferentially absorb infrared light.

Present commercially available devices have fairly broad light sources. Much of the light is scattered and diffused, producing an overall glare that causes poor inherent resolution. Current transillumination techniques should be considered experimental. There is no documented evidence that transillumination has any current role in screening.[93]

Magnetic Resonance Imaging. Magnetic resonance imaging (MRI) takes advantage of the interaction between the susceptible atoms in a magnetic field and radio waves to portray the structure of biological tissue. This new imaging technique has been applied to diseases of the breast. Relaxation times have been calculated for various types of breast tissue. Breast cancer appears to be characterized by longer T_1 and T_2 relaxation times in contrast to normal mammary tissue. McSweeney et al.[73] found excellent discrimination of benign from malignant samples in fatty or fibrofatty breasts. However, in fibrocystic disease there is considerable overlap of the re-

laxation time values for benign and malignant tissue. The presumed role of MRI in breast cancer diagnosis is currently based on anecdotal clinical data and animal experiments. Its ultimate clinical application must await further equipment development and subsequent human trials. System cost will preclude its application to screening and probably limit the use of MRI to clinical research, staging, and follow-up.

Heavy Particle Mammography. Heavy particle mammography has been used in only a few centers but apparently can detect minute differences in density between carcinoma and benign tissue that cannot be detected by conventional mammography.[90] Satisfactory heavy particle mammograms can be produced with radiation doses as low as 100 mrad per exposure. Again, system cost and complexity will probably preclude the widespread application of this imaging procedure.

Localization Procedures and Specimen Radiography. The ability of mammography to detect many nonpalpable cancers represents the greatest contribution of diagnostic imaging to the ultimate control of this perplexing disease. However, the biopsy of the nonpalpable lesions presents a challenge that requires the coordination and cooperation of the surgeon, pathologist, and radiologist. Before using a localization technique for biopsy of nonpalpable abnormalities at our institution, 10% of the patients returned with the mammographic abnormality still present following biopsy.

Numerous techniques are being utilized for directing the surgeon to the abnormality. The choice of technique should be by the consensus of surgeon and radiologist. We have used a variation of the "spot" method[96] (Figure 11-15). In this method the mammogram is repeated without compression to reduce distortion. The distance between the abnormality and the nipple is measured on the image, and coordinate measurements are made on the breast. The location of the abnormality is then estimated by triangulation. The skin overlying the suspicious area is prepared with antiseptic solution. No local anesthetic is usually necessary. A mixture of equal amounts of iodinated radiographic contrast and vital dye (e.g., Evans blue) totaling 0.1 mL is injected through a needle. A trail of dye is then created by injection on withdrawal of the needle. A second set of mammograms is obtained and the distance between the contrast "spot" and the abnormality is measured. If the contrast is within 2.5 cm of the abnormality, it can serve as a reference point for the surgeon. With experience, more than one injection is rarely necessary. To minimize the diffusion of the vital dye, the biopsy should occur within one or two hours of the localization. Since the radiographic contrast is rapidly absorbed by the lymphatics, it does not interfere with any subsequent radiograph on the specimen.

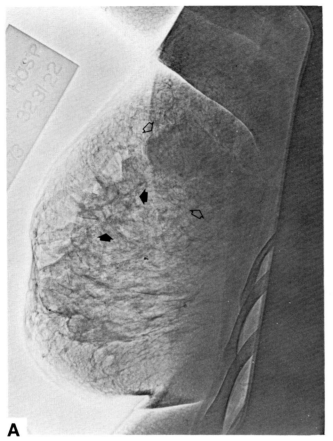

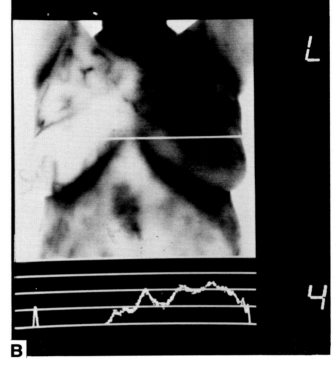

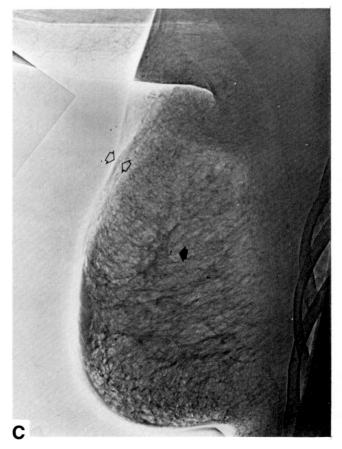

FIG. 11-11. (A) Xeromammogram of left breast showing scirrhous carcinoma (closed arrows) containing microcalcification. Large axillary
nodes (open arrows) can be easily visualized. (B) Thermogram showing
increased heat throughout entire left breast with increased vascularity.
especially in upper inner quadrant. (C) Xeromammogram following incisional biopsy and radiation therapy shows extensive skin thickening
(open arrows) but enlarged axillary nodes are no longer seen. Some
residual tumor calcifications (closed arrows) are unchanged from prebiopsy image. Scattered benign calcifications are seen both before and
after therapy.

With the other common localization method, a stainless steel hooked wire is introduced through an introducing needle that has been positioned in or immediately
adjacent to the abnormality.[61] When the introducing needle is withdrawn, the hook reforms, anchoring the wire
in place. The protruding end of the wire can be affixed
to the skin. The surgeon can then cut down on the wire,
taking care to avoid cutting the wire or contacting it with
electrocautery.

A roentgenogram of the biopsy specimen may verify
that the nonpalpable lesion has been removed. This
technique is particularly useful if a single cluster of calcifications was biopsied. In our institution, biopsy specimens suspected of containing calcifications are immediately taken to the radiology department where an image
of the biopsy specimen is taken and compared with the
original mammogram. The surgeon is then notified wheth-

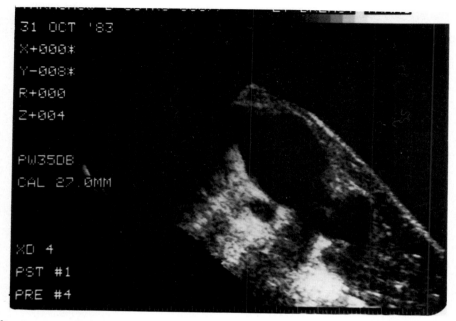

FIG. 11-12. Ultrasonogram revealing cystic nature of masses. Note the cysts are anechoic with well-defined anterior and posterior borders associated with an increased transmission typical of cysts. 143 mL of clear fluid was subsequently aspirated with disappearance of the masses.

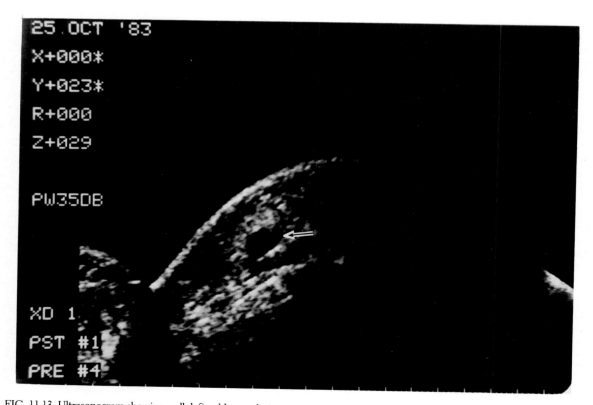

FIG. 11-13. Ultrasonogram showing well-defined hypoechoic mass (arrow) with smooth prominent anterior and posterior borders typical of a fibroadenoma.

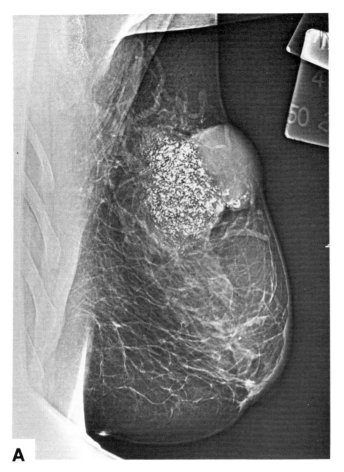

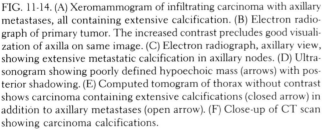

A

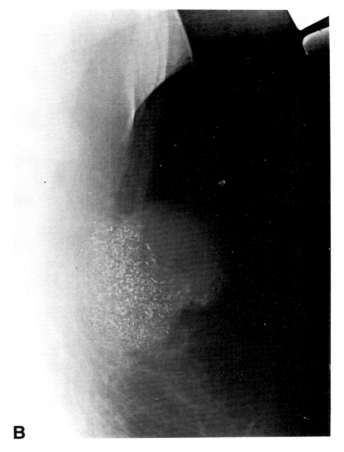

B

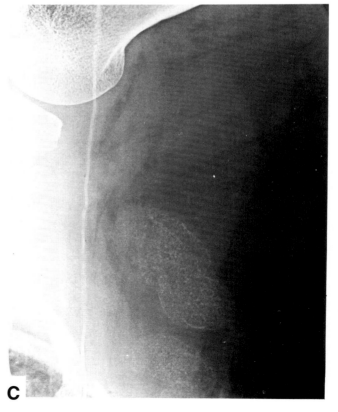

C

FIG. 11-14. (A) Xeromammogram of infiltrating carcinoma with axillary metastases, all containing extensive calcification. (B) Electron radiograph of primary tumor. The increased contrast precludes good visualization of axilla on same image. (C) Electron radiograph, axillary view, showing extensive metastatic calcification in axillary nodes. (D) Ultrasonogram showing poorly defined hypoechoic mass (arrows) with posterior shadowing. (E) Computed tomogram of thorax without contrast shows carcinoma containing extensive calcifications (closed arrow) in addition to axillary metastases (open arrow). (F) Close-up of CT scan showing carcinoma calcifications.

er or not the suspicious calcifications are contained in the specimen. The specimen then is sent to the pathology department, where it is sliced "bread-loaf" style into sections 2–3 mm thick. The slices are then arranged in sequence on a sheet of clear film for support and a second roentgenogram is obtained—this time in a self-contained X-ray unit located in the surgical pathology laboratory. The radiologist then marks areas of suspicion on the films to guide the pathologist in selecting areas to examine histologically.

Specimen radiography is most useful when a biopsy is done for suspicious calcifications discovered on a mammogram or when the entire specimen is so large that it cannot be conveniently examined histologically. It is also helpful when blind biopsies have been done on the contralateral breast.[98]

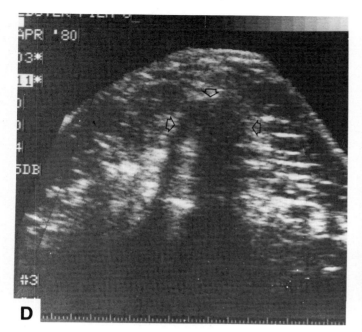

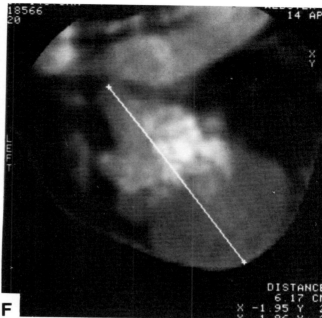

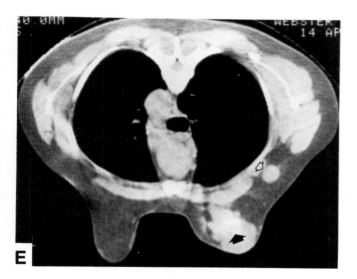

Needle Aspiration Biopsy. Needle aspiration of a cyst is now a generally accepted method for both diagnosis and treatment.[47]

If aspiration is performed, a 21-gauge needle is placed in the mass under sterile technique. If the fluid is clear and yellow in color, it can be safely discarded. Otherwise, cytologic examination is performed. The patient is then seen for follow-up in 6 months.

Martin first reported on needle aspiration biopsy for the diagnosis of solid breast masses in 1930, but it remained a little-used procedure until recent reports by Franzen and Zajicek in Europe and Kline and Frable in the United States.[37,38,60,68] Fine-needle aspiration biopsy is an easily performed out-patient diagnostic method for determining the nature of a breast mass. It is free of complications, convenient, cost effective, and enables a full discussion of treatment options with a breast cancer patient before intervention.[37]

Most of our patients with a palpable mass noted to be solid on ultrasound examination undergo a needle biopsy. A 21-gauge needle is attached to a disposable 20-mL syringe fitted into a commercially available syringe holder, and the needle is filled with saline. After the skin is sterilized, the needle is passed through the mass six to ten times with constant suction maintained. No anesthetic is required. The fluid in the needle is then smeared onto frosted slides and fixed with 95% ethanol. The syringe and needle are then flushed with 40% ethanol and all samples are sent to the cytology laboratory. If the cytologic diagnosis confirms a benign impression, the patient is re-evaluated in 6 months. Occasionally insufficient material is obtained for cytologic evaluation, in which case the procedure is repeated. If a benign diagnosis is obtained on cytologic examination of a lesion thought to be cancer, the patient is referred for excisional biopsy.

Galactography. The use of galactography or mammary duct contrast examination with a water-soluble medium is a valuable procedure in the evaluation of women with needle discharge or bleeding. After sterile preparation of the breast, the secreting duct is identified by gently squeezing the breast and nipple. The identified duct is then cannulated with a number 25 or 27 blunt-nosed needle attached to a small syringe containing water-soluble contrast material. After cannulation of the duct, contrast is injected until the patient experiences mild discomfort or pressure. Mammograms are then obtained in

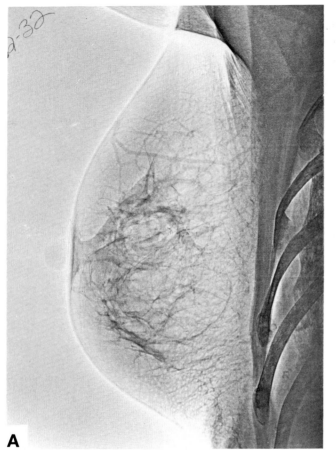

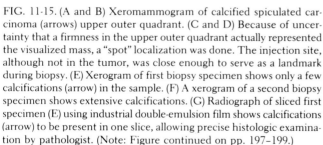

A

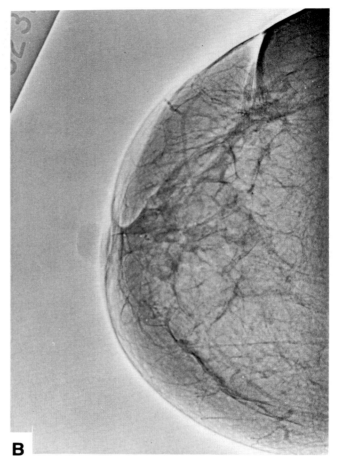

B

FIG. 11-15. (A and B) Xeromammogram of calcified spiculated carcinoma (arrows) upper outer quadrant. (C and D) Because of uncertainty that a firmness in the upper outer quadrant actually represented the visualized mass, a "spot" localization was done. The injection site, although not in the tumor, was close enough to serve as a landmark during biopsy. (E) Xerogram of first biopsy specimen shows only a few calcifications (arrow) in the sample. (F) A xerogram of a second biopsy specimen shows extensive calcifications. (G) Radiograph of sliced first specimen (E) using industrial double-emulsion film shows calcifications (arrow) to be present in one slice, allowing precise histologic examination by pathologist. (Note: Figure continued on pp. 197–199.)

craniocaudal and mediolateral projections. Some authors have found that microfocus magnification techniques improve the demonstration of pathologic findings. With this technique it is possible to identify intraductal papillomas, intraductal papillomatosis and hyperplasia, secretory disease, and carcinoma. In the case of carcinoma, the ducts may be irregular in outline, encased and straightened, or distorted and obstructed. Repeat galactography with a mixture of methylene blue dye and contrast material just before surgery is helpful in identifying the duct to the surgeon.

Detection of Metastases. The choice of diagnostic procedures for the workup of a patient with suspected breast

cancer has been confusing and contradictory. Fortunately, the tendency toward less radical surgery has relieved some of the burden on the medical imager to detect metastatic disease before surgery. Furthermore, there is no clear evidence that the treatment of asymptomatic metastasis of the breast affects survival.

A recommendation for a diagnostic workup is dependent on our understanding of the spread of breast cancer and the accuracy of the various diagnostic tests (Table 11-12).

The most frequent sites for initial metastatic dissemination are the bones, lungs, and pleura. The liver and brain are less frequent sites of metastatic spread.

All patients with suspected breast cancer should have a complete physical examination. Bilateral mammography is imperative, not only to detect the presence of an unsuspected cancer in the opposite breast but also to guide the biopsy of the affected breast. In those patients in whom the breast will not be removed, the initial mammogram also is an important baseline in following the progress of chemotherapy and radiation therapy.

The PA and lateral chest film is an essential procedure in the evaluation of the thorax in the breast cancer pa-

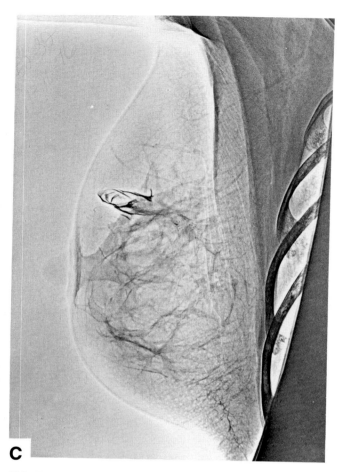

C

FIG. 11-15, continued.

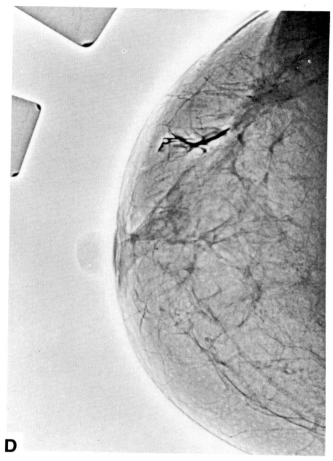

D

FIG. 11-15, continued.

tient. It will exclude any co-existing disease that might render a general anesthetic inadvisable. Furthermore, it is the best initial method to detect metastatic disease within the thorax. The patient suspected of having lymphangitic metastatic disease should virtually *always* be symptomatic, usually complaining of a dry, nonproductive cough and dyspnea.

The most frequent radiographic manifestation of intrathoracic metastatic disease is a pleural effusion. Rarely will a pleural mass lesion be visible with either conventional or special (CT or MRI) techniques in this setting. The parenchymal pulmonary patterns of breast metastatic disease are variable and range from a poorly defined, nodular mass lesion to a lymphangitic process. A solitary nodule, hilar, or mediastinal node mass alone is rarely observed. The patient with a solitary coin lesion should be presumed to have a primary lung cancer until proven otherwise.[18]

The accurate characterization of a patient with lymphangitic tumor spread often is difficult. The radiographic manifestations may be either subtle or nonspecific. Often, the features of lymphangitic spread may be confused with those of congestive heart failure. The radiologist occasionally will make the diagnosis of lymphangitic tumor spread in a completely asymptomatic patient—a remarkably rare event.

Computed tomography in staging the patient with breast cancer before treatment can be justified to outline otherwise occult, but involved, internal mammary, hilar, or mediastinal lymph nodes. Both ultrasound and CT may detect the presence of a malignant pericardial effusion, particularly in those patients with tumor cell-positive pleural effusions.

Bone scans using technetium Tc 99m phosphonate and diphosphonate are sensitive tests for the presence of skeleton metastases and should be used rather than radiographic films for surveying the skeleton. A positive bone scan is due to increased osteoblastic activity or vascularity within the bone and is not specific for metastatic disease. Therefore, it is imperative that X-ray films be obtained of the area of concern on the bone scan. The early detection of metastatic disease of the skeleton in an asymptomatic patient has little effect on patient survival but may have very significant impact on patient morbidity. Early treatment either with radiation therapy or with orthopedic appliances may prevent path-

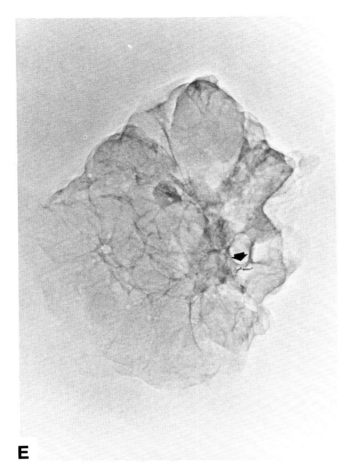

E

FIG. 11-15, continued.

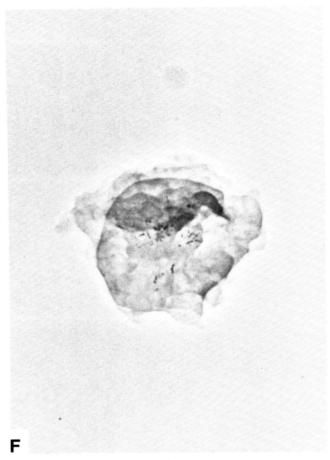

F

FIG. 11-15, continued.

ologic fractures and their very painful, disabling sequel-ae. Therefore, a special effort should be made to detect metastatic disease from the breast to the skeleton as early as possible. There is a great deal of controversy about how the bone scan should be used in the clinical staging of breast cancer patients and in the follow-up of treated patients. Baker and his colleagues found positive bone scans in only one of 64 patients with TNM stage I and II cancers.[8] McNeil, in her review of several series, found true-positive bone scans in 2% of patients with clinical stage I breast cancer, 2% of clinical stage II, and 28% of clinical stage III.[72] Clearly the bone scan is important in evaluating patients with stage III and stage IV breast cancer. An initial baseline bone scan is felt by many to be valuable in patients with stage I and stage II breast cancer.[43,72] Because of the lack of specificity of the bone scan, the appearance of new scan abnormalities is important for accurate interpretation. There is a high rate of conversion from negative to positive bone scans even in those patients with early breast cancer. McNeil quotes a conversion rate for stage I of 7%, for stage II of 45%, and for stage III of 58%. Gerber et al.[43] noted that 5 of 23 women with negative lymph nodes and 2 of 11

women with one to four positive lymph nodes converted from a negative scan to a positive scan. Conversion from negative to positive bone scans usually occurs within two years after diagnosis. Half of the patients who had developed bone metastases within three years after treatment already had positive bone scans by 12 months and 75% developed them by 18 months.[72] The observation that the positive bone scan develops rapidly has an impact in planning the follow-up of the breast cancer patient. McNeil recommends that in addition to a baseline evaluation, the breast cancer patient should have serial bone scans at 6, 12, 18, and 24 months. If the bone scan remains negative after two or three years, follow-up bone scans can be reserved for those patients who develop symptoms. Gerber et al. recommended that patients have bone scans for five years after treatment.[43] Roentgenograms of any bone scan abnormalities are necessary for accurate interpretation.

A radionuclide liver scan is the procedure of choice in the detection of space-occupying lesions of the liver. However, liver function studies are a quite accurate method of detecting hepatic metastases. For example, an abnormally elevated serum alkaline phosphatase level in a

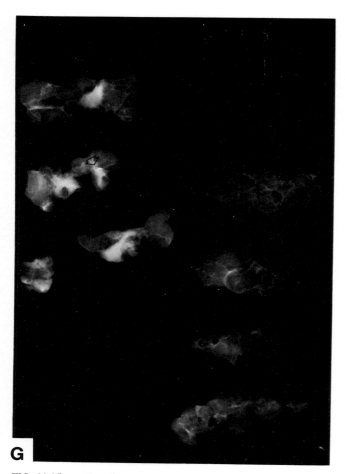

G

FIG. 11-15, continued.

patient with breast cancer indicates hepatic involvement with an 85% accuracy.[26] Radionuclide liver scans should be reserved for those patients who have either abnormal liver chemistry values or in whom a large liver can be palpated. Breast cancer does occasionally spread to the GI tract, but when this does occur, the patient will al-

most always be symptomatic. A survey of the GI tract does not appear warranted in the asymptomatic patient.

Cerebral metastases are almost always symptomatic. Muss found only one abnormal brain scan in 116 patients with metastatic disease of the breast but no symptoms of intracranial disease.[80] Of the 37 patients who had central nervous system symptoms, there were initially 11 abnormal brain scans. Three more patients developed abnormalities in the brain scan at a later date. Although the radionuclide brain scan is highly accurate, detecting 85% to 90% of cerebral metastasis in those breast cancer patients with central nervous system symptoms, the imaging technique of choice is contrast-enhanced computed tomography. The exact extent of the lesion is better shown by CT than by radionuclide brain scans.

Internal mammary lymphoscintigraphy is a noninvasive method of identifying the internal mammary lymph nodes. Radiation therapy fields were revised in 12 of 20 patients with stage I and II breast cancer who were about to undergo radiation therapy planning based on the findings of internal mammary lymphoscintigraphy in patients with breast cancer.[23]

IMAGING STRATEGIES AND DECISIONS

The imaging decision trees for carcinoma of the breast are less complex than in other areas of the body. The (T) or tumor component of the TNM staging is determined by physical examination and mammography. Bilateral mammography should be obtained in all patients with suspected breast cancer. Not only will the mammogram aid in the preoperative determination of the size and extent of the primary tumor but it also provides a road map of the breast to guide the surgeon in his or her biopsy. Other suspicious areas within the breast can be biopsied. If the patient is to be treated by radiation

Table 11-12. Imaging Modalities for Evaluation of Metastatic Breast Cancer

MODALITY	STAGING CAPABILITY	COST/BENEFIT RATIO	RECOMMENDED AS STAGING PROCEDURE	COMMENTS
Chest X-ray film	Essential for all tumor types	High	Yes	
Radionuclide	Essential for baseline verification and evaluation of symptomatic patient	High	Yes	Abnormal bone scans require film
Liver Imaging	Indicated with abnormal chemistries or symptoms	High (when indicated)	Yes (when indicated)	Initial imaging study radionuclide liver scan (requires validation of abnormal scan by ultrasound or CT)
Brain Imaging	Indicated by abnormal physical signs or symptoms	High (when indicated)	Yes (when indicated)	Contrast enhanced CT (or MRI) recommended

Table 11-13. BCDDP/HIP Comparison

	BCDDP				HIP			
	AGES 40–49 AT SURGERY		AGES 50–59 AT SURGERY		AGES 40–49 AT SURGERY		AGES 50–59 AT SURGERY	
SUSPICIOUS MODALITY	NUMBER	PERCENT	NUMBER	PERCENT	NUMBER	PERCENT	NUMBER	PERCENT
Mammography only	270	35.4	540	42.1	6	19.4	27	41.5
Mammography and physical examination	381	50.0	638	49.7	6	19.4	12	18.5
Physical examination only	100	13.1	86	6.7	19	61.3	26	40.0
Unknown	11	1.4	19	1.5	0	0.0	0	0.0
Total	762	100.0	1283	100.0	31	100.0	65	100.0

Reprinted from CA **32**:217, 1982.

therapy or chemotherapy, the initial mammogram can serve as a baseline to measure the progress of therapy. Coexisting carcinomas in the opposite breast can be detected by mammography.

Although ultrasound is not a satisfactory substitute for mammography, in young patients with dense breasts it may provide significant additional information. It is valuable in distinguishing cystic from solid lesions within the breast.

Axillary node involvement is best determined by physical examination and biopsy. The use of lymphoscintigraphy to identify the internal mammary node chain is helpful in planning treatment. In the hands of Ege,[32] the method has a relatively high accuracy in predicting involvement of the internal mammary nodes by tumor.

The decision tree for the detection of distant metastases is the most important in breast disease. For stage I and II tumors, we recommend bilateral mammograms, a chest film, liver function studies, and a baseline radioisotope bone scan (Table 11-15). For stage III and IV breast cancer, a radioisotope bone scan is added to the

diagnostic workup (Table 11-16). When suspicious findings are observed on the radionuclide bone scan, X-ray films of the area in question should be obtained to rule out a process other than metastatic disease.[8]

The follow-up of a patient with treated breast cancer consists of an annual mammogram, chest films, and a liver function study. Radionuclide bone scans should be performed periodically for three to five years. If the scans prove negative for this period of time, additional bone scans should be obtained only if the patient develops symptoms. Computed tomographic scans of the brain are advised only in those patients who are symptomatic. Radionuclide liver scans are reserved for those patients who develop either a large liver or abnormal liver function studies (Table 11-17).

TREATMENT DECISIONS

For many years the approach to treating breast cancer has been based largely on the premise that these tumors begin as a local growth that enlarges and then spreads

Table 11-14.

	YEAR								
RATES	1	1.5	2	2.5	3	3.5	4	4.5	5
Biopsy performance rates	358.1		187.6		173.4		145.9		117.8
Cancer detection rates	55.8		26.5		25.2		25.4		23.6
Minimal cancer detection rates	18.4		8.5		8.6		8.0		7.0
Interval cancer rates		8.0		7.7		8.0		7.5	

Rates are per 10,000 annual screenings.
Reprinted from CA **32**:206, 1982. With permission.

Table 11-15. Imaging Recommendations: Breast Cancer Stage I & II

1. Bilateral mammograms
2. Chest film
3. Baseline bone scan

Table 11-16. Imaging Recommendations: Breast Cancer Stage III & IV

1. Bilateral mammogram
2. Chest film
3. Radionuclide bone scan (with verification X-ray films if abnormal)
4. Radionuclide liver scan (only if liver chemistry values are abnormal)

Liver Scan

Negative	Positive
↓	↓
Stop	CT or Ultrasound

5. CT brain scan (if symptomatic)

Table 11-17. Imaging Recommendations: Breast Cancer Follow-up

1. Mammogram—annual
2. Chest film—annual
3. Radionuclide bone scan (if negative for three years, then only when symptomatic)
4. Radionuclide liver scan (only if liver chemistry values are abnormal)
5. CT brain scan (only if symptomatic)

to regional lymph nodes before the development of systemic metastatic disease. Although this model of tumor spread may be appropriate for many breast cancers, the regional lymph nodes do not serve as a barrier to the distant spread of the tumor. Regional and distant tumor spread may well occur synchronously. It is now felt that tumor characteristics and host defenses determine the pattern of spread of the cancer even though regional lymph node status serves as an important barometer for tumor behavior.

With the reports of comparable survival results from groups of breast cancer patients treated with radical surgery versus conservative surgery with radiation therapy in early stage disease, there has been a gradual shift away from a dependence on surgery as the primary treatment for breast cancer. Excellent cosmetic results from excisional biopsy or "lumpectomy" with axillary lymph node sampling followed by a carefully ordered radiation treatment program have been reported from many centers in Europe and North America. This conservative approach is more effective for both the smaller primary cancer and the patient with larger breast volume. The

classic Halsted radical mastectomy is now infrequently performed. This shift toward more conservative therapy has placed different demands on the mammographer both to localize the cancer, thereby guiding the limited biopsy, and to more accurately stage the patient. Although early stage disease detected by mammography usually results in long-term survival and cure, there remains a significant group of patients, particularly those with positive axillary nodes, who have occult metastases; their survival will not be altered by eradicating the primary tumor earlier. Accordingly, a variety of programs of adjuvant chemotherapy have been designed, and subsets of patients are clearly deriving a benefit from such an approach. Once metastatic disease appears, the chances for long-term control by either chemotherapy or hormonal therapy are diminished, and the possibility for long-term survival or cure becomes remote. Thus, there is a great stimulus to develop more effective combinations of therapy.

Surgery

The surgical management of early breast disease has been gradually shifting from a modified radical mastectomy, which consists of removal of the entire breast and axillary nodes with preservation of the pectoralis muscles, to lumpectomy, tylectomy, or quadrantectomy. These latter procedures preserve the breast and are widely accepted with more conservative dissection of the lower axillary nodes, which is essentially a staging procedure.

Radiation Therapy

There is a considerable amount of literature on the development of radiation therapy as the primary treatment of early stage breast cancer as an alternative to mastectomy. Definitive radiation treatment, when the regional lymph nodes are negative, consists of tangential irradiation of the breast and chest wall following lumpectomy. If the regional lymph nodes are positive, additional fields are added to include the axillary, supraclavicular, and internal mammary node-bearing areas. Utilizing megavoltage irradiation, careful attention to matching of field margins together with electron beam therapy have allowed for individualization and excellent long-term cosmetic results.

Chemotherapy and Hormonal Therapy

The most dramatic change in therapy in the past decade has been the substitution of cytotoxic drugs for hormonal programs and, eventually, the inclusion of the combination of cytotoxic drugs with hormonal alteration in menopausal and postmenopausal women. The concept of adjuvant treatment applies to chemotherapy after primary treatment with surgery or radiation therapy, and essentially refers to any part of treatment that assists another to achieve a desired end result.

The estrogen (ER) and progesterone (PR) receptor status is an important determinant with regard to planning hormonal management of patients. Patients with ER− tumors have higher recurrence rates compared with ER+ patients, who have relatively higher response rates to hormonal treatment. The additional presence of progesterone receptors in tumors is associated with even higher response rates, and such data are helpful in determining whether to employ hormonal manipulation for metastatic disease, particularly in older patients.

It would be beyond the scope to this text to do more than attempt to summarize the principles of treatment by stage (Table 11-18).

1. Stage I and stage II breast cancer are essentially determined by the use of physical examination, mammography, and axillary node sampling with dissection of the first two levels. In stage I disease, treatment with lumpectomy and breast conservation is cosmetically preferred over modified radical mastectomy, which may be necessary in certain circumstances, such as with small-breasted women. Definitive radiation therapy is limited to the breast, with exclusion of nodes, and adjuvant chemotherapy is rarely indicated. It is recommended that patients with stage II disease who have positive axillary nodes have the management plan of the primary tumor essentially the same, with definitive radiation therapy following lumpectomy with breast conservation and treatment of regional axillary, supraclavicular, and internal mammary nodes. Adjuvant multiagent chemotherapy usually consists of a four- or five-drug program in premenopausal women and the addition of tamoxifen in postmenopausal women.

2. In stage III disease the approach to treatment must be more radical, depending upon the advancement of the disease and whether or not modified radical mastectomy is technically feasible. Adjuvant multiagent chemotherapy as defined previously is applied. In stage IIIB disease, where the primary tumor is largely unresectable, multiagent chemotherapy is usually applied first in two to six cycles followed by definitive radiation therapy of the breast and regional nodes.

3. With stage IV patients, where metastatic disease is present along with the discovery of the primary tumor, a "toilette" mastectomy may be considered or, if local-regional disease is sufficiently small and relatively asymptomatic, the primary may be managed along with the metastatic disease by systemic multiagent chemotherapy or hormonal treatment or both. The response of the primary tumor in many instances may be as dramatic as the metastatic disease and may require no surgical or radiation treatment. Radiation treatment in this circumstance is usually reserved for symptomatic areas such as with bone and brain metastases.

There are many nuances of management, but readers are advised to refer to the many standard textbooks.[50]

Mammography can play an important role in monitoring the results of radiation therapy and chemotherapy in the posttreatment breast. Gefter et al.[42] found that 14 of 38 or 37% of mammograms following excisional biopsies provided useful information in treatment planning for early breast cancer. The valuable information in these patients included the presence or absence of gross residual tumor after biopsy and the detection of occult lesions in the opposite breast or axillary nodes. In every case in which a prebiopsy mammogram was available, the postbiopsy study proved to be helpful in the

Table 11-18. Treatment Decisions: Breast

Stage	Surgery		Radiation Therapy		Chemotherapy
I T_1,N_0,M_0	Lumpectomy to modified radical mastectomy	AND AND	Definitive RT of breast NR		NR
II $T_{1,2},N_1,M_0$	Lumpectomy to modified radical mastectomy	AND	Definitive RT of breast and regional nodes		Adjuvant MAC and TAM
IIIa T_3,N_0,N_1	Lumpectomy to modified radical mastectomy	AND	Definitive RT of breast and regional nodes	AND/OR	Adjuvant MAC and TAM
IIIb T_{1-3},N_3 T_4,T_{any}	Unresectable		Definitive RT of breast and regional nodes	AND	MAC±HT
IV T_{any},N_{any},M_1	"Toilette" mastectomy (optional)		Optional		MAC±HT

RT = radiation therapy
NR = not recommended
MAC = multiagent chemotherapy
HT = hormonal therapy
TAM = tamoxifen

evaluation of the extent of residual tumor tissue. In two patients with residual microcalcifications and three with residual masses, gross tumor was confirmed on repeat biopsies. The need for a baseline mammogram cannot be emphasized strongly enough. Not only is it helpful as a guide to biopsy in surgery, but it is imperative information for follow-up of radiation therapy. Nisce et al.[81] found the mammogram to be a valuable addition to the clinical examination of the irradiated breast. The mammogram was found to be more accurate than surgical findings in the recognition of residual disease, in differentiation of radiation fibrosis from persistent disease, and in the detection of reactivation of disease that was not clinically obvious. Timing of the first posttreatment mammogram is important. Radiation will alter the appearance of both normal breast tissue and cancer. Breast changes secondary to radiation usually stabilize at approximately 2 to 4 months after treatment. Therefore, a new baseline mammogram is recommended at this time. Following radiation therapy, tumor masses usually diminish in size or completely disappear (Figure 11-11). A previously palpable mass may become nonpalpable, but a mammogram may show a residual density.

Tumor calcifications may remain the same, diminish, or disappear, but they should not increase. Therefore, the persistence of malignant tumor calcifications does not necessarily indicate persistence of residual viable tumor. Benign-appearing calcifications, usually intraductal, may also be noted following radiation therapy. The skin usually becomes thicker after radiation treatment, often for several months after therapy, but the increased thickness returns to normal in most cases within two or three years.[65] A diffuse increase in the density of the breast that usually occurs after irradiation is caused by skin thickening, fibrosis, and collagenosis. Most patients receiving radiation therapy experience some degree of breast contraction, which may continue over a period of several years. Tumor recurrence usually manifests itself on the mammogram as an increasing mass, occasionally associated with an increase or reappearance of tumor calcifications. Secondary signs of malignancy are of little value in detecting recurrent disease after radiation therapy.

If a patient is primarily treated with radiation therapy, an initial baseline mammogram should be obtained before treatment, preferably before any biopsy, with follow-up examinations at the end of therapy and at 2-month intervals for the first 6 months after treatment. Subsequent mammographic follow-up intervals should be yearly.

Mammography has also been used to evaluate the results of endocrine therapy in breast cancer.[54] Tumor response is characterized by a decrease in the size of the mammographic mass, a change in the pattern of microcalcifications, and occasionally, a more dense radiographic appearance of the tumor mass.

IMPACT OF NEW TECHNOLOGY

Data from breast cancer screening programs worldwide have validated the ability of mammography to detect patients with minimal breast cancer at an acceptable cost and radiation exposure. Further efforts are needed to educate both the population at risk and the referring physician about the efficacy and safety of this detection technique.

Mammographic accuracy is largely a function of radiographic technique and, to a lesser degree, interpretive expertise. Continuing efforts must emerge from within our radiologic specialty to encourage educational programs aimed at both of these professional echelons. Refinements in film-screen combinations will occur in future years; the return in terms of diagnostic yield will be small but the gain in patient radiation dose may well be significant.

Alternate breast screening modalities (diaphanography, sonography, thermography) will probably not be able to challenge the current detection efficiency and accuracy of mammography, even with subsequent modifications. The stimulus to develop these alternate imaging modalities was, in part, a response to the public's concern over radiation, a problem that is now in a more realistic perspective. Hopefully, future breast imaging techniques can be more rationally and scientifically evaluated before being released to the public, a circumstance that has not been true in the past.

Nuclear magnetic resonance imaging represents a research opportunity to study the entire spectrum of the breast cancer problem in vivo. One certainly cannot expect MRI to be used in a screening setting; however, it does have potential in addressing the problem of tissue characterization and in more accurately and specifically staging the patient with breast cancer. Characterizing and understanding the different T_1 and T_2 relaxation times in normal, benign, and malignant breast tissues will be a fertile area for future MRI research.

REFERENCES

1. *Ackerman's Surgical Pathology* Rosai, J., (Ed.). St. Louis, C. V. Mosby Co. Vol. 2, 1981, 1087–1149.
2. American Cancer Society: *Cancer Facts & Figures.* New York, American Cancer Society, 1980.
3. American Cancer Society: Cancer statistics, 1984. CA **34**:1, 1984
4. American Cancer Society: *Nutrition and Cancer and Prevention.* Special Report. New York, American Cancer Society, 1984.
5. American Joint Committee on Cancer: *Manual for Staging of Cancer*, 2nd ed. Philadelphia, J. B. Lippincott, 1983, pp. 127–133.
6. Andersen, J. A.: Lobular carcinoma in situ. A long term follow-up in 52 cases. *Acta Pathol. Microbiol. Scand. [Sect. A]* 82:519, 1974.
7. Baker, L. H.: Breast cancer detection demonstration project: Five-year summary report. CA 32:194–225, 1982.
8. Baker, R. R., Holmes, E. R. III, Alderson, P. O., Curry, N. F., Wagner, H. N.: An evaluation of bone scans as screening pro-

cedures for occult metastases in primary breast cancer. *Ann. Surg.* 186:363, 1977.

9. Bassett, L. W., Gold, R. H.: Breast radiography using the oblique projection. *Radiology* 149:585–587, 1983.

10. Bassett, L. W., Gold, R. H. (Eds.): *Mammography, Thermography and Ultrasound in Breast Cancer Detection.* New York, Grune & Stratton, 1982.

11. Berg, J. W.: Clinical implications of risk factors for breast cancer. *Cancer* 53:589–591, 1984.

12. Berg, J. W., Robbins, G. F.: Factors influencing short and long term survival of breast cancer patients. *Surg. Gynecol. Obstet.* 122:1311–1316, 1966.

13. Betsill, W. L., Rosen, P. P., Lieberman, P. H., Robbins, G. F.: Intraductal carcinoma. Long-term follow-up after treatment by biopsy alone. *J.A.M.A.* 239:1863–1867, 1978.

14. Black, M. M., Barclay, T. H., Cutler, S. J., Hankey, B. F., Asire, A. J.: Association of atypical characteristics of benign breast lesions with subsequent risk of breast cancer. *Cancer* 29:338–343, 1972.

15. Black, M. M., Barclay, T. H., Hankey, B. F.: Prognosis in breast cancer utilizing histologic characteristics of the primary tumor. *Cancer* 36:2048–2055, 1975.

16. Bloom, H. J. G., Field, J. R.: Impact of tumor grade and host resistance in survival of women with breast cancer. *Cancer* 28:1580–1589, 1971.

17. Byrne, R.: The value of breast thermography as a risk indicator. *Acta Thermographica* 2:55, 1977.

18. Cahan, W. G., Castro, E. B.: Significance of a solitary lung shadow in patients with breast cancer. *Ann. Surg.* 181:137, 1975.

19. Carstens, P. H. B.: Tubular carcinoma of the breast. A study of frequency. *Am. J. Clin. Pathol.* 70:204, 1978.

20. Carstens, P. H. B., Huvos, A. G., Foote, F. W., Jr., Ashikari, R.: Tubular carcinoma of the breast. A clinicopathologic study of 35 cases. *Am. J. Clin. Pathol.* 58:231, 1972.

21. Chang, C. H. J., Sibala, J. L., Fritz, S. L., Dwyer, S. J., Templeton, A. W.: Specific value of computed tomographic breast scanner (CT/M) in diagnosis of breast diseases. *Radiology* 132:647–659, 1979.

22. Chang, C. H. J., Sibala, J. L., Gallagher, J. H., Riley, R. C., Templeton, A. W., Beasley, P. V., Porte, R. A.: Computed tomography of the breast. *Radiology* 124:827–829, 1977.

23. Collier, B. D., Palmer, D. W., Wilson, J. R., Greenberg, M., Komaki, R., Cox, J. D., Lawson, T. L., Lawlor, P. M.: Internal mammary lymphoscintigraphy in patients with breast cancer; correlation with computed tomography and impact on radiation therapy planning. *Radiology* 147:845–848, 1983.

24. Cutler, M: Transillumination as an aid in the diagnosis of breast lesions. *Surg. Gynecol. Obstet.* 48:721–729, 1929.

25. Dahl-Iverson, E.: Recherches sur les metastases microscopiques des cancers du sein dans les ganglions lymphatiques parasternaux et susclaviculaires. *Mem. Acad. Chin.* 78:651, 1952.

26. Donegan, W. L., Spratt, J. S.: *Cancer of the Breast, Major Problems in Clinical Surgery,* 2nd ed. Philadelphia, W. B. Saunders, 1979.

27. Egan, R. L.: Experience with mammography in a tumor institution. *Radiology* 75:894–900, 1960.

28. Egan, R. L.: *Mammography,* 2nd ed. Springfield, IL, Charles C. Thomas, 1972.

29. Egan, R. L.: Bilateral breast carcinoma: Role of mammography, *Cancer* 38:931, 1976.

30. Egan, R. L., McSweeney, M. B., Sprawls, P.: Grids in mammography. *Radiology* 146:359–362, 1983.

31. Egan, R. L., Mosteller, R. C.: Breast cancer mammography patterns. *Cancer* 40:2807–2090, 1977.

32. Ege, G. N.: Lymphoscintigraphy-techniques and applications in the management of breast carcinoma. *Semin. Nucl. Med.* 8:26–34, 1983.

33. Farewell, V. T.: The combined effect of breast cancer risk factor.

Cancer 40:931, 1977.

34. Fisher, B., Slack, N. H., Borss, I. D. J.: Cancer and the breast: Size of neoplasm and prognosis. *Cancer* 24:1071–1080, 1969.

35. Fisher, E. R., Gregorio, R. M., Fisher, B.: The pathology of invasive breast cancer. A syllabus derived from findings of the National Surgical Adjuvant Breast Project (Protocol No. 4). *Cancer* 36:1–85, 1975.

36. Fleischer, A. C., Muhletaler, C. A., Reynolds, V. H., Machin, J. E., Thieme, G. A., Bundy, A. L., Winfield, A. C., James, A. E.: Palpable breast masses: Evaluation by high frequency, hand-held real-time sonography and xeromammography. *Radiology* 148:813–817, 1983.

37. Frable, W. J.: Needle aspiration of the breast. *Cancer* 53:671–676, 1984.

38. Franzen, S., Zajicek, J.: Aspiration biopsy in diagnosis of palpable lesions of the breast. *Acta Radiol.* 7:241–262, 1968.

39. Friedrich M., Weskamp, P.: New modalities in mammographic imaging: Comparison of grid and magnification techniques. *Medica Mundi* 23:29–46, 1978.

40. Gallager, H. S., Martin, J. E.: Early phases in the development of breast cancer. *Cancer* 24:1170, 1969.

41. Gallager, H. S., Martin, J. E.: An orientation to the concept of minimal breast cancer. *Cancer* 28:1505, 1971.

42. Gefter, W. B., Friedman, A. K., Goodman, R. L.: The role of mammography in evaluating patients with early carcinoma of the breast for tylectomy and radiation therapy. *Radiology* 142:77–80, 1982.

43. Gerber, F. H., Goodreau, J. J., Kirchner, P. T., Fouty, W. H.: Efficacy of preoperative and postoperative bone scanning in the management of breast carcinoma. *N. Engl. J. Med.* 29:300–303, 1977.

44. Giordano, J. M., Klopp, C. T.: Lobular carcinoma in situ: Incidence and treatment. *Cancer* 31:105–109, 1973.

45. Gisvold, J. J., Reese, D. F., Karsell, P. R.: Computed tomographic mammography (CTM). *A.J.R.* 133:1143–1149, 1979.

46. Greenwald, P., Nasca, P. C., Lawrence, C. E., Horton, J., McGarrah, R. P., Gabriele, T., Carlton, K.: Estimated effects of breast self-examination and routine physical examinations on breast-cancer mortality. *N. Eng. J. Med.* 299:271, 1978.

47. Haagensen, C. D.: *Diseases of the Breast,* rev. 2nd ed. Philadelphia, W. B. Saunders, 1971.

48. Haagensen, C. D., Lane, N., Lattes, R., Bodian, C.: Lobular neoplasia (so-called lobular carcinoma in situ) of the breast. *Cancer* 42:737–769, 1978.

49. Handley, R. S.: Carcinoma of the breast. *Ann. R. Coll. Surg.* 57:59–66, 1975.

50. Hellman, S., Harris, J. R., Canellos, G. P., Fisher, B.: Cancer of the breast. In *Cancer: Principles and Practice of Oncology,* De Vita, V. T., Hellman, S., Rosenberg, S. A. (Eds.), Philadelphia, J. B. Lippincott, 1982, pp. 914–970.

51. Hempelmann, L. H.: *Mammography.* NCRP Report #66, Washington, DC, National Council on Radiation Protection and Measurements, 1980.

52. Henderson, I. C., Canellos, G. P.: Cancer of the breast: The past decade I. *N. Eng. J. Med.* 302:17–30, 1980.

53. Henderson, I. C., Canellos, G. P.: Cancer of the breast: The past decade II. *N. Eng. J. Med.* 302:78–90, 1980.

54. Hill, C. A.: Mammographic evidence of breast cancer control with humoral and chemotherapeutic treatment. *Br. J. Radiol.* 50:674–676, 1977.

55. Hobbins, W. B.: Thermography—highest risk marker in breast cancer. *Acta Thermographica* 2:55, 1977.

56. Humphrey, L. J., Swerdlow, M: Relationship of benign breast disease to carcinoma of the breast. *Surgery* 52:841, 1962.

57. Hutter, R. V. P.: The pathologist's role in minimal breast cancer. *Cancer* 28:1527–1536, 1971.

58. Isard, H. J., Becker, W., Shilo, R., Ostrum, B. J.: Breast thermog-

raphy after four years and 10,000 studies. *A.J.R.* **115**:811–821, 1972.

59. Kern, W. H., Brooks, R. N.: Atypical epithelial hyperplasia associated with breast cancer and fibrocystic disease. *Cancer* **24**:668, 1969.

60. Kline, T. S.: Breast lesions: Diagnosis by fine-needle aspiration biopsy. *Am. J. Gynecol. Obstet.* 1:11–16, 1979.

61. Kopans, D. B., DeLuca, S.: A modified needle-hookwire technique to simplify preoperative localization of occult breast lesions. *Radiology* **134**:781, 1980.

62. Kopans, D. B., Meyer, J. E., Sadowsky, N.: Breast imaging. *N. Eng. J. Med.* **310**:960–967, 1984.

63. Lambird, P. A., Shelley, W. M.: The spatial distribution of lobular in situ mammary carcinoma. Implications for size and site of breast biopsy. *J.A.M.A.* **210**:689, 1969.

64. Lawson, R.: Implications of surface temperatures in the diagnosis of breast cancer. *Can. Med. Assoc. J.* **75**:309, 1956.

65. Libshitz, H. I., Southard, M. E.: Mammography following primary radiation therapy for carcinoma of the breast. *A.J.R.* **120**:62–66, 1974.

66. MacMahon, B., Cole, P., Brown, J.: Etiology of human breast cancer: A review. *J. Natl. Cancer Inst.* **50**:21–42, 1973.

67. MacMahon, B., Cole, P., Lin, T. M.: Age at first birth and breast cancer risk. *Bull. W.H.O.* **43**:209–221, 1970.

68. Martin, H. E., Ellis, E. B.: Biopsy by needle puncture and aspiration. *Ann. Surg.* **92**:169–181, 1930.

69. McDivitt, R. W.: Breast carcinoma. *Hum. Pathol.* **9**:3–21, 1978.

70. McDivitt, R. W., Stewart, F. W., Berg, J. W.: Tumors of the breast. In *Atlas of Tumor Pathology.* Bethesda, Md., Armed Forces Institute of Pathology, 1968.

71. McLeod, R. A., Gisvold, J. J., Stephens, D. H., Beabout, J. W., Sheedy, P. F.: Computed tomography of soft tissues and breast. *Semin. Roentgenol.* **13**:267, 1978.

72. McNeil, B. J.: Rationale for the use of bone scans in selected metastatic and primary bone tumors. *Semin. Nucl. Med.* **8**:336, 1978.

73. McSweeney, B., Small, W. C., Cerny, V., Sewell, C. W., Powell, R. W.: NMR *discrimination of benign and malignant human breast tissue based on multiexponential transverse relaxation parameters.* Presented at the 21st National Conference on Breast Cancer, Hawaii, March, 1984.

74. Meyer, J. E., Kopans, D. B: Stability of a mammographic mass: A false sense of security. *A.J.R.* **137**:595–598, 1981.

75. Monson, R. R., Yen, S., MacMahon, B.: Chronic mastitis and carcinoma of the breast. *Lancet* **2**:224–226, 1976.

76. Moskowitz, M.: The predictive value of certain mammographic signs in screening for breast cancer. *Cancer* **51**:1007–1011, 1983.

77. Moskowitz, M., Gartside, P. S.: Evidence of breast cancer mortality reduction: Aggressive screening in women under age 50. *A.J.R.* **138**:911–916, 1982.

78. Moskowitz, M., Milbrath, J. R., Gartside, P., Zermeno, A., Mandel, D.: Lack of efficacy of thermography as a screening tool for minimal and stage I breast cancer. *N. Engl. J. Med.* **295**:249, 1976.

79. Muir, B. B., Kirkpatrick, A. E., Roberts, M. M., Duffy, S. W.: Oblique-view mammography: Adequacy for screening. *Radiology* **151**:39–41, 1984.

80. Muss, H. B., White, D. R., Cowan, R. J.: Brain scanning in patients with recurrent breast cancer. *Cancer* **38**:1574, 1976.

81. Nisce, L. Z., Snyder, R. E., Chu, C. H.: The role of mammography in evaluating radiation response of inoperable primary breast cancer. *Radiology* **110**:85–88, 1974.

82. Ostrum, B. J., Becker, W., Isard, H. J.: Low-dose mammography. *Radiology* **109**:323–326, 1973.

83. Petrakis, N. L.: Genetic factors in the etiology of breast cancer. *Cancer* **39**:2709–2715, 1977.

84. Robbins, G. F., Berg, J. E.: Bilateral primary breast cancers. *Cancer* **17**:1501, 1964.

85. Rosen, P. P., Lieberman, P. H., Braun, D. W., Jr., Kosloff, C., Adair, F.: Lobular carcinoma in situ of the breast. Detailed analysis of 99 patients with average follow-up of 24 years. *Am. J. Surg. Pathol.* **2**:225, 1978.

86. Saltzstein, S. L.: Clinically occult inflammatory carcinoma of the breast. *Cancer* **34**:382–388, 1974.

87. Schabel, F. M.: Experimental basis for adjunct chemotherapy. In *Adjunct Therapy of Cancer,* vol. 1. Salmon, S., Jones, S. E. (Eds.). New York, North-Holland Publishing Co., 1977, pp. 3–14.

88. Schmidt, A. M., Whitehorn, W. V., Martin, E. W.: Thermography restriction. *FDA Drug Bull.* **6**:32, 1976.

89. Shapiro, S.: Health Insurance Plan of Greater New York Mammography Study. Progress Report December 1, 1977 to November 25, 1978.

90. Sickles, E. A.: Heavy-particle mammography. In *Breast Carcinoma: The Radiologist's Expanded Role.* Logan, W. W. (Ed.). New York, John Wiley & Sons, 1977, p. 239.

91. Sickles, E. A.: Microfocal spot magnification mammography using xeroradiographic and screen-film recording systems. *Radiology* **131**:599–607, 1979.

92. Sickles, E. A.: Further experience with microfocal spot magnification mammography in the assessment of clustered breast microcalcifications. *Radiology* **137**:9–14, 1980.

93. Sickles, E. A.: Breast cancer detection with transillumination and mammography. *A.J.R.* **142**:841–844, 1984.

94. Sickles, E. A., Filly, R. A., Callen, P. W.: Breast cancer detection with sonography and mammography: Comparison using state-of-the-art equipment. *A.J.R.* **140**:843–845, 1983.

95. Silverberg, S. G., Chitale, A. R.: Assessment of significance of proportions of intraductal and infiltrating tumor growth in ductal carcinoma of the breast. *Cancer* **32**:830, 1973.

96. Simon, N., Lesnick, G. J., Lerer, W. N., Bachman, A. L.: Roentgenographic localization of small lesions of the breast by the spot method. *Surg. Gynecol. Obstet.* **134**:572, 1972.

97. Smith, P. G., Doll, R.: Late effects of x-irradiation in patients treated for metropathia haemorrhagica. *Br. J. Radiol.* **49**:224–232, 1976.

98. Synder, R. E., Rosen, P.: Radiography of breast specimens. *Cancer* **28**:1608, 1971.

99. Tabar, L., Dean, P.: Mammographic parenchymal patterns. *J.A.M.A.* **247**:185–189, 1982.

100. Trichopoulos, D., MacMahon, B., Cole, P.: Menopause and breast cancer risk. *J. Natl. Cancer Inst.* **41**:315–329, 1968.

101. Upton, A. C., Beebe, G. W., Brown, J. M.: Report of NCI ad hoc working group on the risks associated with mammography in mass screening for detection of breast cancer. *J. Natl. Cancer Inst.* **59**:479–493, 1977.

102. Valagussa, P., Bonadonna, G., Veronesi, F.: Patterns of relapse and survival following radical mastectomy. *Cancer* **41**:1170–1178, 1978.

103. Von Hansemann, D. P., cited by Haagensen, C. D.: Histological grading of carcinoma of the breast. *Am. J. Cancer* 1933.

104. Wallace, J. D., Dodd, G. D.: Thermography in the diagnosis of breast cancer. *Radiology* **91**:679, 1968.

105. Warren, S. L.: A roentgenologic study of the breast. *A.J.R.* **24**:113, 1930.

106. Wheeler, J. E., Enterline, H. T.: Lobular carcinoma of the breast in situ and infiltrating. *Pathol. Ann.* **11**:161, 1976.

107. Wolfe, J. N.: Xerography of the breast. *Radiology* **91**:231–240, 1968.

108. Wolfe, J. N.: The prominent duct pattern as an indicator of cancer risk. *Oncology* **23**:149–158, 1969.

109. Wolfe, J. N.: Breast parenchymal patterns. *A.J.R.* **138**:113–118, 1982.

12 ESOPHAGEAL CANCER

William Moreau Thompson*

Carcinoma of the esophagus accounts for 1.5% of all cancers and 7% of all gastrointestinal cancer in the United States.[20,100] In spite of recent accomplishments in surgery,[25,28,32,73,75,83,92,94,102,106] radiation therapy,[8,33,53,60,64,86-89,98,125] and chemotherapy,[30,55,114,115] survival of patients with carcinoma of the esophagus remains poor.[14,54,81,90,100,106,107,119,126] The five-year survival for a white population from 1965 to 1969, adjusted to normal life expectancy, was 2% for men and 6% for women.[100] These figures have improved slightly in the United States during the past ten years.[94] Authors from Japan[1,2,44,48] and China[17,39,132] have reported considerably better survival figures, but their patient populations are significantly different than in most other countries. Many of their patients have carcinoma in situ. The form of therapy does not appear to alter survival.[99,100,106,126] In spite of the significant decrease in operative mortality during the past 15 years, the five-year survival for surgically resectable esophageal carcinoma has not dramatically improved.[20,41,90,94]

Based on 122 reports published from 1953 to 1978, Earlam and Cunha-Melo analyzed 83,783 patients who had surgery for esophageal carcinoma.[26] They excluded adenocarcinoma of the gastroesophageal junction from this study because of the differences between this tumor and squamous cell carcinoma. They found that 58% of patients were surgically explored, 39% had their tumors resected, and 13% died in the hospital. Only 4% of the 26% who left the hospital survived five years. They also reviewed 8,489 patients treated with radiation therapy.[27] The five-year survival in these patients was 6%. This is a surprising figure, since most patients treated with radiation therapy are considered inoperable because of extensive tumors or because of medical reasons. Also, comparable data are not available to indicate what would have happened if patients with small, localized lesions were treated with radiation therapy rather than surgery. These authors pointed out that controlled trials comparing these two modalities in similar patients are not available. Some authors have reported improved five-year survival using a combination of preoperative radiation therapy and resection.[33,98,100,125] However, not all reports show a similar increased survival.[61,100]

A weakness of the literature on carcinoma of the esophagus is the failure of researchers and clinicians to use a standard classification or system for staging this cancer, such as the TNM system proposed by the American Joint Committee for staging cancer in 1983.[3] Thus, it is extremely difficult to compare various forms of treatment. Recently, a few authors have suggested using the TNM system of classifying esophageal tumors so that adequate comparisons can be obtained and better data can be accumulated.[8,37] In 1980, Giuli and Gignoux found a significant difference in survival between patients with T_1, T_2, and T_3 lesions.[37] The importance of the N classification for T_1 and T_2 lesions was established then. For T_3 lesions, the N criterion was not important. Beatty et

*The author would like to thank Dr. Reed P. Rice, Dr. Robert A. Halvorsen, Dr. Raymond W. Postlethwait, and Dr. Larry Hedlund for their editorial assistance, and Don Powell for preparation of the illustrations.

al.[8] found that patients with T_1 lesions responded to therapy in 100% of cases, whereas only 68% of patients with T_2 lesions and 50% of patients with T_3 lesions responded to treatment. Patients without lymph node involvement (N_0) and distant metastases (M_0) responded to therapy better than those with lymph node involvement and metastases.[8] In general, patients with lesions less than 5 cm in length (T_1) and without evidence of metastatic lymph nodes (N_0) have a better prognosis than patients with lesions greater than 5 cm in length (T_2).[100] Patients with lesions that extend into the mediastinum (T_3) have the poorest prognosis. The presence or absence of positive nodes and distant metastases also has an influence on survival of patients with T_1 and T_2 lesions.[100]

Presently, accurate radiologic methods for early detection and diagnosis of esophageal carcinoma are not available. American,[56,137] French,[7] Chinese,[17,39,132] and Japanese[20,48,118,131] authors have reported finding early (small) esophageal cancer by double-contrast barium esophagography. Koehler et al.[56] and Suzuki et al.[118] reported an improved five-year survival compared with large tumors, while Zornoza and Lindell[137] found no difference in survival compared with patients with large esophageal cancers. There are reports in areas with a high incidence of esophageal cancer in which esophageal cancer has been detected early. Japanese and Chinese authors, using endoscopic, cytologic, and double-contrast barium esophagographic techniques, reported detecting and diagnosing early lesions and obtaining incredible five-year survival rates of between 35% and 90%.[1,2,17,39,48,59,132] However, many of these lesions are so subtle that they are detectable only by cytologic examination; they would not be identifiable by radiologic methods and may not be seen endoscopically.[7,48] Such lesions would be classified using the TNM system as carcinoma in situ (T_{IS}). A number of reports describing this type of lesion have appeared in the literature in the United States.[12,67,111] It is unlikely that any radiographic modality will ever be helpful in the early detection and diagnosis of these subtle esophageal carcinomas. However, the development of new imaging techniques such as the double-contrast barium esophagogram,[38,56,137] computed tomography (CT),[22,77,120] and magnetic resonance imaging (MRI)[108] may be useful in providing staging information that may help in the choice of therapy and the follow-up of patients with esophageal carcinoma.

A number of authors have described using chest roentgenograms,[23,65,82,96,135,136] barium esophagograms,[38,42] azygos venography,[1,19,76] and CT[18,21,22,44,63,77,121] to help stage and treat[35] carcinoma of the esophagus. Since patients with carcinoma of the esophagus develop symptoms late in the course of their disease, these techniques are only useful for determining if the patient has operable or inoperable disease. The barium esophagogram, azygos venography, and CT have been used to predict operability. In some reports, the esophagogram has been helpful in staging,[1,2] but in others it was not accurate in determining operability.[100] Azygos venography is an invasive procedure that has been used in the past by only a few authors but is not popular today.[1,2,19,76] Preliminary reports indicate CT may be accurate in predicting local invasion and determining the presence of distant metastases in esophageal carcinoma patients.[18,21,22,44,77,121] However, further work is needed to determine the impact of CT on the treatment of patients with esophageal carcinoma.

Because of the potential usefulness of CT, its utility in diagnosis and management will be emphasized throughout this chapter. Unfortunately, the reported experience with CT in patients with carcinoma of the esophagus is small, since less than 200 patients have been evaluated. As mentioned earlier, another problem with esophageal carcinoma is that only a few authors have used a standard classification for staging the lesions. Therefore, it is difficult to compare one series with another, or to evaluate the accuracy of CT in terms of any staging modality. This problem will be put into perspective in terms of using CT to stage the esophageal carcinoma, determine operability, and provide follow-up information.

Bragg[10] has stated that one of the most frequent reasons for unnecessary radiologic procedures in patients with cancer is the referring physician's and radiologist's lack of knowledge regarding the metastatic behavior of the tumor. In order to design an imaging approach for investigating a patient with cancer, an understanding of the behavior of the tumor is needed. Also, each imaging modality has inherent advantages and disadvantages in terms of equipment and operator experience. All of these factors must be taken into account in designing any imaging protocol.[10,95] Thus, in order that an understanding of the current and new imaging modalities be reached, this chapter will cover basic information on the pathology, natural history, and staging of esophageal carcinoma. An imaging scheme for staging carcinoma of the esophagus will be presented, and the results of staging carcinoma of the esophagus from our own work and other reports will be reviewed. The impact of the newer imaging modalities on patients with carcinoma of the esophagus will be discussed. The chapter will emphasize CT, since it appears to be the best radiographic imaging modality available for evaluating patients with esophageal carcinoma. In the final portion of the chapter, tumors of the gastroesophageal junction will be contrasted to tumors in the body of the esophagus.

TUMOR BEHAVIOR AND PATHOLOGY

Histopathology

A classification of malignant tumors of the esophagus based on the World Health Organization (WHO) scheme is listed in Table 12-1. More than 90% of malignant

Table 12-1. WHO Classification of Malignant Esophageal Tumors

Epithelial Tumors
   Squamous cell carcinoma
      Well differentiated
      Moderately differentiated
      Poorly differentiated
   Variants of squamous cell carcinoma
      Spindle-cell carcinoma
      Pseudosarcoma
      Verrucous carcinoma
      In situ carcinoma
   Adenocarcinoma
      Adenoacanthoma
   Adenoid cystic carcinoma (cylindroma)
   Mucoepidermoid carcinoma
   Adenosquamous carcinoma
   Undifferentiated carcinoma
      Oat cell carcinoma
Nonepithelial Tumors
   Leiomyosarcoma
   Carcinosarcoma
   Malignant melanoma
   Lymphoma

esophageal tumors are squamous cell carcinomas.[92–94,100] They originate from the squamous cell epithelium that lines the lumen of the esophagus. Well-differentiated cancers have the characteristic features of keratin formation (epithelial pearls), intercellular bridges, and minimal pelomorphism. Poorly differentiated tumors do not have keratin nor do they demonstrate intercellular bridges, and they have marked nuclear and cellular pleomorphism as well.[92,93,100] In between these two types of tumors are moderately differentiated tumors. The degree of differentiation has been shown by Younghusband and Aluwihare to effect patient survival.[134] Rosenberg et al.,[100] however, did not find the degree of differentiation to effect survival or to correlate with metastases to lymph nodes. Therefore, it is unclear if the distinction among the degrees of differentiation is practically important.

There are variants of squamous cell carcinoma (Table 12-1). Spindle-cell carcinoma, a variant of poorly differentiated squamous cell cancer, is characterized by spindle-shaped cells resembling fibroblasts, which may give the tumor the appearance of a sarcoma. When the tumor contains nests of squamous cells with a spindle-cell stroma, it is classified as a pseudosarcoma.[72,79] Pseudosarcoma is usually a polypoid mass of sarcomatous tissue attached by a pedicle containing squamous carcinoma, either in situ or invasive. This tumor and carcinosarcoma have been grouped together by recent authors because of their common polypoid structure and a similar histologic appearance.[41] A third variant of squamous cell carcinoma, verrucous carcinoma, is well differentiated and has a papillary appearance.[113] Carcinoma in situ, a fourth variant of squamous cell cancer, is rarely encountered in the United States.[12,67,111] It is usually discovered incidentally in patients undergoing endoscopy for dysphagia. It should be differentiated from areas of displasia

of the esophageal mucosa. Displasia has been found in patients who are predisposed to developing esophageal cancer from heavy cigarette smoking.[130]

Primary adenocarcinomas of the esophagus are rare.[24,97,124] They may arise from the submucosal glandular elements within the esophagus or, more frequently, from the columnar epithelium that lines the distal esophagus in patients with Barrett's esophagus.[9,11,15,78,91,100] When a small focus of squamous metaplasia is present, the lesion is called an adenoacanthoma (Table 12-1).

Another variant of epithelial tumors is the cylindroma.[124] These lesions have a characteristic cribriform structure, with glandular and myoepithelial elements as found in the salivary glands and the bronchi. It is rarely present in the esophagus. The mucoepidermoid carcinoma, another rare lesion, is composed of squamous and mucus-secreting cells. It is distinguished from the adenosquamous carcinoma, which has adenomatous and squamous carcinomatous elements.[100]

Undifferentiated carcinomas, resembling oat cell carcinomas, have been found in the esophagus. They originate from argyrophil cells in the esophageal mucosa. This highly malignant tumor occasionally produces paraneoplastic syndromes.[94,100,124]

The leiomyosarcoma is the most common malignant nonepithelial esophageal tumor.[36,84,93] Resection is usually effective but 25% of patients have metastases from this tumor.[36,84,93] Lymphoma may involve the esophagus either as a primary lesion or as contiguous involvement with the stomach.[13,38,116] The radiographic features are similar to those of carcinoma (ulcerated mass, narrowing, and nodularity).

Although uncommon, malignant melanoma of the esophagus can occur as both a primary and a metastatic lesion.[66,110] Like the pseudosarcoma and carcinosarcoma, these are usually large, bulky, ulcerative tumors that do not produce obstruction until they are extremely large.[72] Other extremely rare tumors, such as myoblastomas, choriocarcinomas, and rhabdomyosarcomas, occur in the esophagus, according to some reports.[93,111,124]

A number of primary tumors may metastasize to the esophagus.[4,31] Occasionally, these lesions can mimic a primary esophageal cancer. The most common primary sites are the breast, lung, head and neck, and stomach. Other reported primary sites are the liver, kidneys, prostate, testicles, bone, and skin.[100]

Patterns of Spread

Before becoming widely disseminated, squamous cell esophageal cancers are characterized by extensive local growth and lymph node metastases. As the esophagus courses from the neck to the abdomen, it comes into close proximity with a number of vital structures.[43,50,102] The most notable are the heart, aorta, trachea, and lungs (Figure 12-1). Tumors originating in the esophagus can easily spread into any of these structures, since they have

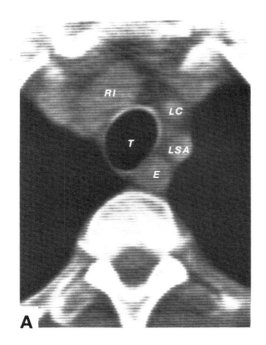

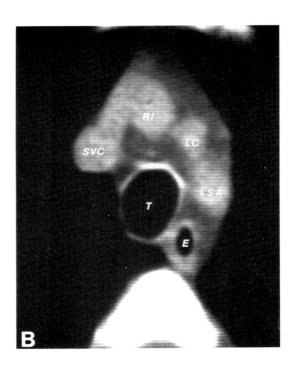

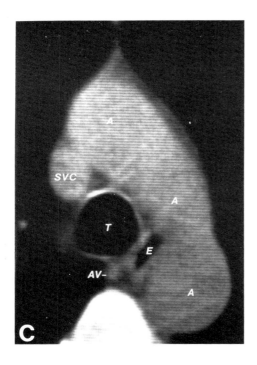

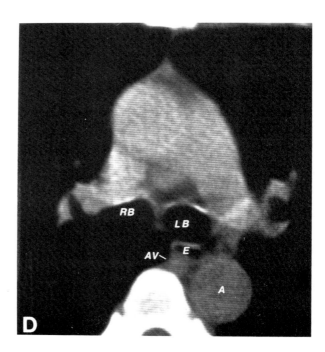

FIG. 12-1. Six computed tomograms showing the relationship of the esophagus to adjacent structures in the mediastinum. Levels of scans: (A) thoracic inlet; (B) above the aortic arch; (C) aortic arch; (D) carina; (E) 4 cm below carina; (F) 2 cm above diaphragm. E = esophagus, T = trachea, A = aorta, AV = azygos vein, LB = left main stem bronchus, RB = right main stem bronchus, LA = left atrium, H = heart, L = liver, SVC = superior vena cava, LSA = left subclavian artery, LC = left carotid artery, RI = right innominate artery.

prognostic significance.[100] The prognosis of squamous cell lesions improves significantly with more distal location.[94,100] Figure 12-2 shows the distribution of carcinoma of the esophagus by location from a number of collected series. In the Duke experience, there were no five-year survivors among patients undergoing curative resection for cervical esophageal cancers.[94] The five-year survival for upper and middle thoracic cancers was 8%, while 17% of patients with lower thoracic lesions were alive five years after surgery.[94]

There is an extensive interconnecting network of submucosal and muscular lymphatics that course the length of the esophagus.[71,100,104] Smaller lymphatics arise within the mucosa and external muscularis and drain into the more extensive network in the deeper layers of the esophageal wall. Thus, lymphatic fluid can flow through many pathways in the wall of the esophagus before emerging from the lymphatic vessels to drain into lymph nodes. Because of this pattern of lymph flow, the spread of tumor cells to adjacent lymph nodes is unpredictable.[1,2,68,70,100,104] Spread of tumor may be in the direction of adjacent nodes or through the above-mentioned network to more distant nodes. There is an extensive network of lymph nodes extending from the neck to the abdomen that receive lymph flow from the esophagus (Figure 12-3).[2,68,94,100,104] Afferent lymphatics draining into these nodes tend to course longitudinally, following the arteries supplying the esophagus (Figure 12-3). The inferior thyroid, bronchial, and esophageal

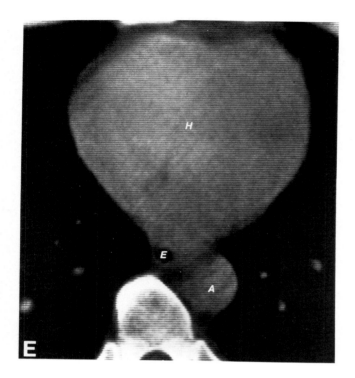

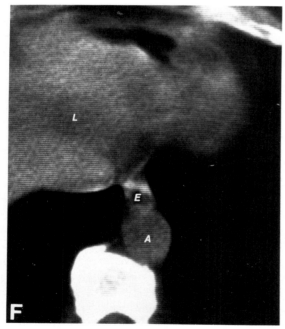

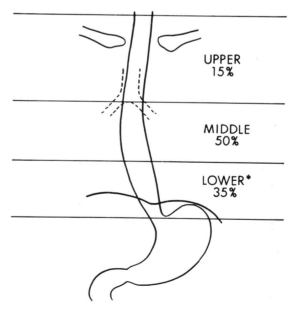

FIG. 12-2. The percentage of primary squamous cell esophageal carcinoma in terms of location: the figure for the lower tract is 50% and 35% for the middle if all gastroesophageal junction tumors including adenocarcinoma are included.

only a mucosal and submucosal layer and no serosa.[89] Thus, esophageal tumors tend to penetrate through the esophageal wall into the mediastinum and invade the contiguous structures early in the course of the disease. This is one of the main reasons why this carcinoma has such a poor prognosis.[89,100,102]

Because this type of carcinoma tends to spread to contiguous structures, the location of the primary tumor has

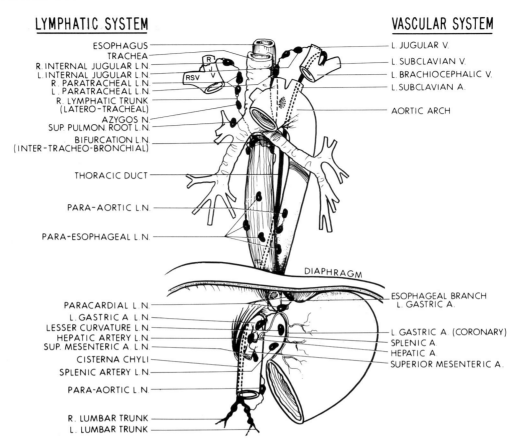

LYMPHATIC SYSTEM   VASCULAR SYSTEM

ESOPHAGUS
TRACHEA
R. INTERNAL JUGULAR L.N.
L. INTERNAL JUGULAR L.N.
R. PARATRACHEAL L.N.
L. PARATRACHEAL L.N.
R. LYMPHATIC TRUNK
(LATERO-TRACHEAL)
AZYGOS N.
SUP. PULMON. ROOT L.N.
BIFURCATION L.N.
(INTER-TRACHEO-BRONCHIAL)

THORACIC DUCT

PARA-AORTIC L.N.

PARA-ESOPHAGEAL L.N.

L. JUGULAR V.
L. SUBCLAVIAN V.
L. BRACHIOCEPHALIC V.
L. SUBCLAVIAN A.

AORTIC ARCH

DIAPHRAGM

ESOPHAGEAL BRANCH
L. GASTRIC A.

PARACARDIAL L.N.
L. GASTRIC A. L.N.
LESSER CURVATURE L.N.
HEPATIC ARTERY L.N.
SUP. MESENTERIC A. L.N.
CISTERNA CHYLI
SPLENIC ARTERY L.N.

PARA-AORTIC L.N.

R. LUMBAR TRUNK
L. LUMBAR TRUNK

L. GASTRIC A. (CORONARY)
SPLENIC A.
HEPATIC A.
SUPERIOR MESENTERIC A.

FIG. 12-3. Anterior view of the vascular structures and lymph nodes in the mediastinum and their relationship to the esophagus. (Adapted from McCort, J. J.; Radiographic identification of lymph node metastases from carcinoma of the esophagus. *Radiology* 59:694–711, 1952).

arteries from the aorta and the left gastric serve as the primary arterial supply to the esophagus. Lymphatics accompanying these arteries drain into lymph node chains as shown in Figure 12-4.[2,68,94] The major lymph node chains include the internal jugular, cervical, supraclavicular, paratracheal, hilar, subcarinal, paraesophageal, para-aortic, paracardial, lesser curvature, left gastric, celiac, hepatic, and splenic.[2,68]

Because of the complex longitudinal interconnections, lymphatic drainage of the esophagus is unpredictable, as is the nature of metastases to nodes from esophageal carcinoma. This is illustrated in Figure 12-5.[1,2,68] Ten percent to 20% of patients with cervical esophageal carcinoma will also have metastatic disease in subdiaphragmatic lymph nodes.[2] Subdiaphragmatic nodal involvement may be found in 40% of patients with cancers in the middle third of the esophagus; patients with lesions in the lower third may have metastases to superior mediastinal and cervical lymph nodes (Figure 12-5).[2] Another important example of the unpredictable lymphatic drainage is the phenomenon of skip areas of involvement.[101,109] As much as 8 cm of normal esophagus may be interposed between

the site of a gross neoplasm and micrometastases within lymphatic vessels of the esophageal wall.[59,94,109]

Studies of the length of the primary esophageal lesion can be directly related to extent of involvement and survival.[100] If the tumor is 5 cm or less in length, approximately 40% of the patients will have localized disease, 25% will have local invasion, and 35% will have distant metastases and the disease will be unresectable for cure. If the tumor exceeds 5 cm, as determined by pathologic examination, only 10% of patients will have localized disease, 15% will have local invasion, and 75% will have distant metastases and the disease will be unresectable for cure. Unfortunately, the routine barium swallow study has not been accurate in assessing the length of the lesion.[100] However, not enough work has been reported with the double-contrast examination to evaluate its accuracy for determining the length of esophageal carcinoma. Thus, the length of the lesion noted on a routine barium swallow study does not correlate well with resectability of the cancer, the degree of lymph node involvement, or the pattern of spread.[68]

Lymph node involvement carries a poor prognosis. A

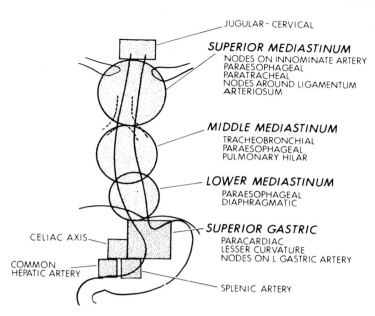

FIG. 12-4. Lymph node groups that drain the esophagus. (Adapted from Akiyama, H., Tsurumaru, M., Kawamura, T., Ono, Y.: Principles of surgical treatment for carcinoma of the esophagus. Analysis of lymph node involvement. *Ann. Surg.* 194:438–446, 1981).

five-year survival of less than 10% can be expected following resection when the lymph nodes are involved.[100] This survival increases two to three times if the nodes are not involved.[100]

The most common visceral metastases occur in the lung and liver. Because there is usually local invasion and lymph node involvement, distant metastases rarely dominate the clinical course of esophageal carcinoma. However, distant metastases are reported in 90% of autopsy cases.[104]

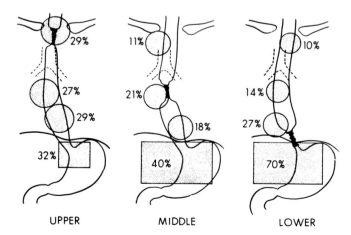

FIG. 12-5. The percentage of positive lymph nodes found at surgery for esophageal carcinoma in the upper, middle, and lower esophagus. (Adapted from Akiyama, H., Tsurumaru, M., Kawamura, T., Ono, Y.: Principles of surgical treatment for carcinoma of the esophagus. Analysisi of lymph node involvement. *Ann. Surg.* 199:438–466, 1981).

CLASSIFICATION AND STAGING

The classification and staging of carcinoma of the esophagus has been slow to evolve and to gain widespread acceptance. The major reason for this is the difficulty of clearly defining the true extent of the tumor by available diagnostic methods. As mentioned previously, CT may be able to provide more specific information than any previous method. Two clinical series, for example, have shown that CT can accurately predict local invasion and distant metastases in patients with known esophageal carcinoma.[21,77] However, additional evaluation is needed before CT can be accepted as a technique for accurate preoperative staging of carcinoma of the esophagus.

Treatment planning requires careful characterization of the extent of involvement of cancer of the esophagus. Information about the extent of involvement can also be used to stage a patient. Staging also aids in comparing the effectiveness of different therapies on homogeneous patient populations.

Since the esophagus is not an accessible organ, clinical staging of disease is difficult and inaccurate. The use of invasive techniques, including biopsies, are important when accurate staging of lesions is attempted. However, these techniques should be performed before radiotherapy or chemotherapy if they are to be reliable, since radiotherapy and chemotherapy will distort the biopsy findings. Because many patients with esophageal cancer are treated with preoperative radiation or chemotherapy, postsurgical evaluation may not accurately define the stage of the cancer before treatment.

The most common method used to stage esophageal carcinoma is the TNM system devised in 1977 by the American Joint Committee (AJC). The TNM system is shown in Figure 12-6 and outlined in Table 12-2.[103] The TNM staging system classifies tumors according to the anatomic extent.[3] Differentiation between T_1 and T_2 primary lesions depends upon whether the tumor is greater (T_2) or less than 5 cm in length (T_1). T_3 lesions extend outside the wall of the esophagus into mediastinal structures. Unfortunately, esophagograms are not precise in differentiating T_1 from T_2 lesions.[100] They also cannot precisely determine T_3 lesions. Computed tomography appears to be accurate in determining the presence of mediastinal invasion, which is, for example, a T_3 lesion.[22,77,121] Prior to CT, surgery was the only useful

method of determining the presence of invasion, lymph node involvement or distant metastases in all patients. Bronchoscopy, mediastinoscopy, and scalene node biopsy are helpful in staging some patients.

A simplified classification of patients with carcinoma of the esophagus is given in Table 12-3. The problem with this classification is that it lacks precision because it allows a wide latitude for interpretation.[100] Prior to CT, it had been difficult to decide whether the malignancy had spread beyond the confines of the esophagus and whether it could be completely resected. A thoracotomy was usually required to determine whether the lesion was a stage II or stage III lesion.

The Japanese Society for Esophageal Diseases has described a more detailed staging system.[40] Its main advantage is that it provides an excellent method for staging esophageal carcinoma for clinical investigators. The system is based on operative findings and uses extension

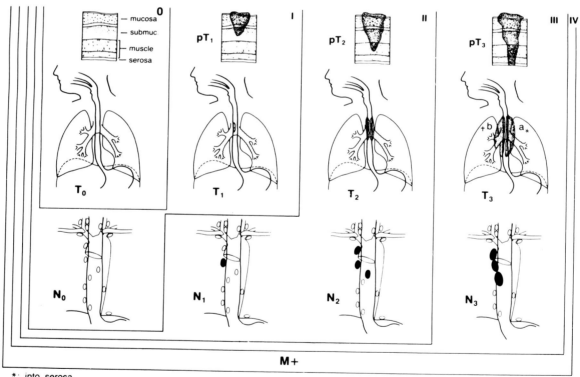

*: into serosa
†: gross invasion of contiguous structures

FIG. 12-6. TNM staging of esophageal cancer. Tumor (T) categories: The major function are size and depth of penetration. Lesions are divided into those less than 5 cm and those greater than 5 cm (T_1 v T_2) and as muscle wall invasion occurs causing obstruction and extension through serosa into the mediastinum (T_2 v T_3). Node (N) categories: This is divided into cervical and thoracic nodes that are essentially negative or positive, established by surgical biopsy. Cervical nodes are defined similarly to head and neck sites, but a number of node-bearing regions and mobility—not size—are the key factors. Stage grouping: This is divided into three stages, each corresponding to a T stage. Positive nodes and metastases are grouped with T_3 and are stage III. AJC v UICC classification: The clinical stages are identical, but UICC has added a pTNM postsurgical stage based upon depth of invasion, which is typical of all alimentary hollow organ viscera. T_1 = muscle and submucosa; T_2 = muscle; T_{3a} = serosa only; T_{3b} = contiguous structures. (Reprinted from Rubin, P. (Ed.): *Clinical Oncology for Medical Students and Physicians: A Multidisciplinary Approach*, 6th ed. New York, American Cancer Society, 1983. With permission.)

Table 12-2. TNM Staging for Esophageal Cancer

Primary Tumor (T)

T_0 No demonstrable tumor
T_{IS} Carcinoma in situ
T_1 Tumor involves 5 cm or less of esophageal length with no obstruction or complete circumferential involvement or extraesophageal spread
T_2 Tumor involves more than 5 cm of esophagus and produces obstruction with circumferential involvement of the esophagus but no extraesophageal spread
T_3 Tumor with extension outside the esophagus involving mediastinal structures

Regional Lymph Nodes (N)

Cervical esophagus (cervical and supraclavicular lymph nodes)

N_0 No nodal involvement
N_1 Unilateral involvement (movable)
N_2 Bilateral involvement (movable)
N_3 Fixed nodes

Thoracic esophagus (nodes in the thorax, not those of the cervical, supraclavicular or abdominal areas)

N_0 No nodal involvement
N_1 Nodal involvement

Distant Metastases

M_0 No metastases
M_1 Distant metastases. Cancer of thoracic esophagus with cervical, supraclavicular, or abdominal lymph node involvement is classified as M_1

Reprinted from American Joint Committee on Cancer: *Manual for Staging of Cancer*, 2nd ed. Philadelphia, J. B. Lippincott, 1983, p. 61–66.

of the tumor to the adventitia of the esophagus rather than the length of the tumor as an index of the primary tumor. Japanese centers also use lymph node involvement, distant metastases, and extension to the pleura as bases for staging.

Another method of staging was described by the Rotterdam Group.[126] They classified esophageal cancer patients as either fit or unfit for surgery and their disease as either curable or incurable. Patients were considered fit for surgery when they could undergo a combined thoracotomy and laparotomy. The tumor was incurable if there was evidence of metastases such as fixation to neighboring structures, proven extension into the respiratory system, or recurrent nerve palsy. Patients thus were classified into four groups: (1) operable-curable, (2) operable-incurable, (3) inoperable-curable, and (4) inoperable-incurable. Of their patients, 42% were in the operable-curable group, 35% were inoperable-curable, and 23% were in the two incurable groups.[126]

Despite the inadequacies of these staging methods, some system must be used. Classification of patients into homogeneous groups is essential when a comparison of different forms of therapy is attempted. There is a real need to perform clinical trials for esophageal cancer that compare the various forms of therapy in similar patient populations.

Akiyama et al.[1,2] recommend that all current techniques, including laparotomy and thoracotomy, be used

to define the anatomic extent of the tumor. They do not, however, advise using the length of the lesion if it has to be based on the esophagograms or on pathologic examination after the use of radiation or chemotherapy. Staging should be based on clinical and pathologic findings that have not been altered by either of these two treatments. A treatment plan should be developed that can be modified as additional data are acquired. Staging should be based on all available correct clinical, radiologic, operative, and pathologic data.

IMAGING PROCEDURES AND ASSESSMENT

Of the many radiographic modalities that have been used to evaluate patients (Table 12-4), none have proved to be accurate in the early detection or staging of esophageal cancer. The newer imaging modalities such as CT

Table 12-3. Stage Grouping from TNM Classification

Stage I

1. $T_{IS}N_0M_0$
   Carcinoma in situ
2. $T_1N_0M_0$
   $T_1N_XM_0$
   Tumor in any region of the esophagus that involves 5 cm or less of esophageal length, produces no obstruction, has no extraesophageal spread, does not involve the entire circumference, and shows no regional lymph node metastases or remote metastases

Stage II

1. A tumor of any size with no extraesophageal spread and with no distant metastasis
   A. Cervical esophagus:
      (1) $T_1N_1M_0$
          $T_1N_2M_0$
          $T_2N_1M_0$
          $T_2N_2M_0$
          Any tumor with palpable, movable, regional nodes
      (2) $T_2N_0M_0$
          A tumor more than 5 cm in length with negative nodes
   B. Thoracic esophagus:
      (1) $T_2N_XM_0$
          Lymph nodes cannot be assessed (clinical-diagnostic evaluation)
      (2) $T_2N_0M_0$
          A tumor more than 5 cm in length or a tumor of any size with obstruction or circumferential involvement with no lymph node involvement (postsurgical treatment–pathologic evaluation)

Stage III

1. Any T_3
2. Any N_3 (cervical)
3. Any N_1 (thoracic)
4. Any M_1
5. Any esophageal cancer at any level with:
   A. Distant metastasis
   B. Extraesophageal spread
      or
   C. Fixed lymph node metastasis
   Any intrathoracic esophageal carcinoma including either upper and midthoracic region or lower thoracic region with any positive findings in regional lymph nodes

Table 12-4. Imaging Modalities for Evaluating Carcinoma of the Esophagus

MODALITY	STAGING CAPABILITY	BENEFIT/ COST RATIO	RECOMMENDED ROUTINE STAGING PROCEDURE
Noninvasive			
Chest films	Good for detecting metastases and second primary. Controversial local invasion.	High	Yes
Bone films	Useful only to confirm metastases.	Low	No
Double-contrast esophagogram	Useful to detect and define primary lesion, occasionally to demonstrate second tumor	High	Yes
Radionuclide studies liver-spleen, brain and bone scans	Useful in evaluation of clinically suspected metastases. CT better than RN scans for liver and brain.	Low	No
Gallium 67	Fairly useful for metastases, good specificity but low, unacceptable sensitivity.	Fair	No
Ultrasound	Useful for evaluating clinically suspected abdominal metastases. CT as good or better than ultrasound.	Fair	No
Magnetic Resonance Imaging	Only one case in which MRI was used to stage carcinoma of the esophagus has been reported. MRI may be a promising new technique.	Unknown	Unknown
Minimally invasive			
CT	Invasive if IV contrast material given. Most useful of all modalities for determining local invasion and distant metastases.	High	Yes
Invasive			
Azygos venography	Very invasive; good for predicting invasion, 86% accurate. False positive 9%, false negative 35%.	Fair	Not now with CT
Transtracheal lymphography	Accurate, but invasive and only preliminary reports from Japan.	Low	Probably not with CT
Percutaneous biopsy guided by imaging technique, usually CT	Invasive but very accurate for squamous cell; will rarely be used in chest, has been used in neck and abdomen.	High	No, only in selected cases

and magnetic resonance imaging (MRI) may prove to be useful for delineation and staging.

Chest and Bone Roentgenograms

The chest film is a standard part of the workup of any patient with a known malignancy, including carcinoma of the esophagus. There is an increased incidence of associated lung cancer in patients with squamous cell carcinoma of the esophagus.[80,94] Also, a number of radiographic abnormalities caused by carcinoma of the esophagus may be detected on chest roentgenograms.[23,42,65,82,96,134,135] The most common of these include an abnormal azygoesophageal line, a widened mediastinum, tracheal deviation, and a widened (>4 mm) tracheoesophageal line or retroesophageal stripe (Figure 12-7). Some authors have indicated that these findings, especially a widened retrotracheal stripe, have prognostic significance.[23,65,82] Recently, however, Lindell et al.[65] found there was no significant difference in survival rates of patients with or without chest film abnormalities. Unexpectedly, the group of patients who had normal films had a lower resectability rate than those with abnormal films. Thus, while the chest film is inexpensive and noninvasive, it is not sufficiently sensitive or accurate enough to be useful for staging the patient with esophageal cancer. However, it is inexpensive and does provide other important information about the cardiovascular and pulmonary systems to warrant routine use. Other plain roentgenograms, such as bone films, are only useful in confirming the presence or absence of metastatic lesions.[94] Since these metastases are rare (<5%) in patients with esophageal carcinoma, bone films are not part of the routine imaging workup.

Esophagogram

The esophagogram is sensitive in detecting the presence or absence of advanced esophageal carcinoma. It cannot detect carcinoma in situ, but has been effective in detecting superficial and early tumors if the double-contrast technique is employed (Figure 12-8).[38,51,52,56,118,131,132,137] Unfortunately, the terminology is not consistently defined. Most authors define "early" as any tumor smaller than 3.5 cm in length. Suzuki et al. reported early tumors ranging from 1.2×0.8 cm to 3.6×3.5 cm.[118] Both Koehler et al.[56] and Suzuki et al.[118] reported an improvement in

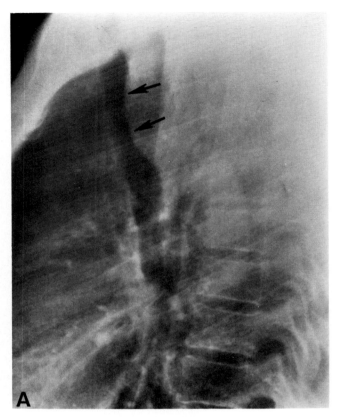

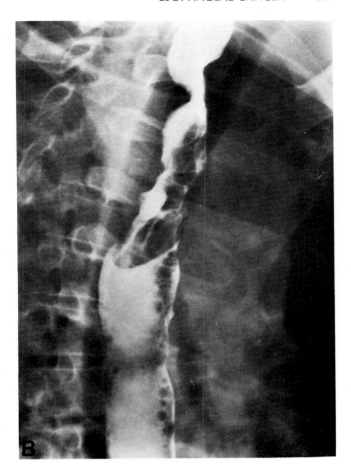

FIG. 12-7. (A) Coned-down view from lateral chest roentgenogram showing anterior displacement of the trachea (arrows). (B) Barium esophagogram of same patient showing large esophageal carcinoma.

overall survival rates in patients with tumors of this size. However, Zornoza and Lindell[137] did not find improved survival in their patients with small lesions compared with patients with "late" tumors (>3.5 cm in length).

In spite of some deficiencies, the esophagogram is important for localizing and characterizing a known or suspected tumor. The majority of these lesions are large and partially obstructing. However, while most esophageal carcinomas are one of the first three types (Figures 12-9 and 12-10), they may occasionally mimic varices,[133] achalasia,[62,70,123] or local inflammatory lesions. Thus, the radiologist should be familiar with all variations of radiographic manifestations of esophageal carcinoma.

Most authors have indicated that routine barium swallow studies cannot accurately define the length of a primary esophageal cancer.[1,2,100] This is an important concern, since in the TNM classification the separation between T_1 and T_2 lesions is based on whether the lesion is less than or greater than 5 cm in length. The tumor length as determined by the routine esophagogram may not be accurate, and some authors question the prognostic significance.[1,2,100] This conclusion, however, is not based on the double-contrast examination that most authors currently believe is significantly better, not only

in terms of detecting early lesions but also in determining the extent of large lesions (Figures 12-8, 12-11, and 12-12).[38,51,56,115,137] Thus the length of involvement on double-contrast studies may prove to be more valuable than the single-contrast examinations that were previously used.[38]

A number of authors have evaluated the "esophageal axis" in patients with carcinoma of the esophagus as defined by single-contrast esophagograms.[1,2,76] The findings, indicating nonresectable tumors, are illustrated in Figure 12-13. Tortuosity of the esophagus results from fixation of the tumor to the surrounding mediastinal structures with prestenotic dilatation and elongation of the structure. The other abnormalities are caused by fixation or traction. In order to adequately evaluate the esophageal axis, the esophagus must be viewed in all 360°. An abnormal esophageal axis cannot be excluded in only one plane. Seventy-five percent to 80% of locally invasive cancers will have a deformed esophageal axis.[1,2,76] Since the latter may also result from inflammatory changes, false positives are reported in 10% to 16% and false negatives in 8% of patients with locally invasive tumors.[1,2,76] To date, only a few authors[1,2,76] employ this type of analysis in patients with proven carcinoma of the esophagus. Mori et al. point

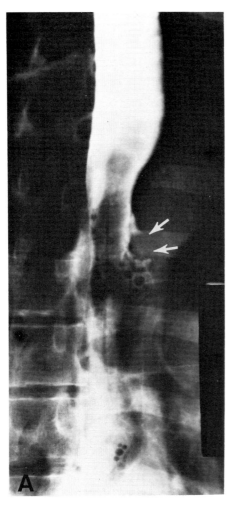

A

FIG. 12-8. (A) Routine barium esophagogram showing a questionable area of irregularity (arrows) along left lateral esophageal wall. (B and C) Double-contrast barium esophagogram showing small (1.5 × 2 cm) primary carcinoma in profile (B) and enface (C). Note subtle polypoid mass (arrow) with infiltrating margins (arrowheads). The patient had undergone a laryngectomy for a laryngeal carcinoma one year earlier. (Reprinted from Thompson, W. M., Oddson, T. A., Kelvin, F. M., Daffner, R., Postlethwait, R. W., Rice, R. P.: Synchronous and metachronous squamous cell carcinoma of the head, neck, and esophagus. *Gastrointest. Radiol.* 3:123–127, 1978).

out that deviation in esophageal axis provides more accurate prognostic information concerning resectability than the type of tumor or its length.[76]

We perform the double-contrast examination in all our patients with known or suspected carcinoma of the esophagus. We also recommend performing this examination in groups at high risk of developing esophageal carcinoma, such as patients with head-neck tumors (Figure 12-14),[80,120] lung cancer,[80,130] a previous history of lye stricture,[5,47,80] or those with known or suspected severe reflux esophagitis.[9,15,80,91] The barium swallow can also

be used to demonstrate a suspected fistula between the esophagus and the tracheobronchial tree (Figure 12-15).

Radionuclide Studies

Radionuclide studies are helpful in determining the presence or absence of abnormalities in the liver, brain, or skeletal system in patients with suspected metastases. However, since CT or some other imaging modality will be needed to confirm the nonspecific finding on the nuclear medicine studies, these are rarely used as screening procedures in our hospitals. A number of authors reported using gallium 67 scans in staging esophageal carcinoma.[57,58,85] The most recent work indicates that gallium 67 studies cannot accurately differentiate between stage I, stage II, and stage III lesions.[57] Thus, these authors concluded that routine performance of gallium 67 scans is probably not justified. Kondo et al. mention that gallium 67 scans may be useful for determining the extent of disease for planning radiotherapy.[57]

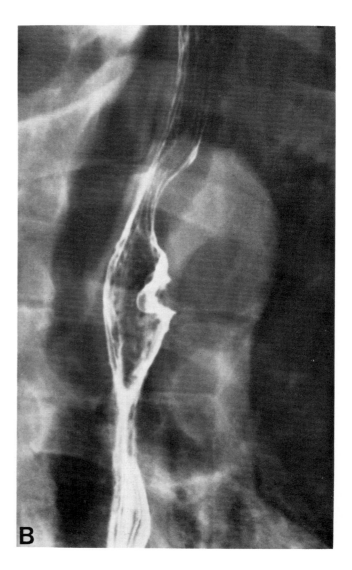

B

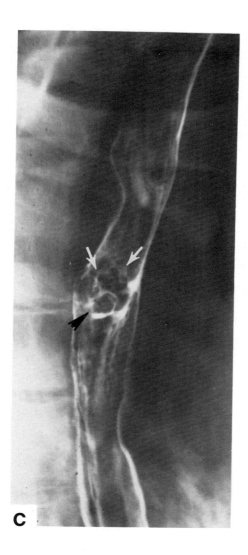

The technique for performing CT scans in patients with esophageal carcinoma is somewhat determined by the status of the patient. Before scanning, most authors recommend administering 200–300 ml of a 1%–2% gastrografin mixture orally to all patients unless there is a severe esophageal stricture or any evidence of a tracheo-esophageal fistula.[22,77,121] Intravenous contrast material is used in some patients to define the mediastinal vascular structures (Figure 12-16). Computed tomographic scans are taken at 1-cm intervals from the sternal notch to the umbilicus with the patient supine. Scans include the neck if the patient has a cervical esophageal lesion. Computed tomographic scans performed with the patient in the left lateral decubitus position can be helpful, especially when evaluating tumors that extend to the gastroesophageal junction.[121]

A number of authors have suggested that CT is an accurate method of assessing extraesophageal spread of carcinoma without surgery (Tables 12-5 and 12-6).[18,22,44,77,121] The important anatomic relationships of structures adjacent to an esophageal tumor can be well defined in over 95% of patients.[22,77,121] This information cannot be obtained by any other current modality. In 1979, Daffner et al. from our institution were the first to report their experience with 30 patients.[22] Of the 23 proven cases of mediastinal invasion, CT correctly identified 21 (91%) with two false negatives and one false positive. Enlarged metastatic abdominal lymph nodes were identified in 13 of 16 (81%) patients with three false negatives and three false positives. Two of three patients with liver metastases were correctly identified by CT with no false-positive studies. This study utilized a GE7800 scanner (General Electric Co.) and the authors stated that a number of mistakes of interpretation were made on the initial reading. In retrospect, the knowledge gained from their experience would have allowed for more successful initial interpretation. One false-positive diagnosis of mediastinal invasion was made in a cachetic patient, and they concluded that "a lack of body fat precludes a reliable CT diagnosis."[22] Overall, CT correctly identified the pres-

Ultrasound

Ultrasound, while noninvasive and inexpensive, is only useful in evaluating patients for the presence of abdominal metastases, especially to the hepatobiliary system. It should not be routinely employed in the staging of patients with carcinoma of the esophagus, but could be used to confirm a suspicious abnormality on liver-spleen scans or to evaluate an abdominal mass, such as might be encountered with liver metastases or massive adenopathy.

Computed Tomography

At present, CT appears to be the single most accurate method of evaluating patients with carcinoma of the esophagus (Tables 12-5 and 12-6).[18,21,22,44,77,121] Computed tomography has the advantage of routinely displaying the anatomy of the esophagus and contiguous mediastinal structures with a high degree of accuracy (Figure 12-1).[43]

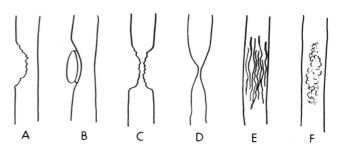

FIG. 12-9. Diagrams of the various radiographic appearances of esophageal carcinoma. (A) Polypoid, (B) ulcerative, (C) circumferential, (D) infiltrative, (E) varicoid, and (F) superficial spreading.

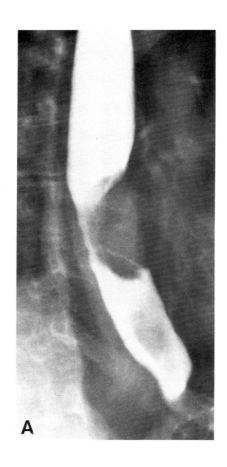

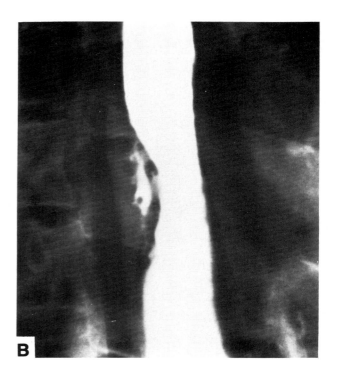

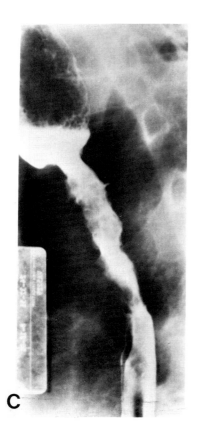

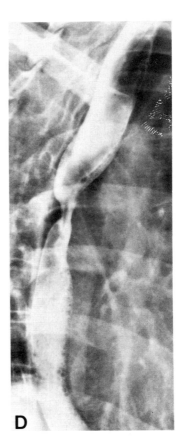

FIG. 12-10. Radiographic examples of various presentations of esophageal carcinoma corresponding to Figure 12-8. (A) Polypoid, (B) ulcerative, (C) circumferential, (D) infiltrative, (E) varicoid, and (F) superficial spreading.

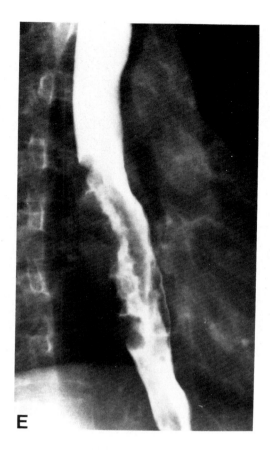

E

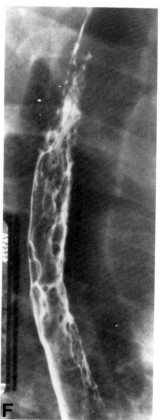

F

ence or absence of mediastinal invasion in 27 of 30 (90%) patients and correctly predicted distant abdominal metastases in 22 of 28 (79%) patients.

Moss et al. used CT to stage 52 patients with carcinoma of the esophagus but surgical confirmation of the CT findings was made in only 17 patients.[77] They recommended a CT staging system that differs from the TNM classification (Table 12-2). Their patients were divided into four groups: stage I—an intraluminal esophageal mass without wall thickening; stage II—wall thickening (>5 mm); stage III—wall thickening (>5 mm) and spread to contiguous mediastinal structures, and stage IV—distant metastatic spread. There were no stage I patients. Seven patients were classified as stage II, 33 as stage III, and 12 as stage IV.

Coulomb et al., in the French literature, reported their experience with CT in staging 40 patients with esophageal carcinoma.[18] Twenty-three of their patients had surgical or autopsy confirmation of the CT results. Their data is analyzed in more detail than the data of Moss et al.,[77] since they separated the ability of CT to define mediastinal invasion, subdiaphragmatic adenopathy, and liver metastases (Table 12-5). They had two false positives and two false negatives for an overall accuracy of 78%. Computed tomography correctly identified six patients with and six patients without abnormal subdiaphragmatic lymph nodes. Two other patients (9%), however, were falsely identified as having adenopathy (Table 12-5).

We have recently analyzed 64 patients with esophageal cancer who had a preoperative CT for staging.[121] All 64 had surgery, autopsy, or bronchoscopy that confirmed the presence or absence of mediastinal invasion. Forty-five of these 64 patients had abdominal CT and surgical or autopsy confirmation of the CT findings. Computed tomography correctly predicted mediastinal invasion in 44 of 47 (94%) patients and there were four false-positive and three false-negative studies (Table 12-5). Computed tomography correctly identified 13 patients with subdiaphragmatic abnormal lymph nodes and 21 patients without metastatic disease to abdominal lymph nodes. There were five false positives (11%) and six false negatives (13%). Liver metastases were correctly identified in four of five patients (Table 12-5).

Table 12-6 shows the combined sensitivity, specificity, and accuracy rates for the four studies described above.[18,22,77,121] Computed tomography can accurately evaluate the mediastinum for the presence or absence of invasion; however, the results in Table 12-5 indicate that there will be a 5% to 6% false-positive and false-negative rate. The error rates are almost twice as high with subdiaphragmatic lymphadenopathy, with 12% false positives and 10% false negatives (Table 12-5). The number of liver metastases is too low for accurate conclusions to be drawn. The ability of CT to accurately determine mediastinal invasion, suggested by these figures, is 90%. Computed tomography is also effective in the diagnosis

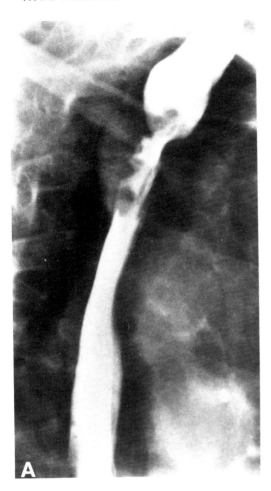
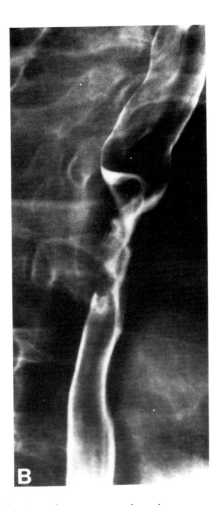

FIG. 12-11. Routine (A) and double-contrast (B) esophagograms showing a 6-cm upper esophageal cancer. The lesion is more visible on the double-contrast study.

of distant metastases but to a lesser degree. The true value of this technique will remain unknown until a significantly greater number of patients are carefully studied. The combined reported world experience to date is less than 200 patients.

Evaluating the tumor and the adjacent mediastinum is easier if the radiologist has reviewed the patient's esophagogram and thus knows the location of the lesion. The CT criteria used to determine the stage of the disease (presence or absence of invasion) are (1) obliteration of tissue fat planes between the esophageal mass and contiguous mediastinal structures (Figures 12-16 and 12-17; see also Figure 12-20B); (2) tumor extension into the trachea or bronchi (Figures 12-17 and 12-20B); and (3) leak of contrast medium outside the confines of the esophageal lumen into mediastinal structures. In our experience, tumor extension into the trachea or bronchus is the most reliable indicator of mediastinal invasion. We have had a number of false-positive and false-negative results using the fat plane criterion.

Moss et al. analyzed esophageal wall thickness, length of the mass, diameter of the tumor, presence of dilata-

tion of the esophagus above the lesion, and location of the air or contrast material in the lumen in relationship to the mass.[77] All of their patients had a thickened wall, which they defined as greater than 5 mm. Our findings suggest that the wall of the normal esophagus is 1 to 2 mm (Figure 12-1). Thus, an abnormally thickened wall is 3 mm or greater. Patients may have a normal chest CT but still have distant metastases. We have evaluated a number of patients with endoscopic and biopsy-proven carcinoma of the esophagus whose esophagograms and CT scans showed a normal esophagus at the level of the lesion (Figures 12-18 and 12-19). However, the abdominal CT showed that the patient had obvious, but clinically silent, distant metastases. These findings in patients emphasize the importance of evaluating the abdomen regardless of the findings in the chest.

Neither Moss et al.[77] nor our group have been able to use CT to determine the exact length of carcinomas of the esophagus as can be done with esophagography. As expected, CT better defines extramucosal extent, while barium esophagography better delineates mucosal abnormalities. Other problems in evaluating the lesion occur when the patient has an obstructing lesion. The esophagus becomes dilated and often filled with fluid above the primary lesion, which can distort the surrounding mediastinal anatomy and obscure the primary tumor (Figure 12-17C). Also, if there is a lack of mediastinal fat, it may be impossible to evaluate the planes separating the esophagus from surrounding structures (Figure 12-20). In this situation, we have adopted the policy of reporting that we cannot evaluate the mediastinum for the presence or absence of local invasion. In our experience, 10% to 15% of patients fall into this category.[121]

Abdominal and thoracic nodes larger than 1 cm are felt to be abnormal. Retrocrural nodes larger than 0.5 cm are abnormal.[105] We have not been as successful in detecting the presence of enlarged lymph nodes in the mediastinum as Moss et al.[77]

The CT criteria used for determining distant metastases are enlargement of lymph nodes that drain the esophagus (Figure 12-18) and evidence of lesions in the liver (Figure 12-19), lung, abdominal structures, and bone. Metastases to the last four areas can be confirmed by CT-guided percutaneous biopsy.[129] A CT-guided biopsy can also be used to evaluate abnormal areas of local invasion, especially in the neck (Figure 12-21).

Azygos Venography

Azygos venography has been used to provide invaluable information regarding extraesophageal invasion and resectability.[1,2,19,76] Although this is an invasive procedure, it has been performed without any major reported complications. When the azygos vein is obstructed, the lesion is almost always unresectable. Occasionally, an obstructed azygos vein will respond to radiation therapy and the tumor can be resected with some chance of a cure.[1,2,19,76] This procedure has not been widely used, and results have been reported from only one group in this country.[19] Since CT is much less invasive, azygos venography probably will not gain wide usage.

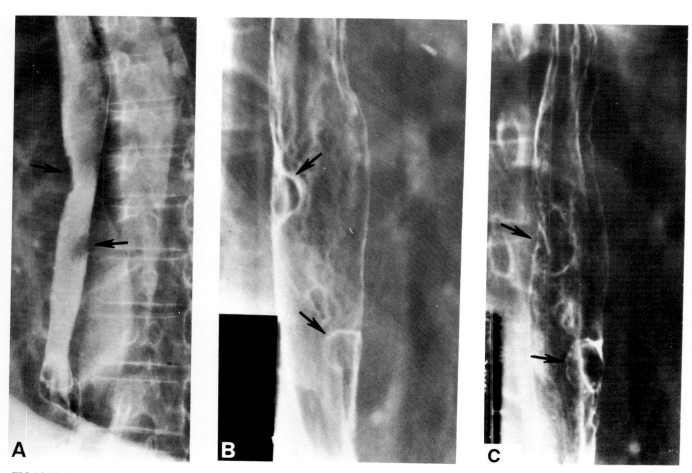

FIG.12-12. (A) Routine esophagogram of a patient with multiple primary sites of squamous carcinoma (arrows). (B and C) Double-contrast esophagograms showing multiple sites (arrows) of primary squamous cell carcinoma. Multiplicity is better demonstrated on the double-contrast studies.

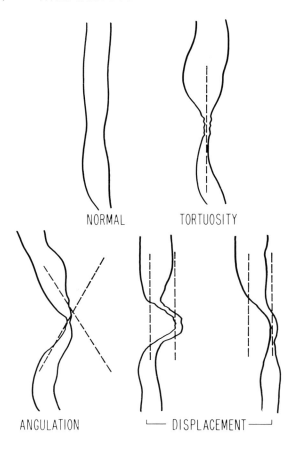

NORMAL   TORTUOSITY

ANGULATION   └─ DISPLACEMENT ─┘

ESOPHAGEAL AXIS

FIG. 12-13. (A) Types of deformities on barium esophagograms of the esophageal axis that may be produced by esophageal carcinoma. (Adapted from Akiyama, H. Surgery for carcinoma of the esophagus. *Curr. Probl. Surg.* 17:55–120, 1980). (B) Barium swallow study of a patient with invasive esophageal carcinoma showing abnormal esophageal axis.

Lymphography

Transtracheal mediastinal lymphography has recently been reported by Sugimachi et al.[117] for use in evaluating patients with carcinoma of the esophagus. The technique diagnosed metastatic nodes from 6 to 16 mm in diameter but failed to detect a 4 × 4-mm focus of tumor. This technique will probably not gain widespread usage because of the difficulties in interpretation as well as the invasiveness of the procedure.

Percutaneous Biopsy

Percutaneous biopsy, using small 22–20 needles, has gained widespread acceptance for confirming both primary and neoplastic lesions in almost every location in the body.[129] The techniques are well described and are becoming accepted as standard, safe, and valuable procedures in virtually every radiology department. This procedure has been used in patients with gastroesoph-

ageal neoplasms (Figure 12-21) and will probably be used even more in the future.

IMAGING STRATEGIES AND DECISIONS

The diagnostic tests for patients with known or clinically suspected esophageal carcinoma are shown in Figure 12-22. Recent reports indicate that authors believe CT is the most effective procedure for staging patients with carcinoma of the esophagus once the diagnosis has been confirmed and characterized by endoscopy and an esophagogram. Computed tomography should be able to determine the potential curability of a lesion by surgery in 85% to 90% of patients.

In our experience, the findings on CT that unequivocally indicate that the patient has an incurable lesion are (1) evidence that the tumor has extended into the trachea or bronchus, producing an esophagotracheal or esophagobronchial fistula (Figures 12-15B, 12-17A, and 12-21B), or (2) evidence that the patient has distant met-

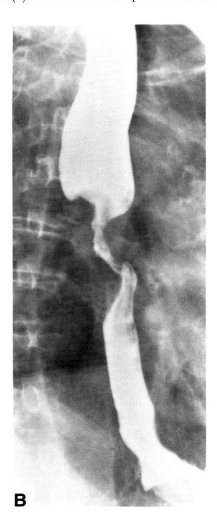

B

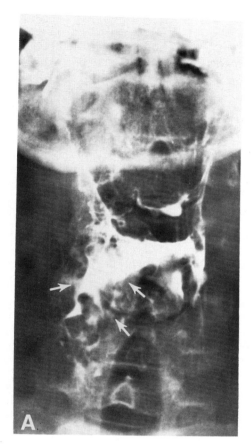

FIG. 12-14. (A) Frontal laryngogram showing a large carcinoma of the right pyriform sinus (arrows). (B) Barium esophagogram during laryngography showing the pyriform sinus tumor (arrows) as well as a separate primary esophageal carcinoma of the upper esophagus (arrowheads). (Reprinted from Thompson, W. M., Oddson, T. A., Kelvin, F. M., Daffner, R., Postlethwait, R. W., Rice, R. P.: Synchronous and metachronous squamous cell carcinoma of the head, neck, and esophagus. *Gastrointest. Radiol.* 3:123–127, 1978.)

astatic lymphadenopathy (Figure 12-18C) or liver metastases (Figure 12-19B). Obvious metastases to lung, pleura, bone, adrenals, or other sites would have the same implication. The loss of fat planes between the tumor and surrounding structures does not have the same accuracy. If CT shows the tumor clearly separated from the surrounding structures, as in Figure 12-16, there is a good chance (approximately 80%) that the tumor is locally confined and surgical resection may cure the patient. The percentage of false-negative CTs is 5% to 6% for predicting the absence of invasion in the chest and 10% to 12% for predicting the absence of distant abdominal metastases.

TREATMENT DECISIONS

As mentioned previously, if a patient is treated with either radiation therapy or chemotherapy before staging, a known esophageal cancer cannot be accurately staged.[1,2,100] Before the advent of CT, this meant that patients receiving either form of therapy before surgery were never reliably staged. Computed tomography should help stage patients, thus avoiding surgery primarily for staging purposes. Most patients should undergo CT scanning before radiation therapy in order for the primary tumor to be reliably evaluated. Both radiation and chemotherapy distort the fat planes in the mediastinum, making it impossible to evaluate the primary tumor and its relationship to the surrounding structures (Figure 12-20).[21,22]

Well-controlled randomized studies comparing radiation therapy and curative surgery in homogeneous patient populations have not yet been reported by many authors. The five-year survival rates reported to date for both forms of treatment in uncontrolled groups are similar.[26,27] However, radiation therapy is usually reserved for patients who are considered inoperable for either medical or surgical reasons. Thus, the data should favor surgery, since these patients should have less advanced cancers. These data show that surgery alone is no better or worse than radiation therapy alone.[26,27] Pearson[88] reported that radiation therapy did show a slightly higher

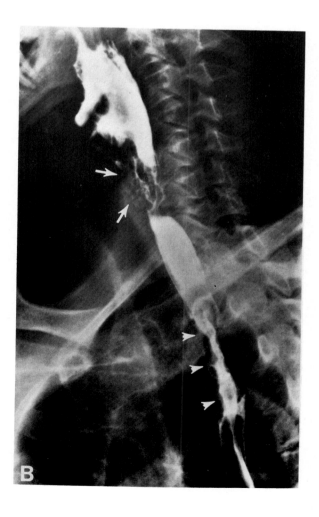

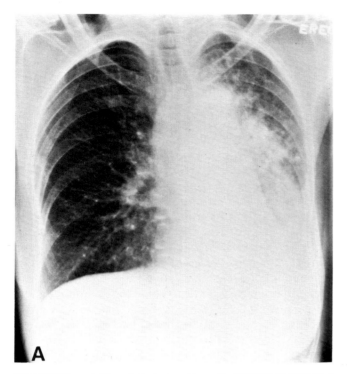

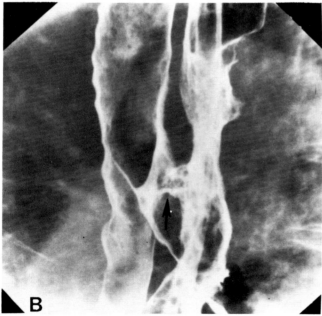

FIG. 12-15. (A) Chest roentgenogram showing aspiration pneumonia left lower lobe. (B) Barium esophagogram in same patient showing large esophageal carcinoma extending into the left mainstem bronchus (arrows).

five-year survival (17%) compared with surgery (11%) in a comparable randomized patient population.

In the last 10 years, there has been little progress in the curative approach to cancer of the esophagus,[94,100] and most authors are therefore pessimistic about treatment.[16,63,74,127] Thus, they often emphasize palliation rather than cure.[16,46,49,64,100,127] Palliation is important in these patients since they usually have advanced lesions. The potential for cure should not be forgotten, however, and both cure and palliation should be integrated into a plan of management. A general plan of management outlined by Rosenberg et al., which incorporates both curative and palliative measures, is shown in Figure 12-23.[100] This is an important concept, since it keeps in focus the three forms of therapy that play an important role in both the curative and palliative approaches to this devastating disease. The various therapeutic options for different stages of esophageal cancer are summarized in Table 12-7.

The pretreatment findings of CT should have important implications for the management of the patient. The demonstration of mediastinal invasion on CT does not always mean that the tumor cannot be removed and an esophagogastrostomy performed. The exact influence on survival of this type of surgery in a patient with a small amount of local mediastinal invasion is unknown. Surgical removal of the tumor will be attempted in most patients at our hospital who display CT evidence of mediastinal invasion. This surgery will include some form of esophageal reconstruction, so that the patient can continue to swallow. If CT shows distant metastases, however, especially in the liver or abdominal lymph nodes, the patient is not usually considered a surgical candidate and will undergo radiation therapy. These patients are stage III in the TNM classification and carry a poor prognosis (Tables 12-1 and 12-2, Figure 12-6).

Before the advent of CT, methods of evaluation of esophageal carcinoma patients after any form of therapy were few and insensitive. Computed tomography should be a better method for posttreatment evaluation of the chest and abdomen, even with the problems of distorted anatomy. To date, however, no data are available on how well CT can evaluate the mediastinum after any form of therapy for esophageal carcinoma. We have evaluated five patients after radiation therapy, chemotherapy, and surgical therapy and have had mixed results. In some cases, we could detect recurrent disease (Figure 12-24) or no response to the nonoperative therapy.[21,22,121] However, CT also failed to show recurrent disease in the mediastinum as well as enlarged nodes in a number of other patients who had undergone curative esophagogastrectomies. Further work is needed to determine if CT will be useful in evaluating patients after treatment.

Table 12-5. Summary of CT Results for Staging Esophageal Cancer

AUTHORS	NUMBER OF PATIENTS	NUMBER CONFIRMED BY SURGERY AUTOPSY OR OTHER MEANS		Normal CT	MEDIASTINAL INVASION		ABDOMINAL LYMPH NODES		LIVER METASTASES	
		Chest	Abdomen		False Positive/ True Positive	False Negative/ True Negative	False Positive/ True Positive	False Negative/ True Negative	False Positive/ True Positive	False Negative/ True Negative
Daffner et al.[22]	30	30	28	6	1/21	2/4	3/13	3/9	0/2	1/25
Moss et al.[77]	52	17	0	0	0/13	0/4	—	—	—	—
Coulomb et al.[18]	40	23	23	1	2/7	2/12	2/6	0/15	0/3	0/20
Thompson et al.[122]	64*	64	45	17	4/44	3/13	5/13	6/21	0/4	1/40
Totals	186	134	96	24	7/85	7/33	10/32	9/45	0/9	2/85

*Includes 30 patients of Daffner et al.[22] but they were reanalyzed by a different group of radiologists.

CARCINOMA OF THE GASTROESOPHAGEAL JUNCTION

The majority of malignant tumors at the gastroesophageal junction are adenocarcinomas.[6,9,11,15,29,34,45,75,112,124,128] They originate either as adenocarcinomas, which start as fundal neoplasms and extend through the gastroesophageal junction into the distal esophagus, or in a columnar epithelium-lined esophagus (Barrett's esophagus).[9,11,15,78,97] The latter is most often the consequence of prolonged reflux esophagitis. Of infrequent primary adenocarcinomas of the esophagus, 86% arise from a Barrett's esophagus.[100] Less than one fourth of the cancers at the gastroesophageal junction have a squamous cell origin. There are a number of similarities and differences between squamous cell lesions and adenocarcinomas.[93,94,100]

Both have a similar roentgenographic appearance (Figures 12-10 and 12-25 through 12-27). The adenocarcinoma from the fundus may be more polypoid and larger than squamous cell lesions mainly because of its gastric component (Figure 12-25). Carcinomas originating in a Barrett's esophagus are usually indistinguishable from squamous cell lesions. Adenocarcinomas associated with a Barrett's esophagus, while rarely congenital, usually show roentgenographic evidence of reflux esophagitis such as a hiatus hernia, abnormal distal esophageal mucosa, a stricture, and fluoroscopic evidence of gastroesophageal reflux. In the presence of these findings and a carcinoma, the diagnosis of Barrett's esophagus in association with an adenocarcinoma should be suggested by the barium esophagogram. However, a number of patients with squamous cell carcinoma at the gastroesophageal junction may also have a hiatus hernia. Regardless of the cell type, malignant tumors at this location have common pathologic features, such as rapid submucosal extension, transmural invasion, and early spread to adjacent lymph nodes. These features result in a low resectability rate and poor prognosis. Late detection is usually responsible for the poor prognosis. Thus, most patients have widespread disease at the time of initial clinical presentation and are not curable by resection. Also adenocarcinomas are radioresistant,[93,100] unlike squamous cell carcinomas, which can be cured by radiation therapy. The five-year survival rate for adenocarcinoma at the gastroesophageal junction therefore is usually worse than for squamous cell carcinoma of the lower esophagus.[100,134]

Recently, a number of authors have reported the accuracy of barium studies for diagnosing carcinomas and CT studies for staging carcinomas at the gastroesophageal junction.[34,63,122] Freeny and Marks found that barium esophagograms detected adenocarcinoma of the gastroesophageal junction in 72 of 77 (94%) patients.[34] In four patients, the diagnosis was felt to be achalasia rather than carcinoma, and one patient initially had a misinterpretation but was correctly diagnosed 6 weeks later. The double-contrast studies were more sensitive than the single-contrast examinations in detecting these abnormalities. These results are significantly better than previous reports, which indicated a 15% to 30% false-negative rate.[6] A properly performed esophagogram, es-

Table 12-6. Accuracy of CT for Staging Esophageal Cancer: Combined Data of Four Studies from Table 12-5*

	MEDIASTINAL INVASION (%)	ENLARGED ABDOMINAL LYMPH NODES (%)	LIVER METASTASIS (%)
Sensitivity	93	78	82
Specificity	83	78	100
Accuracy	90	78	98

*Coulomb et al.,[18] Daffner et al.,[22] Moss et al.,[77] and Thompson et al.[122]

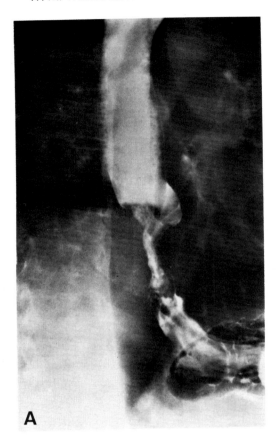

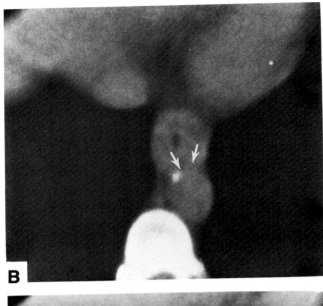

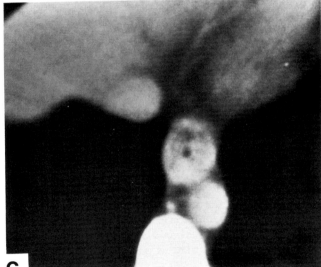

FIG. 12-16. (A) Barium esophagogram showing squamous cell carcinoma in lower esophagus. (B) CT scan without intravenous contrast medium showing poor definitions of fat planes between the esophagus and aorta (arrows). (C) CT scan after intravenous contrast medium showing esophageal mass with normal fat planes surrounding the mass. The patient had no evidence of mediastinal invasion at surgery.

Table 12-7. Treatment Decisions: Esophagus

STAGE	SURGERY	RADIATION THERAPY		CHEMOTHERAPY
I T_1,N_0,M_0	Esophagectomy and anastomosis	Definitive RT 6,000–7,000 cGy cone doses	or	NR
II $T_{1,2},N_{1,2},M_0$	If good PR or CT to RT, then resection attempted	Investigational preoperative RT 4,000 cGy	and/or	Investigational chemotherapy infusion 5-FU and mitamycin C or cisplatin
III T_3,N_3,M_0	Bypass procedure if obstruction is severe	Definitive RT 6,000–7,000 cGy	and	Investigational chemotherapy infusion 5-FU and mitamycin C or cisplatin
IV T_{any},N_{any},M_+	Bypass procedure if obstruction is severe	Palliative RT Doses up to 5,000 cGy		Multiagent chemotherapy

Note that investigational preoperative radiation therapy and chemotherapy infusion during irradiation with 5-FU and mitamycin C or cisplatin is being studied in a number of cooperative groups. For poor responders and unresectable lesions that are more advanced, full doses of radiation therapy are combined with similar chemotherapy infusion programs (p.c., ECOG-RTOG protocols, via Rubin).

RT = radiation therapy; NR = not recommended; PR = partial regression, more than 50%; CR = complete regression

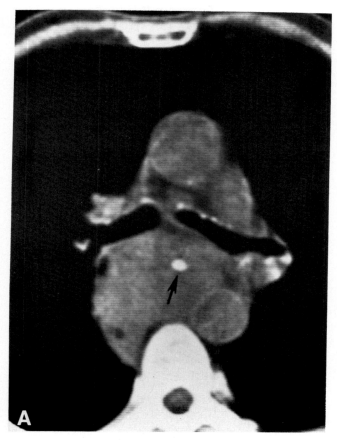

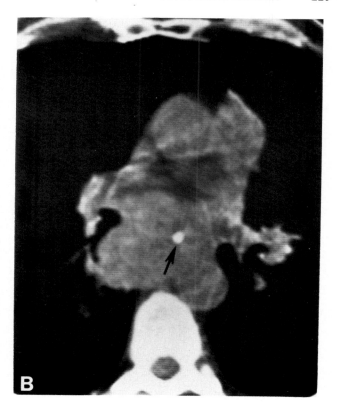

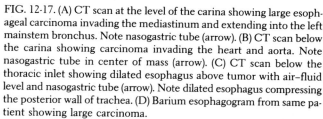

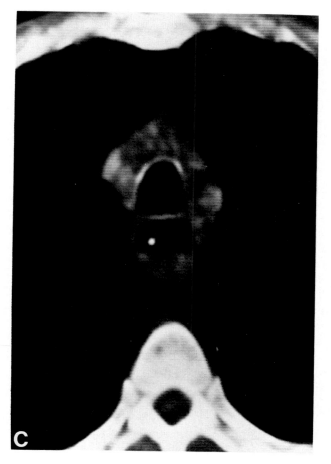

FIG. 12-17. (A) CT scan at the level of the carina showing large esophageal carcinoma invading the mediastinum and extending into the left mainstem bronchus. Note nasogastric tube (arrow). (B) CT scan below the carina showing carcinoma invading the heart and aorta. Note nasogastric tube in center of mass (arrow). (C) CT scan below the thoracic inlet showing dilated esophagus above tumor with air–fluid level and nasogastric tube (arrow). Note dilated esophagus compressing the posterior wall of trachea. (D) Barium esophagogram from same patient showing large carcinoma.

pecially a double-contrast study, should detect tumors at the gastroesophageal junction in 90% of patients.[34]

Computed tomography has been used to stage tumors at the gastroesophageal junction. The majority of these have been adenocarcinomas. Computed tomography accurately staged 18 of 21 (86%) patients (16 unresectable, two resectable) reported by Freeny and Marks.[34] The most reliable CT findings of unresectability were metastases (liver, adrenal) and local tumor extension, both found in 10 of 21 (48%) patients. Regional adenopathy was present in 8 of the 21 (38%) patients. In their experience, the presence or absence of the periesophageal soft tissue planes was not a reliable finding and led to false positives (10%) and false negatives (30%). We found similar results in 10 patients.[122] Computed tomography was used to accurately stage eight of the 10 patients with findings similar to those reported by Freeny and Marks.

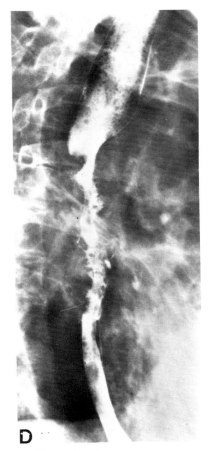

D

FIG. 12-17, continued.

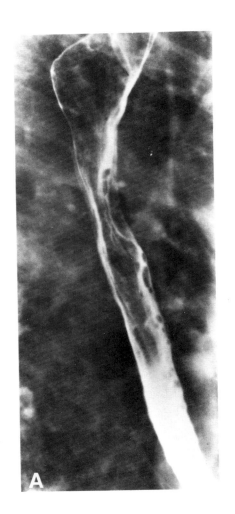

A

Metastases to the liver were encountered in four patients (Figure 12-26) and regional lymph node abnormalities were found in three patients (Figure 12-27). Associated with CT staging of gastroesophageal junction tumors are many of the same problems that are found in staging squamous cell carcinomas of the esophagus. Patients who are cachectic may be difficult to stage with CT. An additional problem is that the normal gastroesophageal junction often produces a pseudomass on CT scans that may be impossible to differentiate from a neoplasm without obtaining decubitus views and using large amounts of water-soluble contrast (Figures 12-25 through 12-28).[69,122] The incidence of a pseudomass or thickening of the wall of the stomach at the gastroesophageal junction in patients who have a normal gastroesophageal junction is 30% to 40% (Figure 12-28).[69,122] In an evaluation of patients with a mass at the gastroesophageal junction, CT scans should be performed with the patient in decubitus positions (Figure 12-28). The left lateral decubitus position has been the most helpful.[122]

As pointed out by Freeny and Marks, if patients with incurable tumors are treated by palliative surgical removal of tumor bulk or a bypass procedure, staging by

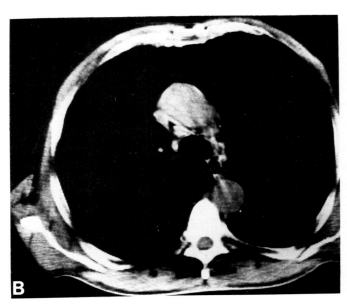

B

FIG. 12-18. Normal barium esophagogram (A) and CT scan (B) of patient with endoscopically proven tumor. (C) CT scan through upper abdomen showing metastatic celiac lymph nodes (arrows).

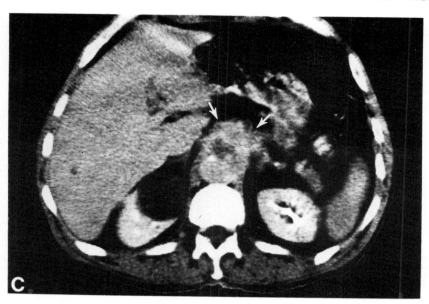

CT is not important since the lesion can be more accurately staged at surgery.[34] However, if patients with a gastroesophageal neoplasm are treated without surgery, then CT staging and, if necessary, fine-needle aspiration biopsy, may obviate the need for exploratory laparotomy.[34] Since many surgical reports show minimal if any improvement in survival after removal of incurable tumors, perhaps the ability to diagnose and stage gastroesophageal junction tumors nonoperatively will result in a diminished need for surgery.

SUMMARY

This chapter summarizes the current concepts of the pathology, natural history, and staging of esophageal carcinoma. The available imaging methods for diagnosing and staging patients with esophageal carcinoma are reviewed and an imaging scheme for evaluation of patients with esophageal carcinoma is presented. More experience is needed to determine the accuracy of CT for staging, but at the present time CT is the best imaging modality for evaluating patients with esophageal cancer. Computed tomography is the only currently available noninvasive imaging modality that can provide accurate staging information. Based on our experience, we feel all patients with carcinoma of the esophagus and gastroesophageal junction should be evaluated by this method. Better understanding by physicians of the natural history, staging, and imaging modalities as outlined in this chapter should lead to more effective patient management and improved survival.

REFERENCES

1. Akiyama, H.: Surgery for carcinoma of the esophagus. *Curr. Probl. Surg.* 17:55–120, 1980.
2. Akiyama, H., Tsurumaru, M., Kawamura, T., Ono, Y.: Principles of surgical treatment for carcinoma of the esophagus. Analysis of lymph node involvement. *Ann. Surg.* 194:438–446, 1981.
3. American Joint Committee on Cancer: *Manual for Staging of Cancer*, 2nd ed. Beahrs, O. H., Myers, M. H. (Eds.). Philadelphia, J. B. Lippincott, 1983.
4. Anderson, M. F., Harell, G. S.: Secondary esophageal tumors. *A.J.R.* 135:1243–1246, 1980.
5. Appelqvist, P., Salmo, M.: Lye corrosion carcinoma of the esophagus. *Cancer* 45:2655–2658, 1980.
6. Balthazar, E. J., Goldfine, S., Davidian, M. M.: Carcinoma of the esophagogastric junction. *Am. J. Gastroenterol.* 74:237–243, 1980.
7. Barge, J., Molas, G., Maillard, J. N., Fekete, F., Bogomoletz, W. V., Potet, F.: Superficial oesophageal carcinoma: An oesophageal counterpart of early gastric cancer. *Histopathology* 5:499–510, 1981.
8. Beatty, J. D., DeBoer, G., Rider, W. D.: Carcinoma of the esophagus. Pretreatment assessment, correlation of radiation treatment of parameters with survival, and identification and management of radiation treatment failure. *Cancer* 43:2254–2267, 1979.
9. Belladonna, J. A., Hajdu, S. I., Bains, M. S., Winawer, S. J.: Adenocarcinoma in situ of Barrett's esophagus diagnosed by endoscopic cytology. *N. Eng. J. Med.* 291:895–896, 1974.
10. Bragg, D. G.: Medical imaging problems in the patient with advanced cancer. *J.A.M.A.* 244:597–599, 1980.
11. Brand, D. L., Ylvisaker, J. T., Gelfand, M., Pope, C. E., II: Regression of columnar esophageal (Barrett's) epithelium after anti-reflux surgery. *N. Engl. J. Med.* 302:844–848, 1980.
12. Burke, E. L., Sturm, J., Williamson, D.: The diagnosis of microscopic carcinoma of the esophagus. *Dig. Dis. Sci.* 23:148–151, 1978.
13. Carnovale, R. L., Goldstein, H. M., Zornoza, J., Dodd, G. D.:

(*References continued on page 239*)

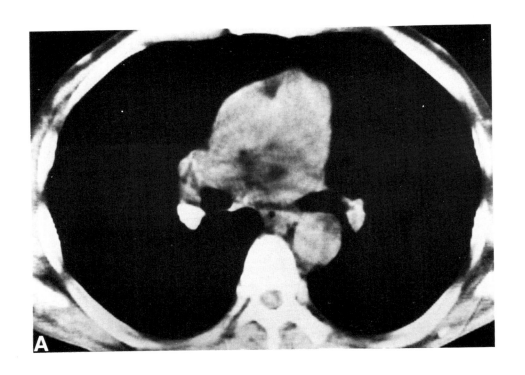

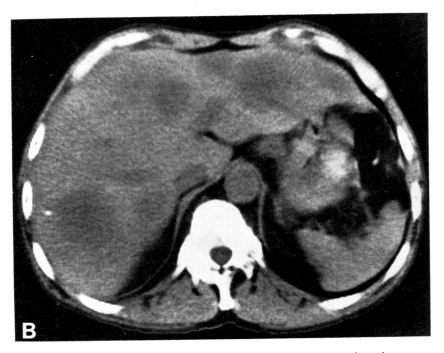

FIG. 12-19 (A) Normal CT scan of a patient with proven esophageal carcinoma who had a normal barium esophagogram. (B) CT scan through liver showing multiple low density metastases.

232

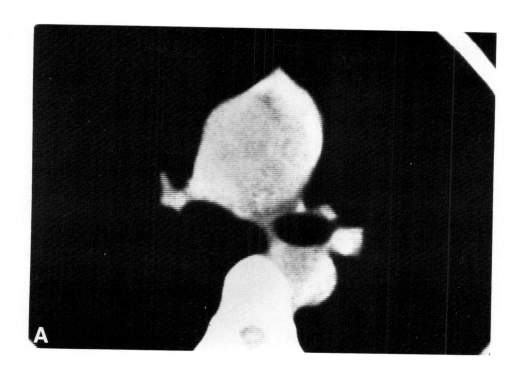

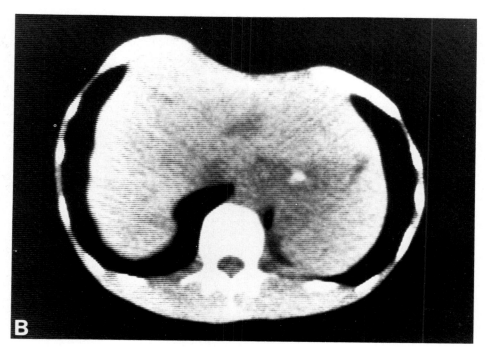

FIG. 12-20 (A) CT scan through chest showing marked loss of fat, making evaluation of the mediastinum impossible. (B) CT scan through the abdomen showing marked loss of retroperitoneal fat.

233

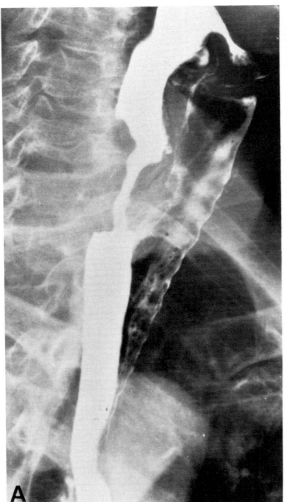

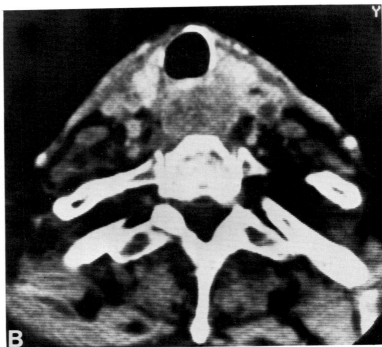

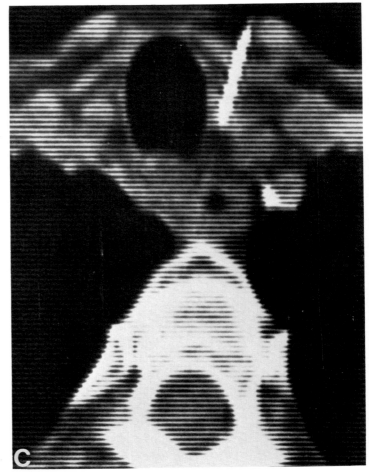

FIG. 12-21 (A) Barium esophagogram showing a mass displacing the cervical esophagus. Numerous endoscopic biopsies were negative. (B) CT scan showing a large esophageal mass invading the trachea. (C) CT scan showing a 22-gauge needle placed in the mass. The biopsy revealed squamous cell carcinoma of the esophagus.

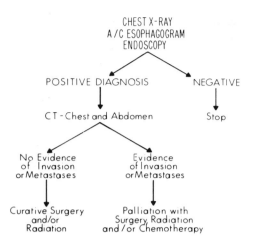

FIG. 12-22. Algorithm for radiologic approach to patients with known or suspected carcinoma of the esophagus.

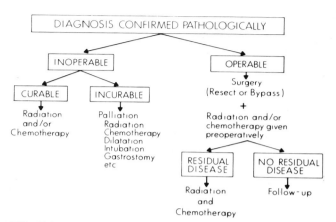

FIG. 12-23. Therapeutic approach for patients with carcinoma of the esophagus. The plan allows for both cure and palliation without compromising either approach. Under OPERABLE, some authors indicate radiation therapy alone will provide similar survival figures when compared with surgery. (Adapted from Rosenberg, J. C., Schwade, J. G., Vaitkevicius, V. K.:[100] Cancer of the esophagus. In Cancer Principles and Practice of Oncology, DeVita, V. T., Jr., Hellman, S., Rosenberg, S. A. (Eds.). Philadelphia, J. B. Lippincott, 1982, pp. 499–533.)

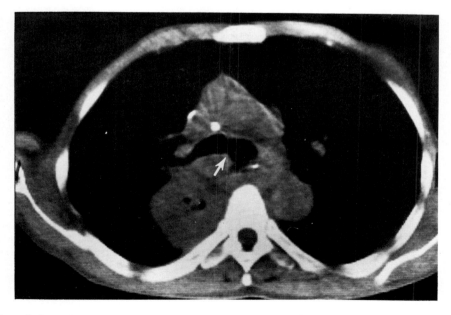

FIG. 12-24. CT scan through the carina in a patient who underwent esophagogastrectomy two years before this study for esophageal cancer. Note recurrent tumor extending into the carina (arrow). The patient had endoscopic proof of an esophagobronchial fistula caused by a recurrent esophageal carcinoma.

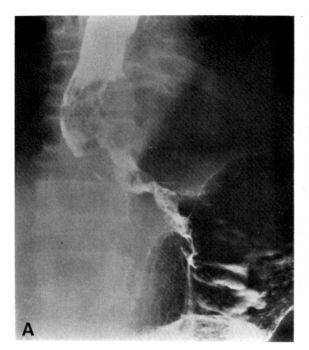

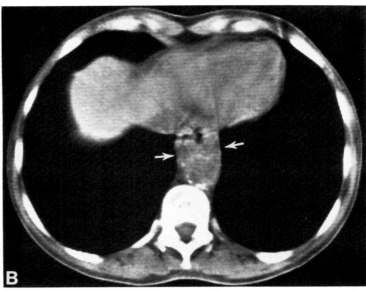

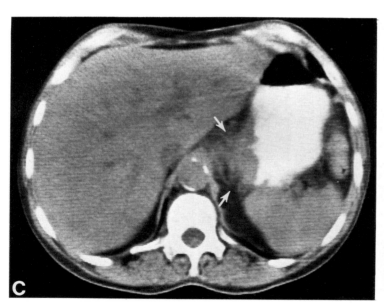

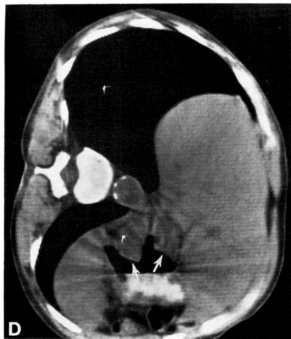

FIG. 12-25. (A) Double-contrast upper gastrointestinal study showing a large adenocarcinoma of the gastric fundus extending up the esophagus. (B) CT scan through the lower esophagus shows gastric adenocarcinoma (arrows) extending up the esophagus and invading the aorta. (C) CT scan shows an abnormal mass at the gastroesophageal junction (arrows). (D) CT scan exposed in the left lateral decubitus position shows the extent of the tumor (arrows). (Reprinted from Thompson, W. M., Halvorsen, R. A., Williford, M. E., Foster, W. L., Jr., Korobkin, M.: Computed tomography of the gastroesophageal junction. *Radio-Graphics* **2**:179–193, 1982. With permission.)

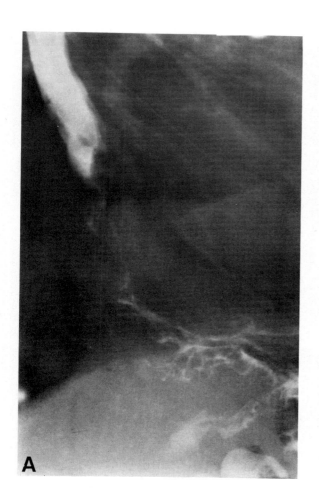

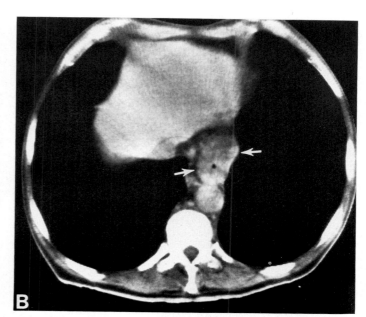

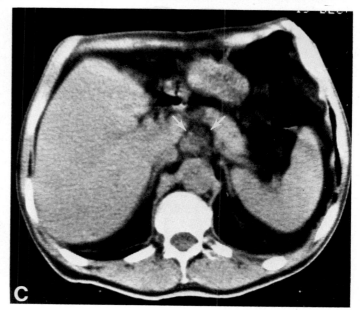

FIG. 12-26. (A) Esophagogram showing partially obstructing gastro-esophageal adenocarcinoma. (B) A CT scan of the same patient showing the adenocarcinoma (arrows) extending up the esophagus. (C) A CT scan showing malignant celiac lymph adenopathy (arrows). (Reprinted from Thompson, W. M., Halvorsen, R. A., Williford, M. E., Foster, W. L., Jr., Korobkin, M.: Computed tomography of the gastroesophageal junction. *RadioGraphics* **2**:179–193, 1982. With permission.)

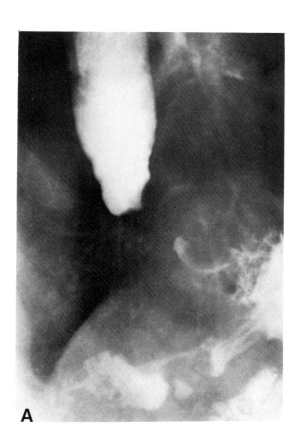

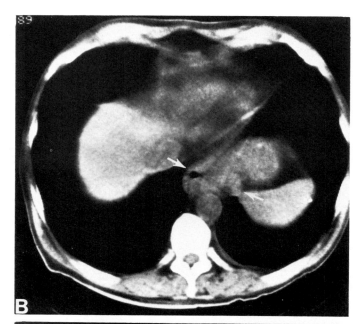

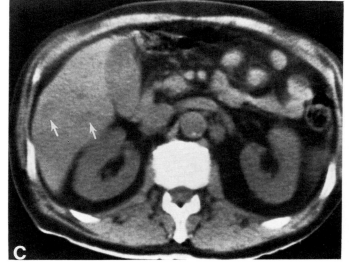

FIG. 12-27. (A) Esophagogram showing mass caused by an adenocarcinoma partially obstructing the gastroesophageal junction. (B) A CT scan of same patient showing the adenocarcinoma at the gastroesophageal junction (arrows). (C) CT scan showing liver metastases (arrows) in same patient. Metastases were confirmed by percutaneous biopsy. (Reprinted from Thompson, W. M., Halvorsen, R. A., Williford, M. E., Foster, W. L., Jr., Korobkin, M.: Computed tomography of the gastroesophageal junction. *RadioGraphics* 2:179–193, 1982. With permission.)

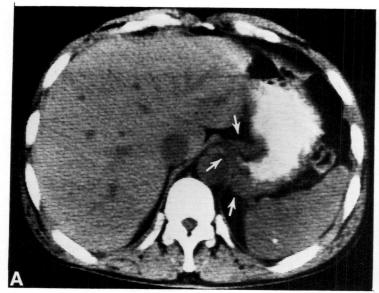
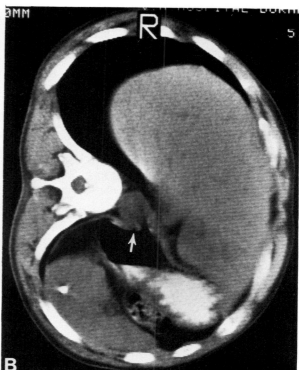

FIG. 12-28. (A) A CT scan through the gastroesophageal junction in a normal patient shows a pseudomass (arrows). (B) A CT of the same patient in the left lateral decubitus position shows a normal gastroesophageal junction (arrow). (Reprinted from Thompson, W. M., Halvorsen, R. A., Williford, M. E., Foster, W. L., Jr., Korobkin, M.: Computed tomography of the gastroesophageal junction. *RadioGraphics* 2:179–193, 1982. With permission.)

Radiologic manifestations of esophageal lymphoma. A. J. R. **128**: 751–754, 1977.

14. Cederqvist, C., Nielsen, J., Berthelsen, A., Hansen, H. S.: Cancer of the oesophagus. I. 1002 cases. Survey and survival. *Acta Chir. Scand.* 144:227–231, 1978.

15. Cho, K. J., Hunter, T. B., Whitehouse, W. M.: The columnar epithelial-lined lower esophagus and its association with adenocarcinoma of the esophagus. *Radiology* 115:563–568, 1975.

16. Cooper, J. D., Jamieson, W. R. E., Blair, N., Todd, T. R. J., Ilves, R., Pearson, F. G.: The palliative value of surgical resection for carcinoma of the esophagus. *Can. J. Surg.* 24:145–147, 1981.

17. Coordinating Groups for the Research of Esophageal Carcinoma, Honan Province, and the Chinese Academy of Medical Sciences. Studies on the relationship between epithelial dysplasia and carcinoma of the esophagus. *Chin. Med. J.* 1:110–116, 1975.

18. Coulomb, M., Lebas, J. F., Sarrazin, R., Geindre, M.: Computed tomography and esophageal carcinoma. *J. Radiol.* 62:475–487, 1981.

19. Crummy, A. B., Wegner, G. P., Flaherty, T. T., Benfield, J. R., Brunette, K. W., Francyk, W. P.: Azygos venography. An aid in the evaluation of esophageal carcinoma. *Ann. Thorac. Surg.* 6: 522–527, 1968.

20. Cukingnan, R. A., Carey, J. S.: Carcinoma of the esophagus. *Ann. Thorac. Surg.* 26:274–286, 1978.

21. Daffner, R. H.: Computed tomography of the esophagus. *CRC Crit. Rev. Diag. Imag.* 14:191–242, 1981.

22. Daffner, R. H., Halber, M. D., Postlethwait, R. W., Korobkin, M., Thompson, W. M.: CT of the esophagus. II. Carcinoma. A. J. R. 133:1051–1055, 1979.

23. Daffner, R. H., Postlethwait, R. W., Putnam, C. E.: Retrotracheal abnormalities in esophageal carcinoma: Prognostic implications. A. J. R. 130:719–723, 1978.

24. Danoff, B., Cooper, J., Klein, M.: Primary adenocarcinoma of the upper oesophagus. *Clin. Radiol.* 29:519–522, 1978.

25. Drucker, M. H., Mansour, K. A., Hatcher, C. R., Jr., Symbas, P. N.: Esophageal carcinoma: An aggressive approach. *Ann. Thorac. Surg.* 28:133–138, 1979.

26. Earlam, R., Cunha-Melo, J. R.: Oesophageal squamous cell carcinoma. 1. A critical review of surgery. *Br. J. Surg.* 67:384–390, 1980.

27. Earlam, R., Cunha-Melo, J. R.: Oesophageal squamous cell carcinoma. II. A critical review of radiotherapy. *Br. J. Surg.* 67:457–461, 1980.

28. Ellis, F. H., Jr., Gibb, S. P.: Esophagogastrectomy for carcinoma. Current hospital mortality and morbidity rates. *Ann. Surg.* 190: 699–705, 1979.

29. Ellis, F. H., Jr., Maggs, P. R.: Surgery for carcinoma of the lower esophagus and cardia. *World J. Surg.* 5:527–533, 1981.

30. Ezdinli, E. Z., Gelber, R., Desai, D. V., Falkson, G., Moertel, C. G., Hahn, R. G.: Chemotherapy of advanced esophageal carcinoma: Eastern Cooperative Oncology Group Experience. *Cancer* 46:2149–2153, 1980.

31. Fisher, M. S.: Metastasis to the esophagus. *Gastrointest. Radiol.* 1: 249–251, 1976.

32. Fleischer, D., Kessler, F., Haye, O.: Endoscopic Nd:YAG laser therapy for carcinoma of the esophagus: A new palliative approach. *Am. J. Surg.* 143:280–283, 1982.

33. Fraser, R. W., Wara, W. M., Thomas, A. N., Mauch, P. M., Fishman, N. H., Galante, M., Phillips, T. L., Buschke, F.: Combined treatment methods for carcinoma of the esophagus. *Radiology* 128:461–465, 1978.

34. Freeny, P. C., Marks, W. M.: Adenocarcinoma of the gastroesophageal junction: Barium and CT examination. A. J. R. 138:1077–1084, 1982.

35. Fullerton, G. D., Sewchand, W., Payne, J. T., Levitt, S. H.: CT determination of parameters for inhomogeneity corrections in radiation therapy of the esophagus. *Radiology* 126:167–171, 1978.

36. Gaede, J. T., Postlethwait, R. W., Shelburne, J. D., Cox, J. L., Hamilton, W. F.: Leiomyosarcoma of the esophagus. Report of two cases, one with associated squamous cell carcinoma. *J. Thorac. Cardiovasc. Surg.* 75:740–746, 1978.

37. Giuli, R., Gignoux, M.: Treatment of carcinoma of the esophagus. Retrospective study of 2,400 patients. *Ann. Surg.* 192:44–52, 1980.

38. Goldstein, H. M., Zornoza, J., Hopens, T.: Intrinsic diseases of the adult esophagus: Benign and malignant tumors. *Semin. Roentgenol.* 16:183–197, 1981.

39. Gua-Qing, W: Endoscopic diagnosis of early oesophageal carcinoma. *J. R. Soc. Med.* 74:502–503, 1981.

40. Guidelines for the clinical and pathologic studies on carcinoma of the esophagus. *Jpn. J. Surg.* 6:69–78, 1976.

41. Gunnlaugsson, G. H., Wychulis, A. R., Roland, C., Ellis, F. H., Jr.: Analysis of the records of 1,657 patients with carcinoma of the esophagus and cardia of the stomach. *Surg. Gynecol. Obstet.* 130: 907–1005, 1970.

42. Haas, L. L., Baker B.: Tumor outline of esophageal carcinoma. *Radiology* 64:241–248, 1955.

43. Halber, M. D., Daffner, R. H., Thompson, W. M.: CT of the esophagus: I. Normal appearance. *A. J. R.* 133:1047–1050, 1979.

44. Hamada, M., Yasuda, Y., Nakayama, S., Kikuchi, S., Akagawa, H., Yano, K., Ohtake, H.: Clinical evaluation of computed tomography in esophageal cancer. *Kurume Med. J.* 28:53–61, 1981.

45. Heck, H. A., Jr., Rossi, N. P.: Esophageal and gastroesophageal junction carcinoma: An evolved philosophy of management. *Cancer* 46:1873–1878, 1980.

46. Hoffmann, T. H., Kelley, J. R., Grover, F. L., Trinkle, J. K.: Carcinoma of the esophagus. An aggressive one-stage palliative approach. *J. Thorac. Cardiovasc. Surg.* 81:44–49, 1981.

47. Hopkins, R. A., Postlethwait, R. W.: Caustic burns and carcinoma of the esophagus. *Ann. Surg.* 194:146–148, 1981.

48. Huang, G. J.: Early detection and surgical treatment of esophageal carcinoma. *Jpn. J. Surg.* 11:399–405, 1981.

49. Hubbard, S. G., Todd, E. P., Dillon, M. L., Griffen, W. O.: Palliation for esophageal carcinoma. *Ann. Thorac. Surg.* 29:551–554, 1980.

50. Isono, K., Onoda, S., Ishikawa, T., Sato, H., Nakayama, K.: Studies on the causes of deaths from esophageal carcinoma. *Cancer* 49: 2173–2179, 1982.

51. Itai, Y., Kogure, T., Okuyama, Y., Akiyama, H.: Diffuse finely nodular lesions of the esophagus. *A.J.R.* 128:563–566, 1977.

52. Itai, Y., Kogure, T., Okuyama, Y., Akiyama, H.: Superficial esophageal carcinoma. *Radiology* 126:597–601, 1978.

53. James, R. D.: Radiotherapy in management of gastrointestinal carcinoma: A review. *J. R. Soc. Med.* 73:659–663, 1980.

54. Kelsen, D. P., Ahuja, R., Hopfan, S., Bains, M. S., Kosloff, C., Martini, N., McCormack, P., Golbey, R. B.: Combined modality therapy of esophageal carcinoma. *Cancer* 48:31–37, 1981.

55. Kelsen, D. P., Bains, M., Hilaris, B., Chapman, R., McCormack, P., Alexander, J., Hopfan, S., Martini, N.: Combination chemotherapy of esophageal carcinoma using cisplatin, vindesine, and bleomycin. *Cancer* 49:1174–1177, 1982.

56. Koehler, R. E., Moss, A. A., Margulis, A. R.: Early radiographic manifestations of carcinoma. *Radiology* 119:1–5, 1976.

57. Kondo, M., Hashimoto, S., Kubo, A., Kakegawa, T., Ando, N.: ^{67}Ga scanning in the evaluation of esophageal carcinoma. *Radiology* 131:723–726, 1979.

58. Kondo, M., Ando, N., Kosuda, S., Lian, S. L., Kubo, A., Masaki, H., Hashimoto, S., Tsutsui, T., Kakegawa, T.: Ga-67 scan in patients with intrathoracic esophageal carcinoma planned for surgery. *Cancer* 49:1031–1034, 1982.

59. Kumagai, Y., Makuuchi, H., Fujita, H., Migoshi, H., Suguro, Y.: "Ebb phenomenon"—diagnosis of submucosal diffuse invasion of esophageal cancer. *Endoscopy* 14:6–8, 1982.

60. Lane, F. W., Jr.: The case for irradiation. *Hosp. Pract.* 11:68–73, 1976.

61. Launois, B., Delarue, D., Campion, J. P., Kerbaol, M.: Preoperative radiotherapy for carcinoma of the esophagus. *Surg. Gynecol. Obstet.* 153:690–692, 1981.

62. Lawson, T. L., Dodds, W. J.: Infiltrating carcinoma simulating achalasia. *Gastrointest. Radiol.* 1:245–248, 1976.

63. Lee, K. R., Levine, E., Moffat, R. E., Bigongiari, L. R., Hermreck, A. S.: Computed tomographic staging of malignant gastric neoplasms. *Radiology* 133:151–155, 1979.

64. Leon, W., Strug, L. H., Brickman, I. D.: Carcinoma of the esophagus. A disaster. *Ann. Thorac. Surg.* 11: 583–592, 1971.

65. Lindell, M. M., Jr., Hill, C. A., Libshitz, H. I.: Esophageal cancer: Radiographic chest findings and their prognostic significance. *A.J.R.* 133:461–465, 1979.

66. Ludwig, M. E., Shaw, R., Suto-Nagy, G. D.: Primary malignant melanoma of the esophagus. *Cancer* 48:2528–2534, 1981.

67. Maimon, H. N., Dreskin, R. B., Cocco, A. E.: Positive esophageal cytology without detectable neoplasm. *Gastrointest. Endosc.* 20: 156–159, 1974.

68. Mandard, A. M., Chasle, J., Marnay, J., Villedieu, B., Bianco, C., Roussel, A., Elie, H., Vernhes, J. C.: Autopsy findings in 111 cases of esophageal cancer. *Cancer* 48:329–335, 1981.

69. Marks, W. M., Càllen, P. W., Moss, A. A.: Gastroesophageal region: Source of confusion on CT. *A.J.R.* 136:359–362, 1981.

70. McCallum, R. W.: Esophageal achalasia secondary to carcinoma. Report of a case and a review of the literature. *A.J.R.* 71:24–29, 1979.

71. McCort, J. J.: Radiographic identification of lymph node metastases from carcinoma of the esophagus. *Radiology* 59:694–711, 1952.

72. McCort, J. J.: Esophageal carcinosarcoma and pseudosarcoma. *Radiology* 102:519–524, 1972.

73. McKeown, K. C.: Resection of midesophageal carcinoma with esophagogastric anastomosis. *World J. Surg.* 5:517–525, 1981.

74. Moertel, C. G.: The case against surgery. *Dig. Dis. Sci.* 23:735–736, 1978.

75. Molina, J. E., Lawton, B. R., Myers, W. O., Humphrey, E. W.: Esophagogastrectomy for adenocarcinoma of the cardia. *Ann. Surg.* 195:146–151, 1982.

76. Mori, S., Kasai, M., Watanabe, T., Shibuya, I.: Preoperative assessment of resectability for carcinoma of the thoracic esophagus. Part 1. Esophagogram and azygogram. *Ann. Surg.* 190:100–105, 1979.

77. Moss, A. A., Schnyder, P., Thoeni, R. F., Margulis, A. R.: Esophageal carcinoma: Pretherapy staging by computed tomography. *A.J.R.* 136:1051–1056, 1981.

78. Naef, A. P., Savary, M., Ozello, L.: Columnar-lined lower esophagus: An acquired lesion with malignant predisposition. *J. Thorac. Cardiovasc. Surg.* 70:826–835, 1975.

79. Nichols, T., Yokoo, H., Craig, R. M., Shields, T. W.: Pseudosarcoma of the esophagus. *Am. J. Gastroenterol.* 72:615–622, 1979.

80. Norton, G. A., Postlethwait, R. W., Thompson, W. M.: Esophageal carcinoma. A survey of populations at risk. *South. Med. J.* 73:25–27, 1980.

81. Orel, J. J., Erzen, J. J., Hrabar, B. A.: Results of resection of carcinoma of the esophagus and cardia in 196 patients. *World J. Surg.* 5:259–267, 1981.

82. Palayew, M. J.: The tracheo-esophageal stripe and the posterior tracheal band. *Radiology* 132:11–13, 1979.

83. Parker, E. F.: Carcinoma of the esophagus: Is there a role for surgery? Edward F. Parker vs Charles G. Moertel. *Dig. Dis. Sci.* 23:730–734, 1978.

84. Partyka, E. K., Sanowski, R. A., Kozarek, R. A.: Endoscopic diagnosis of a giant esophageal leiomyosarcoma. *Am. J. Gastroenterol.*

75:132–134, 1981.

85. Pearlman, A. W.: Gallium imaging in cancer of the esophagus. *Clin. Nucl. Med.* 6: 380–383, 1981.

86. Pearson, J. G.: Value of radiation therapy. *J.A.M.A.* 227:181–183, 1974.

87. Pearson, J. G.: The present status and future potential of radiotherapy in the management of esophageal cancer. *Cancer* 39: 882–890, 1977.

88. Pearson, J. G.: Radiotherapy for esophageal carcinoma. *World J. Surg.* 5:489–497, 1981.

89. Pearson, J. G., LeRoux, B. T.: Malignant tumors of the esophagus. In *Diseases of the Esophagus.* Vantrappen, G., Hellemans, J. (Eds.). New York, Springer-Verlag, 1974, pp. 447–492.

90. Piccone, V. A., Leveen, H. H., Ahmed, N., Grosberg, S.: Reappraisal of esophagogastrectomy for esophageal malignancy. *Am. J. Surg.* 137:32–37, 1979.

91. Poleynard, G. D., Marty, A. T., Birnbaum, W. B., Nelson L. E., O'Reilly, R. R.: Adenocarcinoma in the columnar-lined (Barrett) esophagus: Case reports and review of the literature. *Arch. Surg.* 112:997–1000, 1977.

92. Postlethwait, R. W.: Carcinoma of the esophagus. *Curr. Probl. Cancer* 2:1–44, 1978.

93. Postlethwait, R. W.: Squamous cell carcinoma of the esophagus. In *Surgery of the Esophagus.* Postlethwait, R. W., Sealy, W. C. (Eds.). New York, Appleton-Century-Crofts, 1979, pp. 341–414.

94. Postlethwait, R. W.: *Malignant Tumors Other Than Squamous Cell Carcinoma.* New York, Appleton-Century-Crofts, 1979, pp. 415–438.

95. Potsaid, M. S.: Diagnostic imaging in perspective. *J.A.M.A.* 243: 2412–2417, 1980.

96. Putman, C. E., Curtis, A. M., Westfried, M., McLoud, T. C.: Thickening of the posterior tracheal stripe: A sign of squamous cell carcinoma of the esophagus. *Radiology* 121:533–536, 1976.

97. Reyes, C. V., Wang, T.: Primary adenocarcinoma of the esophagus. A review of 12 cases. *J. Surg. Oncol.* 18:153–158, 1981.

98. Robertson, R., Coy, P., Mokkhavesa, S.: The results of radical surgery compared with radical radiotherapy in the treatment of squamous carcinoma of the thoracic esophagus. The case for preoperative radiotherapy. *J. Thorac. Cardiovasc. Surg.* 53:430–440, 1967.

99. Rosenberg, J. C., Franklin, R., Steiger, Z.: Squamous cell carcinoma of the thoracic esophagus: An interdisciplinary approach: *Curr. Probl. Cancer* 5:3–52, 1981.

100. Rosenberg, J. C., Schwade, J. G., Vaitkevicius, V. K.: Cancer of the esophagus. In *Cancer Principles and Practice of Oncology.* DeVita, V. T., Jr., Hellman, S., Rosenberg, S. A. (Eds.). Philadelphia, J. B. Lippincott, 1982, pp. 499–533.

101. Rosengren, J. E., Goldstein, H. M.: Radiologic demonstration of multiple foci of malignancy in the esophagus. *Gastrointest. Radiol.* 3:1–13, 1978.

102. Rubin, P.: Cancer of the gastrointestinal tract. I. Esophagus: Detection and diagnosis. *J.A.M.A.* 226:1544–1546, 1973.

103. Rubin, P., (Ed.): *Clinical Oncology for Medical Students and Physicians: A Multidisciplinary Approach,* 6th ed. New York, American Cancer Society, 1983.

104. Sannohe, Y., Hiratsuka, R., Koki, K.: Lymph node metastases in cancer of the thoracic esophagus. *Am. J. Surg.* 141:216–218, 1981.

105. Schnyder, P. A., Gamsu, G.: CT of the pretracheal retrocaval space. *A.J.R.* 136:303–308, 1981.

106. Schuchmann, G. F.: Carcinoma of the esophagus. Therapeutic combinations, controversies and compromises. *Chest* 81:400–401, 1982.

107. Schuchmann, G. F., Heydorn, W. H., Hall, R. V., Carter, S. C., Gillespie, J. T., Grishkin, B. A., James, E. C.: Treatment of esophageal carcinoma. A retrospective review. *J. Thorac. Cardiovasc. Surg.* 79:67–73, 1980.

108. Smith, F. W., Hutchinson, J.M.S., Mallard, J. R., Johnson, G., Redpath, T. W., Selbie, R. D., Reid, A., Smith, C. C.,: Oesophageal carcinoma demonstrated by whole-body nuclear magnetic resonance imaging. *Br. Med. J.* 282:510–512, 1981.

109. Solomon, A., Hunt, J.: Multiple squamous carcinomas and the oesophagus. *S. Afr. Med. J.* 55:1028–1030, 1979.

110. Son, Y. H.: Primary mucosal malignant melanoma. Appraisal of role of radiation therapy. *Acta Radiol. Oncol.* 19:177–181, 1980.

111. Sotus, P. C.: Carcinoma in situ of the esophagus. *J.A.M.A.* 239: 335–336, 1978.

112. Spagnolo, D. V., Heenan, P. J.: Collison carcinoma at the esophagogastric junction: Report of two cases. *Cancer* 46:2702–2708, 1980.

113. Sridhar, C., Zeskind, H. J., Rising, J. A.: Verrucous squamous-cell carcinoma: An unusual tumor of the esophagus. *Radiology* 136: 614, 1980.

114. Steiger, Z., Franklin, R., Wilson, R. F., Leichman, L., AsFaw, I., Vaishamapayan, G., Rosenberg, J. C., Loh, J. J., Didogru, A., Seydel, M., Hoschner, J., Miller, P., Knechtges, T., Vaitkevicius, V.: Complete eradication of squamous cell carcinoma of the esophagus with combined chemotherapy and radiotherapy. *Am. Surg.* 47: 95–98, 1981.

115. Steiger, Z., Franklin, R., Wilson, R. F., Leichman, L., Seydel, H., Loh, J. J. K., Vaishamapayan, G., Knechtges, J.: Eradication and palliation of squamous cell carcinoma of the esophagus with chemotherapy and surgical therapy. *J. Thorac. Cardiovasc. Surg.* 82:713–719, 1981.

116. Stein, H. A., Murray, D., Warner, H. A.: Primary Hodgkin's disease of the esophagus. *Dig. Dis. Sci.* 26:457–461, 1981.

117. Sugimachi, K., Okudaira, Y., Ueo, H., Ikeda, M., Inokuchi, K.: Transtracheal mediastinal lymphography for visualization of metastatic lymph nodes in carcinoma of the esophagus. *Surg. Gynecol. Obstet.* 154:34–38, 1982.

118. Suzuki, H., Kobayashi, S., Endo, M., Nakayama, K.: Diagnosis of early esophageal cancer. *Surgery* 71:99–103, 1972.

119. Takita, H., Vincent, R. G., Caicedo, V., Gutierrez, A. C.: Squamous cell carcinoma of the esophagus: A study of 153 cases. *J. Surg. Oncol.* 9:547–554, 1977.

120. Thompson, W. M., Halvorsen, R. A., Foster, W. L., Jr., Williford, M. E., Postlethwait, R. W., Korobkin, M.: Computed tomography for staging esophageal and gastroesophageal cancer. A re-evaluation. *A.J.R.* 141:951–958, 1983.

121. Thompson, W. M., Halvorsen, R. A., Williford, M. E., Foster, W. L., Jr., Korobkin, M.: Computed tomography of the gastroespohageal junction. *RadioGraphics* 2:179–193, 1982.

122. Thompson, W. M., Oddson, T. A., Kelvin, F. M., Daffner, R. H., Postlethwait, R. W., Rice, R. P.: Synchronous and metachronous squamous cell carcinoma of the head, neck and esophagus. *Gastrointest. Radiol.* 3:123–127, 1978.

123. Tucker, H. J., Shape, W. J., Jr., Cohen, S. C.: Achalasia secondary to carcinoma; manometric and clinical features. *Ann. Intern. Med.* 89:315–318, 1978.

124. Turnbull, A. D., Rosen, P., Goodner, J. T., Beattie, E. J.: Primary malignant tumors of the esophagus other than typical epidermoid carcinoma. *Ann. Thorac. Surg.* 15:463–473, 1973.

125. Valente, M., Cataldo, I., Grandi, C., Luini, A., Milani, F., Pizzocaro, G., Ravasi, G.: Preoperative irradiation and surgery for esophageal cancer: Causes of failure. *Tumori* 66:109–116, 1980.

126. van Andel, J. G., Dees, J., Dijkhuis, C. M., Fokkens, W., van Houten, H., deJong, P. C., van Woerkam-Eykenboom, W. M.:Carcinoma of the esophagus. Results of treatment. *Ann. Surg.* 190: 684–689, 1979.

127. Wara, W. M., Mauch, P. M., Thomas, A. N., Phillips, T. L.: Palliation for carcinoma of the esophagus. *Radiology* 121:717–720, 1976.

128. Welvaart, K., Zwaveling, A.: Carcinoma of the oesophagus and gastric cardia. *Clin. Oncol.* 6:203–212, 1980.

129. Wittenberg, J., Muller, P. R., Ferrucci, J. T., Jr., Simeone, J. F., van Sonnenberg, E., Neff, C. C., Palermo, R. A., Islerr, R. J.: Percutaneous core biopsy of abdominal tumors using 22 gauge needles: Further observations. *A.J.R.* **139**:75–80, 1982.

130. Wynder, E. L., Bross, I. J.: A study of etiological factors in cancer of the esophagus. *Cancer* **14**:389–413, 1961.

131. Yamada, A., Kobayashi, S., Kawai, B., Fujimoto, A., Nakayama, K.: Study on x-ray findings of early oesophageal cancer. *Aust. Radiol.* **16**:238–246, 1972.

132. Yanjin, M., Xianzhi, G., Guangyi, L., Wenheng, C.: Detection and natural progression of early oesophageal carcinoma: Preliminary communication. *J. R. Soc. Med.* **74**:884–886, 1981.

133. Yates, C. W., Jr., LeVine, M. A., Jensen, K. M.: Varicoid carcinoma of the esophagus. *Radiology* **122**:605–608, 1977.

134. Younghusband, J. D., Aluwihare, A. P. R.: Carcinoma of the oesophagus: Factors influencing survival. *Br. J. Surg.* **57**:422–430, 1970.

135. Yrjana, J.: The posterior tracheal band and recurrent esophageal carcinoma. *Radiology* **136**:615–618, 1980.

136. Yrjana, J., Kormano, M.: Posterior tracheal band in esophageal carcinoma. *Diag. Imag.* **49**:123–130, 1980.

137. Zornoza, J., Lindell, M. M., Jr.: Radiologic evaluation of small esophageal carcinoma. *Gastrointest. Radiol.* **5**:107–111, 1980.

13 GASTRIC, SMALL BOWEL, AND COLORECTAL CANCER

Wilson S. Wong
Henry I. Goldberg

The majority of gastrointestinal (GI) tract malignancies are adenocarcinomas. In the colon, adenocarcinoma is practically the only clinically significant tumor, and it is the second most common tumor in the small bowel, with carcinoid being the most common. The stomach harbors the greatest variety of malignant neoplasms. Adenocarcinoma, however, is still the predominant cell type, followed by lymphoma and leiomyosarcoma.

Various diagnostic procedures have been used to screen patients for GI tract tumors. Fiberoptic endoscopic examination has been advocated as the study of choice to screen the population at risk of developing stomach and colon cancer because of its ability to directly visualize the mucosa and to permit biopsy of suspicious lesions. However, because fiberoptic endoscopy requires patient sedation, the number of endoscopists is limited, and the number of patients is large, single-contrast and double-contrast roentgenographic examinations of the GI tract remain the most widely accepted screening procedures. As the following section will demonstrate, computed tomography (CT) plays a very important role in the staging of tumors and a relatively minor role in the detection of tumors of the hollow viscus. Ultrasound usually does not play a significant role in the detection of tumors of the GI tract because of the high reflectivity of sound waves by bowel gas. However, because ultrasound is being more frequently employed in recent years for screening patients with nonspecific abdominal complaints, it may be able to detect unsuspected tumor masses before barium contrast studies are done. Needle biopsies guided by CT or ultrasound are additional important diagnostic means of confirming a diagnosis as well as staging a tumor. In addition, CT and ultrasound may demonstrate the presence of metastatic lesions in the liver or lung bases, which would obviate the need for radionuclide liver-spleen scans or other staging procedures. The role of magnetic resonance imaging (MRI) in the detection and staging of GI tract tumors is yet to be defined, although MRI is able to detect liver metastases.[24]

STOMACH

Introduction

Adenocarcinoma accounts for 95% of all gastric malignancies, the remaining 5% being composed of sarcomas.[9,34,92] Adenocarcinoma can occur de novo or it can develop as a complication of partial gastrectomy[23,28,49] or secondary to environmental carcinogens such as asbestos and polyvinyl chloride.[83] An increased incidence of gastric carcinoma in patients with pernicious anemia, chronic atrophic gastritis, adenomatous polyps, or type A blood has been reported.[9,34,92] Gastric carcinomas also occur more frequently in families of patients with gastric carcinoma than in the normal population. It is far more frequent in Japan, Iceland, Finland, Norway, and Chile than it is in the United States, where it is being seen with decreasing frequency.[9,34,106]

Survival Statistics for Primary Stomach Cancers

Although there has been a steady decrease in the incidence of gastric carcinoma in the United States, the survival rates have remained dismally poor. The only types of gastric carcinoma with a good prognosis are the early and the superficial spreading gastric carcinomas, where the five-year survival rates have been reported to be nearly 95%.[9,66] However, these types of tumors account for only 7% of the gastric carcinomas in the United States and for approximately 30% of the gastric carcinomas in Japan.[17] The prognosis for patients with advanced gastric carcinoma depends on the location of the tumor and the extent of tumor spread. The five-year survival rate for localized disease is 47% to 48%, while for disseminated disease it is only 6%.[106] For patients with tumors localized to the antropyloric region who have undergone curative surgery, the five-year survival rate is 15% to 28%, with a median survival time of 18 months.[13,101] The five-year survival rates for patients with tumors located in the fundus, cardia, or gastroesophageal junction and for those with diffuse infiltrating types with penetration of the serosa are only 5% to 15%.[17] As for those patients with tumors considered to be nonresectable, the median survival is 4 to 9 months.[17]

Patients with gastric lymphoma have a better prognosis than those with gastric carcinoma mainly because of the greater radiosensitivity of the tumors. The five-year survival rate for lymphoma in general is about 30% to 50% and the ten-year survival rate is about 13% to 50%.[8] Patients with regional lymph node involvement have a significantly worse prognosis.

Gastric leiomyosarcoma tends to be localized, and greater than 50% of patients with this tumor can be cured surgically.[81] However, patients with metastases to lymph nodes or the liver or with direct extension beyond the confines of the stomach have a poor prognosis.[9]

Tumor Behavior and Pathology

Adenocarcinoma. Over 50% of gastric carcinomas originate in the pyloric and prepyloric region.[92] They have been subdivided into five growth patterns based on their gross morphology: ulcerative (25%), fungating (36%), polypoid (7%), diffuse (26%), and superficial (6%).[92] The ulcerative type can be difficult to differentiate from benign gastric ulcers. Classically, the cancerous ulcer crater is surrounded by heaped up, beaded, overhanging margins, and the crater sits in the center of an elevated mucosal plaque. The fungating type tends to have a broad base with a large cauliflowerlike mass protruding into the lumen. The diffuse type may produce significant wall thickening by permeating the entire wall, producing the classic "linitis plastica" appearance of the

stomach. Mucinous consistency may be seen with any one of the five growth patterns.

Well-differentiated adenocarcinoma is the histologic type common among all five growth patterns. All gastric carcinomas basically are composed of two cell types: metaplastic intestinal globlet cells and gastric mucous cells. Mixtures of these cell types are sometimes observed.[92]

Early gastric carcinoma is one form of gastric carcinoma that deserves special mention. It is defined as carcinoma of the stomach with invasion limited to the mucosa and submucosa.[66,80] It was brought into public attention by Japanese investigators in the 1960s. This form of gastric carcinoma is less often detected in the United States than in Japan, which is a reflection of the attention given to gastric cancer in Japan. The early gastric carcinomas have been classified into three types based upon their macroscopic appearance (Figure 13-1):

Type I: Protruded type
Type II: Superficial type — this is further divided into three subtypes:
   a. Elevated type — surfaces slightly elevated
   b. Flat type — no elevation in the surrounding mucosa
   c. Depressed type — the surface is slightly depressed
Type III: Excavated type

The incidence of submucosal invasion is higher with types IIc and III than with type IIa.

Superficial carcinoma (superficial spreading, surface carcinoma) is a rare form of gastric carcinoma. The gross pathologic appearance of this tumor is that of a slightly depressed or slightly thickened mucosa. These tumors are difficult to detect on gross specimens, and the diagnosis is made mainly by histologic methods. The majority of these tumors are found in the antrum and the tumor may be multicentric.

Although it has not been conclusively proven that early gastric carcinomas or superficial carcinomas eventually become advanced carcinomas, it is generally believed that gastric carcinoma starts as a mucosal lesion and later infiltrates below the submucosa and metastasizes distally.[66] The tumor frequently spreads to involve the celiac, periaortic, and subcrural lymph nodes. Local extension to involve the spleen, pancreas, kidneys, or liver may occur. Gastric carcinomas located in the fundus of the stomach may spread to involve the esophagus. Direct invasion of adjacent bowel loops causes fistula formation, especially to the colon. Seeding of the peritoneum may lead to metastasis to the pelvic cul de sac with development of a mass palpable by rectal examination — a peculiar characteristic of gastric carcinoma.[92] Widespread hematogenous metastases to the lung, brain, bone, and ovaries are very frequent. In general, most of these le-

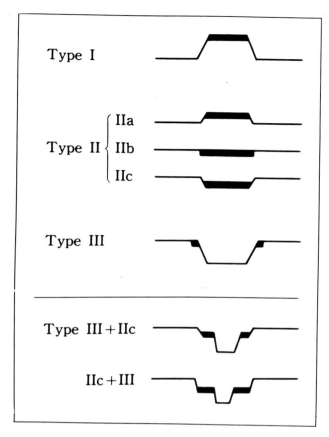

FIG. 13-1. Diagram of the classification of early gastric cancer.

sions are inoperable at the time of detection because of diffused dissemination.[92]

Lymphoma. Lymphomas are the second most common gastric malignancies, and the stomach is the most common site for primary lymphoma of the GI tract. Approximately 80% are of the non-Hodgkin's type and 20% are Hodgkin's type.[120] These tumors may be part of systemic lymphoma with involvement elsewhere in the body, or they may be primary. It is difficult to differentiate by radiographic or histologic means between the primary form of lymphoma originating in the stomach with metastasis elsewhere and the systemic form of lymphoma with secondary involvement of the stomach. However, it is considered to be primary in origin when it is the principal site of disease involvement. The primary form of gastric lymphoma without metastasis is associated with a high rate of curability.[8] The secondary form has a worse prognosis.

Gastric lymphoma may be confined to the stomach (so-called primary gastric lymphoma) or, as in 40% to 50% of cases, it may disseminate to the regional or mesenteric lymph nodes and appear as multiple abdominal masses (so-called secondary lymphoma). The tumor may also spread to the mediastinal lymph nodes, lungs, spleen, liver, kidneys, and bones in about 45% to 50% of patients.[122]

Leiomyosarcoma. Leiomyosarcomas account for 1% to 3% of all gastric malignancies[9,81] and gastric leiomyosarcoma constitutes 60% of all GI tract leiomyosarcomas. They are generally large, bulky, intramural masses that eventually fungate or ulcerate into the gastric lumen. Three histologic types are recognized: spindle cell, epithelioid, and pleomorphic. The histologic type of tumor is not related to the size, the grade of malignancy, or the location of the mass within the stomach.[81]

Leiomyosarcomas are generally large when detected, exhibiting both endogastric and exogastric extension. Twenty-five percent of these tumors spread primarily extrogastrically, with involvement of adjacent organs. Dissemination to the lungs, bones, and other organs may occasionally occur.[80]

Kaposi's sarcoma. Recently, there has been a rise in incidence of Kaposi's sarcoma among young homosexual males,[93] as well as among heterosexual patients. The reason for this sudden increase in frequency of this unusual tumor is still unclear. There are two clinical types of Kaposi's sarcoma. The first type occurs more frequently in elderly men with skin lesions predominately limited to the lower extremities. This type may not have visceral involvement and has a relatively good prognosis. The second type is a more virulent and aggressive systemic disease with generalized lymphadenopathy, hepatosplenomegaly, and anemia; it usually does not have skin manifestations.[93] The GI tract is commonly involved. The latter form has a worse prognosis; this is the form that is rising in incidence. In the early stages, this tumor may resemble simple hemangioma histologically. In the late stages, the tumor may show bundles of spindle-shaped cells in a matrix of vascular structures showing different degrees of differentiation with areas of local necrosis and fibrotic reaction. Focal masses in the submucosa and mucosa of the stomach may be recognized on gross inspection of the stomach and colon.[93]

Kaposi's sarcoma commonly involves the stomach and colon, but may also involve the esophagus and small bowel.[93] The lesions may be limited to one segment or multiple segments of the GI tract. Patients with GI tract involvement tend to have mesenteric or retroperitoneal lymph node involvement.

Other rare malignancies that may originate in the stomach include carcinoid tumors, squamous cell carcinomas, and leiomyoblastomas, liposarcomas, and neurogenic tumors.

Classification and Staging

The clinical-diagnostic classification of gastric carcinoma is based on the extent of disease in terms of three components: (1) T, which defines the degree of penetration of the stomach wall by the primary tumor; (2) N, which defines the extent of involvement of the regional lymph nodes; and (3) M, which defines the presence or absence of metastasis.[4]

T_{is} tumors are limited to the mucosa without penetration into the lamina propria as defined by the American Joint Committee Task Force. T_1 tumors are those which are limited to the mucosa or submucosa regardless of their location. A slight disagreement exists between this task force and the Japanese TNM Committee on this definition. The Japanese TNM Committee members include the area of stomach in which the tumor is located in the staging. T_2 tumors involve the mucosa, the submucosa, and extend to, but do not penetrate the serosa. T_3 tumors penetrate beyond the serosa, but do not invade contiguous organs. A T_{4a} tumor penetrates through the serosa and involves immediately adjacent tissue such as lesser omentum, perigastric fat, regional ligaments, greater omentum, transverse colon, spleen, esophagus or duodenum by way of intraluminal extension. A T_{4b} tumor penetrates through the serosa and involves the liver, diaphragm, pancreas, abdominal wall, adrenal glands, kidney, retroperitoneum, small intestine or esophagus, or duodenum by way of the serosa[4] (Table 13-1).

The major lymphatic channels draining the stomach are parallel to the left gastric artery, the splenic artery, and the hepatic artery. The first major station is the lymph nodes of the lesser curvature, the left gastropancreatic, juxtacardiac, gastroduodenal, gastropyloric, suprapyloric, and pancreatoduodenal, celiac, splenic, and hepatic areas. The second station is the lymph nodes of the periaortic, retropancreatic, and hepatoduodenal areas.

N_0 is defined as no regional lymph node involvement. N_1 is defined as involvement of perigastric lymph nodes within 3 cm of a primary tumor. N_2 is defined as nodal involvement more than 3 cm from the primary tumor. When the periaortic, hepatoduodenal, retropancreatic, and mesenteric nodes are involved, the tumor is classified as N_3.

Distant metastases are staged as M_0 (none known), or M_1 (present). The common sites of metastasis are liver, bone, supraclavicular lymph nodes, and lungs. N_x and M_x apply when minimum requirements to assess the nodal or mediastinal compartments cannot be met.

The clinical-diagnostic staging of gastric carcinoma is based on the TNM system (Figure 13-2; Table 13-2). While this staging system is useful for comparing large population groups, the practical preoperative staging of gastric cancer involves radiographic studies (upper GI series and CT scanning) and endoscopic examination.

Gastric lymphomas are staged similar to lymphomas in other parts of the body, depending upon the extent of regional or distant nodal groups or extralymphatic organ involvement. The TNM system is not suitable for staging lymphomas because of ambiguity with respect to the tumor (T) and node (N) categories. The staging and classification of lymphomas are further explained in the lymphoma chapter.

No staging system has been developed for leiomyosarcomas or Kaposi's sarcomas because of the rarity of these tumors.

Imaging Procedures and Assessment

The major imaging procedures used to detect gastric malignancy are barium radiographic studies and fiberoptic endoscopy because the mucosal and luminal portion of the tumor is best demonstrated by these techniques. Computed tomography is used to stage the tumor once the tumor has been discovered.

Single-contrast and double-contrast upper GI radiography are the primary imaging modalities most widely used for the detection and diagnosis of gastric carcinoma and lymphoma.[85] Although the double-contrast study has been found to have a high diagnostic accuracy, the error rate in one study was found to be significantly reduced when both single-contrast and double-contrast studies were performed.[74] It is important to note, however, that early gastric carcinoma is only detectable by the double-contrast technique.

Technique. The technique of the double-contrast study is described in detail by Maruyama.[66] Special attention to the technique is needed for the evaluation of the stomach in order to detect early gastric carcinoma. About 100 to 200 mL or high-density barium is required to optimally coat the stomach. Effervescent tablets or granules are given orally to obtain gaseous distention of the stomach. Multiple positional changes and multiple filming projections are used to obtain double-contrast views of all parts of the stomach. The single-contrast technique may be added at the end of the double-contrast evaluation, with additional amounts of dilute barium given to distend the stomach. Films are taken with the patient in the prone position with compression to better demonstrate a small ulcer or small shallow depression in the antrum and lesser curvature of the stomach.

Accuracy of Upper Gastrointestinal Series. The sensitivity of the single-contrast or double-contrast studies in detecting various lesions involving the stomach and duodenum is reported to be 70% to 75%.[74] However, the sensitivity for the combination of both procedures is 81% to 84%, which is significantly greater than that of either procedure alone.[74] The specificity for the proce-

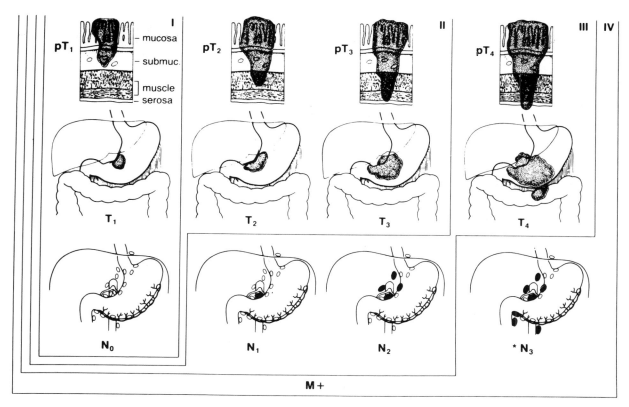

FIG. 13-2. Modified AJC anatomic staging for gastric carcinoma. Tumor (T) categories: This is essentially a postsurgical classification, although with new tumor imaging techniques, it may be possible to determine the depth of penetration. Progression
is through layers of viscera, mucosa, and submucosa, muscle, serosa, and contiguous structures. Node (N) categories: The
distance of nodes from a primary site is used; less than 3 cm or greater than 3 cm (N_1 v N_2) in regional nodal areas of the
lesser and greater curvature; juxtaregional nodes are N_3. Stage grouping: T category determines stage. Positive nodes are stage
III as long as they are resectable (N_1–N_3). Stage IV applies to metastases and unresectable lymph nodes (N_3). AJC v UICC
classification: Differences relate to clinical T categories only. T_1 is similar, but the T_2 and T_3 of the UICC system refer to
occupying more than half of one region or an entire region with deep infiltration that is not defined. T_4 involves more than
one region and invasion to a contiguous structure. The UICC-TNM system[47] is identical to the AJC system[4] and both are
postsurgical. N categories and stage groupings are similar. (Modified from Morton, J. M., Poulter, C. A., Pandya, K. J.: Alimentary tract cancer. In *Clinical Oncology for Medical Students and Physicians: A Multidisciplinary Approach*, 6th ed. Rubin,
P. (Ed.). New York, American Cancer Society, 1983, pp. 154–176. With permission.)

Table 13-1. Tumor (T), Node (N) Classification — Stomach Cancer.

T_{is}	Carcinoma in situ
T_1/pT_1	Mucosa or submucosa only
T_2	Deep invasion $\leq 1/2$ region
pT_2	Extension to serosa
T_3	Deep invasion $> 1/2$ region
pT_3	Extension through serosa
T_4/pT_4	Extension outside stomach
T_{4a}	Immediate tissues
T_{4b}	Other organs
$N_{1/2}$	Regional (operable) nodes
N_3	Other intra-abdominal nodes usually not removed or not removable

p = Pathologic (postsurgical) stage

American Joint Committee on Cancer: *Manual for Staging of Cancer*,
2nd ed. Philadelphia, J. B. Lippincott, 1983. (Modified).

Table 13.2 Stage Grouping — Stomach Cancer

Stage 0	T_{is}	N_0	M_0
Stage I	T_1	N_0	M_0
Stage II	T_2, T_3	N_0	M_0
Stage III	T_1, T_2, T_3	N_1, N_2	M_0
	T_{4a}	N_0, N_1, N_2	M_0
Stage IV	T_1, T_2, T_3	N_3	M_0
	T_{4b}	Any N	M_0
	Any T	Any N	M_1

American Joint Committee on Cancer: *Manual for Staging of Cancer*,
2nd ed. Philadelphia, J. B. Lippincott, 1983.

dures is approximately 90% using endoscopy as a standard.[74] The most common source of error in UGI studies has been shown to be a result of improper techniques, such as an inadequate number of films, residual food material in the stomach, poor coating of stomach by the barium, and over- or underpenetration of the patients.[35]

The accuracy of UGI studies is significantly improved in detecting gastric malignancy. If a lesion is considered to be definitely malignant by radiographic criteria, it has a greater than 95% chance of being malignant.[97,105] The false-negative rate, however, for diagnosing gastric malignancy by UGI studies has been reported to be as high as 25%.[97]

Japanese investigators have been very successful in using the double-contrast technique for diagnosing early gastric cancer. Their accuracy rate has been reported to be as high as 86%.[66]

Angiography. Angiography has also been used in the diagnosis of gastric malignancies. Angiography helps to define the vascular supply, the vascularity, and the extraluminal extent of tumors. However, this imaging modality has been largely replaced by other modalities such as CT and endoscopy.

Ultrasound. Some investigators have suggested that ultrasound be used as a complementary imaging technique after standard UGI radiography for the detection of gastric malignancies.[52,111,120] When patients are discovered to have a palpable mass in the left upper quadrant, an ultrasonogram is frequently requested. Ultrasound may be able to demonstrate a solid mass contiguous with the stomach or thickening of the gastric wall, which would lead to an upper GI study. The sonographic evidence of a malignant gastric mass is an ovoid anechoic mass with dense central echogenicity. This appearance is not specific, however, and may be seen with carcinoma, lymphoma, leiomyosarcoma, or granulomatous disease. Likewise, diffuse thickening of the gastric wall demonstrated by ultrasonography is nonspecific.

Endoscopy. Fiberoptic endoscopy has been advocated as the screening procedure for gastric malignancy because of its ability to visually demonstrate a lesion as well as to obtain a biopsy specimen of it.[104] The technique of endoscopy and complete endoscopic description of gastric tumor are beyond the scope of this chapter. In general, some malignant ulcers cannot be differentiated from benign ulcers on the basis of gross appearance. The irregularity of the margin and the asymmetry of the adjacent folds are features suggestive of malignancy. The endoscopic appearance of gastric carcinoma may also be similar to gastric lymphoma, which may be that of an erosive, hemorrhagic gastritis superimposed on large rugal folds, polypoid lesions, ulcerative lesions, or a com-

bination of the above. The diagnosis can only be confirmed by histologic examination of biopsy specimens. The endoscopic findings of the absence of mucosal folds and the failure of the stomach to distend with air suggest "linitus plastica."[9]

The accuracy of endoscopy in the detection of gastric malignancy is 90% to 95%, which is higher than that of radiography. This accuracy rate is a function of visualization, biopsy, and brush cytology.[55] The accuracy is approximately 100% for diagnosing exophytic lesions; however, it is less than 80% for infiltrating or ulcerating lesions. Lesions located in the body or cardia of the stomach are more likely to be missed by endoscopy.[55,115,117]

Computed Tomography. Recently, CT has been used to examine patients with gastric carcinoma and lymphoma and has been found to be highly accurate and cost effective in the staging of gastric malignancies.[5,12,25,61,77] The method of staging gastric carcinoma by CT has been described by Moss et al.[77] and Lee et al.[61] In preparation for the CT scan, patients are only allowed to ingest water from midnight until the scans are performed in the morning. A 1% to 2% solution of meglumine diatrizoate (Gastrografin, 480 mL) is given to patients to drink approximately 30 minutes before the CT scan. In addition, 250 to 450 mL of the same mixture is administered orally five minutes before the CT examination. The large volumes of oral contrast are needed to adequately distend the stomach. The scans are taken at l-cm intervals from the dome of the diaphragm to the umbilicus with the patient in the supine position. Prone or lateral decubitus scans are obtained to distend the antrum with contrast material. Glucagon may be given intravenously to delay gastric emptying and increase distension of the stomach.

In assessing the extent of gastric carcinoma, the stomach is analyzed by a radiographic imaging technique for gastric wall thickness, ulcerations, and the presence of intraluminal masses, extramural extension, and regional and distant metastasis. Based on these CT findings, the gastric carcinomas are classified into one of four stages. These stages are not related to the stages established by the American Joint Commission for Staging of Gastric Carcinoma.

Radiologic Stage I: The presence of an intraluminal mass without gastric wall thickening and without any evidence of metastasis or tumor extension into the adjacent organs; the normal gastric wall thickness should be less than 1 cm.

Radiologic Stage II: The gastric wall is thicker than 1 cm but without any evidence of metastasis or direct tumor extension (Figure 13-3).

This staging system helps in preoperative management and planning. Since the CT scan can demonstrate the presence of metastases to the liver or kidneys, other imaging modalities such as liver/spleen scans and excretory urograms may be replaced by this single imaging modality.

Computed tomographic scanning is also accurate in the staging of gastric lymphomas (Figure 13-6), since the

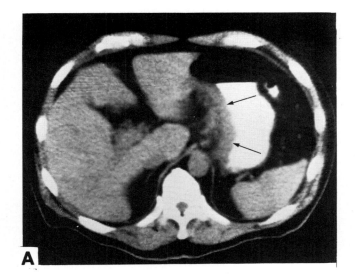

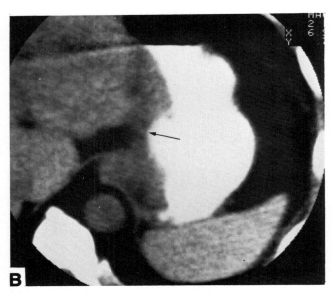

FIG. 13-3. Stage II gastric carcinoma. (A) Notice thickening of the wall along the lesser curvature of the stomach (arrows) in this patient who has undergone a CT scan for staging purposes. (B) Magnified view of the stomach demonstrates a shallow ulceration (arrow).

Radiologic Stage III: There is a thickening of the gastric wall with direct extension of the tumor into adjacent organs or lymph nodes but without any evidence of distant metastasis (Figure 13-4).

Radiologic Stage IV: There is thickening of the gastric wall along with the presence of distant metastasis; direct extension of the tumor into adjacent organs or regional lymph nodes may or may not be present (Figure 13-5)

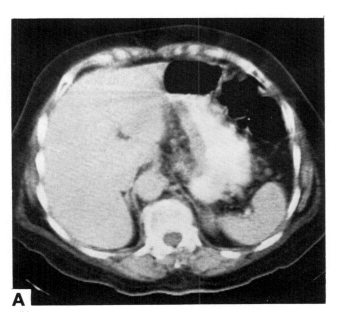

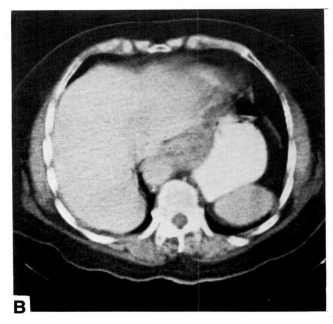

FIG. 13-4. Stage III gastric carcinoma. (A) CT scan shows thickening of the wall of the lesser curvature of the stomach. Also note densities surrounding the stomach which are consistent with adenopathy in the perigastric area extending through the liver. (B) A lesser curvature mass extending to the liver, obliterating the perigastric and subhepatic space.

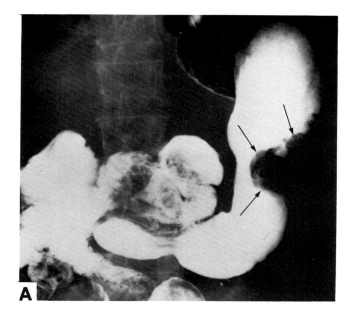

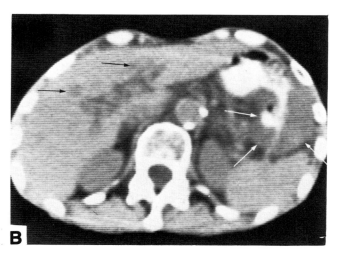

FIG. 13-5. Stage IV gastric carcinoma. (A) Upper GI series shows an ulcerating mass of the greater curvature (arrows). (B) CT scan shows irregularly thickened gastric wall (white arrows) with a small ulceration. In addition, liver metastases are present (black arrows).

CT scan can accurately depict the thickness of the gastric wall and the presence of adenopathy in the regional or retroperitoneal groups.[12,25] In addition, CT can accurately depict the presence of exogastric masses in patients with leiomyosarcomas (Figures 13-7, 13-8)[16] and mesenteric and retroperitoneal lymphadenopathy in patients with Kaposi's sarcomas (Figure 13-9).[93]

Imaging Strategies and Decisions

Screening. The mass screening technique employed by the Japanese to detect early gastric cancer is not necessary in the United States, since the incidence of gastric

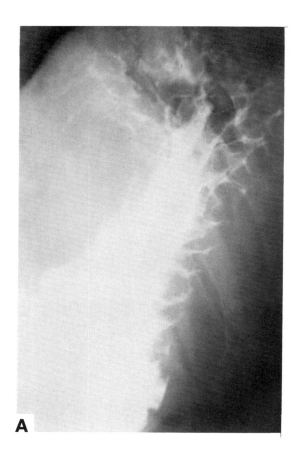

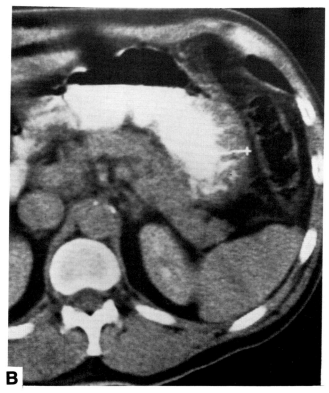

FIG. 13-6. Gastric lymphoma with large folds. (A) Prominent folds in this patient with lymphoma of the stomach. (B) CT scan of the same patient demonstrates marked thickening of the wall of the stomach.

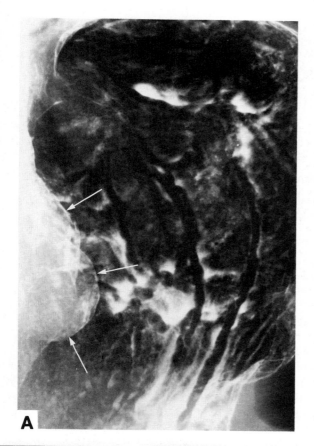

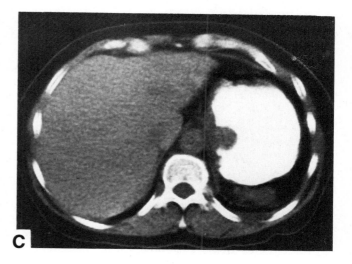

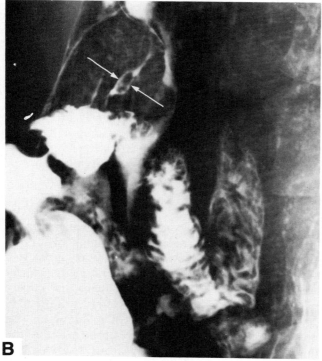

FIG. 13-7. Gastric leiomyosarcoma. (A) A large, smooth tumor projecting into the lumen near the fundus of the stomach has smooth obtuse margins with the gastric walls (arrows). (B) When seen en face (arrows), a central ulceration is present. (C) A CT scan shows the lesion projecting into the gastric lumen.

carcinoma and gastric lymphoma is so low. However, certain patients may be considered at greater risk of developing gastric carcinoma; these include patients who have type A blood or pernicious anemia, who are recent immigrants from high risk countries, who have relatives with gastric carcinoma, who have chronic gastritis, chronic gastric ulcers, or gastric adenomatous polyps, or who have a history of long-term exposure to asbestos or polyvinyl chloride. From the experience gained by the Japanese in screening large numbers of patients with double-contrast radiography for early detection of gastric carcinoma, it seems reasonable that those patients who are suspected of having a gastric malignancy should first be subjected to a good quality double-contrast upper GI examination (Table 13-3). If a lesion is discovered but the signs are not those of classic gastric cancer, the patient should be further examined by fiberoptic endoscopy in

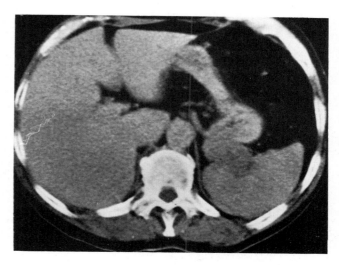

FIG. 13-8. Leiomyosarcoma. A CT scan demonstrates a large extraluminal mass extending from the fundus of the stomach to the spleen.

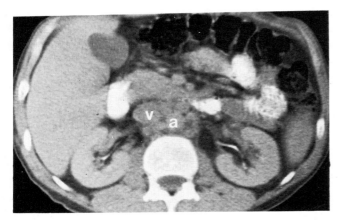

FIG. 13-9. A CT scan of abdominal adenopathy associated with Kaposi's sarcoma. The enlarged lymph nodes surround the aorta (a) and inferior vena cava (v).

Table 13-3. Modalities of Choice for Detecting
Early Gastric Cancer

Double Contrast UGI
↓
Endoscopy with Biopsy
↓
Surgery

The screening examination for detection of early gastric cancer is the double-contrast upper GI examination, or, alternatively, upper GI endoscopy. When a lesion is discovered, it must be biopsied for confirmation of malignancy before surgical resection is performed.

Table 13-4. Modalities of Choice for Detecting
Advanced Gastric Cancer

Single or Double-Contrast UGI
↓
Endoscopy with Biopsy

CT
Liver and Abdomen

Chemotherapy   Surgery

Either single-contrast or double-contrast upper GI radiography is the screening examination for the detection of advanced gastric cancer. Endoscopy and biopsy of the lesion provide confirmation of malignancy. If the tumor has produced gastric obstruction or significant hemorrhage, then surgical excision is indicated immediately. However, in less urgent situations, CT scanning may be performed to determine the presence of hepatic and regional lymph node metastases, as well as determination of the extent of the gastric tumor (invasion of splenic hilum, pancreas, transverse mesocolon). The information from the CT scan is useful in planning the surgical approach or, alternatively, occasionally in recommending chemotherapy rather than surgery in clearly inoperable cases.

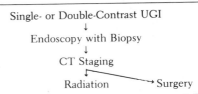

Table 13-5. Modalities of Choice for Detecting Gastric Lymphoma

Single- or Double-Contrast UGI
↓
Endoscopy with Biopsy
↓
CT Staging
↓
Radiation   → Surgery

For evaluation of gastric lymphoma, an upper GI series, either single- or double-contrast, is useful in demonstrating the enlarged gastric folds, ulcerating masses, or nodules characteristic of gastric lymphoma. The diagnosis may be confirmed by obtaining tissue from a mass or nodule using endoscopic biopsy technique. A CT scan should be performed to stage the extent of lymphomatous involvement of the stomach, as well as to detect evidence of abdominal adenopathy.

order to biopsy the lesion. If adequate double-contrast radiography cannot be obtained, then endoscopy should be the first examination. If advanced gastric cancer is suspected, a single-contrast or double-contrast upper GI examination should first be performed, followed by endoscopy with biopsy if tissue is needed for preoperative confirmation (Table 13-4). If the gastric malignancy has not produced partial obstruction or hemorrhage and surgical intervention is considered for cure rather than palliation, then the next step may be a CT scan for staging purposes. If the radiographic studies are normal and the presence of malignancy is strongly suspected because of the patient's history or the clinical findings, the patient should be examined by fiberoptic endoscopy.

Gastric lymphoma is most often detected by single-contrast or double-contrast upper GI examination. However, since many of the radiographic features of gastric lymphoma are not specific for that condition, upper GI endoscopy and biopsy of a visible tumor or of large folds may be necessary (Table 13-5). Occasionally, even endoscopy and biopsy fail to be diagnostic. Computed tomography may be useful in characterizing the size and extent of a tumor, and, more importantly, may act as a method of obtaining histologic material for diagnosis via a CT-guided needle biopsy.

Staging. After diagnosis by contrast examination and endoscopy with biopsy, preoperative staging is possible with CT scanning. It may not be necessary if obstruction or hemorrhage is present, however, because surgery will be necessary to address these problems, and surgery will permit intraoperative staging. However, if immediate surgery is not required, then CT scanning may be useful in providing information about the extent of the tumor and possible surgical approaches. If the patient is in the stage III category, a CT-guided biopsy of the suspicious lesion in the liver or other contiguous organ or enlarged lymph nodes may be needed for proper staging.

Preoperative staging with CT may be particularly use-

Table 13-6. Modalities for Evaluating Carcinoma of the Gastrointestinal Tract

MODALITY	STAGING CAPABILITY	BENEFIT/ COST RATIO	RECOMMENDED ROUTINE STAGING PROCEDURE
Noninvasive			
Chest X-ray films	Good for detecting metastases	High	Yes
Bone films	Useful only for confirming metastases	Low	No
Double-contrast upper GI studies	Very useful in detecting early gastric CA	High	Yes—should be performed along with single-contrast studies
Single-contrast upper GI studies	Useful in detecting and defining primary advanced lesions in stomach	High	Yes—should be performed with double-contrast studies
Small bowel follow-through	Useful in detecting and defining primary lesions in the small bowel	High	Yes
Double-contrast barium enema	Very useful in detecting and defining primary lesions in the colon	High	Yes
Single-contrast barium enema	Less sensitive than double-contrast study in detecting polyps	High	No. Should be used in patients unable to cooperate in double-contrast study
Radionuclide studies liver-spleen, brain, and bone scans	Useful in evaluation of clinically suspected metastases. CT is better than RN scans for liver and brain	Low	No
Ultrasound	May be able to detect primary lesions appearing as abdominal masses. May also be able to detect abdominal metastases	Fair	No
MRI	Unknown at present	?	?
Minimally Invasive			
Enteroclysis	Useful in detecting and defining primary and metastatic lesions when SBFT is negative	High	May be used as substitute for small bowel follow-through. Requires passage of small bowel tube
CT	Invasive if IV contrast is used. Most valuable of all modalities for determining local invasion and distant metastases	High	Yes
Invasive			
Percutaneous biopsy guided by imaging techniques—usually CT	Accurate technique for staging the tumor	High	No. Only in selective cases
Arteriography	Useful in defining vascular supply and vascularity of neoplasms	Low	No
Gastroscopy	Very accurate modality for detecting and defining primary lesions	High	Yes. If used to confirm lesion detected on UGI series and to screen high-risk patients
Colonoscopy	Very accurate modality for detecting and defining primary lesions	High	Yes, if used to confirm lesion detected on BE or to screen high-risk populations

ful in planning radiation ports and field size for radiation therapy of primary gastric lymphomas.

Benefit versus Cost. The benefit versus cost of various imaging modalities is summarized in Table 13-6.

Imaging Strategies by Tumor Types

Early cancer. The earliest radiographic evidence of gastric carcinoma on a single-contrast UGI study includes localized areas of irregularity in the contour and rigidity of the stomach wall. The early phase of gastric cancer is rarely recognized on single-contrast studies. It is most difficult to detect small areas of irregularity in the fundus and body of the stomach on single-contrast roentgenograms. However, the absence of active motility observed fluoroscopically may suggest the presence of a tumor. Lesions located on the anterior or posterior wall at the gastric angulus or in the pyloric area may also influence the gastric motility.

When the double-contrast technique is used, irregularities of the mucosal pattern seen en face are early signs of gastric carcinoma. Early gastric cancers in the phase detected by double-contrast radiography rarely produce evidence of motility abnormalities. The demonstration of a slightly depressed area in the double-contrast study with an irregular margin suggests the presence of early superficial depressed cancer, type IIc (Figure 13-10). Converging folds often surround the depressed area ending at the edge of the depression. This type of lesion is very difficult to demonstrate if it is located on the anterior wall. Double-contrast studies in the prone position may

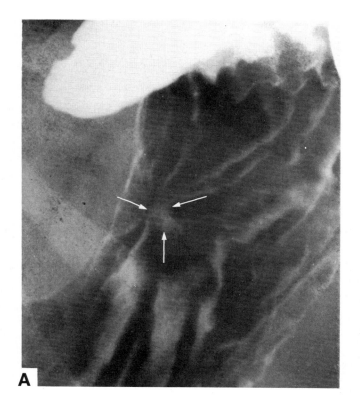

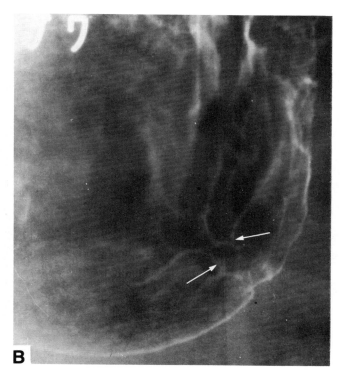

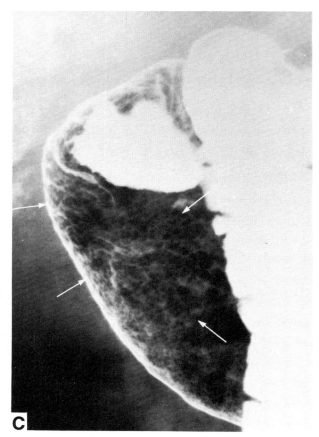

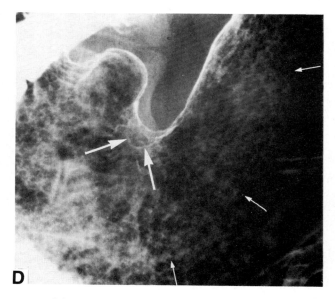

FIG. 13-10. Examples of early gastric cancer. (A) Type IIc. A shallow depression along with converging folds is visible in the posterior gastric wall adjacent to the lesser curvature of the stomach in this double contrast study (arrows). Some of the folds are enlarged at the ulcer margin, indicating malignant infiltration. (B) Type IIa + IIc. Irregularities of the gastric wall with a shallow depression are visible along the greater cur-vature of the stomach (arrows) along with a nodular surface pattern. (C) Type IIa gastric cancer. A large area with a coarse nodular pattern is visible along the greater curvature of the antrum of the stomach on this double-contrast study (arrows). (D) Type IIa + IIc early gastric cancer. A shallow raised plaquelike mass (large arrows) is present at the angulus along with diffuse plaquelike elevation of the mucosa surround-ing this area (small arrows). Irregular areas of barium between these zones of elevation are the shallow depressions of Type IIc.

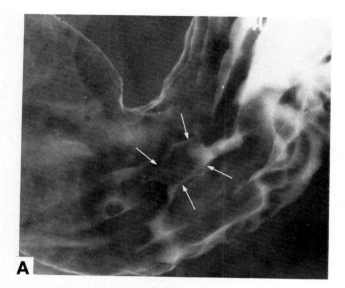

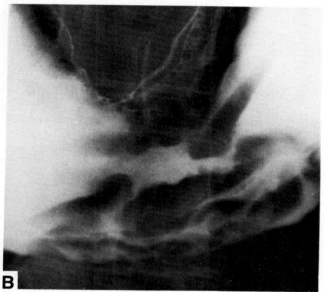

FIG. 13-11. Type III early gastric cancer. (A) A shallow ulceration is visible on the anterior wall of the stomach on this supine view of a double-contrast study (arrows). Note the prominent folds surrounding the ulcerations. (B) A prone view of the stomach shows barium pooling in this ulcer.

be needed to demonstrate it. The presence of a benign ulcer adjacent to the cancerous lesion is a frequent cause of clinical symptoms in a patient with type IIc lesions.[34] Graded distension of the stomach with air and barium is needed to demonstrate a depressed malignant lesion adjacent to a benign ulcer.

Type IIb lesions may be detected by a slight irregularity in the contour with a surrounding area of nodularity created by reaction of adjacent mucosa. It is very difficult to differentiate such a lesion from the scarring secondary to peptic ulcer disease, which is much more

common than type IIb cancer. Endoscopy with biopsy is often required to demonstrate this type of lesion.[34]

The superficial spreading type of carcinoma, also classified in the Japanese classification as type IIa (Figure 13-10), is usually seen in double-contrast studies as a patch of slight nodularity altering the normal surface mucosal pattern of the stomach without significant loss in the elasticity of the wall.[34] This type of lesion is best diagnosed by cytologic evaluation of the contents of fluid obtained by gastric lavage.[9]

Polyp-like type I lesions or the less prominent type IIa lesions can usually be detected by external compression of the barium-filled stomach or by the double-contrast technique. Because these findings are subtle, endoscopy is needed to confirm the presence of malignancy.

Early ulcerated cancer, type III (Figure 13-11), is very difficult to differentiate from a benign ulcer. The presence of an irregular shape of the ulcer niche in the mucosa with surrounding nodularity and without the presence of a uniform ulcer collar suggests the presence of a malignancy (Figure 13-12).[34] Significant rigidity surrounding the cancer may not always be present. Detection of Hampton's line is an important diagnostic aid in differentiating benign from malignant ulcers. Multiple endoscopically directed biopsies in the area of ulceration may be needed to help in differentiating benign from malignant ulcers.

Advanced gastric carcinoma. The detection of advanced gastric carcinoma is relatively easy compared with detec-

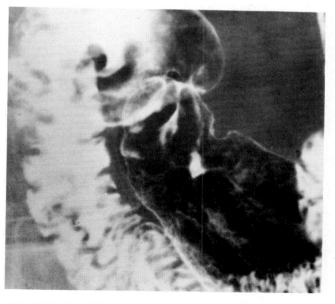

FIG. 13-12. Type III early gastric cancer with nodular folds. A small shallow ulceration is seen in the posterior wall of the antrum. A distinguishing feature of this ulcer is the presence of prominent nodular and blunted folds surrounding the shallow depression.

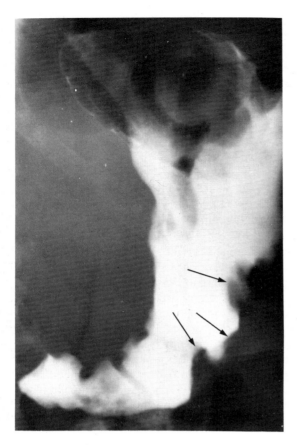

FIG. 13-13. A typical radiographic demonstration of advanced carcinoma appearing as a large mass in the greater curvature with a large, eccentrically placed ulceration (arrows).

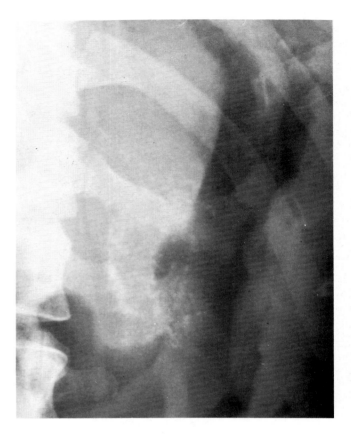

FIG. 13-15. Mucinous adenocarcinoma. A plain film of the left upper quadrant of the abdomen demonstrates multiple stippled calcifications in a mass along the lesser curvature of the stomach.

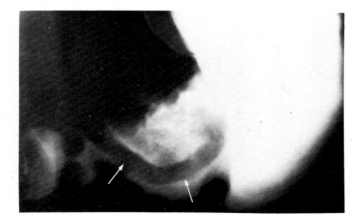

FIG. 13-14. This large ulcerating advanced antral adenocarcinoma demonstrates a Carmen's meniscus sign, with the tumor margin (arrows) separating barium in the ulcerating mass from that in the antral lumen.

tion of early gastric carcinoma. The classic radiographic signs of advanced gastric carcinoma are rigidity, intraluminal filling defects, and amputation of folds with or without ulceration or stenosis (Figure 13-13). An early classification of gastric carcinoma by Shirakabe and Maruyama[103] recognizes a large intraluminal mass as type I, ulceration of varying sizes and extents as types II and III, and diffuse infiltrating tumors as type IV. This classification currently is not often used. In western literature, it is recognized that type IV tumors—the diffuse infiltrating tumors—have a worse prognosis than the other types, which are associated with a mass. In general, the single-contrast study is as accurate as the double-contrast technique in demonstrating advanced gastric carcinoma except for the diffuse infiltrating form. The "Carmen's meniscus" sign (Figure 13-14) is still useful in the diagnosis of a large ulcerating cancer with a mass projecting into the lumen and a large central ulceration. Advanced gastric carcinoma may occasionally be associated with enlarged gastric rugae, presumably because of tumor infiltration and associated edema.

It is difficult to differentiate a large, advanced, proliferating, fungating gastric carcinoma from lymphoma or

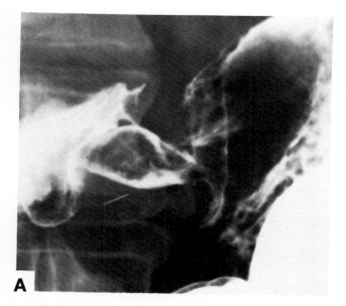

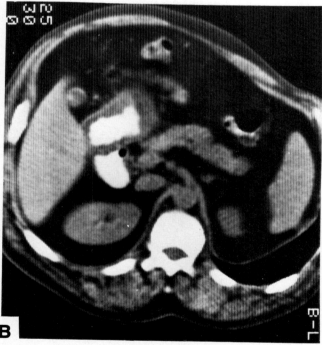

trative form of gastric carcinoma. This appearance is rarely seen in sarcoma of the stomach, but may be encountered in gastric syphilis, tuberculosis, eosinophilic gastroenteritis, Crohn's disease, caustic ingestion, or metastatic carcinoma from the breast.

The demonstration of a carcinoma in the gastric stump (Figure 13-17) following partial gastrectomy may be difficult, since complete filling of the remaining stomach is not always possible. Demonstration of rigidity is also difficult because of a lack of autonomous motility in the stump. The typical gastric cancer occurring in the remaining gastric pouch produces narrowing, lack of distensibility, enlarged folds, and occasionally a well-defined intraluminal mass, usually in the region of the anastomosis. Malignant lesions may be simulated by granulomatous changes in the suture site at the anastomosis.[39] The double-contrast technique is the best technique for detecting gastric stump lesions,[37,38] but gastroscopy with biopsy is indicated in all patients with clinical suspicion of cancer in the gastric stump.[79] Since CT may be able to demonstrate the presence of a mass in the remaining stomach, CT may be used to detect as well as to stage a carcinoma in a gastric stump (Figure 13-18).

FIG. 13-16. (A) Scirrhous adenocarcinoma of the antrum of the stomach. Note the marked narrowing of the antrum, producing the appearance of a pseudo-elongated pyloric channel. (B) A CT scan shows a diffusely thickened antral wall.

leiomyosarcoma purely on radiographic criteria because the presence of a large mass with ulceration is not specific. The presence of calcification in the tumor indicates a mucinous adenocarcinoma (Figure 13-15). Curvilinear calcification may occasionally be seen in leiomyosarcoma.

An area of rigidity encasing and narrowing the entire stomach wall in at least one region is highly characteristic of scirrhous carcinoma (Figure 13-16)—the infil-

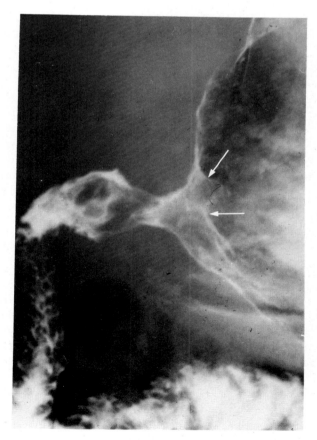

FIG. 13-17. Recurrent gastric carcinoma of the anastomotic zone of a Billroth I resection, producing narrowing and raised tumor margin (arrows).

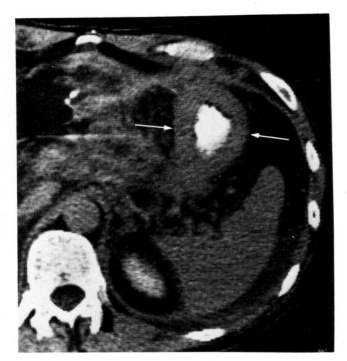

FIG. 13-18. A CT scan of recurrent tumor of the gastric pouch of a Billroth II type gastrectomy. Note the marked thickening of the wall of the gastric remnant (arrows). The patient had a partial gastrectomy for benign ulcer disease 10 years before this CT scan.

Lymphoma. Lymphoma typically produces enlarged gastric rugae because of diffuse infiltration of the wall (Figures 13-6, 13-19). Often the enlarged folds do not lose their pliability. When the antrum is involved, transpyloric extension into the duodenum occurs in approximately 5% to 33% of cases, which is considerably more frequent than adenocarcinoma. Lymphomas may also appear as multiple small nodules studding the mucosal surface (Figure 13-20) or as large ulcerating masses (Figure 13-19B).

Leiomyosarcoma. The majority of the leiomyosarcomas appear as submucosal masses (Figures 13-7, 13-8). These masses are predominately exogastric. Ulcerations are present on the luminal side in 60% of the lesions. Most of the ulcers are small, but a few are large and excavating, occasionally perforating into the chest or peritoneal cavity.[81]

Kaposi's sarcoma. The radiographic findings of Kaposi's sarcoma involving the stomach are those of multiple sessile polyps or submucosal nodules of varying sizes. Ulceration may be seen in the center of these lesions, simulating the appearance of melanoma metastatic to the stomach.[93]

Treatment Decisions[14,21]

Carcinoma. Approximately 80% of all the gastric carcinomas are considered to be operable. Indeed, surgical philosophy stresses the need for surgical removal of a tumor if possible.[69] However, only 50% of all the gastric carcinomas are considered to be resectable at the time of surgery.[17] Of the total number of patients with gastric carcinomas, only 30% actually undergo a curative type of surgery. Since gross gastric carcinoma is generally not responsive to radiation or chemotherapy, both modes have been tried together in a combined modality approach and in adjuvant settings where there is microscopic disease; these techniques have met with limited success (Table 13-7).

Surgery. The location of the tumor is important for determining the type of surgical procedure to be performed. If the tumor is located in the antropyloric region, which is the most common location,[92] a Bilroth II type of op-

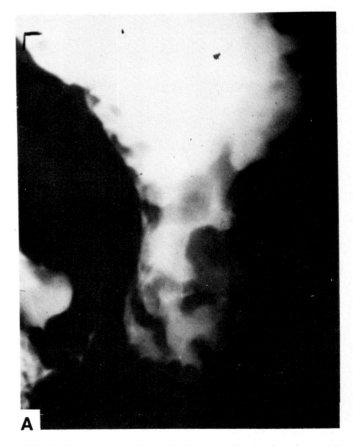

A

FIG. 13-19. Common radiographic features of gastric lymphoma. (A) Large folds. A single-contrast study of the stomach demonstrates prominent folds with multiple mass impression of the stomach. (B) An ulcerating mass is visible here on the greater curvature.

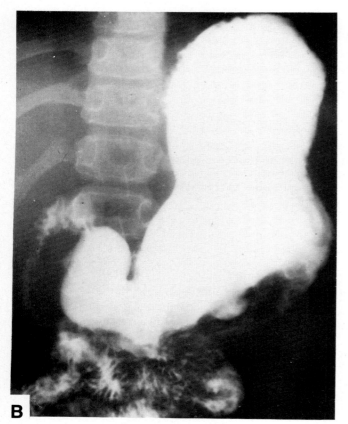

B

FIG. 13-19, continued.

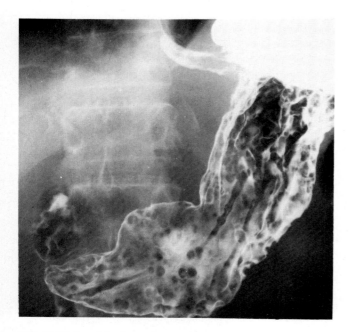

FIG. 13-20. A nodular form of gastric lymphoma with a multiple nodular-polypoid filling defect is visible on this double-contrast view of the stomach.

eration may be performed. A radical subtotal gastrectomy—resection of the distal stomach, greater and lesser curvature, omentum, nodes draining the stomach and spleen—may also be performed for tumors involving the distal half of the stomach.[13] The operative mortality for this procedure is less than 5%.[17] Four fifths of the patients who have undergone curative surgery for antropyloric types of lesions die within five years.

For diffuse infiltrating carcinomas, a total gastrectomy is needed. This type of surgery is associated with a high operative mortality of 20% or more and a low cure rate of 0% to 15%.[17] The five-year survival rate for this type of tumor, if there is no nodal involvement, is about 50%. If there is nodal involvement, however, the five-year survival is less than 10%. If there is no nodal involvement, the degree of mucosal penetration is also important in terms of prognostic significance. If the lesion is restricted to the mucosa, the five-year survival rate is about 85%. However, when there is penetration of the serosa, the five-year survival rate is 15%.[17]

For tumors that are located in the fundus, cardia, or gastroesophageal junction, resection of the tumor requires either a laparotomy or thoracotomy or both approaches. This procedure is associated with a variably high percentage of postoperative morbidity and mortality (6% to 41%).[113] The cardia and the lower esophagus are resected and continuity is usually restored with an esophagogastrostomy or a colonic-interposition procedure. The major postoperative complications are mediastinitis from leakage at the anastomosis and stenosis of the anastomosis.

In those patients who are considered to have nonresectable disease, a palliative resection may be performed. However, there is a 20% operative mortality associated with this type of surgery.

Computed tomographic staging of gastric carcinoma helps to determine the type of surgery required for the patient and may influence the decision not to perform surgery if the patient is considered to have nonoperable disease on the basis of CT (Table 13-7).

Radiation therapy. Unresectable carcinomas causing obstruction or hemorrhage are unlikely to respond to radiation therapy, particularly since the radiosensitivity of surrounding structures such as the stomach, small bowel, and the liver limit the total dose that can be delivered. There are, however, two new concepts whereby the therapeutic ratio may be more favorable for the treatment of microscopic residuum or small deposits.

A carefully shaped field to treat the microresiduum after surgery has been recommended by Gunderson and Sosin[40] based upon the patterns of failure found at elective second-look operations. There is a high tendency for local or regional recurrence to take place in the tumor bed area without remote metastases. The original gas-

Table 13.7. Treatment Decisions: Stomach Cancers[76]

STAGE	SURGERY	RADIATION THERAPY	CHEMOTHERAPY
I (T_1,N_0,M_0)	Radical subtotal gastrectomy and regional lymph nodes	NR	NR
II (T_2,N_0,M_0,T_3,N_0,M_0)	Radical subtotal gastrectomy and regional lymph nodes	NR	NR
III (T_3,N_{1-3},M_0)	Radical subtotal gastrectomy and regional lymph nodes	Postoperative RT	Investigational MAC
IV (T_4,N_3,M_0) (T_4,N_3,M_1, Metastatic)	Radical subtotal gastrectomy and regional lymph nodes and resection of contiguous organs involved if possible	Postoperative RT Palliative RT for selected sites	MAC as FAM
V (Relapse and recurrence)	Palliative if feasible	Palliative RT if feasible	MAC as FAM

NR = not recommended
RT = radiation therapy
MAC = multiagent chemotherapy
FAM = 5-Fluorouacil, doxorubicin, and mitomycin-c

tric barium study and CT examination for oncologic imaging are required to accurately shape this field (Figure 13-21). A dose of 4,500–5,100 cGy is used over 4 to 5 weeks.

Intraoperative treatment has been successfully pioneered by the Japanese.[1] In this technique, the surgeon identifies the residuum after resection and assists the radiotherapist in the placement of a high-energy electron beam cone into the wound, displacing bowel. An intense tumor dose of 1,500–2,000 cGy is delivered in one exposure to the tumor bed. This technique has led to an improvement in five-year survival.

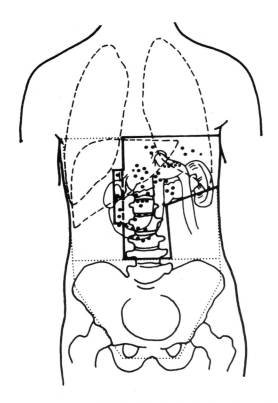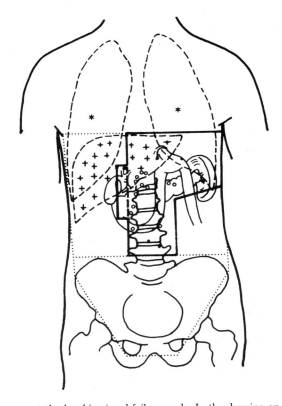

FIG. 13-21. The solid black circles (in the drawing on the left) represent the local/regional failures only. In the drawing on the right are the patterns of failure for both distant liver metastases (+), coupled with lymph node failures ($\bigcirc$). The asterisk (*) represents lung metastases. Encompassing the local/regional failures of both groups (left and right) is a newly designed radiation field that covers the most likely sites of failure following gastrectomy in carcinoma of the stomach. (Reprinted from Gunderson, L. L., Sosin, H.: Adenocarcinoma of the stomach: Areas of failure in a reoperation series (second or symptomatic look) clinicopathologic correlation and implications for adjuvant therapy. *Int. J. Radiot. Oncol. Biol. Phys.* 8:1–2, 1982. With permission.)

Chemotherapy.[7,14] There are some effective combinations of chemotherapy that produce response rates of 30% to 60%. These usually contain 5-fluorouracil (5-FU), which by itself is generally ineffective. The various combinations include cyclohexylchloroethylnitrosurea (CCNU), mitomycin-c, Adriamycin, and cytosine arabinoside. The combination most favored is 5-FU, Adriamycin, and mitomycin-c (FAM).[11] This has been used in settings of both recurrent carcinoma and adjuvant programs with some promise.

The combination of radiation therapy and chemotherapy (5-FU) given concurrently on the first three days of irradiation to inoperable patients leads to an increase in median survival compared with surgery alone.[71] However, the overall survival was not improved, and other controlled studies did not confirm these results. Although reasonable response rates occurred in the majority of patients, none were lasting in nature.

Lymphoma. The therapy for malignant lymphoma is surgical removal of the involved segment of the stomach with wide normal margins and of the lymph node groups draining that portion of the stomach, followed by postoperative radiation therapy.[31] In general, the small cell lymphosarcomas appear to be more radiosensitive than some of the reticulum cell sarcomas.[9] Hodgkin's disease may be radiosensitive and curable when confined to the stomach. The small cell lymphosarcomas have a better prognosis than the reticulum cell sarcomas or Hodgkin's disease. This is most likely related to their better response to radiation therapy.[9] Radiation therapy is applied to the whole abdominal field at 1,500 to 2,000 cGy with kidney and liver shielding, and then a coned-down approach is applied to the residuum with a total dose of 4,000 cGy. In localized stages, long-term cure has been as high as 90%.[71] Regional lymph node involvement is associated with a significantly lower cure rate. Significant advances have been made in the chemotherapy for gastric lymphoma, with the clinical response rate reported to be as high as 70% for non-Hodgkin lymphomas.[41] However, results have not been consistent, and the role of chemotherapy in the treatment of gastric lymphoma remains to be clarified.

Leiomyosarcoma. The only curative treatment for leiomyosarcoma is surgical excision. In patients with tumors confined to the stomach, a partial or subtotal gastrectomy is usually adequate. For tumors located in the proximal stomach, a total gastrectomy or proximal gastrectomy may be necessary.

Impact of New Technology

The early detection of gastric carcinoma with the use of double-contrast upper GI studies has significantly improved the survival rate for patients with this type of tumor.[9,66,80] The massive screening program using this technique in Japan has been justified because there is such a high incidence of gastric carcinoma in that country. However, a massive screening program may not be practical in the United States, since the incidence of gastric carcinoma is low and is decreasing.

Computed tomography has added an additional dimension to the staging of the patient before surgery. Its main impact in management is to separate patients with resectable disease from patients with nonresectable disease and to help plan palliative surgery. Its impact on survival is yet to be determined, however, but it is unlikely to significantly change the survival rate. The role of MRI is yet to be determined in the diagnosis, detection, and staging of gastric tumors.

SMALL BOWEL

Introduction

Malignant tumors of the small bowel are rare, accounting for only a small percentage of all gastrointestinal malignancies.[54,92,95,110] Of these, carcinoid tumors are the most common malignant small bowel tumors. Adenocarcinoma is the next most common tumor and is more likely to produce symptoms than the carcinoid tumors. Primary malignant lymphoma of the small bowel is much less common than adenocarcinoma and carcinoid tumors. However, the small bowel is the second most common site, constituting 30% to 37% of all GI tract lymphomas.[8,110] Leiomyosarcoma is less common than any of the above tumors and constitutes about one tenth of all malignant neoplasms of the small bowel.[95]

Tumor Behavior and Pathology

Carcinoid Tumors. The carcinoid tumors are classified as indeterminate malignant tumors since they cannot be unequivocally classified as benign or malignant. These tumors were originally called "carcinoid" ("carcinoma-like") because they were thought to be unable to metastasize in spite of their locally invasive behavior. It is now well known, however, that they have metastatic potential and can behave like carcinoma. They are slow growing and permit long survival even after dissemination has occurred. Gastrointestinal carcinoid tumors originate from the chromaffin cells of Kulchitsky, which can be found anywhere in the intestinal tract, from the gastric cardia to the anal verge. They are most frequently found in the mid-gut, i.e., from the mid-duodenum to the mid-transverse colon. The appendix is by far the most common location, accounting for 60% of gastrointestinal tract carcinoid tumors. However, carcinoid tumors in this location rarely metastasize. The next most common site is the ileum, with a predilection for the region of the ileocecal valve.[92]

Carcinoid tumors in the small bowel and other extra-appendiceal sites usually appear as small, round-to-plaque-like, submucosal masses up to 4 to 5 cm in diameter with intact overlying mucosa. Multiple lesions are found in 25% of cases. The lesions may become large and ulcerate, appearing as polypoid masses. Upon sectioning, the lesions are usually yellow but may be gray. Gross penetration of the bowel wall with extension into the mesentery may be observed.[6]

Histologic examination of these tumors usually shows masses of epithelial cells with uniform appearance. The nuclei of these cells are round to oval with fine stippling throughout. Granules of yellow-brown lipochrome pigment, which produce the gross coloration, are found in the cytoplasm.[92]

The size of carcinoid tumors correlates well with the likelihood of metastasis. When the tumor is greater than 1 cm but less than 2 cm in size, 50% of the lesions will have metastases. However, when the tumor is greater than 2 cm in size, 80% of the tumors will have metastases.[84]

In the absence of metastasis and the carcinoid syndrome, the majority of small intestinal carcinoid tumors will remain clinically silent. Only those that cause a desmoplastic reaction in the mesentery with adhesions and partial obstruction will become clinically evident. The lesions are usually found incidentally at surgery or autopsy. The carcinoid syndrome is usually a consequence of metastasis to the liver, although occasionally nongastrointestinal neoplasms may produce the carcinoid syndrome. The carcinoid syndrome of abdominal cramps, diarrhea, wheezing, and flushing of the skin is a result of the action of serotonin kallikrein, which liberates bradykinin, antihistamines, and other active hormones from these tumors.[92] In addition, fibrotic changes of the valves of the right side of the heart can occur, leading to pulmonary stenosis and tricuspid insufficiencies.[92]

Most carcinoid tumors discovered incidentally at surgery or at autopsy have not metastasized and are not involved extensively. Those that are invasive generally extend into the submucosa, muscularis, and serosa or even into the mesentery. In the mesentery they incite a very intense fibrotic reaction, initially causing focal deformity of the intestinal wall and later causing kinking of a longer segment of the bowel with resultant obstruction. Massive metastasis to the lymph nodes as well as to the liver may occur, but rarely does the tumor leave the abdominal cavity. The frequency of metastasis is repeatedly shown to be related to the size of the primary lesion.[84] One third of all submucosal primary tumors are multicentric, and there are usually three or more independent primary masses.

Adenocarcinoma. Adenocarcinomas constitute about one fourth of all malignant lesions of the small bowel; 90% of these lesions are located in the duodenum and jejunum (within 20 cm of the ligament of Treitz).[84] Most adenocarcinomas are aggressively infiltrative. A small portion of them may appear as broad-based polypoid masses. The infiltrative form usually extends rapidly around the circumference of the bowel, inciting a fibrotic reaction with narrowing of the lumen that causes small bowel obstruction. About 90% of adenocarcinomas are clinically symptomatic, with pain and obstruction occurring in about 70% of patients. Blood loss and weight loss occur in about one third of the patients.[95]

The adenocarcinomas usually are very aggressive and infiltrative, causing extensive narrowing of a segment of bowel that usually results in obstruction. The tumor may spread to the regional lymph nodes—first the mesenteric nodes and then the periaortic and pericaval nodes. Metastasis to other sites including the liver and lungs may also occur, as can local involvement of contiguous organs such as kidneys or adjacent bowel loops.

Lymphoma. The majority of the malignant lymphomas are located in the ileum, and they are rarely found in the duodenum. There have been reports of association of GI tract lymphomas with ulcerative colitis, Crohn's disease, and celiac disease.[8] The lymphomas usually infiltrate the submucosa and extend longitudinally to form a plaque of tumor. Eighty percent of the tumors are longer than 5 cm, and 20% are longer than 10 cm.[95] The infiltrating tumor usually encircles the bowel. Obstruction, however, usually does not occur because of extensive necrosis, which often takes place on the luminal side of the tumor and has the effect of widening the lumen. This is called aneurysmal dilatation of the small bowel, which is a distinctive feature of lymphoma that occurs in approximately one third of all cases. Not all lymphomas occur as large masses. Approximately one fifth have multiple sites of involvement. Other forms include a single polypoid mass, multiple small nodular or small polypoid masses 3–5 mm in diameter, short extramucosal annular growth, and lesions similar to the annular lesions of adenocarcinoma.[95] Several histologic types are found, including the predominant lymphocytic type, reticulum cell sarcoma, giant follicular lymphosarcoma, and Hodgkin's disease. These tumors cannot be distinguished by gross morphology.[95]

Primary malignant lymphoma of the small bowel usually extends longitudinally, involving long segments. Multicentric involvement of the bowel occurs in about one fifth of all cases. Usually those patients with multiple sites of involvement have widely disseminated disease. Concomitant involvement of the mesenteric nodes and the retroperitoneal lymph nodes is common. Dissemination to other sites including the liver, spleen, and mediastinal lymph nodes can occur.

Leiomyosarcoma. Leiomyosarcomas are found in equal frequency throughout all segments of the small bowel.

The malignant smooth muscle tumors cannot be distinguished from the benign variety by gross examination. In fact, histologic differentiation can also be difficult. Approximately 10% of them are intraluminal and a few of these are pedunculated, while two thirds of these tumors are extraluminal, projecting chiefly into the peritoneal cavity. Like the benign variety, the surface vascularity of these tumors is rich but the central portion of the mass is poorly vascularized and often necrotic. The mass may become very large, the malignant specimen being on average larger than the benign variety.[84,95]

Leiomyosarcomas usually grow extraluminally to involve adjacent loops of bowel. Metastasis occurs most often via the vascular route to the liver and lungs.

Classification and Staging

Because small bowel tumors are so rare, no TNM staging system has been devised for these tumors. However, the staging of lymphoma involving the small bowel is similar to the staging of lymphoma elsewhere in the body. (Please see lymphoma chapter.)

Imaging Procedures and Assessment

The major imaging modalities available for examining the small bowel are the small bowel follow-through procedure and the small bowel enema (enteroclysis). Because of the length of the small bowel, fiberoptic endoscopy usually does not play a significant role in its examination except in the proximal duodenum.

Techniques. The technique of small bowel follow-through is usually that of giving the patient a large volume of a 50% barium suspension, with sequential films documenting the transit of the barium through the small bowel. Sequential films are usually taken at 15-minute or 30-minute intervals until the barium column reaches the terminal ileum. Spot films should be obtained when any suspicious area is seen. However, the proper time sequence should be tailored to the patient's transit time as monitored by the radiologist. Various pharmacologic agents, including neostigmine, cholecystokinin-like drugs, and metoclopramide, are used to accelerate the transit of the barium through the small bowel.[100] Induction of hypotonia can also be performed with the use of anticholingeric agents and glucagon. The small bowel follow-through is usually performed as a latter half of an upper GI study.

The technique of double-contrast small bowel imaging, as described in detail by Sellink[100] and Herlinger,[43] is designed to detect nodules, ulcers, and bowel wall thickening. The technique requires placement of a long tube with its tip at the ligament of Treitz. Twenty milligrams of metoclopramide is often administered orally 15 minutes before the examination to improve the intu-

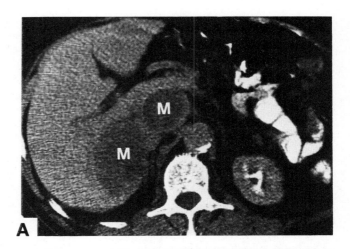

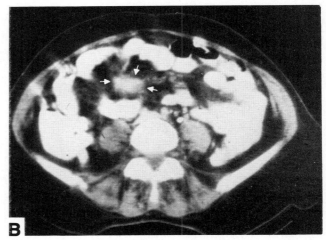

FIG. 13-22. (A) Metastases of a carcinoid tumor to the liver (M). (B) Carcinoid tumor in small bowel mesentery on a CT scan (arrows).

bation of the patient. A long tube is placed through the mouth and the patient is positioned in the right decubitus position with the aim of placing the tube beyond the duodenal-jejunal junction. Barium, barium and water mixed with methylcellulose, or barium and air is then injected rapidly through the tube. The examination is monitored continually with fluoroscopy, and spot films of the distended bowel are obtained when segments are seen to be distended.

Computed Tomography. Similar to the case with the stomach, the major role of CT in evaluating the small bowel is that of staging the above tumors before surgery. Computed tomography is very sensitive in the detection of metastases of these small bowel tumors to the liver and retroperitoneum (Figures 13-22A, 13-23B). However, the demonstration of these small bowel tumors by CT is difficult because of various locations of these neoplasms and their small sizes.

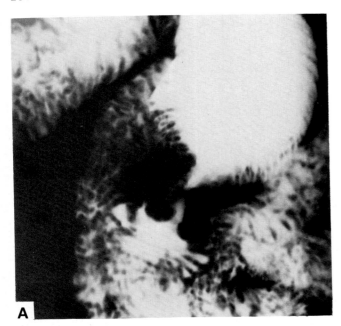

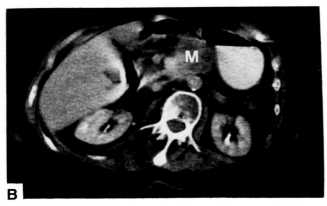

FIG. 13-23. (A) Adenocarcinoma of the jejunum. An annular lesion of the proximal jejunum has caused partial obstruction of the small bowel. (B) A CT scan of a jejunal adenocarcinoma shows the tumor mass extending into the mesentery (M).

Imaging Strategies and Decisions

For patients suspected of having small bowel malignancies, a small bowel follow-through series as part of an upper GI study should be the initial imaging modality. If a tumor is detected, the next image modality may be CT to help define the stage of the malignancy and to detect abdominal and liver metastases (Table 13-8, 13-9). A CT-directed needle biopsy of the mass involving the small bowel may also help in defining the histopathology and stage of the tumor. A chest X-ray film should be obtained to exclude the presence of obvious chest metastases. However, if the small bowel follow-through procedure is negative and a small bowel malignancy is still strongly suspected, a double-contrast study of the small bowel by the methods described above is

Table 13-8. Modalities of Choice for Detecting Suspected Small Bowel Carcinoma

Small Bowel Enema
or Conventional Small Bowel
Follow-Through with Peroral
Pneumocolon
↓
CT For Staging
Liver and Abdominal Extent
↓
Surgery

Although small bowel carcinoma is rarely suspected clinically, its appearance, producing partial small bowel obstruction, usually leads directly to a radiographic study of the small bowel, either a conventional small bowel barium study or a specialized small bowel enema. These positive contrast studies are essential for the detection and characterization of the carcinoma. Once detected, presurgical staging for the presence of liver metastasis and extent of spread in the mesentery and involvement of other segments or organs utilizing CT is very helpful.

recommended. When clinical evidence for carcinoid tumor is strong but the small bowel enema study is normal, a CT scan or ultrasonogram of the liver should be performed to determine if liver metastases are responsible for the carcinoid syndrome. If surgical resection of hepatic carcinoid is contemplated, an hepatic arteriogram should be performed to provide information about the hepatic vascular anatomy. If small bowel lymphoma

Table 13-9. Modalities of Choice for Detecting Suspected Small Bowel Leiomyosarcoma

Single-Contrast or Double-Contrast UGI and
Small Bowel Barium Study
↓
CT   (US)
With Biopsy
↓
Surgery

When a mobile, firm abdominal mass is palpated, and the possibility of leiomyoma or a leiomyosarcoma is considered, a single-contrast or double-contrast upper GI series and small bowel barium study are almost always performed in order to determine the relationship of the suspected mass to the stomach or the small bowel. Smooth muscle tumors characteristically produce smooth indentations into the column of barium, indicating they are mural or extramural in location. Occasionally these will also result in ulceration of the overlying mucosa, which can also be detected by conventional radiographic studies. However, to determine the true nature of the lesion, a CT scan or, alternately, ultrasonography, can be performed to demonstrate the classic appearance of leiomyoma or leiomyosarcoma—namely a solid lesion with generally homogeneous appearance, and occasionally with calcifications seen in the periphery. Once the lesion is discovered by either CT or ultrasound, a percutaneous CT or ultrasound-guided needle biopsy may be performed to confirm the diagnosis. Since leiomyosarcomas occasionally metastasize to the liver, CT or ultrasound can also be used to determine the presence of liver metastasis prior to surgery.

Table 13-10. Modalities of Choice for Detecting
Small Bowel Lymphoma

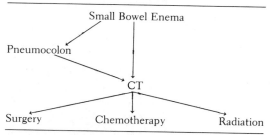

In patients suspected of having lymphoma involving the small bowel, the diagnostic imaging study of choice is the small bowel enema because this study is designed to demonstrate the presence of small nodules — one of the manifestations of small bowel lymphoma. The small bowel enema is also capable of demonstrating the strictures and ulcerating masses seen in intestinal lymphoma. An integral part of the evaluation is the performance of a pneumocolon study to determine whether colonic involvement is present with small bowel involvement. In either case, a CT scan should next be performed because it is capable of demonstrating the presence of mesenteric masses, the extent of masses that involve small bowel and their relationship to other organs, the presence of pericaval, periaortic and mesenteric lymphadenopathy, and involvement of the spleen or liver. Depending upon the findings with the small bowel enema and the CT examination, various courses of therapy may be carried out. For instance, an ulcerating mass producing partial obstruction may require surgery. Focal involvement of an area of bowel without the complications that might require surgery may be treated with radiation therapy; in most instances, however, chemotherapy will be used following the diagnostic workup.

sit time of the barium may be observed because of the action of serotonin and other hormones secreted from metastases.[84,95] However, approximately one half of the patients with carcinoid syndrome will have a normal small bowel examination.

If a carcinoid tumor is suspected on the basis of the small bowel series, selective mesenteric arteriography may lead to more accurate identification. The characteristic findings are that of narrowing of the arteries in the mesentery and a mass of abnormal stellate vessels in the region of the involved mesentery (Figure 13-25). The differential diagnoses of this finding include diffuse fibrous peritonitis, diffuse carcinomatosis of the mesentery from the breast or pancreas, and lymphoreticular malignancy of mesenteric lymph nodes.[98] While the primary lesion is not detected by CT, the effect on the mesentery results in the appearance of a mass or soft-tissue density surrounded by mesenteric fat with strands leading to kinked segments of bowel (Figure 13-22B).[98] The demonstration of a well-defined low-density mass in the right lower quadrant with a stellate or concentrated pattern of neovascularity was reported to be suggestive of carcinoid tumor of the ileum. More importantly, the CT scan may provide information about the presence and size of liver metastases (Figure 13-22B).

Adenocarcinoma. The sensitivity of small bowel examination in the detection of adenocarcinoma is approximately 90%.[95] The most common and most characteristic

is suspected on the basis of lymphoma elsewhere, or previous sprue, then a small bowel enema study should be the initial examination because it is designed to detect small nodules as well as other features of lymphoma (Table 13-10). A pneumocolon should be included to detect colon involvement. A CT scan is an important additional imaging procedure to determine the extent of extraluminal components of small bowel involvement and abdominal lymphadenopathy so that radiation therapy can be planned if this mode of therapy is to be used.

Imaging Strategies by Tumor Type

Carcinoid. The radiographic appearance of carcinoid tumors may be that of a small, rounded, smooth, filling defect suggesting a submucosal tumor. The mucosal folds over these lesions may be thickened or effaced. There may also be multiple areas of constriction and dilatation of the small bowel. Since carcinoid tumors commonly involve the mesentery and cause severe desmoplastic reactions, angulation, kinking of the bowel wall, partial small bowel obstruction, stretching, and rigidity of the small bowel folds are commonly seen (Figure 13-24). In addition, rapid motility of the small bowel and rapid tran-

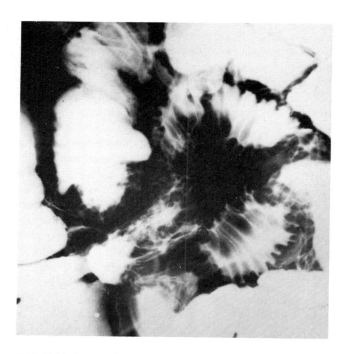

FIG. 13-24. Carcinoid tumor of the small bowel mesentery. The loops of small bowel are separated, the folds thick, with retraction toward the area of mesenteric infiltration.

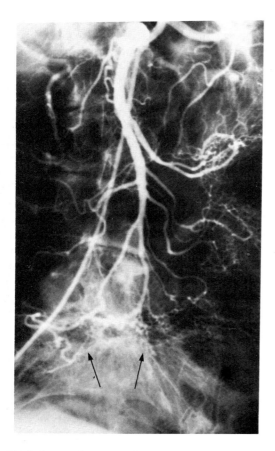

FIG. 13-25. Carcinoid tumor of the small bowel mesentery. Selective injection into the superior mesenteric artery demonstrates hypervascularity with a stellate vascular pattern (arrows).

finding of adenocarcinoma is a short, sharply demarcated, annular filling defect with dilatation of the small bowel proximal to the lesion (Figures 13-23, 13-26). There may be oval or lobulated sessile polypoid masses protruding into the lumen.

Lymphoma. Malignant lymphoma of the small bowel has the greatest variety of radiographic appearances.[8,10,94,110] The most common finding is that of a long growth encircling the bowel lumen, which is extensively ulcerated with aneurysmal dilatation (Figure 13-27). The tumor also may appear as a constrictive form with a short segment of narrowing in the small bowel and alternating areas of constriction and dilatation. Multiple small nodules may be present. The tumor may also be primarily nodular in form with submucosal infiltration by numerous small nodules measuring a few millimeters throughout the entire length of the small bowel. In addition, the tumor may also grow exophytically, with a mass growing towards the retroperitoneum.

Leiomyosarcoma. Leiomyosarcoma frequently projects into the peritoneal cavity with the main roentgenograph-

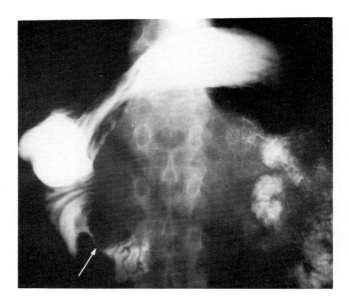

FIG. 13-26. Adenocarcinoma of the duodenum. A large annular lesion encases the descending portion of the duodenum (arrow). A large mass caused by tumor involvement of the retrogastric and gastric lymph nodes presses upon the posterior wall of the stomach, displacing the stomach superiorly and laterally.

ic finding being displacement of adjacent bowel loops. Approximately 5% of the lesions are intraluminal pedunculated masses.[95] Ulceration of the mucosa covering the lesion occurs in approximately 50% of cases,[95] and fistula may form through the mass. However, differentiation between the benign and the malignant forms of the smooth muscle neoplasm cannot be made by radiographic criteria.

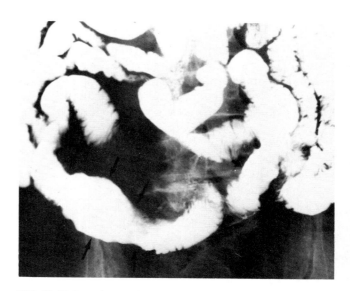

FIG. 13-27. Lymphoma of the small bowel. Note dilatation of a segment of the ilium (arrows) caused by penetration of the bowel wall by lymphoma. This is the so-called "aneurysmal dilatation" of the small bowel, which is characteristic of lymphomatous involvement.

Treatment Decisions[7,14,65,73,76]

Since two thirds of carcinoid tumors do not produce the carcinoid syndrome and are found incidentally on small bowel roentgenograms at surgery or at autopsy, the discovery of a carcinoid tumor on a small bowel follow-through series or a double-contrast small bowel series should lead to complete surgical removal of the tumor along with the involved mesentery. These patients have a much more favorable prognosis than those with evidence of metastases to the liver and carcinoid syndrome. It is important to localize the lesion by a barium study and the extent of involvement of the tumor by CT for proper surgical planning. If resection of a hepatic lesion is planned, hepatic angiography may also be necessary. The use of methylsergide and antihistamines has been shown to be useful in controlling some of the symptoms of carcinoid syndrome; radiotherapy and chemotherapy have not been found to be beneficial.

The treatment of choice for adenocarcinoma of the small bowel is complete surgical resection of the tumor. However, if there is extension to contiguous bowel loops or to adjacent organs, a bypass procedure may be considered rather than complete resection. Hence, CT scans and a small bowel series are useful for planning the extent of the surgical procedure.

The management of the patient with intestinal lymphoma varies and depends, in part, upon the extent of the intestinal involvement and the presence or absence of extraintestinal tumor involvement. If the lymphomatous involvement is confined to a single small segment of small bowel without nodal involvement, surgical resection is the treatment of choice. This type of lesion has by far the best prognosis. The cure rate under these circumstances is on the order of 50% to 75%.[8,110] However, if there is adjacent tissue involvement, such as the mesentery, lymph nodes, or adjacent organs, surgical resection should be followed by postoperative radiotherapy or chemotherapy, or both, since these have been shown to be useful in the general treatment of lymphoma. Radiopaque surgical clips placed at the site of possible residual tumor at the time of surgery help to localize the site for radiotherapy, and CT scans for radiotherapy field and dose determination are useful. There is a significant drop in the survival rate if disease has extended to extraintestinal sites. If there is a long segment of small bowel involvement by the lymphomatous tumor, definitive surgery may be precluded because of the length of the involved segment. In such cases, radiotherapy would then be the treatment of choice. However, its effectiveness in prolonging survival has not been proven. Chemotherapy may also be added to the treatment of such a diffuse tumor. However, treatment with radiation or with chemotherapy may predispose the patient to intestinal perforation by causing necrosis of the primary tumor, leading to development of intra-abdominal abscesses.

The five-year survival rate for this type of tumor is less than 10%. Palliative surgery may be needed to manage complications such as intestinal obstruction, perforation, or intractable bleeding.[110]

Surgery is the treatment of choice for leiomyosarcoma because these tumors are notoriously resistant to radiotherapy and chemotherapy. An aggressive surgical approach is recommended when distant metastases are not identified. Since these tumors generally metastasize hematogenously rather than by the lymphatic route, extensive lymph node dissection is not necessary.

Impact of New Technology

The sensitivity of the small bowel series has been considered to be poor in detecting small bowel tumors when it is used as a screening test without specific clinical indications.[33,88] When the small bowel follow-through procedure is used specifically to detect a tumor that is causing obstruction or cramps or pain, the detection rate increases. There is no specific data on the sensitivity of the small bowel enema study in the detection of small bowel tumors. However, the general superiority of the small bowel enema study in detecting disease has been documented.[30,41] Since most small bowel tumors are not discovered incidentally by radiography, but only after symptoms develop, most are discovered late in their course. Because primary small bowel tumors are rare, it is unlikely that screening programs will be instituted, using small bowel enema studies, to detect early cancer in this viscus.

Although CT has significantly influenced the management of these patients, its impact on survival is still to be defined. The role of MRI in the detection and management of small bowel malignancies is unknown at present.

Survival Statistics on Primary Small Bowel Cancers.

Because of the scarcity of these tumors, the survival statistics of small bowel cancers are generally based upon series of small patient populations. The median survival for patients with primary carcinoid tumor of the small bowel has been reported to be 28.4 months. In one report, eight of nine patients who received surgery for small bowel carcinoid survived five or more years. However, because of the slow growth of these tumors, the five-year survival rate may not be adequate to assess cure.[67]

Although the cure rate for patients with adenocarcinoma of the small bowel is very poor, five-year survival rates as high as 20% have been reported. The prognosis for carcinoma located in the duodenum is slightly worse than for carcinoma located elsewhere in the small bowel.[110] Patients with small bowel lymphomas usually do not do as well as those with gastric lymphomas. However, significant advances have been made in recent years in the therapy of lymphoma, and the five-year survival rate has been reported as high as 50%.[8] Those patients with generalized lymphomatous nodal involvement generally have a worse prognosis than those without nodal involvement. As for leiomyosarcoma, the five-year survival rate has been reported to be about 50%, similar to that of the gastric leiomyosarcoma.[84]

COLON AND RECTUM

Introduction

Adenocarcinoma is by far the most frequent primary malignancy of the colon, accounting for 97% of all colonic malignancies. It was second only to lung carcinoma in incidence in the United States in 1980. It accounts for 12% of all cancer-related deaths in men and 15% in women.[106] The incidence of colonic cancer is approximately the same in each sex. However, carcinoma of the rectum tends to occur more frequently in men than in women at a ratio of approximately 2:1.[41] A significantly higher incidence of colonic carcinoma occurs in North America and Northwest Europe and a very low incidence is found in Mexico, Japan, East Africa, Asia, and South America.[48,106] For example, a sixfold difference in incidence is demonstrated between Canada and Japan.[48,106] Immigrants going from low-incidence countries to high-incidence countries acquire the prevalence and mortality rate of their new locations.[42,48,92] In general, carcinoma of the colon tends to occur in countries where there is a higher standard of living. The differences in incidence between these countries have led to the speculation that the etiology for colonic carcinoma may be environmentally related. There have also been reports of increased risk for colonic carcinoma in workers who have been exposed to coke and asbestos.[89,99] Although it has not been conclusively proven, a dietary intake composed of low fiber, high beef, and saturated fat is believed to be associated with a higher likelihood of developing carcinoma of the colon.[48,92] Differences in the bacterial flora in the different countries are also believed to be related to the differences in the incidence of cancer.[45]

Hereditary factors are undoubtedly important in determining the likelihood of developing carcinoma of the colon. An increase in incidence of colonic or rectal cancer in relatives with the disease has been noted.[64] A definite hereditary relationship in the development of colonic and rectal cancer has been demonstrated with patients with familial polyposis and Gardener's syndrome.[48,92] Patients with familial polyposis usually develop numerous adenomas of the large bowel at an early age. Almost all of these patients will develop colonic carcinoma within 20 years after the development of the adenomas.[48,92] Gardener's syndrome is manifested by epidermoid cysts, osteomas of the skull, and polyps of the small and large

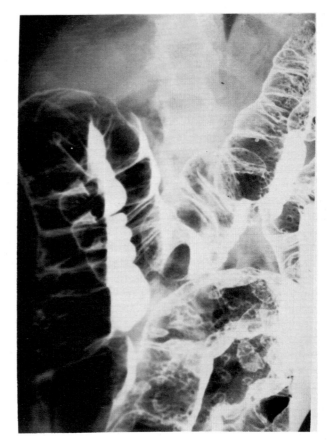

FIG. 13-28. Gardner's syndrome. A double-contrast view of the colon demonstrates multiple polypoid filling defects throughout the colon.

bowel (Figure 13-28). Like those patients with familial poplyposis, these patients invariably will develop adenocarcinoma of the colon and rectum. However, colonic cancer may occur somewhat later in life in Gardener's syndrome than in familial polyposis. In addition, patients with active ulcerative colitis for a long period of time are at a much greater risk than the normal population of developing colonic carcinoma.[20,29]

Approximately three quarters of colonic carcinomas are discovered in the sixth, seventh, and eighth decades of life, with the peak age being 67 years.[48] However, those patients with familial polyposis, Gardener's syndrome, and chronic ulcerative colitis usually develop colonic carcinoma at a much earlier age.

The rectum and the sigmoid colon were previously reported to be the most common sites of colonic carcinoma, with approximately 70% to 80% of the tumor located in those segments of the bowel.[48,92] However, for unknown reasons, an increasing proportion of colonic carcinomas have been observed in recent years arising above the rectosigmoid junction. Presently, only 50% to 60% of colorectal carcinomas are within reach of the rigid sigmoidoscope.[90] Hence, the traditional methods for detecting colonic malignancy by rectal examination and rigid proctosigmoidoscopy are less effective than before. There is now a greater reliance on other techniques such as the testing of stools for occult blood, radiography, and colonoscopy. Infrequently, multiple carcinomas arise concurrently, most often in patients with familial polyposis or ulcerative colitis.[71,86]

Besides adenocarcinoma, carcinoid tumors, leiomyosarcoma, lymphoma, and epidermoid carcinoma compose the remainder of colonic malignancies. These tumors are, in general, rare in the colon.

Tumor Behavior and Pathology

Adenocarcinoma. The gross morphology of colonic carcinoma is slightly different depending upon the site in the colon in which the tumors are located. Carcinoma of the left side tends to grow in an annular encircling fashion. These tumors usually produce early symptoms of obstruction and "napkin ring" constriction of the bowel. On the right side, the tumors tend to grow as polypoid fungating masses that extend along one wall of the cecum and ascending colon. Obstruction is uncommon. Hence, tumors of the left and right colon behave as two distinct types from the viewpoint of morphology and clinical behavior.

Lesions on the left side of the colon usually begin as sessile masses. As the tumor grows, it forms a flat plaque that continues to increase in size, eventually extending circumferentially to encircle the wall in approximately one to two years.[92] The tumor tends to remain superficial for a long period of time with late invasion of the deeper layer. Ulceration may take place in the middle of the encircling mass as penetration of the bowel wall encroaches on the blood supply. Less frequently, left-sided lesions can produce an infiltrative type of tumor with very little luminal growth. As these tumors grow, they invade the bowel wall and penetrate into the pericolic fat and regional lymph nodes.[92]

Carcinomas in the right colon also begin as sessile lesions, but usually progress to polypoid fungating masses or large, irregularly spreading papillomatous plaques that protrude into the lumen. These tumors eventually penetrate the bowel wall and extend into the mesentery, regional lymph nodes, or distant sites. Colonic carcinomas of the right side may also grow in an invasive infiltrating fashion, with mucosal flattening and ulceration without luminal projections. Because the lumen of the cecum and descending colon is much more spacious than the left colon, tumors of the right colon usually do not cause obstruction. They may remain clinically silent for a long period of time before causing significant anemia, weight loss, or pain.[92]

The gross appearance of adenocarcinoma of the colon can be divided into four types: ulcerating, polypoid, colloid, and scirrhous. The polypoid type of adenocarcinoma is more frequent in the right colon, whereas the ulcerating or scirrhous type is more frequent in the left colon. Ulcerating carcinoma is the most common form of colonic cancer and is often associated with obstruction. Polypoid cancer is the next most common form. This type of tumor is usually well-differentiated and slow growing. The colloid type of carcinoma is characterized by an abundance of mucus-secreting cells. Scirrhous carcinoma is uncommon and it occurs most frequently in the rectum or rectosigmoid junction. The scirrhous form produces a "linitis plastica" type of colonic cancer,[48] similar to that seen in the stomach.

Unlike the gross morphology, the microscopic appearance of colonic carcinomas is similar for both right-sided and left-sided tumors. Ninety-seven percent of all carcinomas of the colon are adenocarcinomas. Many of these produce mucin. Other types of carcinoma include squamous, colloid, and villous adenocarcinoma. Occasionally, undifferentiated adenocarcinoma is observed.[92]

Adenocarcinomas of the large bowel arise in the mucosa and extend proximally or distally in the bowel wall. Some tumors extend directly from the mucosa, penetrating through the bowel wall and the serosa. They may invade adjacent organs or seed peritoneal surfaces. They may spread via the regional lymphatic channels draining the colon. These channels characteristically accompany the blood supply and drain into the mesenteric nodes and further on into the periaortic nodes. Tumors of the left transverse colon, descending colon, sigmoid colon, and rectum drain into the nodes around the inferior mesenteric artery from the left colonic, sigmoid, or superior hemorrhoidal nodes. However, tumors located in the cecum, ascending colon, and right transverse colon drain into nodes around the superior mesenteric artery from the ileocolonic and right colonic nodes. Drainage of the anus is usually into the inguinal nodes. However, proximal anal lesions may drain superiorly into the perirectal nodes. For some anal-rectal lesions there may be bidirectional lymphatic drainage. Some of the colonic and rectal tumors disseminate by invading the venous channels. Invasion of the tributaries of the portal vein accounts for hepatic metastasis from colonic and rectal carcinomas. Metastasis to the lungs, bone, brain, and occasionally the adrenal glands also occurs.[48]

Carcinoid Tumors. Large bowel carcinoid tumors are most common in the rectum. The rectal carcinoid tumors appear as rounded, yellowish nodules, which are submucosal or intramural with a smooth appearance. The carcinoid syndrome is rarely observed in carcinoid tumors arising in the rectum. Most patients with rectal carcinoid tumors are reported to be asymptomatic. These tumors are usually slow growing with low-grade malignant potentials, however, 10% of these patients have metastases.[6] The tumors are usually treated by local excision.[48]

Leiomyosarcoma. Colonic leiomyosarcomas also occur more frequently in the rectum. These tumors are rare, constituting 0.01% to 0.1% of all rectal malignancies. It is difficult to differentiate the malignant from the benign variety of smooth muscle tumors by radiographic, gross, or histologic means. Histologically, these tumors appear as interlacing spindle cells and arise from rectal smooth muscles.[48] They may spread by local extension and by metastasizing to the liver.

Lymphoma. Lymphoma rarely arises in the colon or rectum, constituting less than 0.5% of colonic malignancies. Approximately 10% of patients with gastrointestinal tract lymphoma have colonic involvement. The most common site of involvement is the cecum. There are two forms of colonic lymphoma: (1) a localized form, which appears as a large polypoid mass, and (2) a diffuse form, which appears as multiple small nodular lesions.[122] These tumors may be part of a systemic lymphoma or lymphoma of the GI tract. They may spread via the lymphatic channels as described for the colonic carcinomas.

Epidermoid Carcinoma. Epidermoid carcinomas constitute about 2% of all colorectal cancers and are largely limited to the anal region (Figure 13-29). Several histologic types have been described, including squamous cell, basal cell, and cloacogenic. They behave like squamous cell carcinomas located elsewhere in the body, producing plaquelike thickening that eventually fungates and ulcerates. These tumors tend to be locally invasive, extending directly to sphincters, perianal tissue, vagina and prostate, and eventually metastasize to regional lymph nodes.[96] They may also spread via lymphatic channels of the rectum or groin or hematogenously via the portal vein or systemic veins.

Classification and Staging

There are two systems currently in use for staging colonic carcinoma: the Duke's system and the TNM system. The original Duke's staging system has undergone many modifications. Stage A tumors are those limited to the mucosa. A patient with this type of tumor is usually considered cured after resection of the involved colonic segment. The five-year survival rate for this type of tumor is close to 100%. Stage B_1 tumors are those that extend to the muscularis propria but do not penetrate the muscle layer. Stage B_2 tumors are those that have penetrated the muscularis propria layer. Both B_1 and B_2 tumors have a 70% five-year survival rate. Stage C tumors are those with nodal involvement. The tumors are considered to be C_1 or C_2 depending upon whether primary tumor has penetrated the bowel wall or not. Pa-

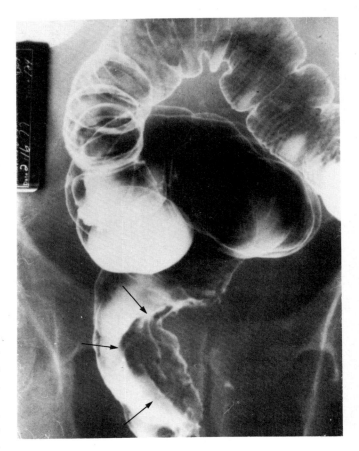

FIG. 13-29. Cloacogenic carcinoma of the rectum. Note the large lesion (arrows) involving the left side of the rectum on this double-contrast view of the colon.

tients with only one lymph node involved by tumor have a five-year survival rate of approximately 60%. However, patients with two to five lymph nodes involved have a five-year survival rate of only 35%. If there are more than six lymph nodes involved, the five-year survival rate drops to 20%. The Duke's stage D tumors are those tumors which have metastasized to the liver, lungs, bone, peritoneum, or bowel segments, are unresectable because of parietal peritoneal invasion or involvement of the adjacent organs. The five-year survival rate for this type of tumor is very low.[19]

The American Joint Committee on Cancer redefined the TNM categories for colon and rectal cancer in 1983 (Table 13-11). A T_0 lesion defines a situation when metastases are found but no primary tumor is evident. T_{is} refers to carcinoma in situ (without invasion of the lamina propria). A T_1 lesion is confined to the mucosa or submucosa whereas a T_2 lesion extends into the lamina propria but not beyond. T_{2a} and T_{2b} distinguish between cancers which just penetrate and extend through the muscularis propria. A T_3 cancer extends through all layers of the bowel wall including the serosa and a T_4 lesion extends to contiguous tissue or adjacent organs.

As stated earlier, the first nodal drainage stations are those that are immediately proximal to the colonic segments at the base of the mesocolon, namely the ileocolic, the right colic, the middle colic, the left colic, the inferior mesenteric, the perirectal, the superior and the inferior hemorrhoidal nodal groups. The second drainage station is the periaortic lymph nodes. The tumor is classified as N_0 if the nodes are not involved. The tumor is classified as N_1 if there are one to three regional nodes adjacent to the primary region. In N_2 disease, involved regional nodes extend to the line of resection or to the ligature of the blood vessels. In N_3 disease, nodes contain metastasis, location not identified. N_x and M_x designations are used when insufficient or minimum criteria to assess the N or M compartment have not been satisfied.

Similar to the classification for gastric carcinomas, distant metastases are staged as M_0 (none known) or M_1 (present). Sites of distant metastasis may include the lungs, liver, bone, brain, extra-abdominal lymph nodes, intra-abdominal lymph nodes proximal to the mesocolon, and inferior mesenteric artery or peritoneal implants. The tumors are further grouped into four stages (Figure 13-30; Table 13-12).

Laboratory studies may aid in detection and staging of colon carcinoma. Examining the stool for occult blood is the most important screening test for colorectal cancer. The patient should be on a meat-free, high residue diet for three days before the hemoccult test. Those patients who have positive results on duplicate samples taken from different parts of the stool each day for three consecutive days should be carefully examined by barium contrast study or endoscopy or both. The hemoccult test is very accurate, with few false negatives and approximately 1% false positives.[86]

Carcinoembryonic antigen (CEA) is a circulating glycoprotein molecule produced in variable amounts by most colorectal cancers. It has been reported that those patients who have an elevated preoperative level of CEA have a worse prognosis. Carcinoembryonic antigen has also been found to be useful in monitoring postoperative patients for recurrence of cancer. A rising CEA level is strongly suggestive of recurrent disease, particularly in the absence of other diseases that produce an elevated CEA level such as cirrhosis and pancreatitis.[48]

Imaging Procedures and Assessment

The primary radiographic imaging modality for the detection and diagnosis of carcinoma of the colon is the single-contrast or double-contrast barium examination of the colon. Plain roentgenograms usually do not play a significant role except in cases where a mass is outlined by colonic gas. Plain roentgenograms may also demonstrate evidence of colonic obstruction or perforation. A double-contrast barium enema is the study of choice for detection of colonic carcinoma. However, single-contrast barium enemas are used in those patients who are debilitated or who are unable to cooperate in a double-contrast study.

Techniques. The technique of the double-contrast barium study is described in detail by Laufer.[56] The patient's colon should be clean, without significant residue that would compromise the interpretation of the study. Barium sulfate of high density should be used, which would provide good coating of the colon. When the contrast material has reached the splenic flexure and the distal transverse colon, the patient may be placed in an upright position in order to drain excess barium from the rectosigmoid colon. Air is usually introduced after the barium column has reached the splenic flexure. The head of the column of barium is monitored by fluoroscopy. The patient is placed in various positions, taking advantage of the effects of gravity to keep the column of barium ahead of the air. Instillation of large amounts of air is essential to adequately distend the colon. Views of the flexures and the sigmoid colon are usually taken in the upright or semierect position. Spot views of the sigmoid colon and also the cecum are taken with the patient in the supine and prone positions and in a slight reverse Trendelenburg position. Routine overhead views should include bilateral decubitus and lateral view of the rectum. Glucagon should be used in instances where colonic spasm is encountered.

A single-contrast barium enema study may be required for patients unable to undergo a double-contrast study or for patients suspected of having colonic obstruction due to tumor. Careful palpation of the barium-filled sigmoid and other portions of the colon with fluoroscopic monitoring will result in detection of plaquelike and polypoid lesions. A post-evacuation roentgenogram is usually obtained to permit identification of intraluminal lesions.

Accuracy of Barium Enema Studies. The double-contrast barium enema examination repeatedly has been found to be an accurate diagnostic procedure in detecting colonic polyps. Various studies have shown the sensitivity to vary between 88% and 91% for polyps greater than 1 cm in size.[27,32,87,109] Most of the missed polyps were located in the sigmoid colon. The redundancy of the sigmoid and the frequency of associated diverticula and muscle hypertrophy distorting the contour result in problems in radiographic detection of colonic polyps.

Endoscopy. Anoscopy, sigmoidoscopy, and colonoscopy are components of complete endoscopic examination of the large bowel. The most commonly used instrument

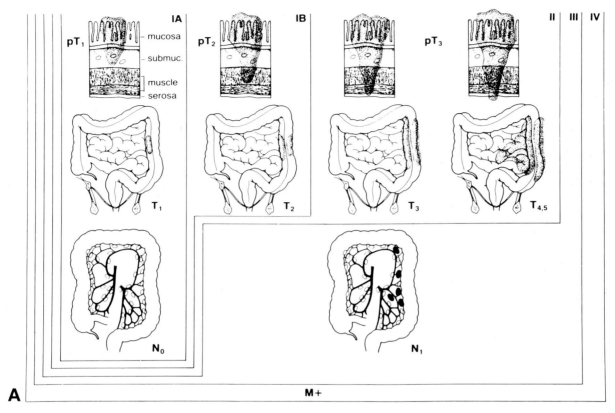

FIG. 13-30. Modified AJC anatomic staging for (A) colon cancer and (B) rectal cancer. Tumor (T) categories: The depth of penetration is the most important criterion and is here carried to five categories. The order of progression for hollow viscera is a stage for each layer: mucosal, muscle, serosa (T_1 to T_2 to T_3). Extension to extramural structures may also be present in T_3. The additional presence of fistula is here defined as T_4 and extension beyond immediately adjacent organs is T_5. Node (N) categories: The regional nodes are either negative or positive and confined to the course of the inferior mesenteric artery and vein. Stage grouping: Favorable T lesions (T_1 and T_2) are grouped as stage I because of ease of resection. Unfavorable T_3 lesions are stage II. Positive nodes of extension beyond immediately adjacent organs are stage III, and metastases that

is a 25-cm rigid sigmoidoscope. Because of the rigidity of the sigmoidoscope, poor patient tolerance, and the tortuosity of the sigmoid colon, it is difficult to pass the scope a full 25 cm into the sigmoid colon in some patients. Recently, a flexible sigmoidoscope has been developed, which allows easier passage of the scope and more complete examination of the sigmoid colon. Several studies have shown that the flexible sigmoidoscope is superior to the conventional rigid sigmoidoscope.[54,116] A significant increase in the detection of the number of adenomatous polyps and cancers was achieved through visualization of greater length of the colon with the flexible instrument. In the majority of studies a 60-cm examination results in complete visualization of the entire sigmoid colon.[62]

The fiberoptic colonoscope varies in length from 105 cm to 185 cm, and may reach all areas of the colon. The

Table 13-11. Tumor (T) Node (N) Classification — Colo-rectal Cancer

T_{is}	Carcinoma in situ
T_1/pT_1	Mucosa or submucosa
T_2/pT_2	Muscle
T_{2a}	Into m. propria
T_{2b}	Through m. propia
T_3/pT_3	Serosa
T_4	Beyond contiguous structures
N_0	No regional nodes
N_1	Regional nodes 1–3 positive
N_2	Nodes positive to line of resection or ligature of vessels
N_3	Nodes positive, number and site undetermined

From American Joint Committee on Cancer: *Manual for Staging of Cancer*, 2nd ed. Philadelphia, J. B. Lippincott, 1983.

Table 13-12. Stage Grouping — Colo-rectal Cancer

Stage 0	Carcinoma in situ			
	T_{is}	N_0	M_0	
Stage I$_a$	T_1	N_0	M_0	
Stage I$_b$	T_2	N_0	M_0	Dukes A
Stage II	T_3	N_0	M_0	Dukes B
Stage III	Any T	N_1,N_2,N_3	M_0	Dukes C
	T_4	N_0	M_0	
Stage IV	Any T	Any N	M_1	

From American Joint Committee on Cancer: *Manual for Staging of Cancer*, 2nd ed. Philadelphia, J. B. Lippincott, 1983.

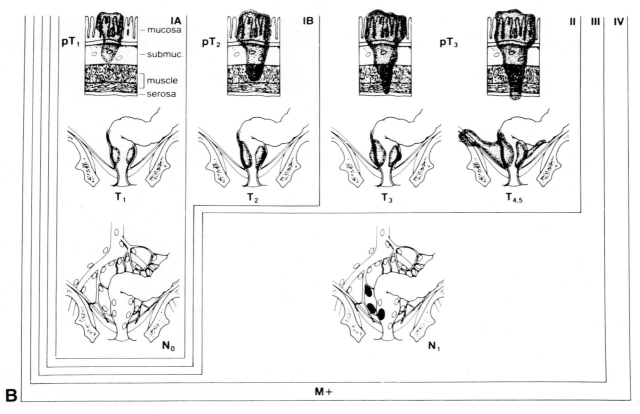

B

include nodes beyond the inferior mesenteric nodes, or include distant involvement, are stage IV. AJC v UICC classification: The UICC[47] has approximately four categories, but confuses the standard categories of visceral organs by lumping muscle and serosal invasion into T_2. The UICC T_3(a and b)[107] is equivalent to T_4 and T_5 in the AJC system[4]. The UICC's T_4 category has primary tumor extending to the immediately adjacent organs, which would be a T_6 in the AJC system. There is an additional UICC N_4 category for juxtaregional nodes, whereas N_2 and N_3 are noted as not applicable. (Modified from Morton, J. M., Poulter, C. A., Pandya, K. J.: Alimentary tract cancer. In *Clinical Oncology for Medical Students and Physicians: A Multidisciplinary Approach*. Rubin, P. (Ed.). American Cancer Society, 1983, pp. 154–176, with permission.)

technique of colonoscopy and the full endoscopic description of colorectal neoplasia are beyond the scope of this chapter.

The endoscopic criteria for diagnosing a malignant polyp are similar to those of double-contrast barium enema studies. Deformity of the head of the polyp and a wide-based sessile polyp that shows deep ulceration on the surface are indications of advanced cancer. These polyps should not be excised endoscopically.[102] However, the pedunculated polyp that shows ulceration can be amenable to endoscopic resection. Pedunculated polyps with invasive cancer tend to have concave surfaces with an irregular nodular appearance. Other features that indicate that a polyp is malignant are a granular, friable surface, disproportion in size between the head and the stalk of the polyp, and areas of discoloration on the head of the polyp. However, colonic appearance of the surface features of a polyp is not sufficiently specific to permit accurate diagnosis of benign or malignant nature.

Advanced colonic carcinomas generally appear as large masses, which may be annular, constricting the lumen of

the colon. Ulceration is a common feature of advanced carcinoma.

The accuracy of colonoscopy and sigmoidoscopy is a function of both visualizing and biopsying lesions. Most studies that compared barium contrast enema examination and colonoscopy have shown that colonoscopy is superior in terms of diagnostic accuracy. The overall accuracy of colonoscopy has been reported to range from 89% to 95%.[32,51,53,63,118] However, the barium double-contrast enema study has several advantages over colonoscopy, including better patient acceptance, lower potential for morbidity, more universal availability and less expense than colonoscopy. In addition, false-negative colonoscopic diagnosis also occurs, primarily in the cecum, rectum, and flexures.[58,109] All factors considered, we believe that even with the improved diagnostic accuracy of colonoscopy and advantages of biopsy, a well-performed double-contrast barium enema is still the primary diagnostic modality for detecting abnormalities of the colon. Colonoscopy has a complementary, not competitive, role in detecting and following colon disease.

Lesions detected with double-contrast barium enema studies are often subsequently evaluated by colonoscopy and biopsy. A negative barium enema study in the face of hemoccult positive stools is an indication for colonoscopic investigation. In one study the sensitivity of colonoscopy alone was 78%, with an accuracy rate of about 76%. However, in combination with the double-contrast barium enema, the two methods had an accuracy rate of 97%.[109]

Use of CT Scanning for Detection and Staging. Similar to gastric carcinoma, CT has been suggested as the imaging modality for staging colorectal carcinomas. Several investigations have shown that CT is a highly accurate method for staging carcinoma of the rectum and sigmoid.[68,108,121] The abdomen is scanned from the dome of the liver to the anal verge at 1-cm intervals. The patient is given 450 mL of 1% iodinated contrast material orally 30 minutes before the examination. About 200 mᵗ of a 1% solution of contrast material is given per rectun occasionally, air can be used alone for maximal rectal distension. In general, intravenous contrast material is not needed. Not only does CT provide transaxial images of the pelvis and perirectal area, but direct coronal images may also be obtained, providing added information on local extension and lymphadenopathy (Figure 13-31).[119] The tumors are classified into four stages based upon computed tomographic findings, with stage III divided into two substages. These are different from the AJC staging system:

stage I: Intraluminal polypoid mass
stage II: Thickening of the bowel wall (greater than 0.5 cm) (Figure 13-32)
stage IIIA: Invasion of surrounding tissue (without extension to pelvic sidewalls) (Figure 13-33)
stage IIIB: Extension to the pelvic sidewalls (Figures 13-32, 13-33)
stage IV: Presence of distant metastases

The CT staging system is not comparable with the Duke's staging system, which cannot be used because CT cannot distinguish between extension of tumor to or through the muscularis or serosa and is less accurate than lymphangiography in assessing lymph node metastases from pelvic tumors.[112] It is possible that a tumor staged I by CT may be Duke's C. In the study by Thoeni et al.,[108] CT detected all 39 primary rectal or rectosigmoid tumors found with barium studies for a sensitivity of 100% and had an overall staging accuracy of 92% when compared with surgical findings. A CT-guided biopsy further adds to the specificity and accuracy of the staging method.

The use of CT in staging carcinoma of the colon other than that of the rectum and sigmoid colon has yet to be

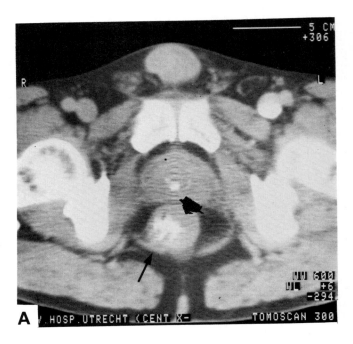

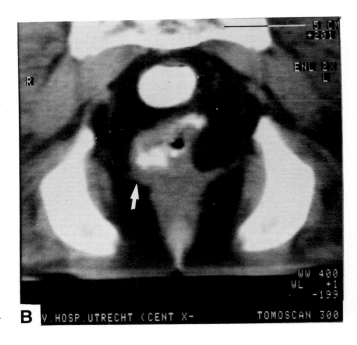

FIG. 13-31. Rectal carcinoma evaluated by direct coronal CT scanning. (Courtesy Dr. Paul Van Waes, Department of Radiology, University of Utrecht, The Netherlands.) (A) A conventional transaxial CT scan of the pelvis shows a rectal tumor (large arrow) narrowing the rectal lumen and producing irregularity in the contour of the contrast material in the lumen. The tumor appears to be invading the levator ani muscle on the right (small arrow). (B) A direct coronal CT scan clearly demonstrates the entire rectal and perirectal anatomy and shows definite invasion of the right levator ani (arrow). (C) A direct coronal CT scan of a different patient with rectal cancer (T) without invasion of the levator ani muscle (arrows).

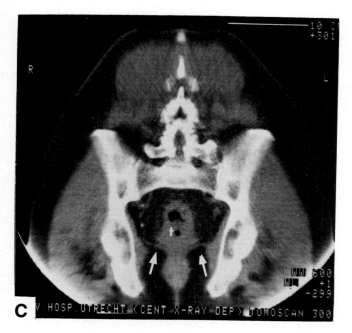

evaluated. Unlike the sigmoid and rectal carcinomas, carcinomas elsewhere in the colon are somewhat difficult to detect by CT because of the relative mobility of the colon (Figure 13-34). However, CT is accurate in determining whether there are any metastases to the liver or enlargement of mesenteric and periaortic lymph nodes.

We believe that CT will also be accurate in staging carcinoma of the colon, similar to the rectal and rectosigmoid colons.

Detecting the Recurrence of Carcinoma. Recurrence of tumor following surgery for rectal carcinoma may be detected by imaging both the lumen and the wall and pericolonic tissue. Thirty percent of the patients who have surgery for rectal carcinoma are found to have recurrence of tumors. Sixty percent of the patients with recurrent rectal carcinoma have only local tumor recurrence and 92% of local recurrences are found to be contiguous to the area of surgical incision.[15] Hence, the detection of tumor recurrence while the tumor is still localized to the operative area may lead to institution of curative therapy. Barium enema examination may detect narrowing at the anastomotic site, plaquelike or polypoid changes indicative of recurrence. However, in patients who have undergone abdominal-perineal (A-P) resection, barium studies cannot be used. Computed tomography has also been found to be valuable in the detection and staging

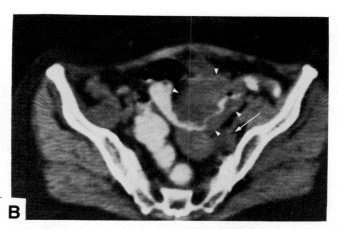

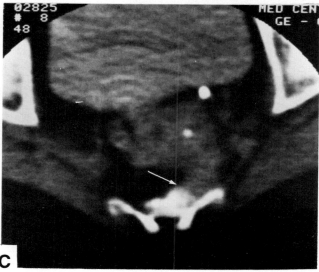

FIG. 13-32. (A) A primary adenocarcinoma of the rectum, stage II according to CT classification. Although the tumor narrows the lumen (outlined by contrast material,*) it has not spread to involve the pelvic side walls or adjacent organs. (B) Primary rectosigmoid adenocarcinoma, stage IIIa. The lesion (arrowheads) has not only encased the sigmoid, but has extended to involve a large area of mesentery and pelvic lymph nodes (arrow). (C) Primary rectal carcinoma, stage IIIb. Although the tumor mass is not enormous, it has extended in the perirectal space to involve the sacrum (arrow).

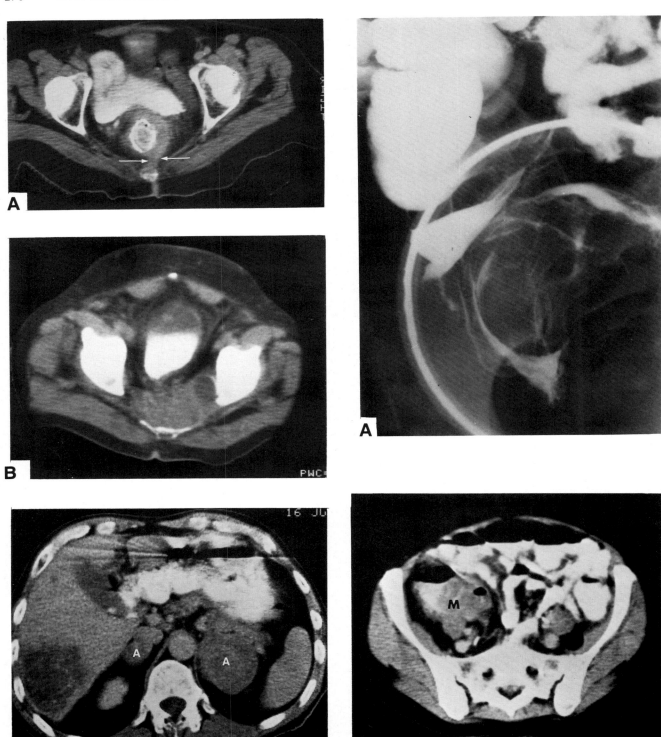

FIG. 13-33. (A) Recurrent rectal carcinoma at the site of previous simple resection. The tumor (arrows) has extended to involve the coccyx — stage IIIb. (B) Recurrent rectal carcinoma at the site of A-P resection. The tumor occupies the entire perirectal fossa and extends to the pelvic side walls — stage IIIb. (C) A CT scan of the liver and upper abdomen of the patient in Fig. 13-37B shows liver metastasis and bilateral adrenal metastases (A) — stage IV.

FIG. 13-34. (A) A large mass is present in the cecum of this patient, deforming the lumen and elevating the terminal ileum. (B) A CT scan shows this mass (M) to be extending widely into the mesentery and merging with the right psoas muscle. The lesion was a primary adeno-carcinoma of the cecum.

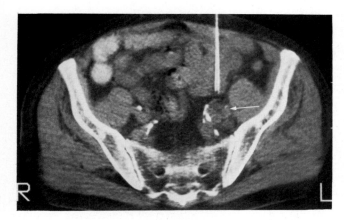

FIG. 13-35. This CT scan of a patient with a small rectal recurrence of carcinoma at the site of previous simple resection shows a soft tissue mass (arrow) in the region of the left common iliac lymph nodes. A CT-guided needle biopsy (two needles shown) confirmed the presence of tumor in lymph nodes.

of recurrent rectal carcinomas.[26,46,78] This is particularly true for patients with A-P resection.[60] In the study by Moss et al.,[78] the overall accuracy of CT in the detection of recurrent rectal carcinoma was 95%, with 100% sensitivity and 95% specificity. The method of study is similar to that of staging primary carcinoma described above. Recurrent rectosigmoid lesions may occupy the entire perirectal fossa, extending to pelvic sidewalls and local lymph nodes (Figure 13-33). A CT-guided needle biopsy is an important adjunct in confirming the diagnosis (Figure 13-35).

Imaging Strategies and Decisions

A double-contrast barium enema examination is the imaging examination of choice for the detection of primary colorectal carcinoma (Table 13-13). However, in those patients who are unable to cooperate in the double-contrast study, either a carefully performed single-contrast barium enema study using compression of the barium or colonoscopy is recommended. Sigmoidoscopy or fiberoptic colonoscopy then may be indicated to confirm the presence of a lesion detected on the single- or double-contrast study and to obtain tissue from the lesion if possible. If colonoscopy cannot confirm the presence of a lesion seen on the double-contrast study, the double-contrast barium enema should be repeated. If the lesion is again seen, colonoscopy should also be repeated. If the double-contrast study is of good quality and is completely normal, the patient can probably be followed clinically. However, if there is a strong clinical suspicion of the presence of a lesion such as persistence of occult blood per rectum, colonoscopy should be performed. Colonoscopy may not be needed in those instances where the lesions seen on the single-contrast or double-contrast study are highly characteristic of colonic carcinoma. Af-

ter the tumor is detected on the barium study and confirmed on the sigmoidoscopic or fiberoptic colonoscopic examination, CT may be of use in staging the primary tumor and in detecting liver metastases. This information may aid in planning preoperative radiation therapy, operative approach, and postoperative chemotherapy usage.

For those patients who are suspected of having recurrent colorectal carcinomas, CT scans should be used to examine the surgical site for possible recurrence as well as the liver and retroperitoneum for presence of metas-

Table 13-13. Modalities of Choice for Detecting Primary Colon Carcinoma

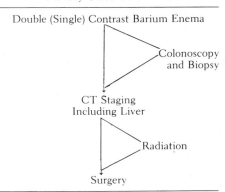

In evaluating a patient with a primary colon carcinoma, the current first diagnostic test is the barium enema. It is possible that in the next decade colonoscopy may assume a more important screening role, but at this time the barium enema, either single or double-contrast, still constitutes the major screening examination. Since it has been clearly shown that double-contrast studies detect more polypoid lesions than single-contrast studies, this approach is recommended for those patients who are properly prepared and are capable of undergoing the maneuvers necessary for a double-contrast colon study. The single-contrast study may be used for those patients who are not able to undergo a pneumocolon and is an effective screening study if properly performed with adequate attention to detail and compression of the barium-filled colon during fluoroscopy.

If a suspicious lesion is discovered, then colonoscopy should be performed, with biopsy of the lesion if necessary.

If a lesion is demonstrated on single-contrast or double-contrast but is clearly malignant in appearance, then a decision may be made about the next level of diagnostic imaging. In some cases, regardless of whether metastases are present or not, surgery is indicated and no more diagnostic tests are required. However, CT scanning, along with ultrasonography, may be used to evaluate the presence of liver metastasis before surgery. Recently CT has been utilized to stage the extraluminal and extramural extent of primary tumors in the rectosigmoid region, providing information about the local and distant extent of the primary tumor, which may be of use to the surgeon planning a local resection or designing radiation ports.

Table 13-14. Modalities of Choice for Detecting
Recurrent Colon Adenocarcinoma (AP Resection)

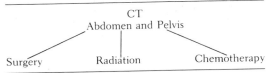

Since the rectum has been removed as part of the initial surgery for colon carcinoma, a barium enema cannot be used to detect recurrent disease. A CT scan of the pelvis is the most useful technique for detecting recurrent colon carcinoma after AP resection. This technique will detect changes in the perirectal fat and indicate the extent of recurrence with relationship to the prostate, bladder, pelvic sidewalls, and lymph nodes. In any situation where recurrent disease is suspected clinically or on the basis of elevated CEA levels, CT scanning should be utilized. On the basis of the information on the scan, surgery for recurrence can be considered, or alternatively, radiation therapy. In addition, since evaluation of the liver by CT during the scanning procedure will reveal the presence of metastases, the metastatic disease may then be considered for chemotherapeutic control.

tases (Table 13-14). For patients suspected of having recurrence after local resection, a double-contrast or single-contrast barium enema should first be performed. If a luminal lesion is seen, endoscopy with biopsy can then be performed. Computed tomographic scanning of the pelvis and abdomen is then recommended (Table 13-15),

Table 13-15. Modalities of Choice for Detecting
Recurrent Colon Adenocarcinoma

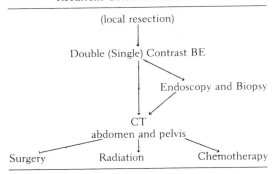

After local resection of a primary colon cancer, recurrence can be monitored either by performance of a barium enema or colonoscopy. Double-contrast radiography is more sensitive than single-contrast for the detection of minor changes in the mucosal pattern and wall contour indicating early recurrent disease, and both techniques are sensitive in the detection of advanced recurrence. In cases where the findings are suspicious on the barium enema studies, colonoscopy can be used to directly visualize the area and obtain tissue for histologic examination.

For recurrence located particularly in the rectosigmoid region, CT scanning is useful in staging the recurrence to detect the extent of extramural tumor and its relationship to other organs and lymph nodes. In addition, the liver can be scanned for the presence of metastases. Depending upon the information gained from the CT scan, reoperation can be considered. The information obtained about liver metastases may determine the institution of chemotherapy.

as in the case of abdominoperineal resections, for surgical and nonsurgical treatment planning.

The benefit versus cost of the various imaging modalities is summarized in Table 13-6.

Colonic Polyps. It is widely believed that most colonic carcinomas arise from benign polyps. Hence, the detection of early carcinoma of the colon is basically the detection of polyps 5 mm and larger. The double-contrast technique is more sensitive for detection of colonic polyps.[57] There are three technical factors that are important for the detection of polyps: (1) a clean colon, (2) good mucosal coating, and (3) adequate colonic distension. The demonstration of a stalk is conclusive proof of the presence of a polyp (Figure 13-36).

A number of radiographic signs may aid in the diagnosis of malignancy in a polyp. Polyps greater than 2 cm in size have an incidence of malignancy close to 50%.[75] If there is definite evidence of growth of a polyp on serial examination, malignancy should be suspected. Malignant polyps tend to have short and thick pedicles. The

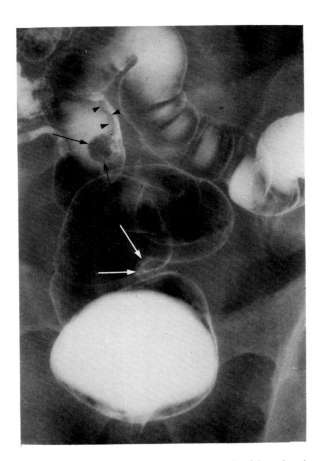

FIG. 13-36. Colonic polyp. A double-contrast study of the colon shows a polyp in the sigmoid colon outlined by the barium pool. The polyp (black arrows) is on a long stalk (arrowheads). In addition, a second smaller sessile polyp (white arrows) is present on the rectal valve.

head of a malignant polyp tends to be irregular and lobulated. Indentation or puckering of the base of the polyp is thought to be a reliable sign of malignancy.[57] Some of the above signs have been disputed in terms of specificity for malignancy. Skucas et al.[107] have shown that many of the above criteria are unreliable for diagnosing malignancy when the polyp is between 1 and 2 cm in size. They found that a carcinoma in an adenomatous polyp 1 to 2 cm in diameter was the most common type of early carcinoma, and these tumors rarely exhibit irregular or lobulated heads. By the time that they have an irregular or lobulated head, they have already grown beyond the 2-cm size and may have already metastasized. These investigators also found that a cancerous polyp rarely metastasizes if it is less than 1.5 cm in diameter, while 23% of those polyps between 1.5 and 2.5 cm in diameter have already had regional lymph involvement. The incidence of metastasis further increases to 53% for cancerous polyps 5.0 to 6.9 cm in diameter.[107] Similarly, the sign of retraction at the base of the polyp as an indication for malignancy has been found to be unreliable by Ament et al.[2] Using a hollow viscous model, they found that such an indentation may be the result of geometric projection rather than invasion of the stalk by the cancer. Colonoscopy has been considered to be more sensitive in detecting small colonic lesions than barium enema studies. However, at times the presence of polyps demonstrated on barium studies may not be seen on endoscopy. There are areas of the colon that are considered to be endoscopic blind spots. These areas include the base of prominent folds, such as in the rectum or cecum, the site of sharp angulation of the bowel, such as at the junction of the sigmoid and the descending colon, and at the flexures. In these areas, polyps may not be detected because they lie behind a fold or just beyond an area of angulation. Hence, if radiographic evidence of a polyp is present while the colonoscopy does not demonstrate one, a repeat barium enema may be needed.[114] In addition, failure to visualize the cecum colonoscopically may result in false-negative determinations.[109]

Detection and Assessment of Advanced Carcinoma. The majority of the patients who are symptomatic from their colorectal carcinoma have advanced lesions. These tumors are generally large annular (Figure 13-37) or polypoid lesions (Figures 13-38, 13-39) that are easily diagnosed on either single-contrast or double-contrast studies. Radiographically, the transition from the tumor to normal or adjacent mucosa is often abrupt, producing overhanging edges of tumor. Infiltrating types of tumors often produce slightly elevated masses with smooth surfaces that stiffen and indent the walls of the colon. However, in the early stages, scirrhous carcinoma and carcinoma associated with inflammation often are difficult to detect because the transition from normal to abnor-

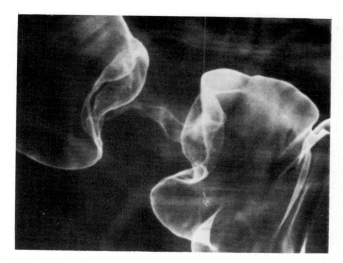

FIG. 13-37. Adenocarcinoma of the colon. A double-contrast view shows a characteristic annular lesion with overhanging edges caused by tumor mass.

mal bowel is indistinct. It is important to note that approximately 5% of the patients with advanced carcinoma have multiple synchronous carcinomas of the colon and also that these tumors are frequently associated with "sentinel polyps" (Figure 13-40).[57] Hence, it is important to examine the entire colon whenever possible. Occasionally, adenocarcinoma of the colon may contain calcification, which may be detected on the plain film in the expected course of the colon. The calcifications are curvilinear, mottled, or both. There may also be calcification in the metastatic lesions to the lymph nodes and to

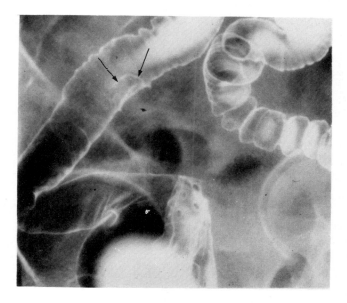

FIG. 13-38. Colonic adenocarcinoma, sessile-polypoid form. The tumor projects into the lumen and is outlined by the barium (arrows), producing a second line in addition to the colon wall.

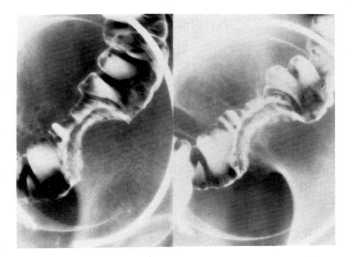

FIG. 13-39. Large sessile adenocarcinoma of the sigmoid with slightly irregular surface features compared with the normal wall.

the liver. Calcified lesions are generally mucoid carcinomas.

Treatment Decisions[14,21,22,91]

Surgery. The management of local and regional colon carcinoma is primarily surgical (Table 13-16). The operative objective is en bloc resection of the primary tumor along with intervening lymphatics and regional lymph nodes in a single specimen. This is easier to achieve with cancer of the colon than with cancer of the rectum because of the limitation of excision by the pelvic sidewalls—a main reason for the higher frequency of local recurrence with resection of rectal cancer (Table 13-17).

In rectosigmoid carcinoma, determination of the lower margins of the tumor is extremely important for planning the approach of the surgical procedure. For those tumors that are located greater than 12 cm away from the anal verge, a simple intra-abdominal approach is used. For those tumors that are located less than 7 cm from the anal verge, an abdominal perineal approach is needed. However, for those tumors that are located between 7 and 12 cm from the anal verge, the surgical approach is variable.[19]

Fifty percent of those patients with rectal carcinoma who had surgery will die of local recurrence with hematogenous metastasis. Thirty percent will have pelvic recurrence. Of these, half will be evident in the first postoperative year and 80% will be evident at the end of the second postoperative year. The site is usually in the posterior pelvic and presacral area for men. In women, the posterior vaginal wall and the rectal-vaginal pouch are the common sites of recurrence.[19] Computed to-

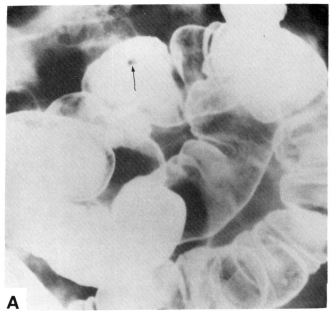

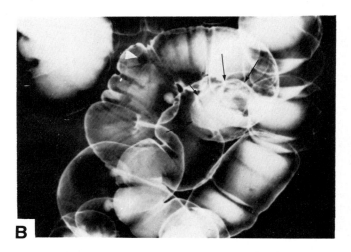

FIG. 13-40. Colonic carcinoma associated with a single polyp. (A) A polypoid filling defect is visible in the barium pool on this double-contrast study of the sigmoid colon (arrow). (B) Oblique view of the colon demonstrates a large polypoid adenocarcinoma (arrows) near the region of the polyp, which was obscured in A by barium in an overlapping portion of the sigmoid. The single polyp visible in A is also demonstrated (white arrow).

mography is the best imaging modality available for the evaluation of these areas.

Greater than 90% of the patients with colorectal carcinoma undergo surgery. Of these, 70% undergo resection for cure. The remaining 20% have palliative operations, often combined with radiotherapy.

Radiation Therapy. There are advocates for both preoperative and postoperative irradiation and both together are under study in different cooperative groups.[50,72] Cur-

Table 13-16. Treatment Decisions: Colon[76]

STAGE	SURGERY	RADIATION THERAPY	CHEMOTHERAPY
IA (T_1,N_0,M_0)	Wide segmental resection and regional nodes in mesentery and primary anastomosis	NR	NR
IIB (T_2,N_0,M_0) (Duke B)	Wide segmental resection and regional nodes in mesentery and primary anastomosis	NR	NR
II (T_3,T_4,N_0,M_0) (Duke C)	Wide segmental resection and regional nodes in mesentery and primary anastomosis	Investigational adjuvant RT 5,000 cGy	Investigational adjuvant MAC
II* (T_5,N_0,M_0) III* (T_5,N_1,M_0)	By-pass colostomy Palliative resection	Palliative RT 4,000–5,000 cGy	Investigational MAC
IV (T_{any},N_{any},M_+) (Duke D)	By-pass colostomy Palliative resection	NR	Investigational MAC

NR = not recommended
RT = radiation therapy
MAC = multiagent chemotherapy

rently, the evidence is mixed for the true role of adjuvant radiation therapy or chemotherapy in its ability to reduce local regional recurrence and in turn have an impact upon survival (Tables 13-16, 13-17).

Preoperative radiation. Many different schedules have been used ranging from 2,000 to 6,000 cGy with little agreement on optimum dose. Low doses of 2000 cGy are unsuccessful, but it has been shown that higher fractionated doses of 4000 cGy preoperative radiation improves the survival rate.[103] Another approach is to utilize 500 cGy in one exposure before surgery and postoperative irradiation if residual disease is left behind.

Postoperative radiation. Based upon patterns of failure in second-look operations, Gunderson and Sosin[40] advocated a wide pelvic field with a para-aortic extension. Although some studies showed a large reduction in relapse, controlled studies, both reported and in progress, suggest gains will be modest. Other trials using combinations of chemotherapy (5-FU and methyl-cyclohexylchloroethylnitrosurea) and radiation have likewise not been impressive in their ability to improve survival.[44,59,70] A new approach is to attempt infusion chemotherapy

(5-FU and mitomycin-c) in conjunction with irradiation, to see if the dramatic improvement in results achieved with anal squamous cell cancers will occur with rectal adenocarcinomas.

Chemotherapy. The chemotherapeutic agent most commonly used in the treatment of colorectal cancer is 5-fluorouracil (5-FU). It has not been shown to have a significant impact on the survival of patients with local or regional colonic cancer. However, it is the mainstay of treatment of unresectable colorectal carcinomas, with a response rate of approximately 20%. There have been recent reports of improved response rate with the use of combination chemotherapy using 5-FU, methyl-CCNU, and other agents. However, further studies are needed to confirm these findings.[82]

The prognosis for patients with adenocarcinoma of the colon depends heavily upon the stage of the tumor. Unlike gastric carcinoma, a significant portion of patients with colorectal cancer have localized disease, hence, the overall survival rates for these patients are significantly better than for those with gastric cancer, i.e., 33% to 47% five-year survival rate for colorectal compared with 12% to 13% for gastric cancer. Forty-

Table 13-17. Treatment Decisions: Rectum[76]

STAGE	SURGERY	RADIATION THERAPY		CHEMOTHERAPY
IA	Abdominoperineural or anterior resection and regional nodes	NR		NR
IB	Abdominoperineural or anterior resection and regional nodes	Postoperative adjuvant RT 5,000 cGy		Investigational MAC
II III	If unresectable, colostomy	Preoperative RT 2,000–5,000 cGy with surgical reassessment	and/or	Investigational MAC or Infusion during RT
IV	If unresectable, colostomy	Palliative RT 5,000–6,000 cGy		MAC

NR = not recommented
RT = radiation therapy
MAC = multiagent chemotherapy

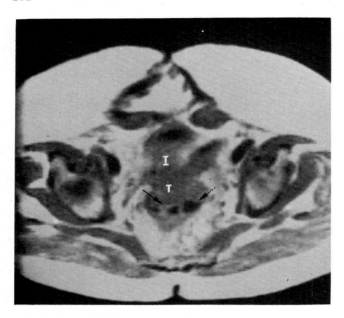

FIG. 13-41. An MRI image of the pelvis of a patient with rectal carnoma. The tumor (T) can be seen invading the seminal vesicles above and the base of the bladder (I) and deforming the rectal air below (arrows).

four percent of patients with colorectal carcinoma have tumors involving only the bowel wall; 26% of the tumors involve the adjacent organ structures, while 25% are disseminated diseases. Those patients with localized disease have a five-year survival rate of 59% to 77% compared with those with disseminated disease, who have a five-year survival rate of only 20% to 29%.[106]

Impact of New Technology

The improvements in the methods of diagnosis of colonic carcinoma over the past 25 years have not resulted in a significant increase in survival in patients with colonic carcinoma. However, it has been shown that the systematic removal of benign polyps during routine proctosigmoidoscopy has resulted in a lower incidence of rectal carcinoma.[18,36] Hence, it is apparent that a decrease in mortality from colorectal carcinoma will depend on the early detection and treatment of carcinoma or premalignant lesions in asymptomatic patients. The routine screening of patients for presence of occult blood in the stool may lead to earlier examination with double-contrast studies, which may lead to the diagnosis of early colonic carcinoma.

Computed tomography probably will not have a significant impact on survival rates. However, it will have a definite impact on the management of the patients with suspected recurrent tumor.

With the advent of MRI and its inherent ability to examine the pelvis in a sagittal or coronal projection as well as axially, the degree of tumor extension may be better defined in that region. At present, no data are available on the MRI appearance of colorectal cancer (Figure 13-41). However, the impact of MRI on survival and staging of rectal carcinoma is yet to be evaluated.

REFERENCES

1. Abe, M., Takahashi, M.: Intraoperative radiotherapy: The Japanese experience. *Int. J. Radiat. Oncol. Biol. Phys.* 7:863–868, 1981.
2. Ament, A. E., Alfidi, R. J., Rao, P. S.: Basal indentation of sessile polypoid lesions: A function of geometry rather than a sign of malignancy *Radiology* 143:341–344, 1982.
3. American Joint Committee on Cancer: Staging of cancer of the colon and rectum. In *Manual for Staging of Cancer*, 2nd ed. Philadelphia, J. B. Lippincott, 1983, pp. 73–80.
4. American Joint Committee on Cancer: Staging of cancer of the stomach. In *Manual for Staging of Cancer*, 2nd ed. Philadelphia, J. B. Lippincott, 1983, pp. 73–80.
5. Balfe, D. M., Koehler, R. E., Karstaedt, N., Stanley, R. J., Sagel, S. S.: Computed tomography of gastric neoplasms. *Radiology* 140:431–436, 1981.
6. Balthazar, E. J.: Carcinoid tumors. In *Radiology of the Colon*. Marshak, R. H., Lindner, A. E., Maklansky, D. (Eds.). Philadelphia, W. B. Saunders, 1980, pp. 561–582.
7. Boros, L.: Gastrointestinal cancers. In *Practical Cancer Chemotherapy*. Rosenthal, S. N., Bennett, J. M. (Eds.). Garden City, N.J., Medical Examiners Publishing Co., 1981, pp. 226–262.
8. Brady, L. W.: Malignant lymphoma of the gastrointestinal tract. *Radiology* 137:291–298, 1980.
9. Brandborg, L. L.: Polyps, tumors and cancer of the stomach. In *Gastrointestinal Diseases—Pathophysiology, Diagnosis, Management*, 2nd ed., Sleisenger, M. H., Fordtran, J. S. (Eds.). Philadelphia, W. B. Saunders, 1978, pp. 752–775.
10. Burgener, F. A., Hamlin, D. J.: Histiocytic lymphoma of the abdomen: Radiographic spectrum. *A.J.R.* 137:337–342, 1981.
11. Bush, R. S.: The compleat oncologist: Franz Buschke lecture. *Int. J. Radiat. Oncol. Biol. Phys.* 8:1019–1027, 1982.
12. Buy, J. N., Moss, A. A.: Computed tomography of gastric lymphoma. *A.J.R.* 138:859–865, 1982.
13. Cady, B., Ramsden, D. A., Choe, D. S.: Treatment of gastric cancer. *Surg. Clin. North. Am.* 56:599–605, 1976.
14. Carter, S. K., Glatstein, E., Livingstone, R. B. (Eds.): *Principles of Cancer Treatment*. New York, McGraw-Hill, 1982.
15. Cass, A. W., Million, R. R., Pfaff, W. W.: Patterns of recurrence following surgery alone for adenocarcinoma of the colon and rectum. *Cancer* 37:2861–2865, 1976.
16. Clark, R. A., Alexander, E. S.: Computed tomography of gastrointestinal leiomyosarcoma. *Gastrointest. Radiol.* 7:127–129, 1982.
17. Comis, R. L.: The therapy of stomach cancer. In *Principles of Cancer Treatment*. Carter, S. K., Glatstein, E., Livingston, R. B. (Eds.). New York, McGraw-Hill, 1982, pp. 420–425.
18. Dales, L. G., Friedman, G. D., Ramcharan, S., Siegelaub, A. B., Campbell, B. A., Feldman, R., Collen, M. F.: Multiphasic check-up evaluation study. 3. Outpatient clinical utilization, hospitalization and mortality experience after seven years. *Prevent. Med.* 2:221–235, 1973.
19. Decosse, J. J.: The management of local and regional large bowel cancer. In *Principles of Cancer Treatment*. Carter, S. K., Glatstein, E., Livingston, R. B. (Eds.). New York, McGraw-Hill, 1982, pp. 390–396.
20. De Dombal, F. T.: Ulcerative colitis: Definition, historical backgrounds, etiology, diagnosis, natural history and local complications. *Postgrad. Med. J.* 44:684–692, 1968.
21. del Regato, J. A., Spjut, H. J.: *Cancer: Diagnosis, Treatment, and*

Prognosis, 5th ed. St. Louis, C. V. Mosby, 1977.

22. DeVita, V. T., Hellman, S., Rosenberg, S. A. (Eds.): *Cancer Principles and Practice of Oncology*. Philadelphia, J. B. Lippincott Co., 1982.

23. Dougherty, S. H., Foster, C. A., Eisenberg, M. M.: Stomach cancer following gastric surgery for benign disease. *Arch. Surg.* 117:294–297, 1982.

24. Doyle, F. H., Pennock, J. M., Banks, L. M., McDonnell, M. J., Bydder, G. M., Steiner, R. E., Young, I. R., Clarke, G. J., Pasmore, T., Gilderdale, D. J.: Nuclear magnetic resonance imaging of the liver: Initial experience. *A.J.R.* **138**: 193–200, 1982.

25. Ellert, J., Kreel, L.: The role of computed tomography in the initial staging and subsequent management of the lymphomas. *J. Comput. Assist. Tomogr.* **4**:368–391, 1980.

26. Ellert, J., Kreel, L.: The value of CT in malignant colonic tumors. *CT* **4**:225–240, 1980.

27. Evers, K., Laufer, I., Gordon, R. L., Kressel, H. Y., Herlinger, H., Gohel, V. K.: Double-contrast enema examination for detection of rectal carcinoma. *Radiology* 140:635–639, 1981.

28. Feldman, F., Seaman, W. B.: Primary gastric stump cancer. *A.J.R.* 115:257–267, 1972.

29. Felsen, J., Wolarsky, W.: Chronic ulcerative colitis in carcinoma. *Arch. Intern. Med.* 84:293, 1949.

30. Fleckenstein, P., Pederson, G.: The value of the duodenal intubation method (Sellink technique) for the radiological visualization of the small bowel. *Scand. J. Gastroenterol.* 10:423–426, 1975.

31. Fleming, I. D., Mitchell, S., Dilawari, R. A.: The role of surgery in the management of gastric lymphoma. *Cancer* 49:1135–1141, 1982.

32. Fork, F. T.: Double-contrast enema and colonoscopy in polyp detection. *Gut* 22:971–977, 1981.

33. Freid, A. M., Poulos, A., Hattfield, D. R.: The effectiveness of the incidental small-bowel series. *Radiology* 140:45–46, 1981.

34. Frik, W.: Neoplastic diseases of the stomach. In *Alimentary Tract Roentgenology*, 2nd ed. Margulis, A. R., Burhenne, H. J. (Eds.). St. Louis, C. V. Mosby Co., 1973, pp. 662–709.

35. Gelfand, D. W., Ott, D. J., Tritico, R.: Causes of error in gastrointestinal radiology. I. Upper gastrointestinal examination. *Gastrointest. Radiol.* 5:91–97, 1980.

36. Gilbertsen, V. A.: Procto-sigmoidoscopy and polypectomy in reducing the incidence of rectal cancer. *Cancer* 34:936–939, 1974.

37. Gohel, V. K., Laufer, I.: Double-contrast examination of the postoperative stomach. *Radiology* 129:601–607, 1978.

38. Gold, R. P., Seaman, W. B.: The primary double-contrast examination of the postoperative stomach. *Radiology* 124:297–305, 1977.

39. Gueller, R., Shapiro, H. A., Nelson, J. A., Bush, R.: Suture granulomas simulating tumors; a preventable post-gastrectomy complication. *Dig. Dis. Sci.* 21:223–228, 1976.

40. Gunderson, L. L., Sosin, H.: Adenocarcinoma of the stomach: Areas of failure in a reoperation series (second or symptomatic look), clinicopathologic correlation and implications for adjuvant therapy. *Int. J. Radiat. Oncol. Biol. Phys.* 8:1–12, 1982.

41. Gurian, L., Jendrzejewski, J., Katon, R., Bilbao, M., Cope, R., Melnyk, C.: Small bowel enema: An underutilized method of small bowel examination. *Dig. Dis. Sci.* 27:1101–1108, 1982.

42. Haenszel, W., Correa, P.: Cancer of the colon and rectum and adenomatous polyps: A review of epidemiologic findings. *Cancer* 28:14–24, 1971.

43. Herlinger, H.: Double contrast enteroclysis. In *Alimentary Tract Radiology*, 3rd ed. Margulis, A. R., Burhenne, H. J., (Eds.). St. C. V. Mosby Co., 1983, pp. 890–902.

44. Higgins, G. A., Jr., Conn, J. H., Jordan, P. H., Humphrey, E. W., Roswit, B., Keehn, R. J.: Preoperative radiotherapy for colorectal cancer. *Ann. Surg.* 181:624–631, 1975.

45. Hill, M. J.: Bacteria and the etiology of colonic cancer. *Cancer* 34:815–818, 1974.

46. Husband, J. E., Hodson, N. J., Parsons, C. A.: The use of computed tomography in recurrent rectal tumors. *Radiology* 134:677–682, 1980.

47. *TNM Classification of Malignant Tumors*, 3rd ed., Geneva, Switzerland, International Union Against Cancer, 1978.

48. Jones, R. S., Sleisenger, M. H.: Cancer of the colon and rectum. In *Gastrointestinal Diseases—Pathophysiology, Diagnosis and Management*. Sleisenger, M. H., Fordtran, J. S. (Eds.). Philadelphia, W. B. Saunders Co., 1978, pp. 1784–1800.

49. Klarfeld, J., Resnick, G.: Gastric remnant carcinoma. *Cancer* 44: 1129–1133, 1979.

50. Klassen, D. J., Cotton, G. E.: Treatment of locally unresectable cancer of the stomach and pancreas. An Eastern Cooperative Oncology Group study, (abstracted). *Proc. Am. Soc. Clin. Oncol.* 21:416, 1980.

51. Knutson, C. O., Max, M. H.: Diagnostic and therapeutic colonoscopy: A critical review of 662 examinations. *Arch. Surg.* 114: 430–434, 1979.

52. Komaiko, M. S.: Gastric neoplasm: Ultrasound and CT evaluation. *Gastrointest. Radiol.* 4:131–137, 1979.

53. Kronborg, O., Ostergaard, A.: Evaluation of the barium-enema examination and colonoscopy in diagnosis of colonic cancer. *Dis. Colon. Rectum.* 18:674–677, 1975.

54. Kurtz, R. C., Lightdale, C. J., Winawer, S. J., Sherlock, P.: Endoscopy and gastrointestinal neoplasia: Diagnosis and management. *Curr. Probl. Cancer* 5:4–48, 1980.

55. Landres, R. T., Strum, W. B.: Endoscopic techniques in the diagnosis of gastric adenocarcinoma. *Gastrointest. Endosc.* 23:203–205, 1977.

56. Laufer, I.: Double contrast enema: Technical aspects. In *Double-Contrast Gastrointestinal Radiology with Endoscopic Correlation*. Laufer, I. (Ed.). Philadelphia, W. B. Saunders Co., 1979, pp. 495–516.

57. Laufer, I.: Tumors of the colon. In *Double-Contrast Gastrointestinal Radiology with Endoscopic Correlation*. Laufer, I. (Ed.). Philadelphia, W. B. Saunders Co., 1979, pp. 517–560.

58. Laufer, I., Smith, N. C. W., Mullens, J. E.: The radiological demonstration of colorectal polyps undetected by endoscopy. *Gastroenterology* 70:167–170, 1976.

59. Lavin, P., Mittelman, A., Douglass, H., Engstrom, P., Klaassen, D.: Survival and response to chemotherapy for advanced colorectal carcinoma. An Eastern Cooperative Oncology Group Report. *Cancer* 46:1536–1543, 1980.

60. Lee, J. K. T., Stanley, R. J., Sagel, S. S., Levitt, R. G., McClennan, B. J.: CT appearance of the pelvis after abdomino-perineal resection for rectal carcinoma. *Radiology* 141:737–741, 1981.

61. Lee, K. R., Levine, E., Moffat, R. E., Bigongiari, L. R., Hermreck, A. S.: Computed tomographic staging of malignant gastric neoplasms. *Radiology* 133:151–155, 1979.

62. Lehman, G. A., Buchner, D. M., Lappas, J. C.: Anatomical extent of fiberoptic sigmoidoscopy. *Gastroenterology* 84:803–808, 1983.

63. Loose, H. W. C., Williams, C. B.: Barium enema versus colonoscopy. *Proc. R. Soc. Med.* 67:1033–1036, 1974.

64. Lynch, H. T., Guirgis, H. A., Lynch, P. M., Lynch, J. F., Harris, R. E.: Familial cancer syndrome. A survey. *Cancer* 39:1867–1881, 1977.

65. MacDonald, J. S., Gunderson, L. L., Cohn, I., Jr.: Cancer of the stomach. In *Cancer: Principles and Practice of Oncology*. DeVita, V. T., Hellman, S., Rosenberg, S. A. (Eds.) Philadelphia, J. B. Lippincott Co., 1982, pp. 534–561.

66. Maruyama, M.: Early gastric cancer. In *Double-Contrast Gastrointestinal Radiology with Endoscopic Correlation*. Laufer, I. (Ed.). Philadelphia, W. B. Saunders Co., 1979, pp. 241–287.

67. Mason, G. R.: Tumors of the duodenum and small intestine. In *Davis-Christopher Textbook of Surgery, The Biological Basis of Modern Surgical Practice*. Sabiston, D. C. (Ed.). Philadelphia, W.

B. Saunders Co., 1977, pp. 969–976.

68. Mayes, G. B., Zornoza, H. J.: Computed tomography of colon carcinoma. *A.J.R.* 135:43–46, 1980.

69. McFee, A. S., Aust, J. B.: Gastric carcinoma and the CAT scan. *Gastroenterology* 80:196–198, 1981.

70. Mittelman, A., Holyoke, P. R. M., Thomas, C. G., et al.: Adjuvant chemotherapy and radiotherapy following rectal surgery: An interim report from the Gastrointestinal Tumor Study Group (GITSG). In *Adjuvant Therapy of Cancer III*. Salmon, S. E., Jones, S. E. (Eds.). New York, Grune & Stratton, 1981, pp. 547–558.

71. Moertel, C. G., Bargen, J. A., Dockerty, M. B.: Multiple carcinoma of the large intestine: A review of the literature and a study of 261 cases. *Gastroenterology* 34:85, 1958.

72. Moertel, C. G., Childs, D. S., Reitemeier, R. J., Colby, M. Y., Holbrook, M. A.: Combined 5-FU and supervoltage radiation therapy of locally unresectable gastrointestinal cancer. *Lancet* 2:865–867, 1969.

73. Montagne, E. D., Votava, C., Jr., Gunderson, L. L.: Gastrointestinal tract. In *Textbook of Radiotherapy*, 3rd ed. Fletcher, G. H. (Ed.). Philadelphia, Lea & Febiger, 1980, pp. 704–719.

74 Montagne, J. P., Moss, A. A., Margulis, A. R.: Double-blind study of single and double contrast upper gastrointestinal examination using endoscopy as a control. *A.J.R.* 130:1041–1045, 1978.

75. Morson, B.C.: The polyp-cancer sequence in the large bowel. *Proc. R. Soc. Med.* 67:451, 1974.

76. Morton, J. M., Poulter, C. A., Pandya, K. J.: Alimentary tract cancer. In *Clinical Oncology for Medical Students and Physicians: A Multidisciplinary Approach*, 6th ed. Rubin, P. (Ed.). New York, American Cancer Society, 1983, pp. 154–176.

77. Moss, A. A., Schnyder, P., Marks, W., Margulis, A. R.: Gastric adenocarcinoma: A comparison of the accuracy and economics of staging by computed tomography and surgery. *Gastroenterology* 80:45–50, 1981.

78. Moss, A. A., Thoeni, R. F., Schnyder, P., Margulis, A. R.: Value of computed tomography in the detection and staging of recurrent rectal carcinomas. *J. Comput. Assist. Tomogr.* 5:870–874, 1981.

79. Nagase, M., Tanigawa, N., Hikasa, Y.: Case report: Primary carcinoma of the remnant stomach – report of three cases. *Gastroenterol. Jpn.* 15:527–531, 1980.

80. Nagayo, T., Yokoyama, H.: Early phases and diagnostic features. *J.A.M.A.* 228:888–889, 1974.

81. Nauert, T. C., Zornoza, J., Ordonez, N.: Gastric leiomyosarcomas. *A.J.R.* 139:291–297, 1982.

82. Neefe, J. R., Schein, P. S.: The management of disseminated large bowel cancer. In *Principles of Cancer Treatment*. Carter, S. K., Glatstein, E., Livingston, R. B. (Eds.). New York, McGraw-Hill, 1982, pp. 402–407.

83. Nicholson, W. J.: Cancer following occupational exposure to asbestos and vinyl chloride. *Cancer* 39:1972–1801, 1977.

84. O'Brien, T. F.: Primary tumors and vascular malformations. In *Gastrointestinal Diseases – Pathophysiology, Diagnosis, Management*. 2nd ed. Sleisenger, M. H., Fordtran, J. S. (Eds.). Philadelphia, W. B. Saunders Co., 1978, pp. 1124–1136.

85. Ominsky, S. H., Margulis, A. R.: Radiographic examination of the upper gastrointestinal tract. A survey of current techniques. *Radiology* 139:11–17, 1981.

86. Ostrow, J. D., Mulvaney, C. A., Hansel, J. R., Rhodes, R. S., Weigand, P.: Sensitivity and reproducibility of chemical tests for fecal occult blood with an emphasis on false-positive reactions. *Am. J. Dig. Dis.* 18:930–940, 1973.

87. Ott, D. J., Gelfand, D. W., Wu, W. C., Kerr, R. M.: Sensitivity of double-contrast barium enema: Emphasis on polyp detection. *A.J.R.* 135:327–330, 1980.

88. Rabe, F. E., Becker, G. J., Besozzi, M. J., Miller, R. E.: Efficacy

study of the small bowel examination. *Radiology* 140:47–50, 1981.

89. Redmond, C. K., Strobino, B. R., Cypress, R. H.: Cancer experiences among coke by-product workers. *Ann. N.Y. Acad. Sci.* 271:102–115, 1976.

90. Rhodes, J. B., Holmes, G. G., Clark, G. M.: Changing distribution of primary cancers in the large bowel. *J.A.M.A.* 238:1641–1643, 1977.

91. Rider, W. D.: The 1975 Gordon Richards Memorial Lecture: Is the Miles operation really necessary for the treatment of rectal cancer? *J. Can. Assoc. Radiol.* 126:167–175, 1975.

92. Robbins, S. L.: The gastrointestinal tract. In *Pathologic Basis of Disease*, 2nd ed. Robbins, S. L., Cotran, R. S. (Eds.). Philadelphia, W. B. Saunders Co., 1979, pp. 946–952.

93. Rose, H. S., Balthazar, E. J., Megibow, A. J., Horowitz, L., Laubenstein, L. J.: Alimentary tract involvement in Kaposi sarcoma: Radiographic and endoscopic findings in 25 homosexual men. *A.J.R.* 139:661–666, 1982.

94. Schlaeger, R.: Examination of the small bowel. In *Alimentary Tract Roentgenology*, 2nd ed. Margulis, A. R., Burhenne, H. J. (Eds.). St. Louis, C. V. Mosby Co., 1973, pp. 799–815.

95. Schlaeger, R.: Neoplasms of the small bowel. In *Alimentary Tract Roentgenology*. 2nd ed. Margulis, A. R., Burhenne, H. J. (Eds.). St. Louis, C. V. Mosby Co., 1973, pp. 883–902.

96. Schrock, T. R.: Diseases of anorectum. In *Gastrointestinal Diseases – Pathophysiology, Diagnosis, and Management*, 2nd ed. Sleisenger, M. H., Fordtran, J. S. (Eds.). Philadelphia, W. B. Saunders Co., 1978, pp. 1875–1888.

97. Segal, A. W., Healy, M. J. R., Cox, A. G.: Diagnosis of gastric cancer. *Br. Med. J.* 2:669–672, 1975.

98. Seigel, R. S., Kuhns, L. R., Borlaza, G. S., McCormick, T. L., Simmons, J. L.: Computed tomography and angiography in ileal carcinoid tumor and retractile mesenteritis. *Radiology* 134:437–440, 1980.

99. Selikoff, I. J., Bader, R. A., Bader, M. E., Chung, J., Hammond, E. C.: Asbestos and neoplasia. *Amer. J. of Med.* 42:487–496, 1967.

100. Sellink, J. L.: Single contrast enteroclysis. In *Alimentary Tract Radiology*, 3rd ed. Margulis, A. R., Burhenne, H. J. (Eds.). St. Louis, C. V. Mosby Co., 1983, pp. 871–889.

101. Serlin, D., Keehn, R. J., Higgins, G. A., Harawer, H. W., Mendeloff, G. L.: Factors related to survival following resection for gastric carcinoma: Analysis of 903 cases. *Cancer* 40:1318–1329, 1978.

102. Shinya, H.: Neoplastic polypoid lesions. In *Colonoscopy – Diagnosis and Treatment of Colonic Disease*. New York, Igaku-Shoin, 1982, pp. 124–169.

103. Shirakabe, J., Maruyama, M.: Neoplastic disease of the stomach. In *Alimentary Tract Radiology*, 3rd ed. Margulis, A. R., Burhenne, H. J., (Eds.). St. Louis, C. V. Mosby Co., 1983, pp. 721–765.

104. Showstack, J. A., Schroeder, S. A., Steinberg, H.: Evaluating the costs and benefits of a diagnostic technology. The case of upper gastrointestinal endoscopy. *Med. Care.* 19:498, 1981.

105. Shulman, A., Simpkins, K. C.: The accuracy of radiological diagnosis of benign, primary and secondary malignant ulcers and their correlation with three simplified radiologic types. *Clin. Radiol.* 26:317, 1975.

106. Silverberg, E.: Cancer statistics, 1983. *CA* 33:9–25, 1983.

107. Skucas, J., Spataro, R. F., Cannucciari, D. P.: The radiographic features of small colon cancers. *Radiology* 143:335–340, 1982.

108. Thoeni, R. F., Moss, A. A., Schnyder, P., Margulis, A. R.: Detection and staging of primary rectal and rectosigmoid cancer by computed tomography. *Radiology* 141:135–138, 1981.

109. Thoeni, R. F., Petras, A.: Double-contrast barium enema examination and endoscopy in the detection of polypoid lesions in the cecum and ascending colon. *Radiology* 144:257–260, 1982.

110. Trier, J. S.: Lymphoma. In *Gastrointestinal Diseases – Pathophysiology, Diagnosis, Management*, 2nd ed. Sleisenger, M. H., Ford-

tran, J. S. (Eds.). Philadelphia, W. B. Saunders Co., 1978, pp. 1115–1123.

111. Walls, W. J.: The evaluation of malignant gastric neoplasms by ultrasonic B-scanning. *Radiology* **118**:159–163, 1976.

112. Walsh, J. W., Amendosa, M. A., Karsten, F. K., Tisnado, J., Hazia, T. A.: Computed tomographic detection of pelvic and inguinal lymph-node metastases from primary and recurrent malignant pelvic disease. *Radiology* **137**:157–166, 1980.

113. Welvaart, K., Zwaveling, A.: Carcinoma of the esophagus and gastric cardia. *Clin. Oncol.* **6**:203–212, 1980.

114. Weyman, P. J., Koehler, R. E., Zukerman, G. R.: Resolution of radiographic-endoscopic discrepancies in colon neoplasms. *J. Clin. Gastroenterol.* **3(suppl.** 1):89–93, 1981.

115. Winawer, S. J., Posner, G., Lightdale, C. J.: Endoscopic diagnosis of advanced gastric cancer: Factors influencing yield. *Gastroenterology* **69**:1183–1187, 1975.

116. Winnan, G., Berci, G., Panish, J., Talbot, T. M., Overholt, B. F., McCallum, R. W.: Superiority of the flexible to the rigid sigmoid-oscope in routine proctosigmoidoscopy. *N. Engl. J. Med.* **302**: 1011–1012, 1980.

117. Witzel, L., Halter, F., Greillat, P. A., Scheuer, U., Keller, M.: Evaluation of specific value of endoscopic biopsies and brush cytology for malignancies in the esophagus and stomach. *Gut* **17**:375–377, 1976.

118. Wolff, W. I., Shinya, H., Geffen, A., Ozoktay, S., De Beer, R.: Comparison of colonoscopy and the contrast enema in five-hundred patients with colorectal disease. *Am. J. Surg.* **129**:181–186, 1975.

119. van Waes, P. F. G. M., Zonneveld, F. W.: Direct coronal body computed tomography. *J. Comput. Assist. Tomogr.* **6**:58–66, 1982.

120. Yeh, H. C., Rabinowitz, J. G.: Ultrasonography and computed tomography of gastric wall lesions. *Radiology* **141**:147–155, 1981.

121. Zaunbauer, W., Haertel, M., Fuchs, W. A.: Computed tomography in carcinoma of the rectum. *Gastrointest. Radiol.* **6**:79–84, 1981.

122. Zornoza, J., Dodd, G. D., Jr.: Lymphoma of the gastrointestinal tract. *Semin. Roentgenol.* **15**:272, 1980.

14 MALIGNANT NEOPLASMS OF THE PANCREAS, LIVER, AND BILIARY TRACT

Thomas L. Lawson
Lincoln L. Berland
W. Dennis Foley

CARCINOMA OF THE PANCREAS

Ductal adenocarcinoma of the pancreas is of increasing medical importance in the United States. The age-adjusted mortality rate has risen from 2.9 to 9.0 per 100,000 population between the years 1920 and 1970.[85] This represents an increase of over 300%. Since the mean survival from time of diagnosis is only 4.3 months, the mortality and incidence rates essentially are equal.[103,104,189]

Pancreatic carcinoma now accounts for 3% of all cancers and 5% of all cancer deaths in the United States. It is the fourth most common cause of death from cancer in men and the fifth most common in women.[83] Despite advances in chemotherapy and radiation therapy, these modalities are primarily palliative and have not been shown to alter survival significantly.

Epidemiology and Survival

Ductal adenocarcinoma of the pancreas generally is more common in men and in older age groups. Blacks have a 30% to 40% higher risk of developing pancreatic cancer than whites.[16] Age-adjusted incidence rates indicate an increase of 43% for black men and 48% for black women; the mortality rates are also higher, 38% and 47%, respectively. It is not known why blacks have such a high pancreatic cancer rate.

Cigarette smoking has been established as a chief risk factor in pancreatic carcinoma. Although the excess risk in the United States is not as high as with lung carcinoma, there is no question that there is a strong and consistent effect.

Although there is a definite association between diabetes mellitus and pancreatic carcinoma, there are a number of uncertainties in the interpretation of the data. On one hand, pancreatic carcinoma may produce diabetes; on the other hand, diabetics usually die from complications of their diabetes. Probably less than 1% of the deaths in diabetic patients is attributable to pancreatic cancer. However, diabetics in the United States have up to a threefold increased risk of developing pancreatic carcinoma.[14,97,118]

The results of surgical treatment of carcinoma of the pancreas are also poor. The classic operation for pancreatic carcinoma has long been a partial pancreaticoduodenal resection (Whipple procedure). Operative mortality has averaged 20%, however, and five-year survival rates have been only 4%. More recently, total pancreatectomy has been recommended as a better procedure for treating pancreatic carcinoma. This recommendation is based upon three observations: (1) pancreatic carcinoma is often multicentric; (2) pancreatic carcinoma metastasizes to regional lymph nodes early in its course; and (3) total pancreatectomy eliminates the need for a pancreatic-enteric anastomosis.

Ductal adenocarcinoma of the pancreas remains a discouraging clinical problem. Despite advances in pancreatic imaging and early diagnosis and improved chemotherapy, radiation therapy, and surgical treatment, there has been no increase in overall survival. However, the combination of computed tomography (CT) and percutaneous needle aspiration biopsy has dramatically diminished the amount of time required to establish the diagnosis, and this has diminished the amount of patient hospitalization. With the short mean survival after diagnosis, even a shortening of the hospital stay by a week or 10 days may be significant to these patients.

While ductal adenocarcinoma is the most common pancreatic neoplasm, metastatic disease to the pancreas and lymphoma involving the peripancreatic nodes may mimic primary adenocarcinoma symptomatically and radiologically. In these cases, the diagnosis is established by biopsy of the pancreatic mass and occasionally of the known primary or peripheral lymphadenopathy for comparison of all types.

Cystic pancreatic neoplasms are uncommon lesions; they are also slow growing and may be effectively treated by total surgical excision. The two types of cystic pancreatic neoplasms include malignant mucinous cystic tumors and benign microcystic adenomas. The mucinous cystic tumor was formerly termed cystadenocarcinoma. This tumor usually has large unilocular cysts, but they may be multilocular or septated. Occasionally, there is peripheral or rim calcification. It may be difficult to differentiate these clinically from a simple inflammatory pseudocyst. The second type of cystic pancreatic neoplasm is benign and is termed microcystic adenoma. This tumor is usually multicystic, with the cystic areas varying in size. There may be central or stellate calcifications. While there are gross anatomic features that might allow differentiation of a benign from a malignant tumor before surgery, practically all of these patients will have the tumor resected so that the histologic diagnosis can be made with certainty.

Carcinomas of the endocrine portions of the pancreas are uncommon and are usually diagnosed by the symptoms they produce. These tumors originate in the endocrine portion of the gland and are classified according to the cell types involved and the symptoms produced. While these tumors may be benign, they are frequently malignant, and hepatic metastases are usually present by the time of diagnosis. These tumors include the glucagonomas, insulinomas, and gastrin-producing tumors. Frequently, pancreatic endocrine tumors may be found in patients with other associated endocrine adenomas and are part of the multiple endocrine adenoma syndromes.

Tumor Behavior and Pathology

Cubilla and Fitzgerald recently reviewed their experience at Memorial Sloan-Kettering Cancer Center and proposed a comprehensive classification of nonendocrine pancreatic carcinoma.[40-43] Duct cell adenocarcinoma was the most common type, representing 75% of cases. The tumor was found in the head of the pancreas

in 61% of patients, the body in 13%, the tail in 5%, and in a combination of sites in 21%. Tumors in the head of the pancreas tended to be smaller (about 5 cm in diameter) than those in the tail (average of 10 cm in diameter).

Lymph node metastases were most common in the superior head and posterior pancreaticoduodenal groups. Some degree of desmoplastic response was present in all cases of ductal adenocarcinomas, while foci of hemorrhage and necrosis were seen to a lesser degree.

Sommers et al.[183] have noted the relationship between pancreatic carcinoma and pancreatic duct hyperplasia. Hyperplasia was found in 41% of their patients with pancreatic carcinoma, but in only 9% of nonneoplastic control patients. Cubilla et al.[43] also noted this relationship and found that in situ changes of pancreatic carcinoma usually were associated with areas of papillary hyperplasia or marked atypia. More recently, Kozuka et al.[102] have noted that ductal hyperplasia is more frequent in pancreatic carcinoma than noncancerous pancreas and have suggested that there is quite likely a sequential change from nonpapillary and atypical hyperplasia to carcinoma.

Mucinous cystic tumors are large neoplasms that may be found in any part of the pancreas, but are most common in the body and tail.[64,91] They are usually encapsulated and have lobulated external surfaces. Internally, they may be unilocular or, less commonly, multilocular, with the cyst lining thrown into numerous folds and papillary excrescences.[34,35] Microscopically, the epithelium of these tumors is composed of tall mucin-producing columnar cells. There is frequent concurrence of or juxtaposition with apparently benign and obviously malignant epithelial cells. This has led to the concept of transformation of benign cystadenomas into their malignant counterpart. However, it is now felt that all mucinous cystic tumors are malignant and that an initial biopsy result of a benign tumor that is subsequently shown to be malignant probably only reflects inadequate sampling of these complex tumors.

Microcystic adenomas represent a distinctive type of cystic pancreatic tumor with no malignant potential. They are large and occur predominantly in women. They are lobulated neoplasms with thick, well-defined fibrous capsules and internal architectures that consist of numerous cysts of varying sizes. These tumors frequently have a central stellate fibrous scar that may calcify. These tumors may occur in any portion of the pancreas and in a small percentage of patients may have multiple areas of involvement. Microscopically, the epithelium lining the multiple cysts is of a single type of flat epithelial cell. The cytoplasm of these cells has been found to be rich in glycogen and hence the term "glycogen-rich cystadenomas."

The pathologic classification of endocrine tumors of the

pancreas depends on the endocrine cell type involved. A significant number of these tumors are malignant. The biologic behavior of these tumors, however, is poorly understood and is quite variable. Some tumors grow rapidly and metastasize widely, while others grow slowly; there are reports of patients with known metastases surviving for long periods.[110,116,152]

Classification and Staging

Staging of pancreatic cancer has not received much attention because in the past it was detected in an advanced stage and little if any effective therapy was available. Therefore, accurate staging and classification was of little practical value. Now, however, with the aggressive use of combined diagnostic modalities leading to earlier diagnosis and aggressive treatment, including surgical, chemotherapeutic, and radiation therapy, accurate tumor staging has gained importance. Current tumor staging is based on the TNM classification as defined by the American Joint Committee on Cancer[8] (Figure 14-1; Tables 14-1, 14-2).

No specific staging or classification has been devised for cystic pancreatic neoplasms or for the endocrine tumors of the pancreas.

Imaging Procedures and Assessment

Plain Roentgenography. Pulmonary metastases from pancreatic adenocarcinomas may arise from direct extension from mediastinal nodes or from hematogenous dissemination. Both types occur late and are found more frequently in patients with tumors in the body or tail. The roentgenographic appearance of pancreatic metastases to the chest is nonspecific.

Osseous involvement from pancreatic carcinomas may result from hematogenous spread or from direct tumor extension into the contiguous lumbar or thoracic vertebral bodies. The incidence of bone metastases in autopsy series ranges from 6% to 20%.[1,72,92,145,200] Typically, pancreatic metastases have been described as lytic.

Large pancreatic tumors may cause displacement or

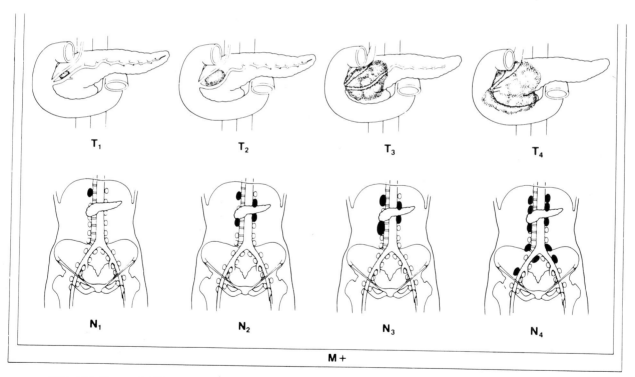

FIG. 14-1. Proposed AJC anatomic staging for cancer of the pancreas. T_1 and T_2 tumors are arbitrarily designated as surgically resectable; T_1 lesions are confined to the pancreas, while T_2 tumors may extend to the duodenum, bile ducts, or stomach, but resection is still possible. T_3 tumors are extensive and are incompatible with surgical resection. The N category is simply determined by whether regional nodes are involved or not (N_0 vs. N_1). Stage grouping: Stage I includes T_1 or T_2 lesions which are confined within the pancreas or extend only to immediately adjacent organs and can be resected en bloc with the primary tumor (T_{1-2}, N_0, M_0). Stage II tumors are unresectable but have no apparent lymph node involvement (T_3, N_0, M_0). Stage III lesions include all with regional node involvement but no distant metastases (T_{1-3}, N_1, M_0), and Stage IV lesions are those which have metastasized distantly (any T, any N, M_1).

Table 14-1. Tumor (T) Node (N) Classification—
Cancer of the Pancreas

T_x	Cannot be assessed
T_0	No primary; regional or distant disease present
T_1	Confined to pancreas
T_2	Limited extra-pancreatic extension, resectable
T_3	Extensive, unresectable
N_x	Cannot be assessed
N_0	Regional nodes not involved
N_1	Regional node involvement
M_x	Cannot be assessed
M_0	No known distant metastases
M_1	Distant metastases present

Modified from American Joint Committee on Cancer: *Manual for Staging of Cancer*, 2nd ed. Philadelphia, J. B. Lippincott, 1983.

compression of the gastric air bubble. This finding may be recognized on abdominal or chest roentgenograms, but should be confirmed with barium studies.

Pancreatic adenocarcinomas may obstruct the common bile duct and produce marked distention and enlargement of the gallbladder; this is classically referred to as a Courvoisier gallbladder. Courvoisier noted that malignant obstruction of the bile duct distal to the origin of the cystic duct frequently produced a palpably enlarged gallbladder, whereas obstruction caused by bile duct stones was usually associated with chronic cholecystitis and a small or normal-sized gallbladder.[38] Marked enlargement of the gallbladder may be recognized on plain films of the abdomen, but it is more often noted during transhepatic cholangiography or sonographic examination of the abdomen of jaundiced patients.

Ascites may result from either neoplastic or inflammatory disease of the pancreas.[49,151] Malignant ascites is most often the result of abdominal carcinomatosis with diffuse peritoneal tumor implantation. Pancreatitis may also cause ascites because of peritoneal irritation by the inflammatory exudate. More rarely, disruption of the pancreatic duct may result in direct extravasation of pancreatic fluid into the peritoneal cavity. This may be caused by either neoplastic or inflammatory disease.

Pancreatic calcifications may be easily recognized on

Table 14-2. AJC Stage Grouping—
Pancreas Cancer

Stage I	T_1, T_2, N_0, M_0
Stage II	T_1, T_2, T_3, N_0, M_0
Stage III	T_1, T_2, T_3, N_1, M_0
Stage IV	$T_1, T_2, T_3, N_0, N_1, M_1$

From American Joint Committee on Cancer: *Manual for Staging of Cancer*, 2nd ed. Philadelphia, J. B. Lippincott, 1983.

abdominal plain films. Most often they are intraductal calculi resulting from chronic pancreatitis. Although there appears to be an increased incidence of pancreatic carcinoma in patients with chronic calcific pancreatitis, pancreatic calcifications per se are indicative of benign disease in over 95% of cases. The roentgenographic disappearance of pancreatic calcification has been observed in both carcinoma and pancreatitis.[12,51] This phenomenon, however, is so infrequent that no special significance should be ascribed to it. Calcification virtually never occurs within adenocarcinoma of the exocrine pancreas. However, a pattern of tumoral calcification has been described in about 10% of cystic neoplasms of the pancreas.

Barium Roentgenography. The increasing utilization of new cross-sectional imaging modalities such as sonography and computed tomography has decreased the use of barium studies for evaluation of the pancreas. Barium examinations may provide important information about patients with nonspecific abdominal pain, or they may be used to define gastroduodenal anatomy before performing ERCP or PTC. Inflammatory and neoplastic disease of the stomach and duodenum may mimic the symptoms of pancreatic carcinoma and identification of these abnormalities on barium studies may obviate examinations directed specifically towards the pancreas.

Primary pancreatic neoplasms may produce a variety of changes of the esophagus and stomach that can be detected by barium roentgenography.

The esophagus is rarely involved directly by pancreatic carcinoma. However, some authors have reported contiguous invasion of the region of the gastroesophageal junction by tumors arising in the tail of the pancreas.[190] Perhaps more frequently seen is extrinsic involvement of the distal esophagus or gastric fundus by metastatic disease to perigastric lymph nodes.

Although large tumors arising in the body or tail of the pancreas may displace the stomach anteriorly and widen the retrogastric space, there has been considerable controversy about the interpretation of this finding.[158,184,190]

Pancreatic carcinomas may also directly invade the stomach, producing extensive areas of mural irregularity. In some cases, roentgenographic differentiation from primary gastric malignancy may be difficult.[30]

Splenic vein obstruction by direct tumor invasion is a frequent finding in carcinomas arising in the body and tail of the pancreas. Venous return from the spleen is then diverted by one of several collateral pathways involving the short gastric or left gastric veins. As these collateral veins enlarge, extensive varices may be produced in the stomach.[70,94,128,143,193] Although varices may also arise in the esophagus and colon, occurrence at these locations is distinctly less common than at the gastric cardia.

The duodenum reflects both inflammatory and neoplastic disease of the pancreas because of the relationship of the duodenum to the head of the pancreas.[159,166,175] However, the diagnostic sensitivity of the conventional barium examination of the duodenum was disappointing. Although the figures vary considerably, it seems that the prospective detection of pancreatic cancer is possible in only 25% of cases.[55]

These poor results led to the development of hypotonic duodenography, which resulted in a threefold increase in diagnostic accuracy. The most recent series utilizing hypotonic duodenography indicates a detection rate for pancreatic disease in the head of the pancreas of 85% to 95%. More recently, the use of high density barium suspensions, effervescent agents, and glucagon has decreased the need for selective intubation of the duodenum. Excellent hypotonic duodenography may now be performed as part of the routine UGI examination.[111,150]

The classic roentgenographic duodenal changes produced by pancreatic carcinoma include (Figure 14-2):

1. Enlargement or displacement of the duodenal loop.
2. Extrinsic pressure on the lesser duodenal curve.
3. Mucosal invasion (nodularity, spiculation).
4. Barium reflux into the pancreatic or biliary duct or into a necrotic tumor cavity.

The pancreas and colon are intimately related via the transverse mesocolon. Pancreatic carcinoma may involve the inferior aspect of the colon by direct spread along the transverse mesocolon. In addition, tumors in the tail of the pancreas may involve the splenic flexure of the colon by direct spread along the splenocolic ligament.

Urography. The head and tail of the pancreas are intimately related to the right and left kidneys, respectively. Tumors arising in either location may extend posteriorly and directly invade the kidney or its collecting system or vascular pedicle.[74,128]

Sonography. There are two primary indications for pancreatic sonography. Sonography is a low-cost noninvasive screening procedure for patients with nonspecific abdominal pain for whom the clinical suspicion of pancreatic disease is low; it may be used as the initial evaluation technique for patients with jaundice of unknown cause that is not felt to be the result of pancreatic carcinoma. Both jaundiced and nonjaundiced patients with a high probability of pancreatic carcinoma should be evaluated initially by modern, high resolution computed tomography unless factors related to computed tomography, such as limited scanner availability and time delay, favor sonography.

The primary sonographic criteria to be evaluated in patients with suspected pancreatic disease include the size and configuration of the pancreas, the parenchymal texture pattern, the caliber of the pancreatic duct, and the appearance of the liver, bile ducts, and gallbladder.

The most common sonographic manifestation of pancreatic adenocarcinoma is a focal or diffuse mass.[93,113] In general, pancreatic masses must be greater than 2 cm in diameter to be detected reliably by sonography. Tumors in the body and tail of the pancreas are most often identified as focal masses and are recognized as contour abnormalities that cause abrupt and obvious changes in the normal configuration of the gland (Figure 14-3). Tumors arising in the head of the pancreas also usually appear as focal masses. They may, however, cause diffuse enlargement of the gland by obstructing the periampullary portion of the pancreatic duct. The ductal obstruction produces distal pancreatitis and results in inflammatory enlargement of the body and tail. Thus, although the tumor is focal, the pancreas may appear to be diffusely enlarged.

A focal or diffuse pancreatic mass is a nonspecific finding; it may be a variant of normal, it may reflect the presence of acute or chronic inflammatory disease, or it may represent a primary or metastatic tumor. A specific diagnosis of neoplasm can be made only if ancillary findings indicative of tumor are recognized, such as hepatic metastases or regional lymphadenopathy. In some cases, masses arising in organs adjacent to the pancreas, such as renal tumors or lymphomas, may be difficult or impossible to differentiate from a primary pancreatic mass on the basis of the sonogram.

Initial sonographic reports characterized pancreatic carcinomas as relatively echo-poor compared with the normal pancreas.[10,37,210] (Figure 14-4) Echogenicity may be variable, however, and heavy reliance on texture patterns should be avoided.

The parenchymal texture of the normal pancreas shows considerable variation, ranging from levels equivalent to that of the normal liver to levels that are so highly echogenic as to render the gland inseparable from surrounding tissue.[127] Thus, the variations of normal and the overlap between neoplastic and inflammatory disease significantly limit the diagnostic specificity of texture patterns.

Although pancreatic duct dilatation has been detected by conventional sonographic equipment, consistent identification of both normal and dilated pancreatic ducts was not achieved until the development of high resolution real-time scanners.

The normal pancreatic duct has an echo-free center and smooth, parallel walls, which are sharply marginated. It is commonly identified in the body of the pancreas anterior to the splenic vein. The inner diameter of the normal duct is 1 or 2 mm and should not exceed 2 mm.[112]

Dilatation of the pancreatic duct may be seen in both pancreatitis and tumor. Tumors cause dilatation by obstructing the duct (Figure 14-5). The contour of the duct

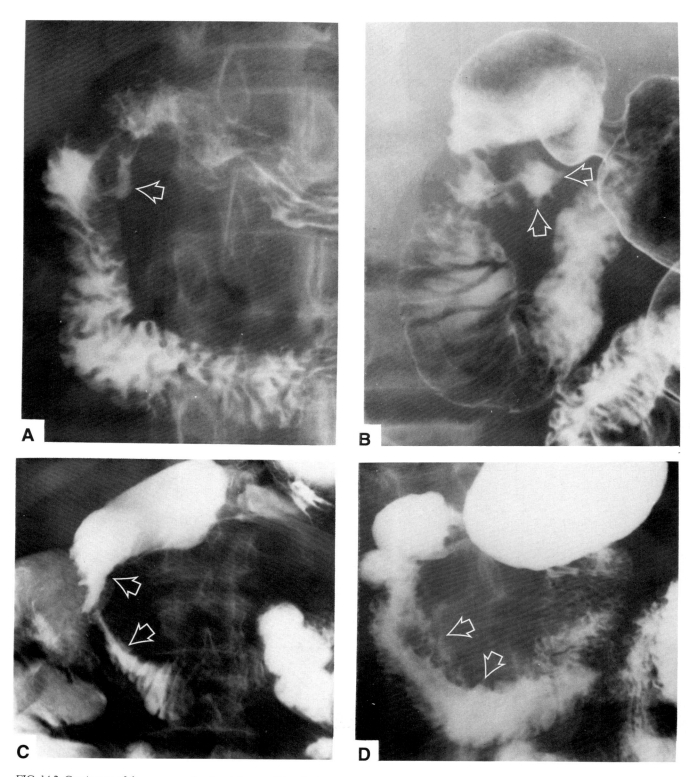

FIG. 14-2. Carcinoma of the pancreas, duodenal abnormalities. Barium upper gastrointestinal roentgenograms of four different patients with carcinoma of the pancreas demonstrate (A) ulceration secondary to tumor invasion (arrow); (B) constriction and invasion with filling of a necrotic tumor cavity (arrows); (C) compression and narrowing secondary to enlargement of the pancreatic head (arrows); and (D) mucosal nodularity and spiculation (arrows).

wall in patients with adenocarcinoma is usually smooth but may be irregular. In most patients, the inner diameter of the obstructed, dilated duct is greater than 3 mm. In some cases, ductal dilatation may be the only manifestation of tumor, particularly small carcinomas in the head of the pancreas or ampullary neoplasms. Occasionally, both a dilated pancreatic and common bile duct ("double duct" sign) may be identified. Although bile duct dilatation can result from chronic pancreatitis, in the absence of pancreatic calculi or a clinical history of pancreatitis, carcinoma is more likely.[156]

One of the advantages of sonography is its ability to evaluate the liver and biliary ducts in conjunction with examination of the pancreas. Identification of hepatic metastases in a patient with a pancreatic mass is a primary criterion for a diagnosis of pancreatic adenocarcinoma.

Sonography is quite sensitive in detecting focal hepatic masses or metastases when clinically suspected.[182,192] Hepatic metastases may produce a variety of sonographic patterns, including a focal echogenic or echo-poor mass, an echogenic mass with a peripheral echo-poor rim, or a diffusely abnormal parenchymal echo pattern.[73,132,182,215] Although liver metastases from pancreatic carcinoma are usually more echodense than the surrounding hepatic parenchyma, the sonographic patterns are nonspecific

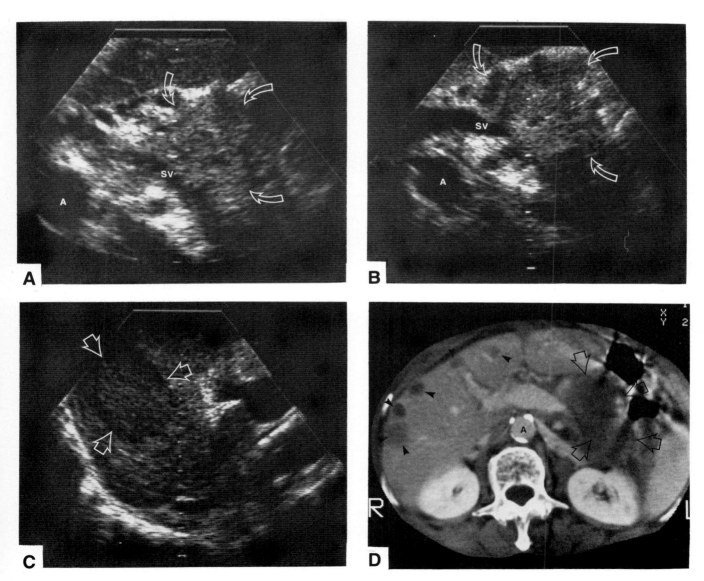

FIG. 14-3. Carcinoma of the pancreas, sonography. Axial sonograms (A,B) demonstrate a mass (arrows) involving the body of the pancreas ventral to the splenic vein (sv). The echo texture of the mass is nonhomogeneous. A sagittal sonogram through the liver (C) demonstrates a large hepatic metastasis (arrows). A computed tomogram (D) confirms the hepatic metastasis (arrowheads) and mass in the pancreatic body (arrows). Diagnosis was confirmed by percutaneous needle biopsy. A = aorta.

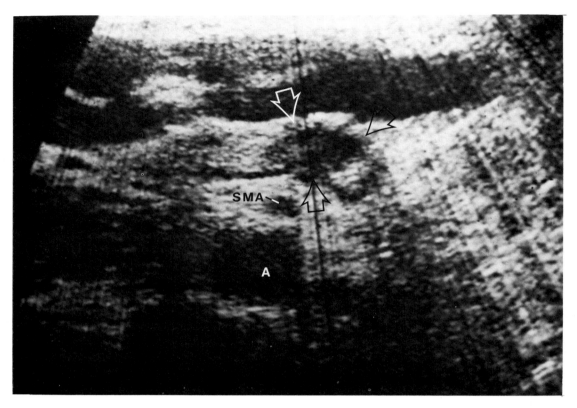

FIG. 14-4. Carcinoma of the pancreas, sonography. An axial pancreatic sonogram demonstrates a small focal mass of decreased echogenicity in the body of the pancreas (arrows). The overall size of the pancreas is normal. A = aorta, SMA = superior mesenteric artery. (Courtesy of Dr. Arthur Rosenfield, New Haven, Connecticut.)

and show no correlation with specific tumor types. Ultrasound also may be used for following the response of hepatic metastases to radiotherapy or chemotherapy. Occasionally, the echo pattern of a metastatic focus will change during therapy, most often becoming less echogenic than the surrounding liver or developing a necrotic, cystic center.

Jaundice has been found to be present at some time in approximately 70% of patients with pancreatic adenocarcinoma.[15] It may be the earliest finding in patients with carcinoma of the head of the pancreas or the ampulla of Vater. In these instances, sonography is an excellent diagnostic modality for detecting the dilated biliary system.

Pancreatic adenocarcinoma often metastasizes to regional lymph nodes, infiltrates into the retropancreatic fascial planes, and directly invades surrounding structures and organs such as the gastrointestinal tract, kidneys and adrenal glands, spleen, and blood vessels. Although high-resolution computed tomography usually is required to visualize these processes, they occasionally may be demonstrated by sonography.

Peripancreatic lymphadenopathy secondary to primary pancreatic adenocarcinoma or metastatic disease is char-

acterized by irregular, nodular soft tissue masses in the paracaval and para-aortic regions (Figure 14-6). The echogenicity of the nodal metastases may be either similar or more echo-free relative to the normal retroperitoneal tissues.

The differential diagnosis of metastatic disease to the pancreas or lymphoma involving peripancreatic lymph nodes may be difficult by sonography. Focal metastatic disease may mimic a primary carcinoma of the pancreas in all respects. Lymphoma, which involves and enlarges peripancreatic nodes, may cause a difficult diagnostic problem. However, sonographically, these nodes are usually somewhat less echogenic than the adjacent pancreas, although they may have the same echogenicity as the adjacent pancreas (Figure 14-7). When lymph node involvement is extensive and nodes are seen above and below the level of the pancreas in the paracaval and para-aortic region, the diagnosis can usually be suggested.

Cystic pancreatic neoplasms may be identified sonographically. The benign microcystic adenoma, because of the usual numerous septations and small cysts as well as the occasional stellate central calcifications, usually appears sonographically as an echogenic mass. If some of the cystic regions are large, the cystic components are

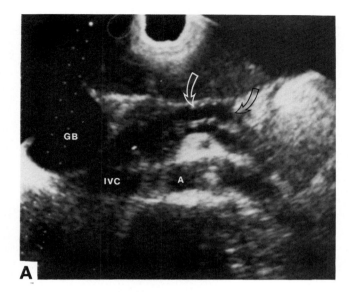

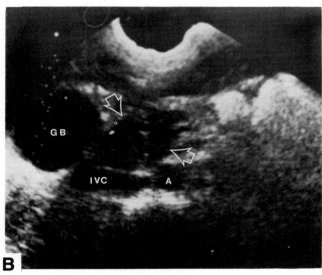

FIG. 14-5. Carcinoma of the head of the pancreas, sonography. Axial pancreatic sonograms demonstrate a dilated pancreatic duct (arrows) in the body of the gland (A). Note the dilated (Courvoisier) gallbladder (GB). An axial sonogram through the head of the pancreas (B) demonstrates enlargement by a relatively echo-poor mass (arrows). A = aorta, IVC = inferior vena cava.

identified as echo-free regions. The malignant mucinous cystic tumor may mimic a pancreatic pseudocyst because it may be unilocular. Septations or eccentric calcifications may be present, which may be a clue to the correct diagnosis (see Figure 14-8).

Endocrine tumors of the pancreas may be visualized sonographically when they are large, or hepatic metastases may be seen even when the primary tumor is small and undetectable by sonography. In general, sonography has not been accurate, and results have been disappoint-

ing in the evaluation and detection of disease in patients with suspected endocrine tumors.

Computed Tomography. High resolution computed tomography has become the major imaging modality for evaluation of the pancreas, and it is the initial procedure of choice for evaluating patients in whom there is a high clinical suspicion of pancreatic carcinoma.[84] In many patients, a diagnosis of pancreatic carcinoma can be made or excluded by computed tomography without the use of any additional imaging procedures. Computed tomography also can reliably assess resectability and precisely guide percutaneous fine-needle aspiration biopsy.

The most common abnormality produced by pancreatic adenocarcinoma is a mass.[57] Most neoplastic masses are focal and produce an abrupt change in the contour of the gland. The margins are usually well-defined, but occasionally may be somewhat indistinct.

Pancreatic masses usually must be at least 2 cm in diameter to produce a recognizable contour abnormality and hence be detectable by computed tomography. However, the requisite size also depends upon the size of the pancreas and upon the location of the tumor within the gland. Tumors that develop in the center of the gland must grow to larger dimensions to be detected by computed tomography than those that arise on the periphery or in the tail of the pancreas.[28] The uncinate process is small and usually has a characteristic wedge-shaped tongue that protrudes beneath the superior mesenteric artery and vein. Tumors that arise in this location cause rounding of the uncinate processes (Figure 14-9).

Tumors that arise in the head or body of the pancreas frequently produce ductal obstruction and atrophy of the tail of the gland.[56,187] In some cases, the tail simply appears small relative to the tumor mass; in other cases, the tail undergoes obstructive atrophy, and the dilated pancreatic duct may be seen as an irregular tubular lucency in the center of the atrophic tail.

The attenuation values of pancreatic tumors and normal pancreatic parenchyma are similar in about half of cases in a noncontrast enhanced or conventionally enhanced scan and, thus, neoplastic and normal pancreatic tissue often cannot be differentiated.[140,180] In many cases, however, bolus injections of intravenous contrast with rapid-sequence computed tomograms accentuate the attenuation differences between normal and neoplastic pancreatic tissue. The technique produces marked enhancement of the pancreatic vasculature and parenchyma. Pancreatic ductal adenocarcinoma is an infiltrating, serous tumor that is very hypovascular. With this contrast bolus technique tumors therefore appear as areas of decreased attenuation relative to the normal surrounding contrast-enhanced pancreatic parenchyma (Figure 14-10).

Normal and dilated pancreatic ducts can be visualized

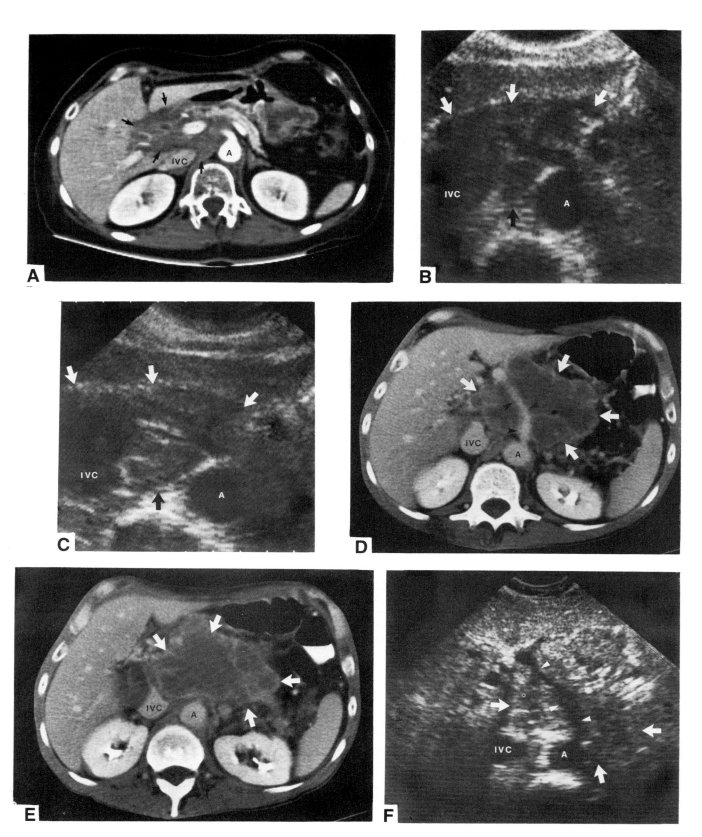

FIG. 14-6. Primary and metastatic carcinoma of the pancreas, retroperitoneal extension. (A) A pancreatic computed tomogram demonstrates extension of tumor into the liver hilum and the retroperitoneum between the aorta and inferior vena cava (arrows) (A). Axial sonograms (B,C) demonstrate extension of tumor to surround the aorta and celiac artery (arrows). Computed tomograms (D,E) and axial sonograms (F,G) of another patient with metastatic cancer to the pancreas demonstrate a large mass destroying the pancreas and invading the retroperitoneum (arrows). The celiac artery is elongated by the tumor mass (arrowheads). A = aorta, IVC = inferior vena cava.

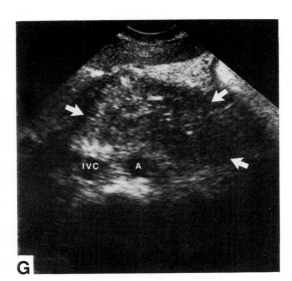

G

FIG. 14-6, continued.

by computed tomography in most patients if optimal scanning techniques are employed; these include 3-mm to 5-mm slice collimation, fast scan speed, high radiographic technique, and intravenous contrast enhancement.[17]

Pancreatic duct dilatation can occur in both chronic pancreatitis and carcinoma[58,81] (Figure 14-11). Carcinoma usually causes a mass with abrupt occlusion of the pancreatic duct. Within the mass, the duct usually is encased or obliterated and cannot be seen; proximal to the mass, the duct may dilate to a large caliber and the walls are often smooth and parallel.[95] Chronic pancreatitis may result in abrupt ductal dilatation proximal to a focal inflammatory stricture and produce pancreatic duct dilatation morphologically that is indistinguishable from carcinoma. More often, however, the entire duct is irregularly dilated, the caliber is usually less than that seen with carcinoma, and the walls tend to be beaded and nonparallel. Focal and diffuse masses may occur in chronic pancreatitis, but often the dilated duct may be seen within the mass. Intraductal debris or calculi and pseudocysts also are frequent findings in chronic pancreatitis and may aid in differential diagnosis.

Pancreatic duct dilatation occasionally may be the only finding indicative of an abnormality. In this case, and in the absence of other ancillary computed tomographic criteria of either tumor or inflammatory disease, ductal dilatation is nonspecific and the patient should be evaluated further with endoscopic retrograde cholangiopancreatography (ERCP). If the ductal dilatation is caused by a tumor, a small carcinoma of the head of the pancreas or an ampullary carcinoma are the primary considerations.

In patients with suspected pancreatic carcinoma, computed tomography also can provide precise information regarding the presence of hepatic metastases, dilated intrahepatic or extrahepatic biliary ducts, and gallbladder dilatation.

The presence of a pancreatic mass and liver metastases indicate malignant disease. While this combination is caused by pancreatic carcinoma in the vast majority of patients, similar findings may be seen with neoplasms metastatic to both the pancreas and liver. None of the available imaging modalities can differentiate primary from metastatic pancreatic carcinoma.

Pancreatic carcinoma frequently extends through the thin fascial covering of the gland and infiltrates into the peripancreatic soft tissues. The most common site of tumor extension is into the retropancreatic space (Figure 14-12). This is identified on computed tomograms by obliteration of the normal posterior fat planes. However, loss of the fat planes may be seen in pancreatitis and in normal patients with minimal retroperitoneal fat. In the latter instance, the use of bolus enhancement of the peripancreatic vascular structures may be helpful for evaluation. Thus, while obliteration of the retropancreatic fat plane is a frequent finding in pancreatic carcinoma, it is nonspecific, and the presence of tumor can only be inferred from the computed tomogram. A specific diagnosis of tumor extension can be made only by biopsy.

Pancreatic adenocarcinoma may extend into the root of the small bowel mesentery and encase the superior mesenteric artery. The computed tomographic appearance of vascular encasement is a halo of slightly increased attenuation or soft tissue collar surrounding the proximal portion of the celiac or superior mesenteric artery (Figure 14-13). The borders of the collar are indistinct. In some cases, the superior mesenteric vein also may be obstructed and venous collateral channels (varices) may be recognized by computed tomography.

Pancreatic adenocarcinoma also may involve the mesentery of the small or large bowel. Mesenteric invasion may be seen by computed tomography as thickening of the soft tissues or as numerous irregular linear areas of increased attenuation extending from the tumor into the mesentery. This finding also indicates that the tumor is unresectable.

Pancreatic adenocarcinoma may metastasize to regional lymph nodes. Enlarged nodes greater than 1.5 cm in diameter are easily detected by computed tomography and appear as focal areas of nodularity in the retropancreatic periaortic-pericaval region. Lymph node enlargement is a nonspecific finding, since lymphadenopathy may be a result of reactive changes, inflammatory disease, or metastatic disease. A nonoperative diagnosis of nodal metastases can be made by CT-guided percutaneous biopsy (Figure 14-14).

The proximity of the pancreas to the spleen, kidneys and adrenal glands, lumbar spine, and gastrointestinal tract accounts for the frequent involvement of these structures by direct tumor extension.[87,129]

Pancreatic adenocarcinoma associated with ascites is a late finding, often detected on follow-up scans. Although ascites may be caused by tumor obstruction of the portal vein and subsequent portal hypertension, it most often results from diffuse peritoneal metastases (Figure 14-15). Computed tomography accurately detects small amounts of peritoneal fluid, but the actual peritoneal metastases are not identified because they are too small.

Cystic pancreatic neoplasms are identified on computed tomograms as masses in the head, body, or tail of the gland, which are unilocular or multilocular.[214] The benign microcystic adenoma appears as a mass with numerous small cysts. While the malignant mucinous cystic tumor is usually unilocular, it may be multilocular and contain numerous small cystic regions and mimic its benign counterpart (Figure 14-16). Classically, the malignant mucinous cystic tumor is large and unilocular with a few septations (Figure 14-8). Calcifications may occur in either tumor and may be detected by computed

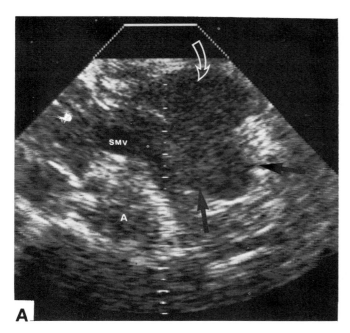

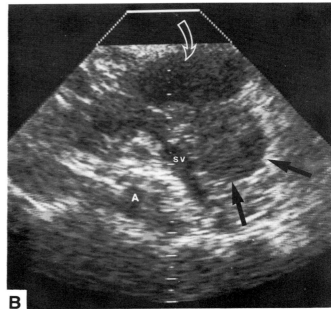

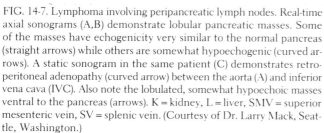

FIG. 14-7. Lymphoma involving peripancreatic lymph nodes. Real-time axial sonograms (A,B) demonstrate lobular pancreatic masses. Some of the masses have echogenicity very similar to the normal pancreas (straight arrows) while others are somewhat hypoechogenic (curved arrows). A static sonogram in the same patient (C) demonstrates retroperitoneal adenopathy (curved arrow) between the aorta (A) and inferior vena cava (IVC). Also note the lobulated, somewhat hypoechoic masses ventral to the pancreas (arrows). K = kidney, L = liver, SMV = superior mesenteric vein, SV = splenic vein. (Courtesy of Dr. Larry Mack, Seattle, Washington.)

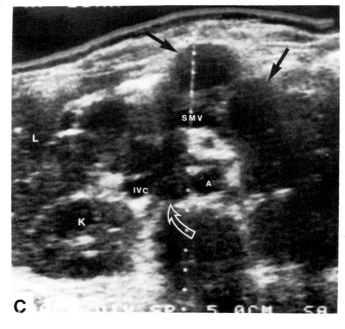

tomography. Characteristically, in benign microcystic adenomas, the calcification is central and stellate, while in malignant mucinous tumors the calcification is focal, amorphous, and peripheral. Final diagnosis, however, rests with the pathologist and careful histologic evaluation.

Detectability of pancreatic endocrine tumors depends on the tumor size, tumor location within the pancreas, and degree of vascularity or enhancement following administration of intravenous contrast. Large but relatively avascular tumors may be detected by their tumor bulk (Figure 14-17). However, very small pancreatic endocrine tumors may be identified with careful, high resolution computed tomography if they enhance following administration of intravenous contrast (Figure 14-18). Results in tumor detection with computed tomography are variable, and at best, only approximately 25% of these pancreatic endocrine tumors are identified by computed tomography.

Endoscopic Retrograde Cholangiopancreatography. The majority of pancreatic neoplasms are adenocarcinomas that arise from the ductal epithelium. Alterations in the main pancreatic duct or small lateral side branches are thus among the first recognizable changes produced by pancreatic carcinoma. Endoscopic retrograde cholangiopancreatography (ERCP) precisely displays these ductal changes and has been shown to have an accuracy rate approaching 95%.[61,163,164,170,171]

The high diagnostic accuracy of ERCP resulted in its use as one of the first major procedures for evaluation of patients with suspected pancreatic adenocarcinoma. The subsequent introduction of computed tomography and refinements in the techniques of sonography have changed the role of ERCP. The primary indications for ERCP now include (1) further investigation of a patient with a normal or technically unsatisfactory computed tomogram or sonogram in whom there is a high clinical suspicion of pancreatic disease or pancreatic carcinoma; (2) evaluation of an equivocal computed

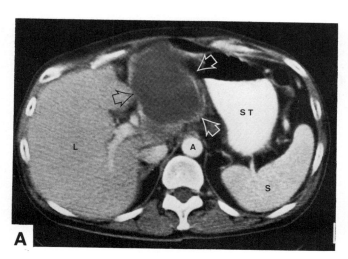

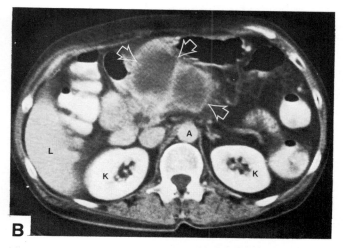

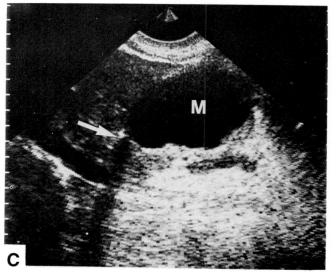

FIG. 14-8. Malignant mucinous cystic tumor. Pancreatic computed tomograms (A,B) of this older woman demonstrate a large bilocular cystic mass involving the body of the pancreas (arrows). The sagittal pancreatic sonogram in this patient (C) demonstrates the cystic mass (M) as well as a focal area of echogenicity and distal sonic shadowing, indicating the presence of peripheral or rim calcification (arrow). K = kidney, A = aorta, L = liver, S = spleen, ST = stomach.

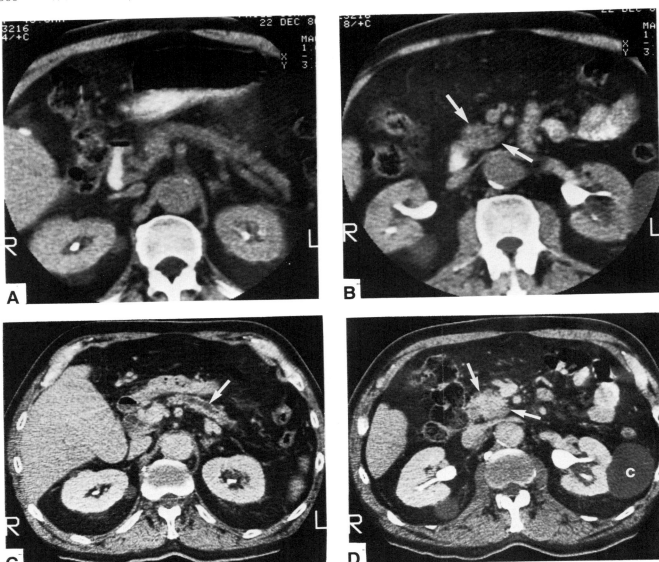

FIG. 14-9. Carcinoma of the uncinate process. Initial pancreatic computed tomograms through the body (A) and head (B) of the pancreas demonstrate an essentially normal gland, although the uncinate process (arrows) is perhaps slightly bulbous. Follow-up computed tomograms approximately 6 months after the initial study now demonstrate dilatation of the pancreatic duct (arrow) in the body of the pancreas (C) and enlargement of the head of the pancreas and uncinate process (arrows) (D). Incidentally noted is a left renal cyst (C).

tomographic or sonographic finding; (3) precise diagnosis of an isolated pancreatic mass demonstrated by computed tomography or sonography; (4) guidance for percutaneously directed pancreatic biopsy or for direct aspiration of pancreatic juice for cytologic examination.

Pancreatic adenocarcinoma causes a variety of changes in both the pancreatic and common bile ducts. These include ductal obstruction or encasement, acinar (field) defects and tumor cavities that communicate with the pancreatic ducts (Figure 14-19).[14–19,66,69,105,169,186] Although these changes may be limited to the pancreatic duct, they are only rarely limited to the bile duct. Biductal abnormalities involving both the pancreatic and common bile duct are quite frequent and have been reported in 30% to 60% of cases of pancreatic carcinoma.[56,63,156]

Pancreatic duct obstruction is the most common abnormality produced by pancreatic adenocarcinoma. The ductal terminus in cases of tumor obstruction is usually irregular, nodular, or eccentric. This is contrasted to a smoother, nonspecific terminus in cases of inflammatory disease. The main duct and lateral side branches between the papilla and point of obstruction are normal in cases of tumor and usually show diffuse changes of pancreatitis in cases of inflammation.

In some cases, focal inflammatory disease may mimic the changes of tumor, and differentiation may not be possible on the basis of the pancreatogram alone. In other cases, pancreatic carcinoma may cause or may coexist with chronic pancreatitis, and accurate preoperative diagnosis may be impossible.

Pancreatic duct encasement is the second most common finding in pancreatic adenocarcinoma. The segment of encased duct is usually short (1 to 2 cm) and ir-

regular. The main duct and side branches on the papillary side of the point of encasement are normal and the transition is abrupt. The main duct and side branches proximal to the area of encasement are dilated and have the appearance of chronic pancreatitis.

Acinar (field) defects are infrequent findings in pancreatic adenocarcinoma. Acinar defects are caused by small carcinomas arising in the periphery of the gland. The tumors cause focal obliteration of the small lateral

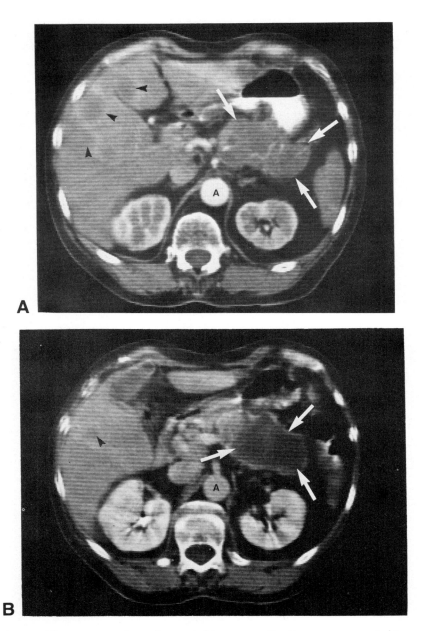

FIG. 14-10. Carcinoma of the pancreas, enhanced computed tomograms. Rapid sequence computed tomograms through the body of the pancreas (A) following bolus injection of intravenous contrast demonstrate enhancement of the aorta (A). There is a mass in the body of the pancreas (arrows), and hepatic metastases are present (arrowheads). A computed tomogram at a slightly lower level (B) demonstrates the tumor in the body of the pancreas (arrows) to be of lower attenuation than the surrounding normal pancreas in the head of the gland, liver parenchyma, and renal parenchyma.

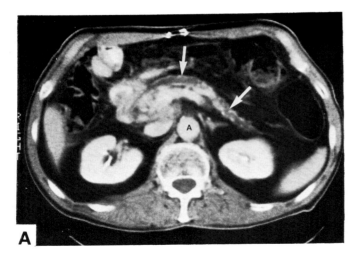

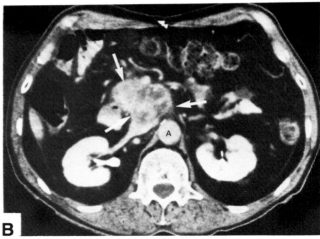

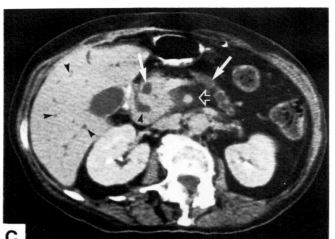

FIG. 14-11. Carcinoma of the head of the pancreas—dilated pancreatic duct. A computed tomogram through the body of the pancreas (A) demonstrates a dilated pancreatic duct (arrows). A computed tomogram through the head of the pancreas (B) demonstrates the tumor mass that has invaded dorsally into the inferior vena cava (arrows). A computed tomogram of another patient (C) demonstrates dilatation of the pancreatic duct (arrows) as well as the common bile duct (arrowheads) and intrahepatic biliary radicles. There is perivascular extension of tumor revealed by a hazy cuff of increased attenuation surrounding the superior mesenteric artery (open arrow). A = aorta.

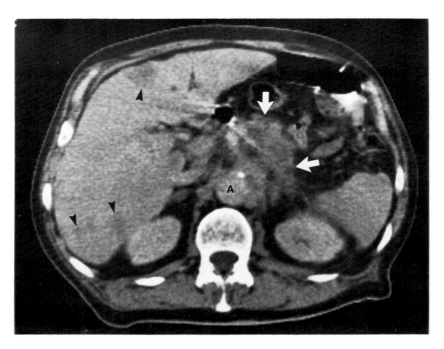

FIG. 14-12. Carcinoma of the pancreas, dorsal extension. A computed tomogram demonstrates a mass in the body of the pancreas (arrows) that has extended dorsally to invade the tissues surrounding the aorta (A) and left adrenal gland. Note the loss of the fat plane that normally surrounds the aorta. There are hepatic metastases (arrowheads).

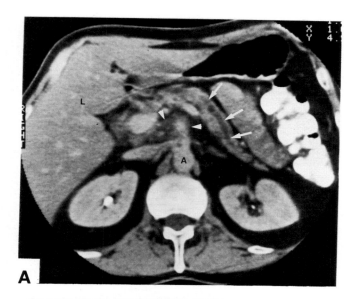

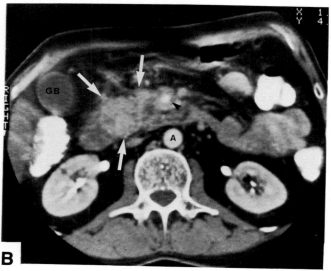

FIG. 14-13. Carcinoma of the pancreas, perivascular extension, and venous occlusion. A computed tomogram through the body of the pancreas (A) demonstrates dilatation of the pancreatic duct (arrows) and a halo of increased attenuation surrounding the celiac artery (arrowheads). A computed tomogram of the head of the pancreas (B) demonstrates a mass (arrows) with a soft tissue mantle surrounding the superior mesenteric artery (arrowhead), and no evidence of enhancement in the superior mesenteric vein. A = aorta, L = liver, GB = gallbladder.

side branches without altering the main pancreatic duct and are seen as defects in the pancreatograms. These small defects can only be appreciated when the entire ductal system is well filled.

Tumor cavities may form in the central portion of neoplasms as a result of necrosis. Most often there is no communication with the pancreatic ductal system. In some cases, however, the cavity may fill with contrast

during pancreatography. The contrast assumes an amorphous configuration as it fills the interstices of the necrotic cavity. This is in contrast to the usual appearance of a pseudocyst, where the walls are smoother and more precisely defined.

There is no clear-cut role for ERCP in the evaluation of patients with cystic pancreatic neoplasms or suspected endocrine tumors. If the tumor mass is large and compresses the biliary ductal system, however, ERCP may be helpful in evaluating the degree and site of ductal obstruction.

Percutaneous Cholangiography. Percutaneous cholangiography is indicated for precise diagnostic evaluation of the bile ducts in patients with obstructive jaundice or for establishment of biliary drainage.

Jaundiced patients with suspected pancreatic adenocarcinoma are best evaluated with sonography or computed tomography. Once a diagnosis of obstructive jaundice has been established, percutaneous transhepatic cholangiography may be used to define the precise nature and location of the obstruction.[173,202]

The range of applicability of transhepatic cholangiography has been extended by the logical development of the techniques of percutaneous biliary drainage.[85,146,167] Biliary drainage may be performed to temporarily decompress the biliary ducts before curative or palliative surgery, thereby decreasing operative mortality. It may also be performed in place of a surgical drainage procedure for palliation of an unresectable carcinoma, thus eliminating the expense and morbidity of major surgery for a patient with a short life expectancy.

Interpretation of percutaneous cholangiograms involves analysis of the location of the abnormality and the morphology of the ductal abnormality (Figure 14-20).[26,59,88,98,109,144]

Pancreatic carcinoma can involve the intrahepatic and extrahepatic ducts by direct contiguous invasion or by metastatic spread. Detectable involvement of the intrahepatic ducts by metastatic tumor is infrequently detected by percutaneous cholangiography, even when known liver metastases are present.

The common hepatic duct may be involved extrinsically by enlarged nodes in the porta hepatis as a result of metastatic tumor or by direct tumor extension into the porta. The findings are nonspecific and differential diagnosis of porta hepatis involvement includes other primary tumors, which may metastasize to the porta, as well as primary carcinoma of the gallbladder or bile duct.

The common bile duct may be divided into three segments; periampullary, intrapancreatic, and suprapancreatic. Each of these segments may be involved by pancreatic carcinoma. Tumors that involve the periampullary segment of the common bile duct may be primary ampullary neoplasms or pancreatic carcinoma. In many cases the origin of the tumor cannot be determined even by careful microscopic evaluation of the surgical specimen.

The distal segment of the common bile duct passes through the pancreas for several centimeters and is completely surrounded by pancreatic tissue. Carcinomas arising in the head of the pancreas frequently involve this segment of the common bile duct. This may be seen as a discrete segment of involvement or as complete obstruction of the intrapancreatic segment. Rarely, the intrapancreatic portion of the common bile duct may be involved by other tumors metastatic to the pancreas. In these cases, differentiation from primary pancreatic carcinoma cannot be made radiographically.

Pancreatic carcinoma can produce a variety of mor-

phologic appearances of the terminus of the obstructed common bile duct. These include round, square, tapered, and irregular (rattailed).

Pancreatic Angiography. Although angiography is a sensitive technique for the diagnosis of pancreatic carcinomas, its role has become more limited as less invasive but similarly accurate techniques have been developed.[71,165,172] These include sonography, computed tomography, endoscopic retrograde cholangiopancreatography (ERCP), and percutaneous cholangiography. Most investigators now employ a combination of these procedures for initial evaluation of patients suspected of having pancreatic carcinoma.

Angiography has been shown to be helpful in the

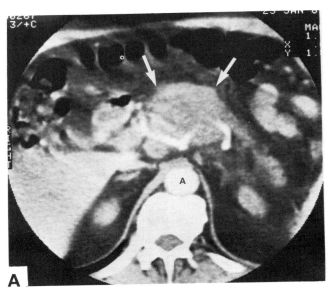

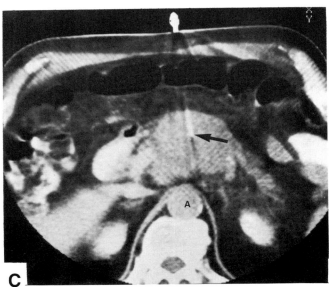

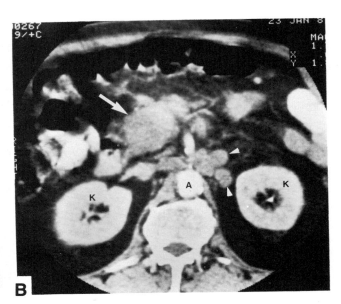

FIG. 14-14. Carcinoma of the lung metastatic to the pancreas and peripancreatic region. A computed tomogram through the body of the pancreas (A) demonstrates a soft tissue mass that encases the celiac artery and its branches (arrows). A computed tomogram at the level of the head of the pancreas (B) demonstrates enlargement of the pancreatic head (arrow) and numerous enlarged retroperitoneal (para-aortic) lymph nodes (arrowheads). The question of primary pancreatic tumor versus metastases from a known carcinoma of the lung was determined by percutaneous needle aspiration biopsy (C). A computed tomogram demonstrated the biopsy needle within the mass (arrow). A = aorta, K = kidney.

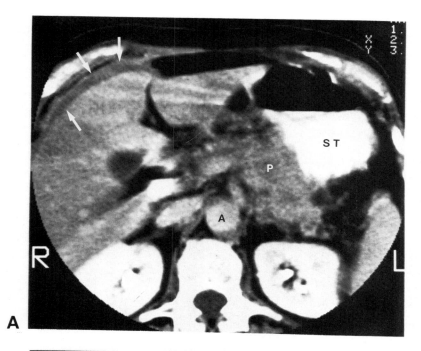

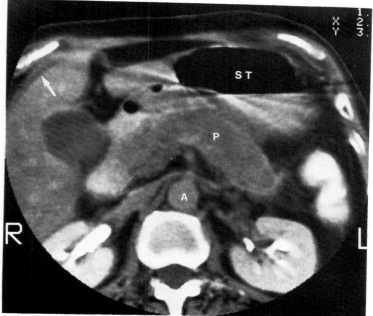

FIG. 14-15. Carcinoma of the pancreas, diffuse glandular involvement. Pancreatic computed tomograms (A,B) demonstrate generalized pancreatic enlargement and a small amount of ascites (arrows), which is most prominent peripheral to the liver. At the time of surgery, diffuse involvement of the pancreas was present with numerous peritoneal metastases. A = aorta, St = stomach, P = pancreas.

diagnosis of patients in whom there is a high clinical suspicion of pancreatic disease but in whom the initial procedures are normal, equivocal, or technically unsatisfactory.

Although computed tomography may reliably indicate the unresectability of a pancreatic neoplasm by demonstrating evidence of metastatic disease or contiguous organ invasion, in many patients these findings are absent. Angiography, however, has been shown to be highly accurate in assessing tumor resectability and thus may have a significant impact on patient management by obviating exploratory laparotomy in cases of unresectable tumors.[53]

Pancreatic adenocarcinoma is an infiltrating neoplasm. It is essentially hypovascular, and the identifiable arteriographic changes are caused by direct tumor involve-

ment of intrapancreatic and peripancreatic vessels (Figure 14-21).[201]

Arterial encasement denotes tumor invasion of the vessel wall with consequent luminar narrowing. Encasement is the most common finding seen in pancreatic carcinoma and denotes tumor infiltration of the vessel wall. Encasement may involve major extrapancreatic vessels or small intrapancreatic arteries.

Arterial occlusions may be abrupt or gradual. Although nonneoplastic diseases, such as atherosclerosis, can result in arterial occlusions, in most cases abrupt vessel occlusion denotes tumor. This is particularly true if the changes are focal; are associated with other findings in contiguous vessels, such as encasement or angulation; or are adjacent to venous occlusions.

Angulation refers to abrupt, acute changes in vessel

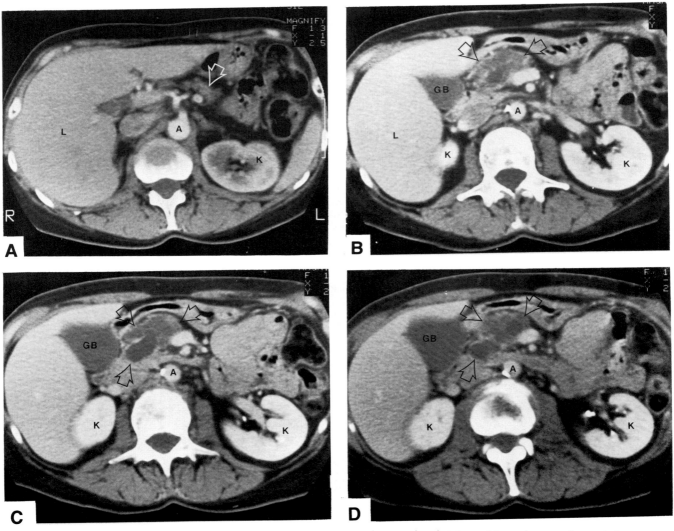

FIG. 14-16. Malignant mucinous cystic tumor. A pancreatic computed tomogram (A) of this middle-aged woman demonstrates a normal body of the gland (arrow). However, images through the head of the pancreas (B, C, D) demonstrate a multiloculated cystic mass (arrows). There is no calcification present within the mass. A = aorta, L = liver, K = kidney, GB = gallbladder.

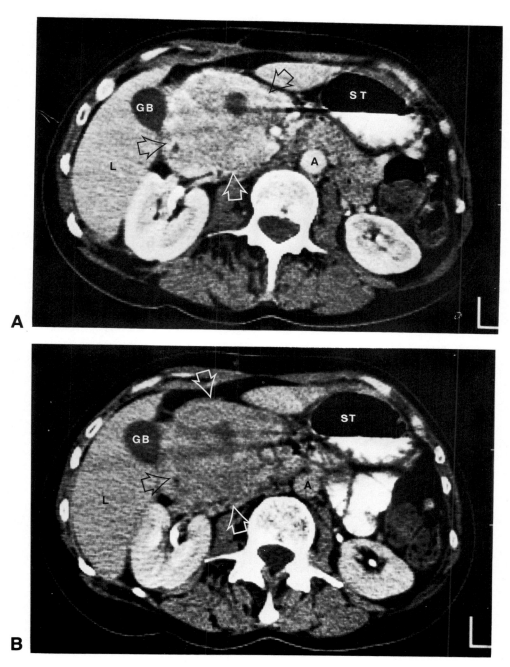

FIG. 14-17. Malignant gastrinoma (Zollinger-Ellison syndrome). Pancreatic computed tomograms (A,B) of this patient with Zollinger-Ellison syndrome demonstrate a large solid mass in the head of the pancreas (arrows). While this mass does not enhance with intravenous contrast, its large size allows identification by computed tomography.

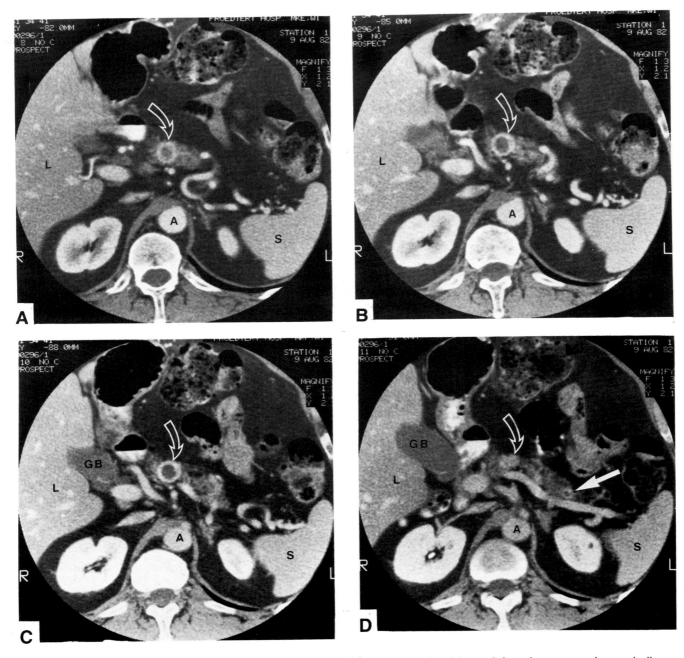

FIG. 14-18. Enhancing small gastrinomas. High resolution pancreatic computed tomograms (A,B,C,D) of this middle-aged man with known Zollinger-Ellison syndrome demonstrate two small enhancing tumor masses. A larger mass in the body (curved arrows) and a smaller mass in the tail of the pancreas (arrow) are identified. While these endocrine tumors are small and do not deform the pancreas, they markedly enhance after the administration of intravenous contrast, which allows their identification by computed tomography. L = liver, S = spleen, A = aorta, GB = gallbladder.

course. Both angulation and displacement of vessels are nonspecific findings that may be caused by neoplasms or inflammatory masses within the pancreas.

The importance of venous involvement by pancreatic carcinoma has been recognized and has been estimated to occur in over half of the cases of pancreatic carcinoma.[22,82,96,122,147] The frequency of involvement depends upon two factors: the clarity of the venous phase, and the size of the pancreatic tumor. Venous changes are also frequently seen in pancreatitis and thus must be correlated with contiguous arterial findings.

Cystic pancreatic neoplasms may be diagnosed and defined by angiography. The primary angiographic manifestations include arterial displacement, dilatation, neo-

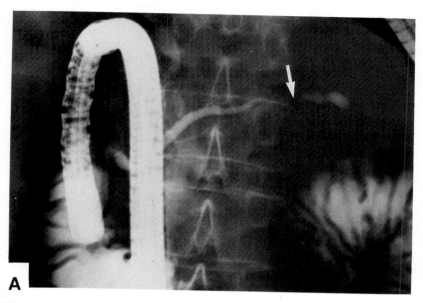

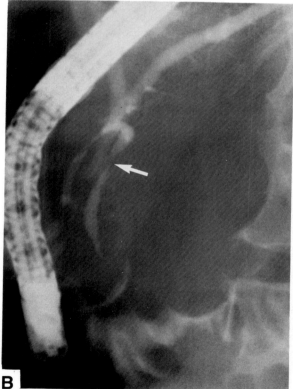

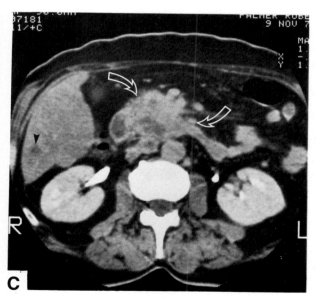

FIG. 14-19. Carcinoma of the pancreas, ductal changes. Retrograde ductography (A) demonstrates narrowing and irregularity of the pancreatic duct in the body of the pancreas (arrow) with dilatation of the pancreatic duct proximal to the obstructing lesion. Retrograde ductography in another patient (B) demonstrates narrowing and irregularity of the pancreatic duct in the head of the pancreas (arrow). A computed tomogram (C) of this patient demonstrates a mass in the head of the pancreas (curved arrows) with a central area of lower attenuation. Hepatic metastases are noted (arrowhead).

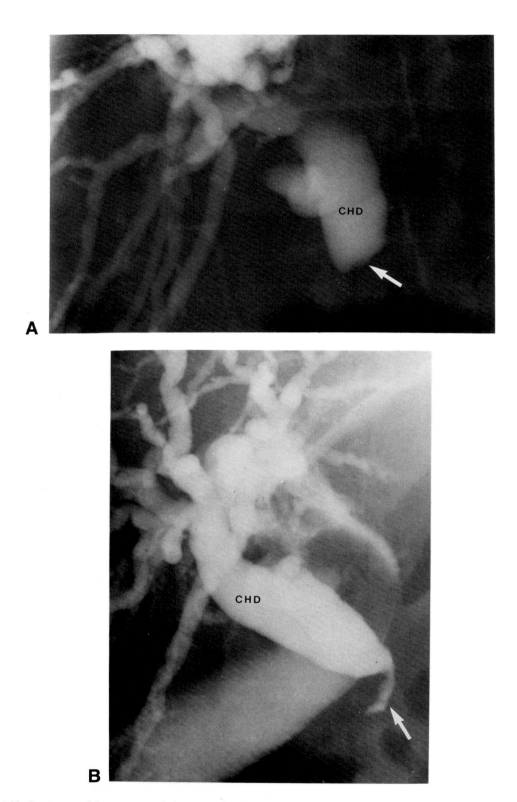

FIG. 14-20. Carcinoma of the pancreas, cholangiographic abnormalities. Percutaneous transhepatic cholangiograms demonstrate a squared or flattened (A) and an irregularly tapered obstruction (B) of the distal common bile duct (arrows). The common hepatic duct (CHD) and intrahepatic bile ducts are dilated.

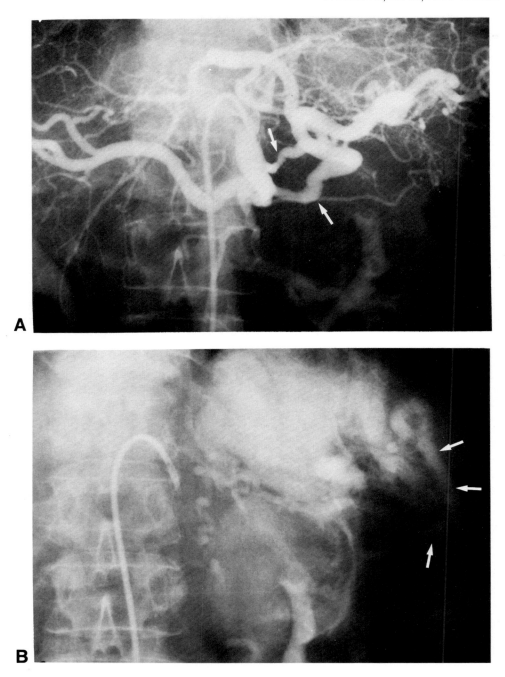

FIG. 14-21. Carcinoma of the pancreas, celiac arteriogram. During the arterial phase (A), there is narrowing and irregularity of the splenic and left gastric arteries (arrows) secondary to tumor encasement. On the delayed venous phase (B), no opacification of the splenic vein is present, indicating splenic vein thrombosis. Perisplenic collateral channels are opacified (arrows).

vascularity, and hypervascularity. Obstruction or compression of the mesenteric venous system occasionally is present, usually involving the splenic vein.

Endocrine tumors of the pancreas may be diagnosed by angiography if the tumor mass is focal, larger than a centimeter, and hypervascular. The overall results of angiographic localization of gastrinomas in patients with Zollinger-Ellison syndrome has been disappointing. Lack

of success probably is related to the fact that many tumors are hypovascular, as well as to a lack of focal tumors with the elevated gastrin levels caused by diffuse islet cell hyperplasia. However, insulinomas are frequently hypervascular and, while small, they may be diagnosed with a 75% to 80% accuracy if careful technique, subselective injections, and magnification techniques are used. Venous sampling has been used in the case of endocrine pancreatic tumors to help localize the site of the tumor within the pancreas. This has been helpful when surgical resection is contemplated. The benefit/cost ratios of the various imaging procedures are given in Table 14-3.

Imaging Strategies and Decisions

A wide variety of techniques are available for patients suspected of having pancreatic disease and carcinoma. These include sonography, computed tomography, transhepatic cholangiography (PTC) endoscopic retrograde cholangiopancreatography (ERCP), pancreatic angiography, magnetic resonance imaging (MRI) and percutaneous fine-needle pancreatic biopsy (Figure 14-22). While the use of these new modalities has increased diagnostic accuracy and the speed of diagnosis, adenocarcinoma of the pancreas is almost invariably incurable at the time of initial diagnosis. Nevertheless, these new techniques have increased the speeed of diagnosis, which has had a positive economic and psychologic impact.[60]

Clinical. The initial symptoms of adenocarcinoma of the pancreas frequently are vague and do not suggest a specific etiology. Tumors arising in the body and tail of the pancreas may grow to enormous size before the onset of symptoms. Tumors in the head of the pancreas often appear earlier because they obstruct the common bile duct and thus produce jaundice.

For nonjaundiced patients. For the nonjaundiced patient, pancreatic cancer should be suspected in the following circumstances:

1. Mental symptoms of depression often are present early and may predate the onset of pain.[216] If mental symptoms are associated with abdominal pain and weight loss, they should suggest the presence of pancreatic carcinoma.
2. Pain usually located in the epigastrium is the most common symptom of pancreatic carcinoma. Initially, it may be vague and poorly defined. As the tumor grows, the pain becomes more intense and frequently radiates to the back. The pain is often made worse by lying down and may be partially relieved by sitting forward in a crouched position.[120]
3. Weight loss is invariably present and is most likely due to a combination of the tumor per se and the associated symptoms of early satiety, anorexia, and poor nutrition. Other contributing factors that may be associated with pancreatic carcinoma include diabetes mellitus and malabsorption.
4. Malabsorption and steatorrhea usually are late manifestations of pancreatic carcinoma. They result from pancreatic duct obstruction and subsequent lack of secretion of pancreatic enzymes. In addition to mal-

absorption, obstruction of the pancreatic duct may also cause surrounding inflammation and lead to an erroneous primary diagnosis of pancreatitis.[67,68,149,205] The association of pancreatitis and carcinoma may significantly delay the diagnosis of carcinoma.

5. Diabetes mellitus occurs in 25% to 50% of patients with pancreatic adenocarcinoma.[135] The onset of acute diabetes in an adult with abdominal pain should alert the physician to the possibility of pancreatic carcinoma.[14,32] Although the pathway by which diabetes results from pancreatic carcinoma is not entirely understood, it is thought to be related to pancreatic duct obstruction by the tumor. Work by McBee et al. has shown that neoplastic obstruction of the pancreatic duct may cause hypoglycemia (Herxheimer-Mansfeld phenomenon) as a result of both hypertrophy and hyperplasia of the obstructed pancreatic islets.[133]
6. Spontaneous venous, or rarely, arterial thrombi may occur in about 25% of cases of pancreatic carcinoma. Although this phenomenon is suggestive of carcinoma, it is nonspecific and has been shown to be unrelated to the size or extent of the tumor.[106,117,185]
7. Hematemesis also may occur. Pancreatic carcinoma often obstructs the splenic, portal, or superior mesenteric veins by direct invasion, which may cause portal hypertension and subsequent gastrointestinal hemorrhage from varices.[108,126,134] Less frequently, direct tumor invasion of the stomach or duodenum may result in ulceration and bleeding.[207]

In the nonjaundiced patient in whom pancreatic carcinoma is suspected, computed tomography is the procedure of choice for initial evaluation. If computed tomograms are normal and carcinoma is still strongly suspected, ERCP should be performed. If this is also normal, follow-up examinations are usually performed. If the computed tomograms demonstrate a mass, fine-needle aspiration biopsy may be performed to confirm diagnosis, followed by surgery if resection of the tumor is felt to have a reasonable chance of success. However, if the mass is identified with extensive metastatic disease, fine-needle aspiration biopsy should be performed to confirm the diagnosis, and palliative procedures should be considered.

For patients with jaundice. Jaundice is present in a large percentage of patients with carcinoma of the pancreas. Tumors arising in the head of the pancreas or periampullary region frequently cause obstruction of the contiguous common bile duct; in these patients, jaundice may be the initial symptom. However, jaundice is usually a late finding in patients with tumors arising in the body or tail; in these cases, jaundice often results from bile duct obstruction caused by metastases to lymph nodes in the porta hepatis or by numerous hepatic metastases.[23]

Table 14-3. Imaging Modalities for Evaluating Carcinoma of the Pancreas

MODALITY	STAGING CAPABILITY	BENEFIT/ COST RATIO	RECOMMENDED ROUTINE STAGING PROCEDURE
Noninvasive			
Chest roentgenograms	Good for detecting pulmonary parenchymal metastases, which are generally late and usually seen only terminally	Moderate	Yes
Bone roentgenograms	Useful to confirm the uncommon bone metastasis	Low	No
Barium—upper gastrointestinal roentgenogram with or without double contrast and hypotonic duodenography	Useful to define effect on stomach and duodenum. Helpful to rule out other causes of upper gastrointestinal symptoms such as ulcer disease.	Moderate	Yes
Radionuclide studies (liver spleen scan)	May be useful in evaluating clinically suspected hepatic metastasis.	Moderate	No (Selected cases only)
Upper abdominal ultrasound	Useful for evaluating suspected abdominal metastases, especially hepatic metastases. May be helpful in defining the primary tumor as well as evaluating for dilated bile ducts and ascites.	High	Yes
Pancreatic MRI	A promising new technique with ability to morphologically image the pancreas and peripancreatic tissues and to evaluate for local as well as distant metastases. Additional diagnostic information may be present with tissue-specific MRI variables.	? High	? Yes
Minimally Invasive			
Computed body tomography	Minimally invasive with intravenous contrast, which is strongly recommended for optimal CT technique. Most useful and beneficial of all imaging modalities in determining local invasion and distant metastases.	High	Yes
Intravenous urography	May be used to assess for metastatic invasion into the kidney.	Low	No
Invasive			
Lymphangiography	May be used to evaluate involvement of retroperitoneal lymph nodes. However, will miss mesenteric and peripancreatic lymph nodes.	Low	No
ERCP/PTC	Very accurate in defining deformity of bile and pancreatic duct and localizing site of obstruction. May be useful in the jaundiced patient or the patient with diagnostic uncertainty or questionable diagnosis.	High	No
Percutaneous biopsy (guided by CT and/or ultrasound and/or ERCP and/or PTC)	Very invasive but very accurate for diagnosis of carcinoma of the pancreas.	High	No (Selected cases only)
Selective pancreatic angiography	Accurate and may be helpful in the patient with diagnostic uncertainty	Moderate	No (Selected cases only)

Painless jaundice is the classic finding in pancreatic adenocarcinoma; however, jaundice may also be caused by pancreatitis, and differentiation from carcinoma may be difficult.[206]

In patients with jaundice, sonography is usually the first imaging procedure performed. This will allow a diagnosis of obstructive versus nonobstructive jaundice to be made. If the sonogram demonstrates dilated bile ducts but no evidence of a pancreatic mass, computed tomography, PTC, or ERCP should next be performed. These procedures will define ductal anatomy and the site and cause of the obstruction. If a mass is identified, percutaneous fine-needle aspiration biopsy may be performed to confirm the diagnosis. Computed tomography has an advantage over PTC or ERCP in that it will also evaluate the liver for possible metastatic disease as well

as the peripancreatic regions for vascular invasion and lymphadenopathy.

Angiography may be performed if additional information is desired for presurgical evaluation or if the diagnosis remains in doubt. The role of MRI in the evaluation of the pancreas has yet to be defined. Plain roentgenograms or barium contrast roentgenograms have a very limited role in the work up of patients with suspected carcinoma. However, they may be helpful in defining causes of patient symptomatology that may be unrelated to the pancreas, such as peptic ulcer disease, renal disease secondary to calculi, or inflammatory or neoplastic disease in the chest.

Other situations that should lead to suspicion of pancreatic neoplasms and need for CT imaging. Pancreatic carcinoma may involve the gastrointestinal tract by direct extension or intraperitoneal spread. Direct extension into the stomach, duodenum, or colon can produce obstruction, ulceration, or hemorrhage.[136,137,211]

Cystic neoplasms of the pancreas are rare. They are somewhat more frequent in women than in men. The initial clinical symptoms are nonspecific and may be vague. Symptoms are usually secondary to the large size of the mass and its location. When the lesion is located in the head of the pancreas, jaundice may be an initial symptom.

The initial clinical symptoms of endocrine or islet cell tumors of the pancreas are related to the endocrine function of the cells in the tumor and the hormone produced. Insulinoma is the most common endocrine tumor of the pancreas, and it produces a hypoglycemic syndrome. Gastrinomas, which release gastrin and cause the Zollinger-Ellison syndrome, are the second most common pancreatic islet cell tumors. The gastrinomas of Zollinger-Ellison syndrome have been associated with the MEA Type I syndrome. The MEA (Multiple Endocrine Adenomatosis) Type I syndrome is an autosomal dominant disorder characterized by pituitary, pancreatic, and parathyroid adenomas. Occasionally a carcinoid syndrome may be found in these patients. Because over 60% of gastrinomas are malignant, many have already metastasized either to regional nodes or to the liver by the time of initial diagnosis. Occasionally, these tumors can become quite large and produce symptoms by their mass effect.

Laboratory Procedures that Lead to Diagnostic Imaging. Serum amylase and lipase values generally are normal in pancreatic adenocarcinoma.[80] However, occasionally lipase may be elevated during the early course of carcinoma and may lead to diagnostic confusion with pancreatitis. Pancreatic function tests (secretin-pancreozymin test) have been used for a number of years to detect pancreatic disease.[50] Impairment of pancreatic function occurs in both carcinoma and chronic pancreatitis and is characterized by a decrease in the volume of fluid and quantity of enzymes and bicarbonate recovered from the duodenum. Although this test is quite sensitive in the detection of pancreatic disease, it is usually nonspecific and only rarely is useful for differentiation of carcinoma and pancreatitis.

DiMagno et al. have measured carcinoembryonic antigen (CEA) levels in duodenal secretions from patients with pancreatic carcinoma.[45] Carcinoembryonic antigen levels did not help to differentiate pancreatic cancer patients from those with nonmalignant disease. However, they found abnormal pancreatic enzyme outputs in almost 90% of patients with carcinoma of the head and in 75% of patients with carcinoma of the body and tail of the pancreas.[44] Subsequent work by DiMagno et al. correlated pancreatic secretion tests with the site of

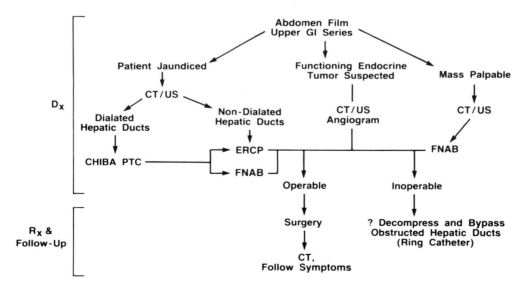

FIG. 14-22. Decision tree for pancreatic tumors. The three most common problems associated with a possible pancreatic neoplasm are shown as different arms of the decision tree. With the jaundiced patient, a CHIBA percutaneous cholangiogram (PTC) will outline the dilated hepatic ducts, which in combination with endoscopic retrograde cholangiopaneraetography (ERCP) will define the location and length of the tumor. Many centers still rely on angiography, both to characterize the suspected functioning pancreatic tumor and to aid in the preoperative assessment of the pancreatic tumor. Fine-needle aspiration biopsy (FNAB) may be performed to confirm diagnosis before any planned surgery. The follow-up of pancreatic tumors and assessment of response to therapy is best performed by CT.

pancreatic duct obstruction as determined by ERCP.[46] This study demonstrated that a decrease in exocrine pancreatic secretion cannot be detected until more than 60% of the total length of the main pancreatic duct has been obstructed.

The discovery and determination of tumor markers in patients with pancreatic carcinoma recently have received considerable attention. Carcinoembryonic antigen, which is the most easily measured, has not been shown to be a reliable indicator of the presence or absence of pancreatic carcinoma.[213]

Pancreatic oncofetal antigens were first identified by Banwo et al.[13] Although initial work was promising, their clinical efficacy has not yet been established.[86] Future work in the area of tumor markers is needed for discovery of a low-cost, noninvasive screening test capable of detecting pancreatic carcinoma at an early resectable stage.

Treatment Decisions

Despite improved understanding of pancreatic disease and the newer imaging modalities of high resolution real-time sonography, dynamic contrast-enhanced computed tomography, and, most recently, MRI, the long-term prognosis of carcinoma of the pancreas remains dismal. There has been no improved survival with these new imaging techniques.

Unfortunately, most patients have highly advanced lesions when their cancer is detected. There is no effective screening procedure for pancreatic cancer and, therefore, although en bloc surgical resection is relatively accurate, it only applies to a very small group of patients who have the cancer discovered in the localized state.

Surgery of lesions of the head of the pancreas consists of an en bloc excision of the distal stomach, common bile duct, and duodenum, i.e., the Whipple procedure.[25] Total pancreatectomy has been advocated when tumors are multicentric and does offer a possibility of cure to 25% of the patients on whom it is performed.[130] Unfortunately, resection is rarely applicable to cancers of the body and tail of the pancreas.

Radiotherapy is favored by some oncologists, particularly with the introduction of linear accelerator high-dose precision radiation therapy by Dobelbower et al.[47,48] This requires careful definition of the tumor volume by surgery and CT scans, which precede use of a shrinking-field technique that allows tumor doses of 6,500 cGy to be delivered in 7 to 8 weeks using megavoltage photon and/or electron beams ranging from 10 to 40 MeV. Split course irradiation also has its advocates. It consists of three courses of 2,000 cGy delivered in 200-cGy fractions at 2-week intervals, resulting in a dose of 6,000 cGy in 10 weeks.[79] Some of the more innovative approaches to treating pancreatic cancer include neutron beam therapy and intraoperative techniques using interstitial implants, iodine 125 seeds or electron beams carefully placed through operative wounds.[33,70] Mixed beam radiation therapy with neutrons is being advocated with some improvement in one-year survival figures.[4]

Table 14-4 summarizes the therapeutic options according to whether the disease is localized, advanced, or metastatic using the TNM classification system.[2]

The cystic neoplasms of the pancreas are slow growing and with radical surgical excision offer a good prognosis for long-term survival. However, because many of these patients are elderly and complete surgical excision requires a major pancreatic resection, the operative mortality and morbidity may be significant. Complete surgical resection is recommended; partial resection or marsupialization are not recommended.

The behavior of pancreatic endocrine tumors is poorly understood. While many are malignant and have metastasized at the time of diagnosis, they may be slow growing. Although radical surgery has met with limited success, a number of these tumors respond favorably to the chemotherapeutic agent streptozotocin.

Impact of New Technology

Magnetic Resonance Imaging. Magnetic resonance imaging (MRI) is a multiplanar cross-sectional imaging modality that utilizes the magnetism inherent in several nuclei normally found in the human body. The technique of MRI has been described elsewhere.[161,162] Pre-

Table 14-4. Treatment Decisions: Pancreas

STAGE	SURGERY		RADIATION THERAPY		CHEMOTHERAPY
Localized T_1,T_2,N_1,M_0	Whipple procedure	or	High dose precision RT 6,500 cGy		NR
Advanced T_3,T_4,N_2,M_0	Unresectable		High dose precision RT 6,500 cGy Split course RT	and/or	Investigational MAC
T_{any},N_{any},M_+	NR		Palliative RT		MAC

RT = Radiation Therapy
NR = Not Recommended
MAC = Multiagent Chemotherapy

OI-K

liminary evaluation of pancreatic imaging with MRI has been promising.[188] The pancreas and retroperitoneal structures can be easily identified, and pathologic morphologic changes can be seen (Figure 14-23). It is hoped that in the future, characteristic MRI tissue variables will be identified that will allow improved diagnostic accuracy.

PRIMARY AND METASTATIC CARCINOMA OF THE LIVER

The presence of either primary or metastatic malignancy within the liver is a grave prognostic sign. The techniques for detecting such neoplasms have undergone radical changes during the past several years, and further significant advances in diagnosis and detection are on the horizon. The improved ability to detect tumors with new imaging techniques has had little scientifically demonstrable impact upon survival statistics.[203] However, the perfection of diagnostic techniques and the routine integration of such techniques into diagnostic evaluation and posttherapeutic follow-up, which will lead to improved treatment results, is the goal of all oncologic imaging.

The goal of liver imaging is to detect malignancy, to discriminate malignancy from benign disease, and to find lesions while they are still isolated to resectable portions of the liver. Radiologic techniques are also valuable in assessing the response of tumor to various therapeutic methods.

In this section, we will consider both primary and metastatic carcinoma of the liver. We will emphasize particularly the most common varieties of liver malignancy in adults—primary hepatocellular carcinoma and metastatic colorectal carcinoma. The role that imaging may play with specificity of diagnosis, guidance for percutaneous biopsy, and for the operative management of disease will be discussed. The potential impact of new imaging technology and contrast agents and the interaction of imaging techniques with new therapeutic methods will be outlined.

Tumor Behavior and Pathology

Hepatocellular Carcinoma. In adults, the most common primary malignancy is hepatocellular carcinoma—hepatoma. About one half of cases of hepatoma in adults in the United States arise in patients with pre-existing cirrhosis.[121] Rarely, angiosarcoma, leiomyosarcoma, fibrosarcoma, or lymphoma may originate within the liver.[168] In children, hepatoblastoma occurs, usually under the age of three years. Rhabdomyosarcoma may also occur within the liver. Hepatoma also occurs in children and is often associated with one of several congenital syndromes or congenital metabolic diseases.[181] There are several discrete manifestations of hepatoma in adults. In about two thirds of cases, the liver is extensively studded with nodules. In about 5% of the cases, the liver is diffusely infiltrated with tumor. These latter cases are universally found in patients with cirrhosis. About 30% of hepatomas are characterized by the presence of a mass, often with multiple satellite lesions. A fourth type is an encapsulated form of hepatoma. This accounts for only a few percent of hepatomas in the United States, but it is much more common in Japan. These latter two types are the only forms that are considered potentially curable.

Hepatoma metastasizes within the liver by parasinusoidal extension, by invasion into the portal and hepatic venous system, and by invasion of lymphatics. This tumor metastasizes distantly most frequently to nodes, the lungs, and bones, but also spreads to the adrenal glands and brain. The male-to-female ratio is about 3 : 1 and the peak age of occurrence is 50 to 60 years of age. Hepatocellular carcinoma may directly invade the adjacent diaphragm, but this does not necessarily indicate incurability because en bloc resections can be performed if the tumor is limited to a resectable portion of the liver. These tumors also have a tendency to cause neuroendocrine and hematopoietic syndromes, such as polycythemia, thrombocytosis, hypercalcemia, hyperglycemia, and ectopic ACTH production.

In the absence of resectable disease, hepatomas are virtually always fatal. Survival statistics are variable following surgical resection. In one series of 46 patients who underwent hepatic resections for hepatoma, 65% survived for three years, 36% survived for five years, and 33% survived for ten years. In another series of 137 patients, 27% had resections, but only five survived for five years.[121]

The initial symptoms of hepatoma are usually pain or jaundice. However, tumors are often quite large before causing such symptoms. Palliative treatment may be directed towards temporary relief of the symptoms. Ascites may suddenly develop because of hepatic vein thrombosis—the Budd-Chiari Syndrome. Hemorrhage is the direct cause of death in 50% of patients with hepatoma.

Metastatic Liver Disease. Liver metastases are often a component of disease leading to death in patients with carcinoma of the colon.[203] There is a 60% one-year survival of patients with solitary untreated liver metastases, but only about a 6% one-year survival with widespread disease. Liver metastasis occurs in about 60% to 70% of patients with metastatic disease from carcinoma of the colon. Tumors arising from the colon, excluding the rectum, most commonly metastasize to the liver. Rectal tumors may metastasize to the lungs or liver first. Thus, in most cases, lung metastases occur subsequent

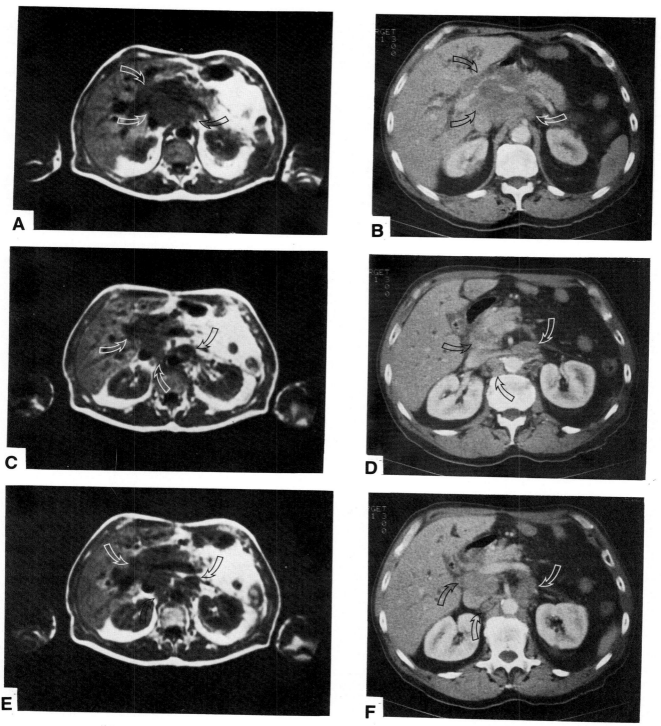

FIG. 14-23. Retroperitoneal metastases. Comparative magnetic resonance (MR) imaging (A,C,E) and computed tomographic (B,D,F) images of the retroperitoneum at the level of the pancreas and porta hepatis. Scans demonstrate a soft tissue mass (arrows) in the region of the head of the pancreas invading into the porta hepatis in this patient with adenocarcinoma of the esophagogastric junction with regional and retroperitoneal metastases. MRI images were obtained at 0.5 Tesla, 10-mm slice thickness, partial saturation recovery with a repetition time of 200 msec.

to and probably as a result of liver metastasis.[191] Depending on the location of the primary tumor, local nodal disease or spread to the spine or peritoneal implantation may occur early. About 15% to 25% of patients have metastases at the time of initial surgery.

Although colon carcinoma accounts for a large fraction of metastatic liver lesions, numerous other tumors metastasize to the liver, including pancreatic, stomach, lung, breast, renal, and ovarian tumors, melanomas, carcinoid tumors, insulinomas, and glucagonomas. However, detecting and determining the extent of liver lesions is most crucial in colon carcinoma because of the possibility of curative resection of isolated disease. Such a possibility does not usually exist in the other tumors mentioned.

Classification and Staging

No specific staging system has been offered for hepatocellular carcinoma. This is presumably because of the usually extensive nature of the disease when first found, the very low cure rate, and very poor survival statistics. Also, it has been difficult to determine the anatomic extent of disease preoperatively.

Malignancies metastatic to the liver are indicated as M_1 lesions, or tumor with distant metastases present. This automatically increases the tumor stage of any primary neoplasm.

Imaging Procedures and Assessment

A variety of biochemical tests are used to screen for liver dysfunction. Serum liver function tests, however, may not be sufficiently sensitive to detect hepatic involvement by tumor. Also, these tests are often not specific enough to distinguish between hepatic tumor and biliary obstruction or diffuse hepatic parenchymal disease.[203] Several imaging studies are available to assess the liver. These include radionuclide liver/spleen scanning, hepatic angiography, sonography, and computed tomography.

Nuclear Medicine. Hepatic radionuclide imaging has long been considered the standard screening test for patients suspected of having metastatic disease to the liver. It involves little risk of exposure to ionizing radiation and is widely available and relatively inexpensive. However, it has low spatial resolution, is only about 70% sensitive in detecting disease, and has a significant percentage of falsely abnormal studies. Hepatic anatomic variations are common, and these variations may cause considerable interpretative difficulty. For example, a prominent porta hepatis, renal or rib impression, or unusually thin right or left lobe may all be misinterpreted as a significant abnormality or at least require further study. Because masses are usually detected by the lack of uptake in the hepatic Kupffer's cells, no specific information is available about the nature of the mass itself. For example, cysts, hemangiomata, and abscesses may be misinterpreted as tumors. However, cases of focal nodular hyperplasia and regenerating nodules do result in radionuclide uptake and thus may be recognizable. Also, the presence of tumor or abscess may be indicated by gallium or indium scanning. Overall, the above features create serious limitations to the utility of radionuclide liver/spleen scanning in the diagnosis of liver disease.[100,119,182,212]

Angiography. Angiography is a valuable method in studying the liver. Excellent spatial resolution in the identification of hepatic vascular anatomy is a particular advantage of angiography. Sensitivity, however, is affected by the vascularity and size of the lesions. Hypovascular lesions such as melanomas, leiomyomas, and metastatic endocrine tumors, which are too small to displace arteries, may go undetected. Angiography is also more time consuming, risky, and expensive than radionuclide scanning, thus relegating angiography to a limited role in diagnosing and managing hepatic malignancy. More recently, intra-arterial digital subtraction angiography (DSA) has proven useful in evaluating the liver for hepatic metastases. The technique involves catheterization of the celiac or hepatic artery and injection of a small amount of iodinated contrast material, usually 20 to 30 mL of a 30% solution. Small peripheral metastases are easily seen with this technique because of the marked improvement in contrast resolution of digital subtraction angiography over standard film recording.

Sonography. Hepatic sonography is a modality often used to evaluate liver disease. Sonography is the preferred screening test for differentiating biliary obstruction from hepatic parenchymal disease in the jaundiced patient but is less valuable for detecting tumors. Neoplasms may be strikingly more or less echogenic than surrounding normal hepatic parenchyma, or may manifest themselves as a disorganization of echo architecture from the usual fine homogeneous pattern (Figure 14-24). However, lesions may also be of equivalent echogenicity to the liver, and lesion borders may be ill defined. Unless the lesions are sufficiently large or inhomogeneous, they may go undetected. The sensitivity of sonography is difficult to ascertain, because of the lack of well-controlled comparative studies, but sensitivity has been most often reported to be in the range of 70% to 80%.[100,182] These data are supported by our own unpublished comparative study of sonography with computed tomography. Nevertheless, some do advocate the use of ultrasound for screening because of its lower expense and easy availability, particularly when high resolution computed tomography is not available.[20]

While we believe that sonography is probably not ade-

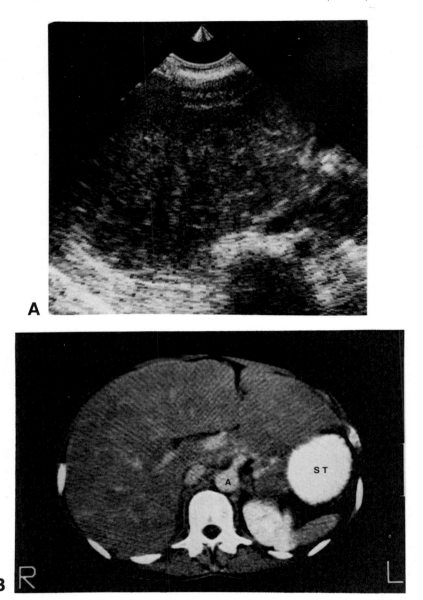

FIG. 14-24. Diffuse hepatic metastases. (A) A real-time sonogram of a patient with diffuse metastatic disease to the liver from oat cell carcinoma. Metastases appear as a disruption of the normal fine homogeneous echo texture of the liver. No discrete masses are visible. (B) A computed tomogram of the same patient showing hepatomegaly with diffuse but mild inhomogeneity. A = aorta, St = stomach.

quate as a screening technique for liver masses because of limited sensitivity, it has a very useful complementary role to play with other methods. When directed to assess specific areas brought into question by other imaging modalities or as an adjunct to other technically suboptimal examinations, sonography performs well. For example, ultrasound is well suited to assess marginal defects on radionuclide liver/spleen scans or to distinguish cystic from solid lesions.[217] Because the computed tomographic and sonographic detections of mass lesions are based on different physical properties, a lesion that is easily detected by computed tomography may be difficult to detect by sonography and vice versa (Figure 14-25). Like radionuclide scanning, sonography has the advantage of relatively low cost and low risk. However, the quality of the sonogram is dependent on the quality of the sonographic unit and the technical expertise of the operator.

Computed Tomography. Hepatic computed tomography combines both high sensitivity to focal lesions and high specificity regarding the nature of these lesions. Most primary and metastatic neoplasms within the liver are lower in attenuation (density) than the adjacent normal hepatic tissue.[141] When of nearly equivalent density, they may be detected by slight inhomogeneities or displacement of normal hepatic structures. Intravenous contrast creates various patterns of enhancement and often improves detectability of lesions by demonstrating tumor vascularity or increasing the attenuation difference between enhancing parenchyma and less enhancing or irregularly enhancing tumor.[18,27,125,141,218] Most primary and metastatic neoplasms are accurately and easily identified by computed tomography. The difficulty arises in the differential diagnosis of malignant neoplasms from several benign lesions that may occur in the liver. Cysts and cavernous hemangiomata are identified and perhaps specifically diagnosed by computed tomography with bolus contrast enhancement.[62,90] One group of investigators has suggested that some hepatomas may have a characteristic appearance by contrast-enhanced computed tomography (Figure 14-26).[89] However, in cases where the diagnosis is difficult or in doubt, angiography or needle biopsy is recommended.

The advantages of computed tomography are its relatively low risk, low patient discomfort, and availability in most centers. Scans confined to the liver provide useful information about the other major upper abdominal organs and retroperitoneum as well as an assessment of biliary dilatation. Disadvantages include the use of intravenous contrast material, significant expense, and the presence of streak artifact. Computed tomography may have difficulty in demonstrating diffuse diseases of the liver, such as cirrhosis and diffuse hepatoma.[77] These entities and their severity may be better assessed by radionuclide scanning. Computed tomography may not allow accurate discrimination of benign from malignant lesions (Figure 14-27). Computed tomography and sonography may also be disadvantageous because of their ability to detect benign lesions so small that they are undetectable by other techniques. This leads to potential confusion with metastatic disease and the possibility of unnecessary laparotomy or therapy. The newest versions of CT scanners produce high quality images with scan times under 3 seconds and have largely eliminated troublesome artifacts, thus improving diagnostic sensitivity and reducing diagnostic errors. Table 14-5 provides the benefit/cost ratio for evaluating carcinoma of the liver.

Accurate identification of hepatic segmental and subsegmental anatomy is important when extensive hepatic resection is contemplated for either primary or metastatic disease. Both sonography and contrast-enhanced computed tomography are accurate, and both have been used to define hepatic anatomy. At the cephalad aspect of the liver, the hepatic veins serve to identify the hepatic segments by cross-sectional imaging.[29] The right hepatic lobe is separated into its anterior and posterior segments by the right hepatic vein. The middle hepatic vein

separates the right from the left lobe, and the left hepatic vein separates the medial and lateral segments of the left lobe. At a more caudad level, the fissure for the ligamentum teres borders the medial and lateral segments of the left lobe. The gallbladder fossa is located between the right and left lobes. At many levels, however, there are no recognizable segmental landmarks. Also, in the presence of a mass effect, the normal anatomy may be so distorted by invasion and displacement of the landmarks that accurate lesion localization may not be possible. This may have an impact on the decision to perform a resection for localized tumor.

Imaging Strategies and Decisions

We believe that in most patients, high resolution computed tomography is the preferred method for evaluating suspected liver masses because of its accuracy, specificity, and the additional information it provides about other organ systems (Figure 14-28).[5,100] Sonography may be used to clarify questions remaining or arising after CT. Angiography may be required to help exclude bilobar disease in patients being considered for hepatic resection or may be performed on patients receiving intra-arterial chemotherapy.

The benefit of lower expense of sonography and radionuclide scanning is often erased by the lower sensitivity and specificity and the necessity of performing further studies and incurring greater delays. However, if high resolution computed tomography is unavailable and expense is a consideration or the index of suspicion is quite low, then these other imaging studies remain quite valuable (Figure 14-29).

Treatment Decisions[2,45]

After the detection of intrahepatic neoplasm, the most crucial judgment concerns the extent of disease. In recent years, aggressive hepatic resection has been more frequently performed. Resection is most often reserved for selected cases of colorectal carcinoma with disease that has metastasized to the liver. Other indications for resection are to reduce tumor bulk in patients symptomatic from endocrine tumors in efforts toward palliation and to debulk tumors in children with neoplasms responsive to chemotherapy or radiation therapy.

It is often feasible to resect as much as three of the four major hepatic segments because the liver may regenerate its former mass within three weeks. Such trisegmentectomies may involve the left lobe and anterior segment of the right lobe or the right lobe and medial segment of the left lobe. The challenge of imaging studies then is to determine the segmental location of isolated masses and to ensure that the remaining liver is free of disease.

When major hepatic resection is considered, multiple imaging modalities should be used to optimize localiza-

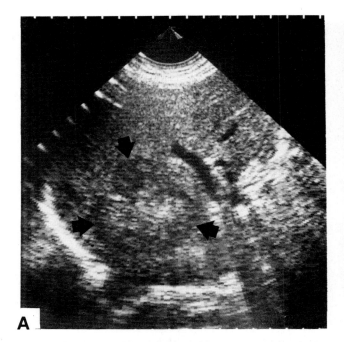

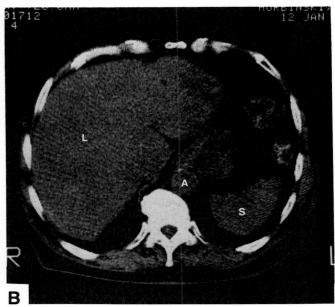

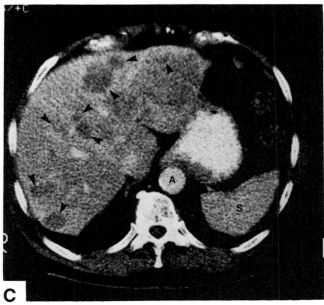

FIG. 14-25. Focal metastases. (A) A real-time sonogram of a patient with metastatic carcinoma of the colon. A hepatic mass (arrows) is apparent, but portions of it are very similar in echogenicity to adjacent liver. (B) A computed tomogram of the same patient before the injection of intravenous contrast. No clearly identifiable masses are visible. (C) A computed tomogram at the same level as in B after the injection of a bolus of intravenous contrast. Liver metastases are now clearly defined (arrowheads). L = liver, S = spleen, A = aorta.

tion and sensitivity, to potentially avoid fruitless surgery. Also, the examination technique should be carefully optimized for this specific purpose.

Sonography has the advantage of intrinsic high resolution image contrast between vessels and parenchyma.

Also, particularly with real-time sonography, vessels may be traced over considerable distances and the relationship to adjacent lesions may be ascertained. Nevertheless, because of the high position of the liver under the ribs, localization using vascular landmarks may still be difficult. Sonography done during surgery with high frequency transducers placed directly on the liver surface may detect small occult lesions. Surgery may then be terminated before extensive resection.

Because of the importance of vascular landmarks for localization, CT should be performed on patients being considered for hepatic resection both before the administration of intravenous contrast and after bolus injection of contrast. Slow infusions of intravenous contrast tend to obscure the hepatic veins and lead to lesions becoming isodense. Computed tomography and sonography are used extensively to localize lesions for percutaneous biopsy. This improves accuracy over blind biopsy techniques.

Angiography may provide helpful indications about the vascular supply and vascularity of lesions and the possible presence of anomalies. Arteriograms may occasionally lead to the detection of lesions missed by other studies. A computed tomographic arteriogram can also be performed in which the CT scan is done with the angiography catheter remaining in place while bolus injections are administered.[138,160]

Imaging studies are most frequently used to monitor the effectiveness of palliative therapy in order to determine whether a specific regimen should be pursued (Figure 14-30).[19,215] A choice of which imaging modality to employ for follow-up depends upon several factors, such as which imaging method best depicted the tumor before

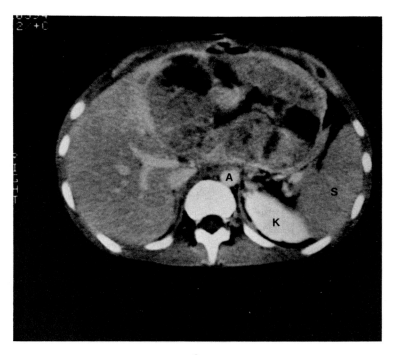

FIG. 14-26. Hepatoma, rapid sequence computed tomography. A focal mass is present in the left lobe of the liver. A contrast-enhanced rapid sequence computed tomogram demonstrates sharp definition of the mass from surrounding liver, bulging of tumor from the hepatic surface, and areas of intense enhancement. A = aorta, S = spleen, K = kidney.

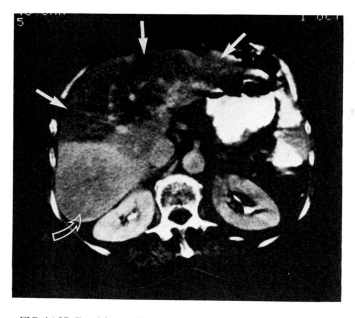

FIG. 14-27. Focal fatty infiltration and hepatoma. A computed tomogram of a patient with two liver abnormalities. The ventral portion of the liver shows regional fatty infiltration (arrows). The posterior segment of the right hepatic lobe demonstrates an inhomogeneous mass, which proved to be a hepatoma (curved arrow).

therapy; whether numerous surgical clips are present, which might limit the utility of CT; how cooperative the patient might be for breath-holding; or the presence of obesity. If diagnosis of alterations in tumor size is attempted, radionuclide liver/spleen scanning may suffice as long as very subtle alterations are not sought. If contrast-enhanced CT is employed, contrast administration techniques should be standardized, because such techniques often affect the apparent size of lesions.

Patients undergoing intra-arterial chemotherapy may have periodic contrast injections through the indwelling arterial catheter that will indicate tumor response and the effect of chemotherapy on the hepatic vessels (Figure 14-30).

In our institution, CT is most frequently used in the follow-up of malignant hepatic masses because it accurately and specifically depicts lesions, it provides ease of comparison between examinations, it demonstrates subtle changes, it can demonstrate associated findings, and it is the test most often performed as the baseline examination.

A recent review article on the management of hepatomas indicates the importance of therapeutic approaches and vaccines in this disease.[65] Intra-arterial infusion chemotherapy with 5-Fluoro-2-deoxyuridine (FUDR) and Adriamycin, totally implanted infusion systems, hepatic artery embolization, and combinations of whole liver ir-

Table 14-5. Imaging Modalities for Evaluating Primary Carcinoma of the Liver

MODALITY	STAGING CAPABILITY	BENEFIT/ COST RATIO	RECOMMENDED ROUTINE STAGING PROCEDURE
Noninvasive			
Chest roentgenograms	Good for detecting pulmonary metastases.	High	Yes
Bone roentgenograms	Useful to confirm the rare metastasis.	Low	No
Barium contrast upper gastro-intestinal roentgenograms	May be helpful to define deformity from metastatic lesions or varices.	Low	No
Radionuclide liver/spleen scans	Extremely helpful in evaluating focal mass and extent of tumor. Combined use of technetium sulfur colloid and gallium scans extremely helpful.	High	Yes
Hepatic ultrasound	Useful for defining focal mass as well as metastases. Helpful in evaluating for metastatic spread into the portal and hepatic veins.	High	Yes
MRI	May be helpful in defining the hepatic mass and vascular metastases. Possible tissue-specific MRI variables may be defined in the future.	?	?
Minimally Invasive			
Hepatic computed tomography	Invasive if intravenous contrast is used, which is strongly recommended for evaluation of tumor, and mandatory for evaluation of vascular metastases. May be the most useful of all imaging modalities for determining local invasion and distant metastases.	High	Yes
Invasive			
Hepatic angiography	Accurate and extremely beneficial in defining hepatic-anatomy and tumor vascularity as well as portal vein and hepatic vein metastases. The combined use of digital subtraction angiography is extremely helpful	High	Yes
ERCP/PTC	Invasive and may not be particularly useful, since bile ducts are rarely directly involved.	Low	No
Percutaneous biopsy guided by imaging technique	Invasive but extremely accurate in establishing diagnosis.	High	No (Selected cases only)

radiation with chemotherapy are considered promising treatments for this type of cancer.[65] Further research on isotopic immunoglobulin may also lead to improved treatment.[65]

Impact of New Technology

Both the diagnosis and treatment of hepatic diseases continue to undergo great changes. A controversy currently surrounds the effectiveness of intra-arterial chemotherapy or its value relative to intravenous chemotherapy. We believe that such questions may be amenable to study with the sophisticated imaging techniques mentioned above and with new techniques currently being developed. The ability to assess the impact of new drugs and new treatments, such as intra-arterial radiation therapy, in which radioactive materials are attached to substances that localize in tumors; enhancement of radiation sensitivity by injection of cell sensitizers; portal vein infusion; and immunotherapy, can only be accurately assessed with the new imaging technology.[124]

One technique currently available but improved upon by the newest scanners is dynamic scanning with intravenous contrast injection following bolus injection of contrast. For example, 15 slices at contiguous levels with 2-second scans may be obtained in less than two minutes, allowing a scan to be made of the complete liver during the brief phase of maximum vascular and hepatic parenchymal enhancement. This not only improves diagnosis, but, because of the brevity of the scan, may permit greater patient volume with a resultant decrease in costs and an improved competitive position with other imaging modalities.

Two promising hepatospecific contrast agents are currently undergoing investigation. EOE-13 is a lipid-soluble, iodine-containing agent that localizes in liver cells and produces intense enhancement, which permits discrimination of normal liver from even very small lesions.[204] Perfluorocytlbromide (PFOB) is in the very early stages of investigation and has the property of creating an enhancing rim around neoplasms visualized both by CT and sonography.[131]

Because of its fundamentally different properties from roentgenography and ultrasound, magnetic resonance imaging (MRI) is likely to find and characterize lesions not seen by conventional imaging. While the resolution of MRI may be limited by motion from long data acquisition times, newer MRI units with stronger magnets (1.5 Tesla) may overcome the time problem. Work is also being done in the area of paramagnetic contrast agents, which may also increase the resolution and specificity of MRI.

New developments in sonographic tissue characterization are underway but have not yet demonstrated convincing clinical efficacy. Dedicated units for intraoperative ultrasound are already commercially available but not in widespread use. The technique of intraoperative ultrasound will certainly affect patient management decisions in surgical planning.

The pressing needs of improved sensitivity and specificity for liver lesions are thus currently being addressed; the problem of segmentally localizing lesions may prove more difficult. We can look forward to upcoming years of dramatic developments as creative imaging and therapeutic techniques are coordinated to work towards prolonged life in patients with hepatic malignancy.

Magnetic resonance imaging (MRI) has shown promise in the evaluation of the liver and in the detection of focal and diffuse hepatic disease (Figure 14-31). It is hoped in the future that with the use of specific MRI tissue variables and with higher resolution MRI imaging, a specific diagnosis can be made. Research is currently underway in this area.[139]

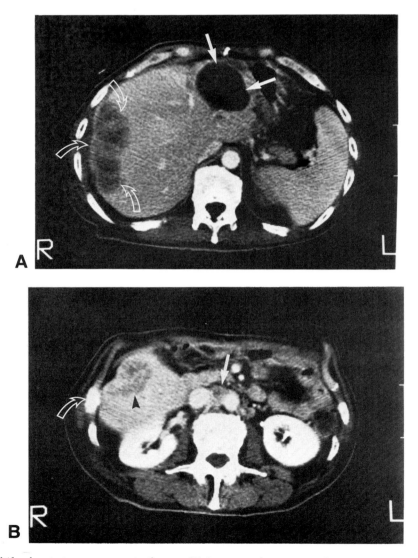

FIG. 14-28. Multifocal metastases, response to therapy. (A) A computed tomogram of a patient with metastatic colon carcinoma. This patient was treated with intra-arterial chemotherapy and developed stenosis of a right lobar arterial branch. Thus, the metastasis to the left lobe is largely necrotic and well-defined (arrows), while the right lobe metastasis (curved arrows) is inhomogeneous and enhances irregularly, indicating probable continued activity. (B) A more caudal computed tomogram demonstrates another area of metastasis in the caudad aspect of the right hepatic lobe (arrowhead). There are nodal metastases between the inferior vena cava and aorta (arrow) and a blastic metastasis to a right rib (curved arrow).

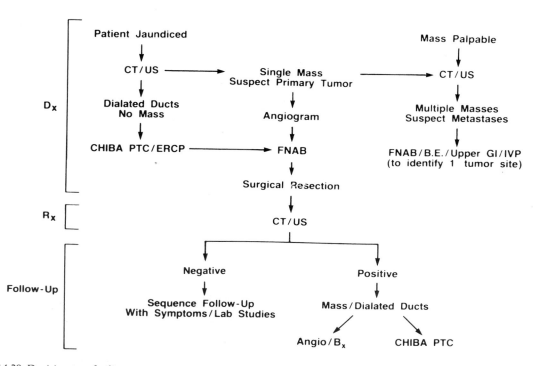

FIG. 14-29. Decision tree for liver tumors. The two arms of the decision tree correspond to patients with jaundice and with a palpable mass. In either setting, the primary and metastatic tumor work-up will differ. Before attempted resection of a primary hepatic neoplasm, both CT and angiography will usually be required to map the vascular bed and determine the likelihood for resectability. Fine-needle aspiration biopsy (FNAB) or core biopsy may be preferred to confirm the suspected diagnosis.

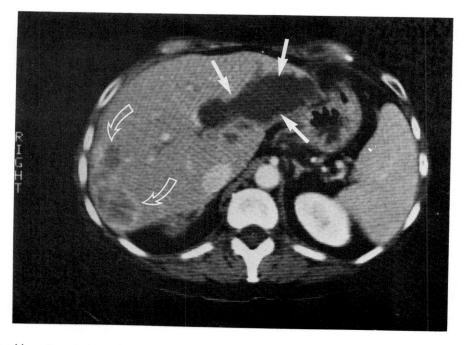

FIG. 14-30. Focal hepatic metastases. A computed tomogram of a patient with metastatic colon carcinoma. The left lobe metastasis is sharply defined and of low density, indicating probable necrosis (arrows). A metastatic lesion to the right lobe shows rim enhancement and inhomogeneous texture (curved arrows).

CARCINOMA OF THE GALLBLADDER AND BILIARY DUCTAL SYSTEM

Primary cancers of the gallbladder and biliary ductal system are relatively uncommon tumors. Cancer of the gallbladder is found in 1.4% of all biliary tract surgical procedures and is somewhat more common than carcinoma of the biliary ductal system. Carcinoma of the gallbladder is more common in women and in patients with cholelithiasis.[31,75,153,154,194] No such relationship exists for cholangiocarcinoma, however.

The tendency of carcinoma of the gallbladder is to spread initially by local invasion to the liver bed and then by metastases to regional lymph nodes. Despite recent advances in cancer detection and management, no improvement in survival has resulted for patients with this disease, and five-year survival continues to be rare. The poor prognosis for patients with this tumor is a result of advanced patient age, lack of specific symptoms, and an inability to establish an early diagnosis, as well as a propensity for early local invasion.[24,76,155,177]

Carcinoma of the gallbladder is the fifth most common gastrointestinal malignancy. Peak incidence occurs in the sixth and seventh decades of life, with a female-to-male ratio of 4 : 1. Most cases are associated with gallstones, and the majority are also associated with cholecystitis, suggesting chronic irritation as a cause. Oral cholecystography typically fails to demonstrate the gallbladder in cases of carcinoma. Sonographically, gallbladder carcinoma usually appears as a complex mass in the right upper quadrant.[6] Less commonly, irregular thickening of the gallbladder wall is present. Occasionally, a distinct polypoid mass may be identified.

Biliary cancer affects more women with the relatively common gallbladder cancer, whereas 60% of the patients with the less frequent bile duct cancers are men. Cholangiocarcinomas are usually slow growing, with death secondary to hepatic failure and cholangitis secondary to biliary obstruction. Because of the slow rate of growth and the difficulties posed by resection of these tumors, surgical treatment usually consists of exploration only or palliative decompression. No improvement in survival has been noted in these patients despite improved methods of diagnosis.

Tumor Behavior and Pathology

The modes of spread of gallbladder cancer are (1) local invasion; (2) lymphatic spread to the cystic node, peridocal nodes, and to superior and posterior pancreaticoduodenal and periaortic nodes; (3) vascular spread, although uncommon, leading to adjacent liver involvement via penetrating vessels in the gallbladder bed and later to diffuse vascular infiltration of the liver and other organs; (4) intraperitoneal spread, which is common and involves

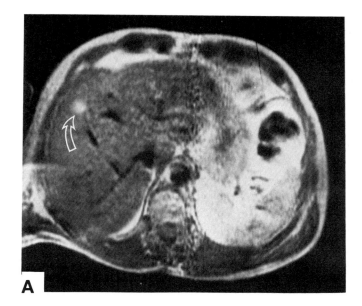

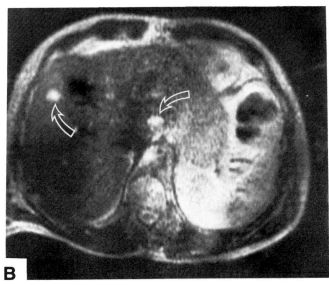

FIG. 14-31. Hepatic metastases, carcinoid tumor, MR images of the liver (A and B) in a patient with hepatic metastases from carcinoid tumor demonstrate high intensity signals representing the metastases (curved arrow). The MR images were obtained with a magnetic field strength of 0.5 Tesla and a spin echo pulsing sequence.

adjacent organs well before the development of disseminated intraperitoneal metastases; (5) neural spread, which occurs relatively frequently and is associated with more aggressive tumors; (6) intraductal spread, which is least common but is most frequently seen in cases of papillary adenocarcinoma of the gallbladder.

Direct invasion to regional tissues from both cholangiocarcinoma and gallbladder carcinoma is common. Direct invasion into the liver is most common although invasion may occur into the stomach, the greater or lesser omentum, the colon, the pancreas, and the duodenum.

Initial tumor lymph drainage is to the cystic and common bile duct nodes, with further drainage into the peripancreatic system, including the celiac axis, superior mesenteric or para-aortic nodes. In one series, regional nodal involvement was noted in 42% of patients at the time of surgical exploration and 52% of patients at autopsy, while retroperitoneal nodal involvement was noted in 23% and 26%, respectively.

Hematogenous spread of tumor may occur, with involvement of the liver, peritoneum, or lung. While liver involvement is most common, it is difficult to determine if involvement from gallbladder carcinoma is hematogenous or via direct extension.

Carcinomas of the extrahepatic bile ducts metastasize early to regional lymph nodes in part because of the rich lymphatic network that covers their thin walls. Extension through the bile duct wall and to lymph nodes in the porta hepatis and celiac axis occurs relatively early. Peripancreatic nodes are involved more frequently in cholangiocarcinoma than in carcinoma of the gallbladder, while intra-abdominal spread and peritoneal metastases are less common than in carcinoma of the gallbladder.

Cholelithiasis has been clearly implicated as a pre-existing pathologic condition that predisposes patients to gallbladder carcinoma. In addition, gallbladder carcinoma is more frequent in women older than 55 years, and who have abnormalities in lipid metabolism. In a series of gallbladder carcinoma, the incidence of cholelithiasis varied between 70% and 90%. In patients with a calcified or porcelain gallbladder secondary to chronic cholelithiasis, the incidence of gallbladder carcinoma has been estimated to be as high as 60%.

There are several predisposing factors to cholangiocarcinoma, with the most common on a worldwide basis being liver fluke (*Clonorchis sinensis*) infestation. The mechanism by which liver fluke infestation results in bile duct carcinoma is unclear, although this may be secondary to the inflammatory reaction in the periductal tissues that is caused by the parasitic infection, or it may be that the parasites incite an inflammatory reaction in the bile ducts, promoting the action of carcinogenic agents excreted in the bile.

Cholangiocarcinoma has also been associated with chronic ulcerative colitis. The incidence of bile duct cancer in these patients is estimated to be approximately 0.4%. The mechanism responsible for this association is unknown. It is known that ulcerative colitis is associated with sclerosing cholangitis, and perhaps there is a relationship between sclerosing cholangitis and bile duct carcinoma.

The signs and symptoms of primary gallbladder carcinoma are similar to those associated with benign disease of the gallbladder. The most common symptom is pain in the right upper quadrant, with nausea, vomiting, and weight loss the next most common symptoms. Approximately one half of patients will have jaundice secondary to early direct invasion of the liver or biliary ductal system.

The clinical appearance of cholangiocarcinoma is similar to that of primary carcinoma of the gallbladder in the sense that the symptoms are frequently vague and similar to those of benign disease. The most common clinical symptomology in patients with cholangiocarcinoma is jaundice. This may be preceded by pruritus, weight loss, and anorexia. The liver may be enlarged and tender. Liver function studies demonstrate elevated bilirubin and alkaline phosphatase levels. There may be a nonspecific anemia or leukocytosis.

Cholangiocarcinoma usually appears in one of three ways: obstruction of a major duct leading to jaundice, local invasion of the liver or adjacent organs causing symptomology, or, rarely, as distant metastases.[9,115,199] Because of these nonspecific presentations, early detection is difficult, and the disease is frequently widespread at the time of diagnosis.

The prognosis of cholangiocarcinoma is poor, since symptoms of the disease only appear after virtually complete occlusion of the bile duct and since the tumor invariably has already invaded locally.[7,54,198] The median survival of patients with surgically unresectable cholangiocarcinoma is approximately 5 months. A four-year survival following surgery is reported to be 6%.

Classification and Staging

To date, no tumor staging pattern has been developed for cholangiocarcinoma or carcinoma of the gallbladder.

Primary cancer of the gallbladder is most commonly an adenocarcinoma, which arises in the body or fundus. Rarely, it develops in the cystic duct. Less common forms of gallbladder carcinoma include anaplastic carcinoma, squamous cell carcinoma, and adenoacanthoma.

Cholangiocarcinomas arise in the bile ducts themselves.[52] Approximately 30% of tumors are found in the midportion of the extrahepatic biliary system, the proximal common bile duct and common hepatic duct. Approximately 20% of the tumors occur in the region of the porta hepatis or an intrahepatic location, and in this location they may be extremely difficult to diagnose. Tumors that arise at the junction of the right and left hepatic ducts have been termed *Klatzkin tumors*.[3,99] Microscopically, these tumors are almost always adenocarcinomas. However, squamous cell and mesenchymal tumors have been reported. As with gallbladder cancer, local extension to regional lymph nodes and to adjacent tissues is common at the time of diagnosis. It is also known that these cancers may be multicentric in origin, although it is unknown if this represents multiple primary tumors or intraluminal spread of tumor from a single primary site. Diagnosis is usually made at the time of percutaneous needle or surgical biopsy. Cytologic evaluation of the bile obtained via a T tube or percutaneous needle aspiration may also be diagnostic.[78]

Imaging Procedures and Assessment

Routine Roentgenography. Plain roentgenograms are nonspecific and usually are not helpful (Figure 14-32). Routine cholecystography also is of little value. It demonstrates a nonfunctioning gallbladder in approximately two thirds of patients with carcinoma of the gallbladder. Barium upper gastrointestinal studies may demonstrate abnormalities of the duodenum, such as extrinsic pressure defects from the tumor mass or direct invasion (Figure 14-33). If the tumor mass is very large with extensive local invasion and fistula formation, necrotic areas may be outlined by internal gas and identified on abdominal roentgenograms (Figure 14-34).

Sonography. Patients with cholangiocarcinoma and advanced carcinoma of the gallbladder frequently have jaundice. Sonography is an excellent method of evaluation. The diagnosis of biliary obstruction may be made, and depending on the clinical situation and the sonographic findings, the correct diagnosis may be suggested.

Sonography may detect the presence of biliary dilatation secondary to obstruction even before liver function tests become abnormal. As a general guideline, the normal internal diameter of the common bile duct in the region of the head of the pancreas and the common hepatic duct in the porta hepatis or hepatoduodenal ligament is approximately 5 to 7 mm. The segment of the right intrahepatic duct just proximal to the common hepatic duct bifurcation often can be seen immediately anterior to the right portal vein and should measure no more than 2 to 3 mm in internal diameter. These size criteria are generally reliable in differentiating a normal duct from an abnormal or dilated duct.[107,114,123,142,148,176,195,209]

Chronic or complete obstruction is characterized by the presence of marked dilatation of the extrahepatic or intrahepatic biliary ducts and gallbladder. Dilated intrahepatic bile ducts may be identified when branch ducts adjacent to portal veins dilate. The dilated bile duct and adjacent vein radicle appear as "double channels."[36,208]

A distal common bile duct obstruction, such as a carcinoma of the head of the pancreas, ampullary carcinoma, cholangiocarcinoma, or obstructing common duct stone will cause the intrahepatic and extrahepatic biliary system to dilate proximal to the obstruction. Both computed tomography and sonography are approximately 95% accurate in the detection of these dilated ducts.

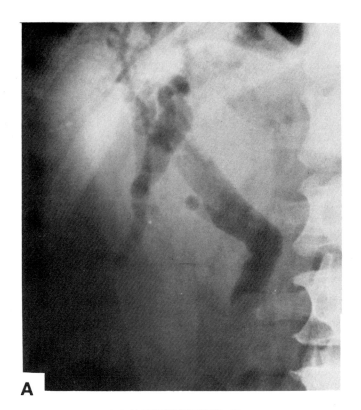

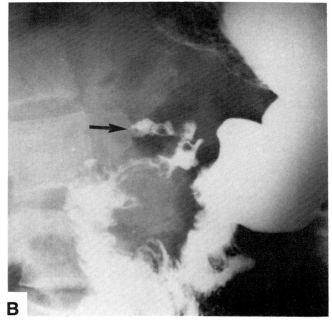

FIG. 14-32. Carcinoma of the gallbladder, standard roentgenography. A plain film of the abdomen (A) demonstrates air in the biliary system. A follow-up barium upper gastrointestinal study (B) demonstrates irregularity of the first and second portion of the duodenum with a small tract of extraluminal barium (arrow). Gas within the biliary system is again noted. Carcinoma of the gallbladder had invaded and eroded into the duodenum, creating a cholecystoduodenal fistula.

The dilated bile ducts can usually be followed down to the region of the obstruction. It may not always be possible to identify the cause of the obstruction on a sonogram because of obscuring gas in the duodenum or gastric antrum. In these cases, computed tomography may be helpful in further delineating the nature of the obstruction.

Longitudinal sonograms obtained through the right flank, with the patient in the decubitus position, may be extremely helpful in visualizing the head of the pancreas and the dilated bile duct near its terminus at the papilla of Vater. The right lobe of the liver acts as a sonic window and usually permits good visualization of the retroperitoneal area in the right upper quadrant. While it may not always be possible to identify normal ductal structures, dilated ducts may be commonly identified using this technique.

The normal extrahepatic bile ducts are less than 5 to 7 mm in internal diameter. On occasion, a nonobstructed duct may be larger. Biliary dilatation in these individuals may be secondary to prior stone disease, common duct surgery, or simply a normal large duct. Conversely, an obstructed or partially obstructed duct may be within the normal range. This is particularly true in cases of sclerosing cholangitis or acutely obstructed ducts.

Experimental study has demonstrated that following acute obstruction, bile ducts expand centrifugally from the obstructing point, with dilatation of the intrahepatic ducts occurring several days after the onset of obstruction.[179] After surgical release of the obstruction, the bile ducts contract centripetally, with the common duct requiring 30 to 50 days to return to normal size. These experimental data help explain why acutely obstructed ducts, especially the intrahepatic bile ducts, will initially appear to be of normal caliber and, conversely, after release of a duct obstruction such as passage of a small stone, the extrahepatic ducts may remain enlarged for several days.

Sonographically, carcinoma of the gallbladder has a variable appearance, from a relatively normal gallbladder with stones to a large invasive poorly defined mass.[21,39,174,216,219] The gallbladder when visualized is variable in size, and there may be internal focal or diffuse echoes. If the carcinoma is relatively localized and small, simply a polypoid soft tissue mass or focal gallbladder wall thickening will be identified (Figure 14-35). Gallstones are invariably present, and early carcinoma of the gallbladder is usually overlooked and a diagnosis of chronic cholecystitis is made. In more advanced cases, a large mass in the region of the gallbladder bed will be noted (Figure 14-36). If the soft tissue mass is seen in conjunction with some strong focal echoes with distal sonic shadowing, suggesting gallstones, a presumptive diagnosis of carcinoma of the gallbladder may be made. However, when widespread tumor distorts the anatomy of the right upper quadrant, a definitive diagnosis and organ of origin of the tumor mass may be difficult.

Occasionally, inflammatory disease and disease metastatic to the gallbladder may mimic a primary gallbladder cancer. Simple chronic cholecystitis usually thickens the gallbladder wall in a generalized fashion, but occasionally this may be focal and simulate a carcinoma. An unusual chronic inflammatory process, xanthogranulomatous cholecystitis, may mimic carcinoma of the gallbladder. This disease produces gallstones and a lobulated mass that fills the gallbladder. The diagnosis can usually not be made preoperatively. Rarely, metastatic disease to the gallbladder may mimic carcinoma of the gallbladder. This most commonly occurs with metastatic malignant melanoma or diffuse organ involvement by leukemia. Metastatic disease from other sites such as carcinoma of the lung or breast may cause a similar appearance.

Sonographic evaluation of cholangiocarcinoma is usually nonspecific and simply demonstrates dilatation of the biliary ductal system proximal to the obstructing tumor (Figure 14-37). Usually there is no associated soft tissue mass at the site of obstruction, and the correct diagnosis is only suggested. The differential diagnosis is usually between inflammatory disease with stones or stricture and cholangiocarcinoma. Rarely, hepatic metastases or metastases to regional lymph nodes may be detected, and this may suggest the correct diagnosis.

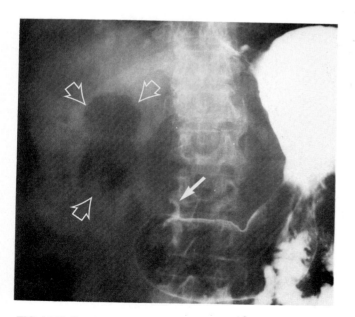

FIG. 14-33. Carcinoma of the gallbladder, hepatic invasion. An abdominal roentgenogram obtained during a barium upper gastrointestinal examination demonstrates narrowing of the first portion of the duodenum (arrow), and an irregular collection of gas later proved to be in the liver (open arrows). Carcinoma of the gallbladder had invaded the liver and duodenum, creating a necrotic liver metastasis and fistula with the duodenum.

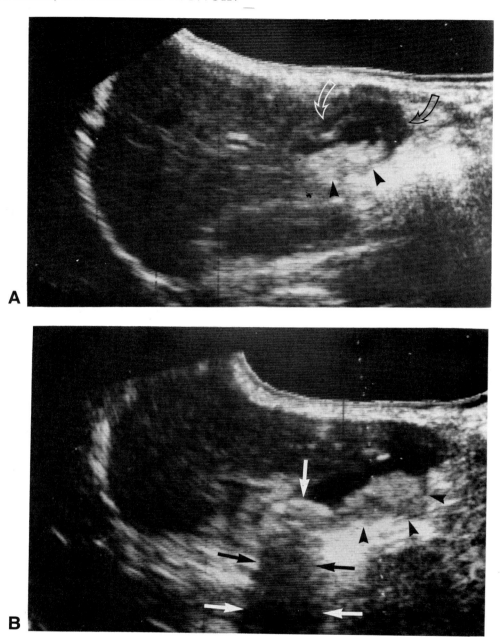

FIG. 14-34. Focal carcinoma of the gallbladder. Sagittal sonograms through the liver and right upper quadrant (A,B) demonstrate thickening of the gallbladder wall (curved arrows) and a polypoid mass (arrowheads). A strong focal echo and distal sonic shadowing (arrows) represent gallstones (B).

Computed Tomography. Computed tomograms of patients with carcinoma of the gallbladder demonstrate a variety of abnormalities.[197] Focal or diffuse thickening of the gallbladder wall may be identified (Figure 14-38). More commonly at the time of initial examination, the disease is widespread, and a bulky tumor mass can be identified in the region of the gallbladder bed with local extension into the liver or along the hepatoduodenal ligament to the region of the head of the pancreas and ret-roperitoneum. In patients with extensive disease, the computed tomographic findings are nonspecific, and metastatic disease from distant sites, carcinoma of the pancreas, or lymphoma cannot be excluded.

Computed tomograms in patients with cholangiocarcinoma will demonstrate dilatation of the biliary ducts proximal to the tumor. Dilated intrahepatic bile ducts are confidently identified on contrast-enhanced computed tomograms as focal areas of low attenuation adjacent to portal vein radicles.[178] The common hepatic and common bile ducts are identified in their characteristic locations in the hepatic duodenal ligament and deep to the head of the pancreas, respectively. In most patients, a focal mass will not be identified. This is either because of the small size of the tumor or because of the lesions being isoattenuating with the surrounding tissues. Occasionally, intravenous administration of large amounts of contrast will cause tumor enhancement (Figure 14-39). Metastases to the liver or regional lymph nodes may be demonstrated in advanced disease (Figure 14-40). Percu-

taneous needle aspiration biopsy directed by computed tomography to the point of biliary ductal narrowing frequently provides the correct diagnosis.

Percutaneous Transhepatic Cholangiography and Endoscopic Retrograde Cholangiopancreatography. For definition of the biliary ductal system and complete delineation of tumor involvement, antegrade or retrograde cholangiograms are frequently performed (Figure 14-41). This procedure allows mapping and definition of the site of obstruction, and at the time of the procedure, biliary

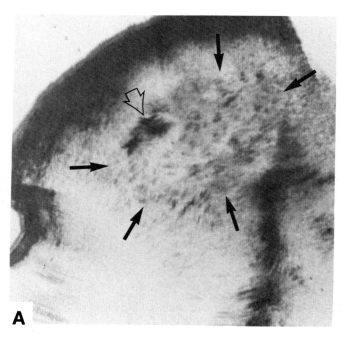
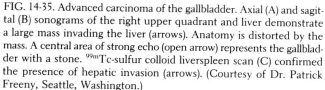
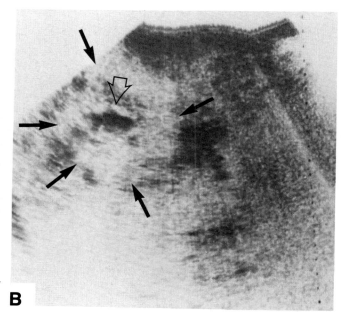
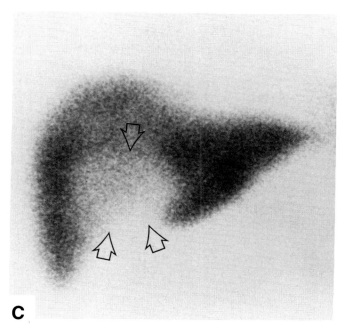

FIG. 14-35. Advanced carcinoma of the gallbladder. Axial (A) and sagittal (B) sonograms of the right upper quadrant and liver demonstrate a large mass invading the liver (arrows). Anatomy is distorted by the mass. A central area of strong echo (open arrow) represents the gallbladder with a stone. ^{99m}Tc-sulfur colloid liverspleen scan (C) confirmed the presence of hepatic invasion (arrows). (Courtesy of Dr. Patrick Freeny, Seattle, Washington.)

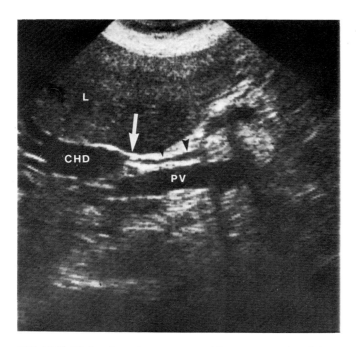

FIG. 14-36. Cholangiocarcinoma, sonographic appearance. A real-time oblique sonogram of the right upper quadrant demonstrates a dilated common hepatic duct (CHD) above a stricture (arrow) with a normal caliber common bile duct (arrowheads). There is no mass identifiable at the site of the malignant stricture. PV = portal vein, L = liver. (Courtesy of Dr. Peter Cooperberg, Vancouver, British Columbia, Canada.)

drainage catheters may be left in place. Cholangiography may also be used as a localization procedure for percutaneous needle aspiration biopsy.

Table-14-6 outlines the benefit/cost ratio of the above imaging modalities.

Imaging Strategies and Decisions

Carcinoma of the biliary tree is an insidious disease and usually produces clinical symptoms secondary to local or diffuse spread of disease, including pain, jaundice, or weight loss. Plain roentgenograms are usually of no help, and the best first examination to perform is a hepatic and biliary sonogram (Figure 14-42). This will identify dilated bile ducts in patients with jaundice, and perhaps pinpoint the site of obstruction. Hepatic metastases can frequently be identified by sonography, and spread to local lymph nodes in the para-aortic or celiac lymph node region occasionally can be identified. If sonography demonstrates the dilated bile ducts but not the location or cause of the obstruction, contrast-enhanced computed tomography will usually provide answers to these questions. Computed tomography is very accurate in identifying the site of the obstruction and in evaluating regional tissues for metastatic spread. If the patient does not appear to be a surgical candidate, percutaneous needle aspiration biopsy can then be performed to document the disease. If surgery is contemplated, transhepatic or retrograde cholangiograms are necessary and beneficial. This will pinpoint the site of the obstruction, and catheters can be left in place for either temporary or long-term biliary drainage.

Treatment Decisions

Despite new imaging modalities and new diagnostic techniques (percutaneous needle aspiration biopsy), the long-term outlook for patients with carcinoma of the biliary tree remains dismal. Because of the usual local metastases, strategic location (which prohibits extensive surgical resection), and resistance to chemotherapeutic agents, the prognosis for these patients is poor and long-term survival has not been increased.[2]

Patients with primary carcinoma of the gallbladder in whom the diagnosis has been made incidentally at the time of cholecystectomy have a good prognosis. Survival in these patients without any further treatment is excellent. However, in the majority of patients where the tumor is invasive at the time of surgery, the prognosis is poor. The five-year survival rate in these patients is approximately 2% to 3%. Even in patients who undergo radical surgical resection, frequently including hepatic lobectomy, the five-year survival rate is only approximately 6%. Chemotherapy and radiation therapy are palliative, but there is no evidence that this therapy increases long-term survival.[11,154]

A recent analysis of the role of radiation therapy[101] in the management of gallbladder and extrahepatic biliary duct cancer suggests that significant palliation can be obtained in the majority of patients treated. A few long-term survivors among patients receiving postoperative irradiation after surgical resection of localized disease have been reported, but advanced lesions usually produce dismal results.[196]

Impact of New Technology

To date, there has been only limited experience using MRI as a diagnostic modality in patients with biliary tract carcinoma. Extension of tumor into the liver may be identified with MRI, and perhaps this modality will more easily demonstrate direct extension of tumor, which is difficult to identify by both computed tomography and sonography.

(References continue on p. 337.)

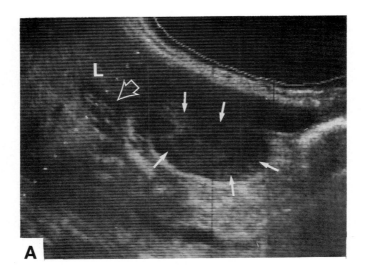

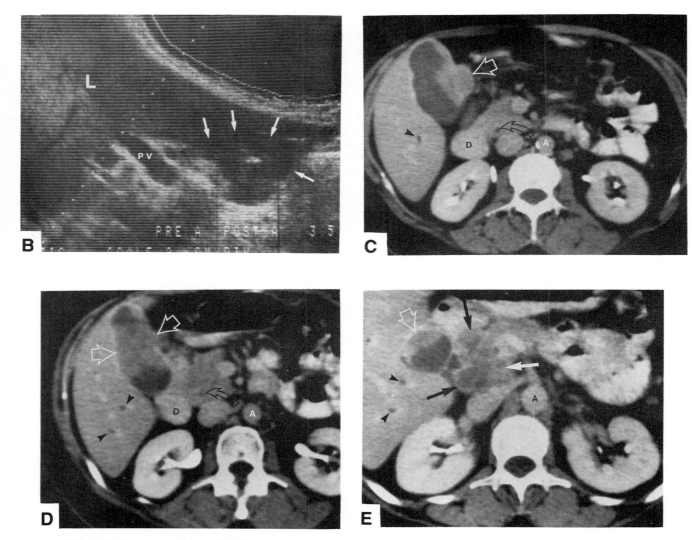

FIG. 14-37. Carcinoma of the gallbladder. Sagittal sonograms of the right upper quadrant (A,B) demonstrate an ill-defined mass partially filling and distorting the gallbladder (arrows). The common hepatic duct is slightly dilated (open arrow). Computed tomograms (C,D) demonstrate the mass partially filling the gallbladder and thickening its wall (arrows). The intrahepatic bile ducts are dilated (arrowheads), although the distal common bile duct is normal (curved arrow). The cause of the biliary obstruction was tumor extension along the hepatoduodenal ligament (E) with involvement of the pancreatic head (arrows). L = liver, PV = portal vein, D = duodenum, A = aorta.

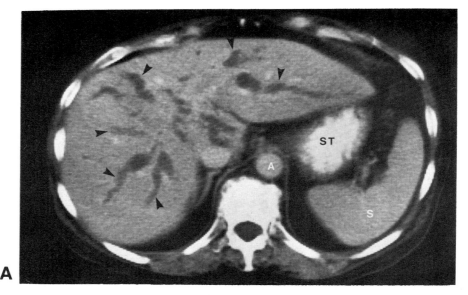

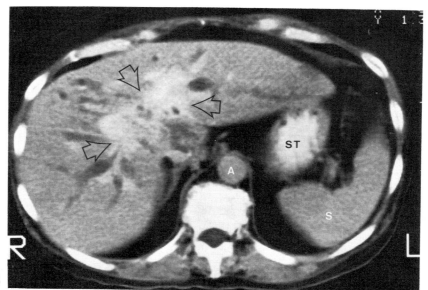

FIG. 14-38. Cholangiocarcinoma after contrast enhancement. An initial computed tomogram after a small amount of iodinated contrast (A) demonstrates dilated bile ducts (arrowheads) but no mass. A repeat computed tomogram after a large amount of contrast (B) now demonstrates an enhancing mass (arrows). A subsequent transhepatic cholangiogram (C) demonstrates an obstructing lesion at the level of the pora hepatis with involvement of the common hepatic duct (arrows). St = stomach, A = aorta, S = spleen.

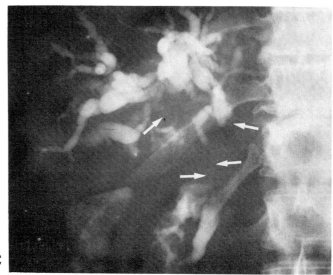

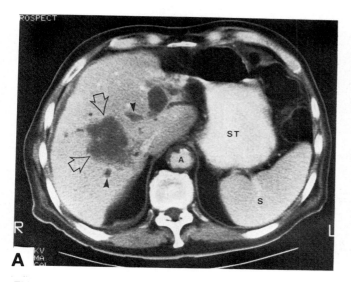

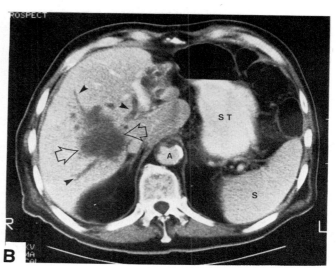

FIG. 14-39. Cholangiocarcinoma; advanced disease with local extension to liver. Computed tomograms (A,B) at the level of the liver demonstrate an irregular area of low attenuation (arrows) secondary to liver metastases. Focal dilation of the intrahepatic bile ducts is present (arrowheads). S = spleen, St = stomach, A = aorta.

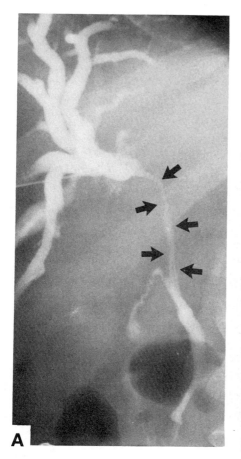

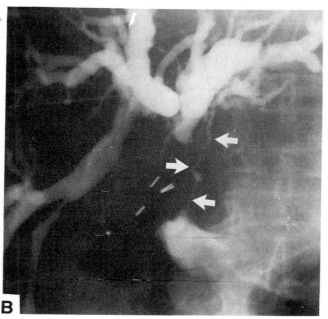

FIG. 14-40. Cholangiocarcinoma; cholangiographic abnormalities. Percutaneous transhepatic cholangiograms of two patients (A,B) with cholangiocarcinoma demonstrate narrowing and irregularity of the common hepatic duct secondary to tumor encasement (arrows). The proximal ducts are dilated.

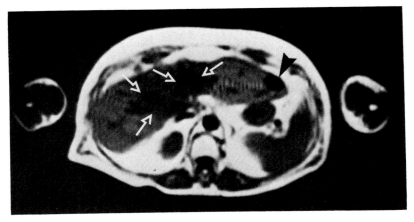

FIG. 14-41. Cholangiocarcinoma. An MR image of a patient with a cholangiocarcinoma demonstrates a slight but real signal difference between the infiltrating tumor and the adjacent liver (arrows). Incidentally noted is a cyst in the lateral segment of the left lobe of the liver (arrowhead). The MR image was obtained with a 0.5 Tesla field strength and a partial saturation pulse sequence with a repetition time of 150 msec.

Table 14-6. Imaging Modalities for Evaluating Cholangiocarcinoma and Carcinoma of the Gallbladder

MODALITY	STAGING CAPABILITY	BENEFIT/ COST RATIO	RECOMMENDED ROUTINE STAGING PROCEDURE
Noninvasive			
Chest roentgenograms	Good for detecting pulmonary parenchymal metastases that are uncommon and late.	Moderate	Yes
Bone roentgenograms	Useful to confirm the very rare osseous metastasis.	Low	No
Barium contrast—upper gastrointestinal roentgenograms	May be used to define mass affect on the stomach or duodenum secondary to metastatic disease.	Moderate	No (Selected cases only)
Oral cholecystogram	Not useful because biliary system usually does not opacify	Low	No
Radionuclide liver/spleen and hepatobiliary scans	May be useful in evaluating for hepatic metastases. Biliary radionuclide scanning may demonstrate level of obstruction.	High	No (Selected cases only)
Hepatobiliary sonography	Excellent for evaluating metastatic disease of the liver and for evaluating the biliary tract. Even when the primary tumor is not seen, dilated bile ducts may be visualized.	High	Yes
MRI	May be useful in staging and evaluating primary spread of tumor as well as distant metastases.	?	?
Minimally Invasive			
Computed tomography	Minimally invasive with intravenous contrast, which is strongly recommended for optimal scanning technique. Most useful of all imaging modalities for determining local invasion, extent of tumor, defining site of biliary ductal obstruction and evaluating for distant metastases.	High	Yes
Invasive			
Lymphangiograms	May be used to evaluate for retroperitoneal lymphadenopathy but almost always does not adequately visualize the high abdominal lymph nodes, which are most commonly involved in this disease.	Low	No
ERCP/PTC	Extremely accurate in localizing the site of obstruction, and evaluating the type of obstruction.	High	Yes
Percutaneous biopsy guided by imaging technique	Accurate in confirming malignant nature of identified mass. Usually peripheral mass in the liver is biopsied. Biopsy of the gallbladder should not be performed percutaneously. Cholangiocarcinoma may demonstrate no mass.	High	No (Selected cases only)
Selective hepatic angiography	Accurate to define hepatic metastases, and may be helpful in selected cases.	Moderate	No (Selected cases only)

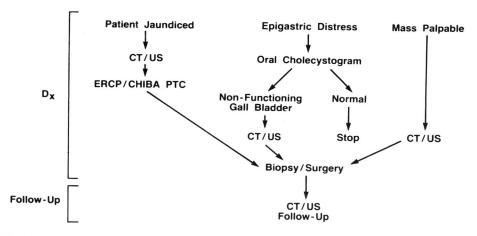

FIG. 14-42. Decision tree for the bile duct/gallbladder cancer. Patients with bile duct/gallbladder cancers either have mass lesions, jaundice, or nonspecific, vague upper GI complaints. In the nonjaundiced patient, oral cholecystography or ultrasound is employed to evaluate the gallbladder, and if these studies are normal, the diagnosis is virtually excluded. In the patient with a nonfunctioning gallbladder, the efforts should be directed at localization of a mass or the site of biliary obstruction in order to direct subsequent biopsy and surgery.

REFERENCES

1. Abrams, H. L., Spiro, R., Goldstein, N.: Metastases in carcinoma. Analysis of 1000 autopsied cases. *Cancer* 3:74–85, 1950.

2. Adams, J. T., Poulter, C. A., Pandya, K. J.: Cancer of the major digestive glands: Pancreas, liver, bile ducts, gallbladder. In *Clinical Oncology for Medical Students and Physicians: A Multidisciplinary Approach*, 6th ed. Rubin, P. (Ed.). New York, American Cancer Society, 1983, pp. 178–189.

3. Akwari, D. E., Kelly, K. A.: Surgical treatment of adenocarcinoma. Location: Junction of the right, left, and common hepatic biliary ducts. *Arch. Surg.* 114:22–25, 1979.

4. Al-Abdulla, A. S. M., Hussey, D. H., Olsen, M. H., Wright, A. E.: Experience with fast neutron therapy for unresectable carcinoma of the pancreas. *Int. J. Radiat. Oncol. Biol. Phys.* 7:165–172, 1981.

5. Alderson, P. O., Adams, D. F., McNeil, B. J., Sanders, R., Siegelman, S. S., Finberg, H. J., Hessel, S. J., Abrams, H. L.: Computed tomography, ultrasound and scintigraphy of the liver in patients with colon or breast carcinoma: A prospective comparison. *Radiology* 149:225–230, 1983.

6. Allibone, G. W., Fagan, C. J., Porter, S. C.: Sonographic features of carcinoma of the gallbladder. *Gastrointest. Radiol.* 6:169–173, 1981.

7. Altemeier, W. A., Gall, E. A., Zinninger, M. M., Hoxworth, P. E.: Sclerosing carcinoma of the major intrahepatic bile ducts. *Arch. Surg.* 75:450, 1957.

8. American Joint Committee on Cancer: *Manual for Staging Cancer*, 2nd ed. Beahrs, O. H., Myers, M. H. (Eds). Philadelphia, J. B. Lippincott, 1983, pp. 95–98.

9. Andersson, A., Bergdahl, L., van der Linden, W.: Malignant tumors of the extrahepatic bile ducts. *Surgery* 81:198–202, 1977.

10. Arger, P. H., Mulhern, C. B., Bonavita, J. A., Stauffer, D. M., Hale, J.: An analysis of pancreatic sonography in pancreatic disease. *J. Clin. Ultrasound.* 7:91–97, 1979.

11. Arnaud, J. P., Graf, P., Gramfort, J. L., Adloff, M.: Primary carcinoma of the gallbladder: Review of 25 cases. *Am. J. Surg.* 138:403–406, 1979.

12. Baltaxe, H. A., Leslie, E. V.: Vanishing pancreatic calcifications. *A.J.R.* 99:642–644, 1967.

13. Banwo, O., Versey, J., Hobbs, J. E.: New oncofetal antigen for human pancreas. *Lancet* 1:643–645, 1974.

14. Bell, E. T.: Carcinoma of the pancreas. I. A clinical and pathologic study of 609 necropsied cases. II. The relation of carcinoma of the pancreas to diabetes mellitus. *Am. J. Pathol.* 33:499–523, 1957.

15. Berg, J. W., Connelly, R. R.: Updating the epidemiologic data on pancreatic cancer. *Semin. Oncol.* 6:275–284, 1979.

16. Berk, J. E.: Diagnosis of carcinoma of the pancreas. *Arch. Intern. Med.* 68:525–559, 1941.

17. Berland, L. L., Lawson, T. L., Foley, W. D., Geenan, J. E., Stewart, E. T.: Computed tomography of the normal and abnormal pancreatic duct: Correlation with pancreatic ductography. *Radiology* 141:715–724, 1981.

18. Berland, L. L., Lawson, T. L., Foley, W. D., Melrose, B. L., Chintapalli, K. N., Taylor, A. J.: Comparison of pre- and postcontrast CT in hepatic masses. *A.J.R.* 138:853–858, 1982.

19. Bernardino, M. E., Green, B.: Ultrasonographic evaluation of chemotherapeutic response in hepatic metastases. *Radiology* 133:437–441, 1979.

20. Bernardino, M. E., Thomas, J. L., Maklad, N.: Hepatic sonography: Technical considerations, present applications, and possible future. *Radiology* 142:249–251, 1982.

21. Bluth, E., Katz, M., Merrit, C., Sullivan, M., Mitchell, W. T., Jr. Echographic findings in xanthogranulomatous cholecystitis. *J. Clin. Ultrasound* 7:213–214, 1979.

22. Bookstein, J. J., Reuter, S. R., Martel, W.: Angiographic evaluation of pancreatic carcinoma. *Radiology* 93:757–764, 1969.

23. Braganza, J. M., Howat, H. T.: Cancer of the pancreas. *Clin. Gastroenterol.* 1:219–237, 1972.

24. Brandt-Rauf, P. W., Pincus, M., Adelson, S.: Cancer of the gallbladder: A review of forty-three cases. *Hum. Pathol.* 13:48–53, 1982.

25. Brunschwig, A.: *The Surgery of Pancreatic Tumors*. St. Louis, C. V. Mosby Co., 1942.

26. Buonocore, E.: Transhepatic percutaneous cholangiography. *Radiol. Clin. North Am.* 14:527–542, 1976.

27. Burgener, F. A., Hamlin, D. J.: Contrast enhancement in abdominal CT: Bolus vs. infusion. *A.J.R.* 137:351–358, 1981.

28. Callen, P. W., Breiman, R. S., Korobkin, M., De Martini, W. J.,

Mani, J. R.: Carcinoma of the tail of the pancreas: An unusual CT appearance. *A.J.R.* **133**:135–137, 1979.

29. Carlsen, E. N., Filly, R. A.: Newer ultrasonographic anatomy in the upper abdomen: I. The portal and hepatic venous anatomy. *J. Clin. Ultrasound* **4**:85–90, 1976.

30. Chait, H., Faegenburg, D. H.: Illusory neoplasms of the stomach and duodenum as a manifestation of carcinoma of the pancreas. *Radiology* **74**:771–777, 1960.

31. Chitwood, W. R., Jr., Meyers, W. C., Heaston, D. K., Herskovic, A. M., McLeod, M. E., Jones, R. S.: Diagnosis and treatment of primary extrahepatic bile duct tumors. *Am. J. Surg.* **143**:99–106, 1982.

32. Cohen, G. F.: Early diagnosis of pancreatic neoplasm in diabetics. *Lancet* **2**:267–269, 1965.

33. Cohn, I., Jr. (Ed.): *Pancreatic Cancer: New Directions in Therapeutic Management.* New York, Masson, 1980.

34. Compagno, J., Ortel, J. E.: Microcystic adenoma of the pancreas (glycogen rich cystadenoma). A clinical pathological study of 34 cases. *Am. J. Clin. Pathol.* **69**:289–298, 1978.

35. Compagno, J., Ortel, J. E.: Mucinous cystic neoplasms of the pancreas with overt and latent malignancy (cystadenocarcinoma and cystadenoma). A clinical pathological study of 41 cases. *Am. J. Clin. Pathol.* **69**:573–580, 1978.

36. Conrad, M. R., Landay, M. J., Jones, J. O.: Sonographic "parallel channel" sign of biliary tree enlargement in mild to moderate obstructive jaundice. *A.J.R.* **130**:279–286, 1978.

37. Cotton, P. B., Lees, W. R., Vallon, A. G., Cottone, M., Croker, J. R., Chapman, M.: Gray-scale ultrasonography and endoscopic pancreatography in pancreatic diagnosis. *Radiology* **134**:453–459, 1980.

38. Courvoisier, L. G.: *Kasvistisch-Statistische, Beitrage zur Pathologie und Chirurgie der Gallenwege.* Leipzig, F. C. W. Vogel, 1890.

39. Crade, M., Taylor, K. J., Rosenfield, A. T., Ulreich, S., Simeone, J., Sommer, F. G., Viscomi, G. N.: The varied ultrasonic character of gallbladder tumor. *J.A.M.A.* **241**:2195–2196, 1979.

40. Cubilla, A. L., Fitzgerald, P. J.: Morphological patterns of primary nonendocrine human pancreas carcinoma. *Cancer Res.* **35**:2234–2248, 1975.

41. Cubilla, A., Fitzgerald, P. J.: Pancreas cancer. 1. Duct adenocarcinoma: A clinical-pathologic study of 380 patients. *Pathol. Ann.* (Part I) 241–287, 1978.

42. Cubilla, A. L., Fitzgerald, P. J.: Classification of pancreatic cancer (nonendocrine). *Mayo Clin. Proc.* **54**:449–458, 1979.

43. Cubilla, A. L., Fortner, J., Fitzgerald, P. J.: Lymph node involvement in carcinoma of the head of the pancreas area. *Cancer* **41**:880–887, 1978.

44. DiMagno, E. P., Malagelada, J.-R., Go, V. L. W.: The relationships between pancreatic ductal obstruction and pancreatic secretion in man. *Mayo Clin. Proc.* **54**:157–162, 1979.

45. DiMagno, E. P., Malagelada, J.-R., Moertel, C. G., Go, V. L. W.: Prospective evaluation of the pancreatic secretion of immunoreactive carcinoembryonic antigen, enzyme, and bicarbonate inpatients suspected of having pancreatic cancer. *Gastroenterology* **73**:457–461, 1977.

46. DiMagno, E. P., Malagelada, J.-R., Taylor, W. F., Go, V. L. W.: A prospective comparison of current diagnostic tests for pancreatic cancer. *N. Engl. J. Med.* **297**:737–742, 1977.

47. Dobelbower, R. R., Jr.: Current radiotherapeutic approaches to pancreatic cancer. *Cancer* **47**:1729–1733, 1981.

48. Dobelbower, R. R., Jr., Borgelt, B. B., Strubler, K. A., Kutcher, G. J., Suntharalingam, N.: Precision radiotherapy for cancer of the pancreas: Techniques and results. *Int. J. Radiat. Oncol. Biol. Phys.* **6**:1127–1133, 1980.

49. Donowitz, M., Kerstein, M. D., Spiro, H. M.: Pancreatic ascites. *Medicine* **53**:183–195, 1974.

50. Dreiling, D. A.: The early diagnosis of pancreatic cancer. *Scand. J. Gastroenterol.* **5** (Suppl 6):115–122, 1970.

51. Eaton, S. B., Jr., Ferrucci, J. T., Jr.: *Radiology of the Pancreas and Duodenum.* Philadelphia, W. B. Saunders, 1973.

52. Edmondson, H. A.: Tumors of the liver and intrahepatic bile ducts. Section VII, Fascile 25, Armed Forces Institute of Pathology, Washington, D.C., 1958.

53. Eisenberg, H.: Pancreatic angiography. In *Small Vessel Angiography: Imaging, Morphology, Physiology and Clinical Applications.* Hilal, S. K. (Ed.). St. Louis, C. V. Mosby Co., 1973, pp. 405–433.

54. Evander, A., Fredlund, P., Hoevels, J., Ihse, I., Bengmark, S.: Evaluation of aggressive surgery for carcinoma of the extrahepatic bile ducts. *Ann. Surg.* **191**:23–29, 1980.

55. Eyler, W. R., Clark, M. D., Rian, R. L.: An evaluation of roentgen signs of pancreatic enlargement. *J.A.M.A.* **181**:967–971, 1962.

56. Fawcitt, R. A., Forbes, W. S., Isherwood, I., Braganza, J. M., Howat, H.: Computed tomography in pancreatic disease. *Br. J. Radiol.* **51**:1–4, 1978.

57. Wittenberg, J., Simeone, J. F., Ferrucci, J. T., Jr., Mueller, P. R., van Sonnenberg, E., Neff, C. C.: Nonfocal enlargement in pancreatic carcinoma. *Radiology* **144**:131–135, 1982.

58. Fishman, A., Isikoff, M. B., Barkin, J. S., Friedland, J. T.: Significance of a dilated pancreatic duct on CT examination. *A.J.R.* **133**:225–227, 1979.

59. Fleming, M. P., Carlson, H. C., Adson, M. A.: Percutaneous transhepatic cholangiography: The differential diagnosis of bile duct pathology. *A.J.R.* **116**:327–336, 1972.

60. Freeny, P. C., Ball, T. J.: Rapid diagnosis of pancreatic carcinoma. An algorithmic approach. *Radiology* **130**:682–691, 1978.

61. Freeny, P. C., Bilbao, M. K., Katon, R. M.: "Blind" evaluation of endoscopic retrograde cholangiopancreatography (ERCP) in the diagnosis of pancreatic carcinoma: The "double duct" and other signs. *Radiology* **119**:271–274, 1976.

62. Freeny, P. C., Vimont, T. R., Barnett, D. C.: Cavernous hemangioma of the liver: Ultrasonography, arteriography, and computed tomography. *Radiology* **132**:143–148, 1979.

63. Frick, M. P., O'Leary, J. F., Walker, H. C., Goodale, R. L.: Accuracy of endoscopic retrograde cholangiopancreatography (ERCP) in differentiating benign and malignant pancreatic disease. *Gastrointest. Radiol.* **7**:241–277, 1982.

64. Friedman, A. C., Lichtenstein, J. E., Dachman, A. H.: Cystic neoplasms of the pancreas: Radiological-pathological correlation. *Radiology* **149**:45, 1983.

65. Friedman, M. A.: Primary hepatocellular cancer — present results and future prospects. *Int. J. Radiat. Oncol. Biol. Phys.* **9**:1841–1848, 1983.

66. Fukumoto, K., Nakajima, M., Murakami, K., Kawai, K.: Diagnosis of pancreatic cancer by endoscopic pancreatocholangiography. *Am. J. Gastroenterol.* **62**:210–213, 1974.

67. Gambill, E.: Pancreatic and ampullary carcinoma: Diagnosis and prognosis in relationship to symptoms, physical findings and elapse of time in 252 patients. *South. Med. J.* **63**:1119–1122, 1970.

68. Gambill, E.: Pancreatitis associated with pancreatic carcinoma: A study of 26 cases. *Mayo Clin. Proc.* **46**:174–177, 1971.

69. Garabedian, M., Shanszad, M.: Pancreatography in the diagnosis of carcinoma of the pancreas. *Med. Clin. North Am.* **59**:239–246, 1975.

70. Goldson, A. L., Ashaveri, E., Espinoza, M. C., Roux, V., Cornwell, E., Rayford, L., McLaren, M., Nibhanupudy, R., Mahan, A., Taylor, H. F., Hemphill, N., Pearson, O.: Single high-dose intraoperative electrons for advanced stage pancreatic cancer: Phase I pilot study. *Int. J. Radiat. Oncol. Biol. Phys.* **7**:869–874, 1981.

71. Goldstein, H. M., Neiman, H. L., Bookstein, J. J.: Angiographic evaluation of pancreatic disease. A further appraisal. *Radiology* **112**:275–282, 1974.

72. Graver, F. W.: Pancreatic carcinoma: A review of 34 autopsies. *Arch. Intern. Med.* **63**:884–898, 1939.
73. Green, B., Bree, R. L., Goldstein, H. M., Stanley, C.: Grey scale ultrasound evaluation of hepatic neoplasms: Patterns and correlations. *Radiology* **124**:203–208, 1977
74. Guerrier, K., Persky, L.: Pancreatic disease simulating renal abnormality. *Am. J. Surg.* **120**:46–49, 1970.
75. Gupta, S., Udupa, K. N., Gupta, S.: Primary carcinoma of the gallbladder: A review of 328 cases. *J. Surg. Oncol.* **14**:35–44, 1980.
76. Hamrick, R. E. Jr., Liner, F. J., Hastings, P. R., Cohn, I. Jr.: Primary carcinoma of the gallbladder. *Ann. Surg.* **195**:270–273, 1982.
77. Harbin, W. P., Robert, N. J., Ferrucci, J. T.: Diagnosis of cirrhosis based on regional changes in hepatic morphology. *Radiology* **135**:273–283, 1983.
78. Harell, G. S., Anderson, M. F., Berry, P. F.: Cytologic bile examination in the diagnosis of biliary duct neoplastic strictures. *A.J.R.* **137**:1123–1126, 1981.
79. Haslam, J. B., Cavanaugh, P. J., Stroup, S. L.: Radiation therapy in the treatment of irresectable adenocarcinoma of the pancreas. *Cancer* **32**:1341–1345, 1973.
80. Haubrich, W. S., Berk, J. E.: Tumors of the pancreas. I. Medical aspects of exocrine tumors. In *Gastroenterology*, Vol. III. Bockus, H. L. (Ed.). Philadelphia, W. B. Saunders, 1976, pp. 1102–1121.
81. Hauser, H., Battikha, J. G., Wettstein, P.: Computed tomography of the dilated main pancreatic duct. *J Comput. Assist. Tomog.* **4**:53–58, 1980.
82. Herlinger, H., Finlay, D. B. L.: Evaluation and follow-up on pancreatic arteriograms. A new role for angiography in the diagnosis of carcinoma of the pancreas. *Clin. Radiol.* **29**:277–284, 1978.
83. Hermann, R. E., Cooperman, A. M.: Current concepts in cancer. Cancer of the pancreas. *N. Engl. J. Med.* **301**:482–485, 1979.
84. Hessel, S. J., Siegelman, S. S., McNeil, B. J., Sanders, R. C., Adams, D. F., Alderson, P. O., Finberg, H. J., Abrams, H. L.: Prospective evaluation of computed tomography and ultrasound of the pancreas. *Radiology* **143**:129, 1982.
85. Hoevels, J., Lunderquist, A., Ihse, I.: Percutaneous transhepatic intubation of bile ducts for combined internal-external drainage in preoperative and palliative treatment of obstructive jaundice. *Gastrointest. Radiol.* **3**:23–31, 1978.
86. Holyoke, E. D., Douglass, H. O., Jr., Goldrosen, M. H., Chu, T. M.: Tumor markers in pancreatic cancer. *Semin. Oncol.* **6**:347–356, 1979.
87. Isherwood, I., Fawcitt, R. A.: Computed tomography of the pancreas. In *The Exocrine Pancreas*. Howat, H. T., Sarles, H. (Eds.). Philadelphia, W. B. Saunders, 1979, pp. 227–242.
88. Isley, J. K., Schauble, J. F.: Interpretation of the percutaneous cholangiogram. *A.J.R.* **88**:772–777, 1962.
89. Itai, Y., Araki, T., Furui, S., Tasaka, A.: Differential diagnosis of hepatic masses on computed tomography, with particular reference to hepatocellular carcinoma. *J. Comput. Assist. Tomogr.* **5**:834–842, 1981.
90. Itai, Y., Furui, S., Araki, T., Yashiro, N., Tasaka, A.: Computed tomography of cavernous hemangioma of the liver. *Radiology* **137**:149–155, 1980.
91. Itai, Y., Moss, A. A., Ohtomo, K.: Computed tomography of cyst adenoma and cyst adenocarcinoma of the pancreas. *Radiology* **145**:419, 1982.
92. Joffe, N., Antonioli, D. A.: Osteoblastic bone metastases secondary to adenocarcinoma of the pancreas. *Clin. Radiol.* **29**:41–46, 1978.
93. Johnson, M. L., Mack, L. A.: Ultrasonic evaluation of the pancreas. *Gastrointest. Radiol.* **3**:257–266, 1978.
94. Johnston, F., Myers, R. T.: Etiologic factors and consequences of splenic vein obstruction. *Ann. Surg.* **177**:736–739, 1973.
95. Karasawa, E., Goldberg, H. I., Moss, A. A., Federle, M. P., Lon-

don, S. S.: CT pancreatogram in carcinoma of the pancreas and chronic pancreatitis. *Radiology* **148**:489, 1983.
96. Keller, F. S., Niles, N. R., Rosch, J.: Retrograde pancreatic venography: Autopsy study. *Radiology* **135**:285–293, 1980.
97. Kessler, I. I.: Cancer mortality among diabetics. *J. Natl. Cancer Inst.* **44**:673–686, 1970.
98. Kittredge, R. D., Baer, J. W.: Percutaneous transhepatic cholangiography. Problems in interpretation. *A.J.R.* **125**:35–46, 1975.
99. Klatzkin, G.: Adenocarcinoma of the hepatic duct at its bifurcation within the porta hepatis. *Am. J. Med.* **38**:241, 1965.
100. Knopf, D. R., Torres, W. E., Fajman, W. J., Sones, P. J., Jr.: Liver lesions: Comparative accuracy of scintigraphy and computed tomography. *A.J.R.* **138**:623–627, 1962.
101. Kopelson, G., Harisiadas, L., Tretter, P., et al.: The role of radiation therapy in cancer of the extrahepatic biliary system. *Int. J. Radiat. Oncol. Biol. Phys.* **2**:883–894, 1977.
102. Kozuka, S., Sassa, R., Taki, T., Masamota, K., Nagasawa, S., Saga, S., Hasegawa, K., Takeuchi, M.: Relation of pancreatic duct hyperplasia to carcinoma. *Cancer* **43**:1418–1428, 1979.
103. Krain, L. S.: The rising incidence of carcinoma of the pancreas—real or apparent. *J. Surg. Oncol.* **2**:115–124, 1970.
104. Krain, L. S.: The rising incidence of cancer of the pancreas—further epidemiologic studies. *J. Chron. Dis.* **23**:685–690, 1971.
105. Kruse, A., Thommesen, P., Frederiksen, P.: Endoscopic retrograde cholangiopancreatography in pancreatic cancer and chronic pancreatitis. *Scand. J. Gastroenterol.* **13**:513–517, 1978.
106. Lafler, C. J., Hinerman, D. L.: A morphologic study of pancreatic carcinoma with reference to multiple thrombi. *Cancer* **14**:944–949, 1961.
107. Laing, F. C., London, L. A., Filly, R. A.: Ultrasonographic identification of dilated intrahepatic bile ducts and their differentiation from portal venous structures. *J. Clin. Ultrasound* **6**:90–94, 1978.
108. La Monte, C. S., DeCosse, J. J., McPeak, C. J.: Carcinoma of the pancreas presenting with gastrointestinal bleeding. *J.A.M.A.* **180**:974–976, 1962.
109. Lang, E. K.: Percutaneous transhepatic cholangiography. *Radiology* **112**:283–290, 1978.
110. Larsson, L. I.: Endocrine pancreatic tumors. *Hum. Pathol.* **9**:401–416, 1978.
111. Laufer, I.: *Double Contrast Gastrointestinal Radiology with Endoscopic Correlation*. Philadelphia, W. B. Saunders, 1979.
112. Lawson, T. L., Berland, L. L., Foley, W. D., Stewart, E. T., Geenan, J. E., Hogan, W. J.: Ultrasonic visualization of the pancreatic duct. *Radiology* **144**:865–871, 1982.
113. Lee, J. K. T., Stanley, R. J., Melson, G. L., Sagel, S. S.: Pancreatic imaging by ultrasound and computed tomography. A general review. *Radiol. Clin. North Am.* **16**:105–117, 1979.
114. Lee, T. G., Henderson, S. C., Ehrlich, R.: Ultrasound diagnosis of common bile duct dilatation. *Radiology* **124**:793–797, 1977.
115. Lees, C. D., Zapolanski, A., Cooperman, A. M., Hermann, R. E.: Carcinoma of the bile ducts. *Surg. Gynecol. Obstet.* **151**:193–198, 1980.
116. Levin, M. E.: Endocrine syndromes associated with pancreatic islet cell tumors. *Med. Clin. North Am.* **52**:295–3412, 1968.
117. Lieberman, J. S., Borrero, J., Urdaneta, E., Wright, I. S.: Thrombophlebitis and cancer. *J.A.M.A.* **177**:542–545, 1961.
118. Lin, R. S., Kessler, I. I.: A multifactorial model for pancreatic cancer in man. Epidemiologic evidence. *J.A.M.A.* **245**:147–152, 1981.
119. MacCarty, R. L., Stephens, D. A., Hattery, R. R., Sheedy, P. F.: II. Hepatic imaging by computed tomography: A comparison with 99mTc-sulfur colloid, ultrasonography, and angiography. *Radiol. Clin. North Am.* **17**:137–155, 1979.
120. Macchia, B., Bobruff, J., Groissier, V. W.: Positional relief of pain;

important clue to clinical diagnosis of carcinoma of the pancreas. *J.A.M.A.* **182**:6–8, 1962.

121. Macdonald, J. S., Gunderson, L. L., Adson, M. A.: Cancer of the hepatobiliary system. In *Cancer: Principles and Practice of Oncology.* DeVita, V. T., Jr., Hellman, S., Rosenberg, S. A. (Eds.). Philadelphia, J. B. Lippincott, 1982, pp. 590–615.

122. Mackie, C. R., Noble, H. G., Cooper, M. J., Collins, P., Block, G. E., Moossa, A. R.: Prospective evaluation of angiography in the diagnosis and management of patients suspected of having pancreatic cancer. *Ann. Surg.* **189**:11–17, 1979.

123. Malini, S., Sabel, J.: Ultrasonography in obstructive jaundice. *Radiology* **123**:429–433, 1977.

124. Mantravadi, R. V. P., Spigos, D. G., Tan, W. S., Felix, E. L.: Intraarterial yttruim 90 in the treatment of hepatic malignancy. *Radiology* **142**:783–786, 1982.

125. Marchal, G. J., Baert, A. L., Wilms, G. E.: CT of noncystic liver lesions: Bolus enhancement. *A.J.R.* **135**:57–65, 1980.

126. Marks, L. J., Weingarten, B., Gerst, G. B.: Carcinoma of tail of pancreas associated with bleeding gastric varices and hyperplenism. *Ann. Intern. Med.* **37**:1077–1079, 1952.

127. Marks, W. M., Filly, R. A., Callen, P. W.: Ultrasonic evaluation of normal pancreatic echogenicity and its relationship to fat deposition. *Radiology* **137**:475–479, 1980.

128. Marshall, J. P., Smith, P. D., Hoyumpa, A. M.: Gastric varices. Problem in diagnosis. *Am. J. Dig. Dis.* **22**:947–955, 1977.

129. Marshall, S., Lapp, M., Schulte, J. W.: Lesions of the pancreas mimicking renal disease. *J. Urol.* **93**:41–45, 1965.

130. Matsui, Y., Aoki, Y., Ishikawa, O., Iwanaga, T., Wada, A., Tateishi, R., Kosaki, G.: Ductal carcinoma of the pancreas: Rationale for total pancreatectomy. *Arch. Surg.* **114**:722–726, 1979.

131. Mattrey, R. F., Long, D. M., Multer, F. K., Mitten, R. M., Higgins, C. B.: Liver-spleen specific contrast material for computerized trans-axial tomography. *Investigative Radiology,* **17**:523, Abstract #92.

132. McArdle, C. R.: Ultrasonic diagnosis of liver metastases. *J. Clin. Ultrasound* **4**:265–268, 1976.

133. McBee, J. W., Lanza, F. L., Erickson, E. E.: Hypoglycemia due to obstruction of pancreatic excretory ducts by carcinoma. *Arch. Pathol.* **81**:287–291, 1966.

134. McDermott, W. V., Jr.: Portal hypertension secondary to pancreatic disease. *Ann. Surg.* **152**:147–149, 1960.

135. Melnyk, C. S.: Carcinoma of the Pancreas. In *Gastrointestinal Disease.* Sleisenger, M. H., Fordtran, J. S. (Eds.). Philadelphia, W. B. Saunders, 1973, pp. 1198–1205.

136. Meyers, M. A.: *Dynamic Radiology of the Abdomen. Normal and Pathologic Anatomy.* New York, Springer-Verlag, 1976.

137. Meyers, M. A., Volberg, F., Katzen, B., Abbott, G.: Haustral anatomy and pathology: A new look. II. Roentgen interpretation of pathologic alterations. *Radiology* **108**:505–512, 1973.

138. Moss, A. A., Dean, P. B., Axel, L., Goldberg, H. I., Glazer, G. M., Friedman, M. A.: Dynamic CT of hepatic masses with intravenous and intraarterial contrast material. *A.J.R.* **38**:847–852, 1982.

139. Moss, A. A., Goldberg, H. I., Stark, B. D., Davis, P. L., Margulis, A. R., Kaufman, L., Crooks, L. E.: Hepatic tumors: Magnetic resonance and CT appearance. *Radiology* **150**:141–147, 1984.

140. Moss, A. A., Kressel, H. Y.: Computed tomography of the pancreas. *Dig. Dis. Sci.* **22**:1018–1027, 1977.

141. Moss, A. A., Schrumpf, J., Schnyder, P., Korobkin, M., Shimshak, R. R.: Computed tomography of focal hepatic lesions: A blind clinical evaluation of the effect of contrast enhancement. *Radiology* **131**:427–430, 1979.

142. Muhletaler, C. A., Gerlock, A. J., Jr., Fleischer, A. C., James, A. E., Jr.: Diagnosis of obstructive jaundice with nondilated bile ducts. *A.J.R.* **134**:1149–1152, 1980.

143. Muhletaler, C., Gerlock, A. J., Jr., Goncharenka, V., Avant, G. R., Flexner, J. M.: Gastric varices secondary to splenic vein occlusion: Radiographic diagnosis and clinical significance. *Radiology* **132**:593–598, 1979.

144. Mujahed, Z., Evans, J. A.: Percutaneous transhepatic cholangiography. *Radiol. Clin. North Am.* **4**:535–545, 1966.

145. Murray, R. O., Jacobson, H. G.: *The Radiology of Skeletal Disorders. Exercises in Diagnosis.* Baltimore, Williams & Wilkins, 1972; pp. 1098.

146. Nakayama, T., Ikeda, A., Okuda, K.: Percutaneous transhepatic drainage of the biliary tract: Techniques and results in 104 patients. *Gastroenterology* **74**:554–559, 1978.

147. Nebesar, R. A., Pollard, J. J.: A critical evaluation of selective celiac and superior mesenteric angiography in the diagnosis of pancreatic disease, particularly malignant tumor: Facts and "artifacts." *Radiology* **89**:1017–1027, 1967.

148. Neiman, H. L., Mintzer, R. A.: Accuracy of biliary duct ultrasound; comparison with cholangiography. *A.J.R.* **129**:979–982, 1977.

149. Niccolini, D. G., Grahm, J. H., Banks, P. A.: Tumor-induced acute pancreatitis. *Gastroenterology* **71**:142–145, 1976.

150. Op den Orth, J. O.: Hypotonic duodenography without the use of a stomach tube. *Radiol. Clin. Biol.* **42**:173–174, 1973.

151. Paloyan, D., Skinner, D. B.: Clinical significance of pancreatic ascites. *Am. J. Surg.* **132**:114–117, 1976.

152. Pearse, A. G. E.: The APUD concept and its implications in pathology. *Pathol. Annu.* **9**:27–42, 1974.

153. Pemberton, L. B., Diffenbaugh, W. F., Strohl, E. L.: The surgical significance of carcinoma of the gallbladder. *Am. J. Surg.* **122**:381, 1971.

154. Perpetuo, M. D., Valdivieso, M., Heilbrun, L. K., Nelson, R. S., Connor, T., Bodey, G. P.: Natural history study of gallbladder cancer: A review of 36 years experience at M.D. Anderson Hospital and Tumor Institute. *Cancer* **42**:330–335, 1978.

155. Piehler, J. M., Crichlow, R. W.: Primary carcinoma of the gallbladder. *Arch. Surg.* **112**:26–30, 1977.

156. Plumley, T. F., Rohrmann, C. A., Jr., Freeny, P. C., Silverstein, F. E., Ball, T. J.: The double duct sign.: An analysis of its significance in evaluating the abnormal endoscopic retrograde cholangiopancreatogram. *Am. J. Roent.* **138**:31–35, 1982.

157. Plumley, T. F., Rohrman, C. A., Jr., Freeny, P. C.: Double duct sign: Reassessed significance in ERCP. *A.J.R.* **138**:31, 1982.

158. Poole, J. G.: A new roentgenographic method of measuring the retrogastric and retroduodenal spaces: Statistical evaluation of reliability and diagnostic utility. *Radiology* **97**:71–81, 1970.

159. Poppel, M. H.: *Roentgen Manifestations of Pancreatic Disease.* Springfield, Charles C. Thomas, 1951.

160. Prando, A., Wallace, S., Bernardino, M. E., Lindell, M. M.: Computed tomographic arteriography of the liver. *Radiology* **130**:697–701, 1979.

161. Pykett, I. L.: NMR imaging in medicine. *Sci. Am.* **46**:78–88, 1982.

162. Pykett, I. L., Newhouse, J. H., Buonanno, F. S.: Principles of nuclear magnetic resonance imaging. *Radiology* **143**:157–168, 1982.

163. Ralls, P. W., Halls, J., Renner, I., Juttner, H.: Endoscopic retrograde cholangiopancreatography of ductal abnormalities in differentiating benign from malignant disease. *Radiology* **134**:347–352, 1980.

164. Reuben, A., Cotton, P. B.: Endoscopic retrograde cholangiopancreatography in carcinoma of the pancreas. *Surg. Gynecol. Obstet.* **148**:179–184, 1979.

165. Reuter, S. R., Redman, H. C.: *Gastrointestinal Angiography.* Philadelphia, W. B. Saunders, 1977.

166. Rigleer, L. G.: Diagnosis of extra-gastrointestinal abdominal masses. *Radiology* **21**:229–238, 1933.

167. Ring, E. J., Oleaga, J. A., Freiman, D. B., Husted, J. W., Lundquist, A.: Therapeutic applications of catheter cholangiography. *Radiology* **128**:333–338, 1978.

168. Robbins, S. L.: Liver and biliary tract. In *Pathology*, Robbins, S. L. (Ed.). Philadelphia, W. B. Saunders, 1967, pp. 897–962.

169. Roberts-Thomson, I. C.: Endoscopic retrograde pancreatography. Analysis of the normal pancreatogram and changes which are associated with chronic pancreatitis and pancreatic carcinoma. *Med. J. Aust.* 2:793–796, 1977.

170. Rohrmann, C. A., Jr., Silvis, S. E., Vennes, J. A.: Evaluation of the endoscopic pancreatogram. *Radiology* 113:297–304, 1974.

171. Rohrmann, C. A., Jr., Silvis, S. E., Vennes, J. A.: The significance of pancreatic ductal obstruction in differential diagnosis of the abnormal endoscopic retrograde pancreatogram. *Radiology* 121:311–314, 1976.

172. Rosch, J., Judkins, M. P.: Angiography in the diagnosis of pancreatic disease. *Semin. Roentgenol.* 3:296–390, 1968.

173. Rosch, J., Lakin, P. C., Antonovic, R., Dotter, C. T.: Transjugular approach to liver biopsy and transhepatic cholangiography. *N. Engl. J. Med.* 289:227–231, 1973.

174. Ruiz, R., Teyssou, H., Fernandez, N., Carrez, J. P., Gortchakoff, M., Manteau, G., Ter-Dautian, P. M., Tessier, J. P.: Ultrasonic diagnosis of primary carcinoma of the gallbladder: A review of 16 cases. *J. Clin. Ultrasound* 8:489–495, 1980.

175. Salik, J. O.: Pancreatic carcinoma and its early roentgen recognition. *A.J.R.* 86:1–28, 1961.

176. Sample, W. F., Sarti, D. A., Goldstein, L. I., Weiner, M., Kadell, B. W.: Gray-scale ultrasonography of the jaundiced patient. *Radiology* 128:719–725, 1978.

177. Sato, T., Koyama, K., Yamauchi, H., Matsuno, S.: Early carcinoma of the gallbladder. *Gastroenterology* 16:459–464, 1981.

178. Shanser, J. D., Korobkin, M., Goldberg, H. I., Rohlfing, B. M.: Computed tomographic diagnosis of obstructive jaundice in the absence of intrahepatic ductal dilatation. *A.J.R.* 131:389–392, 1978.

179. Shawker, T. H., Jones, B. L., Girton, M. E.: Distal common bile duct obstruction: An experimental study in monkeys. *J. Clin. Ultrasound* 9:77, 1981.

180. Sheedy, P. F. II, Stephens, D. H., Hattery, R. R., MacCarty, R. L.: Computed tomography in the evaluation of patients with suspected carcinoma of the pancreas. *Radiology* 124:731–737, 1977.

181. Simone, J. V., Cassady, J. R., Filler, R. M.: Cancers of childhood. In *Cancer—Principles and Practice of Oncology.* DeVita, V. T., Jr., Hellman, S., Rosenberg, S. A. (Eds.). Philadelphia, J. B. Lippincott, 1982, pp. 1254–1330.

182. Snow, J. H., Goldstein, H. M., Wallace, S.: Comparison of scintigraphy, sonography, and computed tomography in the evaluation of hepatic neoplasms. *A.J.R.* 132:915–918, 1979.

183. Sommers, S. C., Murphy, S. A., Warren, S.: Pancreatic duct hyperplasia and cancer. *Gastroenterology* 27:629–640, 1954.

184. Sorabella, P. A., Campbell, W. L., Seaman, W. B.: Comparative detection of pancreatic body-tail enlargement using the supine translateral and axial pancreatic views: A prospective statistical study. *A.J.R.* 125:143–153, 1975.

185. Spain, D. M.: Minute pancreatic tumor associated with arterial thrombi. *Gastroenterology* 43:104–106, 1962.

186. Stadelmann, O., Safrang, L., Loffler, A., et al.: Endoscopic retrograde cholangiopancreatography in the diagnosis of pancreatic cancer. *Endoscopy* 6:84–93, 1974.

187. Stanley, R. J., Sagel, S. S., Levitt, R. G.: Computed tomography of the pancreas. *Radiology* 124:705–712, 1977.

188. Stark, B. D., Moss, A. A., Goldberg, H. I., Davis, P. L., Federle, M. P.: Magnetic resonance and CT of the normal and diseased pancreas: A comparative study. *Radiology* 150:153–162, 1984.

189. Statistical Research Service: *Cancer Mortality Statistics.* New York, American Cancer Society, 1970.

190. Strang, C., Walton, J. N.: Carcinoma of the body and tail of the pancreas. *Ann. Intern. Med.* 39:15–37, 1953.

191. Sugarbaker, P. H., Macdonald, J. S., Gunderson, L. L.: Colorectal cancer. In *Cancer—Principles and Practice of Oncology.* DeVita, V. T., Jr., Hellman, S., Rosenberg, S. A. (Eds.). Philadelphia, J. B. Lippincott, 1982, pp. 643–723.

192. Sullivan, D. C., Taylor, K. J. W., Gottschalk, A.: The use of ultrasound to enhance the diagnostic utility of the equivocal liver scintigraph. *Radiology* 128:727–732, 1978.

193. Sutton, J. P., Yarborough, D. Y., Richards, J. T.: Isolated splenic vein occlusion. *Arch. Surg.* 100:623–626, 1970.

194. Takasan, H., Kim, C. I., Arii, S., Takahashi, S., Vozumi, T., Tobe, T., Honjo, I.: Clinicopathologic study of seventy patients with carcinoma of the biliary tract. *Surg. Gynecol. Obstet.* 150:721–726, 1980.

195. Taylor, K. J. W., Rosenfeld, A. T.: Gray scale ultrasonography in the differential diagnosis of jaundice. *Arch. Surg.* 112:820–825, 1977.

196. Thorbjarnarson, B.: Carcinoma of the bile ducts. *Cancer* 12:708–713, 1959.

197. Thorsen, M. K., Quiroz, F., Lawson, T. L., Smith, D. F., Foley, W. D., Stewart, E. T.: Primary biliary carcinoma: CT evaluation. *Radiology* 152:479–483, 1984.

198. Todoroki, T., Okamura, T., Fukao, K., Nishimura, H., Otsu, H., Sato, H., Iwasaki, Y.: Gross appearance of carcinoma of the main hepatic duct and its prognosis. *Surg. Gynecol. Obstet.* 150:33–40, 1980.

199. Tsuzuki, T., Uekusa, M.: Carcinoma of the proximal bile ducts. *Surg. Gynecol. Obstet.* 146:933–943, 1978.

200. Turner, J. W., Jaffe, H. L.: Metastatic neoplasms. *A.J.R.* 43:479–492, 1940.

201. Tylen, U.: Accuracy of angiography in the diagnosis of carcinoma of the pancreas. *Acta Radiol.* 14:449–466, 1973.

202. Tylen, U., Hoevels, J., Vang, J.: Percutaneous transhepatic cholangiography with external drainage of obstructive biliary lesions. *Surg. Gynecol. Obstet.* 144:13–18, 1977.

203. Ultmann, J. E., Phillips, T. L., Foster, J. H.: Treatment of the metastatic cancer to liver. In *Cancer: Principles and Practice of Oncology.* DeVita, V. T., Jr., Hellman, S., Rosenberg, S. A. (Eds.) Philadelphia, J. B. Lippincott, 1982, pp. 1153–1563.

204. Vermess, M., Doppman, J. L., Sugarbaker, P. H., Fisher, R. I., O'Leary, T. J., Chatterji, D. C., Grimes, G., Adamson, R. H., Willis, M., Edwards, B. K.: Computed tomography of the liver and spleen with intravenous lipoid contrast material: Review of examinations. *A.J.R.* 138:1063–1071, 1982.

205. Waes, L. V., Maele, V. M., Demeulenaere, L., Lamssens, C.: Carcinoma of the pancreas presenting as relapsing pancreatitis. *Am. J. Gastroenterol.* 68:88–90. 1977.

206. Wapnick, S., Hadas, N., Purow, E., Grosberg, S. J.: Mass in the head of the pancreas in cholestatic jaundice. Carcinoma or pancreatitis. *Ann. Surg.* 190:587–591, 1979.

207. Warren, K. W., Jefferson, M. F.: Carcinoma of the exocrine pancreas. In *The Pancreas.* Carey, L. C. (Ed.). St. Louis, C.V. Mosby Co., 1973, pp. 243–294.

208. Weill, F., Eisencher, A., Zelther, F.: Ultrasonic study of the normal and dilated biliary tree. The "shotgun" sign. *Radiology* 127:221–224, 1978.

209. Weinstein, B. J., Weinstein, D. P.: Biliary tract dilatation in the nonjaundiced patient. *A.J.R.* 134:899, 1980.

210. Weinstein, D. P., Wolfman, N. T., Weinstein, B. J.: Ultrasonic characteristics of pancreatic tumors. *Gastrointest. Radiol.* 4:245–251, 1979.

211. White, R. J.: Carcinoma of pancreas presenting as acute duodenal obstruction without jaundice. *Ann. Surg.* 153:769–775, 1961.

212. Wiener, S. N., Parulekar, S. G.: Scintigraphy and ultrasonography of hepatic hemangioma. *Radiology* 132:149–153, 1979.

213. Williams, R. R., McIntire, K. R., Waldmann, T. A.: Tumor-associ-

ated antigen levels (carcinoembryonic antigen, human chorionic gonadotropin, and alpha-fetoprotein antedating the diagnosis of cancer in the Framingham study).

214. Wolfman, N. T., Ramquist, N. A., Karastaedt, N., Hopkins, M. B.: Cystic neoplasms of the pancreas: CT and sonography. *A.J.R.* **138**:37–41, 1982.

215. Wooten, W. B., Green, B., Goldstein, H. M.: Ultrasonography of necrotic hepatic metastases. *Radiology* **128**:447–450, 1978.

216. Yeh, H.: Ultrasonography and computed tomography of car-cinoma of the gallbladder. *Radiology* **133**:167, 1979.

217. Yeh, H., Rabinowitz, J. G.: Ultrasonography and computed tomography of the liver. *Radiol. Clin. North Am.* **18**:321–338, 1980.

218. Young, S. W., Turner, R. J., Castellino, R. A.: A strategy for the contrast enhancement of malignant tumors using dynamic computed tomography and intravascular pharmacokinetics. *Radiology* **137**:137–147, 1980.

219. Yum, H. Y., Fink, A. H.: Sonographic findings in primary car-cinoma of the gallbladder. *Radiology* **134**:693, 1980.

15 ADRENAL AND RETROPERITONEAL TUMORS

P. Ruben Koehler

The adrenal glands and retroperitoneum are areas of great difficulty for radiologists. Because the adrenal glands are located deep within the abdomen, tumors originating from the adrenals or from retroperitoneal tissue are difficult to detect by physical examination or by radiographic methods. Neoplasms are suspected only if the disease is advanced enough to cause symptoms or if it creates abnormalities related to hormone secretion. There have been, therefore, few areas in the body in which the newer imaging techniques of computed tomography and, to a lesser degree, ultrasonography, have had as profound an impact on diagnosis as on detection of neoplasms originating in the adrenal glands and retroperitoneum. These imaging modalities not only aid in identification of tumors of a smaller size, but also help in assessing the extent of the cancer and its relationship to neighboring organs and assist in detecting the presence or absence of distant metastases.

Primary malignant tumors of the adrenals or retroperitoneum are rare. Adrenal tumors account for only 0.2% of all cancer deaths in the United States;[41] the frequency of primary (nonlymphomatous) retroperitoneal tumors is of similar magnitude. The etiology of these tumors remains an enigma; many theories have been suggested but none as yet have been proven. No relationship to a specific chemical, viral, or other exogenic agent has been established.

Adrenal tumors are rare. Brennan[5] estimated that approximately 130 new malignant cortical tumors occur each year in the United States. Benign tumors are identified in about 300 patients. In about 400 instances the diagnosis of pheochromocytoma is made. Autopsy series show that approximately 2% of adults have nonfunctioning adenomas.

The survival of patients with carcinomas depends on the stage of the disease when it is detected. According to Didolkar et al.,[8] however, even in patients who undergo curative surgery, the median disease-free interval is only approximately two to two and a half years. The five-year survival is estimated at 18% for functioning tumors and 11% for nonfunctioning tumors. The range of survival is from one month to 17 years. The true survival rate is difficult to assess, since histologically it is frequently impossible to differentiate between benign and malignant tumors. It is not rare that a tumor is designated malignant because metastases have been found rather than because the histologic appearance is that of malignant tumor. These patients have advanced disease, and their survival is limited. For patients with tumors that have not yet metastasized and are amenable to resection, survival is much longer. Some of these tumors may be benign.

This chapter first discusses the classification of tumors of the adrenals and retroperitoneum. Pathology, behavior, and modes of spread are then described. Next, types of available imaging modalities, their advantages, disadvantages, and expected sensitivity and specificity are presented. Finally, a recommendation for the most cost-effective imaging workup is suggested.

TUMOR BEHAVIOR
AND PATHOLOGY

The normal adrenal glands are structures covering or closely related to the upper poles of the kidneys. They weigh between 5 and 7 g and are somewhat larger and heavier in men than in women. The adrenal glands are contained within Gerota's fascia. Each gland is composed of an inner core, the medulla, and of an outer shell, the cortex. The medulla, composed largely of chromaffin cells, is derived from ectodermal stem cells that migrate from the neural crest. These chromaffin cells may also be found elsewhere in the body. They are most abundant wherever sympathetic nerve tissue is present, but particularly in the sympathetic nerve ganglia and the organ of Zuckerkandl at the bifurcation of the aorta.

The cortex is composed of large lipid-laden epithelial cells, giving this portion of the gland a yellowish appearance. The cortex is divided into three layers. The first is the outer layer, called the zona glomerulosa, the cells of which primarily produce mineral corticoids. The second zone is the widest one, the zona fasciculata, and the most central one is the zona reticularis. Both inner layers produce glucocorticoids, 17-ketosteroids, and estrogens. Both adrenals are richly supplied with arterial blood through branches arising from the renal artery, the aorta, and the phrenic arteries. Small branches from the capsular arteries of the kidney and the ovarian or spermatic arteries are also present. Drainage of the left adrenal vein is into the left renal vein; the right adrenal vein drains directly into the inferior vena cava. The nerve supply is derived from the celiac and renal plexii.[24]

Nonfunctioning Tumors

Cysts. The nonfunctioning tumors of the adrenal cortex are divided into cysts, adenomas, and carcinomas. Cysts may be congenital and are generally of little clinical significance except when they are bilateral and contribute to adrenal cortical insufficiency. Hemorrhagic cysts may develop after trauma or infection and are sometimes encountered in newborns, probably as a result of the trauma of birth. The nonhemorrhagic cysts are generally considered to be developmental in origin.

Adenomas. Small nonfunctioning cortical adenomas are very common. According to Harrison and Mahoney,[20] they are seen so frequently that in the absence of symptoms, it is questionable whether they should be considered pathologic. Most of these small adenomas are not demonstrated radiographically, being incidentally discovered at autopsy or during CT examination.[35]

Carcinomas. About 50% of carcinomas are hormonally nonfunctioning. They are usually large when detected. They occur primarily in adults, most commonly in the fourth to seventh decades of life. The symptoms are produced by progressive enlargement or by metastases to the periaortic lymph nodes, lungs, and liver. Pain in the abdomen or flank is the most common complaint; malaise, weight loss, and fever are frequently present.[48] Other primary adrenal tumors that have been reported include fibromas, myomas, lipomas, hemangiomas, lymphangiomas, fibrosarcomas, myelolipomas.

Functioning Tumors of the Adrenal Cortex

Most functioning tumors of the adrenal cortex will be either adenomas, which cause the hyperglucocorticoid state, aldosterone-secreting tumors, and tumors or carcinomas of the adrenal cortex. Approximately 50% of the neoplasms are benign; however, any large adenoma should be considered potentially malignant. Histologic differentiation between benign and malignant tumors is difficult. Usually, evidence of vascular invasion of the capsule or distant metastases is needed to establish the diagnosis of malignancy.[32]

Cushing's Syndrome. In Cushing's syndrome, the clinical signs will be identical, whether caused by hyperplasia or by tumor. The syndrome is most common in adults and is the result of increased secretion of glucocorticoid hormones. Clinically, the patients are obese in the face, neck, and trunk, have a cervical dorsal hump, and possibly a protruberant abdomen. The extremities, because of muscle wasting, are thin. Striation of the skin and ecchymosis are common. Many will exhibit hypertension, osteoporosis, hyperglycemia, hirsutism, amenorrhea, or impotence.

Adrenal Genital Syndrome. When the tumors secrete androgenic hormones, the adrenal genital syndrome develops. The syndrome can be either congenital or acquired. In this book we are primarily interested in the acquired syndrome, which is caused by the cortical tumors. It is characterized by virilism in females and by precocious development of secondary sexual characteristics in males. If the tumor develops in adults, no endocrine manifestations are recognizable.

Primary Aldosteronism. Primary aldosteronism is caused by excess secretion of mineralocorticoids. Clinical symptoms primarily are hypertension, hypokalemia, and alkalosis.[16']

Carcinoma. The carcinomas, when functioning, most frequently cause virilizing tumors in females and often estrogen-producing, feminizing tumors in males. The tumors, including the carcinomas, usually have capsules.

Of particular interest are the pheochromocytomas. These usually functioning tumors arise from cells that have a close embryologic relationship with the sympathetic nervous system. Neural crest cells migrate into the adrenal cortex. Similar types of cells may also be found in feti along the abdominal aorta at the origin of the inferior mesenteric artery (organ of Zuckerkandl) and at other sites in the sympathetic nervous system (cervical and thoracic ganglia, GI system, bladder, gonads). After birth these cells are usually replaced by lymphatic tissue. However, they may persist and then give rise to extra-adrenal pheochromocytomas. These cells contain cytoplasmic granules with an affinity for chromatin salt stains, giving rise to the name *chromaffin* tumors.

When a tumor develops, it will increase the production of hormones. As a group they are called catecholamines (dopamine, norepinephrine). Laboratory tests used to identify these tumors utilize identification of increased urinary excretion of metabolites of these hormones, mainly vanillymandilic acid (VMA). Ninety percent of the tumors arise from the adrenals; 10% are extra-adrenal, and 5% are multiple.

The most typical clinical symptoms are episodes of paroxysmal hypertension, although persistent hypertension is also associated with these tumors. The radiologist's main objective is not to make the diagnosis of pheochromocytoma, since this is usually done by laboratory methods, but to locate the tumor.

The pattern of spread of the malignant tumors is into the periaortic lymph nodes. Invasion is also into the capsular vessels and surrounding tissues. Distant metastases are most frequently found in the liver and lung. The pattern of spread of all the tumor types is very similar, and radiographic methods do not help in differentiating one type from another.

CLASSIFICATION AND STAGING

Adrenal tumors can be classified into those arising from the cortex, those arising from the medullary portions, and those secondarily involving the adrenals such as metastatic cancers or lymphomas[39] (Table 15-1). Staging of malignant adrenal lesions according to MacFarlane[32] and Sullivan et al.[48] is based on a combination of size and the TNM system.

Stage I: Tumor less than 5 cm. No nodal involvement or distant metastasis (T_1, N_0, M_0)

Table 15-1. Classification of Tumors Arising from the Adrenal Cortex

Tumors with no endocrine function
    Cysts
    Adenomas of the cortex
    Carcinomas of the cortex
Tumors with endocrine functions
    Adenomas
    Carcinomas
Tumors of the medulla—pheochromocytomas
Metastatic involvement of the adrenals—carcinoma and lymphoma

Stage II: Tumor more than 5 cm. No nodal involvement or distant metastasis (T_2, N_0, M_0)
Stage III: Tumor with local invasion of surrounding structures or local lymph node involvement $(T_3, N_0, M_0$ or $T_{any}, N_1, M_0)$
Stage IV: Any tumor with distant metastasis (T_{any}, N_{any}, M_1)

IMAGING PROCEDURES AND ASSESSMENT

A variety of radiographic examinations can be used when a tumor of the adrenal gland is suspected. As reviewed earlier, tumors may develop from either the medulla or the cortex; however, attempts to radiographically differentiate these sites from one another generally have not been successful. An exception are pheochromocytomas, which frequently have a rather specific radiographic appearance.

The diagnosis of nonfunctioning tumor is usually made serendipitously. These lesions are usually quite large and are identified either on physical examination as an abdominal mass or on an X-ray examination performed for another reason. Diagnosis of hormonally functioning tumor is often made earlier because of the clinical symptoms resulting from the abnormal hormonal secretions which suggest the presence of a tumor. The question of benignancy versus malignancy is not related to hormonal activity. Tumors of both groups may be benign or malignant.

Today, in most instances, imaging studies are confined to CT, ultrasonography, venography, venous sampling and, on occasion, angiography (Table 15-2). Magnetic resonance imaging may prove a sensitive test, but more experience is needed. Because on occasion these modern but relatively expensive tools are not available to all radiologists, standard radiographic methods will also be described here. The examinations and their usefulness are summarized in Table 15-2.

Plain Films of the Abdomen

The use of plain films of the abdomen when adrenal tumors are suspected is of little value. Only a very large tumor or a calcified mass will be recognized. Masses, if seen, are in the upper abdomen and are recognized as such because they displace surrounding structures such as the kidneys or air-filled viscii, i.e., the stomach, the small bowel, and the large bowel. The affected organs are displaced in a manner that reflects the growth vector of a mass with a right or left posterior origin in the upper abdomen. Calcifications may be detected in the larger tumors and are found in approximately 15% of tumors larger than 5 cm. Calcifications are rarer in small tumors. Adrenal calcification in adults should be viewed with suspicion.

Table 15-2. Imaging Methods Used in Examination of Adrenal and Retroperitoneal Tumors

METHOD	EASE OF PERFORMANCE AND SAFETY TO PATIENT	ABILITY TO OUTLINE ADRENAL LESIONS	ABILITY TO OUTLINE RETROPERITONEAL TUMORS	EXPECTED RESULTS AND ESTIMATED YIELD
Plain film	Easy/safe	Only large or calcified lesions	Same	Poor unless tumor is large or calcified
IVP	Easy/safe	Only large or calcified lesions	Same	50% if tumor is larger than 5 cm: not recommended unless CT not available
Retroperitoneal air insufflation	Some skill needed—serious complications possible	3–5 cm lesions seen if exam technically satisfactory	Not useful	Poor—not recommended
UGI and BE	Easy/safe	Nonspecific—only large lesions seen	Nonspecific—only large lesions seen	Poor—not recommended
Ultrasound	Technical skill needed; safe	Lesions are usually larger than 3 cm	Large lesion	70%—recommended if CT is not available
Nuclear medicine	Easy/safe	More experience needed to evaluate results	Not useful	Number of patients too small to draw conclusions
Angiography	Moderately difficult technically; serious complications possible	Only good when vascular tumors are suspected	Not sensitive in small tumors	About 50%—recommended before surgery or when multiple tumors are suspected
Venography	Technically difficult; complications possible	Useful when small tumors are suspected	Not useful	About 60%—recommended if CT not available
CT	Easy/safe	Very accurate even in small tumors	Accurate in small tumors	90%—examination of choice

Intravenous Urography

Of all conventional radiographic examinations, intravenous urography is probably the most cost-effective when tumors of the adrenal glands or retroperitoneum are suspected. However, the sensitivity and specificity of intravenous urograms are poor, and they are generally recommended only if CT or ultrasonography are not available. It should therefore be understood that this examination is only recommended when the other modalities are not easily available, and it also should be understood that a negative finding on an intravenous urogram should not be considered to exclude the presence of an adrenal tumor. The diagnostic criteria rely on the effect of the tumor on the kidney. Because the adrenal gland lies within Gerota's fascia, enlargement of the gland will affect the position and axis of the ipsilateral kidney. Adrenal tumors, at least in their early stages, rarely invade the kidney; the abnormalities seen therefore are those of position rather than intrinsic abnormalities of the kidney itself. Urograms are also useful in the differentiation of upper pole renal masses from adrenal tumors. Adrenal masses, unless very large, will not intrinsically distort the calices.[14]

Because the diagnosis depends on indirect signs rather than the identification of the tumor itself, only relatively large masses will be recognized on intravenous urograms. The radiographic detail can often be enhanced by combining the intravenous urogram with tomography, but even with tomography small tumors will not be seen (Figure 15-1).

Barium Studies

Upper GI studies or barium enema studies have been used to better delineate the displacement of these organs by large tumors. Barium studies are of no value with small tumors, and currently are rarely used to study tumors of the adrenals or retroperitoneum. In the series of Didolkar et al.[8] of 42 patients with adrenal carcinoma, barium contrast studies were positive in only six. Five of these six tumors originated in the left adrenal,

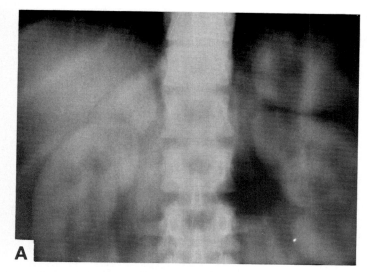

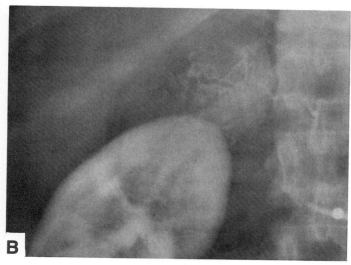

FIG. 15-1. (A) Tomogram done during an intravenous urogram of a patient with hypertension. A 3-cm mass is seen superior to the right kidney. Masses of this size are too small to affect the position of the kidney. The round density above the left kidney is the fundus of the stomach and should not be confused with an adrenal mass. (B) Films taken during the late phase of an arteriogram. Note the tumor vascularity. This is a malignant pheochromocytoma.

suggesting a greater sensitivity with masses on this side.

Retroperitoneal Air Insufflation

Retroperitoneal air (or CO_2) insufflation was used before the advent of angiography and venography as the method that was best suited to identify the adrenal glands. This method is mentioned only for the sake of completeness in the discussion.[33] Gas was injected either directly into perirenal space or presacrally and allowed to dissect through the retroperitoneal tissue planes to the perirenal space. When sufficient amounts of gas

were present, the adrenal gland could be clearly identified and separated from the kidney. Because the examination was inaccurate (there were no objective criteria with which to differentiate hyperplasia from normal size or to identify small tumors) and painful, and because better methods were developed, this type of examination is no longer used.

Arteriography and Venography

As in the identification of many other malignant tumors, selective angiography[2,24] has a distinct role in the diagnosis of adrenal and retroperitoneal malignancies. Angiography and venography (Figure 15-2) were the examinations of choice in adrenal disease until 1978, when CT was shown to be more accurate. Angiography is best suited to the demonstration of vascular tumors such as pheochromocytomas or adrenal carcinomas (Figure 15-3). The radiographic criteria for identification of these tumors are the same as with any other malignant tumor, namely the demonstration of tumor neovascularity or tumor blush on delayed films. The angiographic appearance of adrenal tumors does not allow any conclusions to be made regarding the histologic type of tumor that is visualized.[22] At best, one may speculate that if the vessels appear extremely pleomorphic, one is dealing with a carcinoma. This is only an assumption, however, since such an appearance can be seen in pheochromocytomas and occasionally in adenomas. In adrenal tumors the presence of pathologic vessels does not indicate malignancy. Abnormal vessels are commonly seen in benign adrenal tumors, particularly in pheochromocytomas. Thus, in contrast to most other organs, the presence of tumor vessels does not answer the question of malignancy versus benignancy. Angiography is still being used in patients suspected of having pheochromocytomas and in carcinomas, particularly if surgery is contemplated, in order to better delineate the blood supply to the tumor. If angiography is performed, it is important that a mainstream aortogram injection be done before selective angiography. The reason is that pheochromocytomas may be multiple and in locations other than the adrenal gland. Multiple tumors have been reported in approximately 10% of patients with pheochromocytomas. Therefore, if this tumor is suspected (based on clinical findings), an angiogram is often done before surgical removal so that a second tumor located somewhere else, or possibly even on the opposite side, is not overlooked during surgery.

Because many adrenal tumors are relatively avascular, venography has been used in attempts to identify smaller tumors.[11,23,34,40] Adenomas, benign and malignant, appear as space-occupying lesions within the adrenal glands. Consequently, they are usually devoid of the normal venous plexus of the adrenal gland. Retrograde injection of contrast medium into the veins can outline these

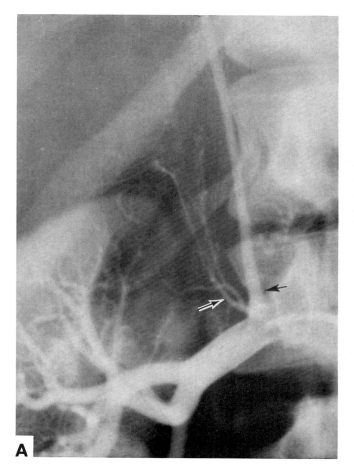

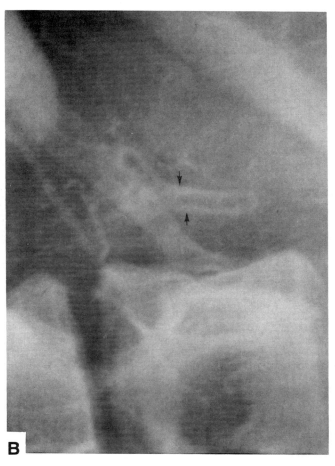

FIG. 15-2. (A) Normal adrenal arteriogram. The catheter is placed in the renal artery. Note the inferior adrenal arteries (arrows) that arise from the proximal aspect of the phrenic artery (arrowhead). (B) Film taken during the capillary phase of the angiogram. The relatively avascular medulla is surrounded by the vascular cortex (arrow). The inverted Y appearance of the gland is quite apparent.

tumors. Lesions as small as 5 mm have been recognized, though generally, accurate diagnosis can only be made if the lesion reaches at least 1 cm in diameter (Figure 15-4). The main disadvantage of venography is the technical difficulty in performing the procedure. While the left adrenal vein is relatively easily entered, the right one is often difficult to negotiate.

During venography, one is able to collect blood samples originating within the gland in addition to demonstrating the anatomy. These can be analyzed for hormonal levels, thus helping identify the location of functioning tumors. Today venography is still used when the diagnosis after CT is equivocal or when hormonal assays are needed.

Venography has been used to treat small adrenal tumors by ablation using retrograde injection of nitrogen mustard or alcohol through the adrenal vein into the tumor. This method has not gained wide acceptance because of the technical difficulties and the potential for incomplete destruction of the tumor.[18]

A note of caution is necessary regarding pheochromocytomas. When catheters are manipulated in the adrenal arteries or veins and particularly when contrast medium is injected into these small vessels, patients with pheochromocytomas may develop a hypertensive crisis. The radiologist must be prepared for this potential complication, and it is advisable to have an intravenous line open so that suitable drugs (phentolamine mesylate or similar drugs) can be infused to counteract this adverse reaction.[24,34]

Nuclear Medicine

Tumors of the adrenal cortex, provided they are functioning, can be identified with ^{131}I-19-iodocholesterol.[30,46] This agent used in dosages of approximately 2_μCi concentrates in adrenal cortex tumors and their metastases and can be visualized between 4 and 14 days after the injection.[15] Usually several scans are obtained using a photogamma camera. New agents such as 6-iodomethyl-19-no cholesterol have been used. With both agents suppression scans can be used. The uptake to both glands as well as to metastases is determined with the use of a microcomputer connected to the gamma camera.

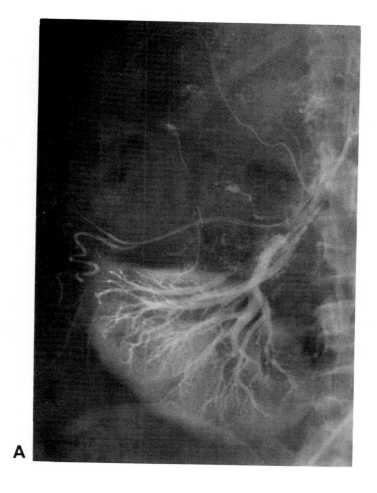

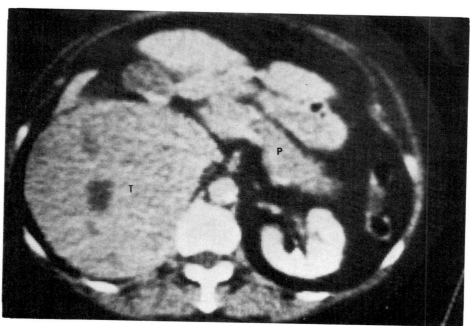

FIG. 15-3. (A) Angiogram of a patient with a large adrenal carcinoma. Note how the kidney is pushed downward and medially by the large suprarenal mass. The tumor is sparsely fed by adrenal and renal capsular vessels. (B) CT scan of the same patient showing the large mass on the right. The lucency in the center represents areas of necrosis (T = tumor, P = pancreas).

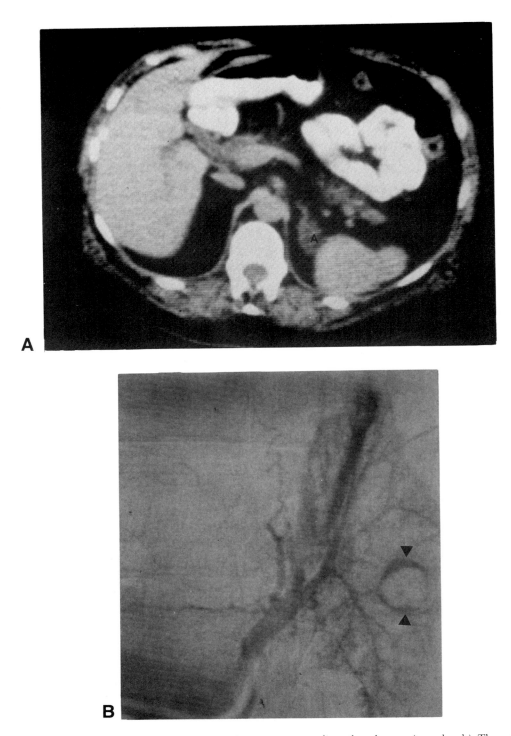

FIG. 15-4. (A) An adenoma of the left adrenal (A). (B) A venogram outlines the adenoma (arrowheads). The catheter tip is in the left adrenal vein.

Ultrasound

It is generally difficult to examine the adrenal glands by ultrasonography.[4,44,54] While large tumors are easy to identify (Figure 15-5), the identification of small adenomas is unreliable because of the difficulty in outlining the normal adrenal gland. According to Abrams et al.,[1] ultrasound had a sensitivity of 79% and a specificity of 61%, or an overall accuracy of 70%. Tumors larger than 2 cm can usually be identified. Because longitudinal scanning is possible, the relationship of a mass to a kidney can generally be more easily appreciated. Sample[44] described a method that allowed identification of the normal adrenal. He felt this technique could demonstrate even small tumors. However, the technique is so difficult and complex that even expert ultrasonographers do not use it. It is therefore fair to state that the role of ultrasonography is that of a screening examination.

Patients will usually be scanned in both the PA and AP positions, since one approach sometimes will be preferential to the other. When the tumors are relatively large or if they are on the right side, the liver can be used as a window, and the tumors are well demonstrated with the patient in the supine position. On the left side, however, gas from the stomach or bowel frequently will limit the usefulness of the supine position. In these cases, it may be possible to better demonstrate this region by scanning the patient while he or she is lying on his or her side or prone. The criteria for identification of masses are the same as for masses elsewhere in the body, namely, cystic structures will appear sonolucent while solid tumors will usually have some echoes within them and will be less sonolucent than cystic masses.[55] The most frequent examination obstacle is the inability of ultrasound waves to penetrate gas or bone.

Computed Tomography

At this time, computed tomography is the examination of choice in the radiologic workup of patients suspected of having adrenal gland tumors. Computed tomography has been successful in identification of the normal gland in 85% to 95% of patients.[1,6,10,13,21,25,26,27,36,50,52,53,55] It is usually advisable to use a CT scan slice thickness of 4 to 7 mm at continuous intervals through the area of the adrenals. The use of intravenous contrast medium is generally not necessary. The position of the normal adrenal gland is described in Figures 15-6 and 15-7. The normal gland has a variety of shapes. On the right it most commonly has the appearance of a comma or an inverted V, while the left adrenal gland most commonly has a triangular shape, i.e., an inverted V or Y (Figures 15-8 and 15-9).

Since the normal structure can be clearly identified, it should not be difficult to recognize abnormalities. Tumors measuring 0.5 cm or larger should be clearly

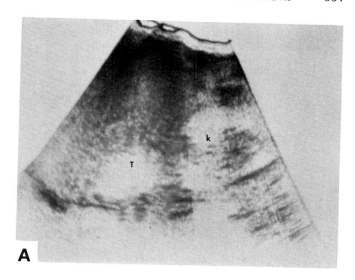

A

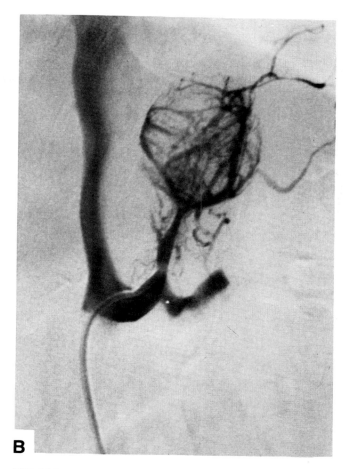

B

FIG. 15-5. (A) Ultrasound of a left adrenal tumor. The tumor (T) is located cranial to the kidney (K). (B) Venogram shows that the adrenal veins are wrapped around a 4–5 cm tumor.

SITE OF ADRENAL GLANDS

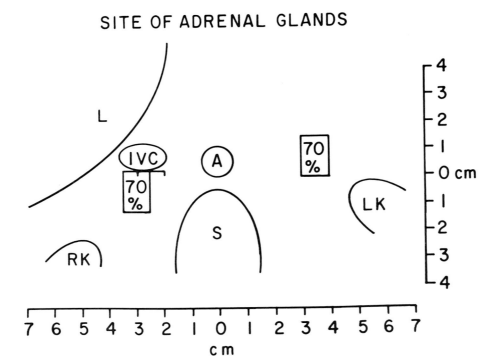

FIG. 15-6. Diagram showing the CT location of the adrenal gland. Seventy percent of right adrenal glands may be found in a 2 cm² space posterior to the inferior vena cava. This space is outlined by an imaginary line drawn between the aorta and the spine. The anterior border of the square will be 0.5 cm anteriorly and 1.5 cm posteriorly behind the line. The square is approximately 3 cm to the right of the midline. The left adrenal gland is found anterior to the imaginary line and 3 to 4 cm to the left of the midline. If one extends the borders of both squares by 1 cm, over 90% of the adrenal glands will be encompassed in these spaces.

identified if the examination is technically adequate (Figure 15-10). Tumors on CT scans appear as an enlargement of either the entire gland or of a part of the organ (Figures 15-4 and 15-11). Abrams et al.[1] report a sensitivity of 84%, a specificity of 98%, and an overall accuracy of 90%. The high sensitivity and specificity of adrenal CT makes this the examination of choice when adrenal tumors are suspected.[52] Not only will the primary lesion be visible, but accurate staging is possible by identification of abnormal para-aortic nodes and invasion of the tumor into the surrounding tissues or organs and distant metastases can be detected in organs such as the liver, spleen, and lung (Figure 15-12). The high degree of accuracy of CT is the reason why CT is today considered by most authorities to be the first and often the only radiographic examination to be done on

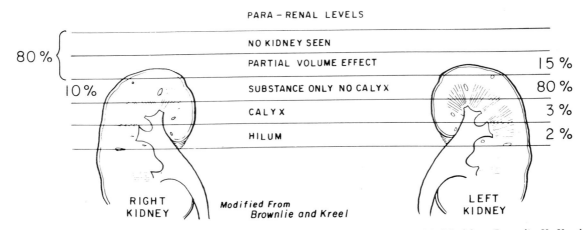

FIG. 15-7. Diagram showing the cranio-caudal position of adrenals relative to the kidney. (Modified from Brownlie, K., Kreel, L.: Computer assisted tomography of normal suprarenal glands. *J. Comput. Assist. Tomogr.* 2:1–10, 1978.)

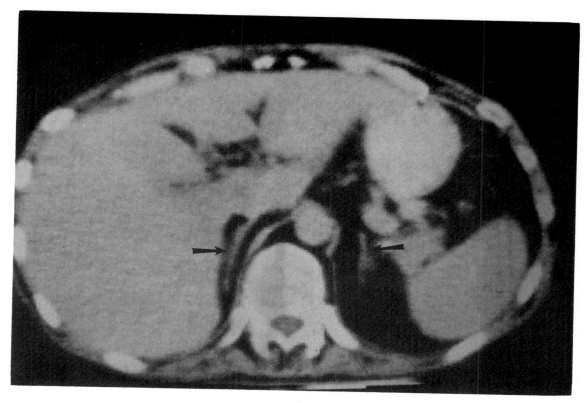

FIG. 15-8. A CT scan of normal adrenal glands. The right has the appearance of a comma (arrow), the left has the appearance of an inverted Y (arrow).

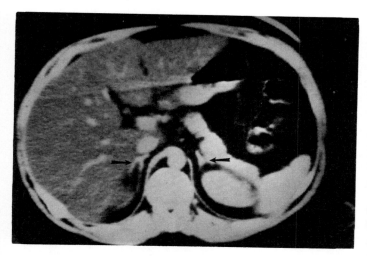

FIG. 15-9. Bilateral normal adrenal scans. Scan is at the most typical level. The right adrenal gland appears as an inverted Y (arrow). Note the relationship of the gland to the inferior vena cava (C). The left gland (arrow) has a triangular shape. Note that the left kidney parenchyma is present at this level but the upper calyces are not visualized.

a patient with a suspected adrenal tumor.[38,45] If normal glands can be visualized on CT, the diagnosis of an adrenal tumor can be excluded with great confidence. Therefore, despite the high cost of a CT, it is probably the most cost-effective examination available.

On occasion an adrenal lesion may be found on CT scans done for other reasons (Figure 15-13). In such instances, a needle biopsy is recommended, since the CT appearance of adrenal tumors is nonspecific; benign adenomas, carcinomas, or metastases all look the same.[12,17,35]

A needle biopsy is easily done and is relatively safe. Generally, an aspiration-type biopsy is performed. After the lesion has been identified, the safest approach is chosen, i.e., a route that does not necessitate penetrating any vital organs, or, in the case of lesions that extend high into the abdomen, an approach that will avoid the deep pleural recesses, thus lessening the chance of pneumothorax formation. After the site has been identified, the skin is cleansed, and approximately 1 to 2 ml of 1%

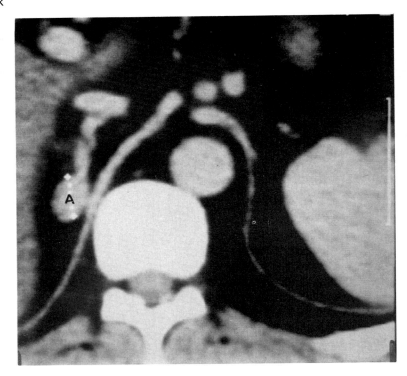

FIG. 15-10. A 1.6-cm adenoma (A) in the most posterior aspect of the right adrenal gland.

xylocaine is injected subcutaneously. A thin, flexible (22-gauge) needle is then advanced into the lesion and a to-and-fro motion is used while vacuum is applied with a syringe, thereby sucking cells into the needle. The material that is obtained in this way is placed in saline and is then examined by the cytologist. The procedure can be done on outpatients, and it is quick, accurate, and relatively safe. Thus, final (pathologic) diagnosis can be reached without subjecting the patient to a battery of expensive tests, and, possibly, invasive exploration and many days of hospital stay.

IMAGING STRATEGIES AND DECISIONS

Adrenal Tumors

As shown in Table 15-2, a variety of radiologic examinations are available. Most are nonspecific, some are difficult to perform, and many carry the risk of poten-

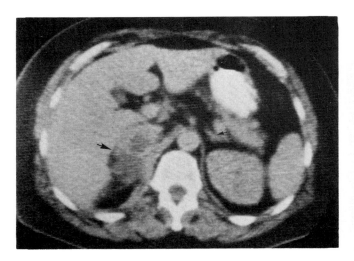

FIG. 15-11. A CT scan of a patient with adrenal carcinoma. Notice the large mass (arrows) with a necrotic center located in the space between the diaphragm and the liver. The inferior vena cava is inseparable from the mass. The unclear posterior borders suggest infiltration into the pararenal fat. The left adrenal is normal (open arrow).

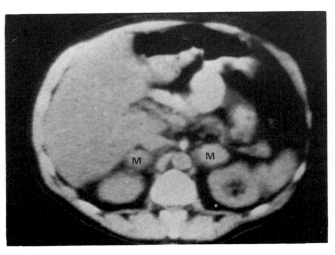

FIG. 15-12. Bilateral adrenal metastases (M). The primary tumor is carcinoma of the lung.

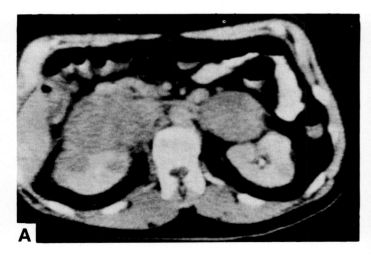

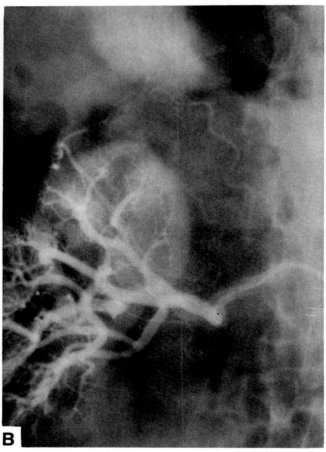

FIG. 15-13. (A) Bilateral masses involving the adrenals and invading the right kidney. The CT scan clearly outlines the masses. The inferior vena cava is encompassed in the mass and cannot be identified. The outline of the aorta is ill-defined because of the presence of retroperitoneal lymph nodes. (B) Despite the extensive disease seen on the CT scan, the angiogram done one day later barely shows any abnormalities. Biopsy showed that it was a histiocytic lymphoma that involved both adrenals and the right kidney and retroperitoneal lymph nodes.

tially serious complications. Therefore, when adrenal lesions are suspected, the most accurate diagnostic study is CT (Figure 15-14). While at first glance it may be tempting to perform less expensive procedures first, such a decision is not cost-effective. Plain films or IVPs are nonspecific; therefore, regardless of the results, the findings will have to be confirmed with CT or ultrasound.

This will often involve additional hospitalization days and consequently increase costs. For these reasons, in this institution, we recommend a CT scan as the first examination. If the results are positive and surgery is contemplated, the vascularity may be mapped by angiography or, in hormonally active tumors, samples of blood may be obtained from the adrenal veins for subse-

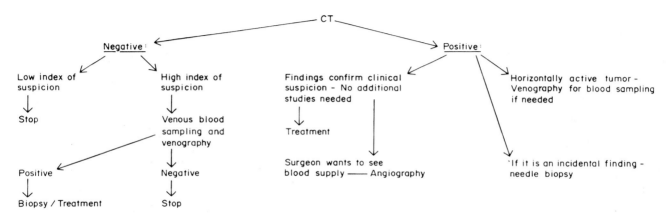

FIG. 15-14. Decision tree for radiologic workup of adrenal lesions.

quent hormonal assays. If the CT scan is normal, no other radiologic tests are needed, since none is likely to show a lesion.

Retroperitoneal Tumors

The most important factor in the differential diagnosis of adrenal tumors is other retroperitoneal tumors, most of which are soft tissue sarcomas. The pathology and behavior and classification patterns of these tumors will be discussed in the soft tissue sarcoma chapter in more detail. Early diagnosis of retroperitoneal tumors is uncommon because the tumors do not generally manifest themselves until they reach significant size. Similarly, because the retroperitoneum is almost inaccessible to physical diagnosis, early changes are not recognized. Etiologic factors in the formation of the soft tissue sarcomas are unknown. Most retroperitoneal neoplasms are malignant from the outset and are not felt to develop from pre-existing benign tumors. Exceptions are malignant neurilemomas, which develop in patients with neurofibromatosis. Angiosarcomas have been reported to develop from benign angiomas after radiation therapy.[37]

Retroperitoneal tumors have been classified according to their tissue of origin. Their much-simplified classification, modified from Stout's, is presented in Table 15-3. When distinct cellular components can be identified, the classification is relatively simple; however, in a significant number of tumors the exact histogenesis is impossible to determine. The reasons suggested by Morton and Eilber[37] are that many tumors are derived from primitive mesenchyma and tend to undergo metaplasia, thereby making classification difficult. This is especially true for fibroblastic cells, which have a great potential for stromal proliferation. Other sarcomas may contain several different types of cells or may vary in histologic appearance in different portions of the same tumor. The more anaplastic neoplasms are often so undifferentiated that the exact histogenesis cannot be determined. These tumors maintain the characteristics of spindle cells and are then classified as spindle cell sarcomas or undifferentiated sarcomas.

Early diagnosis is rare because the tumors usually grow slowly and are only recognized when they reach a large size. Pressure on nerves, the urinary tract, or the GI system may be the first clinical sign. These masses are usually not tender and are frequently well encapsulated. They are firm and hard, although liposarcomas may occasionally be soft. Metastases usually occur through the bloodstream. Another way of spread is through local infiltration and invasion of surrounding organs. Regional lymph node involvement is observed in 5% to 20% of cases.

The clinical behavior of all retroperitoneal sarcomas

is fairly similar. A few specific comments about the more commonly encountered retroperitoneal tumors are included here.

Liposarcoma. Liposarcomas are the most common malignant tumors in the retroperitoneum. They occur with increasing frequency in advanced age. The malignant variety of adipose tumors is usually firmer than the benign, may be multicentric, and often has a pseudocapsule. Nodal metastases occur in about 10% of cases. Microscopically, the degree of differentiation may vary from well-differentiated lesions to the anaplastic variety. Survival rate depends on the types of cells; it is about 80% with surgical treatment of well-differentiated lesions, but there is only approximately a 20% five-year survival in patients with poorly differentiated liposarcomas. Treatment is predominantly surgical.

Fibrosarcoma. According to Morton and Eilber,[37] fibrosarcomas are the second most frequently encountered soft tissue retroperitoneal tumors. These tumors are quite firm and are usually surrounded by a pseudocapsule. They tend to invade locally as well as to metastasize via the bloodstream to the lungs. Regional lymph nodes are involved in approximately 10% of cases. Microscopically, fibrosarcomas may be well differentiated, and these have the best prognosis; however, highly anaplastic lesions may also be found, and these are likely to metastasize early and are highly lethal. The primary treatment is surgical resection. Radiologically, the different retroperitoneal tumors appear identical, and generally one type of tumor cannot be differentiated from the other.

Table 15-3. Retroperitoneal Tumors

TISSUE	MALIGNANT TUMOR
Fibrous	Fibrosarcoma
Adipose	Liposarcoma
Smooth muscle	Leiomyosarcoma
Striated muscle	Rhabdomyosarcoma
Blood lymphatic vessels	Angiosarcoma
	Lymphangiosarcoma
	Hemangiopericytoma
Nervous tissue	Neurolymoma
	Schwannoma
Heterotrophic bone	Osteogenic sarcoma
	Chondrosarcoma
Undifferentiated cells	Myxoma
	Mesenchymoma

Modified from Morton, D. L., Eilber, F. R.: Soft tissue sarcomas. In *Cancer Medicine*, 2nd ed., Holland, J. F., Frei, E. (Eds.). Philadelphia, Lea & Febiger, 1982, pp. 2141–2145.

Exceptions are liposarcomas with large amounts of fat within them, if this is recognized either on plain films as a lucency or on CT scans as tissues with Hounsfield numbers in the range of fat.

The general principles discussed in the diagnosis of tumor of the adrenals also apply to the retroperitoneum.

Imaging Procedures

Conventional studies. Plain films of the abdomen are usually of little value unless the tumor is very large, displaces organs, obliterates the psoas margins, or contains calcifications. As with tumors of the adrenals, the most sensitive conventional radiographic examination is the intravenous urogram. As mentioned earlier in this chapter, intravenous urograms should only be considered as useful examinations if more sensitive examinations such as CT or ultrasound are not available. Because of the retroperitoneal location of the kidneys, tumors arising in this region will affect their position. However, in contrast to adrenal tumors, which almost always dis-

place the kidney downward, the renal displacement of retroperitoneal sarcomas will depend on the location of the tumor; therefore, the kidney may be displaced in almost any direction (Figure 15-15). The tumors may invade the kidneys, pancreas, or diaphragm, and if this occurs it may be difficult to decide if the tumor originated in these organs or if it was a primary retroperitoneal tumor. Barium studies similarly are nonspecific and merely show the displacement of the stomach, small bowel, or colon by an extrinsic mass.

Angiography. Angiography has been of limited value in retroperitoneal sarcomas. Some tumors are quite vascular and in these instances an angiogram will clearly define the tumor. Many of the tumors are almost totally avascular, however, and in these, angiography will be of little or no value. Venography has no value in the workup of retroperitoneal sarcomas.[7,28,29,42]

Computed Tomography. The examination of choice in the diagnosis of retroperitoneal tumors is computed to-

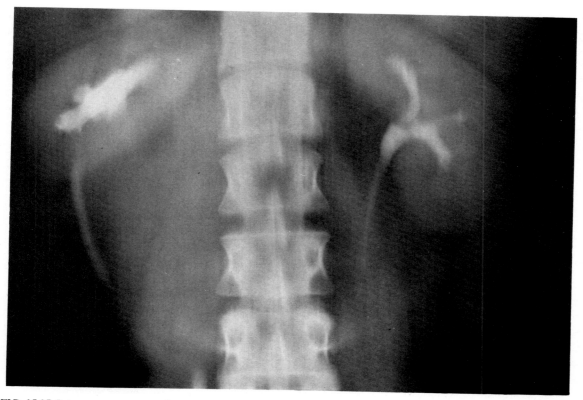

FIG. 15-15. Intravenous urogram of a patient with a large retroperitoneal sarcoma. Notice how the right kidney is pushed laterally and cranially. The right kidney is also rotated along its long axis, affecting the position of the ureter. Despite the presence of a very large mass, there are only minimal changes in the density of the retroperitoneum. The diagnosis would be difficult to make were it not for the grossly abnormal position of the kidney.

mography.[42,47] Because of the abundance of fat and the relatively uncomplicated anatomy, the retroperitoneal space is well suited for examination by computed tomography. In most instances CT diagnosis is obvious and easily made (Figure 15-16). In addition to detecting the tumor and its exact size, location and effect on adjacent structures and organs, the presence or absence of distant metastases can be readily assessed (Figures 15-17 through 15-19). With the exception of liposarcoma, CT is usually not able to differentiate the type of tumor present. The nature of a fatty tumor can be recognized in about 50% of cases, since the absorption coefficient of fat is lower than that of other soft tissue tumors. Many tumors have necrotic centers and these are easily recognized. The necrotic center appears as an area of lower density within the tumor. A CT-guided aspiration biopsy is a quick, safe, and accurate way to rapidly establish a correct histologic diagnosis.

Ultrasound. Ultrasound is capable of detecting many retroperitoneal tumors. However, because the detail and relationship to surrounding organs are so much clearer on CT scans, most clinicians favor CT. In our institution, CT is considered the examination of choice, and is commonly the only radiographic test done on patients with retroperitoneal tumors.

TREATMENT DECISIONS

Since 1960, the advent of o,p'-DDD mitotane has turned the treatment of adrenal cancer into a multimodal venture. The mainstay of treatment is surgery, since this can be curative in approximately 50% of the patients.[51]

Surgery

An aggressive surgical approach should be used for en bloc resection of an adrenal tumor. This may include, depending upon the location of the tumor, the spleen, kidney, and part of the pancreas, which requires a large exposure, often through a thoracoabdominal approach as in the radical removal of renal cancers. This is particularly true for nonfunctioning tumors, which can be large in size. In addition, metastatic deposits, especially in the liver, should be resected, since they may improve survival.[4]

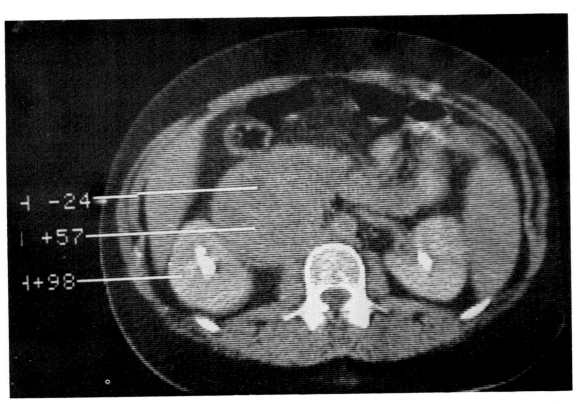

FIG. 15-16. Fibrolipoma of the retroperitoneum. Notice the different densities within the tumor. Some areas show fat density while others show typical soft tissue density. The tumor is less dense than the kidneys. This CT scan shows that the tumor is pushing but not invading the right kidney. There is no clear margin between the tumor and the right psoas muscle, and the inferior vena cava is probably surrounded by the tumor. The tumor reaches the medial aspect of the aorta.

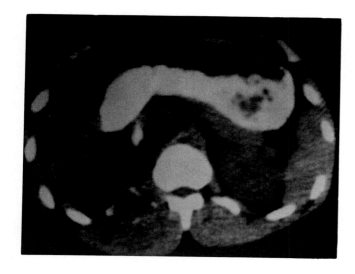

FIG. 15-17. Chondrosarcoma arising from a rib. The tumor invades the psoas muscle and the erector trunci muscles on the right. The kidney is pushed anteriorly and laterally.

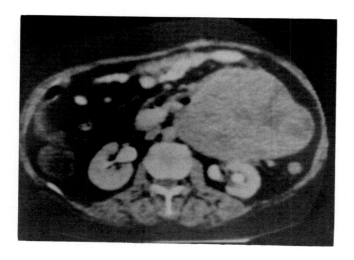

FIG. 15-18. Malignant neurofibrosarcoma in the retroperitoneum. The lucent areas within the tumor are regions of necrosis. The kidney is pushed posteriorly but is not invaded. A thin capsule around the tumor can be identified. The tumor is abutting the aorta, but at surgery it could be separated from the vessel.

Radiation therapy

Retroperitoneal tumors generally are not very radiosensitive. Although preoperative or postoperative radiation therapy has been attempted, it is mainly used for palliative purposes, since, except to very small volumes, this is a difficult area in which to achieve high dose radiation. If such an attempt is made to eradicate residual disease, CT treatment planning is desirable to allow very precise aiming of the radiation.

Chemotherapy

O,p'-DDD (1,1-dichloro-2(o-chlorophenyl)-2-(p-chlorophenyl)ethane) mitotane has induced regression in both primary and metastatic tumor sites.[9,31] The tumor, particularly if it is functioning, may result in atrophy of the contralateral side. When this event is coupled with o,p'-DDD mitotane it could lead to Addisonian syndromes if a response occurs. The major management policy is to monitor the plasma levels carefully and to be sure that full glucocorticoid and mineral corticoid replacements are given in order to prevent adrenal insufficiency. Other chemotherapeutic agents include cyclophosphamides, nitrosourea, doxorubicin, and cisplatin.[19,49]

Retroperitoneal soft tissue sarcomas are managed in a similar fashion to the principles outlined in the soft tissue sarcoma chapter. The major difficulty in the use of preoperative and postoperative irradiation is with regard to the volume of vital viscera that may be included in the retroperitoneal treatment field. Liver and kidney tolerances are below the level of effective tumor doses, which would limit the volume of these organs to be included in the treatment field. Careful imaging of vital structures as well as the tumor bed, particularly through the use of CT scans for treatment planning, is essential to achieve the desired dose levels.[43]

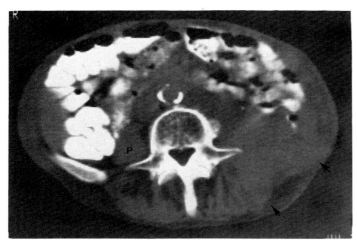

FIG. 15-19. A patient with non-Hodgkin lymphoma diffusely involving the retroperitoneum. Note that in addition to lymph node involvement, the tumor has infiltrated the left psoas muscle and back muscles (arrows). Compare the back muscles on the left with the normal-appearing ones on the right (P = right psoas). Such accurate detail about the extent of the tumor and involvement of adjacent organs could not have been achieved by any other method.

REFERENCES

1. Abrams, H. L., Siegleman, S. S., Adams, D. F., Sanders, R., Finberg, H. J., Hessel, S. J., McNeil, B. J.: Computed tomography versus ultrasound of the adrenal gland: A prospective study. *Radiology* 143:121-128, 1982.

2. Alfidi, R. J., Gill, W. M., Klein, H. J.: Arteriography of adrenal neoplasms. *A.J.R.* 106:635-641, 1969.

3. Bernardino, M. E., Goldstein, H. M., Green, B.: Gray scale ultrasonography of adrenal neoplasms. *A.J.R.* 130:741-744, 1978.

4. Bradley, E. L.: Primary and adjunctive therapy in carcinoma of the adrenal cortex. *Surg. Gynecol. Obstet.* 141:507-511, 1975.

5. Brennan, M. F.: Cancer of the endocrine system: The adrenal gland. In *Cancer: Principles and Practice of Oncology.* DeVita, V. T., Jr., Hellman, S., Rosenberg, S. A. (Eds.) Philadelphia, J.B. Lippincott, 1982, pp. 985-1000.

6. Brownlie, K., Kreel, L.: Computer assisted tomography of normal suprarenal glands. *J. Comput. Assist. Tomogr.* 2:1-10, 1978.

7. Damascelli, B., Musumeci, R., Botturi, M., Petrillo, R., Spagnoli, I.: Angiography of retroperitoneal tumors: A review. *Radiology* 124:565-570, 1975.

8. Didolkar, M. S., Bescher, R. A., Elias, E. G., Moore, R. H.: Natural history of adrenal cortical carcinoma: A clinico-pathologic study of 42 patients. *Cancer* 47:2153-2161, 1981.

9. Dluhy, R. G., Barlow, J. J., Mahoney, E. M., Shirley, R. L., Williams, G.: Profile and possible origin of the adrenocortical carcinoma. *J. Clin. Endocrinol. Metab.* 33:312-317, 1971.

10. Dunnick, N. R., Doppman, J. L., Gill, J. R., Jr., Strott, C. A., Keiser, H. R., Brennan, M. F.: Localization of functional adrenal tumors by computed tomography and venous sampling. *Radiology* 142:429-433, 1982.

11. Dunnick, N. R., Doppman, J. L., Mills, S. R., Gill, J. R., Jr.: Preoperative diagnosis and localization of aldosteronomas by measurement of corticosteroids in adrenal venous blood. *Radiology* 133:331-333, 1979.

12. Dunnick, N. R., Heaston, D. K., Halvorsen, R., Moore, A. V., Korobkin, M.: CT appearance of adrenal cortical carcinoma. *J. Comput. Assist. Tomogr.* 6:978-982, 1982.

13. Dunnick, N. R., Schaner, E. G., Doppman, J. L., Strott, C. A., Gill, J. R., Jr., Javadpour, N.: Computed tomography in adrenal tumors. *A.J.R.* 132:43-46, 1979.

14. Emmett, J. L., Witten, D. M.: *Clinical Urography—An Atlas and Textbook of Roentgenologic Diagnosis.* 3rd ed., vol. 2. Philadelphia, W.B. Saunders, 1971, pp. 1211, 1230-1232.

15. Francis, I. R., Glazer, G. M., Shapiro, B., Sisson, J. C., Gross, B. H.: Complementary roles of CT and ^{131}I-MIBH scintigraphy in diagnosing pheochromocytoma. *A.J.R.* 141:719-725, 1983.

16. Geisinger, M. A., Zelch, M. G., Bravo, E. L., Risius, B. F., O'Donovan, P. B., Borkowski, G. P.: Primary hyperaldosteronism: Comparison of CT, adrenal venography, and venous sampling. *A.J.R.* 141:299-302, 1983.

17. Glazer, H. S., Weyman, P. J., Sagel, S. S., Levitt, R. G., McClennan, B. L.: Nonfunctioning adrenal masses: Incidental discovery on computed tomography. *A.J.R.* 139: 81-85, 1982.

18. Greenfield, A. J.: Transcatheter Embolization of Neoplasms. In *Interventional Radiology.* Athanasoulis, C. A., Pfister, R. C., Greenes, R. E., Roberson, G. H. (Eds.). Philadelphia, W.B. Saunders, 1982, pp. 228-242.

19. Hag, M. M., Legha, S. S., Samaan, N. A.: Adrenal cortical carcinoma: A study of 32 patients. *Cancer* 35:549-554, 1975.

20. Harrison, J. H., Mahoney, E. M.: Adrenal cortex and medulla. In *Cancer Medicine,* 2nd ed. Holland, J. F., Frei, E. (Eds.) Philadelphia, Lea & Febiger, 1982, pp. 1867-1873.

21. Huebener, K. H., Treugut, H.: Adrenal cortex dysfunction: CT findings. *Radiology* 150:195-199, 1984.

22. Jensen, S. R., Novelline, R. A., Brewster, D. C., Bonventre, J. V.: Transient renal artery stenosis produced by a pheochromocytoma. *Radiology* 144:767-768, 1982.

23. Kahn, P. C., Kelleher, M. D., Egdahl, R. H., Melby, J. C.: Adrenal arteriography and venography in primary aldosteronism. *Radiology* 101:71-78, 1971.

24. Kahn, P. C., Nickrosz, L. V.: Selective angiography of the adrenal glands. *A.J.R.* 101:739-749, 1967.

25. Karstaedt, N., Sagel, S. S., Stanley, R. J., Melson, G. L., Levitt, R. G.: Computed tomography of the adrenal gland. *Radiology* 129:723-730, 1978.

26. Korobkin, M., White, E. A., Kressel, H. Y., Moss, A. A., Montagne, J. P.: Computed tomography in the diagnosis of adrenal disease. *A.J.R.* 132:231-238, 1979.

27. Laursen, K., Damgaard-Pedersen, K.: CT for pheochromocytoma diagnosis. *A.J.R.* 134:277-280, 1980.

28. Levin, D. C., Gordon, D. H., Kinkhabwala, M., Becker, J. A.: Arteriography of retroperitoneal lymphoma. *A.J.R.* 126:368-375, 1976.

29. Levin, D. C., Watson, R. C., Baltaxe, H. A.: Arteriography of retroperitoneal masses. *Radiology* 108:543-551, 1973.

30. Lieberman, L. M., Beierwalters, M. D., Conn, J. W., Ansari, A. N., Nishiyama, H.: Diagnosis of adrenal disease by visualization of human adrenal glands with 131-I-19-Iodocholesterol. *N. Engl. J. Med.* 285:1387-1393, 1971.

31. Lubitz, J. A., Freeman, L., Okun, R.: Mitotane use in operable adrenal cortical carcinoma. *J.A.M.A.* 223:1109-1112, 1973.

32. MacFarlane, P. A.: Cancer of the adrenal cortex. The natural history, prognosis and treatment in a study of 55 cases. *Ann. R. Coll. Surg. Engl.* 23:155-186, 1958.

33. McLachlan, M. S. F., Beales, J. S. M.: Retroperitoneal pneumography in the investigation of adrenal disease. *Clin. Radiol.* 22:188-197, 1971.

34. Mikaelsson, C. G.: Epinephro-phlebography of benign tumours. *Acta Radiol.* 8:129-145, 1969.

35. Mitnick, J. S., Bosniak, M. A., Megibow, A. J., Naidich, D. P.: Nonfunctioning adrenal adenomas discovered incidentally on computed tomography. *Radiology* 148:495-499, 1983.

36. Montagne, J. P., Kressel, H. Y., Korobkin, M., Moss, A. A.: Com-

puted tomography of the normal adrenal glands. *A.J.R.* **130**:963–966, 1978.

37. Morton, D. L., Eilber, F. R.: Soft tissue sarcomas. In *Cancer Medicine*, 2nd ed. Holland, J. F., Frei, E. (Eds.). Philadelphia, Lea & Febiger, 1982, pp. 2141–2145.

38. Nielsen, M. E., Jr., Heaston, D. K., Dunnick, N. R., Korobkin, M.: Preoperative CT evaluation of adrenal glands in non-small cell bronchogenic carcinoma. *A.J.R.* **139**:317–320, 1982.

39. Paling, M. R., Williamson, B. R. J.: Adrenal involvement in non-hodgkin lymphoma. *A.J.R.* **141**:303–305, 1983.

40. Reuter, S. R., Blair, A. J., Schteingart, D. E., Bookstein, J. J.: Adrenal venography. *Radiology* **89**:805–814, 1967.

41. Richie, J. P., Gittes, R. F.: Carcinoma of the adrenal cortex. *Cancer* **45**:1957–1964, 1980.

42. Rubinstein, Z., Kreel, L.: Mass lesions of the retroperitoneum (excluding specific organs). *CT* **3**:180–188, 1979.

43. Russell, W. O., Cohen, J., Enzinger, S., Hajdu, S. I., Heise, H., Martin, R. G., Meissnel, W., Miller, W. G., Schmidt, R. L., Suit, H. C.: The clinical pathological staging system for soft tissue sarcoma. *Cancer* **40**:1562, 1977.

44. Sample, W. F.: Adrenal ultrasonography. *Radiology* **127**:461–466, 1978.

45. Sandler, M. A., Pearlberg, J. L., Madrazo, B. L., Gitschlag, K. F., Gross, S. C.: Computed tomographic evaluation of the adrenal gland in the preoperative assessment of bronchogenic carcinoma. *Radiology* **145**:733–736, 1982.

46. Seabold, J. E., Haynie, T. P., De Asis, D. M., Sosmaan, N. A., Glen, A. J., Johns, M. F.: Detection of metastatic adrenal carcinoma using ^{131}I-B-Iodomethyl-19-Norcholesterol total body scans. *J. Clin.*

Endocrinol. Metab. **45**:788–797, 1977.

47. Stephens, D. H., Sheedy, P. F., Hattery, R. R., II, Williamson, A. B., Jr.: Diagnosis and evaluation of retroperitoneal tumors by computed tomography. *A.J.R.* **129**:395–402, 1977.

48. Sullivan, M., Bioleau, M., Hodges, C. V.: Adrenal cortical carcinoma. *J. Urol.* **120**:660–665, 1978.

49. Tattersall, M. H., Lander, H., Bain, B., Stocks, A. E., Woods, R. L., Fox, R. M., Byrne, E., Trotten, J. R., Roos, I.: Cis-platinum treatment of metastatic adrenal carcinoma. *Med. J. Aust.* **1**:419–421, 1980.

50. Thomas, J. L., Bernardino, M. E., Samaan, N. A., Hickey, R. C.: CT of pheochromocytoma. *A.J.R.* **135**:477–482, 1980.

51. Ureles, A. L., Chang, A. Y. C., Sherman, C. D., Jr., Constine, L. S., III: Cancer of the endocrine glands: Thyroid, adrenal and pituitary. In *Clinical Oncology for Medical Students and Physicians: A Multidisciplinary Approach.* 6th ed. Rubin, P. (Ed.). American Cancer Society, 1983, pp. 326–345.

52. Welch, T. J., Sheedy, P. F., vanHeerden, J. A., Sheps, S. G., Hattery, R. R., Stephens, D. H.: Pheochromocytoma: Value of computed tomography. *Radiology* **148**:501–503, 1983.

53. Wilms, G., Baert, A., Marchal, G., Goddeeris, P.: Computed tomography of the normal adrenal glands: Correlative study with autopsy specimens. *J. Comput. Assist. Tomogr.* **3**:467–469, 1979.

54. Yeh, H. C., Mitty, H. A., Rose, J., Wolf, B. S., Gabrilove, J. L.: Ultrasonography of adrenal masses: Usual features. *Radiology* **127**:467–474, 1978.

55. Yeh, H. C., Mitty, H. A., Rose, J., Wolf, B. S., Gabrilove, J. L.: Ultrasonography of adrenal masses: Unusual manifestations. *Radiology* **127**:475–483, 1978.

16 KIDNEY AND URETER

Bruce L. McClennan
Dennis M. Balfe

Malignant tumors of the kidney account for 2% to 3% of all neoplasms in humans. Renal cell carcinomas (hypernephromas, renal adenocarcinomas) account for 85% of all kidney tumors.[91] According to the American Cancer Society, there were to have been 18,400 new cases of kidney and other urinary tract neoplasms and 8,700 subsequent tumor-related deaths in 1984.[86] Renal cell carcinoma is two to three times more prevalent in men than in women and occurs most frequently in the sixth decade of life.[54] Interestingly, renal cell carcinoma is being seen more frequently in younger individuals. Recent data from the M.D. Anderson Hospital computed from a review of 890 cases of renal cell carcinoma showed a significant increase in the proportion of patients with renal cell carcinoma in the 42 to 49 year age range.[77] The diagnosis of renal cell carcinoma is also being made with an increasing frequency in young adults and adolescents.[1,31,60]

A diagnosis of renal cell cancer is often made serendipitously and remains a daily challenge. Between 15% and 30% of cases are discovered as a result of nonurologic symptoms.[52,91] The classic triad of hematuria, pain, and a mass in the flank is present is less than 20% of cases.[52] The existence of this triad confers an ominous prognosis.[88] About a third of patients will have metastatic disease that is clinically apparent at the time of the diagnosis, and close to another 30% of patients will have occult micrometastases.[91]

Renal cell carcinoma is a relatively radioresistant tumor that is treated surgically with or without adjunctive medical therapy.[44] The stage and grade of a tumor are much more significant prognostic features than the choice of treatment.[13,80,91] Survival is definitely related to the extent of the tumor and the presence or absence of distant metastases. Once metastatic disease develops, survival depends on the extent of the disease and the disease-free interval (time from nephrectomy to detection of metastases).[13,80,91] Although renal cell carcinoma may have a peculiar natural history (including isolated spontaneous regression), most patients have a short, progressive downhill course once metastasis occurs.[13,44,52,55,67,80,91]

Overall five-year survival is improved with radical as opposed to simple nephrectomy, since an improvement in the five-year survival rate from 32% to 66.6% has been shown with radical surgery.[80] Complete excision of the tumor is essential because of the high association between local recurrence and lymph node involvement.[91] Local recurrence most likely represents persistent cancer in regional lymph nodes rather than true recurrence.[27,91] On the other hand, palliative surgery, which can carry up to a 6% mortality, has not proved beneficial for patients with distant metastases unless the metastasis is solitary.[27] Increased survival has been reported with solitary pulmonary, bony, and soft tissue metastases.[27,67]

While computerized techniques, i.e., computed tomography (CT), have been recently applied to the imaging of renal cell cancer, computerized analysis of survival has provided useful information for guiding and gauging our oncologic imaging approach. DeKernion et al.[27] reviewed 86 patients with metastatic renal cell carcinoma using computer data banking. Cumulative survival was 43% at one year, 26% at two years, and 13% at five years.[27]

Metastasis confined to the lung only, absence of local recurrence, and a long disease-free interval favorably affected survival. Most of their patients who had local recurrences (86%) died within one year.[27] Boxer et al.,[13] who also used a computer analysis technique, studied a group of 96 patients with renal cell carcinoma treated by nephrectomy. Local or distant metastases were present in 52 patients. Cumulative survival rates for nonmetastatic renal cell carcinoma (stage I–III patients) was 95% at one year, 61% at five years, and 47% at 10 years.[13] Five-year survival for stage IV disease was only 5% in their series.[13]

Other tumors that involve the kidney include transitional cell carcinomas, lymphomas, and a variety of rare benign and malignant neoplasms. Transitional cell carcinomas, although uncommon, account for between 4.5% and 9% of all renal tumors.[35] Transitional cell carcinoma is a disease of the elderly with a mean age at the time of diagnosis of 61.4 years.[73] A male predominance pattern exists, with ratios of between 1.8 : 1 and 3.5 : 1 male-to-female distribution.[35,73] Primary ureteral tumors are even more uncommon, accounting for only 1% of all upper urinary tract neoplasms.[38,78] This amounts to an estimated 850 to 1,700 new cases of transitional cell cancer in the upper urinary tract in 1980 according to the ACS.[29] Like renal cell carcinomas, a significant number of transitional cell carcinomas of the upper urinary tract are advanced at the time of the initial diagnosis (up to 50% have invaded muscle).[30,73] Concurrent bladder or ureteral cancer exists in between 30% and 50% of patients with transitional cell carcinoma of the renal pelvis, and 3% to 4% will have cancer in the contralateral pelvis or ureter. Multiplicity of tumors is an important consideration because patients with multicentric urothelial tumors have a 50% chance of developing invasive cancer.[43,53]

Papillary transitional cell carcinoma is the most commonly encountered renal pelvic tumor and is also the most common ureteral tumor, occurring frequently in the distal ureter.[25] The thin distal ureteral and renal pelvic wall and the rich network of lymphatic channels contribute to early and extensive spread of tumor and, accordingly, very poor survival with high grade and high stage transitional cell tumors.[25] Bloom and associates reported a five-year survival rate for patients with carcinoma of the ureter of only 61.8% for stage I disease, 25% for stage II disease, 33% for stage III disease, and 0% five-year survival for stage IV disease.[12] Stage and grade are as vitally important for transitional cell carcinomas as they are for renal cell carcinomas.[25,48,98] In a recent Mayo Clinic series by Murphy and coworkers of 224 patients with transitional cell carcinomas of the upper urinary tract, 49 (22%) had low grade (I) cancers. Of these 49 patients, 96% had low stage (I) disease. In this select group of patients, survival was identical to age-matched disease-free controls.[74] These data have strong implications both for the choice of treatment options (i.e., local versus radi-

cal surgery) and the diagnostic imaging approach. Conservative surgery seems to be indicated for low grade, low stage disease involving the urothelium.[39,74] In addition, radical surgery seems to be of little benefit in patients with high grade (3 and 4) transitional cell carcinomas when compared with simple nephrectomy or partial ureterectomy.[25,74] While controversy still justifiably exists regarding treatment options, all viewpoints support the contention that accurate and reliable preoperative or intraoperative diagnostic staging techniques are required. An understanding of the natural history of both the primary tumor, particularly for transitional cell carcinoma, and adjacent and distant urothelial involvement is essential to the choice of treatment.[25,65,76]

Survival rates for transitional cell carcinoma of the kidney and ureter are mainly affected by the presence of muscle invasion. The survival rates range from 62% to 91% for stage 0 and A, 43% to 50% for stage B, 23% to 33% for stage C, and 0% for stage D disease.[6,12,74]

The impact of the newer imaging techniques, specifically computed tomography (CT), has been profound on both the diagnosis and management of renal cell carcinomas and transitional cell carcinomas.[7,96,100] Low stage tumors can often be separated from high stage tumors, thereby yielding a more thoughtful and efficacious approach to therapy than was heretofore possible. However, intravenous urography with tomography still remains the backbone of the diagnostic process for detection of renal and ureteral neoplasms. Retrograde pyeloureterography and other interventional procedures often complement urograms and increase diagnostic confidence by providing cytopathologic confirmation. Computed tomography and ultrasonography have enhanced the detection role of intravenous urograms.[24,100] Because of the unique cross-sectional anatomy displayed by CT, the evaluation process for the patient with urologic symptoms of a neoplasm often includes CT at the outset of the diagnostic work up (Figure 16-1). Renal tumors on the anterior or posterior aspect of a kidney may be missed even with excellent urography or angiography.[79] Renal CT is easy to perform, fast, and free from operator dependence. It has met with ready clinician acceptance for both the detection of renal neoplasms and subsequent diagnosis and staging. Early detection and diagnosis of renal tumors can only have a positive effect on patient outcome. Computed tomography, and, to a lesser extent, ultrasonography, appear to be playing just such a positive role. The overall diagnostic accuracy for CT scanning in separating renal cysts from neoplasms is extremely high, approaching 95% in our experience.[96] Valuable staging information and follow-up surveillance now can be provided to clinicians for oncologic evaluation in a nearly noninvasive fashion. Using CT scanning, other more invasive and expensive imaging tests such as arteriography or venography may be obviated. Although insufficient data exist to date on the ultimate impact of CT

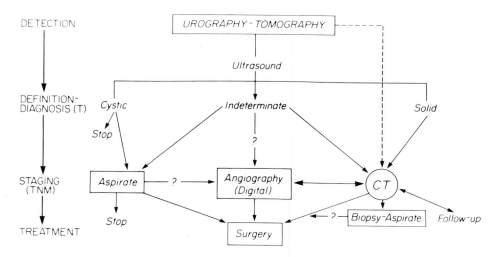

FIG. 16-1. Imaging evaluation for renal tumors. Intravenous urography with tomography is the best screening test for detecting renal cancer. Ultrasonography occupies a major triage position in the decision tree. Computed tomographic scanning can supplement ultrasonography or obviate it in many cases of renal cancer. Interventional procedures such as angiography, although rarely needed, can often be done with digital imaging techniques.

on overall cumulative survival statistics, a review of the myriad articles confirming improved survival with low stage, low grade neoplasms of the upper urinary tract will demonstrate that the role of cross-sectional imaging procedures like CT will continue to be a vital one.

TUMOR BEHAVIOR AND PATHOLOGY

Primary epithelial cancers of the kidney are generally considered to arise from the proximal convoluted tubule in the case of renal cell carcinomas or from the urothelial lining in the case of transitional cell carcinomas.[40] There does not appear to be any convincing evidence that renal cancers originate in the distal nephron or collecting ducts. Synchronous discovery of both types of neoplasms has been reported.[66,87] Multicentric or multifocal occurrence of tumors having the same cell type is not uncommon.[23] Renal cell carcinoma is usually separated by cytoplasmic pattern into (1) a clear cell variety, (2) a granular cell variety, (3) a mixed cell variety, and (4) a sarcomatoid variety. Most (46%) renal cell carcinomas are of the mixed and granular cell types.[91] Clear cell varieties account for another 25%, and pure granular cell types account for another 15%.[1] Sarcomatoid or spindle cell tumors make up the remaining 14% of renal cell carcinomas.[91]

Clear cell carcinomas appear to have a better five-year survival (58%) when compared with pure granular cell or mixed cell renal cell carcinomas (46%).[75,88] This remains controversial, but an increased percentage of clear cells in a renal cell carcinoma seems to improve survival in the first three stages (I–III).[13] Sarcomatoid or spindle cell tumors have a much worse prognosis (23% five-year

survival at best), probably because these tumors are usually of high histologic grade.[91] The same reasoning may apply to mixed or granular cell and clear cell cancers, since the latter are usually of lower histologic grade.[91] Patients with tumors of a granular or mixed histologic type are more likely to have metastases at the time of diagnosis or to later develop metastases than are patients with clear cell cancers.

A variety of tumor growth patterns typically exists: papillary, trabecular, tubular, cystic, or solid. These patterns are unrelated to behavior except for the papillary forms.[6,91] Some authors consider the papillary adenocarcinoma almost unique because of its typical papillary architecture, sparse vascularity, and less aggressive histologic potential (Figure 16-2).[6] A five-year survival rate of up to 85% has been described with papillary tubular adenocarcinomas, which account for between 5% and 15% of all renal cell carcinomas.[6,91] Necrosis and cystic degeneration as well as calcification are common features of papillary adenocarcinomas.[91] Most patients (up to 80%) with papillary adenocarcinomas have low stage (stage I or II) disease compared with only about 50% of patients with nonpapillary architecture.[6]

The ultimate malignant potential of a renal cell carcinoma or a transitional cell carcinoma is determined by its grade. Grading systems for renal cell carcinomas are based on histologic pattern, cell size, cell shape, and nuclear morphology.[6,91] Individual grading is rated according to the most anaplastic area present in the specimen, but interestingly, it is not always the most malignant looking cells that metastasize.[72] The direct relationship of tumor grade and stage is consistently substantiated in the literature. High grade tumors are three times more

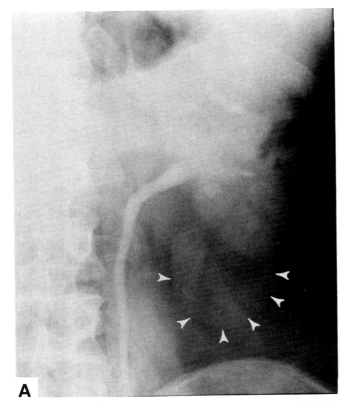

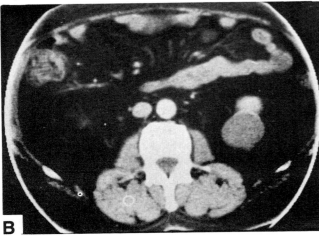

FIG. 16-2. Papillary renal cell carcinoma. (A) Coned-down intravenous urogram of left kidney revealed a renal mass (arrowheads) projecting off the lower pole. No calyceal distortion was noted. (B) CT scan after bolus injection of contrast material showed the lower pole renal mass on the left to be avascular. Note dense opacification of aorta (a). Pathologic examination revealed a papillary renal cell carcinoma.

ett, and others.[15,51,68,95] The concept of urothelial cancer as a "field change" phenomenon was first supported by Melicow, and gained credence with the observation that 30% to 50% of patients who develop renal pelvic transitional cell carcinomas will have cancer elsewhere in the urinary tract.[25,68]

Benign papillomas are tumors of uniform cell size closely resembling normal urothelium without evidence of basement membrane invasion.[25] These are rare lesions, with the more typical transitional cell carcinomas accounting for 90% or more of all upper urinary tract urothelial malignancies.[25] However, 25% of patients with solitary papillomas and 50% of patients with multiple papillomas will eventually develop transitional cell carcinomas. When a transitional cell carcinoma does occur, 50% will already be invasive when diagnosed. The many facets of the natural history of transitional cell carcinomas have serious implications for the imaging process (Figure 16-3).

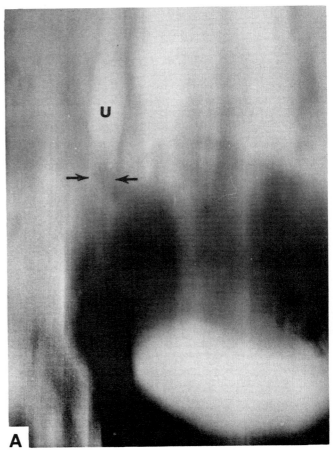

FIG. 16-3. Transitional cell carcinoma. (A) Intravenous urogram revealed delayed visualization of the right kidney and ureter (u). A tomogram showed right ureteral obstruction with an intraluminal mass (arrows). (B) A retrograde pyelogram shows a polypoid, ureteral tumor (arrow) with focal expansion of ureter above an area of sharp angulation, presumably caused by ureteral tethering by the external iliac artery. (C) A CT scan of the ureter at the level of the tumor shows an intraluminal mass (arrow) surrounded by contrast material ("donut sign"). No ex-

apt to have metastasized by the time of initial examination and two times more apt to develop metastases later or to involve the renal vein initially.[13,84,88]

Histopathologic assessment of transitional cell carcinomas is based on the criteria for benignity outlined by Vest and the criteria for malignancy detailed by Broders, Jew-

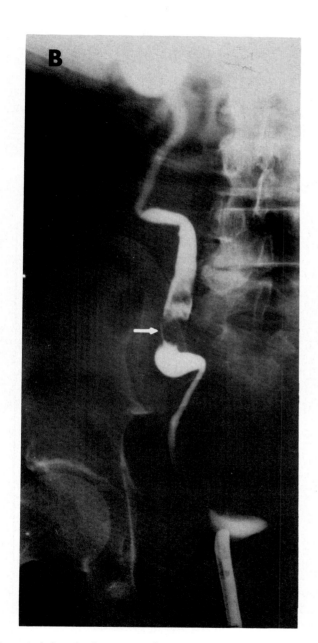

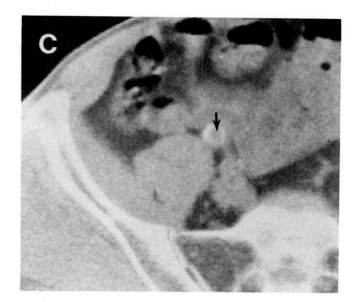

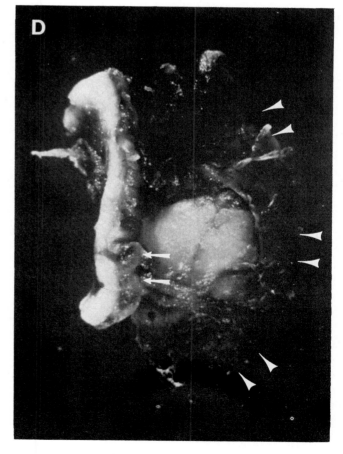

traureteric invasion is present and precise attachment to the ureteral wall is not discernible. (D) The pathologic specimen after local resection showed a low grade, low stage papillary ureteral cancer (arrowheads) arising from the mucosa of the ureter (arrows) but without muscle invasion.

Grading for malignant transitional cell carcinomas is usually done by categories 1 through 4, with well-differentiated papillary types being grade 1 and increasing degrees of anaplasia and infiltration culminating in a grade designation.[15,51,68,95] The character of the mucosa adjacent to known urothelial tumors is also very important.[65] The adjacent mucosal changes are generally not macroscopic and are therefore rarely detected. The incidence of mucosal abnormalities near known urothelial malignancies increases concomitantly with the grade and stage of the tumor. In a recent review of 60 ureteral tumors, all grade 1 tumors were stage 0.[48] All grade 1 and most of all grade 2 lesions were papillary, but grade 3 tumors frequently showed invasion with metastasis while being equally divided between solid and papillary architecture. All grade 1 transitional cell carcinomas had normal adjacent mucosa, but as the grade increased so did adjacent mucosal abnormalities, especially carcinoma in situ (CIS). Likewise, increasing stage of transitional cell carcinomas was associated with increasing mucosal abnormalities in adjacent urothelium.[48] While grade and stage were related to the occurrence of transitional cell carcinomas elsewhere in the urinary tract, abnormal adjacent urothelium was not associated with an increased incidence of additional urothelial tumors.[91] It appears that low grade, papillary transitional cell carcinomas have a much different overall biologic potential than high grade transitional cell carcinomas. This further underscores the need for accurate and early diagnosis.

A variety of other types of neoplasia involve the kidney and ureter (Figure 16-4). These run the gamut from benign adenomas (i.e., oncocytomas) to Wilm's tumors, but most are rare occurrences.[45,46,71] Renal adenomas are small, (less then 3 cm, by definition) and are well-differentiated cortical epithelial tumors arising from the proximal tubular epithelium. They are unencapsulated, with a papillary or solid pattern. Histologically, they are identical to renal cell carcinomas. They rarely metastasize (less than 6%).[91] Their incidence increases with age, and they are three times more common in men. Most are solitary, but 25% can be multiple.[91] Renal adenomas are frequent concomitant findings with renal cell carcinomas. They appear as solid intrarenal masses and are considered by most to be merely small renal cell carcinomas. On the other hand, renal oncocytomas are a separate, distinctive class of cortical adenoma having a larger size and different cellular pattern.[46,71] The cellular picture of an oncocytoma is one of cells with abundant cytoplasm containing large numbers of mitochondria. They have a well-developed capsule and are typically vascular. No cases of metastases have yet been reported, confirming their benign nature.[46,71,91]

Angiomyolipomas (AML) (Figure 16-5) are not uncommon hamartomas composed of varying proportions of fat, smooth muscle, and abnormal blood vessels. They

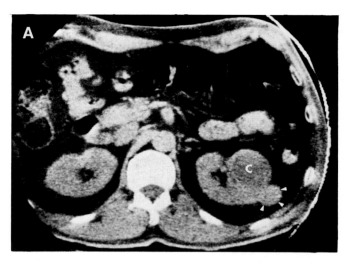

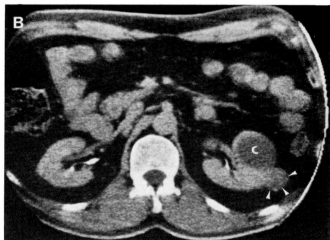

FIG. 16-4. Benign renal tumor (fibroma). (A) Precontrast scan demonstrates a 2-cm mass arising from the lateral surface of the left kidney (arrowheads). The mass has an attenuation value near that of soft tissue and appears solid. A renal cyst (c) is also present but is poorly seen on this scan because of volume averaging. (B) After administration of intravenous contrast, the cyst (c) is better seen. The benign fibroma (arrowheads) showed only minimal contrast enhancement.

tend to bleed but never demonstrate distant metastases. They too are solid renal masses when imaged, but their typical fat content often allows positive preoperative diagnosis.[92,94] Other benign but solid tumors such as leiomyomas and pheochromocytomas occur within the kidney but are extremely rare. They may mimic renal cell carcinomas, making nonoperative diagnosis almost impossible.

Other malignant tumors such as Wilm's tumors, lymphomas (Figure 16-6), and metastatic deposits have been encountered.[3,46,97] Wilm's tumor in adults mimics a renal cell carcinoma but has a worse prognosis than when encountered in children; the three-year survival in adults approaches 29% for all stages.[16,56] Wilm's tumor may be confused with metastatic disease to the kidney, especially small cell tumors such as lung cancer. A host of primary tumors may metastasize to the kidney and ureter, but lung and breast tumors are most common.[3] They are usually avascular and multiple in location. A lymphoma when it involves the kidney is usually part of a more diffuse or systemic disease process.[47] Renal lymphomas are most commonly of the non-Hodgkin variety, appearing as solitary or multiple nodules in and around the kidney. Renal involvement is often secondary and occurs in conjunction with bulky local extranodal disease.[47]

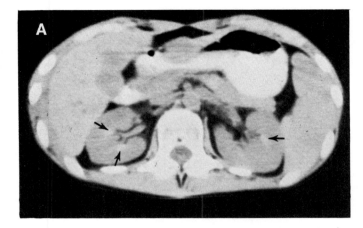

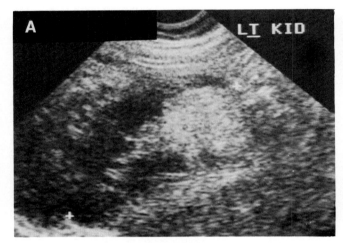

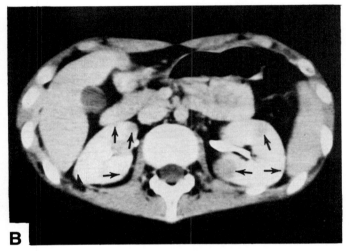

FIG. 16-6. Renal lymphoma. (A) A precontrast CT scan through both kidneys of a patient with known lymphoma shows normal kidneys. The hyperdense areas in the medullary portion of the kidneys (arrows) are thought to represent physiologic hyperconcentration of urine in the pyramids or early nephrocalcinosis. (B) After contrast material was given for enhancement of a suspicious liver lesion, both kidneys revealed focal involvement (arrows) by lymphoma that was undetectable without contrast material.

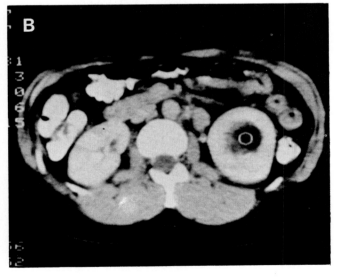

FIG. 16-5. Angiomyolipoma (AML). (A) A markedly echogenic left renal mass is seen on this longitudinal renal ultrasound scan. This finding is virtually pathognomonic of an AML, but some renal cell carcinomas may have this ultrasonic appearance. (B) A CT scan through the left renal mass shows a circular cursor over the fat density mass within the left kidney. Contrast material has been given and no enhancement of the mass is seen on this scan. This is a typical CT/US presentation of an AML.

Patterns of Spread

The pathways of spread for renal cell carcinomas fall into two general categories: one (Figure 16-7) is local extension into the surrounding parenchyma, veins, capsular investments, or perinephric spaces; the other is distant spread via renal lymphatics through hilar lymph nodes and beyond via lymphatic or vascular spread.[1] The size of a renal tumor does correlate with the incidence of metastatic disease, that is, tumors less than 5 to 6.5 cm in diameter uncommonly produce metastatic disease less than 8% of the time.[91] Tumors larger than 10 cm have up to an 80% incidence of metastatic disease at the time of diagnosis.[91]

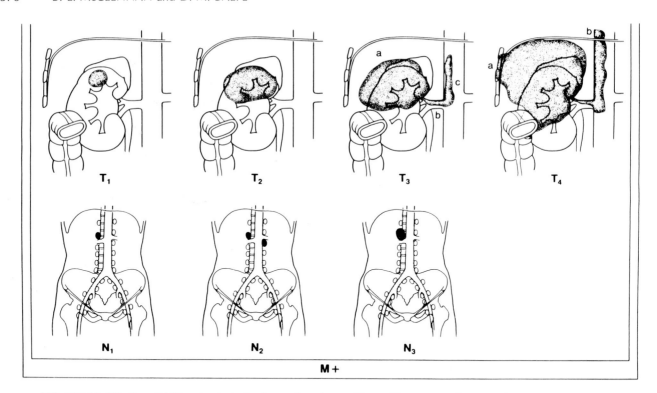

FIG. 16-7. Modification of AJC anatomic staging for renal carcinoma. Tumor (T) categories: Extension through the renal capsule and renal vein is the major type of advancement. Invasion of the calices and deformity of contour (T_2) are the first signs of advancement. Once the perinephric tissue (T_{3a}), the renal vein (T_{3b}), or inferior vena cava (T_{3c}) are infiltrated, the tumor is very advanced. Fixation of tumor to muscle wall, bone, or bowel is T_4. Node (N) categories: Advancement of nodal disease in the regional nodes (para-aortic) is single homolateral (N_1), multiple and bilateral (N_2), fixed (N_3). Stage grouping: No stage grouping is recommended at the present time. AJC *v* UICC classifications: Both committees agree on this classification. The only difference is the degree of venous invasion (V). In the UICC classification, there is only renal vein invasion for T_3 and pTNM adds a V_1 for renal vein and V_2 for vena cava. p = pathologic (postsurgical) stage. (Modified from Frank, I. N., Keys, H. M., McCune, C. S.: Urologic and male genital cancers. In *Clinical Oncology for Medical Students and Physicians: A Multidisciplinary Approach*, 6th Ed. Rubin, P. (Ed.). New York, American Cancer Society, 1983, pp. 198–221.)

Studies of tumor cell turnover demonstrate that in renal cancers, active cell proliferation occurs at the margins of the tumor with normal parenchyma as well as in focal areas within the main tumor mass.[33,83,91] Necrosis seems to stimulate this local cell proliferation.[33,34,83] Local spread, therefore, depends on the morphologic characteristics of the tumor, i.e., cystic, necrotic, or solid, as well as on tumor grade (Figure 16-8). The renal capsule presents a barrier to spread as does the perinephric (Gerota's) fascia once the perinephric fat is involved (Figure 16-9). The capsule itself is involved microscopically in up to 75% of cases, while the perinephric fat has only a 13% to 25% incidence of involvement.[84,91] The vascularity of a tumor (which may be related to the aforementioned factors) also may affect tumor spread and growth, since tumors are unable to grow rapidly if they cannot induce their own blood supply.[33,34] Perhaps this is one reason why papillary adenocarcinomas, which are commonly avascular, grow so slowly and unaggressively. Papillary adenocarcinomas also have a very low incidence of lymph node involvement.[6]

Microscopic intrarenal spread of a renal cell carcinoma into veins is a frequent finding. However, only a portion (30%) of cases involve the main renal vein (Figure 16-10).[49,91] High grade lesions more frequently involve renal veins, and invasion of the main renal vein increases the incidence of subsequent metastases, especially when found in conjunction with perinephric extension or lymph node involvement.[91] Tumor size and lymph node spread do not correlate well with venous invasion. Low grade renal cell carcinomas without renal vein involvement are associated with a favorable survival rate, almost two times that of cases with renal vein involvement.[69] Survival of patients with high grade tumors is more related to tumor grade than to any degree of venous involvement.[69,91] Extension to the main renal vein and subsequently to the inferior vena cava occurs in 5% to 10% of all cases of renal cell carcinoma.[91] Up to 25% of patients with involvement of the main renal vein will have some form of extension to the inferior vena cava, typically a small sliver of tumor thrombus lying free in the vena cava without adherence or direct invasion.[22,62,89] Cases of bland

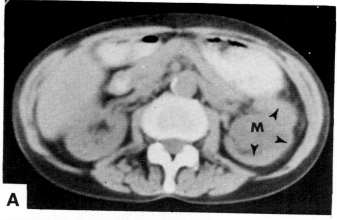

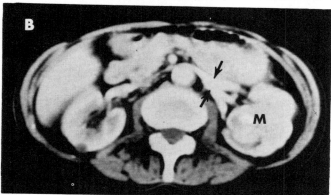

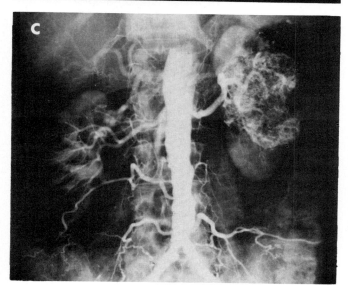

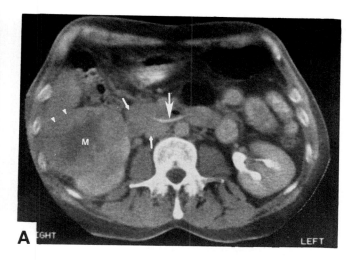

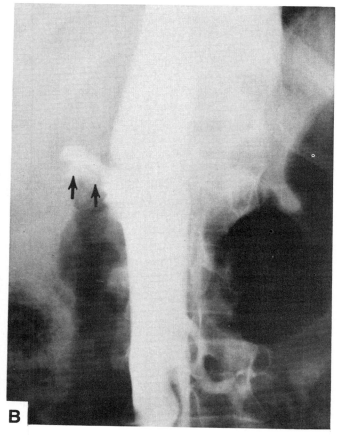

FIG. 16-8. Renal cell carcinoma—stage I; T_2. (A) Precontrast CT scan through both kidneys shows a large mass (M) within the left kidney, expanding the central portion of the kidney (arrowheads). (B) After a bolus injection of contrast material, the mass (M), surrounding parenchyma, and renal vein (black arrows) markedly enhances. (C) Angiography adds little or no diagnostic information but confirms the "CT angiography" findings (B) of a hypervascular tumor. This tumor was confined to the kidney capsule and had no venous or lymph node involvement on CT or at pathologic examination.

FIG. 16-9. Renal cell carcinoma—perinephric spread (stage IIIc; T_{3b}). (A) CT scan through a large tumor (M) in the right kidney. Contrast material has been given by bolus injection. Central necrosis is present within the tumor. The interface between the kidney and liver (arrowheads) is indistinct. This is suggestive of but not pathognomonic for liver invasion. Extensive perinephric hilar invasion (arrows) is present, making precise identification of the right renal vein impossible. The inferior vena cava appeared compressed on other scans. The left renal vein (large arrow) as it enters the inferior vena cava is visible but is surrounded by tumor. (B) An inferior vena cavagram revealed the IVC to be open and the right renal vein to be patent (arrows) but displaced cephalad. At surgery, a perinephric tumor surrounded both renal veins and their junction with the vena cava was found.

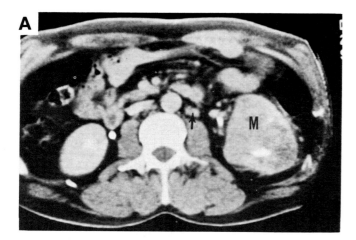

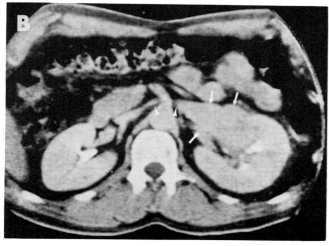

FIG. 16-10. Renal cell carcinoma with renal vein involvement (stage IIIA; T$_{3b}$, N$_1$). (A) A large renal cell carcinoma (M) involving the lower pole of the left kidney is visible. Contrast enhancement shows inhomogeneous areas suggesting areas of necrosis. An enlarged lymph node is present (black arrow). (B) A scan 2-cm cephalad to that in A shows a widened renal vein, which is indicative of tumor invasion of the proximal left renal vein (arrows), but the renal vein is normal (arrowheads) as it crosses under the superior mesenteric artery(s). Renal venography and surgery confirmed these findings.

thrombus may occur that will appear identical to a tumor thrombus with current imaging techniques. Again, high grade renal cell carcinomas will involve the inferior vena cava more frequently; this is more common when the primary tumor is on the right because the right renal vein is shorter and therefore closer to the inferior vena cava. Isolated involvement of the renal vein or involvement of the inferior vena cava in the absence of lymph node or perinephric extension does not preclude curative surgery and prolonged survival.[89]

Lymphatic spread (Figure 16-11) may occur regionally to the renal hilum or nearby periaortic, pericaval, or iliac lymph nodes. Mediastinal lymph node involvement or supraclavicular lymph node involvement may occur. Lym-

phatic extension via lymph nodes to the thoracic duct and then the superior vena cava has been noted, as has hematogenous spread via the inferior vena cava, the gonadal vein, or mesenteric or portal venous shunts.[54,91] The axial skeleton is frequently the site of deposits via Batson's paravertebral plexes. Since the adrenal glands lie within Gerota's fascia, ipsilateral adrenal metastatic involvement occurs about 10% of the time.[91]

Local lymph node involvement is found in 21% of patients undergoing nephrectomy in the absence of distant metastases.[84] In patients with distant metastases, local lymph node involvement is found in 40% of cases.[17] Lymph nodes appear to be an ineffectual barrier to tumor spread, since the incidence of metastasis is 50% higher in patients with positive local lymph nodes.[17] High stage lesions (T$_3$–T$_4$) are more likely to have lymph node involvement than low stage lesions (stage I; T$_1$–T$_2$).[17] As has been mentioned, there is a close correlation between local recurrence and local lymph node involvement.[27] This suggests that local recurrence may be only residual tumor-bearing lymphatic tissue; therefore, there is sound logic to support the radical surgical approach to renal cell carcinomas.

Still, one third of patients with renal cell carcinoma have metastases at the time of diagnosis (Figure 16-12), but 70% of these have single organ involvement with pulmonary or bony metastases predominating.[91] Pulmonary metastases are frequently multiple but may be solitary, lymphangitic, or endobronchial. Excision of such metastases will probably increase survival, particularly if the deposit is solitary and appears late.[93] Aggressive surgical therapy in the face of multiple metastatic deposits only results at best in a prolonged palliative interval, since these patients eventually succumb and long-term cures are rare.[12,71] Osseous metastases commonly seek the vertebrae and bony pelvis. Solitary bony metastases are common, and they are usually lytic in nature (Figure 16-13), with blastic changes occurring infrequently. Metastases from renal cell carcinomas have been found in almost every organ of the body and, strangely enough, even in another primary tumor.[63] About 3% of patients with metastases at the time of diagnosis have a solitary metastasis, but over half soon develop others.[91] Regional recurrence or metastases to the renal bed are frequent. Such patients usually die of distant metastases. In one series with local recurrence, almost all patients were dead within 12 months.[27] At autopsy of patients dying of metastatic renal cell carcinoma, up to 30% had recurrent tumor in the renal fossa.[27] Very late recurrences or metastases (greater than 10 years) do occur, so patients once treated for renal cell carcinoma are always at risk. The surgical scar or the lung are the most frequent sites of late recurrence.[28] The occurrence of a late metastasis is an ominous sign, since most patients are dead within two years from the time of the occurrence of the metastasis even in the best of circumstances.[28]

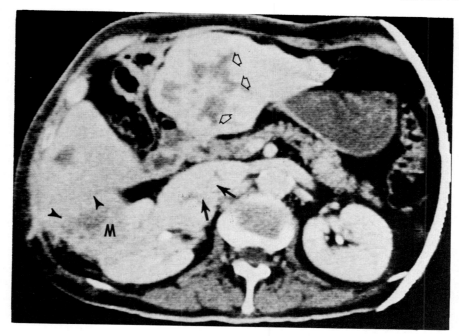

FIG. 16-11. Renal cell carcinoma with inferior vena cava invasion and distant metastasis (stage IVB; T_4, M_{a-d}). A contrast-enhanced CT scan through both kidneys reveals a renal cell carcinoma (M) extending from the lateral surface of the right kidney to invade the liver (arrowheads). Invasion of the right renal vein and IVC are present. Tumor thrombus is seen within the IVC (black arrows). A vascular metastasis is present within the left lobe of the liver (open arrows).

Transitional cell carcinomas gain easy and early access to local lymph nodes largely because of the lack of a thick muscular layer to act as a barrier to spread of tumor (Figure 16-14). The *field theory* has been proposed to account for the wide local spread or involvement of other non-tumor-bearing areas of urothelium.[68] Local mucosal changes of atypia and carcinoma in situ do occur with transitional cell carcinoma of the upper urinary tract.[25,57] The role of carcinoma in situ in the upper urinary tract is unclear at the present; however, local mucosal changes increase as the grade of the tumor increases. Bladder cancer is also associated with upper urinary tract transitional cell carcinomas in up to 48% of some series.[53] This further lends support to the field theory for total urothelial risk from transitional cell carcinomas.[68]

The lymphatic drainage of the renal pelvis and ureter is varied and poorly defined. High grade neoplasms seem to find frequent access to local and regional lymph nodes while low grade papillary transitional cell carcinomas seem to have a much different, more benign biologic potential. Local infiltration is rare, as is direct vascular (venous) involvement, although locally invasive transitional cell carcinoma may appear on occasion as a mass within the kidney, even involving or occluding the renal vein. Since nonvisualization on an intravenous urogram may occur in 31% to 51% of cases, CT plays an important role in defining the cause and site of obstruction in these cases.[7,74] Metastases frequently occur to nearby osseous

structures, i.e., the spine, and to contiguous organs. The renal parenchyma, adrenal glands, pancreas, and spleen may all be sites for metastatic deposits, further supporting a hematogenous mode of spread for transitional cell carcinomas. Distant metastases occur in areas commonly involved by bladder cancer, that is, the lungs, liver, and bones.

Other patterns of spread unique to the type of tumor, stage, and grade can be seen with lymphomatous involvement of the kidney and ureter. Rarer tumors, such as squamous cell carcinoma or adenocarcinoma of the urothelium, display aggressive local behavior and may be superimposed on a picture of chronic infection or obstruction.[99] Aggressive tumor involvement of the kidney or ureter when extensive may present an indeterminate picture when CT is used and may make a definitive diagnosis virtually impossible.[39]

CLASSIFICATION AND STAGING

The stage of a renal tumor, either a renal cell carcinoma or transitional cell carcinoma, is the biologic manifestation of its tumor grade. Therefore, stage more than grade determines outcome with regard to prognosis and survival. The TNM classification (see Figure 16-7) of renal cell carcinoma as proposed by the American Joint Committee on Cancer rightly separates lymph node invasion from venous invasion. The TNM system relies

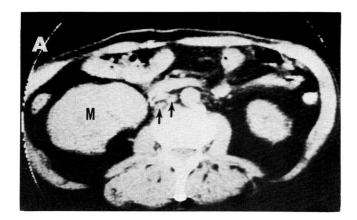

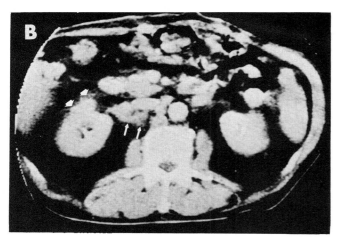

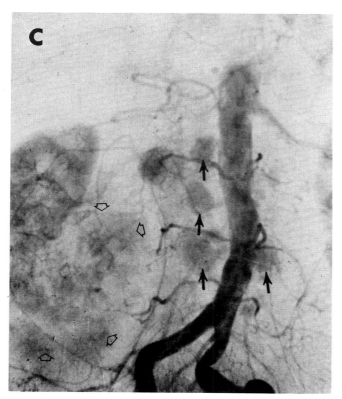

on lymphangiography and angiography, the accuracy of which for staging renal cell cancer is in serious question in the modern CT era.[96,99] Unfortunately, in spite of its comprehensiveness, the TNM system has not gained popularity for staging urinary tract tumors largely because of its many subgroups, which make it cumbersome to use (Table 16-1). A clinical and surgical staging system devised by Flocks and Kadesky in 1958 failed to adequately separate the lesser importance of involvement of the renal vein and inferior vena cava from the ominous consequences of lymph node involvement.[32] Robson and colleagues modified this staging system to reflect the above variations, and their staging system is the one most commonly employed today.[84] Compiling statistics from several large series numbering over 1,500 cases, Sufrin and Murphy found that 33% of all patients with renal cell carcinoma have stage I disease, while 12% have stage II disease, 24% have stage III disease, and 31% have stage IV disease.[91] Even though CT offers the best, most accurate preoperative method for staging renal cell carcinomas, survival still depends on local extent and the presence or absence of distant metastases. Once metastases develop, survival then depends upon the extent of disease and the disease-free interval.[26,91] The survival of 86 patients with metastatic renal cell carcinomas was only 42% at one year, 21% at two years, and 10% at five years in deKernion's series.[27]

Considerable confusion exists regarding a satisfactory and universal staging system for transitional cell carcinomas of the upper urinary tract. Analogies to the staging of bladder cancer exist and various alphanumeric staging and classification systems have been proposed by Grabstald et al.,[43] Batata and Grabstald,[8] and Bloom et al.[12] Unlike the bladder, the very thin muscularis of the renal pelvis and ureter makes the distinction of superficial and deep muscle invasion essentially impossible. In addition, the virtual direct contiguity of the renal pelvis and the renal parenchyma and the aggressive nature (high grade) of tumors that invade the kidney but stay within the capsule is evidence for considering the renal pelvis and kidney as one organ. The TNM classification proposed for bladder cancer when applied to renal pelvic and ureteral cancer is again cumbersome and not widely used. Cummings[25] proposed modifying the TNM and the numeri-

FIG. 16-12. Renal cell carcinoma—lymph node metastasis (stage IIIB; T_{3b}, N_3). (A) A large renal cell carcinoma (M) arising from the lower pole of the right kidney. Retrocaval lymph node metastases are present (black arrows). (B) A CT scan 2-cm cephalad to that in A shows more retrocaval adenopathy (white arrows). The tumor also involves the anterior portion of the right kidney at this level (arrowheads). (C) A subtraction film from an aortogram reveals a moderately vascular right renal tumor (open arrows) and multiple vascular metastases to local lymph nodes (arrows).

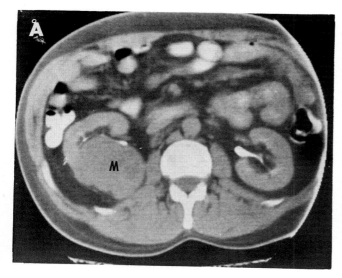

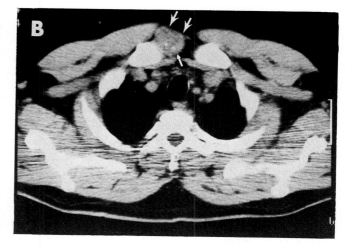

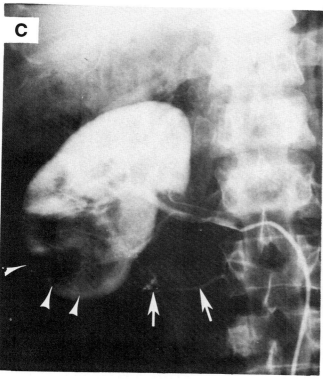

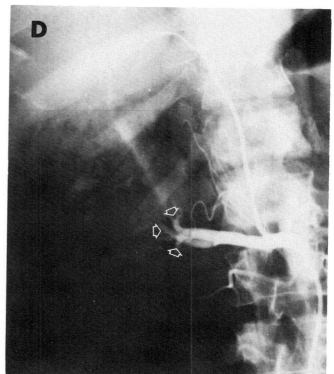

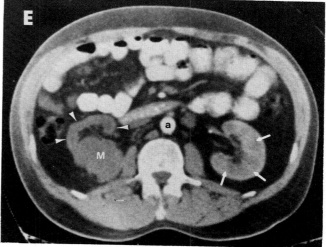

FIG. 16-13. Renal cell carcinoma with distant metastases treated by angioinfarction with alcohol (stage IVB, T_4, N_4). (A) A CT scan through both kidneys shows a right lower pole renal tumor (M). Tumor enhancement is inhomogeneous and slightly less than that of normal parenchyma. (B) A distant metastasis to the right sternal clavicular joint (arrows) plus diffusely positive radionuclide bone scan precludes curative surgery. (C) Late venous phase of a renal angiogram before angioinfarction showed an avascular tumor (arrowheads) with some blood supply from the third lumbar artery (arrows). (D) The renal artery is occluded after intra-arterial alcohol injection (open arrows). (E) Follow-up CT scan 1 month later shows renal atrophy (arrowheads) and decreased tumor (M) size. Note lack of excretion or tumor enhancement on the right after bolus "CT-angiography." Aorta is well opacified and a good corticomedullary junction is present on the left (arrows).

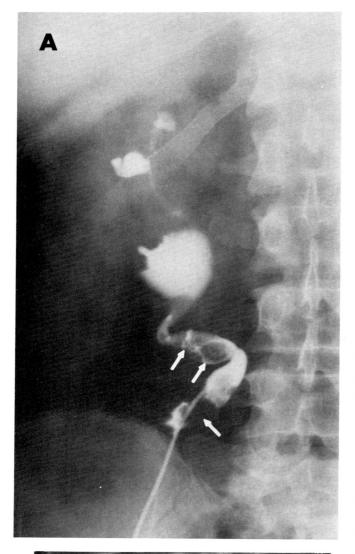

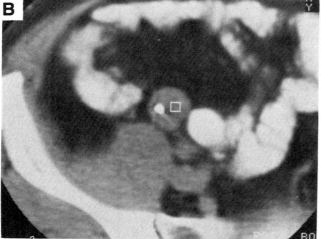

Table 16-1. Staging Renal Cell Carcinoma:
TNM v Robson's[84] Classification

ROBSON	DISEASE EXTENT	TNM
I	Tumor confined to kidney (small, intrarenal)	T_1
	Tumor confined to kidney (large)	T_2
II	Tumor spread to perinephric fat but within Gerota's fascia	T_{3a}
IIIA	Tumor spread to renal vein (T_{3b}) and cava (T_{3c})	T_{3b}, T_{3c}
IIIB	Tumor spread to local lymph nodes (LN)	N_1-N_3
IIIC	Tumor spread to local vessels and LN	T_{3b-c}, N_1-N_3
IVA	Tumor spread to adjacent organs (excluding ipsilateral adrenal)	T_4
IVB	Distant metastasis	M_1

cal staging classification of Bloom et al. to incorporate the limitation of the muscularis layer in the upper urinary tract (Table 16-2). Stage I (T_a) includes noninvasive transitional cell carcinoma (papillomas). Stage II (T_1) includes involvement of the submucosa and lamina propria but not muscle invasion. This is also occasionally called stage A disease. Stage III (T_2, T_{3a}) means muscle invasion of the pelvis and ureteral wall but not through the adventitia. It also includes the kidney parenchyma, with tumor confined within the renal capsule. Occasionally this is called Jewett's stage B disease. Stage IV or stage D (T_{3b}, T_4, N_+) means extension through the adventitia or kidney into adjacent organs or local lymph nodes. This system correlates well with tumor grade and survival and best suits the current imaging trends for transitional carcinoma, which will be addressed subsequently. Multiple tumors and other urothelial changes (i.e., CIS) may occur. In these cases, grade plays the key decisional role. Low grade and low stage tumors can carry an 80% or more five-year survival.[25] High grade, high stage (III or greater) tumors carry a poor prognosis, in the range of 20% five-year survival. Renal parenchymal involvement confined by the capsule does adversely affect overall survival in stage III disease with transitional cell carcinoma.[25] Stage IV disease carries a normal prognosis, with almost no five-year survivors.

Other urothelial tumors such as squamous cell carcinomas or tumors of mesenchymal origin (fibroepithelial polyps) or metastatic disease to the urothelium have no

FIG. 16-14. Transitional cell carcinoma. (A) A right retrograde pyelogram performed because of nonvisualization on a urogram reveals an intraluminal ureteral tumor (arrows). No information regarding tumor stage is evident. (B) A CT scan through the right ureter shows a stent catheter in place. The cursor box is over a solid portion of the ureteral tumor that involves the ureteral wall and compresses the lumen. No extraureteric spread is seen. Pathologic examination revealed ureteral cancer invading the wall of the ureter but no further. (Reprinted from Baron, R. L., McClennan, B. L., Lee, J. K. T., Lawson, T. L.: Computed tomography of transitional cell carcinoma of the renal pelvis and ureter. *Radiology* 144:125–130, 1982. With permission.)

Table 16-2. Staging TCCa of the Pelvis and Ureter:
TNM v Conventional System

CONVENTIONAL STAGE	DISEASE EXTENT	TNM
I;O	No invasion, benign papilloma	T_a
II;A	Submucosa, lamina propria involved, including carcinoma in situ (CIS)	T_1
III;B$_{1-2}$	Muscle invasion, parenchymal involvement, confined by renal capsule or adventitia	$T_2;T_{3a}$
IV;C,D	Extrarenal extension, with or without adjacent organ or LN involvement, distant metastasis	T_{3b},T_4,N_4

conventional staging classification. They are considered as isolated events. The same is true of rare renal parenchymal tumors or renal lymphomatous involvement. Oncologic management decisions are made surgically or as part of an overall systemic approach to the disease, as with lymphomas.

IMAGING PROCEDURES AND ASSESSMENT

Intravenous Urography

The intravenous urogram (IVU) continues to be the best screening test for urinary tract pathologic entities available today. Its role is largely one of detection where renal masses are concerned, since there are better and more accurate techniques available for definition of a renal mass (see Figure 16-1). Proper urography requires the use of routine tomography, otherwise masses, usually less than 4 cm, will be missed.[61] Tomography of the chest may be required as well in cases of real or suspected pulmonary involvement. Adequate plain film examinations will be necessary, along with radionuclide bone scanning for evaluation of real or suspected osseous involvement from renal cancer. A renal mass detected by urography statistically stands an excellent chance of being benign—usually a cyst. Further definition is required even if no clinical symptomatology exists, since signs and symptoms of renal cancer are often protean, subtle, or nonexistent. Other lesions may mimic renal cell cancer such as xanthogranulomatous pyelonephritis, hamartomas (AML), or pseudotumors. In addition, a significant number of renal tumors (up to 10%) will not be visible on a urogram, which further complicates the imaging process.[91] Retrograde pyeloureterography may clarify the nature of an obstructing tumorous process and is commonly employed in the diagnosis of transitional cell carcinoma. Cytologic evaluation and brush biopsy may further enhance the diagnostic process if properly performed.

Computed Tomography and Other Techniques

Ultrasound, angiography, radionuclide scanning, CT, lymphangiography, and magnetic resonance imaging (MRI) are all techniques available for the further definition and diagnosis of renal masses and their extent. Computed tomography has clearly emerged as the imaging procedure of choice for staging renal tumors today.[47] However, modern gray scale ultrasonography, now performed largely by means of high resolution real-time sector scanning, plays a major triage role in the work up of renal tumors (Figure 16-15).[19] Cystic masses are reliably differentiated from solid ones in over 95% of incidences.[19] Very small lesions, less than 2 cm, still present a challenge and approach the resolution limits of ultrasound.[19] When coupled with intravenous urography, ultrasonography can be used to differentiate a cyst from a tumor. An accuracy of approximately 98% for the ultrasonic diagnosis of renal cysts has been reported.[19] Ultrasound will usually detect solid renal tumors and may provide important staging information regarding local spread and involvement of the renal vein or inferior vena cava. Ultrasonography is limited, however, in that extracapsular extension of tumors may be difficult to detect. Local lymph node involvement, which is critical to accurate staging, is rarely detectable. The main impact of ultrasonography on the imaging algorithm for renal tumors is at the T level of staging. Precise tumor identification may be made by ultrasonography in the case of an angiomyolipoma with its typical echodense

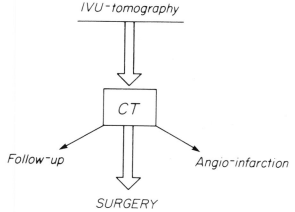

FIG. 16-15. Recommended imaging approach for renal tumors. When intravenous urography suggests a solid renal tumor, a CT scan can effectively become the next imaging study to confirm the tumor (T stage) and stage the tumor by providing a pictorial representation of its true extent. After surgery or angioinfarction, CT can optimally be used to provide important follow-up information.

pattern, although a mixture of echo textures including hypoechoic patterns may be encountered with angiomyolipomas. For adequate tumor staging, other imaging methods are necessary, particularly CT or angiography.[99]

Before the advent of CT, angiography was the major imaging test used to preoperatively diagnose and stage renal cell carcinomas. Selective studies boasted a high degree of accuracy (in the 97% range) for renal cell carcinomas but very low accuracy for transitional cell carcinomas because of their typical avascular nature.[10,59] The need for an angiographic study to diagnose a solid (and therefore usually surgically resectable) renal tumor has been largely obviated by ultrasonography and CT. Additionally angiographic accuracy for the staging and classification of renal cell carcinomas is only 38% to 68% in the best of series.[10,14,37,42,64,82] Futter et al. angiographically examined 54 patients with renal cell carcinomas.[37] The T category correlated with histopathologic stage in only 44.4% of cases.[37] The 55.6% inaccuracy in this series defeats the purpose of TMN classification to provide precise assessment of the primary tumor.[37] The critical weakness of angiographic staging methods for renal cell carcinomas and for transitional cell carcinomas is an inability to detect extracapsular invasion.[11] Frequent parasitic blood supply to renal cell carcinomas results in high false-positive rates (decreased specificity) for local extension (T_3). Furthermore, a significant number of renal cell carcinomas, up to 14%, and almost all transitional cell carcinomas are avascular tumors on conventional selected angiograms.[2] Arteriography has been of some use in clarifying ureteral lesions that are diffuse or stricturelike or in the differential diagnosis of cancer from varices or endometriosis.[58] The role of angiographic procedures for the preoperative staging of renal tumors in the CT era is now much better defined.[14] Angiography is reserved for those patients with renal tumors where the CT scan is equivocal or additional diagnostic or staging information would significantly alter the treatment. This thesis was recently tested in 42 patients with renal cell carcinomas.[14] Of the 42 patients, 24 (57%) underwent CT only, while 18 (43%) underwent angiographic procedures plus CT. Seven of nine venograms and none of 11 arteriograms added any additional information or clarified equivocal CT findings. Twenty-four of 37 patients had surgery with no preoperative angiography. No adverse consequences ensued as a result of the lack of preoperative angiography. Venography proved the most frequently performed study and was particularly useful in detecting bulky lesions on the right side.[14] In a radiologic-pathologic correlation study by Weyman et al. from the same institution, CT was found equal to or better than angiography for overall accuracy and sensitivity in the detection of perinephric extension and lymph node involvement.[99] Computed tomography and venography were equally accurate in detecting involvement of the main renal vein and inferior vena cava.[99] These same investigators found arteriography useful in only 16% of 60 cases of renal masses classed as indeterminate on scans.[5] In the same study group, ultrasonography or cyst aspiration was diagnostic in 84% of these same 60 indeterminate CT cases.[5] Therefore, angiography, specifically venography, may be necessary in a finite number of cases with equivocal CT findings. Other potential indications for arteriography may include (1) questionable contralateral tumor involvement; (2) therapeutic embolization; (3) vascular mapping in solitary or anomalous kidneys where renal-sparing surgery is contemplated, i.e., von Hippel-Lindau disease; (4) definition of suspected arteriovenous malformations (AVM) or rare renal hemangiomas; (5) differentiation of invasive transitional cell carcinomas from renal cell carcinomas if a typical hypervascular pattern is seen.[14] Before the CT era, virtually all patients with renal cell carcinomas and many patients with transitional cell carcinomas who were to undergo surgery had preoperative arteriography with or without venography. Since venography to evaluate the renal vein or inferior vena cava will occasionally be required in spite of state-of-the-art CT scanning, digital vascular imaging (DVI) techniques may well provide the necessary information with a lower dose of contrast material, lower cost, and decreased procedure time (Figure 16-16). Digital vascular imaging techniques for both intravenous and intra-arterial vascular studies are saving time and money while providing the necessary vascular information discussed above.

IMAGING STRATEGIES AND DECISIONS

Renal Cell Carcinoma

Computed tomography has replaced preoperative angiography as the primary staging technique for evaluating renal cancer.[99] No existing technique except perhaps MRI provides such unique anatomic information regarding tumor characteristics and stage. Contrast-assisted CT, usually through bolus techniques, provides accurate staging information for either TNM or Robson's classification of renal cell carcinomas. Renal cell carcinomas are readily recognized when the following CT criteria are fulfilled:

1. An attenuation value close to but usually less than that of normal renal parenchyma, occasionally heterogeneous; rarely attenuation values may be greater than that of normal renal parenchyma.
2. Transient, marked tumor enhancement during bolus contrast administration (CT angiography). More prolonged tumor enhancement may occur but usually this is less dense than the normal renal parenchyma.

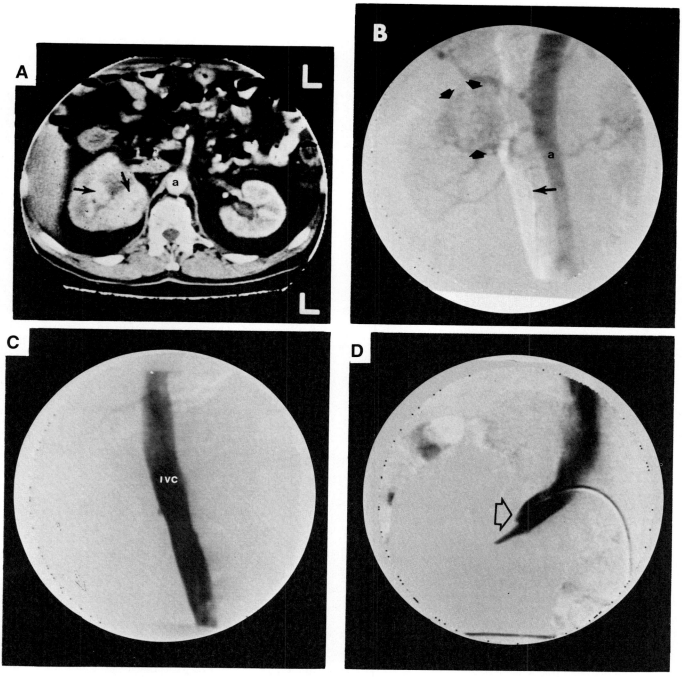

FIG. 16-16. Renal cell carcinoma studied by digital vascular imaging (DVI). (A) A CT scan through a large tumor in the upper pole of the right kidney; bolus injection of contrast medium shows tumor blush (arrows). (B) A DVI study was done to evaluate the right renal vein and the inferior vena cava (IVC). A hypervascular tumor is visible in the right kidney (arrowheads). The injection was made through a pigtail catheter (arrow) in the inferior vena cava. Both the IVC and aorta (a) are visible. (C) Digital recording of injection into the IVC, which is free from tumor. (D) Right renal vein (open arrow) is also free from tumor on this digital image.

3. A poorly demarcated tumor–parenchyma interface, although encapsulation may occur.
4. Calcification may be present, usually centrally (Figure 16-17). Central tumoral calcification with soft tissue mass extending beyond the confines of the calcification is typically malignant. Benign tumoral calcification patterns tend to be peripheral, with the masses having low attenuation centers.
5. Involvement of the renal vein manifest as renal vein enlargement or actual visualization of tumor thrombus by CT. Enlargement of lymph nodes, perinephric tumor extension, and extension to the inferior vena cava may also be seen.[96]

The precise anatomic detail provided by CT gives the best assessment of tumor volume and local extent. In our published series and continued practice, CT is more accurate and more sensitive than angiography for separating stage I from stage II renal cell carcinomas.[96] Computed tomography is limited in this regard, since the small tumor extensions into the perinephric fat are difficult to detect or separate from a parasitic or collateral blood supply within Gerota's fascia. However, standard radical nephrectomy techniques dictate than en bloc excision of Gerota's envelope (kidney, adrenal, and perinephric fat) be performed, so this limitation of the CT imaging process is not critical. With the improved resolution of the newer CT units or MRI, the relationship of the tumor to Gerota's fascia can be determined more accurately. Caution must be exercised, however, in as-sessing adjacent organ invasion because loss of contiguous fat planes may not always mean direct invasion. In our experience, tumors have been adherent to the liver and spleen without pathologic invasion. Direct coronal CT or reconstruction in the sagittal or coronal plane may be of aid in these circumstances. A lack of correlation between tumor size and extracapsular spread has been our experience, and this correlates well with published angiographic series.[15]

Local lymphadenectomy has become part of the radical surgical approach to renal cell carcinomas and transitional cell carcinomas. Positive identification of involved lymph nodes by CT requires that these lymph nodes be enlarged. Computed tomography has a high sensitivity for detecting enlarged perihilar lymph nodes, but the specificity suffers from the fact that lymph nodes may be enlarged because of hyperplasia rather than metastatic involvement. Microscopic lymph node metastases are not detectable by CT. Even lymphangiography fails in this requirement, since bipedal lymphangiography rarely opacifies renal hilar lymph nodes. Juxtaregional nodal involvement (stage III B or C) in the high retroperitoneal or retrocrural areas may be detected by CT, whereas these areas are essentially "blind" to other imaging methods.

Computed tomography optimally displays most main renal vein involvement in cases of renal cell carcinoma except when large bulky disease obscures normal anatomic relationships, particularly on the right side (see Figure 16-9A). Intrarenal venous invasion is not detected by CT but does not affect the treatment alternatives.

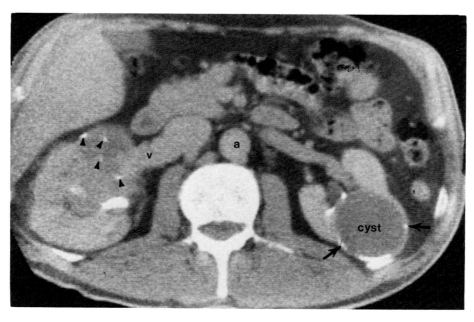

FIG. 16-17. Calcified renal cell carcinoma and calcification in wall of renal cyst. A CT scan through both kidneys shows a right renal tumor with calcification within it (arrowheads). A large right renal vein (v) is noted, suggesting venous invasion. A calcified left renal cyst (arrows) is also present.

Detection of main renal vein involvement is critical to both staging and survival as well as to the surgical approach. With proper scan techniques and bolus administration of contrast material, most renal vein involvement can be adequately assessed with CT. Tumor invasion of the inferior vena cava is likewise frequently detected when present by CT, but contrast material may have to be given via a foot vein or femoral vein to fully evaluate the inferior vena cava when a bulky tumor compresses or invades the vessel. Surgical techniques now allow resection of tumor within the inferior vena cava, so that the staging information CT provides in these cases is crucial.[20] If the CT findings are equivocal, venography with evaluation of the inferior vena cava or superior vena cava must be performed as well as venographic evaluation of the renal veins.[14]

Evaluation of the opposite kidney, adrenal gland, and liver is an important part of the CT staging evaluation of renal cell carcinomas. The chest may be examined with CT to detect potentially resectable metastatic disease. Fine-needle biopsy with computed tomographic, ultrasonic, or fluoroscopic guidance may further enhance the utility of CT for staging renal cell carcinoma. Overall, the impact of CT in the staging of renal cell carcinomas has been profound. Urologic surgeons at our institution are frequently operating on renal cell cancers based on the information provided by CT alone. Other management decisions, vis-à-vis patient operability based on tumor stage, are critically effected by the information provided by CT. More invasive procedures such as angiography are only being done for therapeutic reasons or to evaluate the opposite kidney for tumor involvement or for renal vascular disease as a cause of concomitant hypertension. Venographic studies may be necessary in cases of equivocal CT findings as described above. The follow-up of patients treated for renal cell carcinoma either with embolization or surgery is facilitated with CT scanning.[4,9] Early detection of recurrence in the renal bed may be difficult with ultrasonography, since bowel loops frequently obscure the view. Computed tomography therefore has been the postoperative imaging procedure of choice in these cases.

Transitional Cell Carcinoma

The role of CT scanning in staging transitional cell carcinomas is becoming much better defined.[7] Computed tomography can solve the diagnostic problem of the radiolucent filling defect in the renal pelvis or ureter detected by screening urography or retrograde pyelography. While not histospecific, CT usually differentiates soft tissue masses (tumors) from fresh blood clots or stones. Transitional cell carcinomas of the pelvis and ureter commonly appear as sessile intraluminal masses on CT scans (Figure 16-18).[7] They may be focal or multiple, with attenuation values approaching those of muscle (40–70 Hounsfield units). The surface may be smooth, irregular, or

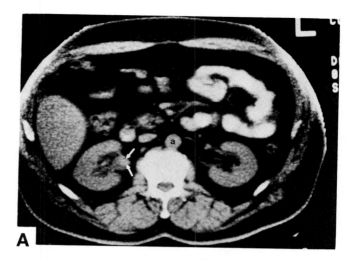

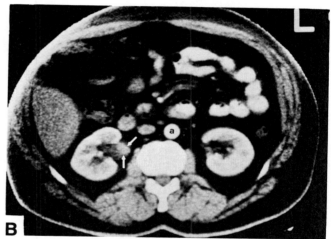

FIG. 16-18. Transitional cell carcinoma. (A) A precontrast CT scan through both kidneys shows a filling defect in the right renal pelvis (arrows). The density of this tumor is higher than that of surrounding urine. (B) After rapid bolus administration of contrast medium, the transitional cell tumor (arrows) enhances, indicating its modest vascularity.

calcified depending on histology, concurrent hemorrhage, and intervening biopsy procedures. When a transitional cell carcinoma invades the renal parenchyma, the urothelium is crossed, and frequently the renal sinus fat plane is lost as the tumor extends into the parenchyma (Figure 16-19). When the degree of parenchymal infiltration is great, CT alone cannot distinguish invasive transitional cell carcinoma from the more common renal cell carcinoma or for that matter any invasive metastatic disease. Precontrast and postcontrast CT scanning is usually necessary when transitional cell carcinomas are evaluated, since minor but real degrees of tumor enhancement may be seen with transitional cell carcinomas, as a result of the excellent contrast resolution inherent in the CT scanning process. Small doses of contrast material—10–20 mL of 50% to 60% solutions—should be used, or urine

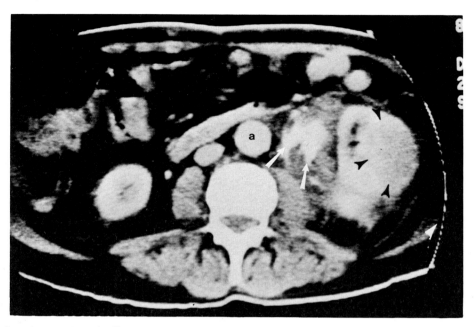

FIG. 16-19. Invasive transitional cell carcinoma. A CT scan through both kidneys after bolus injection of contrast medium shows dense opacification of the aorta (a). The left kidney is displaced laterally by a urinoma. Active extravasation of contrast material is seen (arrows). A poorly enhancing mass (arrowheads) is seen within the left kidney. A transitional cell carcinoma invading the renal parenchyma was found. An obstructing uric acid calculus in the left ureter caused the urinoma.

in the collecting system that is too dense and contrast laden may hide the presence or extent of a tumor.[7]

Intrarenal extension, renal hilar involvement, and periureteric spread of transitional cell carcinomas may be detected and defined by CT. Therefore valuable staging information regarding T characteristics (stages I, II, and III) is available with properly conducted CT scans. Computed tomography cannot differentiate tumors limited to the urothelial mucosa (stage I; T_a–T_l) from those with submucosal or muscle invasion (stage II; T_2, T_3).[7] However, treatment is essentially the same for stage I and stage II disease of the ureter and pelvis. Lymph node involvement (stage IV; T_{3b}, T_4) can be detected but only if the lymph nodes are enlarged. Failure to properly document stage III disease because of the inability of CT to define lymph node metastases is of less importance because stage III and stage IV disease are treated almost the same and carry a dismal prognosis. Extensive stage IV disease (T_3–T_4, N_+) can be successfully imaged, but even with radical surgery these patients rarely do well. Marked involvement of the renal vein or inferior vena cava as is seen with renal cell carcinomas is rare with transitional cell carcinomas. Other tumors such as mucinous adenocarcinomas of the urothelium or squamous cell carcinomas may mimic the CT picture of multifocal or extensive transitional cell carcinoma. Treatment options would rarely be altered, however, and radical surgery is usually performed.[90]

Angiography can offer little staging information for transitional cell carcinomas for reasons similar to those previously outlined for renal cell carcinomas. Further-

more, most transitional cell carcinomas of the upper urinary tract are markedly hypovascular or avascular. Computed tomography is the most effective imaging adjunct to urography for staging transitional cell carcinomas (Figure 16-20). A total of 55% of patients in a recent review of 22 patients with transitional cell carcinomas from our institution were referred for CT evaluation because of a nonfunctioning or poorly visualized kidney on a urogram.

Computed tomography rarely has a direct impact on the early diagnosis or detection of transitional cell carcinomas of the upper urinary tract. Urography, if it demonstrates all the urothelial surfaces, is usually sufficient for initial diagnosis. Retrograde pyelography may be required in some cases to complement the urogram or to aid cytologic evaluations. Precise data regarding sensitivity, specificity, and overall diagnostic accuracy for CT are lacking. Such data as have been accumulated to date for renal cell carcinomas are as yet unavailable for transitional cell carcinomas. Decisions about operability can be based on CT; however, in cases of advanced transitional cell carcinoma, even with the very best radical surgery, the prognostic outlook is extremely grim for patients with high stage, high grade tumors.[25,27]

Other less common tumors, such as metastases to the kidney or even inflammatory disease, may simulate the CT patterns of transitional cell carcinoma or renal cell carcinoma. The ability of CT to assess other organs for involvement, such as the liver and the lung, and to evaluate the renal bed postoperatively are significant advantages over other imaging methods.

The imaging algorithms for renal tumors are best sepa-

PROBABLE UROTHELIAL TUMOR

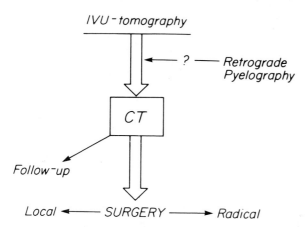

FIG. 16-20. Recommended imaging approach for transitional cell cancers. When transitional cell cancer is suspected after intravenous urography, valuable staging information can be obtained using CT scanning. Retrograde pyelography may be necessary to rule out other sites of involvement or to collect cytologic specimens. Surgical decisions regarding resection may hinge on the staging information provided by CT. A CT scan may provide a definitive diagnosis of a calculus not a tumor, and then only careful follow-up is required.

rated into four steps, the first being the detection process (see Figure 16-1). Subsequently, definition and diagnosis, staging, and treatment considerations will follow. Intravenous urography with tomography remains the primary imaging examination for the evaluation of patients with real or suspected renal tumors. Computed tomography might become the next step for tumor definition and diagnosis (T characteristics) except that most renal masses

are benign cysts. Therefore, ultrasonography occupies a major triage position in the imaging algorithm, particularly regarding renal cell carcinomas. If the diagnostic confidence level is high for renal tumor based on an intravenous urogram, then CT is the best first imaging step (see Figure 16-12). If the ultrasound study reveals confusing results (an indeterminate mass), then CT is also the next best imaging step. Angiography is usually not helpful for diagnostic purposes in cases of an indeterminate mass imaged by ultrasonography or CT.[5] Digital intravenous and intra-arterial vascular imaging may be useful, especially for clarifying suspected involvement of the renal vein or inferior vena cava. Aspiration may yield definitive results, proving the existence of a tumor or an inflammatory mass. Staging (TNM) is best performed using CT for renal cell carcinomas or transitional cell carcinomas as previously outlined. Surgical decisions about operability and type of operation can then be made. Follow-up surveillance is also best done with CT scanning, since ultrasonography may be limited by intervening bowel gas. Other imaging tests such as radionuclide scanning or whole lung tomography or CT may demonstrate metastases and have an impact on the ultimate decision for surgery.

TREATMENT DECISIONS

The treatment decisions by stage of disease are given in Table 16-3.[18,36,81]

The therapeutic maximum seems to have been reached for surgical treatment of renal tumors. Further improvement in survival and disease-free interval must await successful adjunctive therapy or improvement in early detection or prevention of renal neoplasia. Effective

Table 16-3. Kidney: Treatment Decision by Stage

| | TREATMENT MODALITY | | |
STAGE	SURGERY	RADIATION THERAPY	CHEMOTHERAPY IMMUNOTHERAPY
$T_1T_2N_0$	Radical nephrectomy	NR	NR
$T_{3a}N_0$	Radical nephrectomy	If micro- or macroresiduum 5,000–5,500 cGy	NR
$T_{3b}N_0$	Radical nephrectomy	If micro- or macroresiduum 5,000–5,500 cGy	NR
$T_{any}N_1N_2$	Radical nephrectomy includes involved veins	If micro- or macroresiduum 5,000–5,500 cGy	NR
$T_{3b}N_{1-3}$	Radical nephrectomy includes involved veins	If micro- or macroresiduum 5,000–5,500 cGy	NR
T_4M_0	Palliative resection for bleeding	If unresectable	Investigational chemotherapy or IT
M_+	Resect if solitary	If unresectable	Investigational chemotherapy or IT
Relapse	NR	NR	NR

NR = Not recommended
IT = Immunotherapy

chemotherapy or immunotherapy is promising but not yet available.[91] Interest continues in progestational agents, but suitable randomized prospective trials are lacking. At the moment, CT provides optimal diagnostic and staging information for renal tumors and will be the standard against which newer techniques, i.e., MRI, are gauged. Since patients with renal cell carcinomas or transitional cell carcinomas seem to be forever at risk of recurrence of their disease, CT as a follow-up imaging study offers promise, particularly for local recurrence.[4,9] Careful clinical scrutiny, patient screening at suitable intervals using urinalysis, chest radiography, and ultrasound study of the remaining renal unit or units have all become part of the patient follow-up routine in the CT era. However, precise numbers regarding the efficacy of such an approach must await further study (Table 16-4).

Renal adenocarcinomas or hypernephromas are best managed by radical nephrectomy, which includes an envelope of Gerota's fascia, perirenal fat, and kidney in addition to dissection of regional hilar lymph nodes. Resection is feasible for all of the initial stages of renal, capsular, venous, and nodal invasion.[36,81] When metastatic disease exists, radiation therapy to the renal bed is utilized for micro- or macro-residuum and when the disease is unresectable; it cannot, however, totally ablate bulk disease.[36] For metastatic disease and relapse patients, the use of investigational chemotherapy, hormonal therapy, and immunotherapy is reasonable. Since this tumor is known to undergo spontaneous regression, resection of the primary tumor is often attempted to induce possible regression of metastases.[81] This is one of the sites where immunotherapy holds promise and is actively being explored, particularly with attempts at developing some form of antibodies.

IMPACT OF NEW TECHNOLOGY

Computed tomography has become the "gold standard" for the diagnosis and staging of renal tumors. Experience is growing daily with the use of CT, and the availability of the technology is no longer a serious limiting factor. Attention still must be focused, however, on the basics, that is, properly performed urography. If the fundamental screening process is faulty, then the entire imaging work up is weakened and delayed. Confidence in and facility with CT techniques for evaluating renal tu-

Table 16-4. Imaging Methods for Evaluation of Renal Cancer

METHOD	CAPABILITY	COST/ BENEFIT	RECOMMENDED ROUTINE/ STAGING PROCEDURE
Noninvasive			
Chest radiography	Limited usefulness unless tomography used for detection of metastases.	High	Yes
Skeletal radiography	Limited usefulness except to confirm positive bone scan for metastasis.	Low	No
Ultrasound	Useful to exclude simple cysts and confirm primary tumor; limited staging information available, less sensitive and less specific than CT for tumor extent.	Fair	Not usually
MRI	Promising role for tumor detection and staging.	Unknown	Unknown
Nearly non-invasive			
Urography	Best screening test available; limited ability for precise staging.	High	Yes
Radionuclide studies			
Bone scans	Best screening test for skeletal metastasis.	High	Yes
L-S scan	Limited use if liver chemistries normal.	Low	No
CT	Most useful test for TNM staging information.	High	Always
Invasive			
Angiography (digital)			
Arteriography	Limited diagnostic and staging information compared with CT. Arteriography is required for embolization therapy.	Low	No
Venography	Useful if CT indeterminate for renal vein/cava involvement. (N.B. Many arteriographic and most venographic studies can be done digitally.)	Occasionally high	No
Lymphography	Limited or no utility.	Low	No
Biopsy—(CT, US, fluoroscopy)	Percutaneous biopsy requires US, CT, or fluoroscopy. Open biopsy rarely needed. Not necessary for T stage confirmation. May be useful to confirm metastases and determine operability.	Low	No

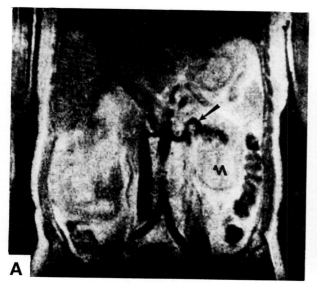
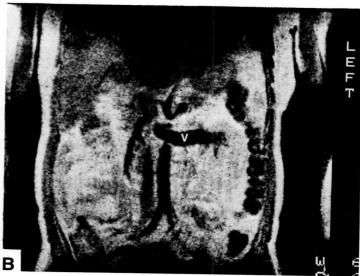

FIG. 16-21. Left renal cell carcinoma—MRI scan (Siemens Magnetom). (A) Coronal projection through left kidney shows lower pole mass (M) of variable intensity. The left renal artery (arrow) is clearly seen. (B) A coronal section at the level of the left renal vein (V) shows no evidence of main renal vein involement.

mors takes time but is well within the grasp of most radiologists and oncologists. When new imaging modalities such as MRI are introduced, they will depend heavily on the knowledge already gathered by CT for the effective implementation. Certainly, the infinite number of projections that MRI can provide will augment the diagnostic and staging process for renal tumors (Figure 16-21).[21,50] If cancers, specifically renal tumors, prove to have a prolonged relaxation time (T_1) as has been suggested, this could represent a major breakthrough in the early detection of renal cancer.[21,41,50,70,85] Research on the development of specific contrast agents for use with MRI may bring further benefits in terms of cancer labeling and more accurate diagnosis. Meanwhile, it is hoped that continued refinement of present imaging techniques, such as CT, in conjunction with research efforts in the field of chemotherapy and immunotherapy will bring about further improvements in the diagnosis, staging, and survival of patients with renal cancer.

REFERENCES

1. Abrams, H. J., Buchbinder, M. I., Sutton, A. P.: Renal carcinoma in adolescents. *J. Urol.* 121:92–94, 1979.
2. Alter, A. J., Uehling, D. T., Zwiebel, W. J.: Computed tomography of the retroperitoneum following nephrectomy. *Radiology* 133: 663–668, 1979.
3. Babaian, R. J., Johnson, D. E., Ayala, A. G., Sie, E. T.: Secondary tumor of ureter. *Urology* 14:341–343, 1979.
4. Balfe, D. M., McClennan, B. L., AufderHeide, J.: Multimodal imaging of two cases of mucinous adenocarcinoma of the renal pelvis. *Urol. Radiol.* 3:19–24, 1981.
5. Balfe, D. M., McClennan, B. L., Stanley, R. J., Weyman, P. J., Sagel, S. S.: Evaluation of renal masses considered indeterminate by computed tomography. *Radiology* 142:421–428, 1982.
6. Bard, R. H., Lord, B., Fromowitz, F.: Papillary adenocarcinoma of kidney. II. Radiographic and biologic characteristics. *Urology* 19: 16–20, 1982.
7. Baron, R. L., McClennan, B. L., Lee, J. K. T., Lawson, T. L.: Computed tomography of transitional cell carcinoma of the renal pelvis and ureter. *Radiology* 144:125–130, 1982.
8. Batata, M. A., Grabstald, H.: Upper urinary tract urothelial tumors. *Urol. Clin. North Am.* 3:79–86, 1976.
9. Bernardino, M. E., deSantos, L. A., Johnson, D. E., Brackan, R. G.: Computed tomography in the evaluation of post nephrectomy patients. *Radiology* 130:183–187, 1979.
10. Bernath, A. S., Addonizio, J. C., Kinkhebwala, M., Thelmo, W.: Renal venography in diagnosis of infiltrating transitional cell carcinoma of renal pelvis. *Urology* 18:164–167, 1981.
11. Blath, R. A., Mancilla-Jimenez, R., Stanley, R. J.: Clinical comparison between vascular and avascular renal cell carcinoma. *J. Urol.* 115:514–519, 1976.
12. Bloom, N. A., Vidone, R. A., Lytton, B.: Primary carcinoma of the ureter: A report of 102 cases. *J. Urol.* 103:590–598, 1970.
13. Boxer, R. J., Waisman, J., Lieber, M. M., Mampasa, F. M., Skinner, D.G.: Renal carcinoma: Computer analysis of 96 patients treated by nephrectomy. *J. Urol.* 122:598–601, 1979.
14. Bracken, B., Jonsson, K.: How accurate is angiographic staging of renal carcinoma? *Urology* 14:96–99, 1979.
15. Broders, A. C.: Epithelioma of the genitourinary organs. *Ann. Surg.* 75:574–604, 1922.
16. Byrd, R. L., Evans, A. E., D'Angio, G. J.: Adult Wilm's tumor and effect of therapy on survival. *J. Urol.* 127:648–651, 1982.
17. Carl, P., Klein, U., Gebauer, A., Schmiedt, E.: The value of lymphography for the TNM classification of renal carcinoma. *Eur. Urol.* 3:286–288, 1977.
18. Chan, R. C.: Renal cell carcinoma. In *Textbook of Radiotherapy*, 3rd ed. Fletcher, G. H. (Ed.). Philadelphia, Lea & Febiger, 1980, pp. 919–921.
19. Charboneau, J. W., Hattery, R. R., Ernst, E. C., James, E. M., Williamson, B., Hartman, G. W.: Spectrum of sonographic findings in 125 renal masses other than benign simple cyst. *A.J.R.* 140:87–94, 1983.
20. Cherrie, R. J., Goldman, D. G., Lindner, A., DeKernion, J. B.: Prog-

nostic implications of vena caval extension of renal cell carcinoma. *J. Urol.* **128**:910–912, 1982.

21. Choyke, P. L., Kressel, H. Y., Pollack, H. M., Arger, P. M., Axel, L., Mamourian, A. C.: Focal renal masses: Magnetic resonance imaging. *Radiology* **152**:471–477, 1984.

22. Clayman, R. V., Gonzalez, R., Fralay, E. E.: Renal cell cancer invading the inferior vena cava. Clinical review and anatomic approach. *J. Urol.* **123**:157–163, 1980.

23. Cromie, W. J., Davis, C. J., Deture, F. A.: Atypical carcinoma of kidney—possibly originating from collecting duct epithelium. *Urology* **13**:315–317, 1979.

24. Cronan, J. J., Zeman, R. K., Rosenfeld, A. T.: Comparison of computerized tomography, ultrasound and angiography in staging renal cell carcinoma. *J. Urol.* **127**:712–714, 1982.

25. Cummings, K. B.: Nephroureterectomy: Rationale in the management of transitional cell carcinoma of the upper urinary tract. *Urol. Clin. North Am.* **7**:569–578, 1980.

26. DeKernion, J. B., Berry, D.: The diagnosis and treatment of renal cell carcinoma. *Cancer* **45**:1945–1946, 1980.

27. DeKernion, J. B., Remming, K. P., Smith, R. B.: The natural history of metastatic renal cell carcinoma. A computer analysis. *J. Urol.* **120**:148–152, 1978.

28. Donaldson, J. C., Slease, R. B., Dufour, R., Saltzman, A. R.: Metastatic renal cell carcinoma 24 years after nephrectomy. *J.A.M.A.* **236**:950–951, 1976.

29. Droller, M. J.: Renal cell carcinoma: An overview. *Urol. Clin. North Am.* **7**:675–676, 1980.

30. Droller, M. J.: Transitional cell carcinoma: An overview. *Urol. Clin North Am.* **7**:519–521, 1980.

31. Fisher, R. G., Granmey, M., Wallace, S., Johnson, D. E.: Renal adenocarcinoma in adolescence and childhood: Emphasis on angiographic findings. *J. Urol.* **118**:83–86, 1977.

32. Flocks, R. H., Kadesky, M. C.: Malignant neoplasms of the kidney: an analysis of 353 patients following five years or more. *J. Urol.* **79**:196–201, 1958.

33. Folkman, J.: Tumor angiogenesis factor. *Cancer Res.* **34**:2109–2113, 1974.

34. Folkman, J.: The vascularization of tumors. *Sci. Am.* **234**:59–73, 1976.

35. Fraley, E. E.: Cancer in the renal pelvis. In *Genitourinary Cancer.* Skinner, D. G., DeKernion, J. B. (Eds.). Philadelphia, W. B. Saunders, 1978.

36. Frank, I. N., Keys, H. M., McCune, C. S.: Urologic and male genital cancers. In *Clinical Oncology for Medical Students and Physicians: A Multidisciplinary Approach*, 6th ed. Rubin, P. (Ed.). New York, American Cancer Society, 1983, pp. 198–221.

37. Futter, N. G., Collins, J. P., Walsh, W. G.: Inaccuracies in angiographic staging of renal cell carcinoma. *Urology* **14**:629–630, 1979.

38. Ghazi, M. R., Morales, P. A., Al-Askari, S.: Primary carcinoma of ureter. Report of 27 cases. *Urology* **14**:18–21, 1979.

39. Gittes, R. F.: Management of transitional cell carcinoma of the upper tract: Case for conservative local excision. *Urol. Clin. North Am.* **7**:559–568, 1980.

40. Glenn, J. F.: Renal tumors. In *Campbell's Urology*, Vol. II. Harrison, J. H., Gittes, R. F., Perlmutter, A. D., Stamey, T. A., Walsh, P. C. (Eds.). Philadelphia, W. B. Saunders, 1979, pp. 983–1009.

41. Goldsmith, M., Koutcher, J., Damadian, R.: NMR in cancer XI. Applications of the NMR malignancy index to human gastrointestinal tumors. *Cancer* **41**:183–191, 1978.

42. Goncharenko, V., Gerlock, A. J., Kadir, S., Turner, B.: Incidence and distribution of venous extension in 70 hypernephromas. *A.J.R.* **133**:263–265, 1979.

43. Grabstald, H., Whitmore, W. F., Melamed, M. R.: Renal pelvic tumor. *J.A.M.A.* **218**:845–854, 1971.

44. Harris, D. T., Maquire, H. C. Jr. (Eds.): Renal cell carcinoma. *Semin. Oncol.* **10**:365–440, 1983.

45. Harrison, R. H., Baird, J. M., Kowierschke, S. W.: Renal oncocytoma: Ten year follow up. *Urology* **17**:596–599, 1981.

46. Hartman, D. S., Davis, C. J., Madewell, J. E., Friedman, A. C.: Primary malignant renal tumors in the second decade of life: Wilm's tumor versus renal cell carcinoma. *J. Urol.* **127**:888–891, 1982.

47. Heiken, J. P., Gold, R. P., Schnun, J. M., King, D. L., Bashist, B., Glazer, H. S.: CT of renal lymphoma with ultrasound correlation. *J. Comput. Assist. Tomogr.* **7**(2):245–250, 1983.

48. Heney, N. M., Nocks, B. N., Daly, J. J., Blitzer, P. H., Parkhurst, E. C.: Prognostic factors in carcinoma of the ureter. *J. Urol.* **125**:632–636, 1981.

49. Hermanek, P., Sigel, A., Chlepas, S.: Renal cell carcinoma—invasion of veins. *Eur. Urol.* **2**:142–144, 1976.

50. Hricak, H., Williams, R. D.: Magnetic resonance imaging and its application in urology. *Urology* **23**:442–454, 1984.

51. Jewett, H. J.: Tumors of the bladder. In *Urology*, Vol. II. Campbell, M. F. (Ed.). Philadelphia, W. B. Saunders, 1963, p. 1027.

52. Jones, G. W.: Renal cell carcinoma. *CA* **32**:280–285, 1982.

53. Kakizoe, T., Fujita, J., Murase, T., Matsumoto, K., Kishi, K.: Transitional cell carcinoma of the bladder in patients with renal pelvis and ureteral cancer. *J. Urol.* **124**:17–19, 1980.

54. Kantor, A. F.: Current concepts in epidermiology and etiology of primary renal cell carcinoma. *J. Urol.* **117**:415–417, 1977.

55. Katz, S. E., Shapira, H. E.: Spontaneous regression of genitourinary cancer—an update. *J. Urol.* **128**:1–4, 1982.

56. Kilton, L., Matthews, M. J., Cohen, M. H.: Adult Wilm's tumor: A report on prolonged survival and review of literature. *J. Urol.* **124**:1–5, 1980.

57. Kutscher, H. A., Trainer, T. D., Fagan, W. T.: Mucinous adenocarcinoma of renal pelvis. *Urology* **20**:94–95, 1982.

58. Lang, E. K.: The arteriographic diagnosis of primary and secondary tumors of the ureter and renal pelvis. *Radiology* **93**:799–805, 1969.

59. Lang, E. K.: Arteriography in the diagnosis and staging of hypernephromas. *Cancer* **32**:1043–1052, 1973.

60. Lieber, M. M., Tomera, F. M., Taylor, W. F., Farrow, G. M.: Renal adenocarcinoma in young adults: Survival and variables affecting prognosis. *J. Urol.* **125**:164–168, 1981.

61. Lloyd, L. K., Witten, D. M., Bueschen, A. T., Daniel, W. W.: Enhanced detection of asymptomatic renal masses with routine tomography during excretory urography. *Urology* **II**:523–528, 1978.

62. Madayag, M. A., Ambos, M. A., Lefleur, R. S., Bosniak, M. A.: Involvement of the inferior vena cava in patients with renal cell carcinoma. *Radiology* **133**:321–326, 1979.

63. Majmudar, B.: Metastasis of cancer to cancer: Report of a case. *Hum. Pathol.* **7**:117–119, 1976.

64. Mauro, M. A., Wadsworth, D. E., Stanley, R. J., McClennan, B. L.: Renal cell carcinoma: Angiography in the CT era. *A.J.R.* **139**:1135–1138, 1982.

65. McCarron, J. P., Chasho, S. B., Gray, G. F.: Systematic mapping of nephroureterectomy specimens removed for urothelial cancer: Pathological findings and clinical correlations. *J. Urol.* **128**:243–246, 1982.

66. McDonald, M. W., Konnak, J. W.: Simultaneous contralateral hypernephroma and renal transitional cell carcinoma. *Urology* **14**:509–511, 1979.

67. McNichols, D. W., Segura, J. W., DeWeerd, J. H.: Renal cell carcinoma: Long term survival and late recurrence. *J. Urol.* **126**:17–23, 1981.

68. Melicow, M. M.: The urothelium: A battleground for oncogenesis. *J. Urol.* **120**:43–47, 1978.

69. Meyers, J. M., Jr., Fehrenbaker, L. G., Kelalis, P. P.: Prognostic significance of renal vein invasion by hypernephroma. *J. Urol.* **100**:420–423, 1968.

70. Mitchell, M. R., Partain, C. L., Price, R. R., Karstaedt, N.: NMR: State of the art in medical imaging. *Appl. Radiol.* 19–25, 1982.

71. Morales, A., Wasan, S., Bryniak, S.: Renal oncocytomas: Clinical,

radiological and histological features. *J. Urol.* **123**:261–264, 1980.

72. Mostofi, F. K.: Pathology and spread of renal cell carcinoma. In *International Symposium on Renal Neoplasm*. King, J. S., Jr. (Ed.). Boston, Little, Brown & Co., 1967, pp. 41–85.

73. Murphy, D. M., Zincke, H., Furlow, W. L.: Primary grade I transitional cell carcinoma of the renal pelvis and ureter. *J. Urol.* **123**: 629–631, 1980.

74. Murphy, D. M., Zincke, H., Furlow, W. L.: Management of high grade transitional cell cancer of the upper urinary tract. *J. Urol.* **125**:25–29, 1981.

75. Murphy, G. P., Mostofi, F. K.: The significance of cytoplasmic granularity in the prognosis of renal cell carcinoma. *J. Urol.* **94**: 48–54, 1965.

76. Nocks, B. N., Heney, N. M., Daly, J. S., Perrone, T. A., Griffin, P. P., Prout, G. R.: Transitional cell carcinoma of renal pelvis. *Urology* **19**:472–477, 1982.

77. Noronha, R. F. X., Johnson, D. E., Guinee, V. F., Borlase, B. C.: Changing patterns in age distribution of renal cell carcinoma patients. *Urology* **13**:12–13, 1979.

78. Ochsner, M. G., Brannan, W., Pond, H. S., Collins, H. T.: Transitional cell carcinoma of the renal pelvis and ureter. *Urology* **4**: 392–396, 1974.

79. Parvay, H. R., Thomas, J. L., Bernardino, M. E., Barnes, P. A., Lewis, E.: Pitfalls in diagnosis of exophytic renal tumors. *Urology* **20**:218–222, 1982.

80. Patel, N. P., Lavengood, R. W.: Renal cell carcinoma: Natural history and results of treatment. *J. Urol.* **119**:722–726, 1978.

81. Paulson, D. F., Perez, C. A., Anderson, T.: Genito-urinary malignancies. In *Cancer—Principles and Practice of Oncology*. DeVita, V. T., Jr., Hellman, S., Rosenberg, S. A. (Eds.). Philadelphia, J. B. Lippincott, 1982, pp. 732–785.

82. Pillari, G., Lee, W. J., Kermari, S., Chen, M., Abrams, H. J., Buchbinder, M., Sutton, A. P.: CT and angiographic correlation: Surgical image of renal mass lesions. *Urology* **17**:296–299, 1981.

83. Rabes, H. M., Carl, P., Meister, P., Rattenhuber, U.: Analysis of proliferative compartments in human tumors. I. Renal adenocarcinoma. *Cancer* **44**:799–813, 1979.

84. Robson, C. J., Churchill, R. M., Anderson, W.: The results of radical nephrectomy for renal cell carcinoma. *J. Urol.* **101**:297–301, 1969.

85. Shepp, L. A.: Computerized tomography and nuclear magnetic resonance. *J. Comput. Assist. Tomogr.* **4**:94–107, 1980.

86. Silverberg, E.: Cancer statistics, 1984. *CA* **34**(1):14–15, 1984.

87. Singh, E. O., Barrett, D. M., Adams, V. I.: Synchronously occurring malignant fibrous histiocytoma of the kidney with contralateral renal cell carcinoma. *J. Urol.* **128**:586–588, 1982.

88. Skinner, D. G., Colvin, R. B., Vermillion, C. D., Pfister, R. C., Leadbetter, W. F.: Diagnosis and management of renal cell carcinoma: A clinical and pathological study of 309 cases. *Cancer* **28**: 1165–1177, 1971.

89. Smith, R. B.: Long term survival of a vena caval recurrence of renal cell carcinoma. *J. Urol.* **125**:575–578, 1981.

90. Sufrin, G.: The challenge of renal adenocarcinoma. *Surg. Clin. North Am.* **62**:1101–1118, 1982.

91. Sufrin, G., Murphy, G. P.: Renal adenocarcinoma. *Urol. Survey* **30**:129–144, 1980.

92. Takeyama, M., Arima, M., Sagawa, S., Sonoda, T.: Preoperative diagnosis of coincident renal cell carcinoma and renal angiomyolipoma in nontuberous sclerosis. *J. Urol.* **128**:579–581, 1982.

93. Tolia, B. M., Whitmore, W. F., Jr.: Solitary metastasis from renal cell carcinoma. *J. Urol.* **114**:836–838, 1975.

94. Totty, W. G., McClennan, B. L., Melson, G. L., Patel, R.: Relative value of computed tomography and ultrasonography in the assessment of renal angiomyolipoma. *J. Comput. Assist. Tomogr.* **5**:173–178, 1981.

95. Vest, S. A.: Conservative surgery in certain benign tumors of the ureter. *J. Urol.* **53**:97–121, 1945.

96. Wadsworth, D. E., McClennan, B. L., Stanley, R. J.: CT of the renal mass. *Urol. Radiol.* **4**:85–94, 1982.

97. Weimar, G., Culp, D. A., Loening, S., Narayana, A.: Urogenital involvement by malignant lymphoma. *J. Urol.* **125**:230–231, 1981.

98. Werth, D. D., Weigel, J. W., Mebust, W. F.: Primary neoplasms of the ureter. *J. Urol.* **125**:628–631, 1981.

99. Weyman, P. J., McClennan, B. L., Stanley, R. J., Levitt, R. G., Sagel, S. S.: Comparison of computed tomography and angiography in the evaluation of renal cell carcinoma. *Radiology* **137**:417–424, 1980.

100. Zimmer, W. D., Williamson, B., Hartman, G. W., Hattery, R. R., O'Brien, P. C.: Changing patterns in the evaluation of renal masses: Economic implications. *A.J.R.* **143**:285–289, 1984.

17 BLADDER CANCER

Dennis M. Balfe
Jay P. Heiken
Bruce L. McClennan

It is expected that in 1983 bladder cancer will be diagnosed in 38,500 patients in the United States, the majority of whom will be men.[57] In the same year, 10,700 patients are expected to die of the disease.[57] Despite rapidly accumulating data on the subject, the overall survival of bladder cancer patients has changed little in the past 40 years.[33] Concluding his editorial on the subject, Prout commented, "It seems that there is more to learn about bladder carcinoma now than there was 25 years ago."[45]

A number of perplexing clinical problems in the management of patients with urothelial tumors remain unsolved. One major difficulty has been in developing techniques that may help characterize patients at risk of developing frankly invasive carcinoma from a pre-existing superficial lesion. Noninvasive superficial carcinomas are relatively common in middle-aged and elderly men, but not all of them will progress to frankly invasive carcinomas. Approximately two thirds of patients with superficial carcinomas will develop recurrence of tumor.[6] The later tumors will be more anaplastic and thus more invasive in 25%.[6] Thus far, no single characteristic pertaining to superficial tumors has proved to be an adequate predictor for judging which patients are at risk of developing invasive transitional cell carcinomas.[29,31]

Clinical staging of invasive carcinomas, which eventually determines the therapeutic choice, is demonstrably erroneous in up to 66% of patients.[48] Superficial tumors are more likely to be correctly staged than deeply invasive neoplasms. Errors of overstaging are far more common in superficial tumors, while understaging is more prevalent in the assessment of invasive tumors.[52] If clinical studies are to provide intelligible data for making rational choices of therapy, much more accurate staging information must become available.

The most important prognostic factor for patients with invasive transitional cell carcinomas is the degree of bladder wall invasion.[21,29-32,46] Thus, the five-year survival for patients with superficial carcinomas is 50% to 80%, while for patients with deeper invasion it is 6% to 23%.[13,43] With current therapeutic techniques, treatment failures are generally the result of widespread metastases rather than local (pelvic) recurrence.[46]

The major goals for an appropriate imaging strategy thus are first to refine the preoperative assessment of local tumor extension, with particular attention to invasion of the adjacent perivesical fat or the nearby visceral structures. Second, a clinically useful imaging method should be able to provide information regarding the presence of metastatic disease. Thus, evaluation of the status of regional lymph node chains assumes paramount importance. Computed tomography (CT), ultrasonography (US), angiography, and lymphangiography all have been used for this purpose. To date, no single imaging technique has successfully met the goals described above. Each method will be discussed separately in a section on imaging and assessment in an effort to evaluate their individual strengths and weaknesses.

As in the case with other pelvic tumors, radiologic methods do not contribute significantly to the detection of bladder carcinoma. The major impact of newer radiologic methods therefore will be to provide more precise preoperative staging and a means for serial postoperative follow-up for the early detection of recurrence. Whether this contribution will significantly alter the survival of patients with transitional cell carcinomas remains to be assessed.

TUMOR BEHAVIOR AND PATHOLOGY

All bladder carcinomas originate from abnormal urothelium. Low grade, papillary types of transitional cell carcinomas probably originate from urothelial hyperplasia; higher grades may arise from carcinoma in situ.[20] The precise etiologic agents that act to produce urothelial neoplasms in humans have not been completely identified. It has been known since the turn of the century that exposure to analine dyes and other aromatic amines is carcinogenic.[44] Epidemiologic studies have indicated that cigarette smokers have an increased risk of developing bladder carcinoma, as do workers in the rubber and leather industries.[11] A specific infectious disease, schistosomiasis, is very closely related to the development of urothelial neoplasms; however, in affected patients, there is a marked tendency for development of squamous cell carcinomas rather than transitional cell carcinomas.[11] While viral particles have been removed from transitional cell tumors, there is as yet no convincing evidence for a viral cause in carcinogenesis.[11]

It is well recognized that many patients with transitional cell carcinomas have widespread urothelial abnormalities peripheral to the obvious tumor.[25] This supports the concept that various carcinogenic agents are present within the urine that induce varying degrees of dysplastic changes within the entire urothelium. In certain areas, this then progresses to frank transitional cell neoplasms. It has been suggested that the extent of such dysplastic changes critically affects the prognosis of bladder cancer patients.[31,44,46,61] For example, Lutzeyer et al.[31] reported 315 patients who had superficial bladder cancer. In this group, 60% developed recurrent carcinoma in other sites within the bladder after transurethral resection; in patients who had already undergone one such recurrence, the likelihood of yet another relapse was 86%. These data strongly suggest that the entire urothelium is at risk in many patients with transitional cell carcinomas.

Clinical predictors proven to be useful in evaluating the likelihood of tumor progression include tumor multiplicity, grade of the initial tumor, invasion of the lamina propria, and the presence of marker chromosomes. The red cell adherence test makes use of the fact that lesions that are biologically more threatening do not express surface antigens of the ABO type.[6] Eighty percent of tumors not expressing the antigen proceed to invasion, whereas only 10% of those not expressing antigen become invasive.[6]

Once patients develop invasive transitional cell tumors, their survival depends greatly on pathologic stage. In a recent series,[43] the five-year survival for T_1 cancer was 65%, while for T_4 it was 10%. Lymph node invasion carries a dire prognosis, although recent studies suggest that the presence of one or two positive pelvic nodes does not categorically rule out the possibility of surgical cure.[59]

Pathologic Patterns

Urothelial tumors may be divided into two major subtypes: papillary and solid. The term papillary refers to the microscopic, not the gross, appearance; 90% of all primary bladder tumors are papillary. They are formed predominantly in men in their sixth or seventh decade. Grading of papillary tumors varies from institution to institution; generally, the higher grade lesions (most anaplastic) have a greater tendency to invade the bladder wall and hence metastasize.

Solid (nonpapillary invasive) urothelial tumors may arise from pre-existing papillary tumors or from nonpapillary carcinoma in situ. Glandular or squamous elements are frequently present. Solid tumors show a marked propensity to invade vesical lymphatics; the presence of such invasion in the pathologic specimens markedly worsens the prognosis.

Patterns of Spread

Local extension. Invasive urothelial cancer initially spreads radially through the wall of the bladder and then circumferentially through the muscular layer. Depending on its point of origin, it may then invade the perivesical fat, the prostate, the seminal vesicles, or the obturator internus muscles (Figure 17-1). In women, it rarely invades the uterus or cervix. Invasion of the ureters or urethra is common when the tumor originates near one of these structures.

Lymphatic metastasis. A rich lymphatic network is present within the bladder mucosa and muscular coat. Anastomoses of lymphatic channels across the midline are common on the posterior wall, less common in the trigone, and rare on the anterior wall. Three major lymphatic trunks have been described.[49]

1. Trunks from the region of the trigone pass medial to the ureters in women and medial to the vasa deferentia in men. They follow the course of the uterine or vas deferens arterial supply to terminate in the medial or middle group of external iliac nodes.
2. Lymphatics from the posterior wall drain into the external iliac or rarely the hypogastric nodes.

3. Channels from the anterior wall drain along the bladder surface posteriorly where they also terminate in external iliac nodes.

Autopsy studies demonstrate that the incidence of nodal metastases in patients dying of bladder cancer is 78%.[29] Metastases to regional lymph nodes increase in proportion to the extent of local tumor (see staging). While in 1972, Prout[44] stated that it was unusual if a patient survived with even one positive node, his more recent surgical series[44] demonstrates some survival if small single nodal metastases are removed.

Another autopsy series[23] bears out the importance of the depth of muscular invasion relative to lymphatic or hematogenous dissemination. Only 23% of patients with superficial tumors had metastases at the time of death; 100% of the 22 patients with deep wall invasion had developed metastatic disease at autopsy. Skinner[60] reported the correlation between local extent of invasive carcinoma and the incidence of lymph node metastases at the time of radical cystectomy. His results are given in Table 17-1.

Distant hematogenous spread. Sites external to the pelvis are usually involved late in the course of the disease

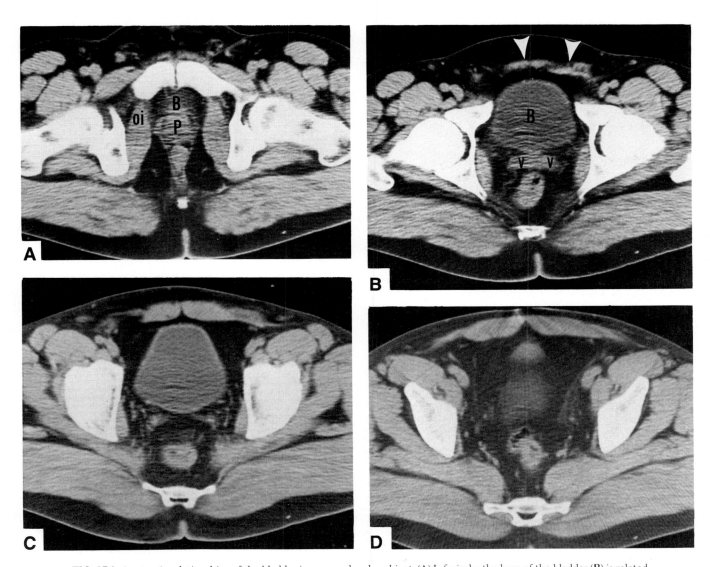

FIG. 17-1. Anatomic relationships of the bladder in a normal male subject. (A) Inferiorly, the base of the bladder (**B**) is related to the symphysis pubis anteriorly, the prostate (**P**) posteriorly, and the obturator internus muscles (**oi**) laterally. (B) the midportion of the bladder is related anteriorly to the prevesical fat and rectus abdominus muscles (arrowheads). Posteriorly lie the paired seminal vesicles (**v**), while posterolaterally the pelvic wall musculature (obturator internus muscles) is present. (C) At a slightly higher level the bladder is almost totally surrounded by perivesical fat. (D) The dome of the bladder is related to the rectum and sigmoid colon posteriorly, to the perivesical fat immediately laterally, and to the vas deferens more laterally.

Table 17-1. Incidence of Lymph Node Metastases by Stage

STAGE	NUMBER OF PATIENTS	PATIENTS WITH LYMPH NODE METASTASES (%)
T_0	17	0 (0)
T_{is}	9	1 (11)
T_1	22	2 (9)
T_2	16	4 (25)
T_{3A}	13	8 (61)
T_{3B}	17	7 (41)
T_3	30	15 (50)
T_4	5	3 (60)

Reprinted from Skinner, D. G.: Management of invasive bladder cancer: A meticulous pelvic node dissection can make a difference. *J. Urol.* **128**:34–36, 1982. With permission.

and confer a dismal prognosis, with survival rarely exceeding a few months.[24,29] The most common sites for distant metastasis include the liver (30% to 38% of autopsied patients), lung (30% to 36%) and the skeleton (24% to 27%).[23,29] The adrenal glands are involved in up to 20% of cases.

CLASSIFICATION AND STAGING

Staging of a patient with bladder cancer begins with careful preoperative clinical assessment. Clinical staging thus includes all efforts to describe total tumor extent short of surgical exploration.

The classic system for staging urothelial tumors was published in 1946 by Jewett and Strong[21] and was modified in 1952 by Marshall.[52] In 1962, the International Union Against Cancer (UICC) developed the TNM staging system and devised its application to urothelial tumors. A comparison of the Jewett-Strong-Marshall and the UICC classification systems is given in Table 17-2 and Figure 17-2. In the Jewett-Strong-Marshall system, carcinomas in situ and papillary, noninvasive carcinomas are both regarded as stage O. In the TNM classification, they are given separate status, and are reported as T_{is} and T_a, respectively. T_1 lesions are equivalent to Jewett-Strong-Marshall A cancers; only the lamina propria is invaded. Invasion of tumor into the superficial layer of bladder musculature defines a B_1 (T_2) carcinoma. B_2 (T_{3a}) cancers have infiltrated the deep muscle layers. Invasion of the perivesical fat is the criterion for Stage C (T_{3b}) disease. If the tumor extends to involve pelvic viscera but no pelvic nodes are involved, it is T_4 (D_1). D_1 lesions also include patients with single homolateral nodes (N_1), contralateral or bilateral regional nodes (N_2), or fixed regional nodes (N_3). Patients with widespread adenopathy (N_4) or distant metastases (M_1) are classed as stage D_2.

The logic of this staging classification relates to the fact that as a transitional cell carcinoma invades deeply into the muscular wall of the bladder or perivesical tissues, the incidence of lymph node metastases increases and the overall patient survival diminishes, regardless of the form of therapy. For example, Prout et al.[46] reported the incidence of lymph node metastases in 151 patients who underwent radical cystectomy. Patients with T_{is}, T_a, or T_1 tumors had only a 10% incidence of nodal metastases. The cancers invading bladder muscle (T_2, T_{3a}) were metastatic to regional nodes in 25%. When the perivesical fat was invaded, 40% had metastatic lymph node involvement. Finally, tumors locally invading surrounding structures (T_4) had a 67% incidence of pathologically involved nodes.

Staging is an important prognostic indicator of patient survival. Patients with "superficial" tumors that do not invade deep muscle (T_{is}, T_a, T_1, T_2) have a five-year survival of 58% to 64%. Patients with deep muscle or immediate extravesical extension have a 20% to 58% survival and patients with advanced tumors (T_4, N_+, M_+) have a 6% to 14% five-year survival.[11]

The degree of cellular differentiation (grade) also affects survival, as reflected by numerous studies. In one recent series,[35] for example, the overall survival of patients with well-differentiated tumors was 39% at one year; of those with poorly differentiated tumors only 14% survived one year.

Despite the importance of accurate clinical staging in assessing the prognosis of patients with urothelial tumors, present clinical methods are difficult to employ and do not in general provide accurate information. In their article on pitfalls in clinical staging of bladder tumors, Schmidt and Weinstein[52] point to a variety of problem areas that contribute to the inaccuracy of clinical staging. These include the insensitivity of commonly employed methods, such as intravenous urography, cystoscopy, and bimanual examination in exactly delineating the extent of the primary tumor. Another important contributor is the inability of any currently available method to detect microscopic metastases within the lymphatic system or metastases disseminated hematogenously. As advances are made in both urologic and radiologic technology, there has been gratifying progress in more precisely defining the total extent of local tumor.[28] As yet, however, the problem of detecting occult metastatic disease has not been solved.

IMAGING PROCEDURES AND ASSESSMENT

Clearly the strategy for staging from the therapeutic point of view is to identify those patients who may benefit from an attempt at curative therapy, i.e., radical surgical extirpation or radiation for cure. This necessitates identifying a subset of patients who have invasive tumors localized to the bladder with, at most, microscopic local

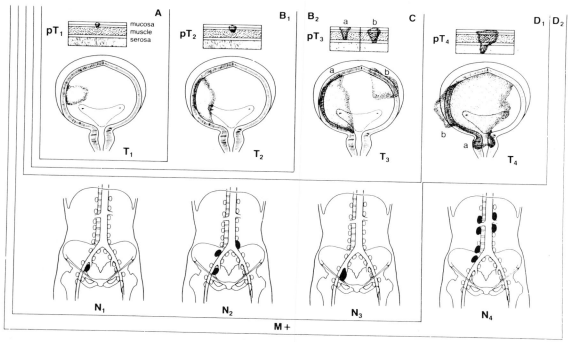

FIG. 17-2. Anatomic staging for bladder carcinoma. Tumor (T) categories: The depth of invasion is the important criterion and follows that of hollow viscera. Size and location, though important, are not critical factors. The progression of invasion is from mucosa to muscle to serosa and then to pelvis or abdominal wall for T_1, T_2, T_3, and T_4, respectively. The clinical criteria are listed, but biopsy proof is required and readily obtained. After transurethral resection (TUR), T_1 and T_2 have no palpable disease. T_3 has palpable induration and nodularity, but is mobile, and T_4 is a mass that is fixed to pelvic viscera (T_{4a}) or to the pelvic or abdominal wall (T_{4b}). Node (N) categories: The regional nodes are defined by single versus multiple, ipsilateral versus bilateral for N_1 versus N_2. Fixed nodes are N_3, and para-aortic nodes are juxtaregional (UICC only). Stage grouping: The American Urologic System (Jewett-Marshall)[21] uses the ABCD stages, which correspond to T categories. The N_1 and M are part of stage D. An AJC staging system exists but is not commonly used. AJC v UICC classification: There is concurrence by the AJC and UICC at this site. The American Urologic System (AUS) (Jewitt-Marshall) uses the letters A, B, C, and D. (Modified from Frank, I. N., Keys, H. M., McCune, C. S.: Urologic and male genital cancers. In *Clinical Oncology for Medical Students and Physicians*, 6th ed. Rubin, P. (Ed.). New York, American Cancer Society, 1983, pp. 198–221.)

Table 17-2. Bladder: Comparison of Jewett-Strong-Marshall with TNM Staging

JSM		TNM
0	Carcinoma in situ	$T_{is}N_0M_0$
	Papillary, noninvasive carcinoma	$T_aN_0M_0$
A	Invasion of lamina propria	$T_1N_0M_0$
B_1	Invasion of superficial muscular layer	$T_2N_0M_0$
B_2	Invasion of deep muscular layer	$T_3N_0M_0$
C	Invasion of perivesical fat	$T_{3a}N_0M_0$
D_1	Extension to pelvic viscera; nodes negative	$T_4N_0M_0$
	Extension to pelvic viscera; single ipsilateral node	$T_4N_1M_0$
	Extension to pelvic viscera; contralateral or bilateral nodes	$T_4N_2M_0$
	Extension to pelvic viscera; fixed regional nodes	$T_4N_3M_0$
D_2	Widespread by lymphadenopathy (UICC only)	$T_xN_4M_0$
	Distant metastases	$T_xN_xM_+$

metastases to pelvic lymph nodes. Patients who are not selected for surgical therapy, whatever the reason, do not require an aggressive evaluation of the status of the pelvic and retroperitoneal lymphatics before institution of therapy, since there is no literature to support that such disease can be eradicated by any currently available means.

A variety of radiologic methods have been used in an effort to more accurately assess the state of patients with urothelial tumors. Their utility in detecting, staging, and postoperatively assessing such patients is the focus of the following sections.

Detection

The cystographic phase of an intravenous urogram is relatively insensitive to all but very large exophytic bladder tumors. Hillman et al.[18] reported 20 cases of known bladder cancers in which the urogram was interpreted as negative in eight (40%). Only one (5%) of 19 negative bladders was misinterpreted as positive. The most useful roles of urography include (1) screening the remainder of the urothelium; and (2) aiding in overall patient assessment, e.g., demonstrating the presence, absence, or degree of hydronephrosis or detecting congenital anomalies (i.e., solitary kidney) that might alter the planned approach.

Cystoscopy with biopsy is the method of choice for confirmation of tumors in the bladder. If there is clinical or urographic suspicion of disease in the upper urinary tract, retrograde pyelograms can be performed at the same sitting. Similarly, bimanual examination while the patient is under general anesthesia should allow smaller lesions to be palpated. Histologic review of the retrieved material completes the detection/confirmation phase.

If the clinician and patient decide that a curative effort is reasonable, a maximum amount of information should be gathered preoperatively. Screening for metastatic disease is based on the most common sites of widespread involvement and has included standard chest roentgenograms and radionuclide scans of the liver, spleen, and skeleton. Recent reports by Berger et al.[3] and Lindner and DeKernion[28] question the effectiveness of obtaining routine liver/spleen and skeletal radionuclide images of patients without chemical abnormalities and with unremarkable histories and physical examinations. This question remains unresolved; at our institution, most patients in whom cystectomy is planned do have radionuclide screening of the skeletal system. The rationale used for obtaining this test is that it provides a baseline for subsequent postoperative evaluation should the patient return with skeletal pain. Liver/spleen radionuclide scans are rarely obtained when individuals are screened before surgery.

Local Extent of Tumor

Assuming the patient remains a candidate for definitive therapy after passing through the screening gamut, he or she may be submitted to a full-scale attempt to define the exact local extent of disease and the nodal status. A variety of radiographic means have been used to assess the actual extent of disease, including CT, sonography (transabdominal, transrectal, or transurethral), and angiography. Less technology-oriented (and less accurate) means, such as fractional cystography, have not been shown to reliably distinguish among the T stages.

Computed tomography,[1,15-17,19,20,22,24,36,37,38,50,51,55,56,67] with its inherent superb contrast resolution would be expected to predict accurately whether tumor (attenuation 20 to 40 Hounsfield units) had infiltrated perivesical fat (-80 to -100 HU) (Figures 17-3, 17-4, and 17-5). However, the recent study of Koss et al[24] shows an overall accuracy of only 60% for CT in T staging. In 20 patients in whom local invasion was predicted, CT agreed with pathologic staging in 12. Five falsely positive examinations were caused by loss of the normal fat plane between the seminal vesicles and the bladder, leading to an er-

roneous diagnosis of invasion. Three false-negative examinations were caused by microscopic invasion of perivesical fat missed on CT. In a smaller series by Ahlberg et al.,[1] CT stage agreed with pathologic T stage in eight of nine (89%) patients; one individual was overstaged when CT predicted deeper muscle invasion than was present. At this stage, the ability of CT to predict invasion of the prevesical tissues or to accurately assess the depth of muscular invasion is limited by the low spatial resolution of CT.

One possible solution to the problem of assessing local extent of invasive urothelial tumor is to use sonography.[39,53,58] Tumors have diminished echogenicity, which allows them to be reliably distinguished from the normal vesical wall. Singer et al.[58] reported an accuracy of 100% in staging deep tumors using transabdominal ultrasound examination. However, more superficial tumors were routinely overstaged by this method, and small tumors may not be successfully imaged. A report by Nakamura and Nijima[39] using transurethral ultrasonography, demonstrated 95% accuracy in assessing the depth of 20 tumors in 12 bladders. Similar accuracy (with less histologic proof) was reported by Schuller et al. using the same method.[53]

Theoretically, angiography can provide information regarding both T stage and tumor grade (highly anaplastic tumors having more primitive vascularity with increased puddling of contrast).[64] This method, however, requires intravesical and extravesical gas insufflation to define the bladder wall in addition to arteriotomy and selective catheterization and can hardly be classed as a noninvasive technique. Accuracy of this method is highest in T_3 and T_4 lesions (90% to 95%) but falls off in low stage tumors (29% to 53% in T_1 and T_2 cancers).[64] As newer noninvasive techniques become perfected, support for this method will likely wane.

Nodal Status

Accurate evaluation of nodal status is critical to selection of appropriate therapy. If an accurate means were available to detect tumor spread, many patients could be spared needless laparotomy and tedious lymph node dissections.

Lymphangiography has been successfully used to determine lymph node status in patients with lymphomas. Its success in staging pelvic malignancies depends on the frequency with which inguinal, external iliac, common iliac, and para-aortic/paracavel nodes are involved with each specific tumor. Since bladder lymphatics drain to the external iliac nodes, lymphangiography should opacify nodes that are at risk (Figure 17-6). Despite this fact, there has been no consistent success in using lymphangiography in studying the bladder.[8,22,62] While Jing et al.[22] reported an accuracy of 91.6% in their series at M.D. Anderson Hospital (false-negative, 9.8%), many investi-

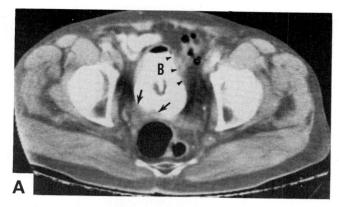

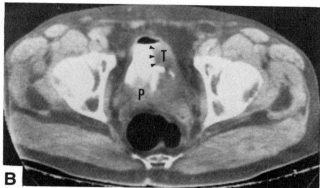

FIG. 17-3. Bladder carcinoma invading superficial muscle only. (A) CT scan near the base of the bladder (B) of a patient with known adenocarcinoma of the prostate (arrows) demonstrates focal bladder wall thickening (arrowheads) involving a segment on the left anterior margin. (B) One centimeter more caudal, in this incompletely distended bladder, the smooth internal margin of the tumor (T), outlined by arrowheads, contrasts with the more irregular margins of the prostatic cancer (P). At surgery, a grade II transitional cell carcinoma of the bladder with superficial muscle invasion was found.

gators have had a more disappointing experience. Farah and Cerny[8] reported 48% correlation between lymphangiographic nodal status and pathologic examination. False-positive diagnoses occur when lymph nodes are enlarged by inflammatory processes; the percentage of false-positive diagnoses can be reduced if strict criteria for the diagnosis of metastatic disease are adopted. False-negative diagnoses are more difficult to avoid, since they are most commonly caused by microscopic metastases in opacified nodes or microscopic deposits in nodes that remain unopacified. A recent small series[62] reported one of seven false-negative and one of 12 false-positive diagnoses by lymphangiography.

The major advantage of CT over lymphangiography is its ability to detect metastatic deposits in nodal groups not opacified by bipedal injection. Its disadvantage lies in the fact that normality is judged by size alone; it is insensitive to infrastructural changes that do not produce gross enlargement. In the series of Koss et al.[24] only three

of five pathologically involved nodes were detected; similarly, three of four positive nodes in the series of Morgan[36] were detected by CT. In both series, all false-negative scans were caused by microscopic metastases.

Jing et al.[22] compared CT and LAG in 26 patients with histologic proof; the accuracy of LAG was superior to that of CT (96% v 88%). All false-negative interpretations were caused by small metastatic deposits except in one of the CT cases, where improper orientation of the transverse slice resulted in an enlarged node being missed. Neither examination yielded a falsely positive diagnosis.

A less invasive (and less accurate) means of providing information regarding nodal status in patients with pelvic malignancies is lymphoscintigraphy.[7] This method involves injection of the ischiorectal fossa and subsequently the dorsum of the feet with a radionuclide designed to be taken up by the lymphatic trunks. If the activity on subsequent images is asymmetric, metastatic

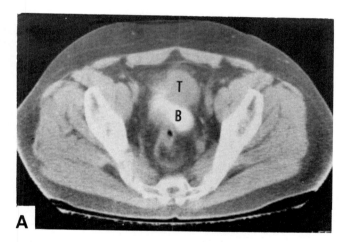

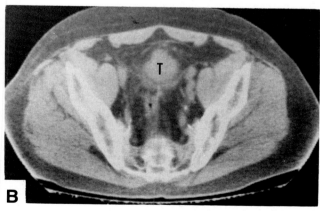

FIG. 17-4. Grade III transitional cell carcinoma invading the serosa of the bladder. (A) Scan through the dome of a contrast distended bladder (B) demonstrates an exophytic tumor (T) arising from the anterior wall of the dome. (B) One centimeter more cephalad, the tumor (T) is totally surrounded by perivesical fat. The fine linear perivesical soft tissue densities looked like tumor extension, but at surgery the perivesical fat was free of tumor.

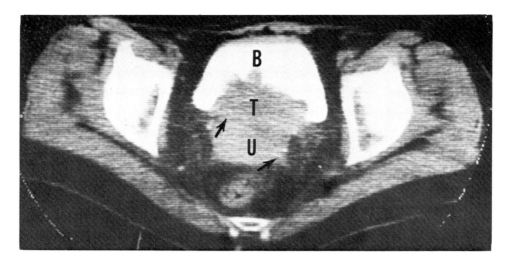

FIG. 17-5. An extensive tumor (T) arising from the posterior surface of the bladder (B) invades the posterior perivesical fat, obscuring the plane between the tumor and the uterus (U) at several points (arrows). This grade III transitional cell carcinoma was inseparable from the uterus at surgery.

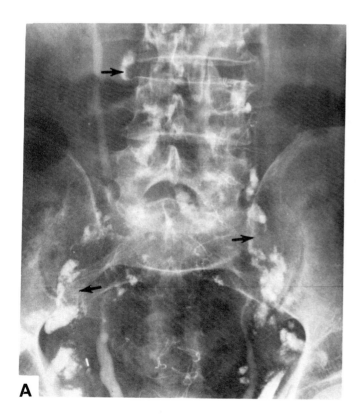

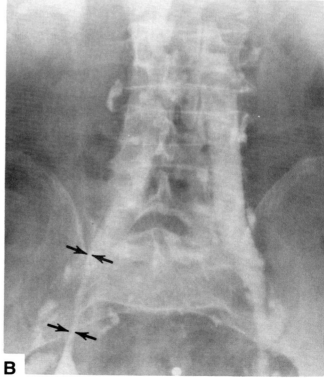

FIG. 17-6. A 70-year-old patient with advanced bladder tumor. (A) A lymphangiogram demonstrates multiple peripheral filling defects within the external iliac, common iliac, and paracaval nodal chains (arrows). Note the absence of filling of the common iliac nodes on the right and the narrowing of the ureter in this region. (B) A venogram performed on the same patient demonstrates extensive narrowing of the common iliac vein (arrows) in the region of the common iliac adenopathy.

adenopathy is suspected. The utility of this technique remains to be evaluated, but it would appear to be most useful in patients with high stage disease.

Distant Metastatic Disease

The sites at greatest risk for distant spread of transitional cell carcinoma are the skeleton, the lungs, and the liver.[11] Obviously, demonstrable spread to any of these sites precludes radical surgery. Thus, patients who are considered candidates for cystectomy and urinary diversion benefit from accurate screening of the target organs.

The chest film stands as the simplest screening procedure for excluding pulmonary metastases. The ability of chest radiology to detect nodules is a function of their size.[27] Uncalcified lesions under 3 mm usually will not be detected. Larger nodules may be missed if they are projected over other high-density areas; thus apical, diaphragmatic, and retrocardiac nodules may be obscured unless they are greater than 1 cm in diameter.

In patients for whom definitive therapy is a consideration, more sensitive methods should be used; yet, very sensitive methods such as CT suffer from their limited ability to distinguish small metastatic nodules from small benign nodules (e.g., granulomata). Conventional whole lung tomography may represent a useful compromise and is often employed in preoperative evaluation at our institution.

There is considerable controversy over the utility of routine liver/spleen or skeletal radionuclide images in cystectomy candidates who have no symptoms of extravesical spread and normal laboratory findings. Liver lesions, for example, must be greater than 2 cm in diameter (larger still, if deeply positioned) to be detected by scintigraphy.[4] Both sonography and CT are far more sensitive and accurate methods for evaluating the liver, and either may be employed in suspicious cases. At present, the incidence of liver metastases in patients thought to be cystectomy candidates who have normal liver function tests appears to be too small to employ routine screening procedures.

For osseous lesions, however, radionuclide scanning has distinct advantages. It is far more sensitive than skeletal survey films in detecting metastatic lesions;[4] such metastases may be seen by radionuclide scan up to 18 months before being apparent on the bone films. The sensitivity of radionuclide imaging is 50% to 80% greater than radiography alone. In addition, in sequential evaluation of patients after radical surgery, bone pain of recent onset may be evaluated by a repeat radionuclide scan.

Screening examinations, by their nature, are highly sensitive and usually are not particularly specific. Thus, a positive finding on any screening examination should be histologically confirmed before hope of definitive cure is abandoned. In this regard, fine-needle aspiration biopsy of soft tissue or lung lesions is a most useful technique.[9,71] For epithelial tumors metastatic to lymph nodes, a success rate above 90% and a diagnostic accuracy with needle aspiration biopsy ranging from 80% to 95% has been reported.[71] Similarly, large-bore needle biopsy of lesions has a 75% to 90% accuracy rate. Lesions seen fluoroscopically (e.g., lymph node metastases seen on lymphangiograms) may be simply evaluated using this technique. For lesions not localized by fluoroscopy, both CT and US have been employed to direct and confirm the appropriate needle placement.

IMAGING STRATEGIES AND DECISIONS

Figure 17-7 outlines the phases through which a patient with suspected bladder cancer will pass. In the detection phase, urography plays a major role in screening the urothelium but not in identifying bladder cancers. Suspicious lesions seen in the kidney or ureter on a urogram can be assessed using retrograde pyelography, cytology, and brush biopsy if necessary. After an initial T stage assessment is made, the candidacy of the patient for radical therapy is evaluated. If the patient has an invasive (T_1–T_4) cancer and is in fair overall condition, he or she is at least potentially a candidate for radical surgery and efforts should be made to exclude patients with unresectable disease. To this end, plain film tomograms or CT of the chest, radionuclide bone scanning, and, when clinical suspicion warrants, liver scanning should be performed, with percutaneous biopsy of probable metastatic lesions. If the patient proves to have no metastatic deposit, the next step depends on the initial T stage obtained by biopsy. Patients with superficial (T_1, T_2) lesions of high grade have an excellent chance that their local tumor can be completely resected; before this procedure, however, evaluation of nodal status should be performed. As discussed, lymphangiography, combined with percutaneous biopsy of suspicious nodes, is the procedure most likely to aid in the selection of operative candidates. Deeper lesions (T_3, T_4) may be locally unresectable and for this reason, further delineation of their precise T stage is necessary. In this regard, transurethral ultrasonography has recently been shown to have a 95% accuracy in assessing the depth of invasion of urothelial tumor.[39] It is not universally available, however, and CT may be used as a substitute in this phase. Assuming the imaging procedures have selected a patient whose local extent of tumor is resectable and who has at most one regional node involved with tumor, operative staging via careful lymphadenectomy is then carried out. This represents an "eleventh hour" staging procedure before the performance of radical cystectomy.

CARCINOMA OF THE BLADDER
INITIAL EVALUATION

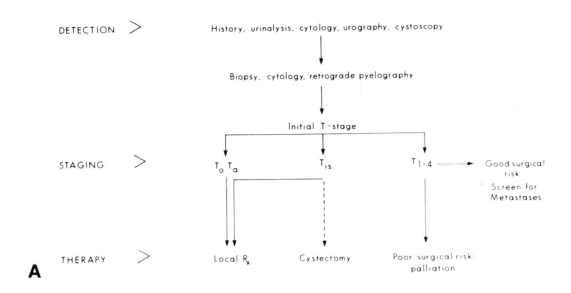

CARCINOMA OF THE BLADDER
SCREENING FOR METASTASES IN SURGICAL CANDIDATES

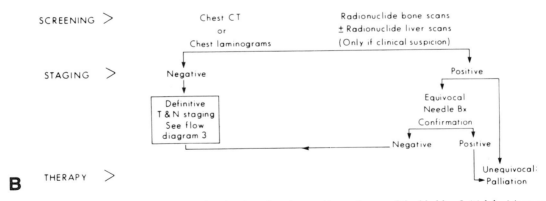

FIG. 17-7. (A) Algorithmic scheme for initial evaluation of patients with carcinoma of the bladder. Initial decisions are made according to the clinical T stage. (B) Algorithmic diagram for screening for metastases in patients thought to be candidates for radical surgery. (C) Algorithmic diagram of further staging procedures in surgical candidates without evidence of metastases. Both the clinical stage and the grade of the tumor are important determinants of the optimal workup.

If no metastases are retrieved in the pathologic material as evaluated by frozen section, the radical cystectomy is performed.

The combination of these imaging procedures should be useful in optimally selecting appropriate patients for radical therapy. To date, however, no large clinical trials prospectively evaluating this imaging strategy have been reported. A comparison of available imaging methods for evaluating carcinoma of the bladder is presented in Table 17-3.

TREATMENT DECISIONS

Survival for patients with invasive carcinoma of the bladder has improved only slightly in the past few decades (Table 17-4).[5,10,42] Evaluation of optimal therapeutic programs is difficult, since clinical staging is highly inaccurate.[52] The foregoing sections make it apparent that radiologic maneuvers are imperfect also, but they are helpful in selecting patients for appropriate management.[37,40]

Therapy of carcinoma of the bladder depends upon

CARCINOMA OF THE BLADDER:
DEFINITIVE STAGING OF T_{1-4} M_0 SURGICAL CANDIDATES

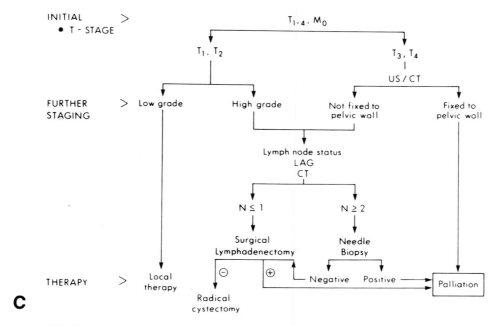

FIG. 17-7, continued.

the clinical stage of disease at the time of initial examination. Superficial carcinoma can be treated adequately with fulguration or transurethral resection in the majority of cases. A certain percentage of patients with carcinoma in situ will not respond to local attempts at therapy, and in view of the high incidence of subsequent development of frankly invasive transitional cell carcinomas, more radical surgical procedures (cystoprostatectomy) have been advocated for medically appropriate patients with unresponsive carcinoma in situ.

For patients with T_2 or T_3 lesions, particularly those of grade III or grade IV cellular architecture, radical cystectomy has been widely advocated. For this procedure to be successful, the tumor must be surgically encompassable; thus, fixation to adjacent visceral structures or to the pelvic wall contraindicates radical surgical therapy. In addition, the presence of pelvic lymphadenopathy is a relative contraindication, and the presence of para-aortic or paracaval adenopathy precludes surgical cure. It is here that the newer imaging methods could have the greatest impact on choice of available therapies by demonstrating clinically inapparent regional extension or lymphadenopathy.

In turn, patients who are not candidates for surgical therapy may be treated with high dose radiation therapy with the intent to cure.[54] Since there are complications to radical radiation therapy, these patients should likewise be evaluated for the presence of para-aortic lymphadenopathy, the presence of which would prevent a curative procedure. In addition to aiding in the selection of appropriate candidates for radical therapy, cross-sectional imaging techniques are also useful in precisely defining the total tumor volume to be irradiated.

A problem that continues to beset both clinical and radiologic evaluation is assessment of patients with previous radiation therapy or segmental bladder resection. Both CT and lymphangiography are known to be unreliable in treated patients and evaluation of both local and nodal disease still remains the province of the surgeon. Clarification of the appropriate preoperative maneuvers in this group of patients awaits further clinical study.

Sequential evaluation of patients after radical surgery is best carried out by CT, since that is the only available method capable of imaging the operative site. Lee et al.[26] reported good results in detecting recurrent carcinoma in postcystectomy patients. A mass effect of any kind following radical cystectomy should raise suspicion about recurrent carcinoma and should be confirmed with needle aspiration techniques (Figure 17-8). Since computed tomography can evaluate masses as small as 1.5 cm, it is hoped that earlier recognition of local recurrence will improve the survival in this group of patients.

In summary, conservative procedures are used for superficial papillary tumors, including transurethral resection or intravesical chemotherapy for recurrent and multiple superficial lesions (Table 17-5). External irradiation is only used when other measures fail or there is a medical contraindication to cystectomy.

Table 17-3. Imaging Methods for Carcinoma of the Bladder

METHOD	STAGING CAPABILITY	COST BENEFIT RATIO	RECOMMENDED ROUTINE/ STAGING PROCEDURE
Noninvasive			
Chest imaging			
Plain films	Capable of detecting large lesions; preoperative screening technique.	High	Yes
Tomography	Capable of detecting smaller lesions (metastases).	Medium	No
CT	Highest sensitivity. Moderate specificity for pulmonary lesions.	Medium	No; only for selected operative candidates
Radionuclide studies			
Bone scan	Sensitive to skeletal metastases.	Medium	No; only in patients clinically at risk for widespread metastases
Liver-Spleen scan	Sensitivity for large intrahepatic metastases.	Low	No
Bone Films	May document skeletal metastases (complements bone scan).	Medium	Only to document lesions detected by RN scanning
Magnetic Resonance Imaging (MRI)	Unknown.	Unknown	Unknown
Minimally invasive			
Urography	Urothelial screening examination.	High	Yes
Cystography	May demonstrate fixation of bladder wall, but insensitive to minimal invasion.	Low	No
CT	Sensitive to local invasion if macroscopic.	Medium	No; only in operative candidates
(Transurethral) Sonography	Capable of imaging local invasion.	Medium	As alternative to CT
Retrograde ureteropyelography	Screens urothelium, evaluates suspicious urographic lesions.	High	Yes
Invasive			
Lymphangiography	Identifies lymph node metastases in external iliac, common iliac and para-aortic areas.	Medium	No; selected operative candidates only
Angiography	May identify gross extravesical extent by abnormal vascularity.	Low	No
Percutaneous Needle Aspiration	Documents presence and character of tumor detected by other methods.	Medium	Selected patients

Table 17-4. Bladder: Survival by Stage

TREATMENT	STAGE	NUMBER OF PATIENTS	FIVE-YEAR SURVIVAL (%)
Radiation only	T_1	43	65
	T_2	117	46
	T_3	218	32
	T_4	42	10
Radiation Followed by Cystectomy			
Skinner[60]	less than T_1		81
	T_2		53
	T_3		37
	T_4		25
Mathur et al.[32]	T_1	11	73
	T_2	8	88
	T_3	29	48
	T_4	7	29

For the more invasive T_2, T_3 (B or C) stage high-grade tumors, a radical cystectomy and ileal loop are performed,[68] usually with preoperative rather than postoperative radiation therapy.[2,34,63,64,66,67] Radiation doses either can be concentrated, delivered in large fractions in one week's time, i.e., 400 cGy × 5, totalling 2,000 cGy, or conventional fractions of 200 cGy, i.e., 4,500 cGy in 4½ weeks. When definitive radiation therapy is used, doses of 6,000 to 7,000 cGy are given usually with a coned-down technique with salvage cystectomy for failures attempting to preserve bladder function in as many patients as possible.[12] For advanced stage T_4 lesions, D_1 disease, or $N_{1,2,3}$ nodal involvement limited to the pelvis, palliative radiation therapy with an ileal loop is a common form of management. There are a number of chemotherapeutic agents,[14,47,70] particularly cisplatin, that have been effectively used in investigational studies, with or without the other modes, or in cases of more advanced or recurrent disease, by themselves.

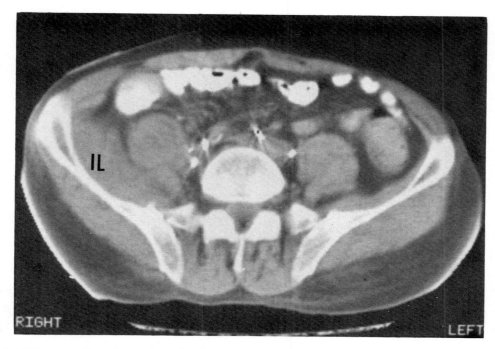

FIG. 17-8. A CT scan performed several months after radical cystectomy for bladder tumor demonstrates marked swelling of the iliacus muscle (IL) on the right. A soft tissue density is present between the psoas and iliacus medially (arrows). At biopsy, this proved to be a metastatic transitional cell carcinoma.

IMPACT OF NEW TECHNOLOGY

Two major problems that continue to plague oncologists in evaluating patients with bladder carcinoma are (1) detection of tumor extension that is below the spatial resolution limits of currently existing methods; and (2) distinguishing between postradiation fibrosis and active tumor in patients who have undergone extensive radiation therapy. Imaging by magnetic resonance (Figure 17-9) can potentially assess the metabolic activity of a selected area of interest. For example, if the rate at which tumor cells metabolize phosphate compounds is known to be distinctly different from the rate at which fibrocytes metabolize the same compounds, it is theoretically possible to distinguish between fibrous tissue and active tumor growth. To date, however, this represents a speculative area that awaits definitive demonstration in human subjects.

Clinical research likewise needs to be performed to evaluate imaging based upon the production of mono-

Table 17-5. Bladder: Treatment Decision by Stage

STAGE	TREATMENT MODALITY					
	SURGERY		RADIATION THERAPY		CHEMOTHERAPY	
T_1N_0 0, A	Transurethral resection		NR		Recurrent, multiple intra-vesical chemotherapy	
T_2N_0 B, Low Grade	Segmental cystectomy		Interstitial implantation		NR	
T_2N_0 B_2 High Grade	Radical cystectomy Ileal loop	and/ or	Pre-operative RT, 2000–4500 cGy Definitive RT, 6000–7000 cGy	and/or	Investigational MAC	
T_3N_0 CN_0	Radical cystectomy Ileal loop	or	Pre-operative RT, 6000–7000 cGy Definitive RT, 6000–7000 cGy	and/or	Investigational MAC	
$T_4D_1N_{1,2,3}$	Ileal division		Palliative RT		MAC	
Relapse	Surgical salvage for RT failure		RT for surgical failure		Investigational MAC	

NR = Not recommended.
RT = Radiation therapy.
MAC = Multiagent chemotherapy.

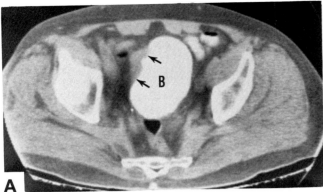

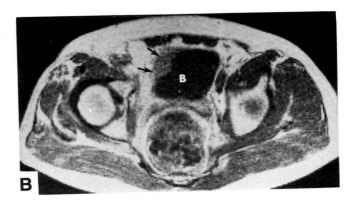

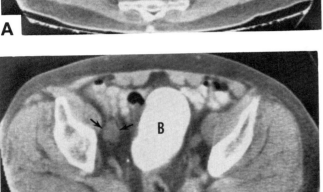

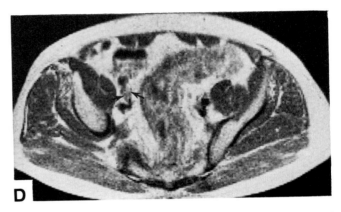

FIG. 17-9. Grade III invasive transitional cell carcinoma imaged by CT and MRI. (A) A CT scan through the midportion of the contrast-filled bladder (B) demonstrates a focal area of wall thickening (arrows) corresponding to a clinically evident carcinoma. (B) An MRI image at the same level shows the high-intensity tumor (arrows) separate from the lower-intensity urine within the bladder (B). (C) A CT scan slightly cephalad shows a soft tissue mass (arrows) in the region of the external iliac artery and vein. A portion of the tumor is still seen in the wall of the bladder (B). (D) An MRI image at the same level demonstrates a high-attenuation lymph node metastasis (arrows) separate from the surrounding vascular structures.

clonal antibodies specific for a tumor antigen. Theoretically, however, microscopic lymph node metastases well below the size observable by computed tomography or lymphangiography could be detected by labeling antibody specific to a tumor antigen and subsequently imaging the target nodal areas. It does, indeed, appear that "there is more to learn about bladder carcinoma now than there was 25 years ago."[45]

REFERENCES

1. Ahlberg, N. E., Calissendorff, B., Wijkstrom, H.: Computed tomography in staging of bladder carcinoma. *Acta Radiol. Diagn.* **23**:47–53, 1982.
2. Batata, M. A., Whitmore, W. F., Jr., Chu, F. C. H., Hilaris, B. J., Unal, A., Chung, S.: Patterns of recurrence in bladder cancer after radiation therapy versus drugs. *Int. J. Radiat. Oncol. Biol. Phys.* **6**: 155–160, 1980.
3. Berger, G. L., Sadlowski, R. W., Sharpe, J. R., Finney, R. P.: Lack of value of routine preoperative bone and liver scans in cystectomy candidates. *J. Urol.* **125**:637–639, 1981.
4. Bernardino, M. E., Thomas, J. L., Barnes, P. A., Lewis, E.: Diagnostic approaches to liver and spleen metastases. *Radiol. Clin. North Am.* **20**:469–486, 1983.
5. Caldwell, W. L.: Carcinoma of the urinary bladder. In *Textbook of Radiotherapy*, 3rd ed. Fletcher, G. H. (Ed.). Philadelphia, Lea & Febiger, 1980, pp. 852–866.
6. Catalona, W. J.: Guest editorial: Bladder carcinoma. *J. Urol.* **123**:35, 1980.
7. Ege, G. N.: Augmented iliopelvic lymphoscintigraphy: Application in the management of genitourinary malignancy. *J. Urol.* **127**:265–269, 1982.
8. Farah, R. N., Cerny, J. C.: Lymphangiography in staging patients with carcinoma of the bladder. *J. Urol.* **119**:40–41, 1978.
9. Ferrucci, J. T., Jr., Wittenberg, J., Mueller, P. R., Simeone, J. F., Harbin, W. B., Kirkpatrick, R. H., Taft, P. D.: Diagnosis of abdominal malignancy by radiologic fine-needle aspiration biopsy. *A.J.R.* **134**: 323–330, 1980.
10. Frank, I. N., Keys, H. M., McCune, C. S.: Urologic and male genital cancers. In *Clinical Oncology for Medical Students and Physicians: A Multidisciplinary Approach*, 6th ed., Rubin, P. (Ed.). New York, American Cancer Society, 1983, pp. 198–221.
11. Gittes, R. F.: Tumors of the bladder. In *Campbell's Urology*, Vol. 2. (Eds.) J. H. Harrison, R. S. Gittes, A. D. Perlmutter, T. A. Stamey, P. C. Walsh. Philadelphia, W. B. Saunders, 1979, pp. 1033–1065.
12. Goodman, G. B., Hislop, T. G., Elwood, J. M., Balfour, J.: Conservation of bladder function in patients with invasive bladder cancer

treated by definitive irradiation and selective cystectomy. *Int. J. Radiat. Oncol. Biol. Phys.* 7:569–73, 1981.

13. Grossman, H. B.: Current therapy of bladder carcinoma. *J. Urol.* 121:1–7, 1979.
14. Hahn, R. G.: Bladder cancer treatment considerations for metastatic disease. *Semin. Oncol.* 6:236–239, 1979.
15. Hamlin, D. J., Cockett, A. T. K.: Computed tomography of bladder: Staging of bladder cancer using low density opacification technique. *Urology* 13:331–334, 1979.
16. Hamlin, D. J., Cockett, A. T. K., Burgener, F. A.: Computed tomography of the pelvis: Sagittal and coronal imaging reconstruction in the evaluation of infiltrative bladder carcinoma. *J. Comput. Assist. Tomogr.* 5:27–33, 1981.
17. Hildell, J. G., Nyman, U. R. O., Norlingh, S. T., Hellsten, S. F. J., Stenberg, P. B. A.: New intravesical contrast medium for CT: Preliminary studies with arachis (peanut) oil. *A.J.R.* 137:777–780, 1981.
18. Hillman, B. J., Silvert, M., Cook, G., Stanisic, T., Bjelland, J., Claypool, H. R., Haber, K., Mellins, H. Z.: Recognition of bladder tumors by excretory urography. *Radiology* 138:319–323, 1981.
19. Hodson, N. J., Husband, J. E., MacDonald, J. S.: The role of computed tomography in the staging of bladder cancer. *Clin. Radiol.* 30:389–395, 1979.
20. Jeffrey, R. B., Palubinskas, A. J., Federle, M. P.: CT evaluation of invasive lesions of the bladder. *J. Comput. Assist. Tomogr.* 5:22–26, 1981.
21. Jewett, H. J., Strong, G. H.: Infiltrating carcinoma of the bladder—relation of the depth of penetration of the bladder wall to the incidence of local extension and metastases. *J. Urol.* 55:366, 1946.
22. Jing, B., Wallace, S., Zornoza, J.: Metastases to retroperitoneal and pelvic lymph nodes. Computed tomography and lymphangiography. *Radiol. Clin. North Am.* 20:511–530, 1982.
23. Kishi, K., Hirota, T., Matsumoto, K., Kakizoe, T., Murase, T., Fujita, J.: Carcinoma of the bladder: A clinical and pathological analysis of 87 autopsy cases. *J. Urol.* 125:36–39, 1981.
24. Koss, J. C., Arger, P. H., Coleman, B. G., Mulhern, C. B., Pollack, H. M., Wein, A. J.: CT staging of bladder carcinoma. *A.J.R.* 137:359–362, 1981.
25. Koss, L. G.: Tumors of the urinary bladder. In *Atlas of Tumor Pathology*, 2nd series, Fascicle II. Bethesda, Md., Armed Forces Institute of Pathology, 1975.
26. Lee, J. K. T., McClennan, B. L., Stanley, R. J., Levitt, R. G., Sagel, S. S.: Utility of CT in evaluation of post cystectomy patients. *A.J.R.* 136:483–487, 1981.
27. Libshitz, H. I., North, L. B.: Pulmonary metastases. *Radiol. Clin. North Am.* 20:437–452, 1983.
28. Lindner, A., DeKernion, J. B.: Cost effective analysis of precystectomy radioisotope scan. *J. Urol.* 128:1181–1182, 1982.
29. Loening, S., Narayana, A., Yoder, L., Slymen, D., Penick, G., Culp, D.: Analysis of bladder tumor recurrence in 178 patients. *Urology* 16:137–144, 1980.
30. Loening, S., Narayana, A., Yoder, L., Slymen, D., Weinstein, S., Penick, G., Culp, D.: Factors influencing the recurrence rate of bladder cancer. *J. Urol.* 123:29–31, 1980.
31. Lutzeyer, W., Rubben, H., Dahm, H.: Prognostic parameters in superficial bladder cancer: An analysis of 315 cases. *J. Urol.* 127:250–252, 1982.
32. Mathur, V. K., Krahn, H. P., Ramsey, E. W.: Total cystectomy for bladder cancer. *J. Urol.* 125:784–786, 1981.
33. McCarron, J. P., Marshall, V. F.: The survival of patients with bladder tumors treated by surgery: Comparative results of an old and a recent series. *J. Urol.* 122:322–324, 1979.
34. Miller, L. S., Johnson, D. E.: Megavoltage irradiation for bladder cancer alone, postoperative or preoperative? In *Proceedings of the 7th National Cancer Conference.* Philadelphia, J. B. Lippincott, 1972, pp. 771–782.
35. Morabito, R. A., Kandzari, S. J., Milam, D. F.: Invasive bladder carcinoma treated by radical cystectomy. Survival of patients. *Urology* 14:478–481, 1979.
36. Morgan, C. L., Phil, M., Calkins, R. E., Cavalcanti, E. J.: Computed tomography in the evaluation, staging and therapy of carcinoma of the bladder and prostate. *Radiology* 140:751–761, 1981.
37. Muir, B. B., Sinclair, D. J., Duncan, W.: The role of radiology in the assessment of bladder cancer. *Clin. Radiol.* 29:479–485, 1978.
38. Murphy, G. P.: Developments in preoperative staging of bladder tumors. *Urology* 11:109–115, 1978.
39. Nakamura, S., Nijima, T.: Staging of bladder cancer by ultrasonography: A new technique by transurethral intravesical scanning. *J. Urol.* 124:341–344, 1980.
40. Nelson, R. P.: New concepts in staging and follow up of bladder carcinoma. *Urology* 21:105–112, 1983.
41. Pagani, J. J., Libshitz, H. I.: Imaging bone metastases. *Radiol. Clin. North Am.* 20:545–560, 1983.
42. Paulson, D. F., Perez, C. A., Anderson, T.: Genito-urinary malignancies. In *Cancer—Principles and Practice of Oncology.* DeVita, V. T., Jr., Hellman, S., Rosenberg, S. A. (Eds.). Philadelphia, J. B. Lippincott, 1982, pp. 732–785.
43. Pilepich, M. V., Perez, C. A.: Does radiotherapy alter the course of genitourinary cancer? In *Genitourinary Cancer 1.* Paulson, D. F., (Ed.). Boston, Martinus Nijhoff, 1982, pp. 215–238.
44. Prout, G. R.: Bladder carcinoma. *N. Engl. J. Med.* 287:86–90, 1972.
45. Prout, G. R.: Bladder cancer. *J. Urol.* 128:284, 1982.
46. Prout, G. R., Griffin, P. P., Shipley, W. U.: Bladder carcinoma as a systemic disease. *Cancer* 43:2532–2539, 1979.
47. Prout, G. R., Jr., Slack, N. H., Bross, I. D.: Irradiation and 5-fluorouracil and adjuvants in the management of invasive bladder carcinoma: A cooperative group report after 4 years. *J. Urol.* 104:116–129, 1970.
48. Richie, J. P., Skinner, D. G., Kaufmann, J. J.: Carcinoma of the bladder: Treatment by radical cystectomy. *J. Surg. Res.* 18:271, 1975.
49. Rouviere, H.: *Anatomy of the Human Lymphatic System.* Ann Arbor, Edwrd Bros, 1938.
50. Sager, E. M., Talle, K., Fossa, S., Ous, S.: The role of CT in demonstrating perivesical tumor growth in the preoperative staging of carcinoma of the urinary bladder. *Radiology* 146:443–446, 1983.
51. Sareczerk, I. S., White, R. D. V., Gold, R. P., Olsson, C. A.: Sensitivity of computed tomography in evaluation of pelvic lymph node metastases from carcinoma of bladder and prostate. *Urology* 21:81–84, 1983.
52. Schmidt, J. D., Weinstein, S. H.: Pitfalls in clinical staging of bladder tumors. *Urol. Clin. North Am.* 3:107–127, 1976.
53. Schuller, J., Walther, V., Schmiedt, E., Staehler, G., Bauer, H. W., Schilling, A.: Intravesical ultrasound tomography in staging bladder carcinoma. *J. Urol.* 128:264–266, 1981.
54. Scott, R. S., Johnson, R. J. R.: Radical radiotherapy in the treatment of transitional cell carcinoma of the urinary bladder. *Urology* (suppl.) 23:48–53, 1984.
55. Seidelmann, F. E., Cohen, W. N., Bryan, P. J., Temes, S. P., Kraus, D., Schoenrock, G.: Accuracy of CT staging of bladder neoplasms using the gas-filled method: Report of 21 patients with surgical confirmation. *A.J.R.* 130:735–739, 1978.
56. Seidelmann, F. E., Temes, S. P., Cohen, W. N., Bryan, P. J., Patil, U., Sherry, R. G.: Computed tomography of gas-filled bladder: Method of staging bladder neoplasms. *Urology* 9:337–344, 1977.
57. Silverberg, E.: Cancer statistics 1983. *CA* 33:9–25, 1983.
58. Singer, D., Itzchak, Y., Fischelovitch, Y.: Ultrasonographic assessment of bladder tumors. I. Tumor detection. *J. Urol.* 126:33–33, 1981.
59. Skinner, D. G.: Current perspectives in the management of high-grade invasive bladder cancer. *Cancer* 45:1866–1874, 1980.
60. Skinner, D. G.: Management of invasive bladder cancer: A meticulous pelvic node dissection can make a difference. *J. Urol.* 128:34–36, 1982.

61. Soloway, M. S.: Bladder cancer—part II. *J. Urol.* **124**:47–49, 1980.

62. Strijk, S. P., Debruyne, F. M. J., Herman, C. J.: Lymphography in the management of urologic tumors. *Radiology* **146**:39–45, 1983.

63. Van der Werf-Messing, B.: Carcinoma of the bladder (T1, NX, MO). Radiation only versus TUR. *Int. J. Radiat. Oncol. Biol. Phys.* 7:299–303, 1981.

64. Van der Werf-Messing, B.: Preoperative radiation therapy followed by cystectomy to treat carcinoma of the urinary bladder, category T3, NX 0-4 MO. *Int. J. Radiat. Oncol. Biol. Phys.* 8:1849–1855, 1981.

65. Weinerman, P. M., Arger, P. H., Coleman, B. G., Pollack, H. M., Banner, M. P., Wein, A. J.: Pelvic adenopathy from bladder and prostate carcinoma: Detection by rapid-sequence computed tomography. *A.J.R.* **140**:95–99, 1983.

66. Whitmore, W. F., Jr., Batata, M. A., Hilaris, B. S., Reddy, G. N., Unal, A., Ghoneim, M. A., Grabstald, H., Chu, F.: A comparative study of 2 preoperative radiation regimens with cystectomy for bladder cancer. *Cancer* **40**:1077–1086, 1977.

67. Whitmore, W. F., Jr., Grabstald, H., Mackenzie, A. R., Iswariah, J., Phillips, R.: Preoperative irradiation with cystectomy in the management of bladder cancer. *A.J.R.* **102**:570–576, 1968.

68. Whitmore, W. F., Jr., Marshall, V. F.: Radical total cystectomy for cancer of the bladder: 230 consecutive cases 5 years later. *J. Urol.* **87**:853–868, 1980.

69. Winterberger, A. R., Wajsman, Z., Merrin, C., Murphy, G. P.: Eight years of experience with preoperative angiographic and lymphographic staging of bladder cancer. *J. Urol.* **119**:208–212, 1978.

70. Yagoda, A.: Chemotherapy of metastatic bladder cancer. *Cancer* **45**:1879–1888, 1980.

71. Zornoza, J.: Needle biopsy of metastases. *Radiol. Clin. North Am.* **20**:569–590, 1983.

18 PROSTATIC CANCER

Dennis M. Balfe
Jay P. Heiken
Bruce L. McClennan

According to estimates of the American Cancer Society, carcinoma of the prostate will be diagnosed in 75,000 American men this year and will be the cause of 24,100 deaths.[67] It is the second most common cancer occurring in men, surpassed only by lung cancer, and it is the third most common cause of male cancer-related deaths. A higher percentage of the black population is afflicted with prostatic cancer, and there is some statistical evidence that the disease is somewhat more virulent in black men and tends to occur at a slightly younger age.[32] That environmental factors play a role in its pathogenesis is suggested by the fact that clinical disease is uncommon in Oriental and Eastern European men; yet, in the American-raised children of immigrants from those geographic areas, its incidence is identical to that of the population at large.[73] The exact dietary or occupational hazards that predispose men to the development of carcinoma of the prostate have not been identified. Some researchers have indicated occupational exposure to cadmium as a carcinogenic agent. Others have drawn attention to the presence of viral particles within cytoplasmic vacuoles in prostate tumors and have concluded that viral agents may play a role in oncogenesis.[73]

The risk of developing prostatic cancer increases with advancing age. Latent tumors (clinically silent carcinomas discovered at autopsy) occur in up to 40% of patients in the eighth decade of life. The overall incidence of clinically significant tumors is much smaller, but shows a similar increase with advancing age: 0.02% at age 50 years, rising to 0.8% at age 80 years.[9,73]

Early detection of prostatic carcinomas remains a complex problem. In view of the fact that the prevalence of latent disease far exceeds that of clinically significant carcinomas, the problem really revolves around detecting carcinomas that have the biologic potential to produce disease. Digital rectal examination is a highly efficient means of detecting posterior prostatic nodules, and in a review of 300 patients reported by Guinan et al.[27] in the *New England Journal of Medicine*, digital rectal examination had a sensitivity of 69% and a specificity of 89%. An indurated nodule within the prostate gland is said to have a 50% chance of being a carcinoma.[73] For a cancer to be discovered by this method, however, the physician must be alert to the possibility of cancer being present, must be scrupulous in performing the examination, and must be experienced in evaluating the prostate. In addition, the tumor must be present within the posterior lobe of the gland and produce a bulge in its contour. In fact, early diagnosis of prostatic carcinoma is uncommon, suggesting that present methods of detection are in need of improvement. Thirty-five percent of patients have locally advanced disease at the time the disease is discovered and up to 45% have evidence of metastases.[73]

Technologic advances have allowed serum screening examinations to be performed for a variety of substances, including acid phosphatase, which is an enzyme produced in prostatic acini and normally secreted in seminal fluid. Its presence in the serum can be measured by enzymatic methods, by radioimmunoassay, or by counterimmunoelectrophoresis. These methods are expensive, and as pointed out in a statistical analysis by Watson and Tang[74], are not effective as screening examinations. Assuming a sensitivity of 70%, a specificity of 94%, and a disease prevalence of 35 per 100,000 individuals, the positive predictive value of the test is 0.41%. This means that only one in 244 patients with a positive test would actually have a prostatic carcinoma.

Radiographic methods likewise do not play a role in the early detection of prostatic cancer. Urography evaluates only the impression by the prostate on the opacified urinary bladder and is insensitive to any variables except overall size. While echo texture changes specific for adenocarcinoma have been described by investigators using transrectal ultrasonography,[34,37] false-positive and false-negative diagnoses continue to occur with significant frequency. The examination is somewhat cumbersome and demands an investment in technical equipment not readily available. At this juncture, it is unlikely that transrectal sonography will develop into a screening examination, but it may have a definite place in staging the local extension of known disease. Similarly, direct injection of the prostate gland with contrast material (prostatography)[60] remains an investigatory method that may be promising in staging known cancer but that has no utility as a screening method.

In summary, the development of an efficient screening program capable of detecting well-confined prostatic cancer remains a challenge for the future.

There has been more interest in using newer technologic methods in staging the overall extent of disease in patients known to have prostatic cancer. Whether the exquisite anatomic information that can be displayed by the new generation of computed tomography and sonographic units will allow more intelligent therapeutic choices and ultimately improve patient survival is not currently known. The impact of the assortment of newer imaging methods in evaluating the local extent of disease will be discussed in the section on imaging procedures and assessment.

TUMOR BEHAVIOR AND PATHOLOGY

Carcinomas of the prostate can be divided into two major groups: adenocarcinoma, which arises within peripheral ducts or gland acini, and carcinomas of the large ducts, a heterogeneous group that includes papillary, endometrioid, transitional cell, and epidermoid cell types.[1,43] The former group constitutes 95% of all prostatic cancers and will be the focus for the remainder of this discussion.

Many of the problems inherent in the clinical staging of prostatic carcinoma stem from the fact that the tumor arises at the periphery of the gland. A fair percentage of tumors arise in the posterior lobe and thus are readily accessible to discovery by digital rectal examination. However, their peripheral location accounts for the clinical observation that the periurethral area is spared until late in the course of the tumor. Thus, many patients do not seek medical attention for symptoms of bladder outlet obstruction until the disease is well advanced. The tumor commonly arises in multiple peripheral sites simultaneously. Ackerman and Rosai cite an 85% incidence of such multiplicity.[1]

Involvement of organs other than the prostate may occur by three means: direct extension, lymphatic spread, or hematogenous dissemination. The prostate is anatomically situated close to the base of the urinary bladder and the seminal vesicles, and extension to these organs by extracapsular carcinoma is common (Figure 18-1). By contrast, direct extension into the rectum is relatively rare because of the strong fascial layer (Denonvillier's fascia) that separates the posterior aspect of the prostate (Figure 18-2) from the anterior rectal wall.[22]

Four lymphatic trunks drain the prostate.[64] The superior margin of the gland is drained by a trunk that extends medial to the seminal vesicle to the external iliac chain. Another trunk follows the course of the middle hemorrhoidal artery to nodes in the internal iliac chains. A third trunk drains to nodes medial to the sacral foramina and then to the promontory of the sacrum. The fourth drains from the inferior aspect of the prostate and follows the internal pudendal artery to the internal iliac chain.

The performance of staging lymphadenectomy has provided a wealth of information regarding the incidence of metastatic disease to each nodal group. In most large series,[11,13,24,34,42,46,59,62,78] the group most commonly involved is the medial chain of the external iliac group, the so-called "obturator" nodal group, so named because of its proximity to the obturator nerve. When single-group nodal metastases are encountered, this group is the most commonly involved. Presacral and presciatic nodes were found to be involved in a high percentage of patients in one report, but were less commonly the only site of metastasis. Common iliac and hypogastric metastases are less commonly encountered than disease in the obturator chain. Para-aortic nodal disease is always associated with pelvic lymph node involvement.

There is a well-documented increase in nodal disease with increasing extent of local tumor and decreasing tumor differentiation. Donohue et al.[14] reviewed the literature and added their own series of 215 patients. Their results are presented in Table 18-1.

Earlier it was believed that metastases to lymph nodes occurred late in the natural history of the disease, well after the occurrence of osseous metastases. However, the weight of evidence currently supports the view that lymphatic and hematogenous dissemination occur independently. Prostatic cancer has a proclivity to metasta-

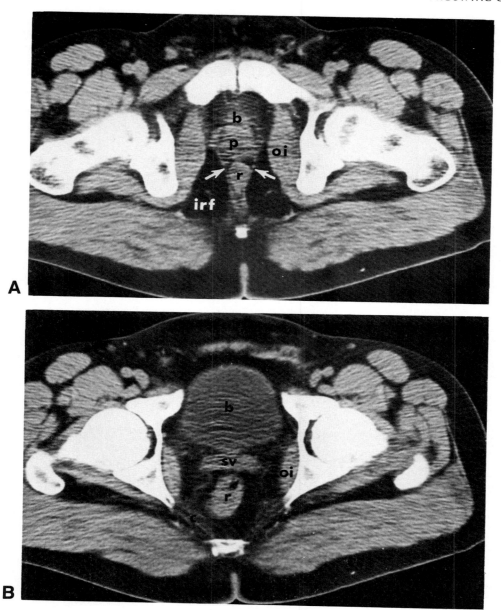

FIG. 18-1. Normal computed tomographic anatomy of the male pelvis. (A) CT scan through the symphysis pubis demonstrates the prostate gland (p) immediately anterior to the rectum (r) within the levator sling (white arrows). The space anterior to the prostate contains the base of the bladder (b) and retropubic fat, in which a rich prostatic plexus of veins is often seen. Posterior and lateral to the prostate is the ischio rectal fossa (irf), the lateral boundary of which is formed by the obturator internus (oi) muscle. (B) Scan 2 cm cephalad to A demonstrates the seminal vesicles (sv) on the superior margin of the prostate. Posterior and lateral to the rectum at this level is the pelvic floor, here formed by the coccygeus muscle (c).

size to the lumbar vertebral bodies. One anatomic explanation offered for this phenomenon is that the prostate is drained by a rich periprostatic venous plexus, which is in communication with the paravertebral plexus. When abdominal pressure is raised, blood (and thus tumor cells) may travel in a retrograde fashion from the prostatic plexus to the vertebral bodies. A report by Dodds et al.[12] casts some doubt on this concept, however, since their review of a large series of bone scans shows that

the distribution of metastases to osseous sites is not appreciably different in prostatic carcinomas than in other malignancies.

Other likely sites of widespread osseous involvement are the pelvis, ribs, and femurs. In autopsy studies, lymphangitic spread to the lungs is present in 25% of patients dying of prostatic cancer, but is radiographically visible in only 10%.[73] Liver metastases occur terminally and are found in approximately 20% of patients dying

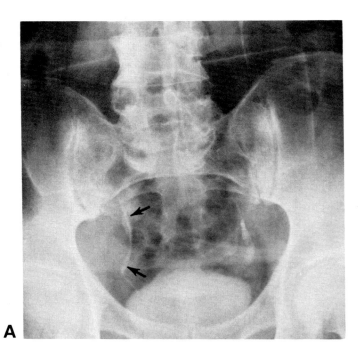

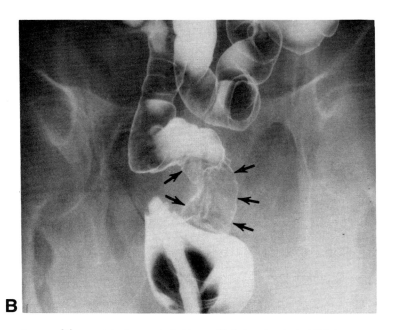

FIG. 18-2. Extensive carcinoma of the prostate demonstrated by multiple imaging tests. (A) Intravenous urogram demonstrates a soft tissue mass in the region of the right obturator internus muscle, with medial deviation of the ureter (arrows) suggesting a large mass in this region. (B) Air contrast enema demonstrates infiltrative narrowing of the rectum (arrows) extending to the level of the peritoneal reflection. (C) CT scan through the symphysis pubis demonstrates enlargement of the prostate (p), as well as thickening (arrows) of the fascial plane surrounding the rectum (r). (D) On a scan 2 cm higher, multiple nodular masses are seen within the perirectal space, and there is infiltration of soft tissue surrounding the rectum (r) and seminal vesicles (arrows). The bladder (b) is not definitely involved. (E) CT scan obtained 2 cm higher than D demonstrates multiple enlarged nodes (n) in the external iliac chain. There is medial displacement of the vas deferens (arrow). This finding accounts for the ureteral deviation seen on the urogram.

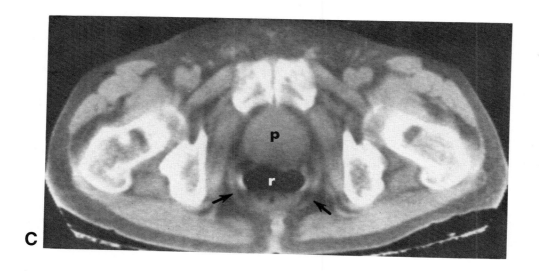

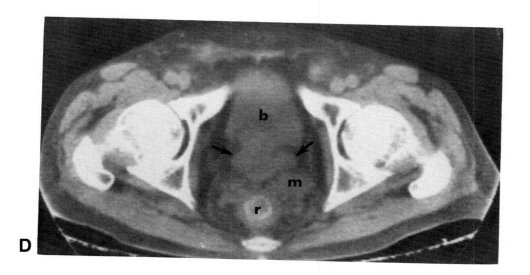

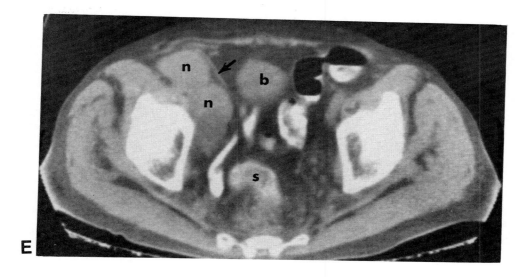

Table 18-1. Prostate: Lymph Node Metastases by Stage and Grade

STAGE	NUMBER OF PATIENTS	POSITIVE NODES (%)
A_2		
well differentiated	29	1 (3.4)
moderately differentiated	19	8 (42.1)
poorly differentiated	13	7 (53.8)
B_1		
well differentiated	72	7 (9.7)
moderately differentiated	55	14 (25.5)
poorly differentiated	15	6 (40.0)
B_2		
well differentiated	28	11 (39.3)
moderately differentiated	46	20 (43.5)
poorly differentiated	24	15 (62.5)

Adapted from Donohue, R. E., Fauver, H. E., Whitesel, J. A., Augspurger, R. R., Pfeister, R. R.: Influence of tumor grade on results of pelvic lymphadenectomy. *Urology* 17:435, 1981.

of disseminated prostatic cancer. It is, however, rare to encounter liver metastases in patients presenting with carcinoma of the prostate.

CLASSIFICATION AND STAGING

Paralleling the biologic potential of prostatic carcinoma, staging follows three separate lines of investigation: evaluation of local extent (T stage), documentation of nodal metastases (N stage), and detection of hematogenous metastases (M stage). The American Urologic System, as proposed by Jewett and Whitmore, is widely used throughout the United States, and all of the currently available information regarding patient survival has been reported using this method. A comparison of this staging system with the TNM system proposed by the UICC is presented in Table 18-2 and Figure 18-3. Stage A encompasses patients who have no clinical evidence of carcinoma but have malignancy discovered incidentally on pathologic review of TUR specimens. If the tumor is well differentiated and is present on fewer than three fragments ("chips") of the resected specimen, it is classified as stage A_1, and is equivalent to Stage T_0. Stage A_2 includes patients without clinical evidence of tumor (thus T_0) who have other than well-differentiated cell types or who have three or more tumor fragments within the specimen. It may be misleading to group these patients within a single stage, since they represent a heterogeneous population in terms of survival. The majority of A_1 lesions probably represent truly latent carcinomas or malignancies with a very low biologic hazard. Their survival parallels that of the tumor-free population. By contrast, patients with stage A_2 disease, despite the fact that a clinically palpable nodule is not present at the time their disease is discovered, often harbor aggressive tumor types or have diffuse disease extent. In the series of Golimbu et

al.[25], 78% of patients with A_2 carcinomas had either moderately or poorly differentiated cancers compared with stage B_1 patients, in whom poorly or moderately differentiated lesions occurred in only 14%. A review by Donohue et al.[13] evaluating the incidence of pelvic nodal metastases revealed that 20 of 44 A_2 patients had poorly or moderately differentiated cancer and 10 of these 20 had proven metastatic lymphadenopathy. A clinical study by Cantrell et al.[8] of 117 patients with stage A carcinomas concluded that both the grade and the total volume of disease in the prostate were good predictors of tumor progression; in their series, the presence of extensive local disease was the single best predictor of recurrence. Accordingly, many clinicians have adopted an aggressive therapeutic approach for patients with stage A_2 carcinomas of the prostate, advising radical surgical or radiotherapeutic methods except for those patients with well-differentiated tumors.[23]

Stage B cancers include all tumors that do not invade the prostatic capsule and are evident on physical examination. If the induration is clinically limited to one lobe, the tumor is categorized as B_1; if both lobes are involved, it falls into the B_2 category. These criteria do not directly correspond to the TNM staging system. In that classification, T_{1a} corresponds to a 1-cm nodule confined to the prostate and surrounded by normal tissue. T_{1b} tumors are larger than 1 cm but confined to one lobe. Both of these would be classified as B_1 in the American Urologic System. T_{1c} is the classification given to a tumor involving both prostatic lobes, and corresponds well to the B_2 stage. T_2 tumors have invaded the prostatic cap-

Table 18-2. Prostate: Comparison of Jewett-Whitmore and TNM Staging

JEWETT-WHITMORE		TNM
A_1	No clinical disease less than three fragments contain tumor	$T_0N_0M_0$
A_2	No clinical disease greater than three fragments contain tumor	
B_1	Palpable nodule confined to one lobe less than 1 cm	$T_{1a}N_0M_0$
	greater than 1 cm	$T_{1b}N_0M_0$
B_2	Tumor involving both lobes	$T_{1c}N_0M_0$
	Invasion of, but not through, the capsule	$T_2N_0M_0$
C_1	Penetration of capsule; minimal extension	$T_3N_0M_0$
C_2	Extensive local disease; ureteral/ bladder obstruction	$T_4N_0M_0$
D_1	Nodal metastases not clinically appreciated	$T_xN_+M_0$
	Widespread metastases not clinically appreciated	$T_xN_xM_+$
D_2	Nodal metastases clinically manifest	$T_xN_xM_0$
	Widespread metastases clinically manifest	$T_xN_xM_x$

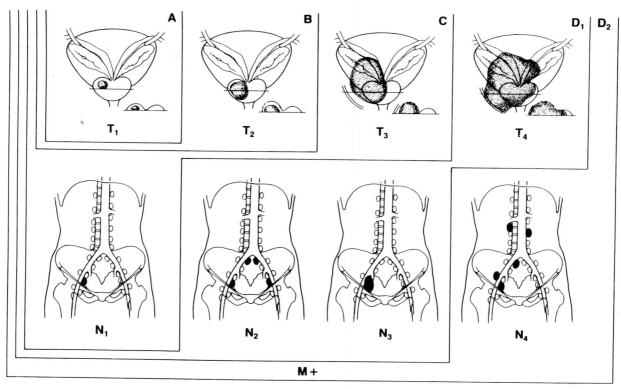

FIG. 18-3. Anatomic staging for carcinoma of the prostate. The *extension* of the cancer beyond the prostate (not size) and to surrounding structures determines the T category. Nodules confined to the prostate depend upon *distortion* of the posterior contour to determine T_1 or T_2 status. Once the cancer spreads beyond the capsule laterally or superiorly into seminal vesicles it becomes T_3; extensive involvement of adjacent organs denotes T_4. Nodal involvement ranges from single (N_1) to multiple homolateral (N_2) to fixed nodules (N_3); in the UICC system, but not in AJC, juxtaregional nodes are classified N_4. The stage grouping shown above follows the T categories and reflects the classic American Urologic system of Jewett and Whitmore. Save for the N_4 category, the AJC and UICC systems are virtually identical. Modified from AJC. Courtesy of Frank, I. N., Keys, H. M., McCune, C. S.: Urologic and male genital cancers. In *Clinical Oncology for Medical Students and Physicians: A Multidisciplinary Approach*, 6th ed. Rubin, P. (Ed.). New York, American Cancer Society, 1983, pp. 198–221.

sule but do not penetrate it, and are also classed as clinical stage B_2.

Stage C tumors have penetrated the prostatic capsule to involve adjacent structures, but the patients do not have distant metastases. If there is minimal extension they are classed stage C_1 (T_3); if extensive disease is palpable, or urography shows ureteral or bladder outlet obstruction, they become C_2 (T_4).

Stage D tumors have metastasized to regional nodes or to distant sites, and are subdivided only by whether the metastatic lesions are clinically apparent before nonclinical staging. If the patient was clinically in stage A, B, or C but nodal metastases were found at surgery or nodal aspiration, he is classed as stage D_1. Patients with clinical evidence of metastases are in stage D_2.

The TNM system attempts to categorize patients with distant metastases by assessing the total extraprimary tumor volume. Single homolateral regional node involvement is classed N_1, multiple regional contralateral metastases are N_2, bulky fixed regional nodes are N_3, and

widespread juxtaregional nodes are N_4. Recent reports support the use of this categorization in terms of patient survival.[31,58,72] The short-term survival of patients with one or two homolateral regional nodes (N_1 or N_2) who undergo radical therapy is better than that of patients with multiple positive nodes undergoing the same treatment. While recent results do not support a significant improvement in long-term survival in N_1 or N_2 patients, the time to disease progression in this group is longer than for patients with N_3 or greater disease. It thus appears to be rational to develop an imaging approach capable of stratifying patients into categories describing both the local tumor extent and the degree of nodal involvement.

Influence of Tumor Grade on Staging

While the local tumor stage has a definite effect on survival, histologic differentiation of the neoplasm undeniably has an impact on prognosis. The effect of local stage and grade on lymph node metastasis (and thus survival) is borne out in a recent report by Donohue et al.[13] (Table 18-1). Their review of the world literature shows only a 3% incidence of nodal metastases in patients with well-differentiated stage A_2 carcinomas, but a 54% incidence of metastases in patients with the same clinical stage who had poorly differentiated neoplasms. Conversely, patients with moderately differentiated tumors have a 25% nodal metastasis rate if they are clinically stage B_1; this rises to 50% in patients with clinical stage B_2 disease who have the same degree of cellular differentiation.

The implications of nodal positivity on disease progression and ultimately patient survival has been thoroughly investigated. Prout et al.[59] encountered 92 patients who underwent pelvic lymphadenectomy, of whom 32 had nodal disease. Progression of disease occurred in 56% of patients with positive nodes but in only 10% of those patients who had no diseased nodes. Nineteen of 23 (83%) of patients with stage T_3 or T_4 local disease and positive nodes had disease progression within the study period, while five of nine (56%) patients with T_0–T_2 cancers developed more extensive disease. Forty-six percent (46%) of patients with metastatic disease died, the mean time of death occurring 22 months after diagnosis. Of the nine patients who had a single positive lymph node, only two (22%) had progression of disease.

The pathologic system of grading used in the Veteran's Administration Cooperative Urologic Research Group (VACURG) was devised by Gleason. In this system, the two predominant histologic types within a given patient's neoplasm were individually graded on a scale of 1 to 5. The sum of the two grades was thus a number ranging from 2 to 10, with 10 representing very anaplastic tumors. When Paulson et al.[46,48] analyzed the data evolving from this cooperative study, they used this information to create an index by which the risk of nodal metastases could be predicted. In their studies, they found that patients with a Gleason sum between 2 and 5 had only 14% nodal positivity, while those with a sum of 9 or 10 had a 100% incidence of nodal metastases. As would be expected, this predictive index is also a function of local disease extent. Thus, T_3 or T_4 carcinomas with a Gleason sum of 2 to 4 have approximately the same incidence (about 30%) of nodal spread as T_1 cancers with a Gleason sum of 8 to 10.

IMAGING PROCEDURES AND ASSESSMENT

It is evident from the foregoing that the challenge of pretherapy staging methods is to select those patients who have disease confined to the prostate and who thus may benefit from radical surgical or radiotherapeutic management. Extracapsular extent and metastatic disease are associated with poor survival and shortened disease-free intervals, and these patients should not be candidates for radical procedures.

The simplest, most universally accessible method of selecting appropriate patients is based on information obtained from physical examination and the pathologic data from prostatic biopsy. Unfortunately, clinical staging is not sufficiently accurate to be useful in determining therapeutic decisions.[10,38] A recent report by Catalona and Stein[10] compared clinical with pathologic staging in 92 patients with clinical A_2 or B cancers. Local staging errors were 11% in stage A_2, 17% in stage B_1, and 39% in stage B_2 tumors. Assessment of lymph node spread was erroneous in 33% of stage A_2, 28% of stage B_1, and 32% of stage B_2 cancers. Twenty-three errors involved clinical understaging of actual tumor extent; of the five early therapeutic failures observed in the entire study, all were in the groups understaged clinically. Furthermore, preoperative clinical grading is based on biopsy material, with the implicit assumption that the cellular differentiation of the biopsied specimen reflects that of the entire tumor. However, in the series of Lange and Narayan,[38] 39% of patients had a significantly less well differentiated tumor in the prostatectomy specimen than was estimated from the needle biopsy.

In view of the difficulties inherent in clinical staging, a variety of imaging techniques have been brought to bear on the accurate assessment of local nodal and distant disease spread.

Local Extension

Assessment of local disease is important for guiding the choice of therapeutic alternatives. If radiation therapy has been decided upon, the choice between internal (^{125}I or ^{198}Au implantation) and external therapy depends on the total volume of disease. For assessment of radical surgical therapy, even minimal invasion of the seminal vesicles, which represents extracapsular local disease, dissuades most clinicians from performing surgery. Thus, one goal of noninvasive staging is to distinguish T_2 from the more extensive T_3 and T_4 disease.

Two methods have been investigated: CT[20,25,33,45,54,58,65,70,71,75] (Figure 18-4) and ultrasonography.[28,29,37,45,49,50,69,70] Both are accurate methods in determining prostatic size as an index of total tumor volume. However, accurate prediction of seminal vesicle invasion has been difficult using conventional computed tomographic methods. While enlargement of one or both seminal vesicles allows confident prediction of extensive tumor invasion, microscopic extension of the primary prostatic tumor may occur without CT findings. Conversely, asymmetry of the seminal vesicular angles may occur in benign prostatic enlargement and is not reliable evidence of extracapsular extension of carcinoma to the seminal vesicles. In Pilepich et al.'s series,[53] as in Golimbu et al.'s,[25] CT was in-

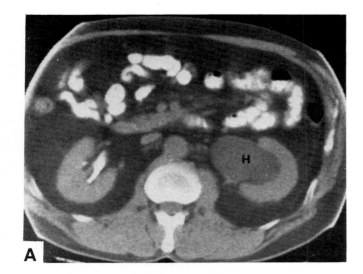

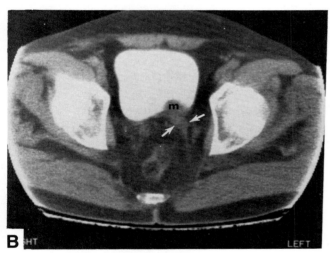

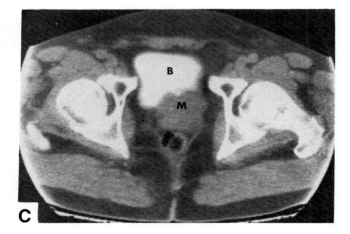

FIG. 18-4. Prostatic cancer producing left ureteral obstruction. (A) Scan through the renal hila demonstrates hydronephrosis (h) affecting the left renal pelvis. (B) Scan at the level of the acetabular roof demonstrates a mass (M) distorting the bladder contour, and causing obstruction of the left ureter (arrows). (C) Contiguity of the mass (M) with the patient's prostate is demonstrated at this level. The tumor directly invades the wall of the bladder (b).

sensitive in predicting extracapsular extent. Two explanations for the poor performance of CT in predicting extracapsular spread have been offered. First, the planes separating the prostate from the base of the bladder or seminal vesicles are curved, so that transverse slices adequately image only that part of the perivesical fat that is perpendicular to the scanning plane. Tumor extension that occurs in a horizontal direction is difficult, if not impossible, to display. Second, microscopic invasion of the perivesical fat may be below the limits of spatial resolution of currently existing machines. VanWaes and Zonneveld[72] have suggested using direct coronal scans or direct sagittal scans of the pelvis in an effort to display the complex anatomy of this region in a plane profiling the fat separating the bladder and prostate (Figure 18-5). This method, while occasionally successful, requires a rather cooperative patient and is often time-consuming. More clinical experience is necessary to establish its efficacy as an adjunct to conventional cross-sectional imaging.

Ultrasonography (US), however, is a promising means of preoperatively establishing a precise T stage. Resnick et al.[63], using transrectal sonography, evaluated 23 patients before radical prostatectomy. Ultrasonography was correct in all 23, including four in whom the clinical impression of totally intracapsular extent disagreed with the ultrasound findings. Only four of the 228 patients undergoing transrectal ultrasonography proved to have prostatic carcinomas in the face of a negative scan (false-negative rate, 1.4%). Kohri et al.[37] investigated 24 patients with known prostatic carcinomas and reported identification of tumor destruction of the prostatic capsule and infiltration of the seminal vesicles. Both investigators noted that transrectal ultrasonography was a simple means of objectively measuring the response of prostatic carcinoma to therapeutic manipulation. These results were obtained using bistable scanning technology and should improve with newer generation equipment. Drawbacks to the use of transrectal ultrasonography include the need for specialized equipment and moderate patient discomfort during the performance of the examination.

In summary, both CT and transrectal ultrasonography can be useful in staging the local extension of prostatic adenocarcinoma, although neither is useful as a screening method. Both methods are undergoing evaluation as to their accuracy, but, at present, ultrasonography appears to have the greater potential to become a routine staging tool.

Lymph Node Status

The "gold standard" for evaluating lymph node status is operative sampling of all available nodes in the external and common iliac chains, including the hypogastric nodes and the presacral nodes. While morbidity from the

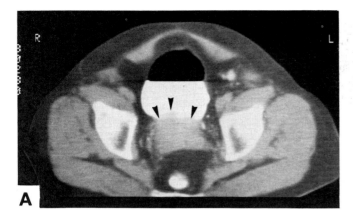

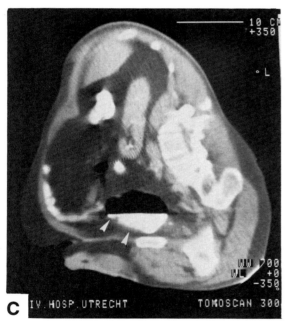

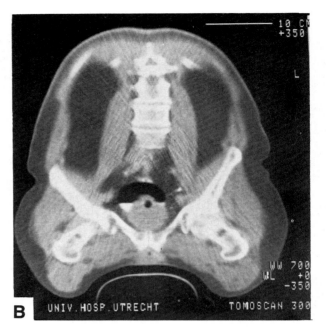

FIG. 18-5. Direct sagittal and coronal CT scans supplementing the transverse images. (A) Transverse CT scan in a patient with prostatic carcinoma demonstrates tumor nodules indenting the base of the bladder (arrowheads). Definite bladder invasion cannot be documented. (B) Direct coronal scan again displays a tumor nodule indenting the base of the bladder. No additional information is available. (C) Direct sagittal scan obtained several centimeters to the left of the midline. Tumor invasion along the anterior surface of the bladder (arrowheads) was the only evidence of Stage T_4 disease (case courtesy of Dr. Paul van Waes, Utrecht, The Netherlands).

lymph node dissection has been reduced because a retroperitoneal, rather than transperitoneal, approach has been adopted, long-term complications from lymphedema do occur and are the stimulus for the search for an accurate noninvasive method.[2,25]

Since many of the major nodal groups at risk of developing metastatic disease from cancer of the prostate are well opacified by bipedal lymphangiography, it seems reasonable to employ this technique to evaluate nodal status (Figure 18-6). Essentially all investigators report a low rate of falsely positive interpretations (specificity of 67% to 92%) but a prohibitively high false-negative rate (33% to 75% sensitivity).[7,34,35,36,40,42,57,62,66,68] Three major reasons are offered for the large number of missed lesions: (1) microscopic nodal metastases, too small to be detected as filling defects within the opacified lymph node, (2) nonfilling of a node completely replaced by tumor, (3) metastatic deposits in nodes in lymphatic chains not routinely opacified by the bipedal route.

The first of these deficiencies plagues any radiologic method. However, methods that do not depend on flow of contrast into an involved node might overcome the second and third obstacles. Thus, there has been considerable interest in using CT to evaluate lymphadenopathy in pelvic malignancy, since essentially any enlarged node can be imaged, regardless of its position in the pelvis or abdomen (Figure 18-7).

Levine et al.[40] reported 15 patients with T_0–T_2 cancers in whom histologic proof of CT prediction was available. Computed tomography was correct in 14 of 15, with one false-positive and no false-negative results. A follow-up study[75] from the same institution reported an accuracy of 81% with false-negative and false-positive rates both equal to 19%. Similar results have been reported from other centers.[33,65] The major difficulty with CT lymph node imaging is its insensitivity to structural changes in normal sized nodes. Thus, if a node is totally replaced by tumor but remains normal in size, CT will assess it as normal. False-positive scans can be the result of technical errors (such as unopacified bowel loops or adjacent vessels) or truly enlarged but histologically benign lymphadenopathy. The report of Golimbu and Morales[21] reflects these difficulties: in 17 patients with proved metastases, only five were detected by CT for a sensitivity of 29%. False-positive diagnoses were much less common in their series (rate, 7%).

While results clearly vary from institution to institution, recent reports reflect improved technology with better spatial resolution as well as more experience in scan interpretation. As with lymphangiography, however, CT does not provide sufficiently accurate information on which to base all therapeutic decisions.

Several investigators have attempted procedures involving direct intraprostatic injections. Lymphoscintigraphy.[19,69,77] is the simplest of these, involving injection of a small quantity of radionuclide (^{99m}Tc antimony sulfur colloid) followed by sequential gamma-camera imaging of the pelvis. Further clinical investigation is necessary before definite conclusions can be drawn, but the limitations in spatial resolution inherent in radionuclide imaging will likely prevent this method from gaining widespread acceptance.

Prostatic lymphography[61,66] with injection of sufficient oily contrast to opacify lymphatics and nodes (including the first-echelon periprostatic nodes, which are seen by no other radiographic method), is likewise under investigation. Vastly improved spatial resolution of the target lymphatics constitutes its advantage over lymphoscintigraphy. Again, limited clinical information is available regarding this method.

Distant Metastases

The skeletal system is the most common site of metastatic disease in patients with disseminated prostate cancer. Sites particularly prone to involvement include the lumbar spine, the osseous pelvis, and the ribs. The most sensitive method for detecting such metastases at an early stage is unquestionably the radionuclide bone scan[56] (Figure 18-8). Up to 15% of patients with metastatic deposits will have positive bone scans despite normal plain roentgenograms.[73] Falsely negative bone scans are extremely uncommon in patients with prostate cancer, since most of such deposits induce intense osteoclastic/osteoblastic activity. The radiopharmaceutical, ^{99m}Tc methylene diphosphonate accumulates avidly in all such areas of increased bone metabolism. This avidity likewise accounts for the high incidence of falsely positive scans: trauma, infection, and other benign processes can induce an identical metabolic response within bone and thus mimic metastases.

Follow-up scanning of patients with known metastases is a helpful means for evaluating the success or failure of therapy. The nonspecificity of radionuclide imaging, however, leads to difficulty in distinguishing between increased metabolic activity caused by healing and similar activity caused by tumor progression. In the series of Levenson et al.,[39] 23% of the scans and 50% of the roentgenograms worsened in patients who were clinical-

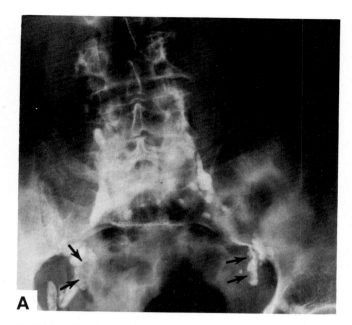
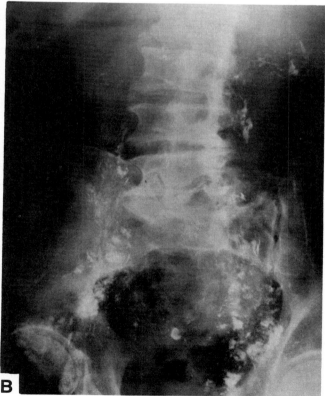

FIG. 18-6. (A) Lymphangiogram of a patient with adenocarcinoma of the prostate demonstrates well-circumscribed filling defects within lymph nodes in the medial portion of the external iliac chain bilaterally (arrows). These nodes correspond to the obturator nodes described in the surgical literature. (B) Lymphangiogram in a patient with extensive metastatic lymphadenopathy demonstrates persistent opacification of lymphatic vessels with filling of multiple collateral branches. While a few classic peripheral filling defects are observed (arrow), the majority of the nodes are totally replaced with tumor, and thus are not opacified.

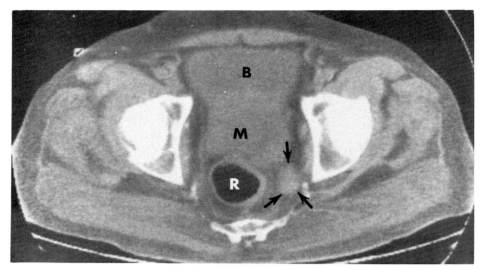

FIG. 18-7. CT demonstration of internal iliac lymphadenopathy. Scan through the acetabular roof demonstrates a large prostatic mass (M) immediately anterior to the rectum (r). A soft tissue density in the left sciatic notch, immediately adjacent to the calcified inferior glutcal artery, represents metastatic disease to lymph node.

ly responding to therapy. Thus, information from both bone scans and roentgenograms should be correlated with overall clinical response before final assessment of the effectiveness of therapy is made.

The other major site at risk for hematogenous metastasis is the lung.[41] While in autopsy studies, lymphangitic spread to the lungs is present in 25% of patients, it is radiographically visible in only 10%.[73] Lymphangitic spread actually implies a hematogenous shower of tumor implants that subsequently drain towards the pulmonary hila via the lymphatic system. Standard chest films are currently employed in screening patients for lung metastases.

IMAGING STRATEGIES AND DECISIONS

Controversy over the appropriate therapy for patients with prostatic carcinoma persists; in part, this is a result of staging information that is insufficient to correctly categorize patients undergoing various treatment methods. Since many therapeutic choices are associated with significant morbidity, it is reasonable to select patients with the best chance for survival to enter radical treatment protocols (Figure 18-9).

A patient may enter the imaging algorithms by one of two routes. In the course of transurethral resection for what is clinically felt to be benign prostatic hypertrophy, tumor may be encountered in the pathologic specimen. If the physical examination is truly normal, the patient is designated stage T_0, and further decisions are based on the differentiation and extent of the tumor. If the tumor is well-circumscribed (present in fewer than three fragments) and of low grade, follow-up may consist of either repeat transurethral resection or clinical observation and digital rectal examination. If these are negative, no further therapy is required. If residual tumor is present, the patient is staged as T_1 (or higher if the physical examination becomes positive). Patients with diffuse or high grade disease may best be considered stage T_1 initially.

Patients with apparently low stage (T_1 or T_2) disease have a good chance of surviving with radical surgical therapy (71% to 75% for stage T_2, 85% for stage T_1).[52] These patients should be aggressively investigated to determine whether they are in fact low-stage and free of metastases. Clinical assessment of the patient's candidacy for radical therapy assumes primary importance. This, of course, includes medical assessment aimed at discovering severe underlying medical disorders that would preclude radical surgical treatment. Urography is a useful adjunct in the overall clinical assessment of patients in this age group. In the course of urographic examination, the urothelium, kidneys, and osseous pelvis are evaluated. A review by Pirck et al.[55] demonstrated abnormal findings in 151 (27%) of 557 patients undergoing prostatectomy for benign prostatic hypertrophy. In 72 patients, the abnormality detected on urograms was considered clinically significant. Invasion of the bladder by extracapsular carcinoma can be suggested by urography, but radiographic methods are not as sensitive as cystoscopy in making this assessment. Thus, many urologists routinely perform cystoscopy before radical surgical therapy.

Assuming that the clinical and early urographic assessments do not preclude radical surgery, screening for

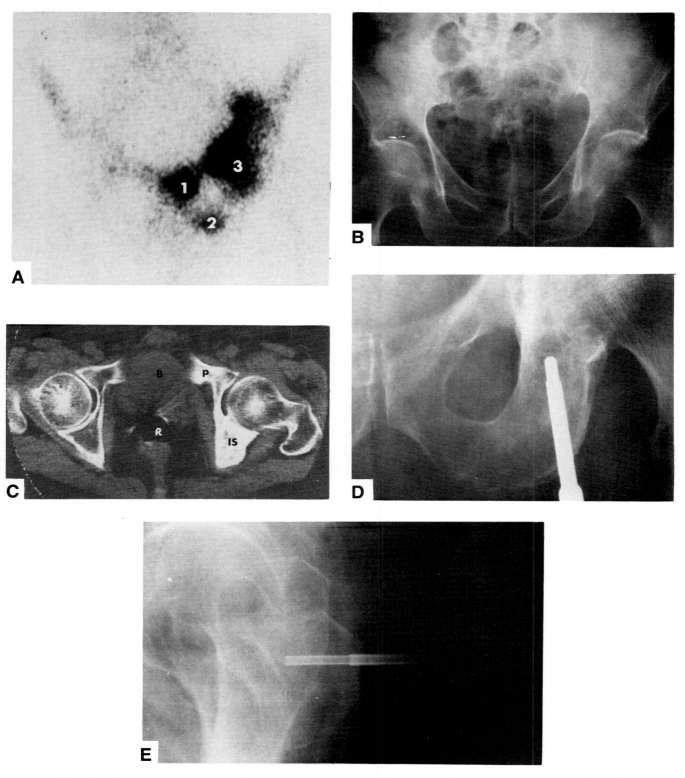

FIG. 18-8. Fifty-five-year-old patient with known adenocarcinoma of the prostrate. (A) An anterior image of a radionuclide scan of the pelvis demonstrates areas of increased radionuclide activity in the left symphysis pubis (1) and supra-acetabular ilium (3). In addition, there is increased uptake in the ischium (2). (B) Plain film of this region shows relatively subtle asymmetry in bony density in the regions imaged scintigraphically. (C) Computed tomographic image demonstrates increased density within the medullary space in the left pubis (p) and ischial spine (IS). (D) An AP film of the pelvis obtained during fluoroscopic positioning of a biopsy instrument. (E) Lateral film of the same patient. Biopsy retrieved metastatic adenocarcinoma.

CARCINOMA OF THE PROSTATE : LOCAL STAGE T_0

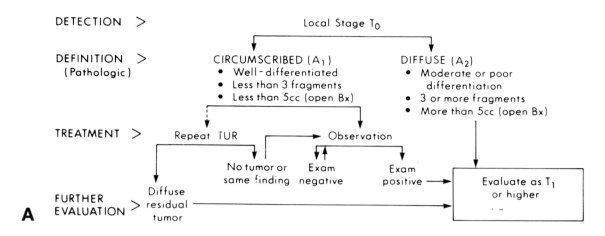

DETECTION > Local Stage T_0

DEFINITION > (Pathologic)

CIRCUMSCRIBED (A_1)
- Well-differentiated
- Less than 3 fragments
- Less than 5cc (open Bx)

DIFFUSE (A_2)
- Moderate or poor differentiation
- 3 or more fragments
- More than 5cc (open Bx)

TREATMENT > Repeat TUR → Observation

No tumor or same finding Exam negative Exam positive → Evaluate as T_1 or higher

FURTHER EVALUATION > Diffuse residual tumor

A

PROSTATE : LOCAL STAGE T_{1-2}

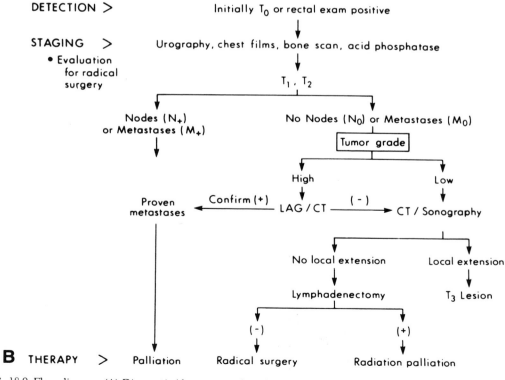

DETECTION > Initially T_0 or rectal exam positive

STAGING >
- Evaluation for radical surgery

Urography, chest films, bone scan, acid phosphatase

T_1 , T_2

Nodes (N_+) or Metastases (M_+)   No Nodes (N_0) or Metastases (M_0)

Tumor grade

High   Low

Proven metastases ← Confirm (+) ← LAG/CT — (-) → CT/Sonography

No local extension   Local extension

Lymphadenectomy T_3 Lesion

(-)   (+)

B THERAPY > Palliation   Radical surgery   Radiation palliation

FIG. 18-9. Flow diagram. (A) Diagnostic/therapeutic algorithm for patients with clinically inapparent (stage T_0) prostatic adenocarcinoma. (B) Diagnostic/therapeutic algorithm for patients with prostatic carcinoma clinically judged to be intracapsular (T_1–T_2). (C) Diagnostic/therapeutic algorithm for patients with locally extensive (T_3–T_4) adenocarcinoma of the prostate.

PROSTATE : LOCAL STAGE T$_{3-4}$

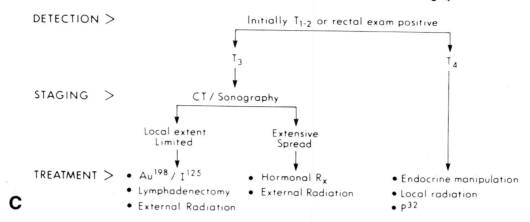

DETECTION >   Initially T$_{1-2}$ or rectal exam positive

T$_3$ T$_4$

STAGING >   CT / Sonography

Local extent   Extensive
Limited   Spread

TREATMENT >   • Au^{198} / I^{125} • Hormonal R$_x$ • Endocrine manipulation
              • Lymphadenectomy   • External Radiation   • Local radiation
C   • External Radiation   • p^{32}

metastatic disease should be undertaken. Chest films, bone scans, and serum acid phosphatase determinations are useful in this regard. While the presence of an elevated serum acid phosphatase level is neither necessary nor sufficient for diagnosing extracapsular disease, it does isolate a group that is at risk of having metastatic disease and thus should raise the clinical index of suspicion.

Positive bone scan findings fall into two general categories. In many cases, the scan exhibits a pattern of multiple focal areas of increased radionuclide accumulation within the osseous pelvis, axial skeleton, and ribs. This pattern is virtually pathognomic of metastatic disease, and further confirmation is unnecessary (Figure 18-10). Alternatively, bone scans may show a pattern of increased radionuclide uptake in one or two areas. This pattern is frequently seen in patients with degenerative disease or focal trauma or infectious processes. In these cases, where clinical doubt exists about the nature of the bone scan findings, confirmation should be obtained before assigning the patient to a palliative group. In such cases, the lesions seen on the scintigraphic study should be evaluated by detailed plain roentgenography. If this is also equivocal, needle aspiration biopsy[79] may be performed before the final therapeutic decision is made.

If the initial metastatic workup is negative for patients with clinically localized (T$_1$ or T$_2$) tumor, the imaging assessment may be influenced by the tumor grade. High grade tumors have up to 45% incidence of nodal metastases, and some way of assessing nodal status is indicated. In this regard, the choice lies between CT and lymphangiography. These methods are complementary, but each is expensive and lymphangiography is invasive. One possible method is to perform CT on patients at particular risk because of high grade tumor; if it is positive, the scan findings should be confirmed with percutaneous fine-needle lymph node aspiration biopsy under CT guid-

ance.[15,17] If it is negative, the patient may be assumed to have, at most, minimal adenopathy and is thus a candidate for staging lymphadenectomy.

Before surgery, for patients in whom the physical examination is difficult or inconclusive, it is rational to precisely define the total regional extent of prostatic tumor. Transrectal ultrasonography is in its infancy, but early reports demonstrate 95% accuracy in determining local disease spread. Further clinical studies are necessary to establish this high accuracy, but transrectal ultrasonography may emerge as the method of choice in firmly establishing the T stage preoperatively.

T$_3$ tumors are generally treated with radiation therapy, and for this method of treatment, nodal assessment is necessary for determining boost field and doses to involved areas. However, the decision to perform ^{125}I seed implantation or external radiation therapy depends on the local extent of tumor, and this can be readily assessed either by CT or transrectal ultrasonography.[68,76] Computed tomography[4] has been useful in judging the adequacy of placement of ^{125}I or ^{198}Au seeds and in calculating the radiation dose distribution.[16,26]

T$_4$ tumors likewise require nodal assessment, since boost field therapy would be determined by this information. Also, pretreatment with hormonal therapy allows imaging of involved nodes to be used to determine response. Response to hormonal manipulation can be judged clinically; or, if there are osseous metastases, by sequential bone scanning or plain roentgenograms of the areas involved.[44] The prognosis of patients with advanced carcinoma can be fairly adequately judged by simple radiographic means. Hovsepian and Byar[30] reported that analysis of plain films of the pelvis and a standard chest film sufficed to place patients in high risk or low risk categories that correlated well with overall survival (Figure 18-11).

A comparison of available imaging methods used to

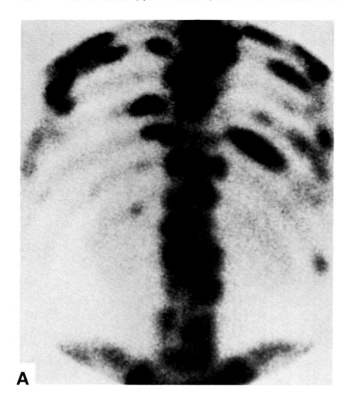

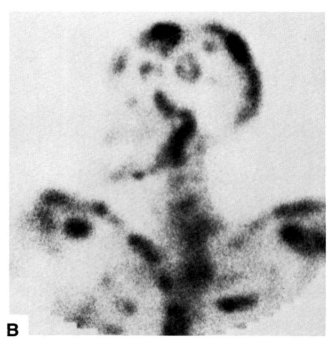

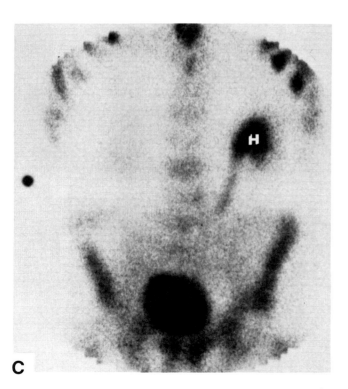

FIG. 18-10. (A–C) Widespread metastatic adenocarcinoma to the skeleton. Posterior image of the thoracic and lumbar spine in this 60-year-old patient demonstrates multiple focal areas of increased radionuclide uptake, diagnostic of diffuse metastatic disease.

evaluate patients with carcinoma of the prostate is given in Table 18-3.

TREATMENT DECISIONS

Radiation therapy is widely used in a definitive fashion, either with ^{125}I seeds or external irradiation for most stages. Bagshaw[3,4] in particular has contributed to the widespread acceptance of external irradiation techniques for prostate cancer and has attempted to define the advantages of extended field techniques. Radical prostatectomy is reserved for localized B lesions as a rule, and hormonal therapy is used for advanced metastatic disease. The use of lymphadenectomy and ^{125}I prostate implantations has been extensively studied by Batata et al.[6] and Whitmore et al.[77] at Memorial Sloan-Kettering Hospital. Hormonal induction therapy with large doses of estrogen is used for the treatment of primary and nodal disease to be followed by radiation therapy. This option currently is undergoing investigation.

Hormonal therapy consists of estrogens or orchidectomy when there are widespread diffuse metastases. Eighty percent of patients receiving this treatment have had good responses. Large doses of estrogen, in the form of diethylstilbestrol diphosphate, may be given intravenously for more refractory cases. Prolonged estrogen administration, particularly at levels of 3 to 5 mg, can lead to an increase in cardiovascular deaths. This higher dose schedule should be used for a limited time to avoid these problems.

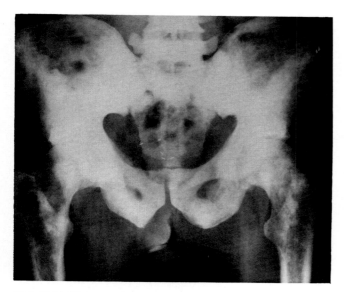

FIG. 18-11. Widespread adenocarcinoma to the pelvis and femurs is demonstrated on this plain AP radiograph.

Some excellent general sources[18,32,47] and a recent review article by Perez[51] are available on the increasingly important role of radiation therapy in the management of this disease. A brief summary of the decisions for different modalities according to TNM staging is found in Table 18-4.

IMPACT OF NEW TECHNOLOGY

Five-year survival in patients with carcinoma of the prostate without clinically appreciable metastases is a function of the clinical stage (Table 18-5). For patients with metastatic disease, the prognosis remains grim; five-year survivals are approximately 10% to 24% in most series. The major areas in which further research is needed are (1) developing more effective methods of treating advanced disease, (2) detecting the disease in its earliest stages, and (3) accurately staging moderately advanced disease to provide the therapist with sufficient information to maximize treatment benefit while minimizing

Table 18-3. Imaging Methods: Carcinoma of the Prostate

MODALITY	STAGING CAPABILITY	COST/BENEFIT RATIO	RECOMMENDED ROUTINE STAGING PROCEDURE
Noninvasive			
Chest films	Detects hematogenous or lymphatic spread.	High	Yes
Bone films	Detects lytic, blastic or mixed metastases in advanced disease.	Medium	No; confirms and follows bone scan findings.
Radionuclide studies:			
Bone scan	Detects early skeletal metastases.	High	Yes
Liver spleen	Detects liver metastases	Low	No; low-yield study.
Magnetic Resonance Imaging (MRI)	Unknown; early reports indicate capability of seeing normal prostatic capsule, and may detect intraglandular tumor.	Unknown	Unknown
Minimally Invasive			
Computed tomography:			
Chest	Capable of assessing lesions seen on chest film; may detect deposits not seen on chest film.	Medium	No; selected patients at high risk for widespread metastases.
Pelvis	Capable of imaging local tumor volume and extension. Capable of imaging pelvic lymph node metastases.	High	No; selected patients at risk for extracapsular and/or lymph node metastases.
Urography	Screens urinary tract for obstruction or coexistent abnormalities.	Medium	Yes
Transrectal Sonography	Capable of assessing T stage.	High	No; but selected patients at risk for capsular penetration may benefit.
Lymphoscintigraphy	Capable of assessing gross lymphatic involvement.	Low	No
Invasive			
Lymphangiography	Capable of assessing nodes in external iliac, common iliac, and para-aortic groups.	Medium	No; selected patients at risk for nodal metastases may benefit.
Prostatography	Theoretically capable of showing direct lymphatic drainage of disease lobe.	Low	No
Percutaneous Aspiration Biopsy	Documents presence and character of tumors seen by other methods.	High	No; selected patients only.

Table 18-4. Prostate: Treatment Decisions by Stage

STAGE/ TREATMENT MODALITY	SURGERY		EXTERNAL RADIATION THERAPY I^{125} INTERSTITIAL IMPLANT		CHEMOTHERAPY HORMONAL THERAPY
A or T_1	Total prostatectomy	or	Definitive ERT or III		NR
B or T_2	Radical prostatectomy	or	Definitive ERT or III		NR
C or T_3, T_4	Transurethral resection if obstructed		Definitive ERT or III 6600 cGy–7000 cGy to prostate and tumor		HT if radiation therapy not used because of age or other reasons
D_1 or $N_{1,2,3}$	NR		ERT	and	HT before radiation therapy
D_2 or N_4	NR		ERT	and	HT
Relapse	NR		RT if surgical failure		HT preferred
Metastatic	NR		Palliative RT		HT preferred

ERT = External radiation therapy
HT = Hormonal therapy
III = ^{125}I interstitial implant
NR = Not recommended
RT = Radiation therapy

risk. In this regard, future technologic advances in radiology should be brought squarely to bear on problem 3. At present, none of the currently available noninvasive methods are sufficiently accurate to guide the choice of therapy in T_1 and T_2 tumors; at best, they can minimize the number of needless staging lymphadenectomies caused by clinical understaging.

The potential impact of magnetic resonance imaging, a method at least theoretically capable of displaying differences in metabolism, is currently unknown. Likewise, developments in immunologic imaging (radionuclide labeling of antibodies specific for the tumor antigen studied),[22] increase the probability that a quantum leap will be made in our ability to preoperatively assess tumor extent.

Accurate follow-up information regarding the total tumor volume provides the therapist with sufficient information to appropriately modify the patient's treatment regime. Although therapeutic choices are somewhat limited at present, advances in management of extensive disease may allow physicians to choose between alternative therapies based on the objectively measured local response of the neoplasm. Both computed tomography and transrectal ultrasonography may be valuable methods in assessing such tumor response. Early results would indicate that ultrasound is somewhat more accurate in assessing tumor volume after radiation therapy.

Table 18-5. Prostate: Survival by Stage

STAGE	NUMBER OF PATIENTS	FIVE-YEAR SURVIVAL (%)	AUTHOR
Radiotherapy			
A	13	88.2	Harisiadis (1978)
A	21	88	McGowan
A + B	19	80	Hill (1970)
A + B	23	95	Lipsett (1976)
B_1	43	90	McGowan (1977)
B_2	30	66	McGowan
B	230	71	Pistenma (1976)
B	21	86.8	Harisiadis B
C	200	41	Pistenma
C	112	58	Harisiadis
C	56	55	Lipsett
C	49	42	Hill
C	13	39	McGowan
C	141	56	Perez
Surgery			
A + B	159	84	Veenema (1977)
B (surgical)	185	78.3	Belt (1972)
B	196	70.6	Vickery (1963)
B	52	75	Williams (1975)
C (surgical)	267	63.3	Belt

Adapted from Pilepich, M. V., Perez, C. A.: Does radiotherapy alter the course of genitourinary cancer? In *Genitourinary Cancer 1*. Paulson, D. E. (Ed.), Boston, Martinus Nijhoff, 1982, pp. 215–238.

REFERENCES

1. Ackerman, L. V., Rosai, J. (Eds.): *Surgical Pathology*, 5th ed. St. Louis, C. V. Mosby Co., 1974, pp. 696–716.
2. Babayan, R., Feldman, M., Krane, R. J., deVere White, R., Olsson, C. A.: Benefits and complications of staging pelvic lymph node dissection in prostatic adenocarcinoma. *Prostate* 1:345–349, 1980.
3. Bagshaw, M. A.: Radiotherapy for cancer of the prostate. In *Genitourinary Cancer*. DeKernion, J. B., Skinner, D. G. (Eds.). Philadelphia, W. B. Saunders, 1978, pp. 213–231.
4. Bagshaw, M. A.: Extended radiation therapy of cancer of the prostate. *Cancer* (suppl) 45:1912–1921, 1980.
5. Barzell, W. E., Bean, M. A., Hilaris, B. S., Whitmore, W. F., Jr.: Prostatic adenocarcinoma: Relationship of grade and local extent to the pattern of metastasis. *J. Urol.* 118:278, 1977.

6. Batata, M. A., Hilaris, B. S., Chu, F. C. H., Whitmore, W. F., Song, H. S., Kim, Y., Horowitz, B., Song, K. S.: Radiation therapy in adenocarcinoma of the prostate with pelvic lymph node involvement on lymphadenectomy. *Int. J. Radiat. Oncol. Biol. Phys.* 1:149–153, 1980.

7. Bergreen, P. W., Antoine, J., Hoffman, H.: Accuracy of lymphangiograms in staging carcinoma of the prostate versus staging pelvic lymphandenectomies. Presented at the 53rd Annual Meeting of the Western Section of the American Urological Association, San Francisco, California, March, 1977.

8. Cantrell, B. B., DeKlerk, D. P., Eggleston, J. C., Boitnott, J. K., Walsh, P. C.: Pathological factors that influence prognosis in state A prostatic cancer: The influence of extent versus grade. *J. Urol.* 125:516, 1981.

9. Catalona, W. F., Scott, W. W.: Carcinoma of the prostate: A review. *J. Urol.* 119:1–8, 1978.

10. Catalona, W. J., Stein, A. J.: Staging errors in clinically localized prostatic cancer. *J. Urol.* 127:452, 1982.

11. Cline, W. A., Kramer, S. A., Farnham, R.: Impact of pelvic lymphandenectomy in patients with prostatic adenocarcinoma. *Urology* 17:129, 1981.

12. Dodds, P. R., Caride, V. J., Lytton, B.: The role of vertebral veins in the dissemination of prostatic carcinoma. *J. Urol.* 126:753–755, 1981.

13. Donohue, R. E., Fauver, H. E., Whitesel, J. A., Augspurger, R. R., Pfeister, R. P.: Influence of tumor grade on results of pelvic lymph-adenectomy. *Urology* 17:435–440, 1981.

14. Donohue, R. E., Mani, J. H., Whitesel, J. A., Mohr, S., Scanavino, D.: Pelvic lymph node dissection. *Urology* 20:559–565, 1982.

15. Efremedis, S. C., Dan, S. J., Nieburgs, H., Mitty, H. A.: Carcinoma of the prostate: Lymph node aspiration for staging. *A.J.R.* 136:489–492, 1981.

16. Elkon, D., Kim, J.-A., Constable, W. C.: Anatomic localization of radioactive gold seeds of the prostate by computer-aided tomography. *Comput. Tomogr.* 5:89–93, 1981.

17. Ferrucci, J. T., Jr., Wittenberg, J., Mueller, P. R., Simeone, J. F., Harbin, W. P., Kirkpatrick, R. H., Taft, P. D.: Diagnosis of abdominal malignancy by radiologic fine-needle aspiration biopsy. *A.J.R.* 134:323–330, 1980.

18. Frank, I. N., Keys, H. M., McCune, C. A.: Urologic and male genital cancers. In *Clinical Oncology for Medical Students and Physicians: A Multidisciplinary Approach*, 6th ed. Rubin, P. (Ed.). New York, American Cancer Society, 1983, pp. 198–221.

19. Gardiner, R. A., Fitzpatric, J. M., Constable, A. R., Cranage, R. W., O'Donoghue, E. P. N., Wickham, J. E. A.: Improved techniques in radionuclide imaging of prostatic lymph nodes. *Br. J. Urol.* 51:561–564, 1979.

20. Giri, P. G. S., Walsh, J. W., Hazra, T. A., Texter, J. H., Koontz, W. W.: Role of computed tomography in the evaluation and management of carcinoma of the prostate. *Int. J. Radiat. Onco. Biol. Phys.* 8:283–287, 1982.

21. Goldenberg, D. M., Deland, F. H., Bennett, S. J., Primus, F. J., Nelson, M. O., Flanigan, R. C., McRoberts, J. W., Bruce, A. W., Mahan, D. E.: Radioimmunodetection of prostatic cancer. *J.A.M.A.* 250:630–635, 1983.

22. Goldfarb, S., Leiter, E.: Invasion of the rectum by carcinoma of the prostate. *Arch. Surg.* 115:1117, 1980.

23. Golimbu, M., Morales, P.: Stage A$_2$ prostatic carcinoma. Should staging system be reclassified? *Urology* 13:592, 1979.

24. Golimbu, M., Morales, P., Al-askari, S., Brown, J.: Extended pelvic lymphadenectomy for prostatic cancer. *J. Urol.* 121:617–620, 1979.

25. Golimbu, M., Morales, P., Al-askari, S., Shulman, Y.: CAT scanning in staging of prostatic cancer. *Urology* 18:305, 1981.

26. Gore, R. M., Moss, A. A.: Value of computed tomography in interstitial ^{125}I brachytherapy of prostatic carcinoma. *Radiology* 146:453–458, 1983.

27. Guinan, P., Bush, I., Ray, V., Vieth, R., Rao, R., Bhatti, R.: The accuracy of the rectal examination in the diagnosis of prostate carcinoma. *New Eng. J. Med.* 303(9):499–503, 1980.

28. Harada, K., Tanahashi, Y., Igari, D., Numata, I., Orisaka, S.: Clinical evaluation of inside echo patterns in gray scale prostatic echography. *J. Urol.* 124:216–220, 1980.

29. Henneberry, M., Carter, M. F., Neiman, H. L.: Estimation of prostatic size by by suprapubic ultrasonography. *J. Urol.* 121:615, 1979.

30. Hovsepian, J. A., Byar, D. P.: Quantitative radiology for staging and prognosis of patients with advanced prostatic carcinoma. *Urology* 14:145, 1979.

31. Huben, R., Natarajan, N., Pontes, E., Metlin, C., Smart, C. R., Murphy, G. P.: Carcinoma of the prostate in men less than 50 years old. *Urology* 20:585–588, 1982.

32. Hussey, D. H.: Carcinoma of the prostate. In *Textbook of Radiotherapy*, 3rd ed. Fletcher, G. H. (Ed.). Philadelphia, Lea & Febiger, 1980, pp. 894–914.

33. Jing, B. S., Wallace, S., Zornoza, J.: Metastases to retroperitoneal and pelvic lymph nodes: Computed tomography and lymphangiography. *Radiol. Clin. North Am.* 20:511–560, 1983.

34. Johnson, D. E., von Eschenbach, A. C.: Roles of lymphangiography and pelvic lymphadenectomy in staging prostate cancer. *Urology* 17 (supp³):66–71, 1981.

35. Kidd, R., Correa, R.: Fine-needle aspiration biopsy of lymphangiographically negative nodes: A negative view. *A.J.R.* 141:1005–1006, 1984.

36. Kidd, R., Crane, R. D., Dail, D. H.: Lymphangiography and fine-needle aspiration biopsy: Ineffective for staging of early prostate cancer. *A.J.R.* 141:1007–1012, 1984.

37. Kohri, K., Kaneko, S., Akiyama, T., Yachiku, S., Kurita, T.: Ultrasonic evaluation of prostatic carcinoma. *Urology* 17:214, 1981.

38. Lange, P. H., Narayan, P.. Understaging and undergrading of prostate cancer. Argument for postoperative radiation as adjurant therapy. *Urology* 21:113–118, 1983.

39. Levenson, R. M., Sauerbrun, B. J. L., Bates, H. R., Newman, R. D., Eddey, J. L., Ihde, D. C.: Comparative value of bone scintigraphy in monitoring tumor response in systematically treated prostatic carcinoma. *Radiology* 146:513–518, 1983.

40. Levine, M. S., Arger, P. H., Coleman, B. G., Mulhern, C. B., Pollack, H. M., Wein, A. J.: Detecting lymphatic metastases from prostatic carcinoma: Superiority of CT. *A.J.R.* 137:207–211, 1981.

41. Libshitz, H. I., North, L. B.: Pulmonary metastases. *Radiol. Clin. North Am.* 20:437–452, 1983.

42. Loening, S. A., Schmidt, J. D., Brown. R. C., Fallon, B., Culp, D. A.: A comparison between lymphangiography and pelvic node dissection in the staging of prostatic cancer. *J. Urol.* 117:752–756, 1977.

43. Mostofi, F. K., Price, E. D., Jr.: Tumors of the prostate. In *Tumors of the Male Genital System, Atlas of Tumor Pathology*, 2nd series, Fascicle 8. Bethesda, Md., Armed Forces Institute of Pathology, 1973.

44. Pagani, J. J., Libshitz, H. I.: Imaging bone metastases. *Radiol. Clin. North Am.* 20:545–560, 1983.

45. Paquette, F. R., Ahuja, A. S., Carson, P. L., Mack, L. A., Ibbott, G. S., Johnson, M. L.: A comparitive study of computerized tomography and ultrasound imaging for treatment planning of prostatic carcinoma. *Int. J. Radiat. Oncol. Biol. Phys.* 5:289–294, 1979.

46. Paulson, D. F.: Assessment of anatomic extent and biologic hazard of prostatic adenocarcinoma. *Urology* 15:537, 1980.

47. Paulson, D. F., Perez, C. A., Anderson, T.: Genito-urinary malignancies. In *Cancer—Principles and Practice of Oncology*. DeVita, V. J., Jr., Hellman, S., Rosenberg, S. A. (Eds.). Philadelphia, J. B. Lippincott, 1982, pp. 732–785.

48. Paulson, D. F., Piserchia, P. V., Gardner, W.: Predictions of lymphatic spread in prostatic adenocarcinoma: Uro-oncology Research Group Study. *J. Urol.* 123:697, 1980.

49. Peeling, W. B., Griffiths, G. J.: Imaging of the prostate by ultrasound. *J. Urol.* **132**:217–224, 1984.

50. Peeling, W. P., Griffiths, G. J., Evans, K. T., Roberts, E. E.: Diagnosis and staging of prostatic carcinoma by transrectal ultrasonography. *Brit. J. Urol.* **51**:565–568, 1979.

51. Perez, C. A.: Presidential Address of the 24th Annual Meeting of the American Society of Therapeutic Radiologists: Carcinoma of the Prostate, A Vexing Biological and Clinical Enigma. *Int. J. Radiat. Oncol. Biol. Phys.* **9**:1427–1438, 1983.

52. Pilepich, M. V., Perez, C. A.: Does radiotherapy alter the course of genito-urinary cancer? *Genitourinary Cancer* **1**:215–238, 1982.

53. Pilepich, M. V., Perez, C. A., Bauer, W.: Prognostic parameters in radiotherapeutic management of localized carcinoma of the prostate. *J. Urol.* **124**:485, 1980.

54. Pilepich, M. V., Perez, C. A., Prasad, S.: Computed tomography in definitive radiotherapy of prostatic carcinoma. *Int. J. Radiat. Oncol. Biol. Phys.* **6**:923, 1980.

55. Pirck, B. D., Corrigan, M. J., Jasper, P.: Pre-prostatectomy excretory urography: Does it merit the expense? *J. Urol.* **123**:390, 1980.

56. Pollen, J. J., Gerber, K., Ashburn, W. L., Schmidt, J. D.: The value of nuclear bone imaging in advanced prostatic cancer. *J. Urol.* **125**:222–223, 1981.

57. Prando, A., Wallace, S., von Eschenbach, A. C., Jing, B. S., Rosengran, J. E., Hussey, D. H.: Lymphangiography in staging carcinoma of the prostate. *Radiology* **131**:641–645, 1979.

58. Price, J. M., Davidson, A. J.: Computed tomography in the evaluation of the suspected carcinomatous prostate. *Urol. Radiol.* **1**:39, 1979.

59. Prout, G. R., Heaney, J. A., Griffin, P. P., Daly, J. J., Shipley, W. U.: Nodal involvement as a prognostic indicator in patients with prostatic carcinoma. *J. Urol.* **124**:226–231, 1980.

60. Raghavaiah, N. V.: Prostatography. *J. Urol.* **121**:174, 1979.

61. Raghavaiah, N. V., Jordan, W. P., Jr.: Prostatic lymphography. *J. Urol.* **121**:178, 1979.

62. Ray, G. R., Pistenma, D. A., Castellino, R. A., Kempson, R. L., Meares, E., Bagshaw, M. A.: Operative staging of apparently localized adenocarcinoma of the prostate: Results in fifty unselected patients. *Cancer* **38**:73–83, 1976.

63. Resnick, M. I., Willard, J. W., Boyce, W. H.: Transrectal ultrasonography in the evaluation of patients with prostatic carcinoma. *J. Urol.* **124**:482, 1980.

64. Rouviere, H.: *Anatomy of the Human Lymphatic System*. Ann Arbor, Edward Bros., 1938.

65. Sawczuk, I. S., White, R. D. V., Gold, R. P., Olsson, C. A.: Sensitivity of computed tomography in evaluation of pelvic lymph node metastases from carcinoma of bladder and prostate. *Urology* **21**:81–84, 1983.

66. Sherwood, T., O'Donoghue, E. P. N.: Lymphograms in prostatic carcinoma: False-positive and false-negative assessments in radiology. *Br. J. Radiol.* **54**:15–17, 1981.

67. Silverberg, E.: Cancer statistics, 1983. *CA* **33**:9–25, 1983.

68. Spellman, M. C., Ray, G. R., Pistenma, D. A., Harrison, G. A., Castellino, R. A.: An evaluation of lymphography in localized carcinoma of the prostate. *Radiology* **125**:637–644, 1977.

69. Stone, A. R., Merrick, M. V., Chisoln, G. D.: Prostatic lymphoscintigraphy. *Br. J. Urol.* **51**:556–560, 1979.

70. Sukov, R. J., Scardino, P. T., Sample, W. F., Winter, J., Confer, D. J.: Computed tomography and transabdominal ultrasound in the evaluation of the prostate. *J. Comput. Assist. Tomogr.* **1**:281, 1977.

71. Van Engelshoven, J. M. A., Kreel, L.: Computed tomography of the prostate. *J. Comput. Assist. Tomogr.* **3**:45–51, 1979.

72. Van Waes, P. F. G. M., Zonneveld, S. W.: Direct coronal body computed tomography. *J. Comput. Assist. Tomogr.* **6**:58–66, 1982.

73. Von Eschenbach, A. C., Johnson, D. E.: Adenocarcinoma of the prostate. *Compr. Ther.* **4**:18, 1978.

74. Watson, R. A., Tang, D. B.: The predictive value of prostatic acid phosphatase as a screening test for prostatic cancer. *Medical Intelligence* **303**:497, 1980.

75. Weinerman, P. M., Arger, P. H., Pollack, H. M.: CT evaluation of bladder and prostate neoplasms. *Urol. Radiol.* **4**:105–114, 1982.

76. Whitehead, E. D., Huh, S. H., Garcia, R. L.: Interstitial irradiation of carcinoma of the prostate with [125]-iodine and simultaneous extraperitoneal pelvic lymphadenectomy in 32 patients: Trials, tribulations and possible triumphs. *J. Urol.* **126**:366, 1981.

77. Whitmore, W. F., Blute, R. D., Kaplan, W. D., Gittes, R. F.: Radiocolloid scintigraphic mapping of lymphatic drainage of the prostate. *J. Urol.* **124**:62–67, 1980.

78. Zincke, H., Utz, D. C., Myers, R. P., Farrow, G. M., Patterson, D. E., Furlow, W. L.: Bilateral pelvic lymphadenectomy for radical retropubic prostatectomy for adenocarcinoma of prostate with regional lymph node involvement. *Urology* **19**:238–247, 1982.

79. Zornoza, J.: Needle biopsy of metastases. *Radiol. Clin. North Am.* **20**:569–590, 1983.

19 TESTICULAR TUMORS

Jay P. Heiken
Dennis M. Balfe
Bruce L. McClennan

Although testicular neoplasms constitute only 1% of all malignancies occurring in men, they are the most common cancers occurring in young adult males (ages 15 to 34), accounting for 8.8% of all cancer deaths in this age group. The overall incidence of testicular cancer is 2 to 3 per 100,000 males per year, but is 62 per 100,000 males per year in the 15 to 34 year age group.[62] An estimated 2,500 new cases of testicular cancer are diagnosed annually.[28]

The extreme radiosensitivity of testicular seminomas plus dramatic recent advances in chemotherapy for non-seminomatous tumors and for advanced seminomas[11] have made long-term survival possible in the large majority of patients. The overall five-year survival rate regardless of stage or histologic type is 62%.[66] However, the five-year survival rate for patients with disease localized to the testis is 75% to 100% and that for patients with lymph node metastases below the diaphragm (stage II) is 65% to 95%, the precise survival rate varying with the histologic type of tumor, the bulk of metastatic disease, and the type of therapy used.[14,16,34,64,66,68] The potential curability of testicular cancer underscores the importance of early detection and accurate staging of these tumors.

Radiology has played and continues to play a central role in the clinical staging of testicular tumors. Imaging methods used in the staging workup vary from institution to institution. Although computed tomography (CT) has supplanted other imaging modalities in the staging and follow-up of certain types of cancer, CT has not had as great an impact on the staging of testicular cancer.

Nevertheless, CT does offer a number of advantages over lymphangiography for the detection of lymphatic metastases and is the initial imaging method of choice for staging testicular tumors. As will be discussed below, however, the decision to perform CT or lymphangiography should be based upon the anticipated method of treatment. In some cases, ultrasonography may be an acceptable alternative primary abdominal imaging method. In addition, ultrasonography may play an important role in the detection of occult testicular neoplasms in patients who have metastatic disease and a normal scrotal examination.[24] Intravenous urography and inferior vena cavography are insensitive methods for the detection of retroperitoneal lymphadenopathy and need not be used routinely for staging. Because the lungs are the major extralymphatic site of metastases in patients with testicular neoplasms, some form of chest imaging should be performed in all patients. In this regard, CT has proved more sensitive than full chest tomography for the detection of both pulmonary and mediastinal metastases.[5,12,25,49,60] Radioimmunoassays for serum alpha-fetoprotein (AFP) and the beta subunit of human chorionic gonadotropin (beta-HCG), although they fall outside the domain of radiology, will be discussed because of their importance in the clinical staging and management of testicular tumors. While radionuclide imaging at present does not play a major role in the staging of testicular tumors, the development of tumor radioimmunodetection techniques using antibodies to HCG and AFP may prove valuable in the future for revealing tumors that are undetectable by other techniques.[30]

425

Because survival is related to the stage of tumor, early detection is critical. The availability of successful methods of treatment adds to the importance of early diagnosis. Unfortunately, the diagnosis of testicular cancer is often delayed, not only because of patient procrastination, but because of initial misdiagnosis by the physician. In the study of Patton et al. of over 500 patients with testicular tumors,[51] an erroneous diagnosis was made in more than one quarter of the cases, epididymitis being the most common misdiagnosis. Donohue also states that more than 50% of patients with cancer of the testis are misdiagnosed initially as having epididymitis.[13] One possible reason for initial misdiagnosis may lie in the fact that almost one-quarter of testicular tumors are associated with pain,[51] which is contrary to the widespread teaching that testicular tumors present as painless masses.

The etiology of testicular tumors is unknown, although genetic and environmental factors, trauma, endocrine abnormalities, and repeated infections have been suggested as causal factors.[47] The incidence of neoplasia appears to be increased in undescended testes.[47] Testicular tumors are rare in Asia, Finland, and New Zealand and are particularly rare among the black population both in America and Africa.[47]

TUMOR BEHAVIOR AND PATHOLOGY

Approximately 93% of tumors of the testis arise from the germ cells and are malignant. Nongerminal tumors of the testis arise from the interstitial cells of Leydig, the Sertoli cells, or the connective tissue stroma and are benign in 90% of cases. The nongerminal tumors are rare and will not be discussed further.

For practical purposes, germ cell tumors of the testis can be divided into two main categories: seminomas and nonseminomatous tumors (Table 19-1). The reason for this dichotomy is that most seminomas are treated by

Table 19-1. Histologic Classification of Germ Cell Tumors of the Testis

Tumors showing one histologic pattern
  Seminoma
    Typical Seminoma
    Anaplastic Seminoma
    Spermatocytic Seminoma
  Nonseminomatous
    Embryonal carcinoma
    Teratoma
    Choriocarcinoma
Tumors showing more than one histologic pattern
  Teratocarcinoma (Embryonal Carcinoma and Teratoma)
  Other combinations

Modified from Mostofi, F. J., Price, E. B., Jr.: Tumors of the male genital system. In *Atlas of Tumor Pathology*, Fascicle 8, Series 2. Washington, D.C., Armed Forces Institute of Pathology, 1973.

radiation therapy while most nonseminomatous tumors are treated by lymphadenectomy (or chemotherapy or both), although chemotherapy is playing a growing role in advanced seminomas.

Seminoma is the most common type of testicular neoplasm, accounting for 40% of all germ cell tumors[5] and 80% of all tumors arising in undescended testes.[56] It is believed to arise from the seminiferous epithelium and is analogous to ovarian dysgerminoma. The peak incidence of seminomas is in the fourth and fifth decades, approximately 10 years later than that of nonseminomatous germ cell tumors. Seminomas are highly radiosensitive and have the most favorable prognosis of the germ cell tumors. The overall five-year survival rate is 90% or better.[16,28] The five-year survival rate for patients with stage I and stage II disease together is approximately 95%.[16,28]

In general, three subtypes of seminomas are recognized: typical or classic, anaplastic, and spermatocytic.[47] Anaplastic seminomas, which constitute 10% of all seminomas, are more aggressive and have a poorer prognosis than the typical seminomas.[43,47] Spermatocytic seminomas constitute about 9% of all seminomas, usually occur in patients over the age of 40 years and have a better prognosis than typical seminomas.[47] Although seminoma is the most common of the germ cell tumors to occur in pure form, 10% to 15% contain nonseminomatous elements.[21] These mixed tumors behave like the more aggressive nonseminomatous tumors and should be treated as such.[21]

Nonseminomatous germ cell tumors are categorized into four types: embryonal carcinomas, teratomas, teratocarcinomas, and choriocarcinomas. This histologic subclassification of nonseminomatous germ cell tumors is of some significance in terms of prognosis but does not influence therapy.[7]

Embryonal carcinomas, which constitute 15% to 20% of all germ cell tumors, are highly malignant tumors composed of multipotential anaplastic cells that are believed to be the stem cells for all nonseminomatous tumors.[38,47] They occur most commonly in the third decade. Approximately one third of patients have distant metastases at the time of diagnosis.[47] Although the overall three-year corrected survival rate is approximately 40%,[53] the five-year survival rate for patients with stage I embryonal carcinomas may be as high as 74%.[33]

Teratomas, which make up approximately 5% to 10% of testicular tumors, contain recognizable elements derived from two or more germ layers. They occur most frequently in the first three decades of life and have the best prognosis of the nonseminomatous germ cell tumors. In contrast to those that occur in adults, teratomas in infants and children are benign neoplasms. In adults, metastasis occurs within five years in about 30% of cases,[47,57] while 24% of patients show evidence of metastasis at the time of diagnosis.[47] The overall five-year survival rate is 71%.[48] However, the five-year survival rate for patients with stage I disease may approach 100%.[33]

Approximately 40% of tumors of the testis contain more than one histologic pattern.[47] The most frequent combination is embryonal carcinoma and teratoma (teratocarcinoma), which accounts for 14% to 32% of all testicular tumors.[47] Although the overall corrected three-year survival rate for patients with teratocarcinoma is 50%,[53] a 93% five-year survival rate has been reported for patients with stage I disease.[33]

Choriocarcinoma is a highly malignant tumor composed of cytotrophoblastic and syncytiotrophoblastic cells. Pure choriocarcinomas are extremely rare, constituting less than 1% of all testicular neoplasms.[57] They occur almost exclusively in the second and third decades and metastasize early through both vascular and lymphatic channels. The prognosis is poor, with death usually occurring within a year after diagnosis. Mixed tumors containing choriocarcinomatous elements usually behave like their less aggressive elements.[21]

Patterns of Spread

The primary route of spread of all germ cell tumors except choriocarcinoma is via the regional lymphatics. The lymphatics draining the testis follow the spermatic cord through the internal inguinal ring and then deviate to follow the spermatic artery and vein. The primary lymphatic drainage from the left testis is to the renal hilar nodes because the left spermatic artery and vein drain into the left renal artery and vein; the primary lymphatic drainage from the right testis is to the paracaval and para-aortic nodes because the right spermatic artery and vein drain directly into the inferior vena cava.[56] The initial retroperitoneal drainage is into a "sentinel" node located lateral to the paralumbar lymphatics; the sentinel node is located in the renal perihilar region on the left (usually at the level of L1 to L2) and in the paracaval region below the renal artery and vein on the right (usually at the level of L1 to L3). A left-sided sentinel node appears to be somewhat less common than its right-sided counterpart.[41] Following spread to the sentinel node, the paralumbar lymphatics become involved. According to Ray et al.,[54] lymphatic spread from left-sided tumors is to the para-aortic, preaortic, left common iliac and left external iliac nodes, in that order of frequency. Subsequent extension involves the interaortocaval, precaval, and paracaval nodes. Right-sided tumors spread to the interaortocaval, precaval, preaortic, paracaval, right common iliac, and right external iliac nodes, in that order, with subsequent extension involving para-aortic, left common iliac, and left external iliac nodes. Donohue et al.[15] have published similar data, showing that the most common site of metastatic tumor deposition from right testis tumors is the interaortocaval zone, just below the left

renal vein (93%), while the preaortic (88%) and left para-aortic (86%) areas are the most common sites of nodal spread from left testis tumors. The suprahilar zones are involved rarely in low stage (IIA) disease.[15]

Although the lymphatic drainage from the testis is predominantly unilateral, crossover may occur. Crossover from right to left is more common than from left to right.[54] If the nodes ipsilateral to the primary tumor are involved with metastasis, the chance of contralateral involvement is 15% to 20%.[54] If no ipsilateral metastatic involvement is present, the incidence of contralateral involvement is very low.[54] When the primary tumor involves the epididymis, metastases may follow the epididymal lymphatics to the external iliac nodes.[46] Invasion of the scrotum with penetration of all layers of the scrotum wall may also change the route of lymphatic drainage. Although it is unusual, aggressive tumors can spread through the tunica albuginea to the tunica vaginalis and into the dartus muscle of the scrotum, altering the lymphatic drainage from the retroperitoneal nodes to the inguinal nodes that drain into the external iliac chain. Inguinal nodal involvement also occurs in patients with massive retroperitoneal disease and in patients who have had disruption of the normal lymphatic pathways by prior scrotal surgery.

From the retroperitoneal lymph nodes, spread may occur through the thoracic duct to the left supraclavicular area, the base of the neck, the mediastinum, and the lungs. Metastases may also take a more direct route to the mediastinum and lungs through transdiaphragmatic lymphatic channels. Although the primary mode of spread of most testicular neoplasms is through the lymphatics, hematogenous metastases also occur, either by direct invasion of the spermatic vein or through venous communications with lymphatics such as those in the supraclavicular region.[46] The thoracic duct drains directly into the venous circulation at the junction between the jugular and subclavian veins; thus rapid dissemination to the lungs occurs commonly. Hematogenous spread occurs more often and earlier with nonseminomatous tumors.[73] Choriocarcinomas are the only germ cell neoplasms to spread predominantly by the hematogenous route. The lungs are the primary site of hematogenous dissemination, followed by liver and brain in that order.

CLASSIFICATION AND STAGING

Despite a large number of proposed classifications for the staging of testicular cancer, no one staging system has gained universal acceptance. Table 19-2 compares four of the systems in use, which show only an approximate stage by stage correspondence. The TNM system proposed by the American Joint Committee on Staging and End Results Reporting (AJC)[1] has not gained widespread use for the staging of testicular cancer. The AJC

Table 19-2. Comparison of Some Staging Systems for Testis Cancer

BODEN AND GIBB[3]	MAIER ET AL.[44]	AJC[1]	UICC[71]
A. No metastases	IA. Tumor confined to one testis. No clinical or radiographic evidence of spread beyond.	T_x. Minimum requirements to assess the primary tumor can not be met T_0. No evidence for primary tumor T_1. Tumor limited to body of the testis T_2. Extension beyond the tunica albuginea T_3. Involvement of the rete testis or epididymis T_{4a}. Invasion of spermatic cord T_{4b}. Invasion of scrotal wall	T_1. Tumor occupying less than half of testis surrounded by palpably normal gland. T_2. Tumor occupying half or more of testis with no enlargement or deformity. T_3. Tumor confined to testis causing enlargement or deformity. T_{4a}. Tumor extending to epididymis. T_{4b}. Tumor invading other local structures.
B. Metastases to retroperitoneum	IB. As in IA but found to have histologic evidence of metastases to iliac or para-aortic lymph nodes at time of retroperitoneal lymphadenectomy. II. Clinical or radiographic evidence of metastases to femoral, inguinal, iliac, or para-aortic lymph nodes. No demonstrable metastases above the diaphragm or to visceral organs.	N_x. Minimum requirements to assess the presence of distant metastases cannot be met N_0. No evidence of involvement of regional nodes N_1. Involvement of a single homolateral regional lymph node that, if inguinal, is mobile N_2. Involvement of contralateral or of bilateral or multiple regional lymph nodes that, if inguinal, are mobile N_3. Palpable abdominal mass present or fixed inguinal lymph nodes	N_0. No deformity of regional lymph nodes on lymphangiography. N_x. Not possible to assess regional lymph nodes. N_1. Regional lymph nodes deformed on lymphangiography. N_2. Fixed, palpable abdominal lymph nodes.
C. Distant metastases	III. Clinical or radiographic evidence of metastases above the diaphragm or other distant metastases to body organs.	M_x. Minimum requirements to assess the presence of distant metastases cannot be met M_0. No (known) distant metastasis M_1. Distant metastasis present	M_1. Metastases to nodes outside abdomen or to viscera.

system shows detailed pathologic stages, and, although it is useful in the evaluation of patients who undergo lymphadenectomy, it is not directly applicable to the radiographic staging of patients with testicular cancer. While the TNM system proposed by the International Union Against Cancer (UICC)[71] is primarily a clinical staging system, it depends upon lymphangiographic examination of the patient, and is thus more limited than other clinical staging systems (Figure 19-1). Most centers have used a modification of either the system proposed by Boden and Gibb[3] or that proposed by Maier et al.[44] One of these two systems has been used throughout most of the current literature dealing with the staging and treatment of testicular tumors. Therefore, although none of the clinical staging systems is ideal, a modification of the Boden and Gibb system will be used in the remainder of this discussion (Table 19-3).

According to this system, stage I lesions are limited to the testis. Stage II tumors show clinical or radiographic evidence of spread beyond the testis but are limited to the infradiaphragmatic lymph nodes. This stage is subdivided into IIA (minimal to moderate sized retroperitoneal metastases) and IIB (bulky retroperitoneal metastases). Stage IIIA tumors show evidence of metastases involving the lymphatics above the diaphragm, and stage IIIB tumors show evidence of extranodal metastases.

IMAGING PROCEDURES AND ASSESSMENT

Many imaging methods applicable to the clinical staging of testicular neoplasms are currently available (Table 19-4). Agreement is not universal on the most productive and cost-effective combination of tests. The imaging procedures used at any particular institution depend to some extent upon their relative accessibility as well as upon the modes of treatment used at that institution.

Nodal Status

For years, bipedal lymphangiography has been the standard imaging procedure used to assess the retroperitoneal lymph nodes in patients with testicular cancer

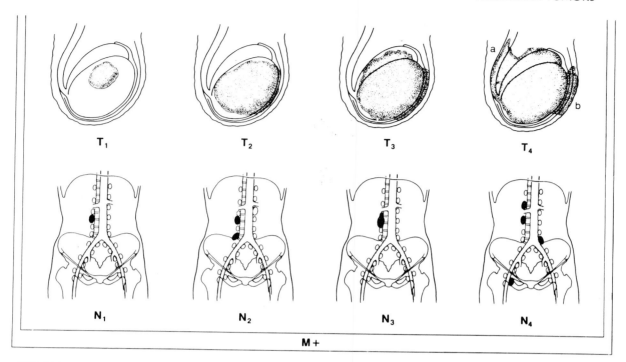

FIG. 19-1. Anatomic staging for carcinoma of the testis. Tumor (T) categories: The depth of invasion through the various layers around the testis determines the stage and requires a surgical specimen. Penetration is into tunica albuginea (T_2), the rete testes and epididymis (T_3), and the spermatic cord (T_{4a}) and scrotal wall (T_{4b}). Node (N) categories: The regional nodes are para-aortic and inguinal if the scrotum is involved. Their progression is from a single homolateral node (N_1) to multiple bilateral nodes (N_2) and clinically palpable nodal masses or fixed nodes (N_3) and juxtaregional nodes (N_4) (UICC only). Stage grouping: AJC places T_{1-3}, N_0 in Stage I; $T_4 N_0$ and N_1 constitute Stage II; N_2 disease is Stage III; and N_3 or M_1 denote Stage IV. AJC v UICC classification: Both systems are in essential concurrence. (Reprinted from Frank, I. N., Keys, H. M., McCune, C. S.: Urologic and male genital cancers. In *Clinical Oncology for Medical Students and Physicians: A Multidisciplinary Approach*, 6th ed. Rubin, P. (Ed.). New York, American Cancer Society, 1983, pp. 198–221. With permission.)

(Figure 19-2). Since the development of computed tomography, however, the number of lymphangiograms performed at most centers has declined considerably. The major advantage of lymphangiography over CT is its ability to detect architectural changes within nonenlarged lymph nodes. This advantage, however, may be more academic than clinically relevant, since many surgeons choose to treat stage I patients as though they have stage II disease (i.e., radiotherapy to the retroperitoneal lymph nodes in patients with seminoma and retroperitoneal lymphadenectomy in patients with nonseminomatous tumors). The reason for this is that 10% to 34% of patients with clinical stage I disease are found to have occult retroperitoneal metastases at lymphadenectomy.[44,70] In addition, tumor marker assays may indicate retroperitoneal lymph node involvement in patients with normal CT scans. On the other hand, lymphangiography has a number of disadvantages: (1) it is a time-consuming and invasive procedure carrying with it the morbidity inherent in such a procedure; (2) it normally does not opacify the sentinel lymph nodes, which are the first sites of retroperitoneal involvement; (3) in patients with extensive retroperitoneal metastases, lymphangiography may fail to demonstrate the upper limits of involvement; (4) reactive hyperplasia and fibrosis of the lymphatic tissues caused by the contrast medium may make subsequent surgery more difficult; and (5) although lymphangiography can detect changes in the internal architecture of nonenlarged nodes, it cannot differentiate between malignant and nonmalignant changes.

Some authors justify the use of lymphangiography in staging seminomas because it outlines the treatment field for the therapeutic radiologist. The problem with this argument is that bipedal lymphangiography does not opacify all of the retroperitoneal nodes. To overcome this deficiency, as well as to opacify the sentinel nodes,

Table 19-3. Clinical Staging System

I. Tumor limited to the testis
II. Clinical or radiographic evidence of spread beyond the testis but limited to the infradiaphragmatic lymph nodes
   A. Minimal to moderate retroperitoneal metastases
   B. Bulky retroperitoneal metastases
III. Supradiaphragmatic metastases
   A. Confined to the lymphatic system
   B. Extranodal metastases

Table 19-4. Imaging Methods for Evaluation of Testis Cancer

METHOD	CAPABILITY	COST/ BENEFIT	RECOMMENDED ROUTINE/ STAGING PROCEDURE
Noninvasive			
Chest radiography	Limited usefulness unless tomography is used for detection of metastases; however, whole lung tomography is less sensitive than chest CT.	High	Yes
Ultrasound	A. Very useful for detection of occult testis cancer.	A. High	B. Yes
	B. For staging and follow-up may be useful in thin patients with sparse retroperitoneal fat but is generally less sensitive and specific than CT.	B. Low	B. No
MRI	Promising role for staging and follow-up.	Unknown	Unknown
Nearly Noninvasive			
Urography	Limited usefulness because of insensitivity in detecting small to moderate-sized retroperitoneal metastases.	Low	No
CT	Method of choice for staging and follow-up (chest and abdomen).	High	Always
Radionuclide Studies			
Routine imaging tests	Limited usefulness.	Low	No
Radioimmunoassay for B-HCG and AFP	Very useful for staging and follow-up; used in conjunction with available imaging tests; has decreased staging errors.	High	Always
Labeled antibodies to B-HCG and AFP	Promising role for detecting occult metastases and residual tumor following therapy.	Unknown	Unknown
Invasive			
Lymphography	Limited usefulness in patients with positive CT scans or in patients with normal CT scans (clinical stage I) who are going to undergo elective treatment of the retroperitoneum.	Low	Recommended only for patients with clinical stage I disease in whom elective treatment of the retroperitoneum is not planned.
Angiography	Limited or no utility.	Low	No
Biopsy (CT, US, fluoroscopy)	Percutaneous biopsy requires US, CT, or fluoroscopy. May be useful in some cases to confirm metastases, but usually is not necessary.	Low	No

some have suggested the routine use of testicular lymphangiography, particularly for left testicular tumors, which drain to the renal perihilar area.[9] However, since four to eight lymphatic channels ascend from each testis,[48] there is no guarantee that the lymphatic vessel being cannulated is the one that drains the tumor.[41] Although testicular lymphangiography provides excellent visualization of the primary draining nodes, it is not widely performed since it must be done at the time of orchiectomy. The use of lymphangiography for nonseminomatous tumors is not widely accepted, since at most centers patients who do not have widespread disease routinely undergo retroperitoneal lymphadenectomy.[69]

The accuracy of bipedal lymphangiography in the detection of nodal metastases from testicular neoplasms has been reported to be 62% to 89%,[10,20,35,36,42,59,61,69,72] with a combined overall accuracy of 77%. The overall sensitivity has been 74% (range, 54% to 88%), and the overall specificity has been 88% (range, 67% to 100%).

The widespread use of CT has brought with it the promise of an accessible, noninvasive, and accurate method for the staging of testicular tumors (Figure 19-3). This promise has not yet been completely realized. Computed tomography does have several important advantages over lymphangiography: (1) it is noninvasive; (2) it can detect disease in adjacent organs and in lymph nodes not opacified by lymphangiography (Figure 19-4); and (3) it can better define tumor margins and true tumor volume. Nevertheless, CT is not without its drawbacks: (1) it cannot detect metastases in nonenlarged lymph nodes (however, as discussed above, this disadvantage may be more academic than clinically relevant; (2) young males tend to have little retroperitoneal fat, which may make CT scans of some patients difficult to interpret; and (3) as with lymphangiography, when nodes are only minimally or moderately enlarged, CT cannot differentiate between benign and malignant enlargement.

A number of studies have compared the utility of CT and lymphangiography in the staging of patients with testicular cancer.[17,18,31,40,45,61,70] Although results have varied, overall CT has not improved upon the accuracy of lymphangiography. The accuracy of CT in the detection of retroperitoneal nodal involvement has ranged from 59% to 89% with an overall accuracy of 76%. The overall sensitivity has been 70% (range, 50% to 93%) and the overall specificity 86% (range, 83% to 100%). The reported

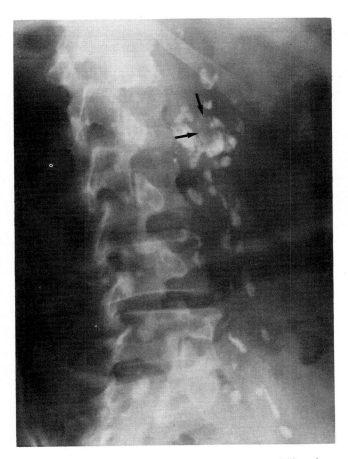

FIG. 19-2. Lymph node metastasis demonstrated by bipedal lymphangiography in a 52-year-old patient with embryonal carcinoma of the right testis. The left posterior oblique view of the abdomen shows a filling defect (arrows) in an enlarged left para-aortic lymph node.

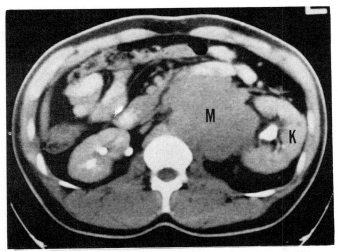

FIG. 19-3. Metastatic seminoma in a 39-year-old patient. A CT scan at the level of the left renal hilum demonstrates a large para-aortic lymph node mass (M) displacing the left kidney (K) laterally.

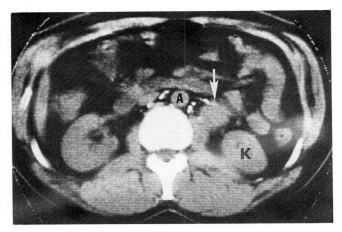

FIG. 19-4. Metastatic retroperitoneal lymphadenopathy in a patient with a seminoma of the left testis. A CT scan at the level of the lower pole of the left kidney (K) demonstrates a large metastatic mass (arrow) not opacified by lymphangiography. Multiple normal-sized lymph nodes surrounding the aorta (A) are opacified. (Reprinted from Lee, J. K. T., Sagel, S. S., Stanley, R. J. (Eds.): Computed Body Tomography. New York, Raven Press, 1983. By permission of the publisher.)

data thus show no improvement in accuracy, sensitivity, or specificity with the use of CT compared with lymphangiography. The unimpressive results with CT are no doubt due, at least in part, to the use of early generation slow (18 second or greater) scanners in almost all of the studies performed to date. It is to be expected that these statistics will improve with the use of state of the art CT scanners with shorter scanning times. Although the combined use of CT and lymphangiography may improve the accuracy of either modality by itself,[17,40] the performance of both of these tests on all patients is not cost-effective.

The above notwithstanding, CT has been shown to have a positive impact on staging and treatment of patients with testicular tumors. In one study CT increased the stages in 22% of a total of 80 patients with testicular teratomas who had been staged by conventional radiographic techniques including lymphangiography.[25] A second study found that the results of CT scans influenced a change in treatment in 36 of 126 patients (29%).[25]

Another important role for CT is in the post-therapy management of patients with bulky retroperitoneal disease. If complete tumor regression occurs in response to chemotherapy, subsequent lymphadenectomy is not performed. If, on the other hand, there is evidence of residual tumor following chemotherapy, an attempt is usually made to excise it.[7] However, approximately one-half of patients with residual masses on CT scans after chemotherapy have no viable tumor remaining. These patients have a good prognosis (approximately 90% long-term survival) and could be spared subsequent lymphadenectomy. Soo et al.[67] have stressed the nonspecificity of CT-detected retroperitoneal and hepatic masses after treatment. However, Husband et al.[26] have shown that it may be possible to differentiate patients with residual malignancy from those without persistent malignancy on the basis of changes in mean CT attenuation values. Their results indicate that a high mean CT number (greater than approximately 30 HU) following chemotherapy with or without irradiation suggests persistent malignancy; a low CT number indicates further tumor differentiation or no evidence of malignancy. However, since seminomas do not undergo cystic degeneration, such separation may not be possible on the basis of the absolute CT numbers alone. Therefore, a change in mean attenuation values may provide further information regarding therapeutic response. A reduction in the mean CT number during treatment of both teratomas and seminomas suggests that the residual mass does not contain active malignant tissue irrespective of the final absolute mean CT number. In patients with solid tumors (those with a high mean CT number), an overall increase in mean CT numbers during treatment suggests the tumor contains active malignant tissue. On the other hand, the estimation of tumor volume is of little value in predicting the presence of viable malignancy in a lesion greater than 20 cc. Tumors less than 20 cc are unlikely to contain viable malignancy. Thus, although much more investigation in this area is needed, the use of CT to direct the management of patients with residual masses after chemotherapy may hold considerable potential.

Several studies have compared the utility of CT and ultrasonography in the staging of testicular tumors.[4,58,74] Although the statistics appear to show that there is no difference in the accuracy of these two modalities (CT, 68% to 87%; ultrasonography, 64% to 81%), closer scrutiny of these studies reveals that ultrasonography is inferior to CT for staging these patients. In one study, while the difference in accuracy was not large (CT 87%; ultrasound 81%) and the sensitivity of each test was the same (93%), the specificity of CT was significantly higher (82% versus 57%).[74] In another study, although accuracy and specificity were similar for both modalities, the sensitivity of ultrasonography was only 25% compared with 50% for CT.[58] In addition, examinations thought to be nondiagnostic were excluded from the statistics, and 17% of the ultrasound studies were considered nondiagnostic, while only 2% of the CT examinations fell into this category. Furthermore, in no case did ultrasonography detect a tumor when the CT scan did not. In a third study, although the accuracy of CT and ultrasonography was equal, the accuracy of CT was considered to be more reproducible.[4] Examinations thought to be inadequate or equivocal were excluded from this study also.

The limitations of ultrasonography include interference by abdominal gas and poor scan quality in obese patients. On the other hand, ultrasonography is well suited for the evaluation of patients with very sparse retroperitoneal fat. Thus, in selected patients, ultrasonography may be an acceptable alternative to CT as the primary method for imaging the retroperitoneum even though CT is preferable.

If CT is used as the primary method for imaging the retroperitoneum, intravenous urography is not needed. Similarly, inferior vena cavagraphy adds no useful information to that provided by CT.

Primary Extension

While abdominal ultrasonography has significant limitations with regard to the staging of testicular tumors, scrotal ultrasonography may allow more accurate assessment of local spread of the primary tumor. Invasion into the epididymis and scrotal wall can be identified using high resolution ultrasound techniques. This additional information is obtained without the risk of additional irradiation of the testes.

An equally important role for ultrasonography is the detection of occult testicular neoplasms (Figure 19-5). Although testicular tumors usually cause local symptoms, the initial clinical appearance in 4% to 14% of patients is secondary to metastatic disease.[32] In a small number of these patients, the testes are normal when palpated. Gray scale ultrasonography has been shown to be useful in the detection of occult testicular neoplasms in these patients.[24,37]

Metastases

Because the lungs are the primary extranodal site of metastatic involvement in patients with testicular cancer, some form of chest imaging is necessary in all patients. Conventional whole lung tomography is capable of detecting pulmonary metastases in approximately 12% to 27% of patients who have negative routine chest films.[2,50,63] In addition, conventional tomography is capable of detecting multiple pulmonary nodules in patients thought to have a solitary nodule on routine chest film.[50] Computed tomography (CT) of the chest is more sensitive still, detecting pulmonary metastases in 18% of testicular cancer patients with normal whole lung tomograms.[8,25] In addition, CT is more sensitive than conventional tomography in detecting mediastinal lymphadenopathy.[12]

Tumor Markers and Dissemination

The development of sensitive and specific radioimmunoassays for human chorionic gonadotropin (HCG) and alpha-fetoprotein (AFP) has added another variable to the staging and management of patients with tumors of the testis. Serum AFP is elevated in approximately two-thirds of patients with advanced nonseminomatous

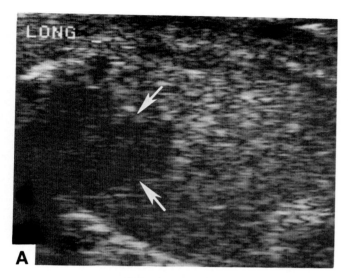

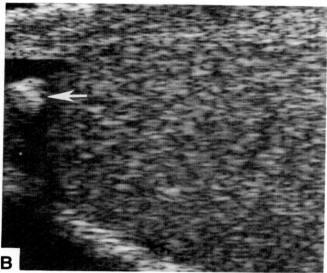

FIG. 19-5. Occult seminoma demonstrated by ultrasonography. This asymptomatic 32-year-old patient had a left supraclavicular mass and a normal physical examination of the testes. Biopsy of the mass produced evidence of metastatic clear cell carcinoma consistent with seminoma. (A) A longitudinal sonogram of the left testis reveals a 1-cm hypoechoic nodule (arrows) in the superior pole. (B) Normal right testis. Epididymis (arrow). A radical left orchiectomy was performed; pathologic examination demonstrated a 1-cm seminoma embedded within the normal testicular tissue beneath the epididymis corresponding to the abnormality shown on the sonogram. (Reprinted from Glazer, H. S., Lee, J. K. T., Melson, G. L., McClennan, B. L.: Sonographic detection of occult testicular neoplasms. A.J.R. 138:673–676, 1982. By permission of the publisher.)

tumors, but is not elevated in patients with pure seminomas or pure choriocarcinomas.[6] Human chorionic gonadotropin is elevated in approximately two thirds of patients with advanced nonseminomatous tumors and in 15% with advanced seminomas.[6] Virtually all patients with choriocarcinomas have elevated HCG. Combining the two tumor markers, approximately

90% of patients with advanced nonseminomatous tumors will have elevation of at least one of the markers, while 15% of patients with seminomas will have elevated HCG. However, tumor markers are less frequently elevated in patients with minimal or low volume disease. In one study, only 50% to 64% of patients with stage II disease had elevated HCG or AFP levels.[65] It is thus possible to have normal AFP and HCG titers and still have metastatic disease. Use of tumor markers, however, has decreased the staging errors in stage I patients to 9% to 14% and the staging errors in stage II patients to 5% to 10%.[29]

Tumor markers are also valuable in the posttreatment management of patients. Several conclusions may be drawn from the available data: (1) persistently elevated serum markers after orchiectomy invariably indicate stage II or III disease; (2) persistently elevated serum markers after positive lymphadenectomy usually suggest stage III disease; and (3) persistently elevated serum markers after lymphadenectomy negative for tumor invariably indicate stage III disease.[29]

IMAGING STRATEGIES AND TREATMENT DECISIONS

The initial staging evaluation as well as subsequent follow-up examinations must be appropriate to the type of treatment used.[22,27,52] Since the optimal method of treatment for any particular stage of the various histologic types of testicular cancer is not a matter of universal agreement, we cannot offer a dogmatic approach to the patient with testicular cancer. The following recommendations are based upon the methods of treatment used at the Washington University Medical Center (Table 19-5, Figures 19-6, 19-7).

Seminomas

The initial workup should consist of computed tomography of the abdomen and chest as well as radioimmunoassays for serum beta-HCG and AFP. Lymphangiog-

Table 19-5. Treatment of Testicular Tumors at the Washington University Medical Center

	Seminoma
Stages I and II:	a. B-HCG and AFP normal: Radiation therapy
	b. AFP elevated: Lymphadenectomy ± chemotherapy
	c. B-HCG elevated: Lymphadenectomy ± chemotherapy or radiation therapy (stage IIA)
Stage III:	Chemotherapy + excision of any residual disease
	Nonseminoma
Stages I and II:	Lymphadenectomy ± chemotherapy
Stage III:	Chemotherapy + excision of any residual disease

Modified from Catalona, W. J.: Current management of testicular tumors. Surg. Clin. North Am. 62:1122, 1982.

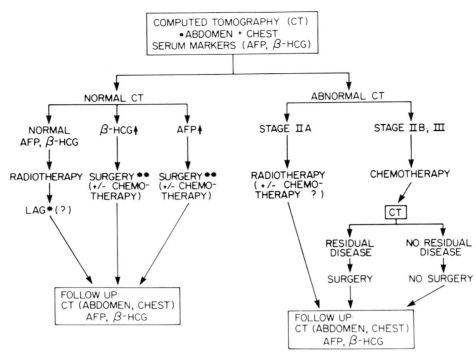

* Lymphangiography (LAG) considered if Stage I disease not to receive Radiotherapy electively
** Radical Retroperitoneal Lymphadenectomy

FIG. 19-6. Seminoma decision tree.

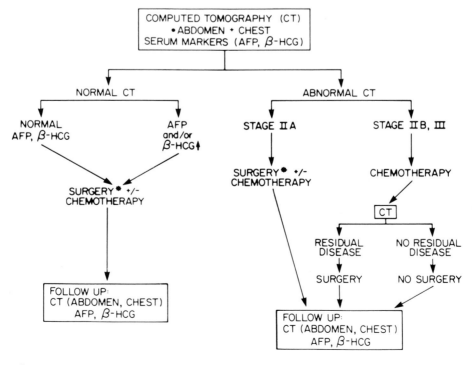

* Radical Retroperitoneal Lymphadenectomy

FIG. 19-7. Nonseminomatous tumor decision tree.

raphy should be performed only in clinical stage I patients in whom elective treatment of the retroperitoneum (i.e., radiation therapy) is not planned. Ultrasonography serves as an acceptable alternative to CT for imaging the abdomen in thin patients with very little retroperitoneal fat.

Stages I and IIA. Patients with pure seminomas and normal HCG and AFP titers are treated with radiation therapy. In general, if CT shows no evidence of lymph node metastases, radiation is given to the retroperitoneum only. If lymph node involvement is evident, radiation is given to the mediastinum and neck as well. If the histologic diagnosis is pure seminoma and the AFP level is elevated, one can be virtually certain that nonseminomatous elements are present, and the patient is treated as though he has a nonseminomatous tumor (lymphadenectomy or chemotherapy or both).

If the histologic diagnosis is pure seminoma and only the HCG is elevated, one is unable to distinguish whether the patient has an HCG-producing seminoma or has nonseminomatous elements present. In this case, the patient probably should be treated with lymphadenectomy or chemotherapy or both, although some patients with elevated HCG titers have been treated primarily with radiation therapy and have done well, particularly those with minimal retroperitoneal disease.[39]

Stages IIB and III. Patients with unresectable subdiaphragmatic disease (IIB) in addition to those with subdiaphragmatic or distant metastases (III) should undergo chemotherapy followed by surgical excision of any residual disease[11] (see comments under nonseminomatous tumors).

Nonseminomatous Tumors

As with seminomas, the initial workup should consist of computed tomography of the abdomen and chest as well as radioimmunoassays for serum beta-HCG and AFP. Lymphangiography should be performed only in clinical stage I patients in whom retroperitoneal lymphadenectomy is not planned. Once again, although CT is preferable, ultrasonography may serve as an acceptable alternative method for imaging the abdomen in thin patients with very little retroperitoneal fat.

Stages I and II. Patients with stage I and II nonseminomatous tumors or mixed tumors containing nonseminomatous elements are treated with lymphadenectomy or chemotherapy or both. Patients with unresectable subdiaphragmatic metastases (stage IIB) are treated initially with chemotherapy (see below).

Stage III. Patients with supradiaphragmatic or distant metastases in addition to those with unresectable subdiaphragmatic disease (IIB) should undergo chemotherapy

before surgical excision is attempted.[7,23,55] Although a smaller tumor burden improves the clinical response rate, surgical debulking before chemotherapy presents practical problems that include prolonged convalescence, which may allow regrowth of tumor before chemotherapy can be initiated. The essential effective drugs producing dramatic and high response rates are cisplatin, vinblastin, and bleomycin, with actinomycin D occasionally added in combined regimens.[52] If chemotherapy produces complete tumor regression as determined by repeat CT scan, subsequent lymphadenectomy is not performed. If, however, residual tumor is present on repeat CT scan, an attempt should be made to excise it. As discussed above, in approximately one half of these patients, the masses persisting after chemotherapy consist of fibrosis, mature teratoma, or cystic degeneration of tumor without viable remaining malignancy. These patients have a 90% long-term survival rate.[22,27,52] On the other hand, patients who after chemotherapy have persistent viable tumor have a 10% long-term survival rate. Further postoperative chemotherapy is needed in this latter group of patients. Preliminary data previously discussed suggest that CT may be able to distinguish these two groups of patients on the basis of mean tumor attenuation values.

Follow-up

The follow-up of patients with testicular cancer (seminomas and nonseminomatous tumors) should include serial radioimmunoassays for serum AFP and beta-HCG levels and periodic CT examinations of the abdomen and chest. The results of these tests along with clinical considerations direct further management of the patient.

Recurrence

Treatment of tumor recurrence depends upon a number of factors, which include the histologic type of tumor, the location and extent of recurrence, and the patient's previous therapy. Although an in-depth discussion of this subject is beyond the scope of this book, several generalizations can be made concerning the treatment of recurrence: patients previously treated surgically are managed with chemotherapy; patients previously given chemotherapy are treated with surgical debulking and further chemotherapy; and patients previously given radiation therapy are also treated with surgical debulking and chemotherapy. Clinical factors relating to each individual patient may alter these general methods of treatment.

IMPACT OF NEW TECHNOLOGY

At present, radiologic staging of testicular cancer is no more than 80% to 90% accurate at best. Computed tomography is currently the imaging procedure of choice for the detection of metastases. Although there are theoretical limits to the ability of CT to detect early metastatic disease, the use of currently available fast (<10 second) scanners should improve the sensitivity, specificity, and accuracy of this method.

The development of sensitive and specific tumor markers has already brought about a decrease in staging errors at most centers. Further experience with the use of tumor markers should help refine our ability to stage and manage patients with testicular tumors. A related technique of great potential value is the use of radioactively labeled antibodies to AFP and beta-HCG to localize areas of metastatic disease. Although still in the early stages of development, this radioimmunodetection technique may be able to detect tumor deposits that are undetectable by currently available methods.

Finally, magnetic resonance imaging (MRI), a technique that uses a magnetic field and pulsed radiofrequency waves to detect differences between normal and abnormal tissues, is a new imaging procedure of potential value. In a study of 25 patients with nonseminomatous germ cell tumors, Ellis et al.[19] found MRI to be nearly equivalent to CT in staging retroperitoneal lymphadenopathies. The use of magnetic resonance as an imaging technique, however, is still in its infancy. Further clinical testing is necessary to determine the role of MRI in the staging and management of patients with cancers of the testis.

REFERENCES

1. American Joint Committee on Cancer: *Manual for Staging of Cancer.* 2nd ed. Beahrs. O. H., Myers, M. H. (Eds.). Philadelphia, J. B. Lippincott, 1983, pp. 165–171.
2. Bergaman, S. M., Lippert, M., Javadpour, N.: The value of whole lung tomography in the early detection of metastatic disease in patients with renal cell carcinoma and testicular tumors. *J. Urol.* **124**:860–862, 1980.
3. Boden, G., Gibb, R.: Radiotherapy and testicular neoplasms. *Lancet* **2**:1195–1197, 1951.
4. Burney, B. T., Klatte, E. C.: Ultrasound and computed tomography of the abdomen in the staging and management of testicular carcinoma. *Radiology* **132**:415–419, 1979.
5. Cameron, K. M.: The pathology of testicular tumors. In *The Management of Testicular Tumours.* Peckham, M., (Ed.). London, Edward Arnold Ltd., 1981.
6. Catalona, W. J.: Tumor markers in testicular cancer. *Urol. Clin. North Am.* **6**:613–628, 1979.
7. Catalona, W. J.: Current management of testicular tumors. *Surg. Clin. North Am.* **62**:1119–1127, 1982.
8. Chang, A. E., Schaner, E. G., Conkle, D. M., Flye, M. W., Doppman, J. L., Rosenberg, S. A.: Evaluation of computed tomography in the detection of pulmonary metastases. *Cancer* **43**:913–916, 1979.
9. Chiappa, S., Uslenghi, C., Bonadonna, G., Marano, P., Ravashi, G.: Combined testicular and foot lymphangiography in testicular carcinomas. *Surg. Gynecol. Obstet.* **123**:10–14, 1966.
10. Cook, F. E., Jr., Lawrence, D. D., Smith, J. R., Gritti, E. J.: Testicular carcinoma and lymphangiography. *Radiology* **84**:420–427, 1965.
11. Crawford, E. D., Smith, R. B., deKernion, J. B.: Treatment of advanced seminoma with pre-radiation chemotherapy. *J. Urol.* **129**:752–756, 1983.
12. Crowe, J. K., Brown, L. R., Muhm, J. R.: Computed tomography of the mediastinum. *Radiology* **128**:75–87, 1978.
13. Donohue, J. P.: Surgical management of testis cancer. In *Testicular Tumors: Management and Treatment.* Einhorn, L. H. (Ed.). New York, Masson Publishing USA, Inc., 1980.
14. Donohue, J. P., Perez, J. M., Einhorn, L. H.: Improved management of non-seminomatous tumors. *J. Urol.* **121**:425–428, 1979.
15. Donohue, J. P., Zachary, J. M., Maynard, B. R.: Distribution of nodal metastases in nonseminomatous testis cancer. *J. Urol.* **128**:320, 1982.
16. Dosoretz, D. E., Shipley, W. U., Blitzer, P. H., Gilbert, S., Prat, J., Parkhurst, E., Wang, C. C.: Megavoltage irradiation for pure testicular seminoma: Results and patterns of failure. *Cancer* **48**:2184–2190, 1981.
17. Dunnick, N. R., Javadpour, N.: Value of CT and lymphography: Distinguishing retroperitoneal metastases from nonseminomatous testicular tumors. *A.J.R.* **136**:1093–1099, 1981.
18. Ehrlichman, R. J., Kaufman, S. L., Siegelman, S. S., Trump, D. L., Walsh, P. C.: Computerized tomography and lymphangiography in staging testis tumors. *J. Urol.* **126**:179–181, 1981.
19. Ellis, J. H., Bies, J. R., Kopecky, K. K., Klatte, E. C., Rowland, R. G., Donohue, J. P.: Comparison of NMR and CT in the evaluation of metastatic retroperitoneal lymphadenopathy from testicular carcinoma. *J. Comput. Assist. Tomogr.* **8**:709–719, 1984.
20. Fein, R. L., Taber, D. O.: Foot lymphography in the testis tumor patient. *Cancer* **24**:248–255, 1969.
21. Fraley, E. E., Lange, P. H., Kennedy, B. J.: Germ-cell testicular cancer in adults. *N. Engl. J. Med.* **301**:1370–1377, 1979.
22. Frank, I. N., Keys, H. M., McCune, C. S.: Urologic and male genital cancers. In *Clinical Oncology for Medical Students and Physicians: A Multidisciplinary Approach*, 6th ed. Rubin, P. (Ed.). New York, American Cancer Society, 1983, pp. 198–221.
23. Garnick, M. B., Canellos, G. P., Richie, J. P.: Treatment and surgical staging of testicular and primary extragonadal germ cell cancer. *J.A.M.A.* **250**:1733–1741, 1983.
24. Glazer, H. S., Lee, J. K. T., Melson, G. L., McClennan, B. L.: Sonographic detection of occult testicular neoplasms. *A.J.R.* **138**:673–675, 1982.
25. Husband, J. E.: Computed tomography in testicular tumours. In *The Management of Testicular Tumours.* Peckham, M. (Ed.). London, Edward Arnold Ltd., 1981.
26. Husband, J. E., Hawkes, D. J., Peckham, M. J.: CT estimation of mean attenuation values and volume in testicular tumors: A comparison with surgical and histologic findings. *Radiology* **144**:553–558, 1982.
27. Hussey, D. H.: Testis. In *Textbook of Radiotherapy*, 3rd Ed. Fletcher, G. H. (Ed.). Philadelphia, Lea & Febiger, 1980, pp. 867–885.
28. Javadpour, N.: The National Cancer Institute experience with testicular cancer. *J. Urol.* **120**:651–659, 1978.
29. Javadpour, N.: Improved staging for testicular cancer using biologic tumor markers: A prospective study. *J. Urol.* **124**:58–59, 1980.
30. Javadpour, N., Kim, E. E., Deland, F. N., Salyer, J. R., Shah, U., Goldenberg, D. M.: The role of radioimmunodetection in the management of testicular cancer. *J.A.M.A.* **246**:45–49, 1981.
31. Jing, B., Wallace, S., Zornoza, J.: Metastases to retroperitoneal and pelvic lymph nodes. Computed tomography and lymphangiography. *Radiol. Clin. North Am.* **20**:511–530, 1982.
32. Johnson, D. E.: *Testicular Tumours.* London, Henry Kimpton, 1972, pp. 48.
33. Johnson, D. E., Bracken, R. B., Blight, E. M.: Prognosis for pathologic stage I nonseminomatous germ cell tumors of the testis managed by retroperitoneal lymphadenectomy. *J. Urol.* **116**:63–65, 1976.
34. Johnson, D. E., Hussey, D. H., Samuels, M. L.: Testis. In *Urology.*

Chisholm, G. D. (Ed.). New York, Appleton-Century-Crofts, 1980.

35. Jonsson, K., Ingemansson, S., Ling, L.: Lymphography in patients with testicular tumors. *Br. J. Urol.* **45**:548–554, 1973.

36. Kademian, M., Wirtanen, G.: Accuracy of bipedal lymphangiography in testicular tumors. *Urology* **9**:218–220, 1977.

37. Kirschling, R. J., Kvols, L. K., Charboneau, J. W., Grantham, J. G., Zincke, H.: High-resolution ultrasonographic and pathologic abnormalities of germ cell tumors in patients with clinically normal testes. *Mayo Clin. Proc.* **58**:648–653, 1983.

38. Kleinsmith, L. J., Pierce, G. B. Jr.: Multipotentiality of single embryonal carcinoma cells. *Cancer Res.* **24**:1544–1552, 1964.

39. Lange, P. H., Nochomoritz, L. E., Rosai, J., Fraley, E. E., Kennedy, B. J., Bose, G., Brisbane, J., Catalona, W. J., Cochran, J. S., Cimosarow, R. W., Cummings, K. B., deKernion, J. B., Einhorn, L. H., Hakala, T. R., Jewett, M., Moore, M. M., Scardinu, P. T., Streitz, F.: Serum alpha-fetoprotein and human chorionic gonadotropin in patients with seminoma. *J. Urol.* **124**:472–478, 1980.

40. Lein, H. H., Kolvenstvedt, A., Talle, K., Fossa, S. D., Klepp, O., Ous, S.: Comparison of computed tomography, lymphography and phlebography in 200 consecutive patients with regard to retroperitoneal metastases from testicular tumor. *Radiology* **146**:129–132, 1983.

41. MacDonald, J. S.: Lymphography in testicular tumours. In *The Management of Testicular Tumours.* Peckham, H. (Ed.). London, Edward Arnold Ltd., 1981.

42. Maier, J. G., Schamber, D. T.: The role of lymphangiography in the diagnosis and treatment of malignant testicular tumors. *A.J.R.* **114**:482–494, 1972.

43. Maier, J. G., Sulak, M. H., Mettemeyer, B. T.: Seminoma of the testis: Analysis of treatment success and failure. *A.J.R.* **102**:596–602, 1968.

44. Maier, J. G., Wittemeyer, B. T., Sulak, M. H.: Treatment and prognosis in seminoma of the testis. *J. Urol.* **99**:72–78, 1968.

45. Maricek, B., Brutschin, P., Triller, J., Fuchs, W. A.: Lymphography and computed tomography in staging nonseminomatous testicular cancer: Limited detection of early stage metastatic disease. *Urol. Radiol.* **5**:243–246, 1983.

46. Merrin, C.: Seminoma. *Urol. Clin. North Am.* **4**:379–392, 1977.

47. Mostofi, F. J., Price, E. B., Jr.: Tumors of the male genital system. In *Atlas of Tumor Pathology*, Fascicle 8, Series 2. Washington, D.C.: Armed Forces Institute of Pathology, 1973.

48. Mostofi, F. K.: Testicular tumors: Epidemiologic, etiologic and pathologic factors. *Cancer* **32**:1186–1201, 1973.

49. Muhm, J. R., Brown, L. R., Crowe, J. K.: Detection of pulmonary nodules by computed tomography. *A.J.R.* **128**:267–270, 1977.

50. Niefeld, J. P., Michaelis, L. L., Doppman, J. L.: Suspected pulmonary metastases: Correlation of chest x-ray, whole lung tomograms and operative findings. *Cancer* **39**:383–387, 1977.

51. Patton, J. F., Hewitt, C. B., Mallis, N.: Diagnosis and treatment of tumors of the testis. *J.A.M.A.* **171**:2194–2198, 1959.

52. Paulson, D. F., Einhorn, L. H., Peckham, M. J., Williams, S. D.: Cancer of the testis. In *Cancer—Principles and Practice of Oncology.* DeVita, V. T. Jr., Hellman, S., Rosenberg, S. A. (Eds.). Philadelphia, J. B. Lippincott, 1982, pp. 786–822.

53. Pugh, R.C.B. (Ed.).: *Pathology of the Testes.* Oxford, Blackwell Scientific Publications, 1976.

54. Ray, B., Hajdu, S. L., Whitmore, W. F.: Distribution of retroperitoneal lymph node metastases in testicular germinal tumors. *Cancer* **33**:340–348, 1974.

55. Richie, J. P., Garnick, M. B.: Changing concepts in the treatment of nonseminomatous germ cell tumors of the testis. *J. Urol.* **131**:1089–1092, 1984.

56. Roberts, K. R., Mettler, F. A.: Diagnostic evaluation of the pelvic and abdominal lymphatic system. *Curr. Probl. Diag. Radiol.* **8**:2–56, 1979.

57. Roth, L. M., Gillespie, J. J.: Pathology and ultrastructure of germinal neoplasms of the testis. In *Testicular Tumors: Management and Treatment,* Einhorn, L. H. (Ed.). New York, Masson Publishing USA, Inc., 1980.

58. Rowland, R. G., Weisman, D., Williams, S. D., Einhorn, L. H., Klatte, E. C., Donohue, J. P.: Accuracy of preoperative staging in stages A and B nonseminomatous germ cell testis tumors. *J. Urol.* **127**:718–720, 1982.

59. Safer, M. L., Green, J. P., Crews, Q. E., Jr., Hill, D. R.: Lymphangiographic accuracy in the staging of testicular tumors. *Cancer* **35**:1603–1605, 1975.

60. Schaner, E. G., Chang, A. E., Doppman, J. L., Conkle, D. M., Flye, M. W., Rosenberg, S. A.: Comparison of computed and conventional whole lung tomography in detecting pulmonary nodules: A prospective radiologic-pathologic study. *A.J.R.* **131**:51–54, 1978.

61. Seitzman, D. M., Halaby, F. A.: Lymphangiography: An evaluation of its application. *J. Urol.* **91**:301–305, 1964.

62. Silverberg, E.: Cancer in young adults (ages 15 to 34). *Cancer* **32**:32–42, 1982.

63. Sindelar, W. F., Bagley, D. H., Felix, E. L., Doppman, J. L., Ketcham, A. F.: Lung tomography in cancer patients: Full lung tomograms in screening for pulmonary metastases. *J.A.M.A.* **240**:2060–2063, 1978.

64. Skinner, D. G.: Management of nonseminomatous tumors of the testis. In *Genitourinary Cancer.* Skinner, D. G., deKernion, J. B. (Eds.). Philadelphia, W. B. Saunders, 1978.

65. Skinner, D. G., Scardino, P. T.: Relevance of biochemical tumor markers and lymphadenectomy in management of nonseminomatous testis tumors. Current perspectives. *J. Urol.* **123**:378–382, 1980.

66. Smith, R. B.: Management of testicular seminoma. In *Genitourinary Cancer,* Skinner, D. G., deKernion, J. B. (Eds.). Philadelphia, W. B. Saunders, 1978.

67. Soo, C.-S., Bernardino, M. E., Chuang, V. P., Ordonez, N.: Pitfalls of CT findings in post-therapy testicular carcinoma. *J. Comput. Assist. Tomogr.* **5**:39–41, 1981.

68. Staubitz, W. J., Early, D. S., Magoss, I. V., Murphy, G. P.: Surgical management of testis tumor. *J. Urol.* **111**:205–209, 1974.

69. Storm, P. B., Kern, A., Loening, S. A., Brown, R. C., Culp, D. A.: Evaluation of pedal lymphangiography in staging non-seminomatous testicular carcinoma. *J. Urol.* **118**:1001–1003, 1977.

70. Thomas, J. L., Bernardino, M. E., Bracken, R. B.: Staging of testicular carcinoma: Comparison of CT and lymphangiography. *A.J.R.* **137**:991–996, 1981.

71. Wallace, D. M., Chisholm, G. D., Hendry, W. F.: TNM classification for urologic tumours (U.I.C.C.)—1974. *Br. J. Urol.* **47**:1–12, 1975.

72. Wallace, S., Jing, B. S.: Lymphangiography: Diagnosis of nodal metastases from testicular malignancies. *J.A.M.A.* **213**:94–96, 1970.

73. Whitmore, W. F., Jr.: Germinal testis tumors in adults. In *Genitourinary Cancer,* Skinner, D. G., deKernion, J. B. (Eds.). Philadelphia, W. B. Saunders, 1978.

74. Williams, R. D., Feinberg, S. B., Knight, L. C., Fraley, E. E.: Abdominal staging of testicular tumors using ultrasonography and computed tomography. *J. Urol.* **123**:872–875, 1980.

20 ONCOLOGIC IMAGING FOR CARCINOMA OF THE CERVIX, OVARY AND ENDOMETRIUM

Dennis M. Balfe
Jay P. Heiken
Bruce L. McClennan

CERVIX

Physicians can take some measure of pride in the fact that the incidence of invasive carcinoma of the cervix is decreasing. This is almost certainly due to the early detection of noninvasive cancer through the widespread cancer screening made possible by Papanicolaou's cytologic method. Nevertheless, 16,000 new cases of invasive clinical cancer are projected for 1984, and the disease will account for 6,800 deaths.[87]

While the primary disease is quite amenable to both radiation and surgical therapeutic measures (provided the local extent is circumscribed), recurrent disease is exceptionally deadly. Of 526 patients reported by Van Nagell,[95] 31% developed recurrence; in this group, the three-year survival was 6%. Improvement in this disheartening statistic can come about through development of better treatment methods, which in turn depend upon proper initial staging. Patients in whom radiation therapy is likely to fail include those with large solid tumors, the hypoxic central zones of which are relatively radioresistant,[24] and those with undetected spread to regional lymph nodes, which may occur in 15% to 22% of patients with clinically low-stage disease.[16,17,43,45,48]

It should be emphasized that the most effective way of reducing the number of cancer deaths from epidermoid carcinoma of the cervix is to intensify efforts to enroll women of all ages in cancer screening programs. Radiographic methods play essentially no role in the detection of carcinoma of the cervix. Once an invasive tumor is identified, however, a variety of methods can be used in staging the disease. Variables that are of the greatest clinical importance are assessment of lymph node status, evaluation of the extent of local disease and detection of recurrence at the earliest possible stage. Appropriate application of newer imaging methods should favorably influence the long-term survival of cervical cancer patients by selecting those individuals most likely to benefit from radical therapeutic measures.

Tumor Behavior and Pathology

Ninety percent of neoplasms of the cervix are epidermoid carcinomas.[15] Most of the remaining 10% is accounted for by adenocarcinomas; sarcomas of the cervix are rare lesions with a very poor prognosis. Grading of the microscopic specimens obtained from patients with epidermoid carcinomas generally follows the standard three-grade system, viz, well, moderately, and poorly differentiated cellular structure. While the degree of differentiation may have less influence on overall survival than does stage and bulk of the primary lesion, there are studies that indicate that patients with high grade lesions have a poorer prognosis. In Chung's series,[16] for example, the incidence of nodal metastases in patients with stage IB squamous cancers was 0% for grade 1, 18% for grade 2, and 50% for grade 3 lesions. Similarly, the two-year survival[17] in the same stage was 100%, 93%, and 77% for grades 1, 2 and 3, respectively.

Biologic Behavior. Cervical intraepithelial neoplasia (CIN) is considered the precursor of invasive epidermoid cancer of the uterine cervix.[15,69] Its origin from metaplasia or dysplasia is less well understood. There is mounting evidence that the agent that incites neoplasia within the cervical mucosa is transmitted during sexual intercourse — epidermoid carcinoma is extremely rare in celibates and quite common in prostitutes. It has been suggested that herpes simplex virus (HSV-2) plays a role in pathogenesis.[15]

Carcinoma in situ (CIS) is the name applied to lesions in which the cytologic features of malignancy extend to the basement membrane of the epithelium. This lesion can be treated locally or with total hysterectomy. That it is a locally confined lesion is borne out by the low (1.2% to 2.5%) rate of recurrent disease.[15]

Microinvasive carcinoma of the cervix represents an extension of carcinoma in situ below the basement membrane; this lesion is also relatively well confined, although some potential for lymphatic spread exists as evidenced by the 2% to 5% incidence of positive nodes in some series.[15]

The natural history of microinvasive cervical cancer, if unchecked, is to become clinically invasive. At this point, it undergoes the usual patterns of spread, namely by direct extension, by lymphatic permeation, and by hematogenous dissemination.

Direct Extension. Organs directly contiguous to the uterine cervix are at risk of becoming involved by direct extension of the neoplastic process (Figure 20-1). These can be enumerated as follows: inferiorly, the upper portion of the vaginal vault; superiorly, the uterine corpus; anteriorly, the base of the urinary bladder; posteriorly, the rectum; and, laterally, the paracervical (parametrial) tissues, including the ureters. In more extensive disease, the obturator internus muscles may be invaded. Invasion of the bladder, rectum, or pelvic sidewall implies extensive disease and is associated with a very poor prognosis. In addition, patients in whom endometrial invasion is observed likewise carry a poorer prognosis than those in whom this finding is not present.

Lymphatic Spread. Lymphatic drainage of the cervix proceeds from a rich cervical plexus and may continue in several directions: (1) into the parametrial nodes superolaterally, (2) anterolaterally into the internal iliac system, (3) posteriorly to the lateral sacral nodes, and (4) into the external iliac nodes. While presence of lymph node metastases does not change the clinical stage, it has long been known that survival and disease-free interval are considerably shortened by the presence of lymphatic metastases.[34,36,76] In the review of Piver et al.,[76] the five-year survival of patients with positive aortic nodes was only 9.6%. Since cervical cancer spreads from primary echelon nodes to secondary nodes, the presence of para-aortic metastases generally indicates extensive disease in the pelvis. Thus, only 2 of 26 patients in the series of Lagasse et al.[59] had positive para-aortic nodes and nega-

tive pelvic nodes; the review of Hammond et al.[42] of 463 patients with cancer confined to the pelvis (stages IB–IIIB) pointed out a survival of more than 92 months in patients with low stage disease with negative lymphangiograms. For the group in whom lymphangiograms showed nodal metastases, the collective survival was 31 months. There is a positive correlation between increasing local stage and the incidence of tumor-bearing pelvic or para-aortic lymph nodes (Table 20-1).[29]

Several other factors influence overall prognosis, however; the bulk of the lesion may be an important predictor of its biologic hazard, and very large lesions with necrotic centers are relatively radioresistant. Similarly, local extension into the uterus, although not specifically mentioned in clinical staging systems, has a definite prognostic significance.[78] In stage I cancer, for example, an overall five-year survival of 85% was reported in patients free of uterine invasion; in those with positive endometrial involvement, the survival was only 68%.

Metastatic Spread. The development of widespread hematogenous metastatic disease likewise parallels the presence of lymph node metastasis. It is probable that lymphatic spread and vascular permeation are independent events related to the size and invasiveness of the primary tumor. In the series of Welander et al.,[100] 55% of patients with positive nodes developed distant metastases while only 25% of those without metastatic adenopathy later developed widespread disease. Common sites of spread include the lung, skeletal system, brain, and liver.

Classification and Staging

Gynecologists have almost universally adopted the staging system devised by the International Federation of Gynecologic Oncology (FIGO) for invasive carcinoma of the cervix. Its relationship to the TNM staging system is presented in Table 20-2 and Figure 20-2. Stage 0, which is specifically excluded from therapeutic statistics for invasive cervical carcinoma, corresponds to carcinoma in situ (T_{is}). Microinvasive carcinoma is stage T_{1a}, while all other carcinomas confined to the cervix are T_{1b}. T_{2a} carcinoma has extended to the vagina (but not the lower third); T_{2b} involves the parametrium (but not the pelvic sidewall). T_3 lesions are a somewhat heterogeneous group, which represents extensive local disease. All patients with hydronephrosis or nonvisualization of a kidney on urograms are placed in stage T_{3b}, as are patients with extension to the pelvic wall. Tumors with predominantly inferior extent, so that the lower third of the vagina is involved, are T_{3a}. T_4 tumors have invaded local viscera (bladder or rectum) or extend beyond the true pelvis.

Nodal status, while clearly a determinant of patient survival and the disease-free interval, is not included in the FIGO system.

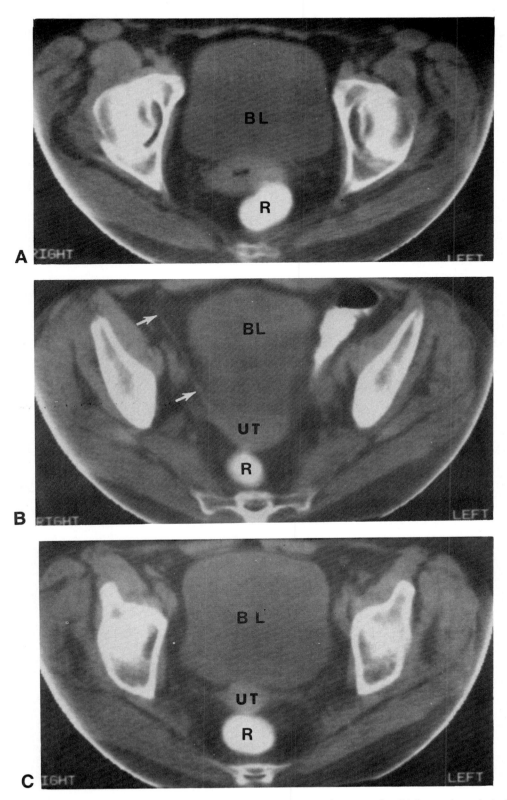

FIG. 20-1. Normal relationships of the cervix demonstrated by computed tomography. (A) A scan through the lower portion of the pelvis demonstrates an oval-shaped cervix (C) in this multiparous patient. Air in the region of the cervical os is present because of insertion of a vaginal tampon. The bladder (BL) lies immediately anterior with the rectum (R) immediately posterior. Laterally, the richly vascular paracervical region is noted. (B) At a slightly higher level, the uterine and cervical vessels follow the course of the broad ligament immediately lateral to the lower uterine segment (UT).

Table 20-1. Carcinoma of the Cervix:
Incidence of Para-Aortic Lymph Node Metastases

AUTHOR	STAGE/LYMPH NODE METASTASES (%)			
	I	II	III	IV
Avarette	8.0	22.0	10.0	50.0
Berman	8.3	23.5	13.6	
Brady		8.3	35.0	50.0
Buschbaum		16.0	46.0	
Delgado	0	44.0	38.0	
Guthrie			35.0	66.6
Nelson		14.9	38.4	
Piver			35.7	66.6
Piver		5.2	37.5	40.0
Sudarsanam	7.0	16.0	19.0	
Wharton	0	21.0	33.0	

Reprinted from Emami, B., Watring, W. G., Tak, W.,
Anderson, B., Piro, A. J.: Para-aortic lymph node radia-
tion in advanced cervical cancer. *Radiat. Oncol. Biol.
Phys.* 6:1237–1241, 1980.

Table 20-2. Comparison of FIGO with TNM Staging of
Carcinoma of the Cervix

FIGO		TNM
Stage IA	Microinvasive carcinoma	$T_{1a}N_xM_0$
Stage IB	Invasive cancer confined to the cervix	$T_{1b}N_xM_0$
Stage IIA	Extension to vagina (not lower one third)	$T_{2a}N_xM_0$
Stage IIB	Extension to parametrium	$T_{2b}N_xM_0$
Stage IIIA	Extension to lower one third of vagina	$T_{3a}N_xM_0$
Stage IIIB	Extension to ureter; hydronephrosis	$T_{3b}N_xM_0$
Stage IVA	Extension to bladder/rectum/beyond true pelvis	$T_4N_xM_0$
Stage IVB	Distant metastases	$T_xN_xM_+$

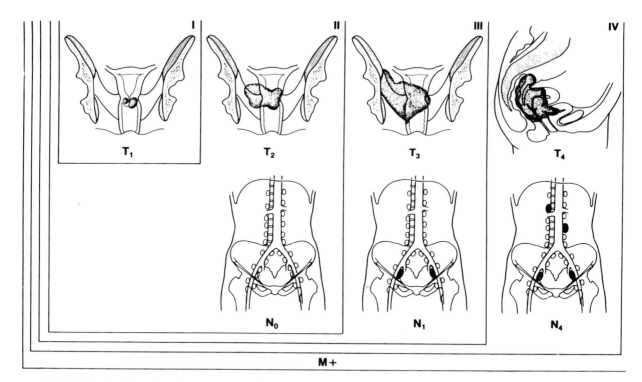

FIG. 20-2. Anatomic staging for cervix cancer. Tumor (T) categories: The extent and depth of invasion are the critical factors.
The extension from the cervix into either the vagina (T_{2a}) or the parametrium (T_{2b}) and further to the lower vagina (T_{3a}) or
to pelvic sidewall (T_{3b}). Anterior and posterior spread is into adjacent viscera or bladder and rectum (T_4). Note that this must
be established histopathologically as in T_{1a} and occult cancers after a cone. Node (N) categories: Only location is considered
and is referred to as regional in pelvic nodes (N_4). There are no N_2 or N_3 categories. Stage grouping: Each T category determines stage, and evidence of involved nodes or metastases indicates stage IV. N_1 is equivalent to T_3 or stage III; N_x to T_x
in stage IV. (Modified from Beecham, J. B., Helmkamp, B. F., Rubin, P.: Tumors of the female reproductive organs. In *Clinical
Oncology for Medical Students and Physicians: A Multidisciplinary Approach,* 6th ed. Rubin, P. (Ed.). New York, American
Cancer Society, 1983, pp. 428–480. With permission.)

It must be emphasized that the FIGO staging classification is a clinical system based on physical examination and adjunctive techniques such as hysteroscopy, cystoscopy, sigmoidoscopy, and colposcopy. Findings at laparotomy do not change the clinical stage. However, the influence of nodal metastases on survival has prompted many investigators[75,78] to perform laparotomies to detect para-aortic nodes. In this way, they hope to modify the radiation therapy portal to treat involved nodes in only those individuals with proven para-aortic disease. Opponents of the technique[42,51] point out that over half of patients with para-aortic metastases will develop widespread metastatic lesions and thus are inappropriate candidates for an extended radiotherapeutic field technique. Thus, there may be no therapeutic benefit to justify the morbidity attendant to staging laparotomy.

It is important in the clinical staging procedure to give patients the benefit of the doubt and place them in a more favorable category or downstage them. It can be misleading if patients are deliberately placed in a higher stage and can lead to the appearance of improved results when actually the only item that is altered is patient selection by the staging procedure. This is demonstrated in Figure 20-3.

Imaging Procedures and Assessment

Intravenous urography is part of the FIGO staging system; indeed, the mere presence of hydronephrosis or nonfunction of a kidney on a urogram places a patient in stage T_3. Most patients also undergo barium examinations of the colon as part of the pretreatment assessment. In young patients with low stage lesions, however, the incidence of positive findings on contrast enemas is quite low, and this examination could be omitted. Theoretically, cross-sectional imaging techniques might be useful to more accurately assess the local extent of tumor in the pelvis. In addition to CT or ultrasonography, lymphangiography has been employed as a noninvasive means of assessing nodal status. Since most distant metastatic deposits from epidermoid carcinomas involve the lung or skeletal system, chest films and radionuclide imaging are frequently useful. A summary of available techniques and an estimate of their cost effectiveness is given in Table 20-3.

Urography (IVP) and Barium Enema.
The FIGO staging system accepts urographic demonstration of hydronephrosis as sufficient criterion to classify epidermoid carcinoma of the cervix as stage III. This fact is a reflection of the biologic behavior of the tumor and its propensity to spread laterally through the parametrial tissues to engulf the ureter. Additionally, gross invasion of the bladder may be detectable by either urography or cystography. Care must be taken, however, not to over-

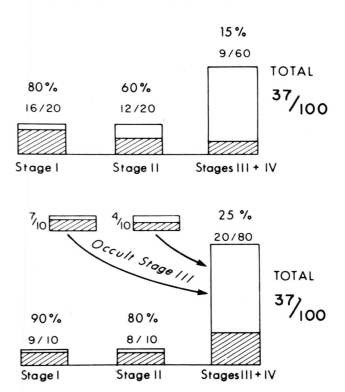

FIG. 20-3. Hypothetical graph of five-year survival (shaded column) by stages of 100 patients with cervical carcinoma. The upper row indicates the original staging, the lower row shows reassignment or one half of each group in stages I and II because of the discovery of occult biopsy-proven extension to either the diaphragmatic peritoneum or the retroperitoneal nodes. Although the overall cure rate is unchanged (37%), the rate in each column is significantly increased. (Reprinted from Ulfelder, H.: Classification systems. *Int. J. Radiat. Oncol. Biol. Phys.* 7:1083–1086, 1981. With permission.)

stage patients with radiographic findings of irregularity or thickening of the bladder wall. Lymphatic obstruction may produce bullous edema of the bladder wall when tumor invasion is, in fact, not present. This phenomenon is also widely appreciated with cystoscopy, and FIGO staging methods demand biopsy evidence of tumor invading the bladder wall in order to place a patient in stage IV.[15,24]

Barium examination of the colon is frequently performed on patients before therapy. In clinically low-stage disease, the yield is quite low, but in older patients, concurrent disease, such as diverticulosis, diverticulitis, or colon neoplasia may be disclosed. In high stage, bulky disease, invasion of the rectum may be demonstrated. Subtle mucosal changes are better demonstrated using air contrast techniques, which have therefore been recommended in evaluating this group of patients.[34]

Computed Tomography Versus Physical Examination (EUA) for Staging Primary Cervical Cancer.
Clinical examination to evaluate the extent of local disease is least

Table 20-3. Imaging Methods for Evaluating Cervical Carcinoma

METHOD	CAPABILITY	COST/ BENEFIT	RECOMMENDATION FOR USE
Noninvasive Chest radiography	Detects soft tissue nodules greater than 15 mm; detects acute/chronic pulmonary disease.	High	Routine
Chest laminography	Detects soft tissue nodules greater than 10 mm.	Moderate	Patients considered for radical surgical therapy
Skeletal radiography	Confirms suspicious findings on radionuclide scans.	Low	When radionuclide scan is equivocal
Sonography Primary tumor	Detects extension in immediate paracervical area.	Low	Not routine
Liver	Detects metastatic deposits greater than 15 mm.	Moderate	Patients with elevated liver enzymes
Barium enema	Detects serosal invasion of primary tumor; screens for diverticulosis, adenomatous polyps.	Low Moderate	Patients with colonic symptoms or guaiac positive stool
MRI	Not yet investigated.	Unknown	Unknown
Minimally invasive Urography	Detects parametrial extension of tumor producing hydronephrosis; screens for unsuspected urinary tract disease.	High	Routine
CT	Detects liver metastases greater than 1 cm in size; detects lymphadenopathy greater than 15 mm in size; detects extension of tumor locally to pelvic sidewall.	High	Patients with high clinical stage
Radionuclide Bone	Sensitive assessment of bone metastases.	Moderate	Operative candidates, patients with elevated alkaline phosphatose or bone pain
Liver	Detects peripheral metastases greater than 20 mm.	Low	Operative candidate; patients with elevated liver enzymes
Invasive Angiography	Detects abnormal vascularity in primary tumor and local extension.	Low	Not routine
Lymphangiography	Detects abnormal lymph node architecture in external iliac, common iliac, para-aortic nodes.	Moderate	Operative candidates
Biopsy	Confirms lesions detected by radionuclide scans, CT scans, or lymphangiograms	High	Patients with suspicious lesions

reliable in the assessment of parametrial tumors: specifically, it is difficult to clinically assess whether a tumor-free plane is preserved medial to the obturator internus muscle.[96] From a therapeutic standpoint, this information is vital to management, since surgical removal cannot be contemplated in patients with actual invasion of the pelvic sidewall. This has stimulated several oncologists to use CT to assess the local pelvic extent of tumor (Figure 20-4). One investigator[55] reported an overall 88% accuracy in staging patients by CT preoperatively; three of the four errors made in local (T) staging were in mistaken evaluations of rectal invasion. There was only one patient in whom assessment of parametrial extension was in error. However, in the series of Walsh et al.,[96] seven of the nine errors made in CT staging were the result of inaccurate assessment of the tumor's relationship to

the pelvic sidewall: in three, CT predicted that the tumor stopped short of the obturator internus muscle, when in fact there was microscopic invasion. In four, the CT prediction of pelvic sidewall invasion was not borne out surgically. Similar difficulties have been reported by Whitley et al.[102] and Grumbine et al.[38] At this time, the ability of cross-sectional imaging techniques to predict the local extent of disease is no better than clinical examination under anesthesia (EUA); thus, routine use of this technique for pretherapeutic local staging is unwarranted. Selected patients, such as those who are very difficult to examine because of obesity or previous radiation therapy, may benefit from preoperative CT evaluation.

Lymphangiography versus CT for Staging Lymph Node Status. Two major techniques have been used to predict

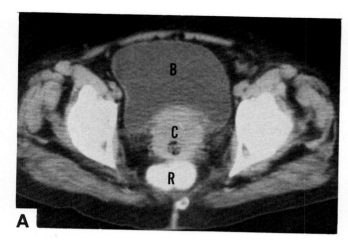

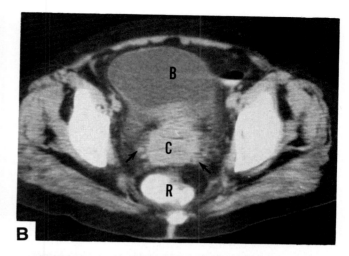

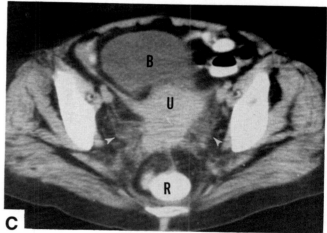

FIG. 20-4. Extensive carcinoma of the cervix demonstrated by CT. (A) Scan through the primary tumor demonstrates an enlarged cervix (C) with extension of tumor into the base of the bladder (B). The rectum (R) is not invaded. Note the increased serpiginous soft tissue densities lateral to the cervix. (B) Nodular densities (arrows) are present within the paracervical soft tissues and represent direct tumor extension into the broad ligament. (C) Scan through the uterine fundus (U) demonstrates some thickening of the attachment of the ligamentum teres. The parametrial tissues are bilaterally infiltrated with tumor (arrowheads). The distal ureters pass immediately adjacent to these regions.

the status of regional lymph nodes: lymphangiography and computed tomography. The rationale underlying the continued search for an accurate means of assessing lymph nodes is simply stated: patients with para-aortic nodal involvement have a dismal prognosis—if they could be accurately identified, radiation therapy, which can achieve moderate improvement in survival,[56] could be used in favor of radical surgical or radiotherapeutic techniques (which cannot hope to bring success).

Theoretical considerations favoring lymphangiography include the fact that direct opacification of nodal architecture gives the best chance of detecting small areas of tumor deposition (Figure 20-5). From a prognostic and therapeutic standpoint, the target nodes are those of the common iliac and para-aortic chains, so the fact that nodes in the internal iliac and parametrial regions are not opacified may be of less importance. However, most investigators agree that lymphangiography is not a sufficiently accurate basis on which to plan therapy. In the series of Lagasse et al.,[59] of 95 patients in whom operative proof was available, there were 16 lymphangiographic errors that would have led to inappropriate therapy if operative staging had not been performed. In seven of these, patients would have been overtreated; in nine, malignant nodes would have been outside the radiation portal. Similar results in other studies have led investigators to search elsewhere for a more accurate imaging procedure.

Computed tomography has proved to be a reliable method for staging and following abnormal lymph nodes in patients with lymphoma; stimulated by this success, similar staging procedures were carried out in patients with solid tumors. Certainly no other currently available procedure can image nodes in the presacral and hypogastric region in addition to the external iliac, common iliac, and para-aortic chains. The major theoretical drawback to CT, however, is that it requires enlargement to diagnose nodal disease; subtle architectural changes, which are visible on lymphangiograms, will go unnoticed on CT scans.

Several studies have borne out the importance of this latter fact. Grumbine et al.[38] reported a series in which CT detected none of six surgically positive lymph nodes; all were less than 2 cm in greatest dimension. Similar problems with reduced sensitivity plague most authors, e.g., Walsh and Goplerud[97] (70%), Whitley et al.[102] (80%), and Kilcheski et al.[55] (70%).

Ginaldi et al.[36] attempted to use CT and lymphangiography as complementary studies in 24 patients. In this

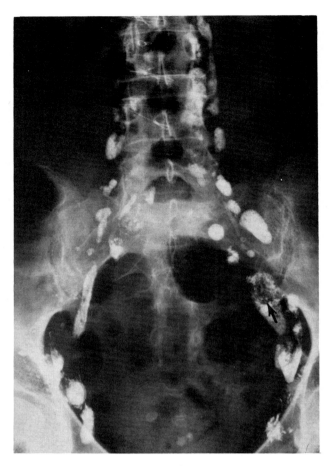

FIG. 20-5. Lymphangiographic demonstration of metastic cervical carcinoma. Peripheral filling defect within an opacified lymph node in the external iliac chain proved to be metastatic epidermoid carcinoma.

group, CT added information in 10 cases; in only one patient did this information affect therapy. In addition, CT failed to detect lymphangiographically positive nodes in 3 of 17 patients (sensitivity, 82%). The kind of information contributed by computed tomography was better definition of overall disease extent, and CT was thus much more useful in high-stage disease. Since no effective treatment regimen has been developed for widespread disease, this information seldom produces a change in therapy.

Fine-Needle Aspiration Biopsy. An adjunctive technique that should reduce the incidence of falsely positive diagnoses by any method is percutaneous fine-needle aspiration biopsy.[31,46,105] Suspicious nodes that are identified by lymphangiography can be approached under fluoroscopic or CT guidance and the needle tip directed into the suspicious area of an opacified node. The success rate in retrieving diagnostic material varies among institutions, but is as high as 95%. The specific accuracy for solid epithelial tumors approaches 85%. This technique thus should refine the ability of CT or lymphangiography

to predict disease extent. Unfortunately, a node must be identified as being suspicious before an aspiration biopsy will be performed. Therefore, the critical problem with either CT or lymphangiography is its low sensitivity.

Surgical experience suggests that extraperitoneal lymph node dissection has fewer complications, particularly when associated with radiation therapy, than the transperitoneal approach. When assessment of lymph node status is necessary, many centers rely on operative staging rather than any radiologic technique.

Metastatic Survey. In patients who died of advanced cervical carcinoma, autopsy studies have shown the lungs to be involved in 25%, the liver in 18%, and the skeletal system in 16%.[15] The appearance of metastatic epidermoid carcinoma in the pulmonary system resembles that of most hematogenous metastases: multiple, spherical nodules of varying sizes that may occupy any segment but are most prevalent in the lung bases. Cavitation is occasionally observed in epidermoid cancers.

In patients with clinically high-stage tumors and abnormalities in alkaline phosphatase levels, screening examination of the liver is warranted. Radionuclide (technetium sulfur colloid) liver/spleen imaging has a sensitivity of approximately 85%. The most sensitive method for detecting intrahepatic metastases is computed tomography, which can detect lesions as small as 0.5 cm. Ultrasonography has an intermediate sensitivity and specificity.[8]

Radionuclide skeletal imaging is exceptionally sensitive in detecting bone lesions from metastatic disease. This method is, however, quite nonspecific. Bones involved by trauma or Paget's disease may produce images identical to those of metastases. When the pattern of skeletal involvement is not a classic one for metastatic disease, plain roentgenography or computed tomography may be useful in confirming the presence of bone destruction.[72] In equivocal cases, needle biopsy should be performed to confirm the presence of a metastatic deposit. Some interesting reports by Fisher[32] and Rubin and Prabasawat[84] describe a characteristic pattern in bony metastases from carcinoma of the cervix. Bony destruction of the left side of low thoracic or high lumbar vertebral bodies was present in seven of eight patients with skeletal metastases from cervical carcinoma.

A review of commonly employed diagnostic methods was recently reported by Cooper et al.;[18] chest roentgenograms and intravenous pyelograms were obtained in nearly all patients in the responding institutions. Barium enemas were performed in roughly half of the preoperative patients, while liver/spleen scans, bone scans, skeletal surveys, and lymphangiograms were performed only in selected cases. The authors point out that the 50% to 60% incidence of lymph node metastases in stage III patients cannot be detected on lymphangiograms performed in only 18% of cases. These data were accumulated before computed tomography gained wide clinical acceptance, and thus no information on the referral pattern for CT in patients with carcinoma of the cervix is available.

Imaging Strategies and Decisions

For all patients, clinical examination under anesthesia, with careful bimanual assessment of the cervix, vagina, and parametrial areas, in addition to the rectovaginal septum and the sidewalls of the pelvis for nodes remains the standard approach to staging before decision making. Unlike cancer of the ovary, clinical staging remains the major assessment and is usually performed by a gynecologic oncologist and a radiation oncologist.

For early in situ disease, which will apply to approximately half of the patients, conization or multiple biopsies may need to be done where an abnormal Papanicolaou smear is found. The major point in the evaluation is the detection of microinvasion or occult carcinoma, and this depends upon the depth of invasion, which varies in different pathologic classifications from 1 to 5 mm. Currently, 3 mm or less is the limit applied to microinvasion.[22,23]

Occult cancers by definition are 3 mm or more below the basement membrane, and gross invasion is often seen throughout the conization specimen. For this very early invasive stage no radiologic examination other than a chest film and routine blood work would be required.

For grossly invasive cancers (stage I and II), once it has been determined by EUA that this could be either a bulky cervix or invasion into the parametrium or vagina, cystoscopy is commonly added at the time of the EUA. A barium enema is usually reserved for symptomatic patients in this stage. Routine radiography includes an intravenous pyelogram; CT and lymphangiography can be added to determine depth of invasion and presence of pelvic and para-aortic nodes. Surgical exploration and selective lymphadenectomy provide a better assessment of pelvic and para-aortic nodes. In addition, cytologic sampling from washings of the abdominal cavity is often possible and the liver can also be palpated and evaluated at the time of surgery.

For stage III and IV carcinomas, once the cancer has become extensive (as determined by EUA), cystoscopy and sigmoidoscopy are added to the studies. Computed tomographic examination is more frequently done for assessment of both primary and nodal disease. Lymphangiography increases the possibility of detecting lymph node involvements, and fine-needle evaluation is often used for verification. Surgical exploration may be used in selected cases, but more often is deferred. Supraclavicular node aspiration or biopsy should be considered for individuals who have positive para-aortic nodes, to be sure that the disease is not beyond the pelvis.

The metastatic workup as outlined should be incorporated definitively in this group of patients to determine whether or not aggressive pelvic treatment is indicated (Figure 20-6).

CERVICAL CANCER : CLINICAL / RADIOLOGIC FLOW DIAGRAM

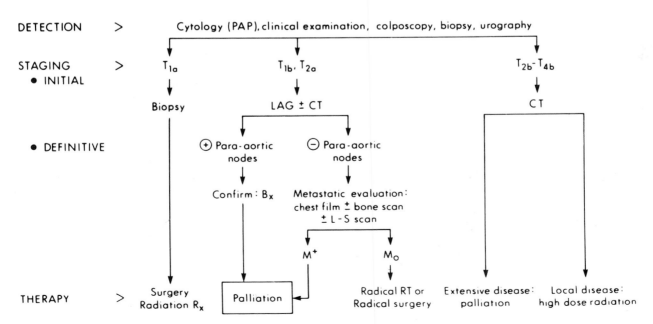

FIG. 20-6. Clinical/radiologic flow diagram. Optimal evaluation of patients with invasive cervical carcinomas depends on the clinical stage of the disease at initial examination (see text).

Treatment Decisions

Traditionally, cancer of the cervix has been managed by different techniques of radiation therapy combining internal and external sources of radiation. The surgical treatment of early stage carcinoma of the cervix has had a renaissance with regard to improved techniques and accomplishments and now yields end results comparable to that achieved with radiation (Table 20-4).[57,58] A standard hysterectomy can be done for microinvasive disease, but once the disease is frankly invasive, a radical hysterectomy should be done that encompasses the upper vagina and cardinal ligaments in addition to pelvic lymphadenectomy. Meticulous attention should be paid to the dissection of the ureters. Selective sampling of the para-aortic nodes is usually also part of this procedure. Readers are referred to standard texts for more details of combining intracavitary sources and external irradiation.[5,33,74] Generally, intracavitary irradiation is used more often during the early stages of cancer of the cervix, in contrast to the advanced stage III and IV disease. In the more difficult advanced cancers, external irradiation is used first with the hope of obtaining sufficient tumor regression so that subsequent intracavitary applications can be planned to encompass the disease more fully. Chemotherapy is mainly reserved for recurrent and disseminated disease and is seldom curative. Agents such as methotrexate, bleomycin, mitomycin C, and cisplatin give the highest response rates.

A brief summary follows according to the initial staging evaluation made by criteria established by the International Federation of Gynecology and Obstetrics, and is sufficient to place patients in one of three groups (Table 20-5).

Microinvasive Cancer. The first group comprises patients with microinvasive (T_{1a}) carcinomas. The incidence of lymphadenopathy or hematogenous metastases is very small in this group, and justifiably, most investigators proceed with standard surgical or radiotherapeutic techniques. A total hysterectomy and bilateral salpingo-oophorectomy and a wide vaginal cuff are sufficient and obviate the need for lymphadenectomy.

Localized and Early Cancer. The second group (T_{1b}, T_{2a}) comprises individuals whose local disease is surgically encompassable.[61] Radical abdominal hysterectomy is the preferred method for patients considered surgical candidates. Radiation therapy is equally curative. The radical abdominal hysterectomy method involves removal of the uterus, tubes, ovaries, parametrial tissue, upper vagina, and all accessible lymph nodes from the bifurcation of the aorta to the inguinal ligaments. Before this procedure, it is common in many institutions to obtain information regarding the status of the pelvic and para-aortic lymph nodes.[40] As previously reviewed, in low stage disease lymphangiography rather than CT is more likely to be useful in identifying suspicious nodes. If positive para-aortic nodes are present, fine-needle aspiration biopsy should be performed for confirmation. If carcinoma is retrieved, radical surgery is obviated. If lymphangiography detects no evidence of para-aortic metastases, patients should undergo a limited screening for the presence of occult metastases. For this purpose, the initial chest films serve to identify pulmonary metastases. For patients with skeletal symptoms or unexplained elevations of alkaline phosphatase levels, radionuclide bone imaging is a reasonable choice. Similarly, patients with elevated liver enzyme values can be evaluated with liver/spleen radionuclide imaging. More expensive means such as CT are more accurate but are more likely not cost effective in this low-stage group, since few T_{1b}–T_{2a} patients will have detectable metastatic disease.

Radiation therapy is highly individualized for each patient. Intracavitary applications with radioisotopic sources are usually loaded to provide certain dose rates to specially designated points in the parametrium. These applications provide very high doses to the cervix itself with rapid fall-off to tissues beyond the uterus. External irradiation gives an even dose throughout parametrium with midline shields to provide lower doses to the rectum and bladder. Attention to treatment planning details and

Table 20-4. Carcinoma of the Cervix: Survival

STAGE	NUMBER OF PATIENTS	FIVE-YEAR SURVIVAL (%)	AUTHOR (YEAR)
Surgery			
IB	116	91 (78.4)	Liu (1955)
IB	168	137 (82.7)	Christensen (1964)
IB	173	141 (81.5)	Brienschwig (1966)
IB	120	105 (87.5)	Masterson (1969)
IB	98	64 (65.5)	Blakley (1969)
IB + IIA	165	119 (72.1)	Liu
IB + IIA	219	168 (77)	Christ
IB + IIA	308	231 (76)	Brienschwig
IB + IIA	150	124 (82.7)	Masterson
IB + IIA	161	96 (59.6)	Blakley
Radiotherapy			
I	101	87 (86.4)	Wall (1966)
I	194	152 (78.0)	Muirhead (1968)
I	183	123 (67.2)	Blakley (1969)
IB	611	547 (89.5)	Kottmeir (1964)
IB	45	37 (81.4)	Kline (1969)
IB	549	Actu. (91.5)	Fletcher (1971)
IB	348	249 (71.6)	Dickson (1972)
IB + IIA	1576	1244 (78.9)	Wall
IB + IIA	64	47 (70.5)	Kline
IB + IIA	973	Actu. (83.5)	Fletcher
IB + IIA	983	589 (60.0)	Dickson

Reprinted from Cavanagh, D., Praphat, H., Ruffolo, E. H.: Carcinoma of the uterine cervix: Some current views. *Obstet. Gynecol. Annu.* 10:193–236, 1981.

Table 20-5. Treatment Decisions: Cervix

STAGE	SURGERY	RADIATION THERAPY		CHEMOTHERAPY
IA (T_{1a},N_0) microinvasive	Standard hysterectomy	Intracavitary RT mainly Pt. A: 7000 cGy; Pt. B: 5000 cGy		NR
IB* invasive (T_{1b},N_0) II A,B ($T_{2a,b}$,N_0)	Radical hysterectomy plus Pelvic node dissection extrafascial	Combined intracavitary and external RT Pt. A: 7500 cGy; Pt. B: 5500 cGy		NR
III A,B (T_3,N_1,M_0) IV (T_4,N_0,M_0)	NR Exteneration for central locations	Combined external, intracavitary and vaginal RT Pt. A: 8000 cGy, Pt. B: 6000 cGy	and	Investigational chemotherapy (hydroxyurea) and radiosensitizers (misonidazole)
IV (T_{any},$N_4$$M_0$)	NR	Combined external and intracavitary and vaginal and para-aortic RT Para-aortic dose: 4500–5000 cGy	and/or	Investigational chemotherapy (hydroxyurea) and radiosensitizers (misonidazole)
IV (T_{any},N_{any},M_+) Metastatic	NR	Palliative RT		MAC

*Bulky and barrel-shaped cervix, stages I, IIA—preoperative irradiation and radical hysterectomy
NR = not recommended
RT = radiation therapy
MAC = multiagent chemotherapy

three-dimensional reconstruction with computerized iso-dose curves has refined radiation delivery and lowered radiation complications.

For bulky or barrel-shaped tumors (T_{1b}), preoperative irradiation and surgery are combined because of the increased incidence of central recurrence and have provided improved results to date without adding significantly to complications.

Parametrial Extensions. The third group comprises patients with parametrial extension (T_{2b}), advanced local disease (T_3), or carcinoma invading viscera locally (T_{4a}) or outside the pelvis (T_{4b}). In this group, most authors recommend radiation therapy techniques mainly for T_{4a}, with extenterative surgery reserved for individuals in whom radiotherapy fails. Patients with para-aortic adenopathy may be improved by extending the radiotherapy portal to this area; this technique is under active investigation by the Radiation Therapy Oncology Group (RTOG). Since involved lymph nodes in the parametrial and pelvic regions will be included routinely, radiation boost fields to achieve high doses require exact determination and mapping of lymph node status to reduce bowel dose to minimum volume. As pointed out by the study of Ginaldi et al.[36] CT added information about the overall extent of disease in 10 of 24 cases. Thus, CT is useful in modifying treatment portals or in identify-

ing patients with systemic disease in whom local therapy is inappropriate.

Recurrent Cases. There is as yet limited information regarding the utility of imaging methods in detecting disease that recurs after therapy. After either radiotherapy or surgery, clinical examination may be difficult and errors in estimating disease extent are frequent. The prognosis in this group of patients is dismal, as reflected by a one-year survival of 15% and a three-year survival of 6%.[95] Early detection of the recurrence is one hope for improving this grim statistic. In the report of Walsh et al.[96] on 33 patients, CT was accurate in predicting recurrence in 82% and had a sensitivity of 93%. The main advantage of CT is its ability to display the total extent of both central and distant tumor and to provide an objective means to evaluate response to therapy (Figure 20-7). Its major disadvantage is its inability to distinguish reliably between radiation fibrosis and recurrent tumor. An assessment of the effectiveness and impact of CT on patient survival awaits further investigation.

Impact of New Technology

The major problem in current imaging techniques is the inability of any radiographic method to detect microscopic foci of metastatic epidermoid carcinoma. It is doubtful that magnetic resonance imaging (MRI) will

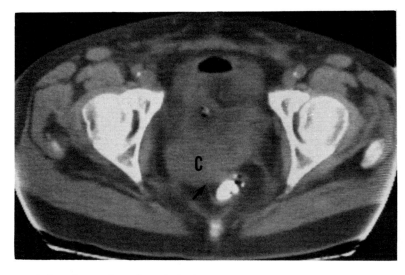

FIG. 20-7. Recurrent cervical carcinoma. Scan through the lower pelvis demonstrates recurrent cervical carcinoma (C) with invasion of the rectum (arrow). Thickening of the soft tissue surrounding the rectum is caused by previous radiation therapy.

contribute significantly to the solution of this problem, since at the moment its spatial resolution is similar to that of CT. However, MRI may be reliable in showing parametrial invasion. Many centers are now investigating radionuclide agents containing antibodies specific to a given tumor antigen. It is feasible but not yet proven that systemic or lymphatic injection of such substances might provide a sensitive means for staging primary disease as well as evaluating recurrence. Time will tell.

OVARY

Ovarian carcinoma is the name applied to a heterogeneous group of neoplasms having in common only their anatomic site of origin. As a group, they represent the most lethal gynecologic neoplasm: the overall five-year survival for the 18,300 women who will be diagnosed this year is in the range of 30% to 35%. Eleven thousand five hundred women were predicted to die of ovarian carcinoma in 1984.[87]

No age group is spared: stromal and sex cord tumors are common in young women, especially the premenarchal ages; epithelial tumors predominate in later decades.[53] Early pregnancy may be protective, and nulliparous women have a greater incidence of developing ovarian malignancies than parous women.[6] There is a geographic/social distribution: Scandinavian, Swiss, and North American women have a high incidence of the disease, whereas it is rare in Latin America.[6] Interestingly, reports from the 19th century rarely mention the diagnosis of ovarian neoplasm, despite the fact that ovariotomies have been performed since 1809. It is possible that ovarian neoplasms are a 20th century problem, re-

lated to carcinogenic agents linked in some way to our industrial society.[69]

In all patients, clinical symptoms occur relatively late in the course of the disease, and no successful solution to the problem of early detection of ovarian carcinoma has been offered. Today, 70% of all patients with ovarian carcinoma have advanced disease at initial examination.[13] Reduction in mortality from ovarian carcinoma thus is more likely to ensue from methods providing early detection than from improved treatment means. Unfortunately, no screening mechanism currently exists.

Tumor Behavior and Pathology

Epithelial Neoplasms. Eighty-five percent of ovarian carcinomas take origin in the celomic epithelial cells.[64,65,69] A mechanism postulated in the development of epithelial carcinoma is metaplasia within the lining of epithelial inclusion cysts, leading eventually to neoplastic proliferation.[66] The epithelial lining of such inclusion cysts has the capacity to recapitulate all müllerian histologic patterns; thus, four major histologic types may be observed.

Serous tumors resemble the ciliated columnar cells found in the fallopian tubes. Extensive papillary cellular architecture is characteristic of this tumor; psammomatous calcification occurs in one third. This cell type accounts for 50% of the malignant epithelial forms. The tumor tends to grow rapidly, especially within the peritoneal cavity. Overall, the five-year survival is approximately 25%.

Endometrioid tumors may be strikingly similar to (often histologically identical with) adenocarcinomas of the endometrium. Indeed, a coexistent carcinoma of the endometrium is present in 15% to 30% of patients. This type accounts for 15% of all cases of epithelial invasive cancer. Since it requires a fair degree of cellular differentiation to be recognized as endometrioid, its growth rate is somewhat slower than that of serous carcinoma, and the five-year survival approaches 50%.

Mucinous tumors also account for 15% of ovarian epithelial cancers. Its cells resemble those of the endocervical canal or even the colon, and elevated serum levels of carcinoembryonic antigen (CEA) may be present in these patients. These tumors are better differentiated and more likely to be confined to the ovary than serous malignancies. The five-year survival, accordingly, approaches 50% for patients with these tumors.

Mesonephroid tumors possess a cellular architecture similar to clear cell carcinomas of the kidney or adenocarcinomas induced by diethylstilbestrol. Approximately 5% of ovarian cancers are of this type. Survival in this group is also close to 50%.

Fifteen percent of ovarian malignant tumors are not sufficiently differentiated to be classified by cell type. As would be expected, patients with these tumors have a poor five-year survival.[26]

A histologic grade may be assigned to any of the four major subtypes of epithelial carcinoma to describe its degree of differentiation. Most institutions use a three-grade (well, moderately, poor) system for such description.

Germ Cell Neoplasms. A wide variety of malignant neoplasms arise from the germinal cells. Dysgerminomas account for 1% to 2% of ovarian neoplasms and are most frequent in the second and third decades of life. The tumor is bilateral in 10% of cases. In addition to potential for spread through the peritoneal cavity, it has a strong predilection for lymphatic permeation. It is now accepted that these tumors take origin in primitive germ cells.[66]

The prognosis for this type of tumor is good if it is confined to a single ovary; the presence of other cellular types, such as choriocarcinoma or gonadoblastoma, worsens the prognosis. Embryonal carcinomas (endodermal sinus tumors, yolk sac tumors) likewise occur almost exclusively in children and young women. The tumor often histologically resembles placental tissue and may have trophoblastic differentiation, in which case chorionic gonadotropin levels may be detectable in the serum.

Choriocarcinoma rarely occurs in pure form; more often, it is part of a mixed germ cell tumor. While some cases of remission have been reported, it is a more lethal tumor than gestational choriocarcinoma, possibly because the fetal tissue present in the latter incites a more intense immunologic response. Gonadoblastomas are actually benign but have a marked propensity to be associated with dysgerminomas. They occur almost exclusively in patients with gonadal dysgenesis.

Stromal tumors are fascinating entities from the standpoint of the variety of endocrine substances they produce. Since they have relatively low malignant potential[26] and are exceptionally rare, they are less important from the standpoint of oncologic staging decisions and will not be further discussed.

Patterns of Spread. Carcinomas of the ovary can involve extraovarian structures in a wide variety of ways, some of which are clinically more important than others. As is the case with all invasive neoplasms, the potential exists for local spread into anatomic structures contiguous to the ovary. Organs at particular risk include the ipsilateral fallopian tube, the uterus and broad ligament, the rectum, sigmoid and perirectal fat, and the lateral pelvic wall (obturator internus muscle). In addition to direct extension, ovarian tumors have a marked tendency to shed cells into the peritoneal cavity and thus disseminate the neoplasm throughout the peritonealized surfaces of the abdomen and pelvis. Thus, the retrouterine pouch (of Douglas), which is the most dependent portion of the peritoneal cavity, is particularly at risk. Other commonly involved areas are the sigmoid colon, the small bowel mesentery, the right lateral colonic "gutter," and the omentum.

As many investigators have observed, the whole peritoneum is at risk when any portion is involved; there is a circulation of peritoneal fluid throughout the entire peritoneal space. The lymphatics of the diaphragm apparently function as a "blotter" for peritoneal fluid, and thus the diaphragm lymphatics are likely sites for peritoneally implanted tumors. In fact, the probable mechanism for the occurrence of ascites in these patients is obstruction of the diaphragmatic lymphatics by tumor implants.[65,66] The anterior surface of the right hemidiaphragm adjacent to the liver is particularly at risk.

Investigators have long postulated that the peritoneal cavity may be at risk for disseminated ovarian neoplasms for a reason other than seeding and subsequent implantation by malignant cells shed into peritoneal fluid.[66] The mesothelial cells of the peritoneum itself retain a pluripotency, and extragonadal müllerian-type tumors may develop directly from the peritoneum. It is attractive to postulate that the same etiologic influences (as yet undefined) that produce malignant change in ovarian epithelium may produce identical changes in peritoneal mesothelium. This remains a theoretical speculation.

The influence of peritoneal spread on survival is undeniable. In one series of stage I, grade 1 tumors,[28] the five-year survival was 90% in patients with totally intracystic disease, 68% when an extracystic excrescence was present, and 56% if the cyst had ruptured.

Lymphatic spread is being recognized as an important prognostic factor in predicting patient outcome. The collecting trunks draining the ovary form a dense plexus in and around the ovarian hilus.[83] From there they ascend with the gonadal vein along the anterior margin of the psoas muscle, then turn medially to cross the ureter. On the right side, the trunks enter precaval and laterocaval nodes at varying levels, stretching from the aortic bifurcation to the renal hilus. On the left, the trunks do not diverge from each other as extensively and terminate in nodes above and below the left renal vein. An accessory pedicle has been described that traverses the broad ligament and terminates laterally in the middle chain of the external iliac group.

For years, it had been considered axiomatic that para-aortic nodal involvement without pelvic nodal disease was more common than pelvic disease without aortic involvement. This would follow logically from the anatomy of lymph node drainage described above. Thus, in a study by Athey et al.[2] 14 of 33 (42%) patients had para-aortic adenopathy only, while 4 of 33 (12%) patients had iliac adenopathy alone. Castellino and Marglin[14] quote Musumeci, however, who reported a series of 365 patients studied with lymphangiography and noted metastases confined to iliac nodes in 27.6%, while the para-aortics were the only site of involvement in 15.5%. These data at least suggest that the lymphatic drainage of the ovary is highly variable and that it is important to assess drainage to both para-aortic and pelvic sites.

Recent information also underscores the importance of lymphatic drainage in apparently low-stage disease. Abnormal para-aortic nodes were found in 10.3% of 58 stage I and 10% of 10 stage II patients reported by Novak et al.[69] This is similar to information by other investigators based on staging laparotomy;[26] a constant 10% to 15% rate of periaortic or pelvic adenopathy is present in clinically low stage disease. In one small series, only those patients with para-aortic nodal metastases had relapsed during the study interval.

Hematogenous spread occurs late in the course of ovarian carcinoma. Clinically, fewer than 1% of all patients with ovarian cancer have liver metastases at initial examination. Other sites such as the skin and lungs may be involved in advanced disease. Autopsy studies demonstrate liver metastases in 34%, lung metastases in 27% and bony lesions in 14% of patients dying of disseminated carcinoma.[26]

Dysgerminomas tend to behave in a similar fashion to seminomas in men, that is, it is not unusual to observe bulky metastatic deposits in the region of the left renal hilum without metastatic disease in the pelvis or lower retroperitoneal nodes. Similarly, nodes in the anterior mediastinum may be involved while abdominal disease is inapparent. Involvement of such nodes does not confer a dismal prognosis, since both the primary and the metastatic tumor are exquisitely radiosensitive.[69]

In summary, ovarian carcinomas have a propensity to spread widely throughout the peritoneal cavity and often involve the retroperitoneum as well; thus the entire abdomen is at risk even in clinically well-localized disease.

Classification and Staging

Clinicians have adopted the staging system of the International Federation of Gynecology Oncology (FIGO) for epithelial carcinomas of the ovary. Each FIGO stage corresponds closely to a T stage in the TNM system (Figure 20-8, Table 20-6). Thus stage I (T_1) cancer includes all cases in which the neoplasm is limited to the ovaries. If only one ovary is involved, it is classed as IA (T_{1a}); if both ovaries have tumors it is classed as IB. A IC classification is applied if the surgeon detects ascites or if there is cytologic evidence of positive peritoneal washing in a tumor that would otherwise be classified as IA or IB.

In stage II disease, there is local pelvic extension, either to the uterus (IIA) or fallopian tubes (IIB). Again, IIC indicates a tumor that would have been classed as IIA or IIB but for the presence of ascites or positive peritoneal washings. Stage III represents advanced disease without distant metastasis. A tumor will be placed in this category if it (1) involves retroperitoneal lymph nodes, (2) has intraperitoneal metastases outside of the true pelvis, or (3) has invaded the omentum or small bowel (even if contained within the true pelvis). Stage IV (M_+ tumors have spread hematogenously (or by lymphatics to extra-abdominal sites) (Figure 20-8).

It is worth mentioning that patients who are assumed to have ovarian cancer but in whom exploration is not performed are reported in a separate category for the purpose of therapeutic survival statistics. Staging does include the histologic and cytologic material retrieved at exploration. Ulfelder[94] cites the recent FIGO report of treatment results in 4,892 patients treated at 45 institutions (Table 20-7). This report supports the utility of the stage grouping because lower stage implies prolonged survival. As Ulfelder points out, refinement in surgical technique will assign more apparent stage I tumors to a stage III category as a more careful search is made at laparotomy for subdiaphragmatic implants and peritoneal lymph nodes. Thus, the number of cases having "true" stage I disease will be smaller and their survival better, as more patients are discovered to have advanced disease. This, in turn, will allow more refined analysis of therapeutic trials in all stages.

The percentage of patients with lymphadenopathy likewise increases by stage. In the series of Marglin and Castellino[63] of patients undergoing lymphadenectomy, 12.8% of stage I patients and 11.8% of stage II patients had retroperitoneal lymph nodes positive for tumor. As the tumor became more advanced, lymphadenopathy increased precipitously, 31% in stage III and 60% in stage

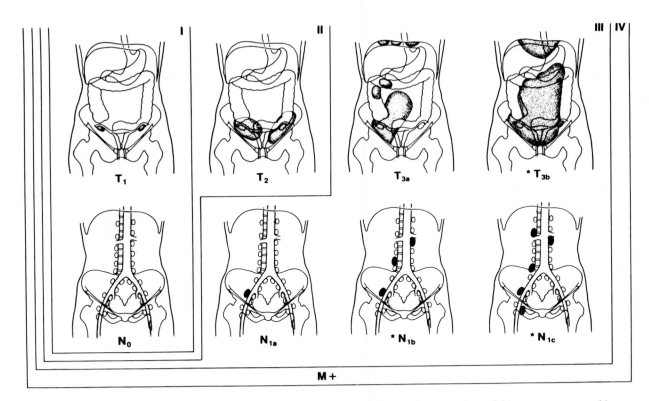

FIG. 20-8. Anatomic staging for ovarian cancer. Tumor (T) categories: The peculiar extensions of this cancer are caused by shedding of cells and developing seedlings into the peritoneal cavity, progressively from the pelvis (T_2) to the abdomen, limited by the diaphragm (T_3). Spread beyond the diaphragm is stage IV. To be favorable, the largest nodule of residual disease should be less than 1 cm. Node (N) categories: This refers only to N_1, positive regional nodes, which are pelvic, although it also can apply to retroperitoneal nodes. N_{1a} is pelvic nodes; N_{1b} is para-aortic nodes below the renal artery; N_{1c} is high para-aortic nodes. Stage grouping: The stage corresponds to the first three T categories. Nodes are not considered. Metastases in the lower peritoneal cavity and beyond indicate stage IV. N_1 is equivalent to T_3 or stage III disease. FIGO v UICC v AJC classifications: There is concurrence among these systems. FIGO has provided the guidelines for stage grouping and the AJC and UICC have translated them into T categories. Wherever T categories determine stage, there is good agreement. The N categories need to be more fully integrated and defined. (AHC has only an N_1 category and UICC adds N_4 for regional and juxtaregional nodal involvement). FIGO = International Federation of Gynecology and Obstetrics. UICC = International Union Against Cancer. AJC = American Joint Committee. (Modified from Beecham, J. B., Helmkamp, B. F., Rubin, P.: Tumors of the female reproductive organs. In *Clinical Oncology for Medical Students and Physicians: A Multidisciplinary Approach*, 6th ed. Rubin, P. (Ed.). New York, American Cancer Society, 1983, pp. 428–481. With permission.)

Table 20-6. Comparison of FIGO and TNM Staging Systems: Carcinoma of the Ovary

FIGO		TNM
IA	Neoplasm limited to one ovary.	T_{1a}
IB	Neoplasm limited to both ovaries.	T_{1b}
IC	Positive peritoneal washings.	T_{1c}
IIA	Local extension to the uterus or to the fallopian tubes.	T_{2a}
IIB	Local extension to other pelvic tissue.	T_{2b}
IIC	Positive peritoneal washings; tumor otherwise would be classed as T_{2a}, T_{2b}	T_{2c}
III	Advanced disease but no distant metastases. May involve retroperitoneal nodes, peritoneal seeding outside true pelvis, omentum/small bowel.	T_3 T_{1-3}, N_+
IV	Widespread metastases.	T_{1-3}, M_+

Table 20-7. Treatment Results by Stage: Cancer of the Ovary

STAGE	FIVE-YEAR SURVIVAL (%)
IA	72.0
IB	62.5
IC	57.4
IIA	52.2
IIB + IIC	37.5
III	10.8
IV	4.6

Reprinted from Ulfelder, H.: Classification systems. *Int. J. Radiat. Oncol. Biol. Phys.* 7:1083–1086, 1981. With permission.

IV. As has been mentioned, there is a positive correlation between lymphadenopathy and cancer recurrence regardless of therapy.

As pointed out by Ozols et al.,[71] there is a definite influence of tumor grade (degree of cellular differentiation) on response to therapy and ultimate patient survival. This influence is most marked in low (I and II) stage tumors.

Imaging Procedures and Assessment

Physical Examination and Laparotomy. Because of the difficulty of arriving at a final stage classification by non-operative means, FIGO has recommended that staging of ovarian cancer include findings of both physical examination and laparotomy. It has been estimated that 25% of patients with ovarian malignancies seek medical attention from physicians who are not gynecologists because of vague or even misleading symptomatology.[103] The initial evaluation thus may be directed toward the alimentary or urinary tract before the exact focus of the disease is discovered. All physicians, radiologists included, should make a special effort to consider the possibility of ovarian neoplasm in perimenopausal or postmenopausal women whom they are examining for any indication (Figure 20-9). Thus, a mass effect on the dome of the bladder seen on a urogram may be a vital clue to the presence of a pelvic mass, which may then be further evaluated.

Once a tumor of the ovary is discovered, the preoperative workup should be individualized. Essentially all patients but the medically unsuitable will undergo laparotomy, and expensive radiologic examinations designed to image the exact extent of tumor spread preoperatively yield little additional information useful to the surgeon.

IVP and Barium Enema. Intravenous urography provides general information regarding the status of the urinary tract, including the presence or absence of ureteral obstruction by the pelvic mass. Information about local spread of disease may be obtained from barium examination of the colon. In the series of Severini et al.,[86] 81 patients with ovarian carcinomas were evaluated with air-contrast enemas. Radiologic signs indicative of serosal involvement included flattening, fixation, and spiculation of colonic fields or nodular intramural filling defects. The study correctly identified colonic involvement by tumor in 9 of 21 patients referred for initial staging. In no case, however, did it change the clinical stage. In most centers, barium examinations are obtained to detect coexisting colonic disease, such as carcinoma or diverticulitis, as well as to detect direct tumor invasion.

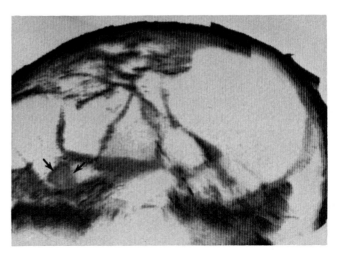

FIG. 20-9. Ultrasound examination performed on a woman clinically believed to have ascites demonstrated a large, chiefly cystic multiseptated mass in which several solid elements (arrows) were found. This appearance is typical for an ovarian cystadenocarcinoma.

Laparotomy versus Lymphangiography. At our institution, as at many others, all patients suspected of having ovarian carcinomas will undergo surgical evaluation. At this time, careful evaluation by inspection and cytologic assessment will be performed to detect small peritoneal or retroperitoneal metastases. An effort is made to remove all disease that can be surgically resected, since the literature strongly supports the contention that patient response and survival are vastly improved when no appreciable disease remains after surgery (Table 20-8).[11,30,49,60,85,88,93] Thus, preoperative staging to identify the exact extent of disease is not particularly useful in our center since it does not modify operative treatment.

In high stage disease, the dominant factor determining patient outcome is generally the total volume of intraperitoneal spread; however, in apparent stage I and stage

Table 20-8. Five-Year Survival by Stage

STAGE	FIVE-YEAR SURVIVAL (%)
Tumor resected	
Stage I	63.0
II	54.0
III	31.0
Tumors not resected	
Stage II	18.0
III	08.0
IV	07.0

Adapted from DiSaia, P. J., Creasman, W. T.: *Clinical Gynecologic Oncology*. London, C. V. Mosby, 1981.

II tumors, there is a small group of patients in whom lymphatic metastases may be present in the absence of widespread peritoneal disease. This may not be apparent to the surgeon, since lymph node sampling is not always performed at the time of the original laparotomy; even if it is performed, a significant sampling error may be present. Thus, lymphangiography (LAG) may be advantageous, since all the nodal groups at risk are routinely opacified by the technique.[2] Since LAG is usually performed after surgical confirmation of ovarian neoplasms, histologic proof of its predictions is not always available. However, in the series of Musumeci et al.[67] of 365 patients, the sensitivity of LAG was 80.5%, the specificity was 100%, and the overall accuracy was 91.7%.

Computed Tomography versus Ultrasonography.

Computed tomography has been used to assess retroperitoneal adenopathy in a wide variety of tumors; it is most efficacious in the staging of lymphomas. In the series of Whitley et al.,[101] CT predicted adenopathy in four patients, but histologic material was obtained in only one. Thirteen negative CT assessments were confirmed and there were no false-negative interpretations. Overall, in most centers, there would appear to be at best limited utility for preoperative CT staging of epithelial cancers.[89]

An exception to this is evaluation of dysgerminoma. This tumor resembles testicular seminoma in its propensity for lymphatic invasion as well as in its radiosensitivity.

Omental involvement is difficult to detect by CT[101] but as omental cakes enlarge and become fixed to the anterior abdominal wall they are more readily detected. Ultrasonography may be superior to CT, since it can distinguished solid tumor from ascitic fluid. Both methods can readily detect ascites. Computed tomography or ultrasonography of the abdomen, if used to detect retroperitoneal nodes, can also be used to assess the liver and diaphragm for metastatic involvement simultaneously.

Approximately 10% of dysgerminomas are bilateral when discovered. The prognosis for this tumor is good as long as adequate radiation therapy is given. Afridi et al.[1] report 92% survival; 70% of patients treated for recurrent disease had remissions and were clinically free of disease. Since dysgerminomas involve renal hilar nodes and often high abdominal and mediastinal nodes, lymphangiography alone is insufficient for diagnostic assessment (Figure 20-10). In patients with dysgerminomas, CT scans of the mediastinum and upper abdomen are recommended in all patients.

Metastatic Survey.

Routine screening for hematogenous metastases to the liver is not warranted unless liver function abnormalities are present.

Chest Films.

Further routine preoperative study includes chest roentgenography. In view of the low prevalence

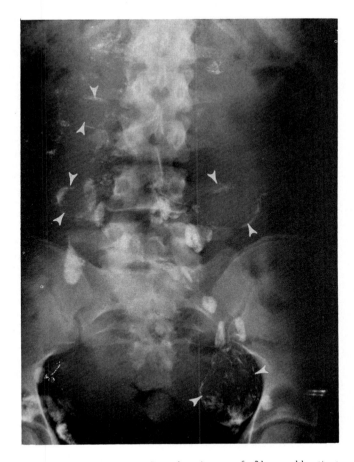

FIG. 20-10. Dysgerminoma. Lymphangiogram of a 31-year-old patient with a dysgerminoma demonstrates multiple enlarged and tumor-replaced lymph nodes in the periaortic, paracaval, and external iliac distribution (arrowheads).

of metastatic disease to the lungs at the time of initial examination, this study is a sufficiently sensitive screen for pleural or parenchymal metastases; in epithelial ovarian carcinoma, thoracic computed tomography is not cost-effective. Table 20-9 indicates the relative cost/benefit correlations between different imaging methods.

Follow-Up Imaging.

A major role that imaging techniques may play in the assessment of patients with ovarian carcinomas is sequential follow-up. Two separate areas of investigation in treated patients include (1) evaluation of patients suspected of recurrent disease, and (2) linear assessment of patient response to chemotherapy or radiotherapy. In our institution, as in most others, the majority of patients studied radiographically for ovarian carcinomas fall into one of these categories. Chemotherapy with alkylating agents has been moderately successful in inducing remissions in patients with ovarian carcinomas. However, continued use of such agents results in an increased incidence of hematologic malignancies,

Table 20-9. Imaging Methods for Evaluating Ovarian Carcinoma

METHOD	CAPABILITY	COST/ BENEFIT	RECOMMENDATION FOR USE
Noninvasive			
Chest radiography	Detects soft tissue nodules greater than 15 mm. Detects acute/chronic lung disease.	Low High	Routine
Sonography			
Primary tumor	May detect unsuspected tumor. Displays overall bulk of primary tumor in pelvis/abdomen. Sensitive to ascites but not small peritoneal implants.	Moderate	Postoperative follow-up Evaluation of suspected ovarian mass
Liver	Detects metastatic deposits greater than 15 mm.	Low	Not routine. Only in patients with high-stage disease.
Barium enema	Detects coincident colon tumor. Detects peritoneal spread of tumor.	Moderate	Routine
MRI	Not yet investigated.	Unknown	Unknown
Minimally invasive			
Urography	Detects ureteral obstruction, bladder invasion. Screens for unsuspected renal disease.	Moderate	Routine
CT	Detects liver metastases greater than 10 mm to ascites and moderate-sized implants. Detects pelvic masses greater than 20 mm in size.	High	Following patients on chemotherapy
Invasive			
Lymphangiography	Detects abnormal lymph node architecture.	Moderate	Not routine
Biopsy	Confirms lesions detected by ultrasound, CT.	High	Patients with suspicious lesions

particularly acute myelogenous leukemia. For this reason, most oncologists perform "second-look" operations on patients clinically free of disease after one year of chemotherapy.[80,90] Since there is some morbidity associated with this operative procedure, noninvasive methods have been evaluated to determine if they can accurately establish the presence or absence of persistent disease.

Computed Tomography. Whitley et al.[101] reported their experience using CT in following patients with known ovarian carcinomas (Figure 20-11). They concluded that CT was 100% accurate in predicting ascites, but missed small (≤ 1 cm or less) tumor nodules within the peritoneum. Thus a 64% sensitivity for peritoneal implants and a 67% sensitivity for omental metastases was reported. Similarly, Walsh and Amendola found CT to be an accurate means of gauging the response of bulky tumors to therapeutic agents, but likewise lamented its insensitivity to peritoneal implants less than 2 cm in diameter (Figure 20-12).[96] Johnson et al.[49] assessed CT in comparison with clinical examination in treated patients and found it to be superior (Figure 20-13). In some cases, it was able to sufficiently demonstrate diffuse disease and thus obviated the need for second-look procedures.

Ultrasonography. Ultrasonography (US) likewise has been used to assess candidacy for reoperation.[20,79,99] Pussell et al.[79] used abdominal ultrasonography in 26 stage III or IV patients who were clinically suitable for reoperation. Ultrasonography was 84% accurate in detecting residual pelvic tumors and 92% accurate in detecting liver and right hemidiaphragmatic metastases. However, unless ascites was present, it was only 36% accurate in detecting peritoneal metastases.

Several investigators have reported an 11% to 17% incidence of lymph node metastases as the only manifestation of recurrent ovarian carcinoma. It thus may be useful to perform lymphangiography or CT on patients clinically free of disease. The relative merits of each study have been reviewed earlier in the section on initial staging. Since we recommend CT on all patients thought to be candidates for second-look operations, and since the sensitivity and accuracy of CT and lymphangiography are approximately comparable, we do not recommend lymphangiography for this group.

The accuracy of noninvasive imaging procedures, including those discussed above, can be enhanced significantly by routine use of percutaneous fine-needle aspiration biopsy to evaluate suspicious lesions.[27,31,46,105]

Imaging Strategies and Decisions

Resectable Disease. Although there are many recommended radiologic imaging procedures, none of them provides the accuracy required for staging and decision making (Figure 20-14). In addition to a regular physical

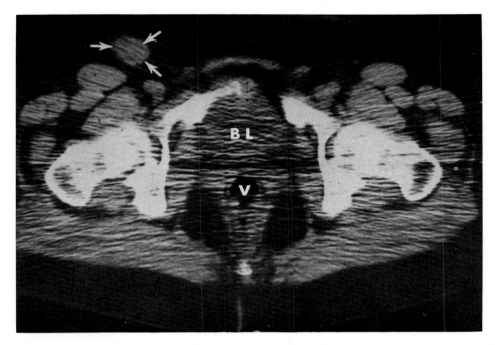

FIG. 20-11. A CT scan through the symphysis publis demonstrates a rounded soft tissue mass within the inguinal canal (arrows). This proved to be metastatic carcinoma from an ovarian primary.

examination of the breasts, abdomen, and pelvis and routine laboratory studies, ultrasound scans and computed tomography of the pelvis are the most widely used in practice. Lymphangiography is used in selected cases, particularly for dysgerminomas. Many other imaging procedures are done, including upper gastrointestinal examination, small bowel follow through, and barium enema, particularly if there are vague, ill-defined abdominal and pelvic pains. But neither these studies nor the intravenous pyelogram, which can be done if the BUN is high, are considered to be part of the standard staging evaluation.

A number of invasive procedures can be done short of laparotomy, and include paracentesis, or thoracocentesis if ascites and pleural effusion are present; such fluid should be sent *in toto* to the cytologic laboratory for evaluation. Laparoscopy and biopsy of suspicious areas have been useful, but are not substitutes for laparotomy.

Unlike most cancers, clinical staging has a very limited value in ovarian cancer. Accordingly, the AJC and UICC recommend this disease be surgically staged; all of the pelvic contents and entire abdominal and peritoneal surfaces need meticulous inspection, including the diaphragmatic nodes, liver, spleen, intestines, mesentery, paracolic gutters, and pelvis. Careful sampling of the periaortic and pelvic lymph nodes is also recommended. Adhesions, any suspicious granularity, any nodularity, and the omentum are frequently included in the staging process. Details of the diagnostic and therapeutic components of the pri-

mary and reassessment surgery for ovarian cancers are shown in Table 20-10. Washings of the peritoneal cavity should always be included as a terminal event and the fluid sent for cytologic evaluation to determine if there are any malignant cells.

Unresectable Disease. Ovarian cancer most often appears as advanced metastatic pelvic and abdominal disease. Even thoracic spread does not in and of itself contradict the need for the same imaging procedures and assessment of the abdominal cavity. Oftentimes the degree of disease in the abdomen is less bulky in stage IV than in stage III patients and the only presence of disease outside the abdomen is pleural effusion. The same tumor debulking procedures in the pelvis and abdomen can be done unless circumstances are unusual. The metastatic workup will first consist of evaluation of the chest films, liver chemistry studies, pelvic-abdominal CT scans, or ultrasonograms. Most often implants tend to be on the surface of the diaphragm or liver, protruding externally rather than spreading in a true hematogenous fashion. A second favorite site is the chest, where pleural effusion is more common than hematogenous spread throughout the lungs, as in other carcinomas. Bone metastases and bone marrow involvement are extremely uncommon in this disease, as are brain metastases. If such hematogenous spread patterns were found, they would be contradictions to laparotomy, and one would need to carefully consider whether one is dealing with a lung, breast, or

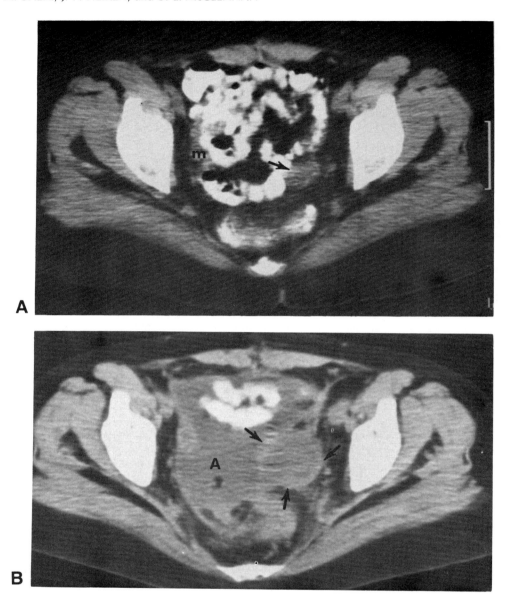

FIG. 20-12. Recurrent ovarian carcinoma. (A) A CT scan through the mid-pelvis demonstrates minimal thickening in the small bowel mesentery (m) and an oval mass (arrow) in the left lower quadrant. These findings were the only evidence of recurrent tumor. (B) Same patient, four months later. Considerable ascitic fluid (A) is now present within the pouch of Douglas. The previously described mass (arrows) is now much larger. This proved to be widespread metastatic carcinoma of the ovary.

gastrointestinal cancer that is producing a Krukenberg tumor of the ovary.

Evaluation of Response: Second Look. Surgical reassessment of second-look operations is commonly done to evaluate treatment because of the limitations of imaging procedures. Although imaging procedures may suggest no evidence of disease, it is well recognized that nodules less than 1 cm to granular deposits may not be detected either by ultrasonography or by CT. Laparoscopy is occasionally helpful when there are no adhesions,

and careful exploration can be done. If the findings are negative, a laparotomy may still be required, since it is the best means of evaluating peritoneal surfaces.

If a clinical response to chemotherapy is observed, a second-look operation is performed, the aim of which is to assess the chemotherapy and determine if there is no residual disease present. If the second-look procedure documents the absence of disease, the chemotherapy is halted and the patient observed; if disease is present but resectable, another debulking procedure is performed and an alternate program of chemotherapy restarted. In some circumstances, imaging procedures can obviate the necessity for a second operation by demonstrating extensive persistence. In addition, in patients who are not clinically responding to chemotherapy, it provides a means to document persistent disease and also suggests whether alternative therapy should be initiated.

Treatment Decisions

The approach to ovarian cancer is often multidisciplinary and includes surgery, radiation therapy, and chemotherapy. The treatment policies are based on surgical staging and the histopathologic evaluation of biopsies.

Surgery. As previously noted, careful exploration and surgical staging at laparotomy is the first step. Omentectomy should always be done, and the specimen should be divided grossly into multiple sections so that the pathologist can carefully search for microscopic disease. Biopsies from the diaphragmatic surfaces and paracolic gutters involving the pelvic peritoneum can be done in addition to selected periaortic and pelvic lymphadenectomy. Debulking surgery can be done since this is usually a lesion that spreads along the surfaces of the peritoneal cavity, and maximum site of reductive surgery allows for more effective use of radiation therapy and chemotherapy in an adjuvant fashion. Even in the most advanced stages of disease, removal of as much tumor as possible must be done to be of benefit when chemotherapy will be used.

Radiation Therapy. As a rule, external beam radiation therapy in the form of either whole abdominal irradiation or a strip field technique allows for complete coverage of the pelvic and abdominal contents. Generally, once an ovarian cancer seeds throughout the abdomen, it cannot be treated as a local regional pelvic disease and conceptually must be considered as a disease of the peritoneal cavity. Pelvic doses up to 4,500 to 5,000 cGy can be delivered safely, but the kidneys and liver need careful shielding, where the dose is usually confined to 1,500 to 2,500 cGy for routine fractional doses.[28] Radioactive isotopes such as phosphorus (^{32}P), and radioactive gold have been used in the early stages of disease. Combinations of radiation therapy and chemotherapy are mainly investigational in nature, particularly if whole abdominal irradiation techniques are used, since considerable bone marrow toxicity develops when both modes are used aggressively.

Chemotherapy. There are a variety of chemotherapeutic agents that can be used in advanced stages as well as in the adjuvant setting where minimal residual disease is left behind or there are positive washings. The alkylating agents have been the most extensively used agents and include chlorambucil and cyclophosphamide as well as L-phenylalanine mustard. Melphalan is the most widely used oral agent but has caused concern when it has been used in one-to-two-year maintenance programs because of the induction of leukemia. The commonly used com-

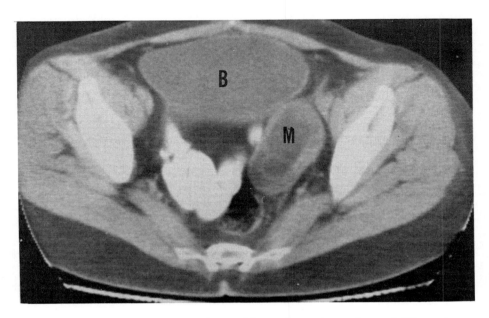

FIG. 20-13. A 65-year-old woman two years after completion of therapy for ovarian carcinoma. A CT scan demonstrates a large mass (M), with central near-water attenuation lying immediately posterior to the bladder (B). An aspiration biopsy revealed metastatic ovarian carcinoma.

A

EPITHELIAL OVARIAN CANCER

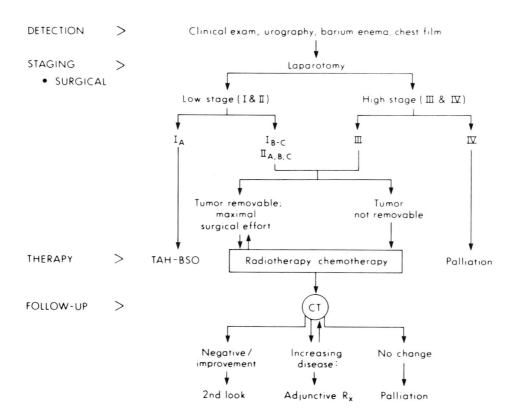

DETECTION   >   Clinical exam, urography, barium enema, chest film

STAGING   >
   • SURGICAL   Laparotomy

Low stage (I & II)   High stage (III & IV)

I$_A$ I$_{B-C}$ II$_{A,B,C}$ III   IV

Tumor removable; maximal surgical effort   Tumor not removable

THERAPY   >   TAH-BSO   Radiotherapy chemotherapy   Palliation

FOLLOW-UP   >   CT

Negative/ improvement   Increasing disease: No change

2nd look   Adjunctive R$_x$ Palliation

B

OVARIAN DYSGERMINOMA

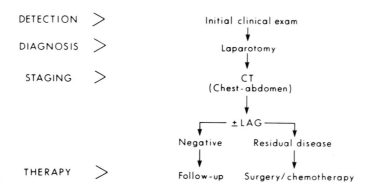

DETECTION   >   Initial clinical exam

DIAGNOSIS   >   Laparotomy

STAGING   >   CT (Chest-abdomen)

±LAG

Negative   Residual disease

THERAPY   >   Follow-up   Surgery/chemotherapy

FIG. 20-14. Radiology plays little role in the preoperative assessment of ovarian carcinoma. Patients undergoing chemotherapy may profit from serial CT examination in the monitoring of tumor response. (B) Postoperative staging of ovarian dysgerminoma includes routine chest and abdominal CT scans.

Reprinted from Beecham, J. B., Helmkamp, B. F., Rubin, P.: Tumors of the female reproductive organs. In *Clinical Oncology for Medical Students and Physicians: A Multidisciplinary Approach*, 6th ed. Rubin, P. (Ed.). New York, American Cancer Society, 1983, pp. 428–481. With permission.

Table 20-10. Diagnostic and Therapeutic Components of Primary and Reassessment Surgery for Ovarian Cancer

Diagnostic
1. Cytologic washings from both diaphragms and pelvis
2. Manual and visual exploration of all peritoneal surfaces: diaphragma, liver, spleen, stomach, small intestine and mesentery, large intestine and mesentery, paracolic gutter, pelvis, umbilicus, and both supra- and infracolic omentum
3. Retroperitoneal pelvic and para-aortic nodes (when no gross peritoneal disease is detected)
4. Multiple biopsies of diaphragmatic, colonic gutter and pelvic peritoneum, as well as any suspicious areas from #2 above
5. Laparoscopy prior to assessment surgery to document visible peritoneal disease and thereby prevent unnecessary laparotomy in cases where positive

Therapeutic
1. Removal of primary tumor in ovaries
2. Removal of other gynecologic organs (unless conservative surgery is indicated)
3. Excision of infracolic omentum from hepatic flexure to splenic flexure
4. Removal of supracolic omentum (gastrocolic) if technically and clinically indicated
5. Removal of other bulk tumor deposits
6. Intestinal resection only if such surgery will result in minimal or no remaining gross tumor

binations include CAP (cyclophosphamide, doxorubicin [Adriamycin], and cisplatin), CHAD (cyclophosphamide, hexamethylmelamine, doxorubicin [Adriamycin], and diaminodichloroplatinum [cisplatin]), and HEXA-CAF (hexamethylmelamine, cyclophosphamide, methotrexate (A-methopterin), and 5-fluorouracil).[5,25,104]

The approach to the treatment of ovarian carcinoma by stage is outlined in Table 20-11.[5,12,19,21,25,26,39,104]

Stage I and II Disease. When the disease is grossly removed, the washings or ascites fluid is negative, there are no external excrescences on the ovary, and the pelvic and periaortic nodes and omentum are negative, no further treatment is advisable in well-differentiated carcinomas. Once the tumor becomes undifferentiated, if there are excrescences on the ovary or if positive washings are found, it is advisable to consider the use of adjuvant treatment. Usually in stage II disease when the disease is confined to both ovaries and the secondary gynecologic structures can be completely removed, conservative treatment such as intraperitoneal radioisotopes or single agent melphalan therapy is advisable. If residual disease exists in the pelvis, total abdominal irradiation is recommended using either a pelvic field within an abdominal field technique or a strip-field technique.

Stage III Disease. Most patients will be in stage III, and they are further divided and subdivided into favorable versus unfavorable patients, depending upon how much residual disease is left after surgery. The optimum situation is considered to be found in those patients in whom there is macroscopic residuum to the largest nodule less than 1 cm; such patients are often vigorously treated with external irradiation to the whole abdomen and pelvis with selected boost fields and doses to targeted tumor areas. This is recommended in the majority of favorable patients until new clinical trials[23] comparing multiagent chemotherapy are established as superior. Suboptimal disease, which is defined as residual disease greater than 1 cm, is treated by combination chemotherapy using one of the multiagent chemotherapy schedules previously noted. Eight cycles of chemotherapy are often considered adequate, particularly if full doses have been given at each cycle and, as

Table 20-11. Treatment Decisions: Ovary

STAGE	SURGERY	RADIATION THERAPY		CHEMOTHERAPY
I (T_1, N_0, M_0)	Oophorectomy with tumor resection, radical HBSO and omentectomy	Intraperitoneal radioisotopes		Melphalan
II (T_2, N_0, M_0)	Oophorectomy with tumor resection, radical HBSO and omentectomy Excise adhesions Biopsy diaphragm and pelvis	Whole abdominal/pelvic irradiation 2500 cGy/5000 cGy	or	MAC
III (T_3, N_1, M_0)	Cytoreductive surgery	Investigational whole abdominal/pelvic irradiation		MAC
IV (T_{any}, N_{any}, M_+)	Debulking optional	Palliative RT		MAC
Relapse and Recurrence	Second look	Palliative RT		MAC

HBSO = hysterectomy and bilateral salpingo-oophrectomy
MAC = multiagent chemotherapy
RT = radiation therapy

noted, re-exploratory laparotomy is done to assess the results. If the surgical findings are that of complete regression, there are investigational studies exploring the use of consolidated, moderate dose radiation therapy to the whole abdomen and pelvis. If the disease is unresponsive to the first line of agents, a second crossover nonresistant group of chemotherapeutic agents may be used since this disease is responsive to a variety of agents.

Stage IV Disease. If the major finding is that of a pleural effusion, the patient should undergo thoracocentesis and then the abdomen should be treated as in stage III disease. The patient should then be treated with chemotherapy and second-look surgery, particularly if the pleural effusion does not recur and there is no clinical evidence of good response to bulk disease.

Relapse or Recurrent Disease. This is most unfortunate for patients who have persistent disease since there are few second-line measures that prove successful. Aggressive radiation therapy is often impossible, particularly if the bulk disease is greater than 1 cm. New combinations of chemotherapy can be attempted, but usually are much less successful. Intraperitoneal isotopic therapy or chemotherapy rarely contains the ascites, since it is associated with bulk disease, and such agents only act topically. Investigative approaches such as adjuvant immunotherapy are best applied when there is less bulk disease, when the patient's condition is optimal, and when appropriate research protocol evaluation has been undertaken. Also, radiolabeled antibodies are being explored in the treatment of this disease. Hormonal receptors have recently been evaluated in ovarian cancer, and there are some reports of the successful use of tamoxifen. There are also some favorable reports on new agents and drugs in patients failing to obtain remission on the standard form of chemotherapy.[70]

Impact of New Technology

It is doubtful that chemotherapy for advanced disease will improve sufficiently to effect a major change in the appallingly low survival of patients with ovarian carcinoma. What leverage physicians may have on the disease will come from improved detection. Although both CT and US are capable of detecting adnexal masses, it is obviously impractical to screen half the population on a regular basis using either modality. Not uncommonly, however, patients are referred to the radiology department for studies designed to image extragonadal organ systems, e.g., urograms, barium studies, abdominal CT scans, or ultrasonograms. It is obvious that we can perform a service by being alert to the presence of pelvic soft tissue masses on any of these examinations so that further evaluation can be optimally performed. At present, no specific tumor marker exists that will permit large-scale screening efforts. MRI needs to be evaluated and holds promise for detecting peritoneal spread.

For postoperative disease assessment, there has already been some interest in instillation of radionuclides into the peritoneal cavity to image small residual tumor nodules. Assuming a specific surface tumor antigen can be isolated, radionuclide-labeled antibodies to this antigen could provide a sensitive means for detection of small peritoneal implants that still escape CT, US, and peritoneoscopy.

ENDOMETRIUM

Endometrial adenocarcinoma is now the most common invasive gynecologic malignancy in the United States, with an estimated incidence of 39,000 new cases yearly.[87] There has been an absolute increase of the disease over the past few decades, a fact that has been attributed to the increased use of exogenously administered estrogen derivatives.[10] At the same time as widespread cancer screening programs have been successful in reducing the incidence of invasive carcinoma of the cervix, there has been a relative increase in endometrial adenocarcinoma as a major cause of morbidity and mortality in women.

The typical patient at risk of developing cancer of the endometrium is either a woman with low parity or, more often, a nulliparous woman; at the time of detection she will be postmenopausal or perimenopausal. Before the menopause, she may well have had a history of infrequent, irregular periods consistent with anovulatory cycles. She may be obese, diabetic, hypertensive or a combination of any of these. A family history of cancer of all types commonly will be elicited. In more than 75% of cases, she will be over 50 years of age.[10]

Fortunately, most patients seek medical attention while the disease is relatively confined, chiefly because of the vaginal bleeding associated with this neoplasm. Up to 75% to 80% of patients have stage I disease at the time of diagnosis.[7,10,27] While 37,000 new cases of endometrial neoplasms are projected for 1985, only 2,900 are expected to die of disease. Five-year survival for patients undergoing treatment for stage I disease is close to 80%.[27]

Radiographic methods only rarely contribute to the detection of carcinomas of the endometrium; clinically silent uterine enlargement may be detectable on urograms, barium enema examinations, or pelvic CT scans. Ultrasonography may specifically suggest the diagnosis in rare instances by demonstrating a mass arising from the endometrial cavity.

The major impact of the new imaging methods, including computed tomography and ultrasonography, lies in refining the accuracy of the currently existing staging methods so that preoperative information regarding the total extent of the neoplasm is maximized. Studies that incorporate this added information into randomized clinical trials have not yet been published; the eventual impact of such improved precision on patient survival is therefore not yet assessed.

Tumor Behavior and Pathology

Ninety percent of invasive carcinomas of the endometrium are epithelial adenocarcinomas.[27] There is a somewhat hazy zone pathologically between atypical adenomatous hyperplasia and well-differentiated adenocarcinoma.[27] This fact, it is speculated, has led to considerable confusion in interpreting cancer therapy statistics;[9] obviously, the success rates of any therapy directed toward hyperplastic lesions (which have no metastatic potential) will be very good. Pathologically, carcinomas that retain glandular patterns while containing some cellular atypia are classed as well-differentiated or grade 1 cancers. A decreasing tendency toward well-defined gland formation is reflected by increasing grade, with poorly differentiated lesions assigned to grade 3.[69]

In some cases, the adenocarcinoma stimulates squamous metaplasia within the endometrial mucosa, leading to an adenocanthoma. This type of squamous metaplasia tends to occur in association with well-differentiated lesions, which accounts for the overall favorable prognosis of uterine adenocanthoma.[69] Adenosquamous carcinoma, by contrast, implies true epidermoid malignancy in association with glandular epithelial adenocarcinoma. This lesion has a tendency to infiltrate extensively and metastasize widely and has a poor prognosis.[69]

The etiology of endometrial adenocarcinoma is not completely understood, but many authors suggest that adenomatous hyperplasia in the postmenopausal years is the precancerous lesion.[69] The stimulus that produces adenomatous hyperplasia and that, if unopposed, proceeds to the development of frank malignancy is thought to be an estrogenic steroid. Associations that tend to support this hypothesis include the high incidence of adenocarcinoma developing in patients with Stein-Leventhal syndrome, in whom there are long periods of unopposed estrogen stimulation. Similarly, feminizing ovarian tumors are associated with a 15% to 25% incidence of fundal adenocarcinoma.[69] Finally, an increasing number of cases of adenocarcinoma have occurred in individuals receiving exogenous estrogen therapy. Most gynecologic pathologists believe that, at the very least, estrogen stimulation conditions the endometrium in a way that permits the evolution of carcinoma in the presence of the appropriate carcinogen.

The incidence of uterine sarcomas is difficult to estimate, since there remains controversy among pathologists in distinguishing between low grade sarcomas and cellular myomas. Major types of sarcoma include those arising from smooth muscle (leiomyosarcoma), those taking origin from uterine stroma (stromal sarcoma) and tumors with mixed mesodermal elements (mixed müllerian tumor).[73] Leiomyosarcomas are usually found incidentally in patients undergoing hysterectomy for benign leiomyomata. These tumors tend to recur locally and spread by direct extension, although some may invade blood vessels and undergo hematogenous dissemination.

Mixed müllerian tumors constitute 2% to 5% of malignant uterine tumors.[4,52,68] Local and hematogenous spread occur relatively early in the course of the disease and confer a poor prognosis. In one series of müllerian tumors, no patient with confirmed disease outside the uterus survived five years.[4] Pathologically, a distinction is made between homologous tumors, the sarcomatous elements of which are normally present in the uterus (smooth muscle, endometrial stroma) and heterologous lesions, the sarcomatous elements of which are foreign to the uterus (rhabdomyosarcoma, osteosarcoma). Heterologous tumors appear to metastasize earlier and more widely and thus have a poorer prognosis than the homologous forms.[4]

Patterns of Spread

Direct Extension. Since the neoplastic cells in uterine malignancy arise on the epithelial surface lining the inner margin of a hollow viscus, it is natural that the initial mode of spread would be radial; thus the myometrium adjacent to the site of tumor origin is most at risk of direct extension.[27,69] Continued growth in the radial dimension will lead to involvement of the serosa of the uterine body, and hence extension to the entire peritoneal cavity may occur (Figure 20-15). Even when the serosa is not involved, deep myometrial extension is associated with a high incidence of lymph node metastasis.[69] Longitudinal growth of tumor proceeds caudally to involve the lower uterine segment and eventually the cervix. When this occurs, the biologic behavior of the tumor resembles that of primary carcinoma of the cervix, and there is an accompanying increase in lymph node metastases and parametrial extension. Eventually the vaginal vault may become involved.

Lymphatic Spread. The uterus is rich in lymphatic networks.[83] The innermost, or mucous, lymph network drains the endometrium. The muscular network drains the myometrium and the serous network drains the peritoneal surface of the uterus. These drain into the subserous network, which then transports lymph to the lateral and superior portions of the uterus.

Three sets of efferent vessels drain the uterus: the utero-ovarian trunk travels within the broad ligament along the uterine artery and joins the lymphatics of the fallopian tube and ovary on each side. From this point, they follow the ovarian pathways previously described

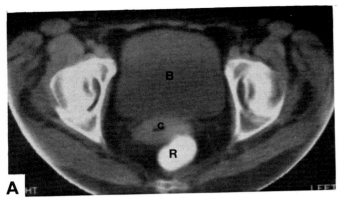

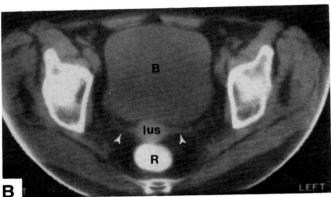

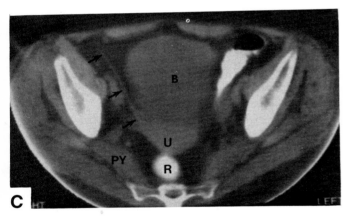

FIG. 20-15 Relationships of the uterus in a normal woman. (A) CT scan through the lower uterine segment demonstrates the oval cervix (c) in this multiparous woman. A small amount of gas is present centrally because of the insertion of a vaginal tampon. Note the relationship of the cervix, with the bladder (B) anteriorly and the rectum (R) posteriorly. The rich vascularity of the paracervical space can be appreciated immediately lateral to the cervix. (B) At a slightly higher level, the paired uterine arteries and veins (arrowheads) are seen supplying the lower uterine segment (lus). (C) A scan through the uterine corpus (U) demontrates the attachment of the ligamentum teres (arrows). Posterior and lateral to the uterus, the internal iliac artery and vein lie on the anterior surface of the pyriformus muscle (PY).

(see section on ovarian tumors), terminating on the right in lateroaortic nodes near the origin of the inferior vena cava and on the left in preaortic nodes near the origin of the inferior mesenteric artery. Another trunk drains across the umbilical artery to end in the middle group of the external iliac chain. Finally, a third trunk drains the uterine wall near the attachment of the ligamentum teres. It follows the course of this structure to terminate in a superficial inguinal node. The first two pathways described above are clinically the most important; the latter is an accessory pathway.

There is a definite relationship between lymph node metastases and local tumor factors, including grade, stage,[77] and depth of myometrial invasion (Table 20-12). In Piver's[75] recent series of 65 patients with stage I, grade 1 cancer of the endometrium, only 3.1% had pelvic adenopathy, but 36% (9 of 25) stage I, grade 3 patients had positive pelvic nodes and 28% had spread to the aortic nodes. In another work,[10] the five-year survival diminished from 91% for grade 1 tumors to 48.1% for grade 2 neoplasms. A number of investigators have further substantiated the relationship of local tumor stage to pelvic adenopathy. In patients whose tumors are clinically confined to the uterus (clinical stage I) there is a 10.6% incidence of lymphadenopathy. If the tumor has grown longitudinally to involve the cervix (stage II), the incidence of adenopathy rises to 36.5%.[27] Similarly, if

Table 20-12. Endometrial Cancer:
Influence of Local Tumor Factors on Survival

LOCAL FACTOR	NUMBER OF PATIENTS	NUMBER SURVIVING FIVE YEARS	PERCENTAGE
Stage			
Boutselis			
Stage IA	328	265	80
IB	92	65	70
II	82	41	50
III	60	17	28
IV	24	2	8.3
Berman et al.			
Stage I	12,655	9,670	76.4
II	2,185	1,089	49.8
III	1,596	480	30.1
IV	585	54	9.2
Grade			
Boutselis			
Grade 1	177	166	91.5
2	160	118	73.7
3	83	40	48.1
Myometrial invasion			
Boutselis			
Endometrium only	81	76	93.8
Inner one third	157	135	86.5
Middle one third	90	71	78.8
Outer one third	92	38	41.3

the disease grows radially, so that the myometrium is extensively involved, the incidence of positive pelvic lymph nodes rises from 2.8% (when there is minimal invasion) to 30.7% (when the myometrium is extensively involved.[69]

Direct Peritoneal Spread. Infrequently, the surgeon encounters peritoneal spread, omental involvement, or extension to the ovaries in clinically confined (low stage) disease (Figure 20-16). Some authors have postulated that cancer cells pass through the rich lymphatic communications connecting the uterus to the fallopian tubes and ovaries to reach the peritoneal cavity. Surwit[91] quotes Creasman's work, which noted a 16% incidence of positive peritoneal cytology in stage I patients. Omental spread is much more common in clinically advanced disease in which the tumor can spread directly from the diseased surface of the uterus to involve intraperitoneal structures.

Hematogenous Spread. Similar to other malignant neoplasms, spread by hematogenous dissemination occurs in advanced disease; target sites include lung, liver, and skeletal structures.

Classification and Staging

The staging system developed by the International Federation of Gynecologic Oncology (FIGO) has been adopted by most cancer researchers in the United States; the TNM staging system is quite comparable to it, so that interpretation of T stage data from data reported in the FIGO system can be done without much difficulty (Figure 20-17, Table 20-13). Carcinoma in situ is assigned stage 0 (T_{is}), and the FIGO system further stipulates that data on cure rates for this stage will not be reported in combination with true invasive carcinoma. Because of the pronounced influence of cellular differentiation (grade) on patient survival, in stage I carcinoma the tumor grade is reported along with the stage. Stage I (T_1) cancer is defined as being limited to the uterus; if sounding of the uterine cavity reveals its length to be less than 8 cm, it is stage Ia (T_{1a}). If greater, it is stage Ib (T_{1b}). In this system, therefore, a patient who had a poorly differentiated but clinically well-confined tumor would be classified in stage Ia grade 3. Stage II (T_2) tumors have spread longitudinally to involve the uterine cervix. Stage III (T_3) neoplasms have spread extensively either in a radial direction to involve the parametrium or longitudinally to involve the vagina. Finally, pronounced extrauterine growth of tumor to involve the rectum or bladder places the patient in stage IVA (T_4). Distant metastasis, using the FIGO classification, is stage IVB; in the TNM system, this would be listed as M_+ (Figure 20-17).

Clinical staging maneuvers include careful physical examination with bimanual palpation of the uterus and adnexae. Careful fractional dilatation and curettage is performed to detect clinically occult disease in the cervix. In patients with extensive disease in whom bladder invasion is suspected, cystoscopy should be performed. It is noted that the mere presence of bullous edema of the bladder is insufficient to assign the patient to stage IVA, since this can occur when vesical lymphatics are obstructed and need not imply actual bladder invasion. Similarly, patients whose clinical presentation suggests invasion of the rectum or sigmoid colon should undergo sigmoidoscopy. Air-contrast enema examination has been recommended to detect serosal invasion of the rectosigmoid,[35] but this examination is rarely positive in clinically low stage disease.

Imaging Procedures and Assessment

In view of the clinical behavior of endometrial carcinoma, a clinically relevant imaging method should attempt to answer three questions concerning the local extent of disease: (1) what is the extent of myometrial invasion; (2) is the cervix involved, and (3) is there parametrial extension of tumor? The imaging modalities that can be brought to bear on these questions include ultrasonography, computed tomography (CT), and angiography (Table 20-14).

Ultrasonography. One advantage of ultrasonography is that it can be used in an oblique scanning axis parallel with the long axis of the uterus. This often makes it easier to resolve problems caused by the complex geometric shapes encountered in the myomatous uterus. A review by Requard et al.[82] however, found ultrasonography insensitive in distinguishing tumor from normal myometrium; likewise, cervical involvement by carcinoma could not be predicted with confidence. They did find that patients with low stage (I and II) disease had normal or somewhat bulbous uterine shapes, while higher stage disease was associated with lobular uterine geometry. However, false-positive diagnoses were caused by leiomyomata creating lobular uterine shapes.

Computed Tomography. Computed tomography (CT) has the potential of displaying differences in attenuation values between tumor and the myometrium, thus making precise staging possible. This was addressed in reports by Hasumi et al.[44] and Hamlin et al.,[41] who documented that the infusion of contrast material reliably increased the attenuation of the myometrium to a greater extent than that of the adenocarcinoma. In the series of Hasumi et al.,[44] prediction of depth of myometrial invasion (inner half versus outer half) by CT was borne out by pathologic examination in 100% of patients. Similarly, using these criteria to predict cervical invasion, CT was accurate in 90% of cases, with two false-negative cases, found at pathologic examination to have micro-

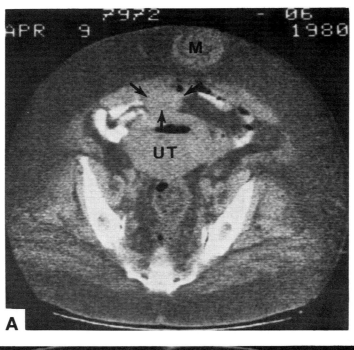

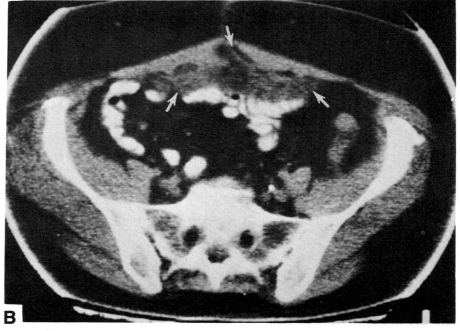

FIG. 20-16. Demonstration of metastatic endometrial carcinoma by CT. (A) A 55-year-old markedly obese woman with clinical stage I, grade 2 endometrial carcinoma. A scan through the uterine fundus (UT) demonstrates a small amount of gas within the uterine cavity as a result of a recent dilatation and curettage. An oval soft tissue density (arrows) is present immediately anterior to the uterus and proved to be mesenteric implantation of tumor. The soft tissue mass (M) in the periumbilical region was metastatic nodal disease. (B) A CT scan through the lower abdomen of a patient with recurrent endometrial carcinoma demonstrates thickening of the omentum (arrows) immediately posterior to the rectus abdominus musculature. This "omental cake" is more common in ovarian carcinoma.

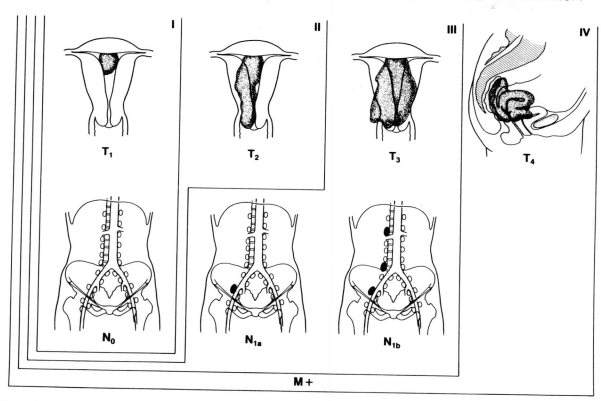

FIG. 20-17. Anatomic staging for uterine fundus cancer. Tumor (T) categories: This is defined according to extension and depth of invasion and follows stage. T_1 is confined to the uterine fundus; extension to cervix signifies T_2; parametrial invasion signifies T_3; and invasion into bladder or rectum denotes T_4. Node (N) categories: This refers only to pelvic regional nodes (N_1). N_{1a} is pelvic nodes; N_{1b} is para-aortic nodes in the above schema; neither AJC nor UICC make this distinction, however. Stage grouping: This, as noted, is identical to the T categories. However, N_1 is grouped with T_3 and both T and N refer to pelvic disease. N_1 is equivalent to T_4 and stage IV disease. (Reprinted from Beecham, J. B., Helmkamp, B. F., Rubin, P.: Tumors of the female reproductive organs. In *Clinical Oncology for Medical Students and Physicians: A Multidisciplinary Approach*, 6th ed. Rubin, P. (Ed.). New York, American Cancer Society, 1983, pp. 428–480. With permission.)

scopic invasion. In identifying local extension of tumor to the parametrium, Walsh and Goplerud[98] reported two of three falsely negative scans as a result of the presence of microscopic metastases. In the same study, a single case of bladder extension was missed with CT. In ad-

Table 20-13. Comparison of FIGO with TNM Staging of Carcinoma of the Endometrium

FIGO		TNM
Stage IA		$T_{1a}N_xM_0$
Grade 1	Tumor confined to the endometrium.	Grade 1
Grade 2	Uterine cavity less than 8 cm.	Grade 2
Grade 3		Grade 3
Stage IB		$T_{1b}N_xM_0$
Grade 1	Tumor confined to the endometrium.	Grade 1
Grade 2	Uterine cavity greater than 8 cm.	Grade 2
Grade 3		Grade 3
Stage II	Tumor invasion of the cervix.	$T_2N_xM_0$
Stage III	Tumor spread to parametrium or vagina.	$T_3N_xM_0$
Stage IVA	Tumor invasion of the bladder or rectum.	$T_4N_xM_t$
Stage IVB	Distant metastases.	$T_xN_xM_t$

vanced disease, CT is capable of detecting metastases to peritoneal and omental surfaces. In our experience,[3] clinical evaluation was slightly better than CT examination in low stage disease, while CT was clearly superior to clinical staging in detecting metastatic carcinoma to omentum and lymph nodes.

Angiography. Angiography has been used in some centers for staging various pelvic malignancies, including carcinomas of the cervix, bladder, and prostate. Angiography is not routinely used to stage pelvic tumors in our institution. In patients with extensive disease, or in whom surgery is contraindicated because of severe medical disorders, angiography may be useful in the treatment of intractable bleeding. Selective catheterization of the hypogastric artery with injection of embolic material has been used to successfully manage severe hemorrhage.

Lymphangiography. Several investigators[47,52,68] have employed lymphangiography in evaluating the lymph nodes status of patients with endomentrial carcinoma (Figure

Table 20-14. Imaging Methods for Evaluating Endometrial Carcinoma

METHOD	CAPABILITY	COST/ BENEFIT	RECOMMENDATION FOR USE
Noninvasive			
Chest radiography	Detects soft-tissue nodules greater than 15 mm; detects acute pulmonary disease.	High	Routine
Skeletal radiography	May confirm suspicious findings on radio-nuclide scans (low probability in low-stage disease).	Low	Only when radionuclide scan is positive
Sonography			
Primary tumor	Rarely detects unsuspected tumor. Not accu-rate in distinguishing stage I or II from stage III.	Low	If CT scan equivocal
Liver	Detects metastatic deposits greater than 15 mm (low probability unless liver enzymes elevated).	Moderate	If enzymes elevated. High grade/stage tumor.
Barium enema	Detects serosal implantation of peritoneal spread; screens for diverticulosis, adematous polyps.	Low Moderate	If high-stage disease, or colonic symptoms, or guiac positive stool
MRI	Not yet investigated. Potentially useful in local tumor staging.	Unknown	Unknown
Minimally invasive			
Urography	Detects ureteral obstruction, bladder inva-sion; screens for unsuspected renal anomaly.	Moderate	All operative candidates
CT	Accurate staging information; assesses myo-metrial invasion. Not known to be accurate in detecting lymph node spread.	High	All patients except those with clinical stage I grade I tumor, or clinical stage IV
Radionuclide scan			
Bone	Sensitive assessment of bone metastases	Low	Only in patients with skeletal pain
Liver	Detects peripheral metastases greater than 20 mm.	Low	When liver enzymes are elevated
Hysterography	Provides gross estimate of tumor size.	Low	Not recommended
Invasive			
Angiography	Detects abnormal vascularity; minimal local staging information available.	Low	Not routine. May be useful for therapy.
Lymphangiography	Detects abnormal lymph node architecture.	Moderate	Preoperative patients with greater than 50% myo-metrial invasion.
Biopsy	Confirms lesions detected by radionuclide scan, CT scan, or lymphangiogram.	High	For patients with suspicious lesions.

20-18). The majority of the patients in these series were treated with radiation therapy, and thus histologic proof was rarely obtained. Therefore, data regarding accuracy and sensitivity of lymphangiography are difficult to ab-stract. Using criteria established for the lymphangiograph-ic diagnosis of nodal metastasis in other tumors, however, these investigators found that patients with positive lymph-angiograms had a survival considerably worse than pa-tients with negative lymphangiograms.

The efficacy of CT in evaluating pelvic or para-aortic adenopathy has not been adequately studied to date. In our own series of 18 patients studied preoperatively,[3] the diagnosis of metastatic disease to lymph nodes was made only three times, with two true-positive assess-ments and one false-positive assessment. We had no false-negative interpretations. Prospective evaluation of unselected patients will be necessary before accuracy and sensitivity rates can be determined.

Metastatic Surveys. Common sites of widespread me-tastases from endometrial carcinomas include the lung parenchyma, liver, spine, and peritoneal surfaces. For pa-tients with symptoms and signs referable to the liver or spine, many imaging procedures can be used, including radionuclide liver or skeletal imaging, CT of the liver or spine, ultrasonography of the liver, and conventional tomography of bone. For detection of skeletal metastases, radionuclide bone scanning remains the initial procedure of choice; it is the most sensitive of all the radiographic imaging procedures. As discussed in previous sections, it is also the least specific. Worrisome lesions detected on radionuclide skeletal imaging thus require confirmation by plain films, tomography, or CT directed to the area of interest. If necessary, needle biopsy should be performed. Less than 1% of patients with endometrial carcinoma will have bone metastases at initial examination, although up to 12% have osseous metastases at autopsy.[72]

The relative merits of CT, ultrasonography, and radionuclide imaging of the liver have been discussed in previous sections on imaging strategy. Basically, radionuclide imaging is the least sensitive and least specific of the imaging methods available, while CT is the most sensitive, most specific, and most expensive modality. Ultrasonography combines relatively low cost, no exposure to ionizing radiation or intravenous contrast, and relatively high sensitivity and specificity. Thus, many authors[8] suggest using ultrasonography in the initial eval-

uation and follow-up assessment of patients suspected of having liver metastases.

From a practical standpoint, chest roentgenograms are a sensitive means for detecting clinically occult metastases to the pulmonary parenchyma.[37] In patients with low stage, high grade disease in whom radical therapeutic measures are being considered with curative intent, it is reasonable to adopt more sophisticated methods. Whole lung tomography and thoracic computed tomography are available methods that will improve sensitivity with the price being poor specificity and greater expense.[62]

Imaging Strategies and Decisions

The application of sophisticated imaging methods to the preoperative staging of neoplasms is futile if it can have no effect on therapeutic decisions (Figure 20-19). Thus, patients should be chosen for such preoperative evaluation who satisfy the following criteria: (1) patients

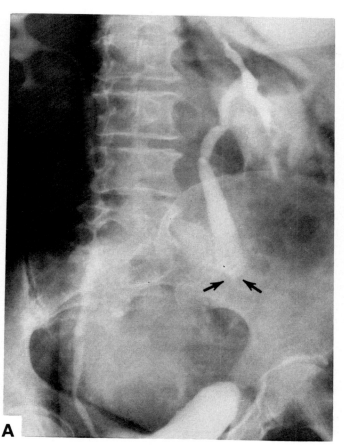

A

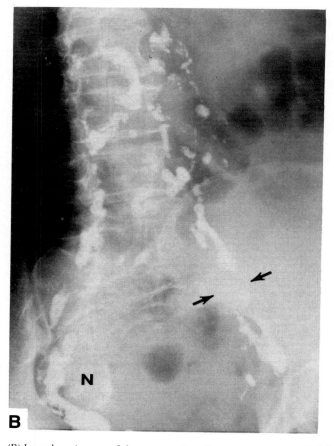

B

FIG. 20-18. Lymphangiographic demonstration of nodal metastases from carcinoma in the endometrium. (A) Urogram of a patient with clinically advanced carcinoma of the endometrium demonstrates abrupt narrowing of the left ureter as it crosses into the true pelvis (arrows).

(B) Lymphangiogram of the same patient demonstrates nonfilling of the left common iliac nodes in the region of the ureteral stricture (arrows). A right external iliac lymph node (N) is likewise evident.

should be at risk of undergoing clinically occult spread of disease; (2) the method chosen should be highly sensitive to the mode of spread at issue; (3) successful detection of such spread will necessitate different therapeutic measures than would be applied if no spread were encountered.

Localized and Early Stage: Confined to Uterus (Stage A).

Patients who are clinically felt to have well-differentiated carcinoma confined to the uterus (FIGO stage IA, grade 1) are at extremely low risk of having occult spread to parametrial or pelvic lymph nodes. The potential yield of CT or lymphangiography in this patient population is too small to justify routine use of these procedures. However, patients with higher grade tumors are at risk of having pelvic or even para-aortic lymphadenopathy; indeed, we have encountered patients in this category who had occult metastases to the omentum detected by CT. It is in this group that preoperative computed tomography may be useful in detecting extrauterine spread.

Depth of Myometrial Invasion.

Computed tomography with intravenous contrast infusion has been shown to be highly accurate in assessing yet another risk factor—depth of myometrial invasion. Hasumi et al.[44] suggest performing contrast-enhanced CT in all patients in whom occult lymph node spread is to be assessed. If, by CT examination, less than half the myometrium is invaded, a simple total abdominal hysterectomy with bilateral salpingo-oophorectomy may be performed. This is based on their data in which none of the 104 patients with less than half the myometrium involved had pelvic adenopathy; in the same series, 13 of 35 patients with more than half the myometrium involved had positive pelvic lymph nodes. Thus, CT could be used as a patient stratification procedure to detect those individuals at greatest risk of having lymph node metastases. Further studies of the type suggested by Hasumi et al.[44] would clarify the exact role of CT in this clinical situation.

Advanced and Spread Beyond Uterus.

In patients with stage III carcinoma of the endometrium, the risks of lymphatic spread are very high (44% in one report).[10] Thus, a patient stratification method based on myometrial invasion is not as helpful in this group of advanced lesions. In some cases, lymphangiography could be useful; if suspicious nodal groups are demonstrated, percutaneous fine-needle aspiration biopsy would be performed to confirm the presence of untreatable disease.[31,46,105] Thus, radiation therapy to the pelvis with intent to cure would be precluded. Patients with disease limited to the pelvis or with no evidence of lymph node spread radiographically could then be treated with high-dose pelvic irradiation.

Surgical staging is more accurate than clinical staging

and can provide the following information: depth of myometrial penetration, degree of tumor differentiation, involvement of the endocervix, uterine size, involvement of the adnexa, presence of malignant cells in the peritoneal fluid, pelvic or para-aortic lymph node metastases, and distant metastases from hematogenous spread, particularly in the liver.[5]

Follow-up Imaging.

Eighty percent of patients who will develop recurrent carcinoma of the endometrium do so within two years. Sites of recurrence depend in part on the treatment used: if radiation is given to the vaginal cuff, recurrences to the vagina are relatively infrequent. In the series of Reddy et al.,[81] eight of the nine recurrences occurring in 94 patients treated with surgery alone were in the pelvis or vagina. In 83 patients treated with combined surgery and radiotherapy, only two of the recurrences were in this anatomic region. Further operative or radiation therapy is feasible for patients with recurrent disease provided it is sufficiently well confined. Thus, there is a premium on early detection of pelvic recurrence. Computed tomography has been quite valuable in detecting recurrent endometrial carcinoma,[3,92] and is recommended for patients with suspicious physical findings occurring after therapy (Figure 20-19).

Treatment Decisions

Endometrial carcinoma is generally found in early stage I and II categories and is very amenable to a combination of surgery and radiation therapy. The vast majority of patients will survive with 90% remaining alive at five years for stage I disease and 80% remaining alive for stage II disease.[5,74] The standard surgical procedure is a radical hysterectomy, often with pelvic lymphadenectomy and sampling of the para-aortic nodes. The role of lymph node dissection is undefined in terms of its true value except in patients with higher grade cancers, where they are more commonly found.

Traditionally, preoperative irradiation has been widely used to reduce implant metastases, to seal lymphatic channels, to reduce operative tumor spill, to decrease uterine size or operability, to decrease the potential for vaginal tumor implants and to sterilize or ablate cancer in a well-oxygenated tumor-containing organ and thereby reduce the likelihood of releasing viable cells at the time of surgery. With the advent of surgical staging in this disease and with the increasing number of investigational studies of the Gynecologic Oncology Group, postoperative irradiation is more commonly offered and has the advantage of precise surgical staging to determine depth of invasion and evidence of spread beyond the pelvis and pelvic lymph nodes or positive washings.

Progestational agents, particularly the oral progestins, i.e, negestrol acetate and medroxyprogesterone acetate

A   ENDOMETRIAL CANCER : CLINICAL / RADIOLOGIC FLOW DIAGRAM

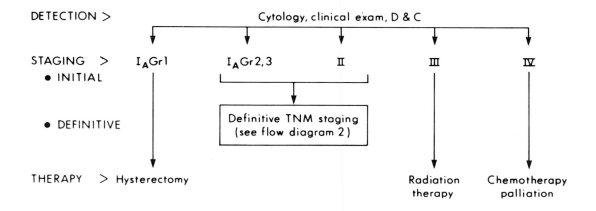

B   ENDOMETRIAL CANCER : DEFINITIVE EVALUATION OF TNM STAGE

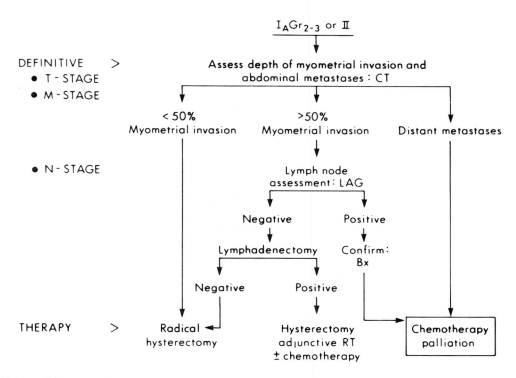

FIG. 20-19. (A) The optimal evaluation of patients with endometrial carcinoma depends upon the initial clinical stage. (B) Patients at risk of nodal or distant metastases should be thoroughly evaluated before radical therapeutic measures.

have proved to be of value in causing regression of neoplasms. Multiagent chemotherapy has generally been disappointing, with agents such as Adriamycin and 5-fluorouracil being used.[54,92]

The approach according to stage can be found in Table 20-15.

For stage IA, IB, grade 1 cancers, total abdominal hysterectomy and bilateral salpingo-oophorectomy with

surgical exploration and washings to determine if cells are positive is used. Generally, no adjuvant radiation therapy or hormonal therapy is used.

Stage IA or IB, grade 2 and 3 neoplasms are generally managed with a similar procedure using total abdominal hysterectomy and bilateral salpingo-oophorectomy with selective para-aortic and pelvic lymphadenectomy. Postoperative irradiation is generally used and limited to

Table 20-15. Treatment Decisions: Endometrium

STAGE	SURGERY		RADIATION THERAPY		CHEMOTHERAPY
I (T_1,N_0)	Radical hysterectomy Selected nodal sampling	and/or	Preoperative or post-operative RT 4500–5000 cGy Intracavitary or external RT		NR
II (T_2,N_0)	Radical hysterectomy Selected nodal sampling Pelvic lymphandenectomy Para-aortic sampling	and/or	Preoperative RT 4500–5000 cGy		NR
III (T_3,N_0,N_{1a}) IV (T_4,N_0,N_{1a})	If feasible, radical hysterectomy	and/or	External and intracavitary RT to higher doses 6000–6500 cGy if only RT	and	Progestational agents
IV (T_{any},N_{1b},M_+)	NR		Palliative RT	and	Progestational agents Investigational MAC

NR = not recommended
RT = radiation therapy
MAC = multiagent chemotherapy

the pelvis. Doses are in the neighborhood of 5,000 cGy in 5 weeks. A vaginal cylinder can be used to treat the vaginal surface with 4,000 to 8,000 cGy and thereby reduce the likelihood of metastatic involvement of this vaginal site to virtually zero. Selection of intracavitary loading of doses depends on how much of the vagina had previous external irradiation.

Most stage III cancers of the endometrium are treated preoperatively in a fashion similar to cervical carcinoma. External irradiation is started with midline shielding introduced in the latter half of the course of treatment to be followed by one application of intracavitary sources yielding tumor doses of 6,000 to 6,500 cGy and 4,000 to 5,000 cGy to the pelvic sidewall. Total hysterectomy and bilateral salpingo-oophorectomy follow and can provide a high degree of survival and control. There is no indication for adjuvant hormonal therapy.

If feasible, radical hysterectomy is performed, removing as much of the disease as possible, particularly if the spread is to other gynecologic organs and structures that lend themselves to resection. If the disease is extensive and cannot be resected, surgery is deferred. Radiation therapy can therefore be definitive and combines external and internal irradiation, often using Heyman's capsules rather than the standard intracavitary applicator in the form of a single stem. This applicator can be used for small uteri but the Heyman's capsules are preferred for large or irregular uterine cavities to obtain better dosage distribution throughout. Progestational agents can be used if the disease is extensive. Table 20-15 summarizes the treatment choices according to stage.

Stage IV, metastatic disease, is best handled by progestational agents, with investigational multiagent chemotherapy, if this is desired. The major role of radiation

therapy is palliative. Seldom is a surgical resection required in the advanced stages of this disease (Figure 20-20).

Sarcomas of the uterus are uncommon and usually consist of endometrial stromal sarcomas or mixed sarcomas of the uterine muscle and of the leiomyosarcomatous type, generally arising in benign leiomyomas and mixed carcinosarcomas. Surgery and radiation are also often combined in this disease.

One unique tumor arising in the uterine cavity that

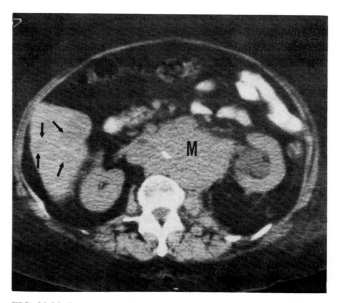

FIG. 20-20. Recurrent endometrial cancer. Note extensive retroperitoneal lymph node metastases (M) surrounding the aorta and vena cava. Hepatic metastases (arrows) are also present.

deserves mention is the placental trophoblastic neoplasm as a hydatidiform mole or choriocarcinoma. This is a very aggressive epithelial cancer of the cytotrophoblasts and syncytiotrophoblasts and is associated with abnormal elevation of human chorionic gonadotropin (HCG) in the blood or urine, which can be assayed quantitatively. Pelvic ultrasonography, amniography, or CT are generally done with a complete metastatic workup, since pulmonary, liver, and brain metastases are all possible. The management of this advanced tumor is one of the major successes of chemotherapy and is among the first of the neoplasms to lead to the use of chemotherapy for other malignancies. Titration of chemotherapy versus hormonal therapy has provided true precision in treatment of metastatic disease.[25] Methotrexate has been the most widely used agent but more recently combinations with actinomycin D and chlorambucil have yielded the best results. Complete remissions will occur in 70% of these cases.[50]

Impact of New Technology

The impact of magnetic resonance imaging (MRI) on staging of endometrial cancer is unknown. However, one property of MRI that might prove useful in pelvic imaging is its ability to display undegraded images in any plane. Computed tomographic images, limited to an axial plane of section, are often difficult to interpret because of the complex curvilinear pelvic anatomy. Thus, it will be theoretically possible to choose the most appropriate plane of section to display pelvic images. Whether this will allow detection of small but macroscopic tumor extension into perivisceral fat planes remains to be seen.

REFERENCES

1. Alfridi, M., Vongtama, V., Tsukada, Y., Piver, M. S.: Dysgerominoma of the ovary: Radiation therapy for recurrence. Am. J. Obstet. Gynecol. 126:190, 1976.
2. Athey, P. A., Wallace, S., Jing, B-S., Gallager, H. S., Smith, J. P.: Lymphangiography in ovarian cancer. Am. J. Roentgenol. Radium. Therapy. Nucl. Med. 123:106–113, 1975.
3. Balfe, D. M., Van Dyke, J., Lee, J. K. T., Levitt, R. G.: Utility of CT in staging endometrial carcinoma. J. Comput. Assist. Tomogr. (in press).
4. Barwick, K. W., LiVolsi, V. A.: Malignant mixed müllerian tumors of the uterus. Am. J. Surg. Pathol. 3:125–135, 1979.
5. Beecham, J. B., Helmkamp, B. F., Rubin, P.: Tumors of the female reproductive organs. In Clinical Oncology for Medical Students and Physicians: A Multidisciplinary Approach, 6th ed. Rubin, P. (Ed.). New York, American Cancer Society, 1983, pp. 428–481.
6. Beecham, J. B., Knauf, S. S.: The quest for a clearer understanding of ovarian carcinoma. Int. J. Radiat. Oncol. Biol. Phys. 7: 1099–1101, 1981.
7. Berman, M. L., Ballon, S. C., Lagasse, L. D., Watring, W. G.: Prognosis and treatment of endometrial cancer. Am. J. Obstet. Gynecol. 136:679, 1980.
8. Bernardino, M. E., Thomas, J. L., Barnes, P. A., Lewis, E.: Diagnostic approaches to liver and spleen metastases. Radiol. Clin. North Am. 20:469–486, 1983.
9. Boronow, R. C.: Staging of endometrial carcinoma. Int. J. Radiat. Oncol. Biol. Phys. 6:355–359, 1980.
10. Boutselis, J. G.: Endometrial carcinoma: Prognostic factors and treatment. Surg. Clin. North Am. 58:109–119, 1978.
11. Bruckner, H. W.: Therapeutic strategies for ovarian cancer. Ann. Intern. Med. 95:653–654, 1981.
12. Bush, R. S.: Malignancies of the Ovary, Uterus, and Cervix. London, Edward Arnold, Ltd., 1979.
13. Cantarow, W. D., Stolbach, L. L., Bhattacharya, M., Chatterjee, S. K., Barlow, J. J.: The value of tumor markers in cancer of the ovary. Int. J. Radiat. Oncol. Biol. Phys. 7:1095–1098, 1981.
14. Castellino, R. A., Marglin, S. I.: Imaging of abdominal and pelvic lymph nodes. Lymphography or computed tomography? Invest. Radiol. 17:433–443, 1982.
15. Cavanagh, D., Praphat, H., Ruffolo, E. H.: Carcinoma of the uterine cervix: Some current views. Obstet. Gynecol. Annu. 10: 193–236, 1981.
16. Chung, C. K., Nahhas, W. A., Zaino, R., Stryker, J. A., Mortel, R.: Histologic grade and lymph node metastasis in squamous cell carcinoma of the cervix. Gynecol. Oncol. 12:348–354, 1981.
17. Chung, C. K., Stryker, J. A., Ward, S. P., Nahhas, W. A., Mortel, R.: Histologic grade and prognosis of carcinoma of the cervix. Obstet. Gynecol. 57:636–642, 1981.
18. Cooper, J. S., Davis, L. W., Diamond, J. J., Sedransk, J., Curley, R. F.: Evaluation of carcinoma of the uterine cervix before radiotherapy. J.A.M.A. 242:1996–1997, 1979.
19. Coppleson, M.: Gynecologic Oncology: Fundamental Principles and Clinical Practice. New York, Churchill Livingstone, 1981.
20. DeLand, M., Fried, A., VanNagell, J. R., Donaldson, E. S.: Ultrasonography in the diagnosis of tumors of the ovary. Surg. Gynecol. Obstet. 148:346–348, 1979.
21. Delclos, L., Dembo, A. J.: Ovaries. In Textbook of Radiotherapy, 3rd ed. Fletcher, G. H. (Ed.). Philadelphia, Lea & Febiger, 1980, pp. 834–851.
22. Delclos, L., Quinlan, E. J.: Malignant tumor of the ovary managed with post-operative megavoltage irradiation. Radiology 93:659–663, 1969.
23. Dembo, A. J., Bush, R. S.: Radiation therapy of ovarian carcinoma. In Cancer Research and Treatment — Gynecologic Malignancy I. Griffiths, C. T. (Ed.). Boston, Martinus Nijhoff, 1981.
24. DiSaia, P. J.: Surgical aspect of cervical carcinoma. Cancer 48: 548–559, 1981.
25. DiSaia, P. J., Creasman, W. T.: Clinical Gynecologic Oncology. London, C. V. Mosby, 1981.
26. DiSaia, P. J., Morrow, C. P., Townsend, D. E. (Eds.): Synopsis of Gynecologic Oncology. New York, John Wiley & Sons, 1975, pp. 136–202.
27. Dunnick, N. R., Fisher, R. I., Chu, E. W., Young, R. C.: Percutaneous aspiration of retroperitoneal nodes in ovarian cancer. A.J.R. 135:109–113, 1980.
28. Eltringham, J. R.: Radiation therapy for ovarian carcinoma. Clin. Obstet. Gynecol. 22:967–992, 1979.
29. Emami, B., Watring, W. G., Tak, W., Anderson, B., Piro, A. J.: Para-aortic lymph node radiation in advanced cervical cancer. Int. J. Radiat. Oncol. Biol. Phys. 6:1237–1241, 1980.
30. Eyre, H. J.: Chemotherapy of ovarian carcinoma. Clin. Obstet. Gynecol. 22:957–965, 1979.
31. Ferrucci, J. T., Jr., Wittenberg, J., Mueller, P. R., Simeone, J. F., Harbin, W. P., Kirkpatrick, R. H., Taft, P. D.: Diagnosis of abdominal malignancy by radiologic fine-needle aspiration biopsy. A.J.R. 134:323–330, 1980.
32. Fisher, M. A.: Lumbar spine metastases in cervical carcinoma. A characteristic pattern. Radiology 134:631–634, 1980.
33. Fletcher, G. H., Hamberger, A. D.: Squamous cell carcinoma of

the uterine cervix. In *Textbook of Radiotherapy*, 3rd ed. Fletcher, G. H. (Ed.). Philadelphia, Lea & Febiger, 1980, pp. 720–772.

34. Fuller, A. F., Elliott, N., Kosloff, C., Lewis, J. L.: Lymph node metastases from carcinoma of the cervix, stages IB and IIA: Implications for prognosis and treatment. *Gynecol. Oncol.* 13:165–174, 1982.

35. Gedgaudas, R. K., Kelvin, F. M., Thompson, W. M., Rice, R. P.: The value of preoperative barium enema examinations in the assessment of pelvic masses. *Radiology* 146:609–613, 1983.

36. Ginaldi, S., Wallace, S., Jing, B-S., Bernardino, M. E.: Carcinoma of the cervix: Lymphangiography and computed tomography. *A.J.R.* 136:1087–1091, 1981.

37. Gordon, R. E., Mettler, F. A., Wicks, J. D., Bartow, S. A.: Chest x-rays and full lung tomograms in gynecologic malignancy. *Cancer* 52:559–562, 1983.

38. Grumbine, F. C., Rosenshein, N. B., Zerhouni, E. A., Siegelman, S. S.: Abdominopelvic computed tomography in the preoperative evaluation of early cervical cancer. *Gynecol. Oncol.* 12:286–290, 1981.

39. Gusberg, S. B., Frick, H. C.: *Corscaden's Gynecologic Oncologic Cancer*, 5th ed. Baltimore, Williams & Wilkins, 1978.

40. Hamberger, A. D., Fletcher, G. H.: Is surgical evaluation of the para-aortic nodes prior to irradiation of benefit in carcinoma of the cervix? *Int. J. Radiat. Oncol. Biol. Phys.* 8:151–153, 1982.

41. Hamlin, D. J., Burgener, F. A., Beecham, J. B.: CT of intramural endometrial carcinoma: Contrast enhancement is essential. *A.J.R.* 137:551, 1981.

42. Hammond, J. A., Herson, J., Freedman, R. S., Hamberger, A. D., Wharton, J. T., Wallace, S., Rutledge, F. N.: The impact of lymph node status on survival in cervical carcinoma. *Int. J. Radiat. Oncol. Biol. Phys.* 7:1713–1718, 1981.

43. Hardt, N., Van Nagell, J. R., Donaldson, E., Yonada, J., Maryama, Y.: Radiology-induced tumor regression is a prognostic factor in patients with invasive carcinoma of the cervix. *Cancer* 49:35–39, 1982.

44. Hasumi, K., Matsuzawa, M., Chen, H. F., Takahashi, M., Sakura, M.: Computed tomography in the evaluation and treatment of endometrial carcinoma. *Cancer* 50:904–908, 1982.

45. Heller, P. B., Lee, R. B., Leman, M. H., Park, R. C.: Lymph node positivity in cervical cancer. *Gynecol. Oncol.* 12:328–335, 1981.

46. Jaques, P. F., Staab, E., Richey, W., Photopulos, G., Swanton, M.: CT-assisted pelvic and abdominal aspiration biopsies in gynecological malignancy. *Radiology* 128:651–655, 1978.

47. Jing, B. S., Wallace, S., Zornoza, J.: Metastases to retroperitoneal and pelvic lymph nodes: CT and lymphangiography. *Radiol. Clin. North Am.* 20:511–530, 1982.

48. Jobson, V. W., Girtanner, R. E., Averette, H. E.: Therapy and survival of early invasive carcinoma of the cervix uteri with metastases to the pelvic nodes. *Surg. Gynecol. Obstet.* 151:27–29, 1980.

49. Johnson, R. J., Blackledge, G., Eddleton, B., Crowther, D.: Abdominopelvic computed tomography in the management of ovarian carcinoma. *Radiology* 146:447–452, 1983.

50. Jones, W. B.: Treatment of chorionic tumors. *Clin. Obstet. Gynecol.* 18:247–265, 1975.

51. Kademian, M. T., Bosch, A.: The value of staging laparotomy in cervical cancer. Letter to the editor. *Am. J. Obstet. Gynecol.* 136:264–265, 1980.

52. Kademian, M. T., Buchler, D. A., Wirtanen, G. W.: Bipedal lymphangiography in malignancies of the uterine corpus. *A.J.R.* 129:903–906, 1977.

53. Katz, M. E., Schwartz, P. E., Kapp, D. S., Luikart, S.: Epithelial carcinoma of the ovary: Current strategies. *Ann. Intern. Med.* 95:98–111, 1981.

54. Kaupplia, A., Janne, O., Kujansuu, E., Kujansuu, E., Vihko, R.: Treatment of advanced endometrial adenocarcinoma with a combined cytoxic therapy. *Cancer* 46:2162–2167, 1980.

55. Kilcheski, T. S., Arger, P. H., Mulhern, C. B., Colman, B. G., Kressel, H. Y. Mukuta, J. I.: Role of computed tomography in the presurgical evaluation of carcinoma of the cervix. *J. Comput. Assist. Tomogr.* 5:378–383, 1981.

56. Kosiak, R., Mattingly, R. J., Hoffman, R. G., Barber, S. W., Satre, R., Greenberg, M.: Irradiation of paraaortic lymph node metastasis from carcinoma of the cervix or endometrium. *Radiology* 147:245–248, 1983.

57. Kottmeier, H., Kolstad, P. (Eds.).: *Atlas of Colposcopy*. Baltimore, University Park Press, 1972.

58. Kottmeier, H., Kolstad, P., McGarrity, K., Petterrson, F., Ulfelder, H. (Eds.): *Annual Report on the Results of Treatment in Gynecologic Cancer*, Vol. 17. Stockholm, Editorial Office. Radiumhemmet, 1979.

59. Lagasse, L. D., Ballon, S. C., Berman, M. L., Watring, W. G.: Pretreatment lymphangiography and operative evaluation in carcinoma of the cervix. *Am. J. Obstet. Gynecol.* 134:219, 1979.

60. Lambert, H.: Treatment of epithelial ovarian carcinoma (commentary). *Br. J. Obstet. Gynecol.* 88:1169–1173, 1981.

61. Lerner, H. M., Jones, H. W., Hill, E. C.: Radical surgery for the treatment of early invasive cervical carcinoma (stage IB): Review of 15 years experience. *Obstet. Gynecol.* 56:413, 1980.

62. Libshitz, H. I., North, L. B.: Pulmonary metastases. *Radiol. Clin. North Am.* 20:437–452, 1983.

63. Marglin, S. I., Castellino, R. A.: Radiologic staging of ovarian carcinoma — necessary or redundant? *Int. J. Radiat. Oncol. Biol. Phys.* 7:1091–1093, 1981.

64. Morales, P. H., Fayos, J. V.: Epithelial carcinoma of the ovary. *Int. J. Radiat. Oncol. Biol. Phys.* 7:1649–1654, 1981.

65. Morrow, P. C.: Classification and characteristics of ovarian cancer. *Clin. Obstet. Gynecol.* 22:925–937, 1979.

66. Mount, P. M.: The pathogenesis of ovarian cancer — developmental aspects and modes of spread. *Int. J. Radiat. Oncol. Biol. Phys.* 7:1087–1089, 1981.

67. Musumeci, R., DePalo, G., Kenda, R., Tesoro-Tess, J. D., DiRe, F., Petrillo, R., Rilke, F.: Retroperitoneal metastases from ovarian carcinoma. *A.J.R.* 134:449–452, 1980.

68. Musumeci, R., Kenda, R., Volterrani, F., Spatti, G. B., Luciani, L., Attili, A., DePalo, G.: Diagnostic and prognostic value of lymphography in patients with cancer of the endometrium. *Tumori* 65:77–85, 1979.

69. Novak, E. R., Woodruff, J. D. (Eds.): *Novak's Gynecologic and Obstetric Pathology*, 8th ed. Philadelphia, W. B. Saunders, 1978, pp. 380–384, 396–436, 476–503.

70. Order, S. E.: Key Note Address to ASTR, 1981. Monoclonal Antibodies: potential role in radiation therapy and oncology. *Int. J. Radiat. Oncol. Biol. Phys.* 8:1193–1202, 1982.

71. Ozols, R. F., Fisher, R. I., Anderson, T., Makuch, R., Young, R. C.: Peritoneoscopy in the management of ovarian cancer. *Am. J. Obstet. Gynecol.* 140:611–619, 1981.

72. Pagani, J. J., Libshitz, H. I.: Imaging bone metastases. *Radiol. Clin. North Am.* 20:545–560, 1982.

73. Perez, C. A., Askin, F., Baglan, R. J., Kao, M.-S., Kraus, F. T., Perez, B. M., Williams, C. F., Weiss, D.: Effects of irradiation on mixed müllerian tumors of the uterus. *Cancer* 43:1274–1284, 1979.

74. Perez, C., Knapp, R. C., Young, R. C.: Gynecologic tumors. In *Cancer — Principles and Practice of Oncology*. DeVita, V. T., Jr., Hellman, S., Rosenberg, S. A. (Eds.). Philadelphia, J. B. Lippincott, 1982, pp. 823–883.

75. Piver, M. S.: Para-aortic node biopsy in staging women with cervical, ovarian and endometrial carcinoma: A review. *J. Surg. Oncol.* 12:365–370, 1979.

76. Piver, M. S., Barlow, J. J., Krishnamsetty, R.: Five-year survival (with no evidence of disease) in patients with biopsy-confirmed aortic node metastasis from cervical carcinoma. *Am. J. Obstet. Gynecol.* 139:575, 1981.

77. Prempree, T., Patanophen, V., Salagar, O. M.: Influence of treatment and tumor grade on prognosis of stage II carcinoma of the endometrium. *Acta Radiol (Rx)* 211:225–229, 1982.

78. Prempree, T., Patanaphan, V., Viravathana, T., Sewchand, W., Cho, Y. K., Scott, R. M.: Radiation therapy of carcinoma of the cervix with extension into the endometrium. *Cancer* 49:2015–2020, 1982.

79. Pussell, S. J., Cosgrove, D. O., Hinton, J., Wiltshaw, E., Barker, G. H.: Carcinoma of the ovary—correlation of ultrasound with second look laparotomy. *Br. J. Obstet. Gynecol.* 87:1140–1144, 1980.

80. Quinn, M. A., Bishop, G. J., Campbell, J. J., Rodgerson, J., Pepperell, R. J.: Laparoscopic follow-up of patients with ovarian carcinoma. *Br. J. Obstet. Gynecol.* 87:1132–1139, 1980.

81. Reddy, S., Lee, M.-S., Hendrickson, F. R.: Pattern of recurrences in endometrial carcinoma and their management. *Radiology* 133:737–740, 1979.

82. Requard, C. K., Wicks, J. D., Mettler, F. A.: Ultrasonography in the staging of endometrial adenocarcinoma. *Radiology* 140:781–785, 1981.

83. Rouviere, H.: *Anatomy of the Human Lymphatic System.* Ann Arbor, Edward Brothers, 1938.

84. Rubin, P., Prabasawat, D.: Characteristic bone lesions in post-irradiated carcinoma of the cervix. *Radiology* 76:703–717, 1961.

85. Schwartz, P. E.: Surgical management of ovarian cancer. *Arch. Surg.* 116:99–106, 1981.

86. Severini, A., Petrillo, R., Kenda, R., DePalo, G.: The value of double-contrast enema in the assessment of ovarian carcinoma's diffusion. *Gynecol. Oncol.* 11:17–22, 1981.

87. Silverberg, E.: Cancer statistics 1984. *CA* 34:7–23, 1984.

88. Smith, W. G.: Surgical treatment of epithelial ovarian carcinoma. *Clin. Obstet. Gynecol.* 22:939–955, 1979.

89. Solomon, A., Brenner, H. J., Rubinstein, Z., Chaitchik, S., Morg, B.: CT in ovarian cancer. *Gynecol. Oncol.* 15:48–55, 1983.

90. Stuart, G. C. E., Jeffries, M., Stuart, J. L., Anderson, R. J.: The changing role of "second-look" laparotomy in the management of epithelial carcinoma of the ovary. *Am. J. Obstet. Gynecol.* 142:612, 1982.

91. Surwit, E. A.: Stage I cancer of the endometrium. *Arizona Med.* 37:29–32, 1980.

92. Thigpen, T., Buchsbaum, H., Mangan, C., Tak, W. K., Anderson, B., Vardi, J. R., Beecham, J. B., Marchant, D. J.: Invasion and hysterography in endometrial carcinoma. *Obstet. Gynecol.* 50:159–165, 1977.

93. Tyler, H., Kardinal, C. G.: Ovarian cancer: Current management. *Missouri Med.* 78:13–16, 1981.

94. Ulfelder, H.: Classification systems. *Int. J. Radiat. Oncol. Biol. Phys.* 7:1083–1086, 1981.

95. VanNagell, J. R., Rayburn, W., Donaldson, E. S., Harrison, M., Gay, E. C., Yoneda, J., Marayuma, Y., Powell, D. F.: Therapeutic implications of patterns of recurrence in carcinoma of the uterine cervix. *Cancer* 44:2354–2361, 1979.

96. Walsh, J. W., Amendola, M. A., Hall, D. J., Tisnado, J., Goplerud, D. R.: Recurrent carcinoma of the cervix: CT diagnosis. *A.J.R.* 136:117–122, 1981.

97. Walsh, J. W., Goplerud, D. R.: Prospective comparison between clinical and CT staging in primary cervical carcinoma. *A.J.R.* 137:997–1003, 1981.

98. Walsh, J. W., Goplerud, D. R.: Computed tomography of primary, persistent, and recurrent endometrial malignancy. *A.J.R.* 139:1149–1154, 1982.

99. Walsh, J. W., Taylor, K. J. W., Wasson, J. F. M., Schwartz, P. E., Rosenfield, A. T.: Gray-scale ultrasound in 204 proved gynecologic masses: Accuracy and specific diagnostic criteria. *Radiology* 130:391–397, 1979.

100. Welander, C. E., Pierce, V. K., Nori, D., Hilaris, B. S., Kosloff, C., Clark, D. G. C., Jones, W. B., Kim, W. S., Lewis, J. L.: Pretreatment laparotomy in carcinoma of the cervix. *Gynecol. Oncol.* 12:336–347, 1981.

101. Whitley, N., Brenner, D., Francis, A., Kwon, T., Villasanta, U., Aisner, J., Wiernik, P., Whitley, J.: Use of the computed tomographic whole body scanner to stage and follow patients with advanced ovarian carcinoma. *Invest. Radiol.* 16:479–486, 1981.

102. Whitley, N. O., Brenner, D. E., Francis, A., Villa Santa, U., Aisner, J., Wiernik, P. H., Whitley, J.: Computed tomographic evaluation of carcinoma of the cervix. *Radiology* 142:439–446, 1982.

103. Wijnen, J. A., Rosenshein, N. B.: Surgery in ovarian cancer. *Arch. Surg.* 115:863, 1980.

104. Young, R., Knapp, R. C., Perez, C. A.: Cancer of the ovary. In *Cancer—Principles and Practice of Oncology.* DeVita, V. T., Jr., Hellman, S., Rosenberg, S. A. (Eds.). Philadelphia, J. B. Lippincott, 1982, pp. 884–913.

105. Zornoza, J.: Needle biopsy of metastases. *Radiol. Clin. North Am.* 20:569–590, 1983.

21 HODGKIN'S DISEASE AND THE NON-HODGKIN LYMPHOMAS

Christian H. Neumann
Bruce R. Parker
Ronald A. Castellino

The lymphomas and leukemias accounted for some 4% of newly diagnosed cancers in adults in the United States in 1985. In 1985, projections were for 6,900 cases of Hodgkin's disease and 26,500 new cases of non-Hodgkin lymphoma, with a sex incidence slightly greater for males. In 1985, 1,500 deaths related to Hodgkin's disease and 13,400 to non-Hodgkin lymphoma were expected.[72,73]

Survival rates for Hodgkin's disease as well as for non-Hodgkin lymphoma have improved considerably over the last 20 years. This dramatic improvement in control over these diseases is ascribed to improvement in histopathologic and staging classifications, clinical and pathologic staging techniques and, most importantly, innovative radiotherapeutic techniques and the emergence of effective multiagent chemotherapy. Thus, 300 years after Malpighi's incidental description of lymphomas involving the spleen, " . . . Medicine has come close to a total therapeutic conquest of a once inevitable fatal malady, at least in the case of Hodgkin's disease . . . "[34,35]

In children aged 1 to 15 years, the lymphomas account for 10.6% of all malignant neoplasms in the white population and 14.2% of the malignant neoplasms in the black population. The lymphomas rank third behind leukemia and neoplasms of the central nervous system in this age group. Approximately 700 children per year are diagnosed as having lymphoma. About 40% of these children have Hodgkin's disease and 60% have one of the non-Hodgkin lymphomas. In children the five-year survival rate for Hodgkin's disease (95%) is better than in adults, with virtually all deaths occurring in children with stage IV disease at initial examination. The long-term survival rate for children with non-Hodgkin lymphoma (>70%) is also distinctly better than survival rates found in the adult population.[55]

This group of diseases, which are defined as primary malignant tumors of lymphoid tissue, consists of two major categories, Hodgkin's disease and the heterogeneous group of diseases collectively referred to as the non-Hodgkin lymphomas. Although much of the diagnostic radiology literature often does not differentiate between Hodgkin's disease and the non-Hodgkin lymphomas, these tumors differ in their histologic structure, patterns of appearance, responsiveness to various therapies, and overall survival. Thus, they must be considered separately. Furthermore, there are sufficient differences between children and adults to warrant separate discussions in these age groups.

The age-specific incidence curve for Hodgkin's disease in the United States is characteristically bimodal, with a peak around 30 years and a second peak around 70 years. Similar statistics are noted in Germany, Denmark, and Israel. Hodgkin's disease appears to be more prevalent in males than in females.[33,72] Both mortality and incidence rates for non-whites (predominantly blacks) are appreciably lower than those for whites. Hodgkin's disease in childhood increases with advancing age.[61]

TUMOR PATHOLOGY AND BEHAVIOR

Jackson and Parker developed a long-used histologic classification for Hodgkin's disease in 1944. The term *Hodgkin's granuloma* was assigned to the typical cases;

Hodgkin's sarcoma was assigned to a much more malignant variant seen in a small proportion of cases and usually characterized by an abundance of Sternberg-Reed cells; and *Hodgkin's paragranuloma* was assigned to another infrequent variant characterized by extremely slow clinical evolution, a relative paucity of Sternberg-Reed cells, and a relative abundance of lymphocytes.

Lukes et al.[44] developed a pathologic classification that appeared to have appreciably greater prognostic relevance and usefulness than the Jackson-Parker classification. In 1966, it was slightly modified at the Rye conference, and is now generally recognized as the standard histopathologic classification for Hodgkin's disease (Table 21-1). Variables in differentiating the types of Hodgkin's disease in this classification are given by the frequency and character of diagnostic Sternberg-Reed cells, Sternberg-Reed cell variants, the character and amount of fibrosis, and the relative frequency of lymphocytes, among others. The most common subtype is nodular sclerosis, with the more favorable lymphocytic predominance and least favorable lymphocyte depletion being somewhat equally divided, but less common than the mixed cellularity subtype.

Although the same histologic classification is used for children, the relative incidence varies somewhat. In children under the age of 10 years, there is an equal incidence (38%) of nodular sclerosis and mixed cellularity subtypes. Lymphocytic depletion is almost never seen in the younger child. In children aged 11 to 15 years, the relative incidence of histologic subtypes is the same as in the adult population.

For the non-Hodgkin lymphomas, the terms *lymphosarcoma, reticulum cell sarcoma* and *giant follicular lymphoma* were in common use until the 1960s. In 1956, Rappaport, Winter, and Hicks proposed a new histopathologic classification, which was revised in 1966.[66] In this classification they developed two broad groupings based upon a nodular or diffuse pattern of lymph node tumor involvement. These were further classified according to the predominate cell type, i.e., well or poorly differentiated small cells (lymphocytes), large cells (histiocytes), mixed or undifferentiated (Table 21-2). In each cytologic class, lymphoma with a nodular architecture tended to have a better prognosis than those with a diffuse pattern, and patients with lymphocytic lymphomas had a longer survival than patients with mixed and histiocytic lymphomas. Rappaport's classification gained wide acceptance and proved to be a useful tool in guiding treatment decisions, advice on prognosis, and comparison of the treatment results between different centers.

More recently, numerous classifications have been proposed to more precisely classify these tumors.[68] Lukes and Collins developed a histologic classification based upon morphologic appearance that categorized tumors according to T and B cell types. The Kiel/Lennert classification, also based on morphologic and functional criteria, placed greater importance on the cytologic type of lymphoma than upon the architectural (nodular or diffuse) pattern. A recent conference[68] adopted a compromise histopathologic classification based upon the above criteria, which is currently gaining increasing acceptance (Table 21-3).

There are certain significant differences between adults and children with non-Hodgkin lymphoma that make a different classification system for children more

Table 21-1. Rye Classifications of Hodgkin's Disease

HISTOLOGY	DISTINCTIVE FEATURES	RELATIVE FREQUENCY IN ADULT (%)
Lymphocytic predominance	Abundant stroma of mature lymphocytes and/or histiocytes; no necrosis, Sternberg-Reed cells may be sparse	10–15
Nodular sclerosis	Nodules of lymphoid tissue separated by bands of doubly refractile collagen; atypical "lacunar" Hodgkin's cells in clear spaces within the lymphoid nodules	20–50
Mixed cellularity	Usually numerous Sternberg-Reed cells and mononuclear Hodgkin's cells in a pleomorphic stroma of eosinophils, plasma cells, fibroblasts, and necrotic foci	20–40
Lymphocytic depletion	Sternberg-Reed cells usually although not always abundant; marked paucity of lymphocytes; diffuse nonrefractile fibrosis and necrosis may be present	5–15

Adapted from Rosenberg, S. A.: Report of the Committee on the Staging of Hodgkin's Disease. *Cancer Research* **26:**1310, 1966. With permission.

Table 21-2. The Rappaport Classification of Non-Hodgkin Lymphoma

NODULAR		DIFFUSE
	Lymphocytic	
	well differentiated	DLWD 8%
NLPD 19%	poorly differentiated	DLPD 14%
NH 3%	Histiocytic	DH 19%
NM 16%	Mixed	DM 7%
	Undifferentiated	
	non-Burkitt	DU 6%
	Burkitt's	BT 8%

Adapted from Garvin, A. J., Berard, C.: Comparative analysis of pathologic classifications: Current recommendations regarding new technical considerations. *Semin. Oncol.* **7:**234–244, 1980. With permission.

Table 21-3. A Working Formulation of Non-Hodgkin Lymphomas for Clinical Usage
(Equivalent or Related Terms in the Kiel Classification are Shown)

WORKING FORMULATION	KIEL EQUIVALENT OR RELATED TERMS
Low grade	
A. Malignant lymphoma	
Small lymphocytic consistent with	ML lymphocytic, CLL
CLL plasmacytoid	ML lymphoplasmacytic/lymphoplasmacytoid
B. Malignant lymphoma, follicular	
Predominantly small cleaved cell	
diffuse areas	
sclerosis	ML centroblastic-centrocytic (small), follicular ± diffuse
C. Malignant lymphoma, follicular	
Mixed, small cleaved and large cell	
diffuse areas	
sclerosis	
Intermediate grade	
D. Malignant lymphoma, follicular	
Predominantly large cell	
diffuse areas	
sclerosis	ML centroblastic-centrocytic (large), follicular ± diffuse
E. Malignant lymphoma, diffuse	
Small cleaved cell	
sclerosis	ML centrocytic (small)
F. Malignant lymphoma, diffuse	
Mixed, small and large cell	ML centroblastic-centrocytic (small), diffuse
sclerosis	ML lymphoplasmacytic/-cytoid, polymorphic
epithelioid cell component	
G. Malignant lymphoma, diffuse	
Large cell	ML centroblastic-centrocytic (large), diffuse
cleaved cell	ML centrocytic (large)
noncleaved cell	ML centroblastic
sclerosis	
High grade	
H. Malignant lymphoma	
Large cell, immunoblastic	ML immunoblastic
plasmacytoid	
clear cell	
polymorphous	T-zone lymphoma
epithelioid cell component	Lymphoepithelioid cell lymphoma
I. Malignant lymphoma	
Lymphoblastic	
convoluted cell	ML lymphoblastic, convoluted cell type
nonconvoluted cell	ML lymphoblastic, unclassified
J. Malignant lymphoma	
Small noncleaved cell	
Burkitt's	
follicular areas	ML lymphoblastic, Burkitt type and other B-lymphoblastic
Miscellaneous	
Composite	—
Mycosis fungoides	Mycosis fungoides
Histiocytic	—
Extramedullary plasmacytoma	ML plasmacytic
Unclassifiable	—
Other	—

Reprinted from Rosenberg, S. A.: The non-Hodgkin's Lymphoma Pathologic Classification Project. National Cancer Institute-sponsored study of classifications of non-Hodgkin's lymphomas. *Cancer* **49**:2112–2135, 1982. With permission.

clinically useful (Table 21-4). In children, the non-Hodgkin lymphomas are typically of a higher grade of malignancy than in adults and have a diffuse appearance in affected nodes rather than the nodular appearance frequently seen in adults. Clinically, the disease in children frequently has an abrupt onset, an extremely rapid and progressive downhill course until therapy is instituted, and a much greater predilection for central nervous system involvement than seen in adults. The currently used histologic classification of greatest value divides the disease into three subtypes: (1) lymphoblastic, convoluted or nonconvoluted; (2) undifferentiated, Burkitt or non-Burkitt; and (3) histiocytic, immunoblastic, or large lymphoid cell type. The lymphoblastic lymphoma in children is more closely related in its clinical manifestations to lymphoblastic leukemia than it is to adult non-Hodgkin

Table 21-4. Histopathologic Classification and Distribution of Diffuse Non-Hodgkin Lymphoma in Childhood

HISTOLOGIC CLASSIFICATION	APPROXIMATE FREQUENCY (%)
Lymphoblastic	30–50
Convoluted	
Nonconvoluted	
Undifferentiated	20–40
Burkitt	
Non-Burkitt, pleomorphic	
"Histiocytic," large lymphoid cell	15–20
Unclassifiable	5–10
TOTAL	100

Adapted from Murphy, S. B.: Classification, staging and end results of treatment of childhood non-Hodgkin's lymphomas: Dissimilarities from lymphomas in adults. *Semin. Oncol.* 7:332–229, 1980. With permission.

lymphoma. Burkitt's lymphoma seems to be specific for children and has a relatively characteristic clinical course as well as histologic appearance. The histiocytic, immunoblastic, and large lymphoid cell types in children are histologically and clinically similar to their adult counterparts.

Regarding non-Hodgkin lymphoma, the incidence of different histologies at initial examination is given in Table 21-2.[24] At initial diagnosis, the non-Hodgkin lymphomas are at a more advanced stage than is Hodgkin's disease. The distribution of involved sites at initial staging is noted in Table 21-8. Initial sites of appearance in children with non-Hodgkin lymphoma are somewhat different than in adults. However, the sites of presentation do correlate with the histologic subtype. Children with undifferentiated non-Burkitt or Burkitt's lymphoma of the North American variety have abdominal involvement (65%), bone involvement (20%), or cervical lymphadenopathy (15%). Lymphoblastic lymphoma involves the mediastinum in almost all cases. The bone marrow is frequently involved either at initial examination or shortly thereafter, and involvement of the meninges is

common if prophylactic CNS treatment is not instituted early in the course of the disease. Histiocytic lymphoma in children typically appears with either mediastinal or abdominal involvement. Skeletal lesions are seen in about 20% of patients. Involvement of the peripheral lymph nodes is common in the advanced stages of the disease.[46]

CLASSIFICATION AND STAGING

A variety of staging systems have been used to anatomically define the extent of disease at presentation. Since 1971, the Ann Arbor staging classification has enjoyed widespread use in Hodgkin's disease (Table 21-5).[7] Although not designed specifically for the non-Hodgkin lymphomas, this classification has been widely adapted to these diseases as well. Exceptions to this are in the childhood non-Hodgkin lymphomas, which some have chosen to stage differently (Tables 21-6, 21-7).[53,54]

In the Ann Arbor classification, a distinction is drawn between the clinical stage (CS), which is based on evidence derived from the initial biopsy, history, physical examination, laboratory tests, radiographic and radioisotopic studies, and bone marrow examination; and the pathologic stage (PS) which, in addition, is based upon gross and microscopic evidence derived from laparotomy, which includes splenectomy, liver biopsy, bone marrow biopsy, and additional lymph node or other tissue biopsies. Certain letter symbols can be used to indicate that tissue specimens were obtained from various organs or tissues, with the added symbol of + or − to indicate the presence or absence, respectively, of histopathologic evidence of involvement: S = spleen, H = liver, M = marrow, N = lymph nodes (para-aortic or others), L = lung, P = pleura, O = bones. A and B indicate the absence or presence of constitutional symptoms (fever, night sweats, weight loss >10%), respectively. The designation E is intended for extralymphatic disease caused by direct invasion from adjacent lymph node involvement, usually readily encompassed within standard radiation therapy fields (Figure 21-1).

Table 21-5. Ann Arbor Staging Classification*

STAGE	DEFINITION
I	Involvement of a single lymph node region (I) or of a single extralymphatic organ or site (I_E)
II	Involvement of two or more lymph node regions on the same side of the diaphragm (II) or localized involvement of an extralymphatic organ or site and of one or more lymph node regions on the same side of the diaphragm (II_E)
III	Involvement of lymph node regions on both sides of the diaphragm (III), which may also be accompanied by involvement of the spleen (III_S) or by localized involvement of an extralymphatic organ or site (III_E) or both (III_{SE})
IV	Diffuse or disseminated involvement of one or more extralymphatic organs or tissues, with or without associated lymph node involvement

The absence or presence of fever, night sweats, and/or unexplained loss of 10% or more of body weight in the 6 months preceding admission are to be denoted in all cases by the suffix letters A or B, respectively.

*Adopted at the Workshop on the Staging of Hodgkin's Disease held at Ann Arbor, Michigan, in April 1971 (Carbone et al., 1971)[7].
Reprinted from Kaplan, H. S.: Clinical staging classification. In *Hodgkin's Disease*, 2nd ed. Kaplan, H. S. (Ed.). Cambridge, Harvard University Press, 1980, pp. 340–365. With permission.

Table 21-6. St. Jude Children's Research Hospital Staging Scheme for Non-Hodgkin Lymphoma in Children

Stage I	A single tumor (extranodal) or single anatomical area (nodal), with the exclusion of mediastinum or abdomen.
Stage II	A single tumor (extranodal) with regional node involvement. Two or more nodal areas on the same side of the diaphragm. Two single (extranodal) tumors with or without regional node involvement on the same side of the diaphragm. A primary gastrointestinal tract tumor, usually in the ileocecal area, with or without involvement of associated mesenteric nodes only.
Stage III	Two single tumors (extranodal) on opposite sides of the diaphragm. Two or more nodal areas above and below the diaphragm. All the primary intrathoracic tumors (mediastinal, pleural, thymic). All extensive primary intra-abdominal disease. All paraspinal or epidural tumors, regardless of other tumor sites.
Stage IV	Any of the above with initial CNS or bone marrow involvement.

Adapted from Murphy, S. B.: Classification, staging and end results of treatment of childhood non-Hodgkin's Lymphomas: Dissimilarities from lymphomas in adults. *Semin. Oncol.* 7:332–229, 1980. With permission.

Table 21-7. Clinical Staging of Burkitt's Lymphoma

STAGE	EXTENT OF TUMOR
A	Single extra-abdominal site
B	Multiple extra-abdominal sites
C	Intra-abdominal tumor
D	Intra-abdominal tumor with involvement of multiple extra-abdominal sites
AR	Stage C but with >90% of tumor surgically resected

Adapted from Ziegler, T. L., Magrath, I. T.: Burkitt's lymphoma. In *Pathobiology Annual.* Joachim, H. L. (Ed.). New York, Appleton-Century-Crofts, 1974, pp. 129–142.

At the Ann Arbor conference, guidelines for the diagnostic evaluation of patients with Hodgkin's disease were established. In July 1969 at the Stanford Medical Center, a policy of submitting all previously untreated patients with Hodgkin's disease (except those with overt stage IV) to staging laparotomy with splenectomy was begun as a clinical investigative tool. The magnitude of the staging error when the stage is based only upon clinical criteria was clearly established and confirmed by others. The clinical stage may be changed by laparotomy findings in 14% to 48% of cases.[32] More often in Hodgkin's disease than in non-Hodgkin lymphoma, the exact determination of the pathologic stage significantly influences treatment decisions and prognosis.

At initial presentation, lymphocytic predominant Hodgkin's disease is usually associated with stages I and II, while lymphocytic depletion is often seen with stages III and IV. Mixed cellularity and nodular sclerosing subtypes are associated with intermediate stages. Anatomic patterns of involvement at initial examination are noted in Table 21-8.

For children, the distribution of patients aged 11 to 15 years at initial diagnosis by stage is similar to that seen in adults. Under the age of 11 years, children are much more likely to have isolated cervical lymph node involvement, occasionally associated with mediastinal masses. These patients with clinical stage I and II disease are equally likely to be affected by nodular sclerosing and mixed cellularity Hodgkin's disease.

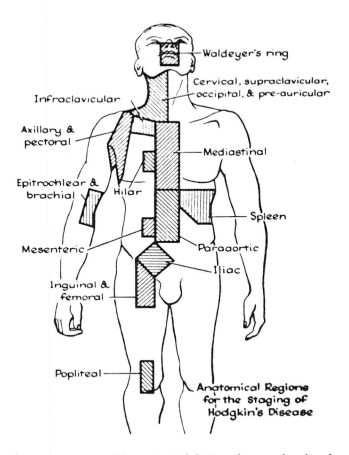

FIG. 21-1. Diagram of the anatomic definition of separate lymph node regions adopted for staging purposes at the Rye (1965) symposium on Hodgkin's disease. (Reprinted, by permission, from Kaplan, H. S. *Hodgkin's Disease,* 2nd Ed., 1980, Cambridge, MA: Harvard Univ. Press.)

Table 21-8. Anatomic Sites Involved at Initial Examination in Adults

	HODGKIN'S DISEASE (%)	NON-HODGKIN LYMPHOMA (%)
Thoracic nodes	65	25
Lung parenchyma	10	4
Pleural effusion	10	7
Para-aortic nodes	34	55
Mesenteric nodes	<5	51
Spleen	34	33
Liver	6	14
GI tract	0	8
Urinary tract	0	3

Note: considerable variation in anatomic sites involved at initial examination occurs in the various histologic subtypes in children (see text).

Reprinted from Castellino, R. A.: Newer imaging techniques for extent determination of Hodgkin's disease and non-Hodgkin lymphoma. In *13th International Cancer Congress, Part D. Research and Treatment* Miraud, E. A., Hutchinson, W. B., Milich, E. (Eds.). New York, Alan R. Liss, 1983, pp. 365–372. With permission.

PROGNOSIS

In 1,225 patients with Hodgkin's disease of all stages admitted and treated at Stanford University Medical Center between 1961 and 1977, the 5-, 10-, and 15-year survival was 80.6%, 66.5%, and 54.5%, respectively. Freedom from relapse was observed in 65.5%, 61.4%, and 60.8%, respectively. In this group of 1,225 patients, five-year survival and freedom from relapse was seen in 90.3% and 78.5% of patients with stage I disease at admission, in 87.6% and 69.1% of patients with stage II disease, in 73.6% and 61% of patients with stage III disease, and in 57.3% and 46.4% of patients with stage IV disease, respectively. Improvement in survival rates has occurred. The latest figures, based on patients treated between 1974 through 1979, show a five-year survival of 90.4% and freedom from relapse in 81.3%. The anatomic extent of the disease appears to be the single most important factor that determines outcome. The best outlook for long-term survival and freedom from relapse appears to be associated with the lymphocytic predominant subtype, followed by nodular sclerosing, mixed cellularity, and, finally, lymphocytic depletion Hodgkin's disease.[38]

According to data published by the National Cancer Institute, the overall five-year survival as of 1984 for the non-Hodgkin lymphomas was 48%.[72,73] Survival data derived from the Stanford experience distinguished between favorable (nodular) and unfavorable (diffuse) histologies. For favorable histologies, stage I and II, which include nodular, lymphocytic, well differentiated (NLWD), nodular, lymphocytic, poorly differentiated (NLPD), nodular, mixed cellularity (NM) and diffuse, lymphotcytic, well differentiated (DLWD), five-year survival was seen in 85% to 100% and five-year relapse-free survival was seen in 77.8% to 100%. For the unfavorable histologies, i.e., diffuse, lymphocytic poorly differentiated (DLPD),

diffuse, mixed cellularity (DM), diffuse histiocytic (DH) and diffuse undifferentiated (DU) of the same stage, the results were 65% to 75% and 41.5% to 66.7%, respectively. In stage III disease, a relatively favorable category was given to NLWD, NLPD, NM, DLWD, NH, and DLPD, which had a 4.5-year survival of 62.75% and relapse-free survival of 55% to 80%. The favorable histologies in stage IV, NLWD, NLPD, NM and DLWD, showed 65% to 95% five-year survival and 20% to 40% 4.5-year relapse-free survival. In the unfavorable histologies of stages III and IV, DM, DH, NH, DLPD and DU, four-year survival was seen in 25% to 50% and relapse-free survival in 10% to 25%.[25]

IMAGING PROCEDURES AND ASSESSMENT

The ability of a diagnostic method to detect or exclude involvement by lymphoma is best evaluated in studies based on pathologic proof. The criteria for the actual value of a diagnostic method includes its sensitivity, specificity, and overall accuracy.[50] Sensitivity is the percentage of patients with proven disease at sites where imaging tests were correctly interpreted as positive. Specificity is the percentage of patients with no disease at sites where imaging tests were correctly interpreted as negative. Overall accuracy refers to the percentage of patients whose imaging studies were correctly interpreted as positive or negative. The diagnostic accuracy of the various imaging tests will be presented in the discussions of the various anatomic sites.

Many diagnostic imaging approaches have been used, evaluated, and advocated. Those tests for which routine application has been replaced in favor of new methods, or because of a better understanding of the disease, will not be discussed (such as inferior venacavograms, gastrointestinal barium studies, and excretory urograms).

Thorax

Lymph Node Bearing Areas. In Hodgkin's disease, the intrathoracic lymph nodes are involved in two thirds of patients at initial examination, and this is most commonly observed in the nodular sclerosing subtype[23] (Table 21-8). The superior mediastinal lymph nodes are virtually always radiographically enlarged in patients who have any manifestation of intrathoracic disease, including lymphadenopathy at other sites. The lymph nodes in the pulmonary hila (bronchopulmonary group) are involved in 22% of patients. At times enlargement of lymph nodes will be noted in other sites, such as in the paravertebral region and cardiophrenic angles.

Radiographic findings in the chest in older children are similar to those in adults. In the age group 1 to 10 years, however, only 36% of patients have intrathoracic abnormalities identified on chest roentgenograms. Over 90% of these patients have anterior mediastinal lymphadenopathy, and 55% have concomitant involvement of the bronchopulmonary nodes.[61]

Intrathoracic lymph node involvement is less common in the non-Hodgkin lymphomas,[23] however, occurring in 25% to 30% of all newly diagnosed cases. Another difference from Hodgkin's disease is that at times intrathoracic lymph nodes, such as those in the pulmonary hilus and paravertebral or cardiophrenic regions, are radiographically enlarged without concomitant superior mediastinal lymphadenopathy.

In children, approximately one third of patients with lymphoblastic lymphoma present with anterior mediastinal lymphadenopathy. Ninety percent of patients with lymphoblastic lymphoma having T cell markers have mediastinal lymphadenopathy, while 10% of patients with B cell or Null-cell markers have such involvement. This presentation is much less common with the other histologic subtypes. Mediastinal disease in children frequently is rapidly progressive, and these patients commonly have or rapidly develop the superior vena caval syndrome or respiratory distress from tracheal compression.

Chest Roentgenograms. Posterior-anterior and lateral chest roentgenograms remain the mainstay of evaluating the intrathoracic lymph nodes as well as the region of the thymus, the lung parenchyma, the pleura, and chest wall. Most intrathoracic lymphadenopathy is readily detected by this method and serves to correctly stage the disease. Thus, demonstration of other enlarged nodes by more sensitive techniques, such as conventional tomography and CT scanning, often does not change stage or treatment.

Tomography. At times the detection of only minimal lymph node involvement or specific sites of nodal involvement within the thorax is of importance. In these cases, conventional chest roentgenograms may not be sufficiently sensitive, and full-lung tomography has been used with success. The latter technique delineates nodal enlargement of the mediastinum, which may not be seen on plain chest roentgenograms, particularly in the subcarinal regions and the pulmonary hilus. Tomography often provides additional information in determining whether there is local extension of lymphadenopathy into adjacent pulmonary parenchyma.

In a group of 243 consecutive patients with newly diagnosed, previously untreated Hodgkin's disease and non-Hodgkin lymphoma, all of whom underwent stereoscopic frontal and lateral chest roentgenograms and full-lung tomograms on the same day, full-lung tomography produced radiographic evidence of additional sites of disease in 21.4% of patients.[10] However, further analysis indicated that although new information was obtained, this information affected staging or treatment planning in only 1.2% of patients. We concluded that full-lung tomography had a low yield of additional valuable information when performed in a routine fashion, and recommended its employment in specific instances, which included evaluation of any equivocal findings on standard chest roentgenograms and further evaluation of the hilus (usually with supplemental oblique or lateral tomograms), if such information would affect treatment.

Computed Tomography. Computed tomography (CT) of the thorax has clearly evolved as the preferred imaging method in evaluating the mediastinum. The cross-sectional images have the advantage of delineating mediastinal anatomy better than conventional tomography, and, most importantly, provide information regarding the contents of the mediastinum, thus explaining what tissues or organs are causing the abnormality of mediastinal contour. Our experience is in agreement with the published results from others that CT indeed more precisely delineates the anatomic extent of lymphadenopathy within the mediastinum when compared with conventional chest roentgenography and tomography.[29] Furthermore, CT will at times reveal enlarged lymph nodes detected only with great difficulty, or not at all, on conventional studies, even when viewed in retrospect (Figures 21-2, 21-3). However, there is relatively little histologic proof confirming these CT results, and the incidence of false-positive (as well as false-negative) CT diagnoses is not known.

Evaluation of the hilus with CT has been viewed by some as being more difficult than conventional tomography, and by others as being as good or perhaps surpassing the information derived from more conventional studies. Once again, the absence of pathologic proof of these observations is unfortunate although understandable.

Gallium 67 Citrate Radionuclide Studies. Gallium 67 citrate radionuclide studies are interpreted as positive when areas of increased uptake cannot be explained by normal anatomy or tracer metabolism. These studies have found success in the hands of some investigators, but not in the hands of others, and their routine use in staging these patients is, at least in our opinion, questioned. It is reported that certain cell types, such as Hodgkin's disease in general and histiocytic lymphomas more specifically, are more amenable to detection with this technique. Gallium scanning appears to be more accurate in evaluating supradiaphragmatic, rather than subdiaphragmatic, disease.[30,63] The remarkable sensitivity of CT scanning in detecting mediastinal lymph node enlargement, as well as the very valid information derived from

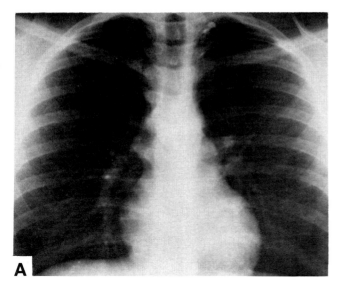

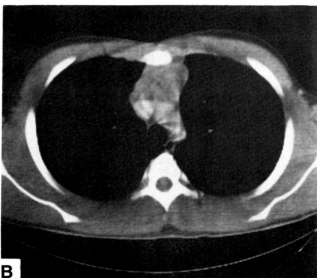

FIG. 21-2. Young man with newly diagnosed Hodgkin's disease. (A) A PA chest roentgenogram shows minimal widening with double contours of the upper mediastinum to the left of the trachea. Although abnormal, the findings are quite subtle. (B) A CT scan at the level of the aortic arch shows a large anterior mediastinal mass.

a critical analysis of conventional standard roentgenograms and full-lung tomograms, leads us to believe that instances where gallium scanning would provide important new information are rare indeed. Thus, our policy is not to use gallium scanning in staging these patients. We must point out, however, that others have found this technique to be of value.

Lungs. In 11.6% of patients with Hodgkin's disease at initial examination, conventional chest roentgenograms and tomograms will provide evidence of pulmonary parenchymal involvement.[23] The majority of such lesions

are identified on standard chest films, but there are those patients in whom full-lung tomograms are required to demonstrate such involvement.[10] In our experience, involvement of the pulmonary parenchyma by Hodgkin's disease at presentation has not been seen without concomitant enlargement of intrathoracic lymph nodes; furthermore, usually there is concomitant ipsilateral hilar lymphadenopathy as well (Figure 21-4).[23] Pulmonary involvement in children aged 1 to 10 years with Hodgkin's disease is unusual, occurring in less than 5% of patients at risk. Pulmonary involvement in older children occurs with frequency similar to that seen in adults.[60]

The incidence of pulmonary parenchymal involvement at initial presentation in non-Hodgkin lymphomas is lower (3.7%).[23] This lung involvement is not always accompanied by intrathoracic lymphadenopathy, at least based upon conventional radiographic and tomographic findings, and may represent the only site of disease in rare cases (Figure 21-5). Pulmonary parenchymal involvement is also uncommon in childhood.[15] In some cases, the pulmonary disease may progress so rapidly that it mimics infection or edema, thus delaying the appropriate diagnosis.[20]

Manifestations of pulmonary parenchymal involvement by nodular lesions, often with surprisingly ill-defined margins, are common. In Hodgkin's disease, radiographic evidence of cavitation is not uncommon. Spread of tumor along the bronchovascular structures can usually be recognized with confidence, as can the massive infiltration of a segment or lobe. A more difficult radiographic evaluation is the interpretation of the ill-defined margins sometimes noted with bulky mediastinal lymphadenopathy, since such findings could be caused by direct lung invasion from adjacent involved lymph nodes or simply by subadjacent atelectasis. We know of no reliable criteria to use to separate these situations, including information derived from tomography and CT scans.

Conventional tomograms certainly detect a greater incidence of parenchymal disease than chest roentgenograms.[10] It appears that CT scanning may detect further instances of pulmonary abnormalities than noted on conventional tomograms. However, there is little histologic proof in those cases reported in the literature, or from our own experience, to prove that these additional observations are in fact caused by histologic parenchymal disease. Studies of CT scanning in patients with solid tumors are somewhat sobering, since a high proportion of "additional lesions" in that patient population were unrelated to the patient's underlying malignancy.[70]

Pleura and Chest Wall. Radiographically detectable pleural effusions are seen in 7% of patients with Hodgkin's disease and 10% of patients with non-Hodgkin lymphoma at initial presentation. Pleural effusions do not nec-

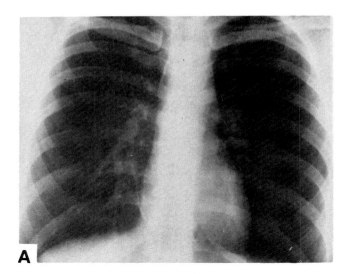

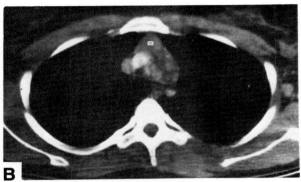

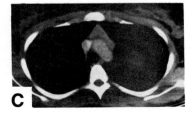

FIG. 21-3. Young woman with newly diagnosed Hodgkin's disease. (A) A PA chest roentgenogram is abnormal, with "fullness" of the superior mediastinum and minimal loss of the normal aortic arch contour. Computed tomographic scans just above (B) and at the aortic arch (C), show enlarged mediastinal lymph nodes. The thymus is also enlarged, presumably because of infiltration.

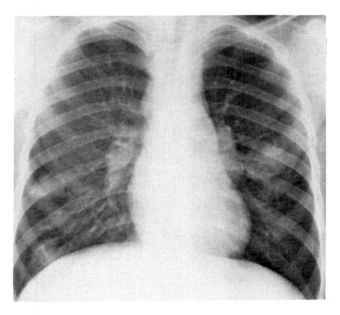

FIG. 21-4. A 14-year-old boy with newly diagnosed Hodgkin's disease. Multiple ill-defined nodular lesions are present in both lungs. There is also associated mediastinal and bilateral hilar lymphadenopathy.

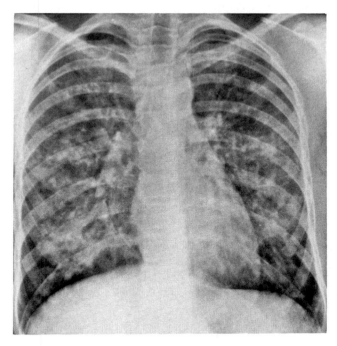

FIG. 21-5. A 30-year-old woman had diffuse, course interstitial infiltrates. Open lung biopsy demonstrated non-Hodgkin lymphoma of the lárge cell, histiocytic subtype. No other evidence of disease was found in the chest or elsewhere.

essarily signify intrinsic involvement by tumor of the pleural space. In fact, malignant cells rarely are recovered from such pleural fluid. Furthermore, the pleural fluid will often decrease following radiation therapy only to the enlarged mediastinal lymph nodes, which almost always accompany such observations. This suggests that in many instances radiographically detectable pleural effusions are related to lymphatic/venous obstruction sec-

ondary to enlarged mediastinal and/or hilar lymph nodes, rather than intrinsic pleural deposits of tumor.[23]

Pleural effusions in children with Hodgkin's disease are almost never found in the preadolescent age group and in only 6% of teenagers.[61] In children with non-Hodgkin lymphoma, however, pleural effusions are quite common and, in fact, represent the single most common roentgenographically demonstrable abnormality in patients with Burkitt's lymphoma, occurring in virtually all cases.[21] In these latter cases, however, the pleural effusions are most frequently associated with intra-abdominal disease, and involvement of the mediastinum or lung is rare. Of the one third of children with lymphoblastic lymphoma with anterior mediastinal lymphadenopathy, virtually each patient has associated pleural effusions.

Chest wall involvement at presentation is usually caused by local invasion from enlarged lymph nodes in the anterior mediastinum. Such invasion of the sternum, ribs, and soft tissues of the anterior chest wall, such as the pectoral muscle and breast tissues, can at times be appreciated on conventional roentgenograms or tomograms. However, the CT scan images clearly demonstrate such involvement with greater ease and precision, with such information at times determining changes in radiation therapy techniques (Figure 21-6). CT scans are particularly useful in demonstrating the subtle lateral extension of tumor in the extrapleural space around the concavity of the chest cage.

Virtually any organ or tissue within the thorax can be infiltrated by these tumors. Despite the many patients with extremely bulky lymphadenopathies, however, the incidence of obstruction of the superior vena cava or other manifestations of organ compromise are quite low. This is because these tumors seem to displace, rather than constrict, adjacent structures when compared with carcinomas. The diffuse histiocytic lymphomas are an exception, since they more frequently will cause obstruction of the superior vena cava.

The recognition of a pericardial effusion may be noted on conventional chest roentgenograms, although CT

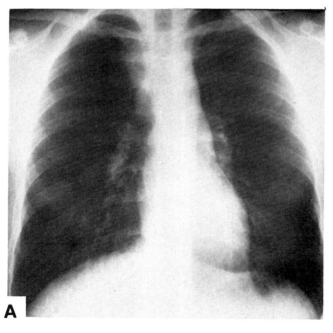

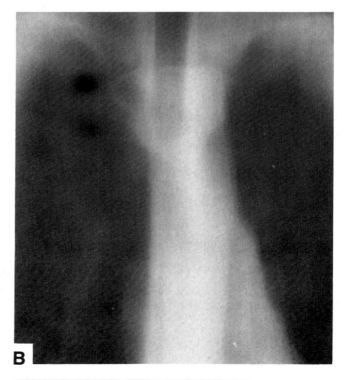

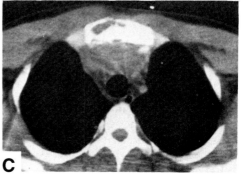

FIG. 21-6. Young man with newly diagnosed Hodgkin's disease. (A) A PA chest roentgenogram shows a superior mediastinal mass. (B) An anterior full-lung tomographic cut shows a destructive lytic lesion in the right portion of the manubrium. (C) A CT scan at the same level shows a large anterior mediastinal mass with invasion into the manubrium.

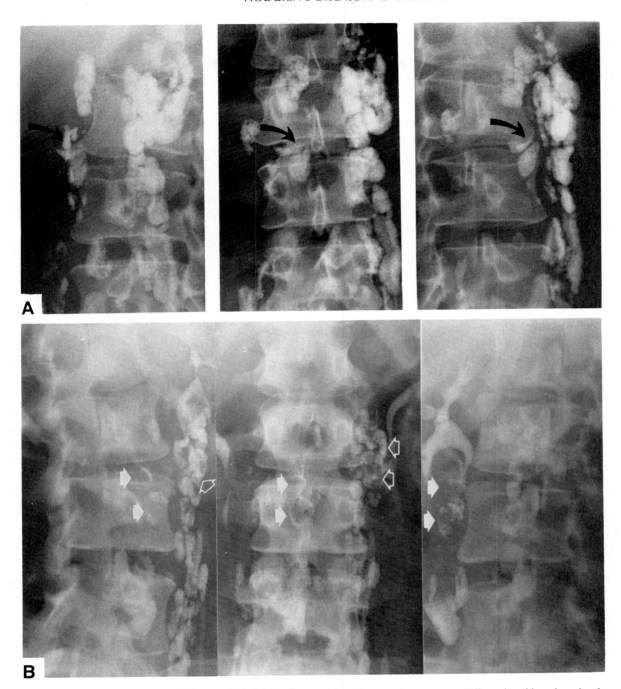

FIG. 21-7. (A) Young woman with newly diagnosed Hodgkin's disease. A lymphogram shows one partially replaced lymph node of normal size (arrows) that was interpreted as positive (biopsy confirmed). The other nodes are evenly opacified and were interpreted as normal (random biopsies were also negative). (B) Young woman with newly diagnosed Hodgkin's disease. A lymphogram shows several nodes of normal size that contain filling defects (closed arrows) or a foamy pattern (open arrows), interpreted as being positive (biopsy proven). Courtesy of Parker and Castellino.[60]

scans are more adept at demonstrating such findings. Echography remains the preferred technique in evaluating the presence of pericardial fluid. Pericardial effusions are usually ascribed to local invasion of the pericardium, which is often seen in the presence of bulky mediastinal masses.

Abdomen and Pelvis

A multitude of sites within the abdomen and pelvis are at risk of becoming involved by Hodgkin's disease and non-Hodgkin lymphoma in patients presenting with these diseases. The introduction of routine staging laparotomies in Hodgkin's disease and limited data from non-Hodgkin lymphoma patients have provided accurate incidences of disease at various sites based upon histopathologic proof. These incidences vary between patients with Hodgkin's disease and non-Hodgkin lymphoma, and between adults and children with these disorders, as indicated in Table 21-8. The following information represents the experience gained at Stanford Medical Center from staging laparotomies and, when appropriate, their correlations with various diagnostic imaging procedures.[27,37]

Lymph Node Bearing Areas. The retroperitoneum, abdomen, and pelvis contain an extensive network of lymphatic channels and lymph nodes that generally accompany major arteries and veins in this portion of the trunk.

1. The "retroperitoneal" lymph nodes lie adjacent to the inferior vena cava, abdominal aorta, and iliac (common, external, and internal) vasculature, as well as other major branches from these vessels. The retroperitoneal lymph nodes are often assumed to be confined to those lymph nodes opacified by bipedal lymphography, which represents a somewhat narrow definition. For example, the so-called "celiac lymph nodes" are those para-aortic nodes at the origin of the celiac artery that lie in the retroperitoneum and are continuous with the more caudal para-aortic lymph nodes but have assumed a somewhat different status simply because they are not routinely opacified by bipedal lymphography.
2. The mesenteric lymph nodes lie within the leaves of the mesentery. This group represents the continuum of the lymphatic network that drains into the para-aortic lymphatics at the origin of the superior mesenteric artery at the mesenteric root. For the purposes of this discussion, *mesenteric lymphadenopathy* will refer to abnormal lymph nodes within the mesentary itself rather than to nodes in the mesenteric root, i.e., at the superior mesenteric artery origin.
3. Perivisceral lymph nodes lie adjacent to major intraabdominal organs such as those nodes that lie in the splenic hilus, porta hepatis, and peripancreatic regions. These lymph nodes are not opacified by pedal lymphography, yet they represent a potential site for intraabdominal involvement.

The incidence of histologically proven lymph node involvement based on staging laparotomy data in patients with these diseases is noted in Table 21-8. Retroperitoneal lymph node involvement, predominantly documented by para-aortic and paracaval lymph node biopsies at and below the level of the renal vessels, occurs in one third to one half of patients with Hodgkin's disease and non-Hodgkin lymphoma. The incidence of mesenteric lymph node involvement in these two diseases at initial examination is, however, significantly different. Patients with Hodgkin's disease rarely (less than 5%) will have mesenteric lymph node involvement, compared with a greater than 50% incidence in the non-Hodgkin lymphomas.[27] Furthermore, when these lymph nodes are involved in Hodgkin's disease, they are usually normal in size, the involvement representing small foci of tumor scattered within lymph nodes of normal size.

In non-Hodgkin lymphoma, involved mesenteric lymph nodes are often moderately to massively enlarged, facilitating their recognition with imaging techniques. Splenic hilar lymph node involvement usually accompanies histologic involvement of the spleen. Extensive perivisceral lymphadenopathy generally is more common in the non-Hodgkin lymphomas (although systematic sampling of these lymph nodes has not routinely been performed in these diseases).

Bipedal Lymphography. Bipedal lymphography had been the preferred routine abdominal imaging study employed in staging these patients. This technique provides opacification of the majority of lymph nodes in the para-aortic and paracaval regions up to but not cephalad to the renal vascular pedicle, as well as the lymph nodes associated with the common and external iliac vasculature. The study provides precise information regarding lymph node size and position. More importantly, however, it provides fine detail images of intrinsic nodal architecture, which permits detection of architectural abnormalities caused by tumor replacement within normal-sized or only slightly enlarged lymph nodes (Figure 21-7), and allows identification of enlarged but otherwise normal hyperplastic lymph nodes in contrast to enlarged tumor containing nodes. This is particularly important in children, since 12% to 20% of children may have significantly enlarged lymph nodes secondary to reactive lymphoid hyperplasia.[14] Furthermore, the nodes retain the particulate oily contrast material for many months, providing a convenient method for serial assessment of lymph node size by surveillance abdominal roentgenograms to determine response to treatment or relapse.

Sensitivity, specificity, and accuracy data for lymphography are very good, with reported rates in the 90th percentile from centers with sufficient experience based upon laparotomy data.[13,31,47] Thus, for assessment of those nodes that are opacified, lymphography remains the most reliable imaging technique.[8] However, the technique is invasive and is a potential source of discomfort to the patient (and of frustration to some radiologists).

As a general rule, lymph nodes involved with Hodgkin's disease usually are only modestly enlarged and the architectural abnormalities are often focal, irregular defects rather than difuse "foaminess" (Figure 21-7). Visualized nodal involvement is often confined to limited sites and, when widespread, usually involves certain nodal sites to a greater extent than others. In contradistinction, patients with nodular non-Hodgkin lymphomas often mani-

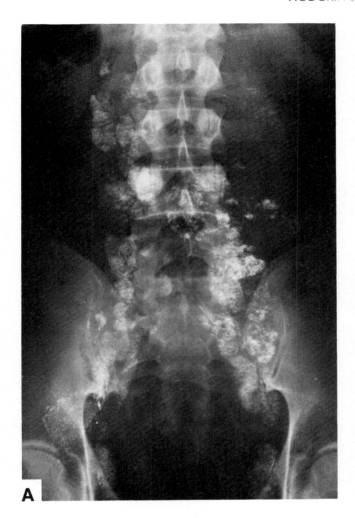

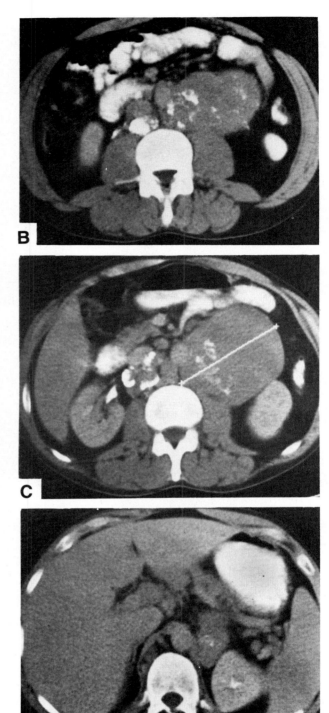

FIG. 21-8. Middle-aged man with newly diagnosed nodular non-Hodgkin lymphoma. (A) An AP lymphogram shows marked enlargement of all nodes, which have a foamy architecture that is characteristic of this disease. In addition, some contrast appears to outline the border of a larger left retroperitoneal mass. (B) A CT scan at the level of the lower right kidney shows a large retroperitoneal mass extending towards the left, with scattered lymphographic contrast. (C) A CT scan at the level of the right renal hilum shows further extent of the bulk of the retroperitoneal mass, with less contrast medium. (D) A CT scan at the level of the upper left kidney shows additional left para-aortic adenopathy. Furthermore, enlarged nodes are also seen in the retrocrural region, the porta hepatis, and possibly the splenic hilum. The precise anatomic extent of the disease is more completely delineated by the CT scan compared with the lymphogram. Reprinted from Castellino, R. A.: Computed tomography, lymphography, and staging laparotomy. In *13th International Cancer Congress. Part D. Research and Treatment.* New York, Allen R. Liss, 1983, pp. 365–372. With permission.

fest large, bulky lymph nodes that demonstrate a generalized involved pattern characterized as being "foamy," with all lymph node groups relatively equally involved (Figure 21-8). The diffuse non-Hodgkin lymphomas lie somewhere between these two generalizations.

Computed tomography (CT) is being used with increasing frequency in the initial staging of these patients.

Since CT scans do not portray lymph node architecture, a CT diagnosis of lymph node metastases depends upon an increase in lymph node size. When such nodes are sufficiently enlarged to produce moderate to extensive bulky masses, the CT findings are readily apparent and convincingly diagnostic (Figure 21-8). Increasing diagnostic difficulties are noted with lymph nodes that are only

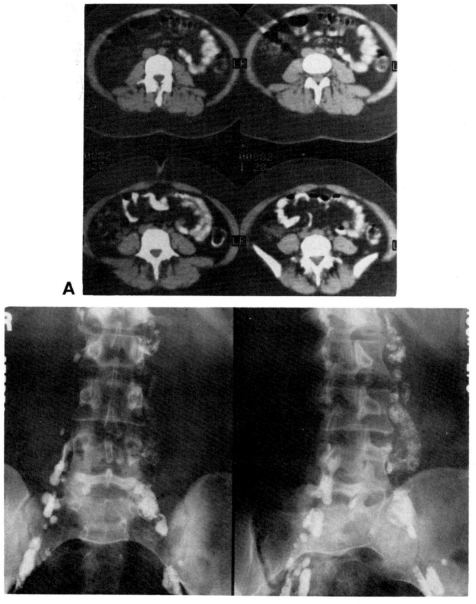

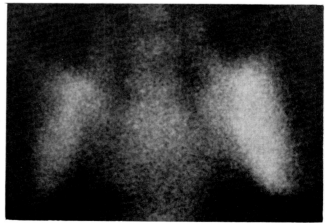

FIG. 21-9. Young woman with newly diagnosed Hodgkin's disease. (A) Contiguous CT scans at 1-cm intervals through the bifurcation of the aorta and IVC. There are moderately enlarged left common iliac nodes, which could be readily mistaken for the bifurcated aorta and IVC. However, careful tracing of the vascular anatomy avoids this trap. (B) Anterior and left posterior oblique lymphograms readily show moderately enlarged nodes with focal areas of replacement and foaminess in the left paraaortic and common iliac sites, interpreted as being involved by Hodgkin's disease (biopsy proven). Note also the dense left medial iliac wing. (C) Radionuclide bone scan with increased uptake in the medial portion of the left ilium, compatible with bony involvement.

minimally enlarged (Figure 21-9); and, nodes that contain tumor but are not enlarged will not be detectable with CT scanning. Computed tomographic scanning requires adequate surrounding fat to delineate the enlarged lymph nodes as well as optimum opacification of bowel to avoid confusing appearances that can lead to false-positive diagnoses. The relative lack of retroperitoneal fat in prepubertal children reduces the efficacy of CT scanning in this age group.

Evaluation of the para-aortic/paracaval lymph nodes is easier than evaluation of the pelvic nodes, since the relationships of the former to the aorta and inferior vena cava are readily identified, with the nodes being sectioned perpendicular to their long axis. In comparison, the pelvic nodes are frequently sectioned obliquely and can thus appear falsely prominent, and their relationship to the adjacent vessels is less well-defined in the pelvis. Mesenteric lymphadenopathy is detected by identification of rounded masses within the mesenteric fat, which must be shown not to represent nonopacified loops of bowel (Figure 21-10). Enlarged lymph nodes in the splenic hilus and porta hepatis are often best identified after administration of intravenous contrast medium to document that they do not represent prominent vascular structures.

Table 21-9 presents accuracy data for CT from a prospective evaluation of intra-abdominal lymph nodes in newly diagnosed patients with Hodgkin's disease and non-Hodgkin lymphoma based upon laparotomy findings.[8,13] The differences in accuracy data between patients with Hodgkin's disease and non-Hodgkin lymphoma are best explained by the fact that patients with non-Hodgkin lymphoma will often have more advanced and bulky lymphadenopathy than those with Hodgkin's disease. The accuracy data are relatively good for the retroperitoneal nodal groups, although not as accurate as lymphography in our experience.

Furthermore, CT appears to be more accurate in as-

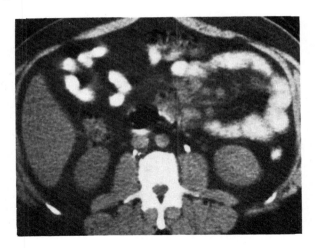

FIG. 21-10. Middle-aged man with newly diagnosed NLPD. A CT scan shows rounded masses (arrows) within the mesenteric fat compatible with enlarged, involved nodes. Note good opacification of surrounding bowel loops.

sessing the retroperitoneal nodes than the mesenteric nodes. This is particularly true in Hodgkin's disease, where mesenteric nodal involvement is rare and, when present, usually is within lymph nodes of normal size. Computed tomographic scanning of the mesenteric lymph nodes in patients with non-Hodgkin lymphoma has a higher yield; however, the value of such information for treatment and prognosis is unclear. Based on data collected on non-Hodgkin lymphoma patients, the sensitivity of CT in evaluating the mesenteric nodes was 67% compared with 86% in evaluating the para-aortic lymph nodes.[8]

Ultrasound evaluation of lymphadenopathy relies upon criteria similar to those employed for CT scanning, i.e., the presence of enlarged lymph nodes in order for a diagnosis of lymph node involvement to be made. The presence of gas and bone often precludes adequate evaluation of the entire retroperitoneum with ultrasound.

Table 21-9. LAG/CT/Laparotomy Correlations

	RETROPERITONEAL NODES		MESENTERIC NODES	SPLEEN	LIVER
	LAG	CT	CT	CT	CT
Hodgkin's Disease (n = 121)					
Sensitivity	14/20 = 85%	13/20 = 65%	Only 1 positive biopsy in	17/51 = 33%	1/4 = 25%
Specificity	85/87 = 98%	80/87 = 92%	92 patients — and that	53/70 = 76%	117/117 = 100%
Accuracy	102/107 = 95%	93/107 = 87%	was missed by CT	70/121 = 58%	118/121 = 98%
Non-Hodgkin Lymphoma (n = 24)					
Sensitivity	14/14 = 100%	12/14 = 86%	10/15 = 67%	5/11 = 45%	2/3 = 67%
Specificity	6/8 = 75%	6/8 = 75%	6/8 = 75%	10/12 = 83%	21/21 = 100%
Accuracy	20/22 = 91%	18/22 = 82%	16/23 = 70%	15/23 = 65%	23/24 = 96%

Adapted from Castellino, R. A.: Computed tomography, lymphography and staging laparotomy. Correlation in initial staging of Hodgkin's disease and newer staging techniques for extent determination of Hodgkin's disease and non-Hodgkin's lymphoma. In *13th International Cancer Congress. Part D. Research and Treatment.* New York, Allen R. Liss, 1983, pp. 365–372.[8,13] With permission.

Thus, in 30% to 50% of ultrasonographic examinations, not all abdominal and retroperitoneal node sites will be evaluable.[58] In addition, ultrasound studies are operator dependent, and results are, at times, difficult to reproduce. Accuracy data for ultrasound studies are scarce, since most reports are not based on laparotomy/biopsy proof; they often do not distinguish between Hodgkin's and non-Hodgkin lymphoma; and they do not specify the distribution of newly diagnosed patients versus patients with relapses.

Nonetheless, experienced ultrasonographers frequently generate imaging data similar to that obtained by CT. The occurrence of incomplete studies as a result of intervening gas and bone and the relative lack of understanding among many clinicians of the generated images have detracted from the routine utilization of this modality in staging these patients.

Gallium 67 citrate isotope studies are of less value below the diaphragm than above it (see section on Intrathoracic Lymphoid Sites). The sensitivity of the method within the abdomen and retroperitonium is reduced because of artifacts caused by the tracer metabolism.

Spleen and Liver. The spleen is involved in approximately one third of patients with Hodgkin's disease and non-Hodgkin lymphoma (Table 21-8).[27,37] Evaluation of splenic involvement using size as a criterion, such as determined by palpation or various imaging techniques (abdominal roentgenograms, CT scans, radionuclide studies), is a suboptimal predictor of histologic involvement.[57] In both Hodgkin's and non-Hodgkin lymphoma, approximately one third of patients with an apparently normal-sized spleen based on these techniques and usually with a normal-sized spleen at laparotomy, do in fact have histopathologic evidence of splenic involvement. Conversely, moderately enlarged spleens frequently do not contain tumor, although massively enlarged spleens almost always are associated with diffuse tumor infiltration. When the spleen is involved, the tumor deposits are frequently less than 1.0 cm in size, which is too small for current imaging studies to detect.

At initial examination, the liver is involved in 6% to 9% of patients with Hodgkin's disease, and in 14% of patients with non-Hodgkin lymphoma.[27,37] Liver involvement is almost never seen without concomitant splenic disease. As with the spleen, the histopathologic evidence of hepatic involvement at presentation is usually small infiltrations of tumor, often only several millimeters in size. Such lesions are usually not detectable with current imaging techniques.[13]

Computed Tomography. Computed tomography both before and after intravenous administration of aqueous contrast medium reliably predicts splenic size, as proved by correlation with spleen weight at laparotomy.[5] As noted above, however, a simple determination of splenic size is fraught with errors when used as a predictor for histologic involvement by tumor. Evaluation of liver size is more difficult and more subjective with CT scans than evaluation of spleen size. Markedly enlarged livers may represent widespread tumor infiltration, when the multiple other causes of liver enlargement can confidently be excluded.

At times, CT scans will demonstrate focal low attenuation defects within the spleen or liver that represent deposits of tumor. This is clearly the exception rather than the rule.[57] Our experience, in which interpretation was based upon an estimation of spleen and liver size or upon the identification of discrete parenchymal defects, yielded the accuracy data presented in Table 21-9, which is based on splenectomy and multiple liver biopsies at staging laparotomy.[8,13] As can be noted, sensitivity is low, reflecting the inability of this technique to detect these relatively small infiltrations by tumor. These data obtained with CT scanning, however, are at least as good as those reported with other imaging techniques, such as radiocolloid liver/spleen scans, and clinical assessment.[17,26,43,74]

An emulsified Ethiodol solution is being evaluated that, when injected intravenously, is taken up by the reticuloendothelial cells of the liver and spleen, thereby opacifying the parenchyma for many hours; this allows superb CT images of these organs to be obtained.[77] Improved lesion detection should certainly result, although some false-positive studies may be caused by visualization of the epithelioid granulomas that are seen in some 9% to 19% of spleens from Hodgkin's disease patients who have otherwise normal spleens.

Radionuclide Liver/Spleen Scans. Radionuclide liver/spleen scans performed with technetium sulfur colloid provide accurate images of liver and spleen size. As with CT scanning, detection of focal defects caused by tumor deposits is unusual, since areas of decreased isotope uptake may be visualized in the spleen or liver only if they are larger than 1 cm, depending upon their depth within the organ, and most tumor deposits are smaller than this size. Our experience with technetium sulfur colloid liver/spleen scans has been sufficiently disappointing so that these studies are not routinely employed in staging these patients.[43,74]

Ultrasonography. Ultrasound evaluation of the liver and spleen suffers from the same drawbacks as those described for CT scanning. Splenic and hepatic size can be predicted from ultrasound scans, and the larger focal lesions can be detected. A potential advantage that ultrasound would have over CT and nuclear medicine studies, however, may result from investigations into tissue characterization.[75] This information, which is based upon reflected waveform analysis rather than image interpretation, may provide a method for detecting tumor involvement that is beyond current image resolution. This work, however, is still investigational and remains to be proven of clinical utility.

Other Abdominal Pelvic Viscera. For all practical purposes, intrinsic involvement of the gastrointestinal tract, kidneys, pancreas, and other organs does not occur in patients with Hodgkin's disease at presentation, either in adults or children. This is not the case for those with non-Hodgkin lymphoma, however, particularly as regards the gastrointestinal tract, which is involved in 8% of adults and 18% of children (Table 21-8).

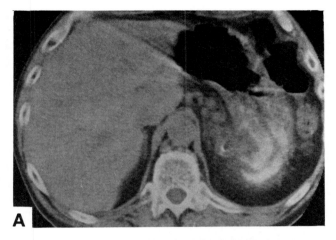

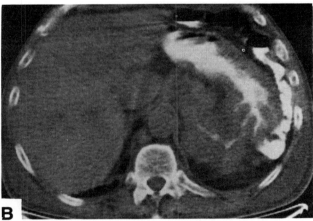

FIG. 21-12. Elderly man with newly diagnosed DHL of the stomach. (A) A CT scan shows celiac axis adenopathy and right retrocrural node enlargement. There is marked thickening of the wall of the stomach. (B) A CT scan several months later after (unsuccessful) therapy shows progression of the gastric and celiac axis disease.

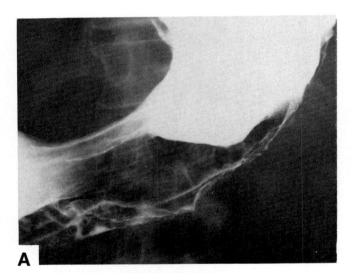

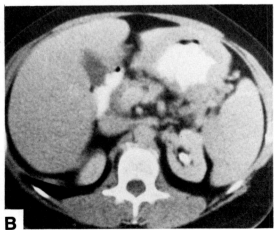

FIG. 21-11. Middle-aged woman with newly diagnosed non-Hodgkin lymphoma. (A) An AP view of the stomach during a double contrast upper GI examination shows an irregular mucosal surface and rigidity of the greater curvature. (B) A CT scan shows markedly thickened gastric walls throughout the entire circumference of the stomach, compatible with gastric lymphoma (biopsy proven).

Gastrointestinal Tract. Intrinsic gastrointestinal involvement with non-Hodgkin lymphoma can be seen in all portions of the digestive tract. Almost without exception, these patients have signs or symptoms that would ordinarily prompt further investigations with barium gastrointestinal studies (Figures 21-11, 21-12). Our experience with routinely performed barium studies of the stomach, small bowel, and colon in patients with Hodgkin's disease and non-Hodgkin lymphoma produced a virtual 0% yield of unsuspected findings.[12] Thus, we do not perform barium studies as a routine screening study.

The gastrointestinal tract of children with non-Hodgkin lymphoma is frequently involved,[9] especially in cases of the undifferentiated histologic subtype, including both Burkitt's and non-Burkitt lymphoma. Most typically, these lesions represent a primary disease process, which may be isolated to the gastrointestinal tract and the adjacent mesentery. Nevertheless, patients with primary gastrointestinal lymphoma should be thoroughly evaluated for manifestations of disease elsewhere in the body. The incidence of involvement with undifferentiated lymphoma in children varies from 35% to 60%.[45] Involvement of the small intestine is most common, and the terminal ileum is the single most common site in the gastrointestinal tract. Ileocolic intussusception occurs with such frequency that non-Hodgkin lymphoma represents the most common cause of intussusception in children over the age of 4 years. Ascites is frequently seen in children with intestinal involvement. The draining mesenteric lymph nodes are frequently involved, while the retroperitoneal lymph nodes are less commonly involved.

Gentio-Urinary Tract.

The Kidneys. The kidneys are intrinsically involved in 1% to 3% of patients with non-Hodgkin lymphoma at presentation, and this involvement is usually observed as an incidental, unsuspected finding. The intraparenchymal mass is readily delineated on excretory urograms, CT scans, or ultrasonograms (Figure 21-13). If the kidneys are diffusely infiltrated, such involvement may go undetected by these techniques unless the filtration is accompanied by nephromegaly, in which case the correct diagnosis can indirectly be suspected.

Urinary tract obstruction may be symptomatic or asymptomatic and should be suspected in the presence of bulky retroperitoneal lymphadenopathy. If hydronephrosis is suspected, evaluation with ultrasound is a highly sensitive, readily available, noninvasive method to provide this information. Excretory urography provides similar data. A caveat in children with non-Hodgkin lymphoma is the high incidence of uric acid uropathy, which may also lead to bilaterally enlarged kidneys.

Gonads. Involvement of the gonads is occasionally noted, particularly in females with non-Hodgkin lymphomas of the Burkitt subtype. Such organ involvement is distinctly unusual and is usually suspected by the presence of appropriate signs or symptoms. Ultrasonographic studies of the pelvis or CT scans readily evaluate these sites. Children with lymphoblastic lymphoma rarely have gonadal involvement, but recurrence in both the testes and ovaries similar to that seen in lymphoblastic leukemia is not uncommon. Ultrasonographic evaluation of the gonads is useful in these patients.

Miscellaneous

Bone. Involvement of bone[62] must be distinguished from bone marrow involvement. The former indicates tumor involvement of the cortical and medullary osteoid structure, whereas the latter indicates cellular infiltration of the marrow cavity. Bone marrow involvement is not detectable with imaging techniques, except perhaps indi-

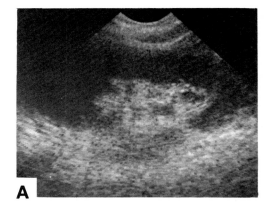

A

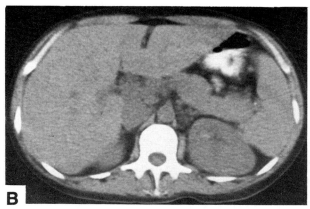

B

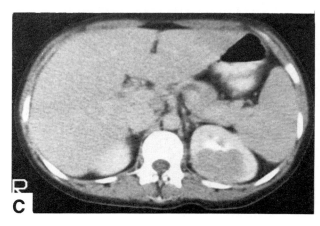

C

FIG. 21-13. Middle-aged woman with newly diagnosed non-Hodgkin lymphoma. (A) A longitudinal real-time ultrasound image through the left kidney shows an echopenic mass within the upper pole of the kidney. (B) An abdominal CT scan before I.V. contrast medium shows some prominence of the posterior parenchyma in the left kidney. (C) After injection of the contrast medium, the lymphomatous mass in the renal parenchyma is readily visible. Incidentally noted is adenopathy in the porta hepatis and probably in the splenic hilum. Reprinted from Castellino, R. A.: Computed tomography, lymphography and staging laparotomy. In *13th International Cancer Congress. Part D. Research and Treatment.* New York, Allen R. Liss, 1983, pp. 365–372.

rectly by indium-labeled bone marrow scans and now with magnetic resonance imaging (MRI). In a small number of cases marrow infiltration may stimulate osetoblastic activity in surrounding bone, causing radiographically demonstrable osteosclerosis. This is most commonly seen with leukemia, particularly acute myelogenous leukemia, but may be seen in non-Hodgkin lymphoma and rarely in Hodgkin's disease.

Cortical and medullary bone involvement may be focal or diffuse, solitary or multifocal, and lytic, blastic, or of a mixed pattern (Figure 21-14). When focal and adjacent to a nodal mass, such lesions are frequently designated as $_E$, indicating local extension rather than a manifestation of widespread (stage IV) disease.

Primary bone involvement is rare in non-Hodgkin lymphoma and probably does not occur in Hodgkin's disease. Although some series report that primary lymphoma accounts for 5% of all bone tumors, this figure is suspect. Careful evaluation of patients with an apparent primary bone lesion usually discloses evidence of tumor involving other organs, especially in the lymphoreticular system. Primary bone lymphoma is rare in children, more common in men than in women, and most frequently found in the femur or pelvis. Since a truly primary bone lesion is stage I, a vigorous search for other sites of disease is necessary to exclude stage IV disease before the initiation of therapy.

Conventional bone roentgenograms can reveal the presence of bony involvement either by Hodgkin's disease or non-Hodgkin lymphoma (Figures 21-9, 21-14). Radionuclide bone scans are more sensitive as an indicator of bone involvement although not as specific (Figure 21-9). Thus, bone scanning supplemented by detailed roentgenograms of those sites that are abnormal or suspicious on the bone scan represents a logical diagnostic sequence. Computed tomographic scans can also demonstrate osseous involvement and might be employed in the unusual case where the above combination provides ambiguous data.

Our experience with routinely performed radiographic skeletal surveys and routinely performed radioisotope bone scans in an attempt to detect asymptomatic, unsuspected bone lesions in Hodgkin's disease and non-Hodgkin lymphoma has been unrewarding. We do not routinely perform these studies on patients with Hodgkin's disease and non-Hodgkin lymphoma. Children with non-Hodgkin lymphoma have a higher incidence of bone involvement (18%) at initial presentation than do adults, but they also rarely, if ever, have asymptomatic disease.[9]

An interesting subtype of childhood lymphoma with common involvement of the facial bones is the endemic or African type of Burkitt's lymphoma.[78] These children typically have clinical manifestations of an enlarging jaw, and involvement of the mandible, maxilla, orbits, and adjacent structures is present in over 50% of affected patients. The incidence of facial bone involvement in children with the nonendemic or American form of Burkitt's lymphoma is no different than that found with the other lymphomas.

Patients with suspected bone involvement, based upon history, physical examination, or laboratory data, should undergo appropriate studies to evaluate the possibility of bone involvement. Once again, care should be taken not to confuse bone marrow involvement with osseous involvement. The former is readily evaluable with bone marrow biopsies, which are routinely employed in the initial staging evaluation of these patients.

Nervous System. Lymphomatous involvement of the central nervous system (CNS) is more common in non-Hodgkin lymphoma (10% to 20%) than in Hodgkin's disease (less than 1%). Among the non-Hodgkin lymphomas, the diffuse variety, especially diffuse histiocytic lymphoma, is more often found to affect the CNS. The most common site of involvement is the leptomeninges. Intraparenchymal and dural involvement is rare. The diagnosis of CNS lymphoma is usually made on clinical

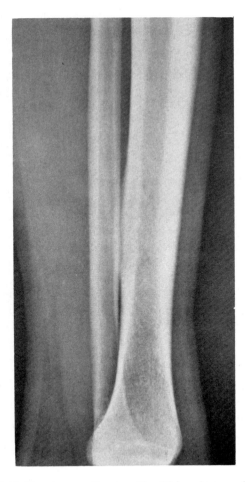

FIG. 21-14. Twenty-year-old man with a lifelong history of Wiskott-Aldrich disease who had a fever, leukocytosis, and redness and swelling over the lower right tibia. Radiographic examination demonstrated irregular lucency, cortical thickening, and periosteal new bone formation. Biopsy demonstrated non-Hodgkin lymphoma, undifferentiated non-Burkitt type. The patient did well for 6 months, following which he developed widespread systemic lymphoma.

grounds with supportive spinal fluid cytologic examination. Computed tomography has a relatively low (16%) yield, since leptomeningeal and dural involvement usually evades detection.[4,22] MRI assessment of brain, cord, and menninges hold great promise to become the imaging modality of choice over CT and myelography.

Involvement of the meninges is so common in children with lymphoblastic lymphoma that routine CNS prophylaxis is typically carried out. Computed tomographic scans and myelography are not routinely performed in asymptomatic children, since they will all undergo prophylactic therapy. Lesions of the brain substance in secondary or rare cases of primary lymphoma, often termed *reticulum cell sarcoma, microglioma,* or *histiocytic lymphoma,* are more readily seen on CT scans.[4] They most commonly involve the basal ganglia and corpus callosum and appear as intrinsically dense masses with homogeneous postcontrast enhancement. Intrathecal or extrathecal lymphoma in the spinal canal can be seen by myelography. Computed tomographic scans often provide similar information, especially for lesions of the lumbar spine.

Retro-bulbar tumors are especially well delineated on CT or MRI scans. Orbital lymphoma can be accurately detected by CT, although the findings are unspecific. In patients with lymphoma, however, diffuse lesions in the orbit or optic nerve enlargement are sufficient evidence of lymphomatous involvement. In the case of detecting intrabulbar lesions and determining their extent, ultrasonography can be of additional help, as it is with large retrobulbar masses.

IMAGING STRATEGIES AND DECISIONS

A multitude of imaging tests can be used to evaluate newly diagnosed, previously untreated patients with Hodgkin's disease and non-Hodgkin lymphoma for staging. A sequential approach is recommended based upon these assumptions.

1. It is valuable to perform imaging studies routinely to screen those sites that are frequently involved with tumor as long as the imaging test is sufficiently sensitive and specific. However, routinely performed imaging studies, even if associated with high levels of accuracy, are of little value when sites that are infrequently involved with tumor are screened.
2. Conversely, routinely performed studies are nonproductive when sites that are frequently involved with tumor are screened if the imaging technique is associated with a low sensitivity.
3. At all times, suggestive symptoms and signs at any site should prompt performance of the appropriate imaging examinations to thoroughly evaluate the possibility of disease involvement.

The imaging evaluation of these patients can thus be approached as follows:

1. Intrathoracic disease is frequently adequately assessed with standard posteroanterior and lateral chest roentgenograms. When further evaluation is desirable, CT scanning is generally the preferred test. A possible exception is in the evaluation of the hilus, which might be equally studied with 55° oblique hilar tomograms. Otherwise, CT is the preferred study when the following situations are being addressed:
   a. Evaluation of a suspicious or equivocal mediastinum.
   b. Evaluation of the "normal" mediastinum (which at times will contain enlarged lymph nodes demonstrable by CT) to pursue whether adenopathy might be present.
   c. Evaluation for chest wall involvement in the presence of bulky mediastinal disease.
   d. Evaluation for pulmonary parenchymal lesions.
   e. More precise definition of the anatomic extent of disease for treatment planning.
2. Bipedal lymphography still represents the most accurate imaging test for evaluating the retroperitoneal lymph nodes. Furthermore, the study provides a convenient means for follow-up regarding response to treatment or relapse.
3. Abdominal and pelvic CT scanning will more precisely delineate the anatomic extent of bulky lymph node disease. However, normal-sized lymph nodes that contain tumor deposits, at times readily demonstrable by lymphography, will not be detected by CT scanning. Mesenteric lymphadenopathy is relatively reliably shown by CT in the non-Hodgkin lymphomas. However, disease at this lymph node site is not sufficiently frequent in patients with Hodgkin's disease to justify CT scanning for this evaluation.
4. The spleen is frequently involved at presentation; however, the tumor deposits are often smaller than 1 cm, and correlation of splenic size with tumor involvement is unreliable unless the spleen is markedly enlarged. No imaging techniques, including CT scanning with a conventional water-soluble contrast medium, have shown sufficient accuracy or sensitivity to warrant their utilization specifically for this purpose.
5. The liver is less frequently involved than the spleen and when involved is usually involved by deposits smaller than those seen within the spleen. The above comments for the spleen are applicable to evaluation of the liver.
6. When bulky lymphadenopathy is present, it is frequently desirable to exclude urinary tract obstruction, which when present may alter treatment plans. Ultrasonography can be used to evaluate this problem unless the kidneys have already been studied as part of a prior CT scan.

7. Routinely performed roentgenographic skeletal surveys or radionuclide bone scans in asymptomatic patients have such a low yield that we no longer routinely perform these studies. In patients with any evidence of bone involvement, however, appropriate studies should be done.

8. Routinely performed barium studies of the gastrointestinal tract for screening purposes in asymptomatic patients have a similarly low yield. Those patients with non-Hodgkin lymphoma who have intrinsic gastrointestinal tract involvement almost invariably have compelling signs or symptoms that prompt an appropriate imaging workup.

IMAGING STUDIES IN THE POST-TREATMENT FOLLOW-UP PERIOD

The choice of imaging modalities for evaluating these patients after their initial diagnosis and staging is complex. The choice of imaging studies is often dependent upon the philosophy of the oncologic physician regarding frequency of such evaluation, as well as upon the availability of various imaging techniques and his or her expertise with such techniques in a clinical setting. Imaging studies are often requested to evaluate the response (or lack thereof) of the tumor to treatment, and, after completion of therapy, to evaluate relapses. The latter, i.e., evaluation of relapse, can be done for patients who are (1) felt to be free of disease based on standard clinical and laboratory assessment but in whom an imaging study might show evidence of unsuspected relapse; (2) suspected of having a relapse based on nonspecific signs or symptoms in whom a routine imaging study might show evidence of disease or for whom a more specific imaging study might be requested based upon the nonspecific clinical and laboratory findings; and (3) known to have relapse but for whom further imaging studies are requested to define the extent of the relapse for further treatment planning. Obviously, the yield of positive imaging studies is greater in the latter two categories than in the former.

Imaging studies to evaluate treatment response are chosen because they delineate the initial anatomic extent of tumor and can be objectively compared, i.e., a decrease in size over time. A common example is the gradual response to treatment of a mediastinal mass based upon a serial decrease in size as determined from conventional chest roentgenograms. Likewise, serial abdominal roentgenograms performed after lymphography will demonstrate a decrease in size of enlarged and abnormal lymph nodes based upon objective measurements on roentgenograms taken with the same technique. Similar information can also be obtained from CT scans (and ultrasound studies), but the significantly greater expense of CT studies and the overburdened schedule of such units makes frequent evaluation with this technique somewhat disadvantageous. On the other hand, if the CT scan is the only modality that clearly defines the area of tumor that is being monitored, then limited serial CT studies might well be indicated.[76]

At Stanford Medical Center, the medical and radiation oncologists generally follow their patients on treatment with frontal and lateral chest roentgenograms and abdominal films after lymphography at monthly intervals. Once a planned course of radiotherapy is administered, a relative radiation therapy "endpoint" is reached, i.e., further radiotherapy is rarely administered because of tissue tolerance limitations. This is not true, however, with many forms of chemotherapy, since cycles beyond the standard number can be administered if the patient can tolerate such further treatment and if there is concern about residual viable tumor. When such chemotherapy is stopped is often based upon observed stability as evaluated by clinical, laboratory, and imaging studies over approximately 3 months.

The radiation therapy and chemotherapy administered to these patients can produce changes observable on various imaging studies. It is important for the diagnostic radiologist to be quite familiar with these expected findings and not mistake them for evidence of tumor.[42] Such changes are not specific to patients with Hodgkin's disease and non-Hodgkin lymphoma and will be noted only to highlight some major observable effects and to serve as a reminder to keep this possibility in the differential diagnosis.

Radiation therapy can cause tissue fibrosis, such as is readily observed in irradiated areas of the lung on conventional chest roentgenograms, lung tomograms, and CT scans. At times there is loss of the normal homogeneity of fat in the mediastinum and retroperitoneum as seen on CT scans following radiation therapy, presumably related to alterations in the normal fat in these areas. Lymph node masses frequently shrink dramatically with radiation or drug therapy; however, residual "mass lesions" remain identifiable on various imaging studies. This is frequently related to the presence of fibrosis within successfully treated tumors.[41] At times, however, presumably viable tumor remains, since subsequent regrowth is noted after cessation of therapy.

Radiation therapy in standard treatment doses can cause calcifications within involved lymph nodes, particularly in patients with Hodgkin's disease. These are more frequently seen in the mediastinum but can be noted subdiaphragmatically as well.[49] Infrequently, the development of an enlarging mediastinum is related not to recurrent tumor but instead to peculiar growths of the thymus gland.[2] Radiation therapy can cause myocardial and pericardial disease; however, refinements of treatment techniques have markedly decreased these important complications induced by radiation therapy. The effects of radiation therapy upon the growing skeleton are well known. Important therapeutic modifications have been made to reduce the dose of radiation to the growing skeleton without sacrificing the excellent survival statistics currently achieved in Hodgkin's disease in childhood.[64]

Certain drugs used in combination chemotherapy can produce pulmonary changes related either to relatively acute "allergic" type responses, or to more chronic deposition of interstitial infiltrates or fibrosis.[52] The immunosuppression associated with chemotherapy (with or without associated radiation therapy) predisposes these patients to the expected increased incidence of infections, with both usual as well as opportunistic organisms, frequently manifested by opportunistic pneumonias. The induced thrombocytopenia might cause hemorrhage in various sites. Cyclic corticosteroid administration as part of combination chemotherapy may induce development of radiation pneumonitis or pericarditis in patients previously irradiated.[11]

The development of second tumors in this patient population deserves comment. There is an increased incidence of lymphoproliferative second tumors, particularly leukemia, in these patients, related in part to their prior treatment with chemotherapy and radiation therapy.[16] Patients with treated Hodgkin's disease are also susceptible to the emergence of tumor with a "changed" histology, i.e., to a non-Hodgkin lymphoma. This is particularly true of patients who have received chemotherapy, often with associated radiation therapy.[40] These patients frequently develop subdiaphragmatic disease. The development of such second tumors should be kept in mind when imaging studies depict new disease that does not quite fit with the familiar patterns of tumor relapse of Hodgkin's disease.

Percutaneous needle aspiration biopsy using imaging techniques such as fluoroscopy, CT, and ultrasound to guide needle placement, is of distinct value in assessing solid tumors, because a pathologic diagnosis of tumor can be made based upon well-established cytologic, rather than histologic, changes. A diagnosis of Hodgkin's disease or non-Hodgkin lymphoma, even in patients with prior established diagnosis of these tumors, is difficult to make on the scant material usually obtained with percutaneous needle techniques. The need for histologic, rather than cytologic, specimens severely limits the utilization of percutaneous needle sampling techniques in this patient population.

REFERENCES

1. Bakemeier, R. M., Zagars, G., Cooper, R. A., Jr., Rubin, P.: The malignant lymphomas: Hodgkin's disease and non-Hodgkin's lymphoma, multiple myeloma and macroglobulinemia. In *Clinical Oncology for Medical Students and Physicians: A Multidisciplinary Approach*, 6th ed. Rubin P. (Ed.). New York American Cancer Society, 1983, pp. 346–369.
2. Baron, R. L., Sagel, S. S., Baglan, R. J.: Thymic cysts following radiation therapy for Hodgkin's disease. *Radiology* 141:593, 1981.
3. Bennett, J. M. (Ed.): *Lymphomas I.* Boston, Martinus Nijhoff, 1981.
4. Brant-Zawadski, M., Enzmann, D.: CT brain scanning in patients with lymphoma. *Radiology* 129:67–71, 1978.
5. Breiman, R. S., Castellino, R. A., Harell, G. S., Marshall, W. H., Glatstein, E., Kaplan, H. S.: CT-pathologic correlations in Hodgkin's disease and non-Hodgkin's lymphoma. *Radiology* 126:159–166, 1978.
6. Canellos, G. P. (Ed.): The lymphomas. *Clin. Haematol.* 8:529–719, 1979.
7. Carbone, P. P., Kaplan, H. S., Musshoff, K., Smithers, E. W., Tubiana, M.: Report of the committee on Hodgkin's disease staging. *Cancer Res.* 31:1860–1861, 1971.
8. Castellino, R. A.: Newer imaging techniques for extent determination of Hodgkin's disease and non-Hodgkin's lymphoma. In *13th International Cancer Congress, Part D. Research and Treatment.* Miraud, E. A., Hutchinson, W. B., Milich, E. (Eds.), New York, Allen R. Liss, 1983, pp. 365–372.
9. Castellino, R. A., Bellani, F. F., Gasparini, M., Musumeci, R.: Radiographic findings in previously untreated children with non-Hodgkin's lymphoma. *Radiology* 117:657–663, 1975.
10. Castellino, R. A., Filly, R., Blank, N.: Routine full-lung tomography in the initial staging and treatment planning of patients with Hodgkin's disease and non-Hodgkin's lymphoma. *Cancer* 38:1130–1136, 1976.
11. Castellino, R. A., Glatstein, E., Turbo, M. M., Rosenberg, S., Kaplan, H. S.: Latent radiation injury of lungs or heart activated by steroid withdrawal. *Ann. Intern. Med.* 80:593–599, 1974.
12. Castellino, R. A., Goffinet, D. R., Blank, N., Parker, B. R., Kaplan, H. S.: The role of radiography in the staging of non-Hodgkin's lymphoma with laparotomy correlation. *Radiology* 110:329–338, 1973.
13. Castellino, R. A., Hoppe, R. T., Blank, N., Young, S. W., Neumann, C. H., Rosenberg, S. A., Kaplan, H. S.: CT, lymphography and staging laparotomy correlations in initial staging of Hodgkin's disease. *A.J.R.* 143:37–41, 1984.
14. Castellino, R. A., Musumeci, R., Markovits, P.: Lymphography. In *Pediatric Oncologic Radiology,* Parker, B. R., Castellino, R. A. (Eds.). St. Louis, C. V. Mosby, 1977, pp. 58–84.
15. Castellino, R. A., Parker, B. R.: Non-Hodgkin's lymphoma. In *Pediatric Oncologic Radiology,* Parker, B. R., Castellino, R. A. (Eds.). St. Louis, C. V. Mosby, 1977, pp. 183–208.
16. Coleman, C. N., Williams, C. G., Flint, A., Glatstein, E. G., Rosenberg, S. A., Kaplan, H. S.: Hematologic neoplasia in patients treated for Hodgkin's disease. *N. Engl. J. Med.* 297:1249–1252, 1977.
17. Czembirek, H., Neumann, C., Haydl, J., et al.: Angiographie, Scintigraphie and Ultraschall zum Nacheis von Milz und Leberbefall bei Morbus Hodgkin. *Fortschr. Rontgenstrahlen* 123:403–408, 1975.
18. DeVita, V. T., Jr., Hellman, S.: Hodgkin's disease and non-Hodgkin's lymphomas. In *Cancer—Principles and Practice of Oncology.* DeVita, V. T., Jr., Hellman, S., Rosenberg, S. A. (Eds.). Philadelphia, J. B. Lippincott, 1982, pp. 1331–1401.
19. DeVita, V. T. Jr., Somon, R. M., Hubbard, S. M., DeVita, V. T., Jr., Simon, R. M., Hubbard, S. M., Young, R. C., Berard, C. W., Moxley, J. H., Frei, E., Carbone, P. P., Canellos, G. P.: Curability of advanced Hodgkin's disease with chemotherapy. Long-term follow-up of MOPP-treated patients at the National Cancer Institute. (In press.)
20. Dunnick, N. R., Parker, B. R., Castellino, R. A.: Rapid onset of pulmonary infiltration due to histiocytic lymphoma. *Radiology* 118:281–285, 1976.
21. Dunnick, N. R., Reaman, G. H., Head, G. L., Shawker, T. H., Ziegler, J. L.: Radiographic manifestations of Burkitt's lymphoma in American patients. *A.J.R.* 132:1–6, 1979.
22. Enzmann, D., Krikorian, J., Norman, D., Kramer, R., Pollock, J.,

Faer, M.: CT in primary reticulum cell sarcoma of the brain. *Radiology* 130:165–170, 1979.

23. Filly, R., Blank, N., Castellino, R. A.: Radiographic distribution of intrathoracic disease in previously untreated patients with Hodgkin's disease and non-Hodgkin's lymphoma. *Radiology* 120:277–281, 1976.

24. Garvin, A. J., Berard, C.: Comparative analysis of pathologic classifications: Current recommendations regarding new technical considerations. *Semin. Oncol.* 7:234–244, 1980.

25. Glatstein, E., Donaldson, S. S., Rosenberg, S. A., Kaplan, H. S.: Combined modality therapy in malignant lymphomas. *Cancer Treat. Rep.* 61:1199–1207, 1977.

26. Glees, T. P., Taylor, K. T. W., Gazet, J. C., Peckham, M. C., McCready, V. R.: Accuracy of gray scale ultrasonography of liver and spleen in Hodgkin's disease and other lymphomas compared with isotope scanx. *Clin. Radiol.* 28:233–238, 1977.

27. Goffinet, D. R., Warnke, R., Dunnick, N. R., Castellino, R., Glatstein, E., Nelsen, T. S., Dorfman, R. F., Rosenberg, S. A., Kaplan, H. S.: Clinical and surgical (laparotomy) evaluation of patients with non-Hodgkin's lymphomas. *Cancer Treat. Rep.* 61:981–992, 1977.

28. Golomb, H. M. (Ed.): Non-Hodgkin's lymphoma. *Semin. Oncol.* 7: 221–356, 1980.

29. Heitzmann, E. R., Goldwin, R. L., Proto, A. V.: Radiological analysis of the mediastinum utilizing computed tomography. *Radiol. Clin. North Am.* 15:309–329, 1977.

30. Johnston, G. S., Go, M. F., Benua, R. S., Larson, S. M., Andrews, G. A., Hubner, K. F.: Gallium-67 citrate imaging in Hodgkin's disease. Final report of cooperative group. *J. Nucl. Med.* 18:692–698, 1977.

31. Kademian, M., Wirtanen, G.: Accuracy of bipedal lymphography in Hodgkin's disease. *A.J.R.* 129:1041, 1977.

32. Kaplan, H. S.: Clinical staging classification. In *Hodgkin's Disease*, 2nd ed. Kaplan, H. S. (Ed.). Cambridge, Harvard University Press, 1980, pp. 340–365.

33. Kaplan, H. S.: Etiology and epidemiology, In *Hodgkin's Disease*, 2nd ed. Kaplan, H. S. (Ed.). Cambridge, Harvard University Press, 1980, pp. 16–51.

34. Kaplan, H. S.: Historical aspects. In *Hodgkin's Disease*, 2nd ed. Kaplan, H. S. (Ed.). Cambridge, Harvard University Press, 1980, pp. 1–15.

35. Kaplan, H. S.: Hodgkin's disease, multidisciplinary contributions to the conquest of a neoplasm. Erskine Memorial Lecture. *Radiology* 123:551–558, 1976.

36. Kaplan, H. S.: *Hodgkin's disease*, 2nd ed. Kaplan, H. S. (Ed.). Cambridge, Harvard University Press, 1980.

37. Kaplan, H. S.: Patterns of anatomic involvement. In *Hodgkin's Disease*, 2nd ed. Kaplan, H. S. (Ed.). Cambridge, Harvard University Press, 1980, pp. 280–359.

38. Kaplan, H. S.: Prognosis. In *Hodgkin's Disease*, 2nd ed. Kaplan, H. S. (Ed.). Cambridge, Harvard University Press, 1980, pp. 548–597.

39. Keller, A. R., Kaplan, H. S., Lukes, R. J., Rappaport, H.: Correlation of histopathology with other prognostic indicators in Hodgkin's disease. *Cancer* 22:487–492, 1968.

40. Krikorian, J. G., Burke, G. S., Rosenberg, S. A., Kaplan, H. S.: The occurance of non-Hodgkin's lymphoma following therapy for Hodgkin's disease. *N. Engl. J. Med.* 300:452–458, 1979.

41. Lewis, E., Bernardino, M. E., Salvador, P. G., Cabanillas, F. F., Barnes, P. A., Thomas, J. L.: Post-therapy CT-detected mass in lymphoma patients. Is it viable tissue? *J. Comput. Assist. Tomogr.* 6:792–795, 1982.

42. Libshitz, H. E. (Ed.): *Diagnostic Roentgenology of Radiotherapy Change*. Baltimore, Williams & Wilkins, 1979.

43. Lipton, M. J., DeNardo, G. L., Silverman, S., Glatstein, E.: Evaluation of the liver and spleen in Hodgkin's disease in the value of hepatic scintigraphy. *Am. J. Med.* 52:356–361, 1972.

44. Lukes, R. J., Butler, J. J., Hicks, E. B.: Natural history of Hodgkin's disease as related to its pathologic picture. *Cancer* 19:317–344, 1966.

45. Magrath, I.: Malignant lymphomas. In *Cancer in the Young*. Levine, A. S., (Ed.). New York, Masson Publishing, 1982, pp. 508–509.

46. Magrath, I. T., Ziegler, J. L.: Bone marrow involvement in Burkitt's lymphoma and its relationship to acute B-cell leukemia. *Leuk. Res.* 4:33–59, 1980.

47. Marglin, S., Castellino, R. A.: Lymphographic accuracy in 623 consecutive, previously untreated cases of Hodgkin's disease and non-Hodgkin's lymphoma. *Radiology* 140:351–353, 1981.

48. McKelvey, E. M., Gottlieb, J. A., Wilson, H. E., Haut, A., Talley, R. W., Stephens, R., Lane, M., Gamble, J., Jones, S. E., Grozea, P. N., Gutterman, J., Coltman, C., Moon, T. E.: Hydroxyldaunomycin (Adriamycin) combination chemotherapy in malignant lymphoma. *Cancer* 38:1484–1493, 1976.

49. McLennan, T. W., Castellino, R. A.: Calcification in pelvic lymph nodes containing Hodgkin's disease following radiotherapy. *Radiology* 115:87, 1975.

50. McNeil, B. J., Keeler, E., Edelstein, S. J.: Primer and certain elements of medical decision making. *N. Engl. J. Med.* 293:211–215, 1975.

51. Million, R. R.: The lymphomatous diseases. In *Textbook of Radiotherapy*, 3rd ed. Fletcher, G. H. (Ed.). Philadelphia, Lea & Febiger, 1980, pp. 584–636.

52. Morrison, D. A., Goldman, A. L.: Radiographic patterns of drug-induced lung disease. *Radiology* 131:299, 1979.

53. Murphy, S. B.: Prognostic factors and obstacles to the cure of non-Hodgkin's lymphoma. *Semin. Oncol.* 4:265–271, 1977.

54. Murphy, S. B.: Childhood non-Hodgkin's lymphoma. *N. Engl. J. Med.* 299:1446–1448, 1978.

55. Murphy, S. B., Hutsu, H.: A randomized trial of combined modality therapy of childhood non-Hodgkin's lymphoma. *Cancer* 45:630–637, 1980.

56. Nathwani, B. N., Kim, H., Rappaport, H., Solomon, J., Fox, M.: Non-Hodgkin's lymphomas—a clinico-pathologic study comparing two classifications. *Cancer* 41:303–325, 1978.

57. Neumann, C. H., Castellino, R. A.: CT-assessment of splenic involvement by Hodgkin's disease and non-Hodgkin's lymphoma. *Tumor Diagnostik and Therapie* 3:113–115, 1984.

58. Neumann, C. H., Robert, N. J., Rosenthal, D., Canellos, G.: Clinical value of ultrasonography for the management of non-Hodgkin's lymphoma patients as compared with abdominal computed tomography. *J. Comput. Assist. Tomogr.* 7:666–669, 1983.

59. Non-Hodgkin's Lymphoma Pathologic Classification Project. National Cancer Institute sponsored study of classifications of non-Hodgkin's lymphomas. *Cancer* 49:2112–2135, 1982.

60. Parker, B. R., Castellino, R. A.: Hodgkin's disease. In *Pediatric Oncologic Radiology*. Parker, B. R., Castellino, R. A. (Eds.). St. Louis, C. V. Mosby, 1977, pp. 160–182.

61. Parker, B. R., Castellino, R. A., Kaplan, H. S.: Pediatric Hodgkin's disease. I. Radiographic evaluation. *Cancer* 35:2430–2435, 1976.

62. Parker, B. R., Marglin, S. I., Castellino, R. A.: Skeletal manifestations of leukemia, Hodgkin disease and non-Hodgkin lymphoma. *Semin. Roentgenol.* 15:302, 1980.

63. Pirushy, St. M., Heutzin, R. E.: Gallium-67 tumor scanning. *Semin. Nucl. Med.* 6:397–408, 1976.

64. Probert, J. C., Parker, B. R., Kaplan, H. S.: Growth retardation in children after megavoltage irradiation of the spine. *Cancer* 32:634–639, 1973.

65. Proceedings of the Symposium on Contemporary Issues in Hodgkin's Disease: Biology, Staging, and Treatment. *Cancer Treat. Rep.* 66:601–1071, 1982.

66. Rappaport, H.: Tumors of the hematopoietic system. *Atlas of Tumor Pathology*, Sec. Fascicle 8. Washington, D.C., Armed Forces Institute of Pathology, 1966.

67. Rosenberg, S. A.: Hodgkin's disease. In *Cecil's Textbook of Medicine*. Beeson, P. B., McDermott, W., Wyngaarden, J. B. (Eds.). Philadelphia, W. B. Saunders, 1982, pp. 954–961.

68. Rosenberg, S. A. (Chairman): The Non-Hodgkin's Lymphoma Path-ologic Classification Project. National Cancer Institute sponsored study of classifications of non-Hodgkin's lymphomas. *Cancer* **49**: 2112–2135, 1982.

69. Santoro, A., Bonfante, V., Bonadonna, G.: Salvage chemotherapy with ABVD in MOPP-resistant Hodgkin's disease. *Ann. Intern. Med.* **96**:139–143, 1982.

70. Schaner, E. G., Chang, A. E., Doppman, J. L., Conkle, D. M., Flye, M. W., Rosenberg, S. A.: Comparison of computed and convention-al whole lung tomography in detecting pulmonary nodules. *A.J.R.* **131**:51, 1978.

71. Schein, P. S., DeVita, V. T. Jr., Hubbard, S., Chabner, B. A., Canel-los, G. P., Berard, C., Young, R. C.: Bleomycin, Adriamycin, cy-clophosphamide, vincristine, and prednisone (BACOP) combina-tion chemotherapy in the treatment of advanced diffuse histiocytic lymphoma. *Ann. Intern. Med.* **85**:417–422, 1976.

72. Silverberg, E.: Cancer statistics, 1985. CA **35**:19–35, 1985.

73. Silverberg, E., Lubera, J. A.: A review of American Cancer Socie-ty estimates of cancer cases and deaths. CA **33**:2–8, 1983.

74. Silverman, S., DeNardo, G. L., Glatstein, E., Lopton, M. J.: Eval-uation of the liver and spleen in Hodgkin's disease. II. The value in splenic scintigraphy. *Am. J. Med.* **52**:362–366, 1972.

75. Sommer, F. G., Joynt, L. F., Carroll, B. A., Macovski, A.: Ultrasonic characterization of abdominal tissue via digital analysis of backscat-tered waveforms. *Radiology* **141**:811, 1981.

76. Thomas, J. L., Barnes, P. A., Bernardino, M. E., Hagemeister, F. B.: Limited CT studies in monitoring treatment of lymphoma. *A.J.R.* **138**:537, 1982.

77. Vermess, M., Doppman, J. L., Sugarbaker, P. H., Fisher, R. I., Chat-terji, D. C., Luetzeler, J., Grimes, G., Girton, M., Adamson, R. H.: Clinical trials with a new intravenous liposoluble contrast material for computed tomography of liver and spleen. *Radiology* **137**:217, 1980.

78. Ziegler, T. L., Magrath, I. T.: Burkitt's lymphoma. In *Pathobiology Annual*. Joachim, H. L. (Ed.). New York, Appleton-Century-Crofts, 1974, pp. 129–142.

22 TUMORS OF THE SKELETAL SYSTEM

Julius Smith
David G. Bragg

Primary tumors of bone are uncommon in the general population, being greatly outnumbered by metastatic lesions and inflammatory conditions, which often thwart the specific diagnosis of primary bone tumor. Metastatic tumors of the skeleton account for approximately 65% of all malignant bone tumors in adults. Of all types of human cancers, primary bone tumors account for only 0.5% excluding multiple myeloma.[10] In spite of their infrequent occurrence, an understanding of the specific tumor types, age at occurrence and anatomic site of predilection, staging requirements, therapeutic options, and clinical course is essential in determining the appropriate management of these lesions.

In the United States, mortality from bone cancer has a bimodal age curve with two relatively well-defined peaks: at ages 15 to 19 years and after age 65 years. The incidence of primary bone cancer is greater for whites and it tends to occur more often in males than females. During the past 10 to 15 years, mortality rates for primary bone cancer have progressively declined in the United States and Europe. The five-year relative survival rate for patients with localized primary bone cancer diagnosed between 1960 and 1973 was 45% in white patients and 33% for black patients. The five-year survival rate during those years was 27% for osteosarcoma, 15% for Ewing's sarcoma, and 60% for chondrosarcoma.[48] At present, many centers are reporting five-year survival rates for osteosarcoma and Ewing's sarcoma of 80% or more.[13,40,41,42] Taylor et al. have reported that the improvement in prognosis for patients with osteosarcoma treated by surgery alone preceded the introduction of the new chemotherapeutic drugs used today. These authors have speculated that a possible change in behavior of this tumor may be occurring analogous to observations on gastric cancer reported in the United States.[56] Ewing's sarcoma, a neoplasm much less common than osteosarcoma, almost always occurs in children and young adults. This tumor is virtually nonexistent in nonwhite children, a racial characteristic that should be remembered when considering the diagnosis of Ewing's sarcoma in a black child.[15,28] Osteosarcoma shows no significant racial predilection in incidence or mortality. The survival statistics for Ewing's sarcoma have dramatically improved over the past 10 years as a result of newer chemotherapeutic agents. Five-year survivals are now being reported between 70% and 80% in contrast to 10% or less 10 years ago.[13,41]

If one accepts multiple myeloma as a primary bone tumor, it should then be listed as the most common primary osseous neoplasm. This lesion shows a striking predisposition toward blacks, suggesting that some genetic error leads to this susceptibility, although environmental factors probably contribute to increased risk. Myeloma accounts for 1.1% of all cancers in whites and 7.2% in blacks. The age-adjusted incidence rate in whites is 4 per 100,000 in males and 2.7 per 100,000 in females. In the black population those rates are 8.1 per 100,000 and 2.65 per 100,000 respectively.[3,6,59]

As with osteosarcoma and Ewing's sarcoma, improved chemotherapeutic agents have allowed longer remissions for patients with myeloma during the past decade, with a median survival at present of approximately 40 months.

Myeloma may appear in a variety of clinical and radiographic forms, often frustrating the clinician in establishing a specific diagnosis, especially if the skeleton merely shows osteopenia on radiographic evaluation. Bone marrow aspiration and serum and urine protein studies for immunoglobulins will usually enable the diagnosis to be established. Myelomatous tumors arising in the axial skeleton are usually more difficult to detect, requiring radionuclide bone scans, computed tomography, and biopsy to define the lesions.

The evaluation of patients suspected of having a primary bone tumor usually begins with plain roentgenographic films, occasionally supplemented either with film tomographic or xeroradiographic evaluation. Before definitive treatment, more sophisticated techniques are required to stage the local tumor, evaluate skeleton and visceral organs for metastatic lesions, and determine whether or not the detected lesions is monostotic or polyostotic. The thorough pretreatment evaluation of primary tumors of bone by the sophisticated newer techniques of computed tomography, magnetic resonance imaging, digital radiography, and, occasionally, angiography, have allowed more precise localization and have been of help in the determination of appropriate treatment. These more sophisticated techniques have also allowed intergroup comparisons and have often made optimal treatment decisions among the principal therapeutic choices of surgery, radiation therapy, and chemotherapy easier.

TUMOR BEHAVIOR AND PATHOLOGY

Myelomatosis

Myeloma (Table 22-1) has its origins in the bone marrow, virtually always in a multicentric fashion.[7,21,36,44] The growth of this process within the marrow frustrates its early radiographic detection because the most frequent appearance on roentgenographic films is either a perfectly normal skeletal image or one of nonspecific, diffuse deossification. As a reflection of its frequency, myelomatosis represented 53% of all malignant skeletal tumors in one large series.[7] Occasionally, a solitary focus of myeloma with normal bone marrow and few if any protein abnormalities in the serum or urine are encountered. With time, these patients usually develop diffuse myelomatosis; however, this may take years to manifest itself.

The disease is more common in males and is not commonly observed before the fifth decade, with a peak incidence during the sixth and seventh decades. It is most commonly found in the bones that harbor hemopoietic marrow in adult life, such as the spine, ribs, skull, pelvis, and, occasionally, long bones. The most common symp-

Table 22-1. Primary Malignant Tumors of Bone

1. Myelomatosis
2. Osteosarcoma
    Conventional Intramedullary (High Grade)
    Parosteal Sarcoma
    Periosteal Sarcoma
    Telangiectatic Osteosarcoma
    Secondary Osteosarcoma
        Paget's Sarcoma
3. Chondrosarcoma
    Primary: Peripheral
                Central
    Secondary: Peripheral
                Central
    Mesenchymal Chondrosarcoma
4. Ewing's Sarcoma
5. Fibroscarcoma
6. Malignant Fibrous Histiocytoma
7. Primary Malignant Lymphoma of Bone
8. Chordoma
9. Malignant Giant Cell Tumor
10. Adamantinoma
11. Angiosarcoma
    Hemangioendothelioma: Solitary
                          Multicentric
    Hemangiopericytoma

tom is pain, which is most often localized to the spine. Nonspecific systemic symptoms such as lassitude, easy fatigability, and loss of weight are frequently present and may precede symptoms of bone pain. Pathologic fractures are common and this may even be the first manifestation of myelomatosis. Neurologic symptoms from spinal cord or nerve compression from fractures of the spine are relatively common. Renal involvement by myeloma may lead to kidney failure; however, this is usually a late complication.

Solitary myeloma initially appears as a monostotic lesion with no systemic symptoms. Extramedullary myeloma is uncommon, but when present is usually found in the head and neck area.

The plasma cells, which constitute much of the tumor process, retain the capacity to synthesize polypeptides. Thus, each clone of cells has a signature, a specific polypeptide chain or intact immunoglobulin molecule that accumulates in the serum. Approximately 60% of patients with myeloma have a monoclonal IgG spike in the serum.[12] The next most common abnormality is the IgA spike, which occurs in more than 20% of cases. IgD myeloma occurs in 1% to 2% of patients, while monoclonal production of IgE and IgM is rare. In as many as 10% to 15% of patients, the serum is devoid of an abnormal accumulation of intact immunoglobulin molecules, but immunoelectrophoresis reveals a homogeneous accumulation of light chain immunoglobulins. More than half of the patients with myeloma excrete monoclonal collections of light chain globulin molecules in the urine (Bence-Jones proteins). In some cases it has been possible to correlate specific immunoglobulin production with the natural history of the clinical disorder. IgD myeloma, for example, represents a more aggressive form of this disease.[12]

Plain films of the skeleton in patients with myeloma typically reveal well-marginated "punched out" areas (Figure 22-1), which vary in size from tiny 5-mm lesions to ones as large as 5 cm and in which there is characteristically no surrounding sclerosis. Expansion of the affected bone may lead to a ballooned out or expanded appearance, especially in the ribs (Figure 22-2). As many as 15% to 25% of patients will have no focal lesions and merely show diffuse osteopenia. The lesions of solitary myeloma are usually destructive and may be expansile as well.

Purely sclerotic changes in myeloma have been well documented in recent years but are extremely uncommon (Figure 22-3). A sensorimotor neuropathy occurs quite frequently in patients with myeloma (10%).[44] The incidence of peripheral neuropathy with the sclerotic form of myeloma is much higher, approximately 30%. Periosteal reaction in a lesion of myeloma is extremely uncommon in the absence of fracture or infection. This is frequently a useful clue in evaluating a solitary bone lesion.

Amyloidosis with myeloma occurs in about 10% of patients.[36] It may be so dominant a process as to mask the underlying myeloma; thus biopsy specimens of lesions thought to represent myelomatosis that are interpreted as amyloidosis need to be treated with skepticism.

Osteosarcoma

Osteosarcoma is the most common primary tumor of bone after myeloma and accounts for 20% of all primary sarcomas of bone.[47,52,54,55,57] It is defined as a primary

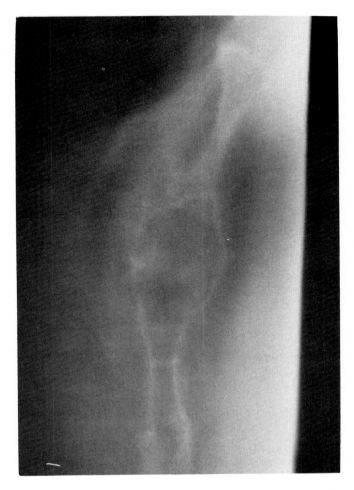

FIG. 22-2. Myelomatosis. Lateral tomogram of the sternum. Note the marked expansion of the upper sternum.

malignant bone tumor, the neoplastic cells of which produce osteoid. The amount of osteoid produced is variable, and this variability is used in the subclassification of osteosarcoma. In some tumors there is predominance of cartilage or fibrous tissue and thus osteosarcoma may be subclassified into osteoblastic, fibroblastic, or chondrosarcomatous osteosarcoma. The vast majority of osteosarcomas occur in the appendicular skeleton. They are high grade tumors and are commonly referred to as *conventional high grade osteosarcoma*. In recent years a number of distinct clinicopathologic varieties of osteosarcoma have been identified.

Conventional Osteosarcoma.
Conventional osteosarcoma is a disease of the young—mainly adolescents and young adults—and is slightly more common in males. The tumor typically arises in the metaphysis of a long bone and rarely occurs in the bones of the hand and feet. Lesions below the knee and elbow tend to be less aggres-

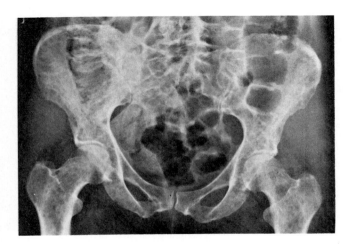

FIG. 22-1. Myelomatosis. An AP view of the pelvis showing multiple tiny punched-out lesions in lumbar spine, pelvis, and upper femora.

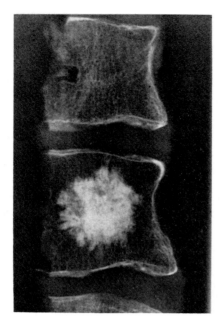

FIG. 22-3. Myelomatosis. Sagittal section of vertebra D-12. Note the unusual spiculated lesion within which myeloma cells in the center of the sclerotic area. (Specimen radiograph).

sive than those situated more centrally. Osteosarcoma is a bulky tumor; its appearance may be purely lytic or sclerotic (Figures 22-4–22-8), but generally a mixed radiographic pattern is seen. While the tumor may be completely intramedullary, it often bursts through the cortex and will have produced a soft tissue mass at the time the patient is first seen. Histologically, the appearance of these tumors is variable. Most have a stroma that is predominantly composed of spindle cells and is cytologically highly malignant. Mitotic figures are easily found; the nuclei are large and irregular and malignant giant cells may be present. The normal trabeculae of the involved bone are usually destroyed by the tumor. The tumor cells may permeate or envelop the residual bony trabeculae.

Telangiectatic Osteosarcoma. Telangiectatic osteosarcoma (Figure 22-9) is a rare tumor characterized by lytic changes on the roentgenograms. There is usually no visible sclerosis, but on occasion minimal sclerotic reaction may be present. Periosteal reaction is uncommon. Histologically, cystlike spaces and osteoid are present in a fine lacelike pattern, but only in limited amounts. Telangiectatic osteosarcoma may be easily mistaken for an aneurysmal bone cyst both histologically and radiographically. The pronounced anaplasia of the cells seen in telangiectatic osteosarcoma, however, is never seen in an aneurysmal bone cyst. In a recent study, 30% of patients with this type of sarcoma had a pathological fracture.[22] There is no significant difference in survival for patients with telangiectatic sarcoma compared with those with conventional osteosarcoma.

Parosteal Osteosarcoma. Parosteal osteosarcoma (Figure 22-10) is an uncommon, low grade tumor affecting the periosteal surface of a bone. It accounts for approximately 1% of all primary malignant tumors of bone. The patients affected are usually adults, and the tumor is particularly common in the lower end of the femur. The lesions tend to be slow-growing and frequently are large in size. On gross inspection, the tumor is attached by a broad base and, as the lesion grows, a clear space develops between the tumor and the underlying bone. Eventually the tumor may encircle the bone shaft. Evaluation of possible medullary involvement is not possible with conventional roentgenograms but CT scans demonstrate the relationship between the tumor and medullary cavity extremely well. The character of some of these indolent, slow-growing tumors may change, with the lesions becoming indistinguishable histologically from high grade osteosarcomas. The medulla may become involved at this stage, and widespread metastases may develop. However, the parosteal osteosarcoma typically is only locally aggressive, with minimal metastatic potential.

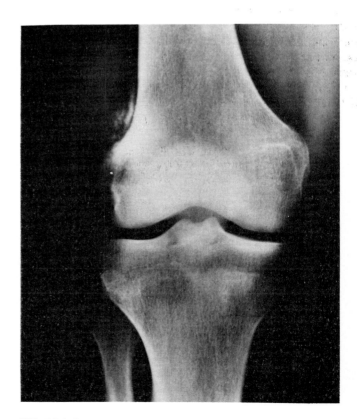

FIG. 22-4. Osteosarcoma. An AP view of the knee. Note the small sclerotic lesion in lower femur with periosteal reaction.

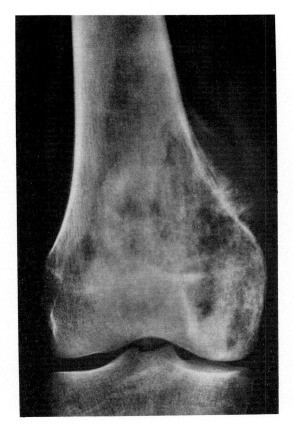

FIG. 22-5. Osteosarcoma. An AP view of the knee. Large lytic lesion with prominent lamellar and spiculated periosteal reaction.

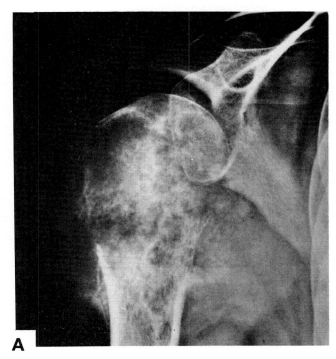

A

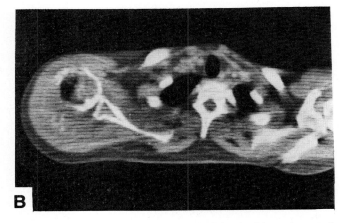

B

FIG. 22-7. Osteosarcoma. (A) An AP view of the shoulder with marked lytic and sclerotic change, a bulky soft tissue mass, and periosteal reaction. (B) A CT scan showing prominent bone destruction and calcifications in the soft tissue masses.

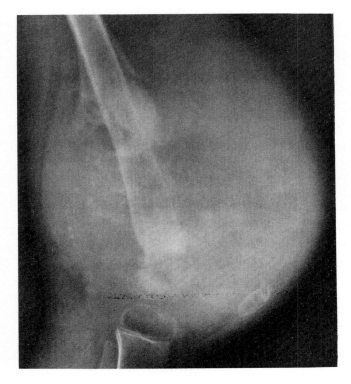

FIG. 22-6. Osteosarcoma. Lateral view of the knee. A bulky soft tissue mass with prominent periosteal reaction. Patchy sclerosis is apparent in the shaft of femur.

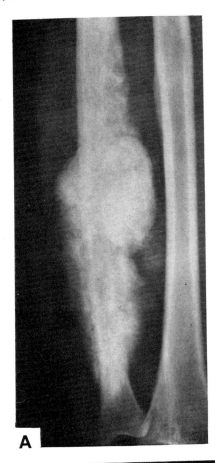

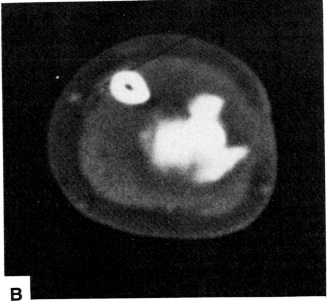

FIG. 22-8. Osteosarcoma. Lateral views of the radius and ulna. (A) Exuberant, bulky bony lesion of distal half of ulna in a 65-year-old who had no evidence of Paget's disease in surgical specimen nor in the rest of the skeleton. (B) A CT scan showing the extent of the bony mass.

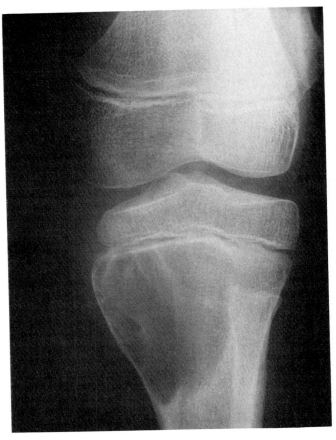

FIG. 22-9. Telangiectatic osteosarcoma. An AP view of the tibia. A slightly expansile lytic lesion originally thought to be an aneurysmal cyst at the referring hospital.

Periosteal Osteosarcoma. Periosteal osteosarcoma is a recently described tumor that, like parosteal osteosarcoma, occurs on the surface of bone and needs to be distinguished from parosteal osteosarcoma.[57] These are much smaller tumors with a predilection for the upper tibial metaphysis. The neoplasm may, however, occur in other bones such as the femur. Roentgenographically, periosteal osteosarcomas are characterized by a relatively shallow lytic area with prominent spiculation perpendicular to the bone shaft. There is usually no involvement of the medullary cavity by the tumor. Histologically the tumor is relatively poorly differentiated and is predominantly chondroblastic. Fine osteoid production is usually seen towards the center. These tumors are fairly high grade and have an aggressive tendency that rests somewhere between parosteal osteosarcoma and conventional osteosarcoma. Some have claimed that these tumors are best classified as juxtacortical chondrosarcomas or periosteal chondrosarcomas.[47]

Secondary Osteosarcoma. Secondary osteosarcoma develops in patients with Paget's disease and also in individuals in whom a bone has been incidentally radiated during treatment for soft tissue cancer. In both these groups of patients, the complication is quite rare.

Paget's Sarcoma. This uncommon complication of Paget's disease is thought to occur in only 0.15% of patients; however, if the Paget's disease is very extensive, it is thought to rise to 10%. These assumptions are based on only limited statistical data. This is a most serious complication of Paget's disease, since the majority of patients are dead within a year (70%). Early diagnosis is difficult because at the time of initial examination, the tumor is well-established clinically and radiographically. A pathologic fracture may be the initial symptom (10%) and needs to be differentiated from a simple fracture, which is not rare in uncomplicated Paget's disease. A gallium 67 radionuclide scan is an extremely useful test and demonstrated the site of the sarcoma in each of our ten most recent patients. The alkaline phosphatase level is increased in uncomplicated Paget's disease and may reach high levels when there is florid polyostotic disease. With the development of Paget's sarcoma, the alkaline phosphatase level may attain significantly higher values. Unfortunately, however, there are usually no previous baseline estimations available for comparison when a patient has a secondary sarcoma. There are also significant fluctuations in the level of alkaline phosphatase in patients with simple Paget's disease as well as with Paget's sarcoma.

Treatment results have been disappointing. Radical surgical ablations and radiation therapy have only rarely resulted in permanent cure. Only 3.5% of 85 patients seen at Memorial Sloan-Kettering Hospital between 1925 and 1982 survived five years. Intensive chemotherapy with high dose methotrexate (the same protocol used in spontaneous osteosarcomas) has been tried recently with varying success.

Radiation-Induced Sarcoma of Bone (RIS). A sarcoma arising in irradiated bone is a well-recognized but uncommon entity.[51,53] A review of the world literature reveals only 300 cases. In earlier decades, the tumor arose most commonly from a bone that was abnormal, usually the site of a benign tumor, cyst, or dysplasia. The recognition that irradiation of a benign lesion, although effective in some cases, might occasionally be associated with a complicating sarcoma led to the abandonment of this form of treatment. As a result, the majority of patients now encountered with RIS have underlying bone that has been incidentally irradiated during the course of treatment of a contiguous cancer. These neoplasms are virtually always malignant and are usually epithelial cancers; however, some soft tissue sarcomas have been reported. Two patients with benign tumors—a cystic hygroma and a hydatidiform tumor—that progressed to malignancy have been documented at Memorial Sloan-Kettering Hospital.

Until 1970, breast cancer was the most common primary tumor occurring in patients with RIS. Since then, there has been a marked increase in the number of patients with lymphoma (primarily Hodgkin's disease) who have developed this complication. Of 46 patients recently studied at Memorial Sloan-Kettering Hospital, 13 were patients with lymphoma. There were only eight patients with breast cancer. The next most common primary tumors were cancer of the cervix and retinoblastoma, with five cases each. The survival of patients with Hodgkin's disease has improved greatly over the past decade. This can be directly related to the more aggressive treatment with radiation therapy and chemotherapy. The direct cellular effects of irradiation combined with the immunosuppressive effects of chemotherapy and greater survival are probably the main factors explaining the occurrence of secondary neoplasms in these patients.

The course of radiation-induced sarcomas of either bone or soft tissue is rapidly progressive in spite of aggressive treatment. Radiation therapy is often selected as the most effective palliative method of treatment. In the 46 patients referred to above only 5 of 46 patients are alive for analysis. Each of the patients with secondary neoplasms as a result of treatment for Hodgkin's lymphoma have died.

Chondrosarcoma

Chondrosarcoma is the third most common primary tumor of bone and accounts for 10% of all malignant tumors of bone.[8,10,23,30,31] This lesion occurs either as malignant cartilaginous tumor arising primarily in a bone or superimposed on a pre-existing benign cartilaginous tumor. Most chondrosarcomas arise de novo and are designated primary chondrosarcoma; those arising from pre-existing cartilaginous tumors such as osteochondromas or enchondromas are considered secondary chondrosarcomas. Another subdivision is based on anatomic site. A large bony tumor that develops on the surface of a bone is termed a peripheral chondrosarcoma. A tumor arising within the medullary space is referred to as a central chondrosarcoma. Approximately 75% of chondrosarcomas are primary with the remainder arising from pre-existing cartilage tumors. Patients with multiple exostoses and enchondromatoses are known to be at risk of developing chondrosarcomas.

The pelvic bones are the most common sites for chondrosarcomas but other skeletal sites such as long bones, short bones, and flat bones may occasionally be involved (Figures 22-11, 22-12). It is curious that chondrosarcomas

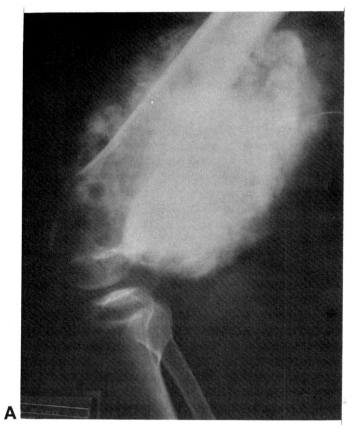

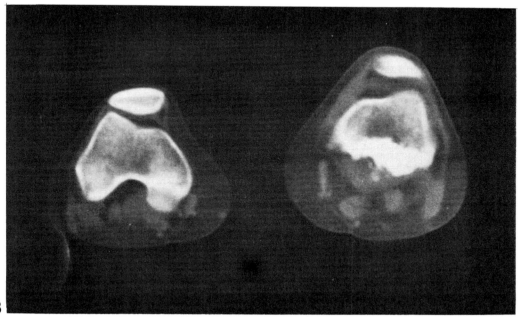

FIG. 22-10. This 22-year-old black man had noted swelling of his thigh for approximately one year before these images were obtained. (A) A lateral roentgenogram of the right knee shows the typical cauliflower-like excrescences surrounding the distal femur that results from the densely productive bone formation characteristic of this tumor. (B) A roentgenogram of the resected specimen that better demonstrates the characteristic appearance of this neoplasm. (C) A CT scan showing the normal left knee in comparison with the involved right knee. Note the largely extracortical nature of this bulky tumor, with only minimal extension inside the medullary canal. (D) A magnetic resonance image of the knee and distal femur revealing the distinct margins of the tumor and the location of the femoral artery, which appears to course through the lesion (arrows). These lesions usually displace the vessels; however, this neoplasm appeared to incorporate the artery.

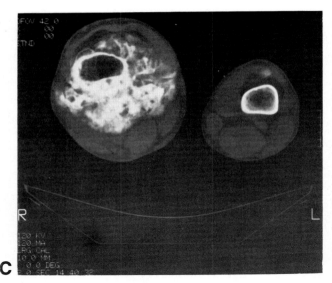

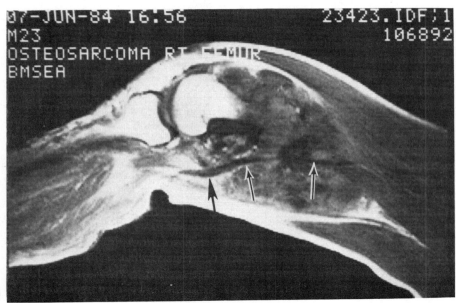

of the hands and feet are exceedingly rare even though benign cartilaginous tumors in these sites are so common.

Mesenchymal Chondrosarcoma. Mesenchymal chondrosarcoma has a distinct histologic pattern with malignant cartilage cells that blend with an undifferentiated mesenchymal component, which in some areas may resemble a small cell tumor. Radiologically they may resemble a conventional chondrosarcoma, but they are somewhat more invasive than the usual chondrosarcoma.

Dedifferentiated Chondrosarcoma. Dedifferentiated chondrosarcoma (Figure 22-13) is a fairly recent designation of a chondrosarcoma that, although mainly well differentiated, shows an area of rapid growth that does not have any characteristics of the other portions of the tumor. These areas may resemble a malignant fibrous histiocytoma or fibrosarcoma. A dedifferentiated chondrosarcoma should be suspected, therefore, when a patient has had a well-differentiated chondrosarcoma over a long period that shows rapid growth.

Ewing's Sarcoma

Ewing's sarcoma is a tumor of the young, most commonly affecting those in the first and second decades of life.[10,48,49] Ewing's sarcoma is very uncommon in persons over the age of 30 years and is rarely observed in children under the age of 5 years. This tumor accounts for 6% of all primary malignant lesions of bone. It is an aggressive, high grade tumor that may affect any bone.

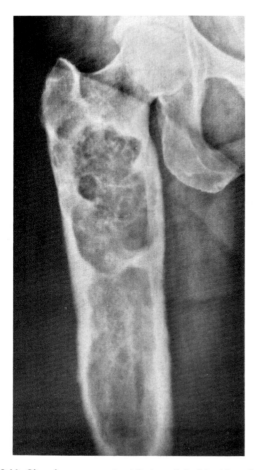

FIG. 22-11. Chondrosarcoma. An AP view of the hip. Note the bulky bony mass typical of chondrosarcoma.

Approximately half of the lesions occur in flat bones, with the innominate bone being the most commonly involved in this group.

On gross pathologic inspection, the tumor is soft and gray in appearance. Following hemorrhage, there may be necrosis, cyst formation, an increase in connective tissue, or focal regression of the tumor. Microscopically, the tumor is made up of broad sheets of polyhedral-shaped cells with very scanty cytoplasm and appears colorless or pale pink. The cells are uniform in size and have nuclei with small nucleoli. There is no intercellular substance; the tumor should never produce osteoid. Glycogen is abundent in the cytoplasm and glycogen stains (PAS) help to differentiate this tumor from other small cell tumors. Unfortunately, not all Ewing's sarcomas are PAS positive. These glycogen granules are well demonstrated under electron microscopy.

In the long bones, the tumor takes origin in the diaphysis and quite rapidly infiltrates the medullary cavity. Primary origin or involvement of the epiphysis is most

uncommon. Radiographically, the tumor has a permeated or moth-eaten appearance (Figures 22-14–22-18). A fine lamellary periosteal reaction may be obvious when the patient is first seen, but prominent onion-skin layering is quite rare in the early lesions. Sclerotic changes are unusual in this tumor, and when they occur they are purely reactive in nature. The sclerosis may occasionally be prominent, leading to radiographic confusion with osteosarcoma.

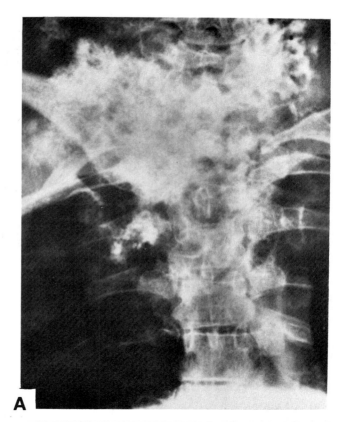

A

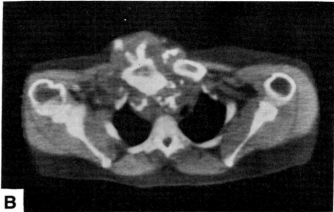

B

FIG. 22-12. Chondrosarcoma. (A) An AP view of the lower neck. A very large tumor arises from the sternum. (B) A CT scan shows a very large soft tissue mass and extensive destruction of the sternum.

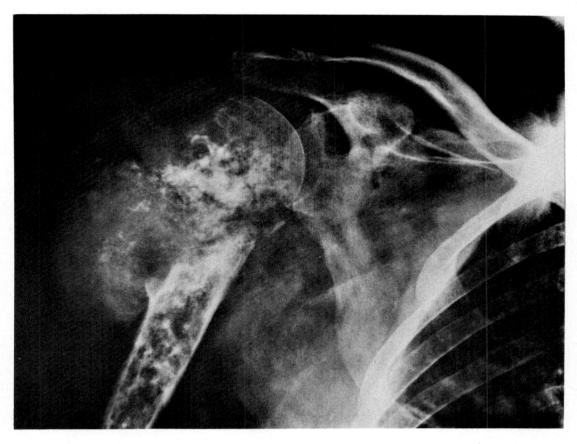

FIG. 22-13. Dedifferentiated chondrosarcoma of the shoulder. Note the typical features of central chondrosarcoma. Unossified area was caused by an unossified malignant fibrous histiocytoma element.

Systemic symptoms such as easy fatigability, lassitude, and fever are common early in the disease. This, in association with leukocytosis and an elevated erythrocyte sedimentation rate, may lead to a clinical suspicion of osteomyelitis. Differentiation of Ewing's sarcoma from osteomyelitis may be extremely difficult, and until biopsy proven the diagnosis may be in doubt.

While Ewing's sarcoma is uncommon, it enters into the differential diagnosis of other small cell tumors such as metastatic neuroblastoma, primary malignant lymphoma of bone and undifferentiated carcinoma metastatic to bone. Neuroblastoma usually occurs in infants and children under five, but it may occur in an older child and even in an adult. The characteristic cytologic feature of the tumor is the presence of tumor cells arranged in rosettes. In a typical case, the rosettes are clustered aggregations of tumor cells enclosing a small central network of filamentous neurofibrils, some of which can be shown to constitute processes of the cells making up the periphery of the rosette.

Primary malignant lymphoma of bone may resemble Ewing's sarcoma, but the cell nuclei are somewhat larger, and, while they are usually round to oval, may be indented. If a reticulin stain is used, delicate threads and strands of reticulum are found to run around groups of cells but also between individual cells. This is not found is Ewing's sarcoma. Undifferentiated metastatic carcinoma may reveal small cells on biopsy and the question of Ewing's sarcoma may be raised. Ewing's sarcoma is so unusual in a mature or elderly patient that the diagnosis is rarely established before death.

Fibrosarcoma

Fibrosarcoma is a malignant tumor of spindle-shaped cells that produces no osteoid material in either the primary or metastatic form. Fibrosarcoma accounts for 3% of all primary malignant bone tumors and is only one sixth as common as osteosarcoma. The tumor tends to be evenly distributed between the second and sixth decades of life and is much more frequently encountered in older patients. This distribution is quite different from that of osteosarcoma. The tumor is most common in the long bones and usually is metaphyseal in location. Radiographically, fibrosarcomas are destructive, radio-

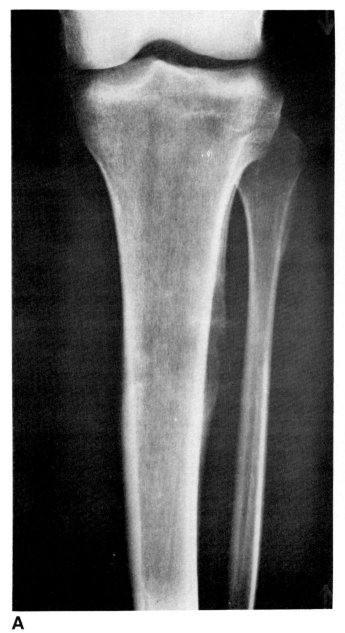

A

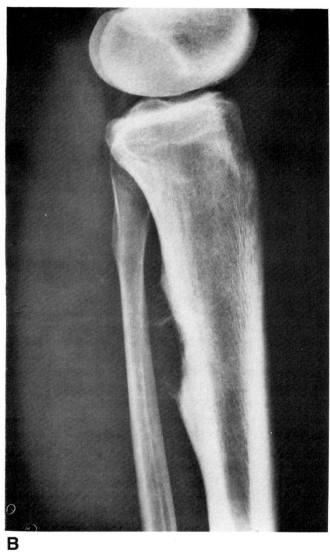

B

FIG. 22-14. Ewing's sarcoma. (A) AP and (B) lateral views of the tibia. Note the typical findings of "saucerization" of the lesion.

characteristically shows a "storiform pattern" with clusters of cells and nuclei that are similar but appear to be histiocytic in type. Many sarcomas of bone may have areas that histologically resemble a malignant fibrous histiocytoma. These usually are only a part of the tumor, however, and the basic nature of the tumor can be easily recognized. The term *malignant fibrous histiocytoma* as primarily a sarcoma of bone is correctly used when multiple sections throughout the lesion demonstrate the histologic pattern described above. The tumors are high grade, appear to be aggressive, and metastasize readily. The lesions are purely lytic radiographically (Figure 22-19), and reactive bone is rarely seen within the tumor. Periosteal reaction may occur but it is rarely very prominent. This tumor is one of the few primary bone tumors that metastasize readily to lymph nodes.

Chordoma

This uncommon tumor, which accounts for approximately 4% of all primary malignant tumors of bone, arises from the primitive notochord. It has a predilection for the ends of the spinal column; thus the sacrococcygeal region and the base of the skull near the spheno-occipital synchondrosis are the sites where almost all of these tumors occur. Chordomas are most commonly found in the sacrococcygeal region. They may, however, be found in any vertebra and occasionally in an extraspinal location. Chordomas occur more frequently in men and are more common in older patients. The tumor is usually purely lytic, but calcification of the matrix of the tumor may occur rarely and may thus superficially resemble a chondrosarcoma radiographically. Pathologically, the tu-

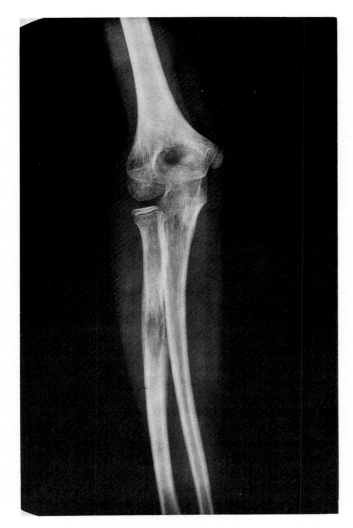

FIG. 22-15. Ewing's sarcoma. A relatively small lytic lesion in the upper radius with periosteal lamellation.

lucent lesions commonly penetrating the cortex of a long bone at the time of initial examination. Histologically, fibrosarcomas are spindle cell tumors with a wide range of histologic differentiation. Some are very anaplastic and high grade, whereas some may be very low grade and very insidious in their growth. Histologically, fibrosarcomas frequently have a herringbone pattern, which is very characteristic but not ubiquitous to all fibrosarcomas.

Primary Malignant Fibrous Histiocytoma

Primary malignant fibrous histiocytoma of bone has only recently been described as a distinctive entity.[9] It is uncommon, but histopathologists are increasingly reporting this tumor, usually at the expense of fibrosarcoma, which has been seen much less commonly during the past decade as a primary sarcoma of bone. The tumor

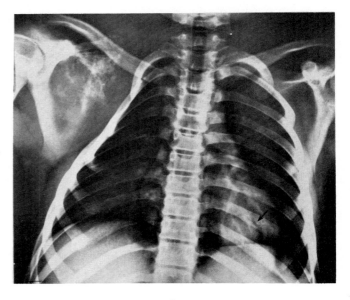

FIG. 22-16. Ewing's sarcoma. A bulky lesion of the scapula with a large soft tissue mass. Note the metastasis in the left lung (arrow) and the deformity of the chest wall.

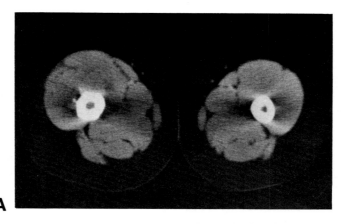

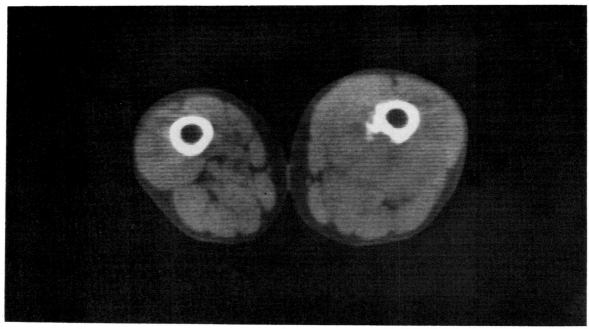

FIG. 22-17. (A) Ewing's sarcoma of bone. CT scan of a 15-year-old boy with a bulky soft tissue mass and associated periosteal reaction. The scan shows increased attenuation in the medullary cavity indicating that the tumor arose from the bone itself and not from the soft tissue. (B) Ewing's sarcoma of soft tissue. A CT scan of a 22-year-old man with a very bulky soft tissue mass. The scan shows the primary tumor and extensive erosion of the cortex. The medullary cavity was totally lucent and there was no evidence of tumor within the medullary space. The tumor was categorized as a Ewing's sarcoma of soft tissue.

mor has a lobulated appearance and the destructive element is the physaliferous cell with a distinctive cytoplasm. The tumors are generally low grade and slow growing. A variety of other patterns may be found histologically. On occasion areas are found that resemble chondrosarcoma, osteosarcoma, or even fibrosarcoma. Distant metastases are not common but when they do occur they may involve the lungs, liver, and other bones.

Primary Malignant Lymphoma of Bone

Primary malignant lymphomas of bone are quite uncommon and account for only 3% of all malignant tumors. The diagnosis should only be entertained if there are no other foci of lymphoma in either the lymph nodes, viscera, or remainder of the skeleton. A lymphangiogram or CT study is essential to exclude retroperitoneal nodal disease. The tumor can occur in persons at any age but is rare in the very young. Skeletal lymphoma may involve any bone but is most common in the axial skeleton. Patients usually have bone pain with associated swelling and weakness.

Radiographically, the lesions are generally quite large (5 to 10 cm), predominantly lytic, and have commonly broken through the cortex at the time of diagnosis. Prominent periosteal reaction is one of the characteristic features of this tumor but, unfortunately, is not present in all cases. Sclerotic changes may be associated with this lytic process, and on occasion the lesion may be densely sclerotic.

Histologically, the basic cell of this tumor is the reticulum cell, but the tumor may contain variable numbers of lymphoblasts and lymphocytes; these cells may dominate the histologic pattern. On occasion there may be a purely lymphocytic pattern. Occasionally, a highly malignant lymphoma of bone may contain Reed-Sternberg cells, in which case it should be correctly termed a Hodgkin's sarcoma.

The differentiation of a primary lymphoma of bone from Ewing's sarcoma may be difficult. The cells of a malignant lymphoma lie in a reticulum framework, and there is a tendency for an alveolar grouping of the cells, a feature that is often prominent. This helps to differentiate primary lymphoma of bone from Ewing's sarcoma in which large masses of cells are associated with no fibrillar, intercellular material. The PAS stain may be useful in differentiating sarcomas, since the glycogen granules are stained in this tumor but not in patients with lymphoma of bone. Most tumors are of moderate histologic grade; however, high grade tumors are not rare.

Adamantinoma

This unusual primary tumor of bone with a distinctive histologic appearance comprises less than 1% of all primary tumors of the bone. The name is derived from a distinct resemblance to the cellular material found in ameloblastoma of the mandible. The histogenesis of adamantinomas is still uncertain, but many believe these tumors are of vascular origin and have suggested the term *malignant angioblastoma*. The overwhelming majority of these tumors arise in the tibia, yet it rarely may occur in other sites. Adamatinomas occur more commonly in men and may be seen in patients of almost any age, yet rarely under age 20 years. The tumor is slow growing, and patients usually have pain and local swelling. The duration of symptoms may vary from a few months to many years. Radiographically, adamantinomas are large lesions, sometimes involving the whole shaft of the tibia, with multiple sharply circumscribed lucent areas of various sizes and interspersed zones of sclerosis. This appearance resembles fibrous dysplasia quite frequently, and this is the most important radiographic differential diagnosis. However, metastatic lesions, chondrosarcomas, and other primary tumors should be considered in the differential. The tumor is low grade and tends to grow slowly. Metastases, however, do occur, usually to the lungs, other bones, or lymph nodes.

Malignant Giant Cell Tumor

This is an uncommon tumor and accounts for less than 1% of all malignant tumors of bone. The majority of giant cell tumors pursue a benign course, although they may be locally aggressive. In 15% to 30% of patients, however, the tumor exhibits an aggressive behavior (Figure 22-20). Predicting which giant cell tumors will behave in a malignant fashion is extremely difficult. Rarely, a giant cell tumor with a classical appearance may be found to be "malignant" at the first examination. Approximately 8% of malignant giant cell tumors will fall into this category. The usual situation, however, is that a benign giant cell tumor recurs and the histologic pattern of the recurrent tumor is found to be frankly malignant. The predominant microscopic pattern in these lesions is that of an anaplastic spindle cell sarcoma with prominent telangiectatic features and a lack of collagenization. In the past, radiation therapy was regarded as

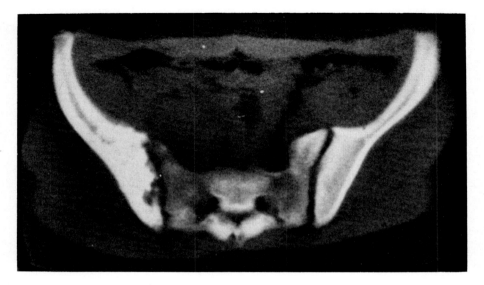

FIG. 22-18. Ewing's sarcoma. A CT scan of the pelvis showing a densely sclerotic tumor invading the SI joint. Reactive sclerosis may on occasion be very prominent and thus make differentiation from osteosarcoma difficult.

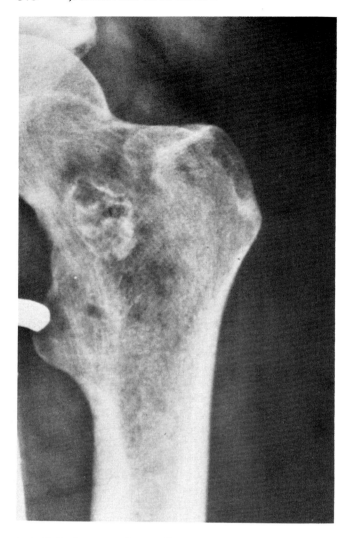

FIG. 22-19. Primary malignant fibrous histocytoma of bone. An AP view of the femur. Note the large area of poorly defined lytic destruction without periosteal reaction. Note also small bone infarct.

the prime etiologic factor in inducing malignant change in what appeared to be benign giant cell tumors. Because of this risk, radiation therapy has been used only rarely in the most common sites of giant cell tumor in the limbs. In inaccessible areas, such as the spine and sacrum, irradiation still plays an important therapeutic role. *Benign metastasizing giant cell tumor* is one of the descriptive labels that describe the course of these neoplasms. The metastases of a malignant giant cell tumor have the characteristics of the primary tumor.

Angiosarcoma

The term *angiosarcoma* is a generic term for the two primary sarcomas of bone of vascular origin, the hemangioendothelioma and the hemangiopericytoma.[37,58] The former is much more common in bone and the latter

more commonly arises as a soft tissue tumor. Angiosarcoma comprises less than 1% of all malignant tumors. The hemangioendothelioma may be found clinically in two forms: as a solitary tumor or as a multicentric lesion. Paradoxically, the multicentric tumor has a more benign course than the solitary tumor. The multicentric lesions have a unique distribution in that they tend to involve multiple bones of the hands, feet, and long bones, all in the same limb (Figure 22-21). This curious distribution of multicentric tumors is found in at least 60% of cases and is presumed to result from a defective limb bud. They may occur at any age and involve any bone. When the lesion is solitary, it appears as a single lytic lesion with no evidence of reaction in the surrounding bone. The appearances of angiosarcoma are nonspecific radiographically and may resemble metastasis, myeloma, and many other lytic lesions. The characteristic histologic appearance is that of pronounced proliferation of capillaries. The cells of the endothelial lining are plump, pleomorphic, and hyperchromatic. Late in the course of this tumor, widespread, anastomising vascular proliferation may occur. On occasion, this tumor will histologically resemble synovial sarcoma, Ewing's sarcoma, or an aneurysmal bone cyst. Hemangiopericytoma shows a characteristic histologic appearance as well, with proliferating vasoformative channels lined by a single layer of attenuating endothelial cells and spindly round or oval cells, the so-called pericytes of Zimmerman. Most of these tumors are of low grade, but when of high grade, the pericytic tumor cells show marked variation in size and multiple mitotic figures may be found. Some metastatic lesions of bone might sometimes exhibit a growth pattern that resembles a hemangiopericytoma.

The radiographic differential considerations when evaluating a solitary bone lesion are considerable. Met-

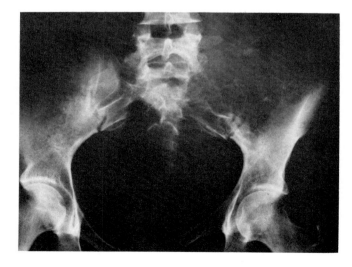

FIG. 22-20. Malignant giant cell tumor. Note the massive destruction of the sacrum and both sacroiliac joints.

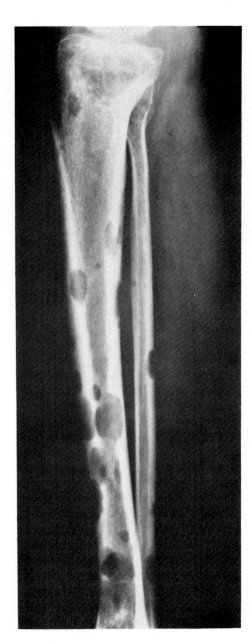

FIG. 22-21. Multicentric hemangioendothelioma of bone. Lateral view of the right tibia. Multiple well-defined lytic lesions in the tibia and fibula. Similar lesions were present in the femur and in the tarsal and metacarpal bones of the right lower extremity. The patient had been NED (no evidence of disease) for 13 years since a hemipelvectomy.

astatic disease to the skeleton may manifest itself as a single area of destruction or as new bone formation (Figures 22-22 through 22-25). Routine roentgenograms or, preferably, a radionuclide scan will usually demonstrate other lesions if present. The radiographic patterns of bony involvement with metastatic disease vary depending upon whether the process is predominantly lytic or blastic. Although some primary cancers produce a con-

stant radiographic pattern, for example, kidney and thyroid cancers, which are nearly always purely lytic, or prostate cancer, which is nearly always sclerotic, there is considerable overlap in the appearance of the metastases, and many cancers may produce similar radiographic patterns in the skeleton. Skeletal metastases may appear as solitary lesions and this may in fact be the initial symptom of an underlying cancer.

Osteomyelitis (Figure 22-26) should be considered, particularly in patients in whom the diagnosis of a small cell tumor is possible. Inflammatory clinical features may stimulate Ewing's sarcoma, since in both instances pyrexia, leukocytosis, and elevated sedimentation rates will occur. The pattern of bone destruction and periosteal reaction may be similar in both conditions.

An aneurysmal bone cyst (Figure 22-27) is generally considered to be a reactive process and radiographically may have the appearance of the very characteristic eccentric ballooning of the involved bone. This reactive change is frequently associated with benign bone tumors such as chondroblastoma, chondromyxoid fibroma, and giant cell tumor. Differentiation of aneurysmal bone cysts from telangiectatic osteosarcoma may on occasion be very difficult, both for the pathologist and the radiologist.

Traumatic lesions may result in bizarre areas of ossification in the soft tissues and in bone. Usually there is a history of trauma to suggest the diagnosis. Healing stress fractures of the lower limbs may occasionally raise the suspicion of a malignant tumor as well. The pattern is usually recognized quite easily, and biopsy should be unnecessary. A biopsy taken from a healing fracture may have a most alarming histologic appearance. Close co-

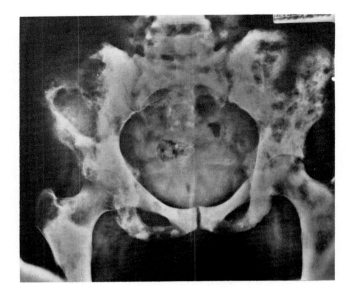

FIG. 22-22. Breast cancer metastases. Mixed lytic and blastic lesions in the pelvis and upper femora.

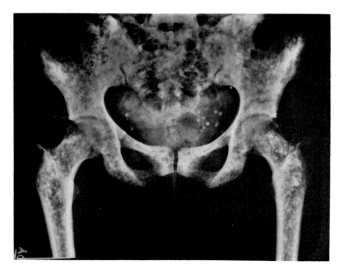

FIG. 22-23. Sclerotic metastases throughout the skeleton, all very tiny.

operation between the pathologist and the radiologist in the diagnosis of bone lesions will reduce the potential for tragic errors.

CLASSIFICATION AND STAGING

Staging and classification is not uniform among institutions worldwide. The considerations and requirements for staging and classification here will be divided between multiple myelomas and solid tumors.

Myelomatosis

The staging system described by Durie and Salmon is the one currently in general use.[12] This is a clinical staging system that groups the patients between stages

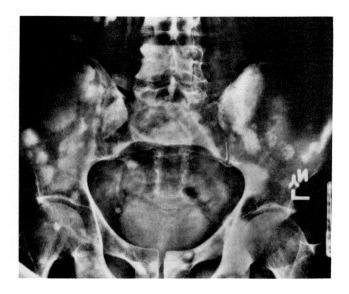

FIG. 22-24. Lung cancer; multiple sclerotic metastases in the pelvis.

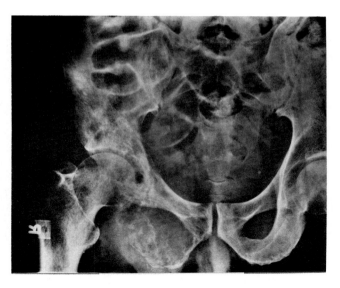

FIG. 22-25. Prostatic cancer; a large area of destruction in the ischium. There are some mottled sclerotic areas in the pelvis.

I and III based on hemoglobin, serum calcium, immune globulin evaluation, and radiographic changes of the skeleton.

Other Solid Tumors of the Skeleton

Classification and staging of nonmyeloma skeletal tumors has not gained wide acceptance. The most recent, the 1983 edition of the *Manual for Staging of Cancer* published by the American Joint Committee on Cancer, suggests an interim TNM classification. This refers to a T_x lesion (minimum requirements to assess primary tumor cannot be met), T_0 (no evidence of primary tumor), T_1 (tumor confined within the cortex of the bone), and T_2 (tumor extending beyond the cortex of the bone). A modification of this system has been made by Rubin et al.,[45] is illustrated in Figure 22-28 and explained in the legend and Tables 22-2 and 22-3. A histologic reading system of G_1 through G_4 arbitrarily divides those lesions that are well-differentiated from those that are poorly differentiated or anaplastic. Ewing's sarcoma and malignant lymphoma are arbitrarily grouped as G_3 and G_4 lesions.

IMAGING PROCEDURES AND ASSESSMENT (TABLE 22-4)

Plain Films

Bone. Good quality plain films of a primary tumor of bone in the appendicular skeleton represent the simplest and perhaps the most valuable single study in the evalu-

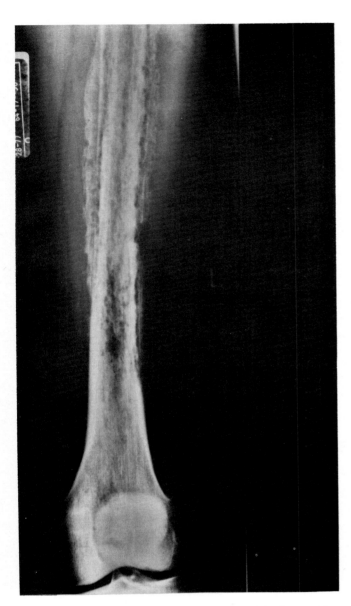

FIG. 22-26. Osteomyelitis. Extensive destruction of the femur with a florid periosteal reaction. This healthy 35-year-old man was referred to our institution with a diagnosis of Ewing's sarcoma.

ation of a primary bone tumor. Films demonstrating good detail in at least two planes with the addition of oblique projections when necessary, together with soft tissue films, are essential. Despite the lack of sensitivity and perhaps a lack of specificity, the pattern of bone involvement and the rate of growth of a bone lesion enable a radiologist who is equipped with good clinical information to predict the nature of an underlying tumor in 70% to 80% of cases. In the axial skeleton, because of complex anatomic arrangements and overlying structures, plain films are somewhat less accurate but nevertheless should never be omitted in the investigation of tumors at this site.

Chest. The most common site for metastases in tumors of bone is the lungs, and adequate evaluation of the chest is essential. Good quality posteroanterior and lateral chest studies are usually adequate, but if these are unable to resolve questionable densities, then tomography needs to be performed.

Computed Tomography

The high resolution of computed tomography makes possible the detection of bony lesions that might not be detected with any other modality.[17,18,20,34] It also delineates the extent of disease in the medullary cavity and cortical bone, the extent of soft tissue spread, and the neurovascular bundle.

Ideally, CT scans should be monitored by a radiologist so that the entire lesion is covered and the upper and lower limits of the tumor adequately shown. Contiguous 1-cm sections are usually adequate for large lesions, but 5-mm overlapping cuts may be necessary for smaller tumors. Symmetrical positioning of the extremities to allow comparison with the opposite side of the body is essential in order to detect subtle changes. Contrast is not given routinely, but when a lesion is not well visualized, contrast enhancement may render the lesion more obvious. For detailed evaluation of the neurovascular bundle, contrast is essential. Contrast may be given intravenously via drip infusion or as a large bolus. If CT is planned immediately after arteriography, the intra-arterial route may be used with optimal effect. If the suspected bone tumor is adjacent to the abdomen, retroperitoneum, or pelvis, dilute Gastrografin (diatrozoate meglumine and diatrozoate sodium) should be given orally. If the lesion involves the sacrum or pelvis, Gastrografin is given 12 to 24 hours before the study to opacify the colon. A dilute Hypaque enema given at the beginning of the examination may serve equally well. This technique is particularly useful when a small lesion of the sacrum is suspected. For good visualization of a soft tissue mass, individual muscles, vessels, and nerves, adequate soft tissue fat is necessary. When patients are emaciated, very thin, or very young, the absence of fat planes may severely compromise the CT study, making interpretation difficult. The distal extremities, as a result of the paucity of fat, are difficult areas to evaluate when soft tissue spread of tumor is suspected. The bony tumors at this site can, however, be well visualized. The combined use of a radionuclide bone scan and skeletal roentgenograms usually allows detection of and confirmation of skeletal metastases. In a small number of patients with abnormal bone scans, however, the plain films may be either normal or reveal nonspecific abnormalities. In patients in whom there is a strong suspicion of malignancy, CT may be the only modality that can demonstrate the tumor. Conservative en bloc surgery with limb preservation is now the primary surgical ap-

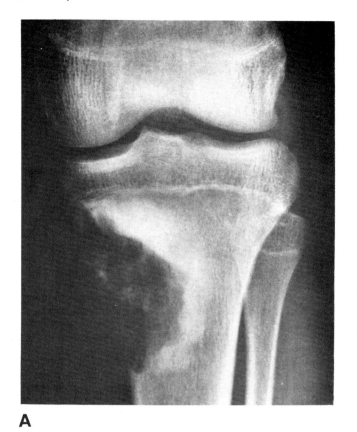

A

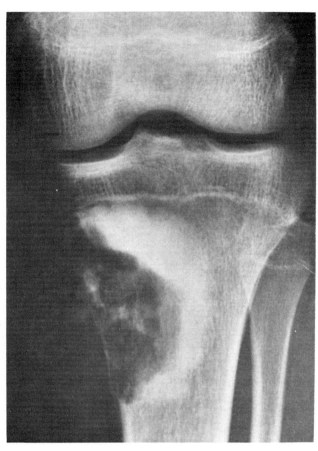

B

FIG. 22-27. Telangiectatic osteosarcoma. (A) A large destructive lesion with a soft tissue mass that is best seen on the lateral films. Note the poorly defined margins with extension of the tumor through the epiphyseal plate. (B) After chemotherapy the margins of bony destruction are very well defined and sclerotic. The soft tissue mass is no longer present. The appearance now suggests a benign lesion.

proach to malignant tumors of the extremities. Detailed information on the extent of disease, possible soft tissue extension, and the status of the neurovascular bundle is required by the surgeon to assess the possibility of en bloc resection. The relationship of the tumor to the main arterial supply and whether there is invasion of the vessel, compression, or simple displacement can usually be determined from high resolution CT scans.

After surgery, CT will frequently demonstrate postoperative hematoma or abscess formation. Residual tumor can usually be differentiated from these complications with contrast enhancement. However, interpretation may on occasion be difficult because of distortion and obliteration of soft tissue planes. In the long-term follow-up of patients with malignant tumors of the extremities, in particular, CT is the most reliable means of demonstrating recurrence. Patients who have been started on chemotherapy and are being followed at regular intervals for evaluation of response are best assessed with CT. Unfortunately, plain roentgenograms, bone scans, and alkaline phosphatase estimations may have to suffice in

large bone tumor centers because of limited access to CT. The former studies, however, have proved adequate in assessing response to chemotherapy in most cases.

Other Tomographic Techniques

Skeletal Tomography. Film tomography of the involved portion of the skeleton is an invaluable technique in more clearly defining the extent of bone tumors. This is particularly true in the axial skeleton, where elimination of overlying intestinal gas and other camouflaging structures is an essential part of the conventional evaluation of a primary bone tumor. Multidirectional film tomography should be used when available, since linear tomography will create "parasite" linear artifacts on the image, which degrade the film and limit the diagnostic yield. The soft tissue penetration of primary bone tumors may be clearly visible on film tomograms, offering another baseline for follow-up of subsequent treatment. In the assessment of primary appendicular lesions before

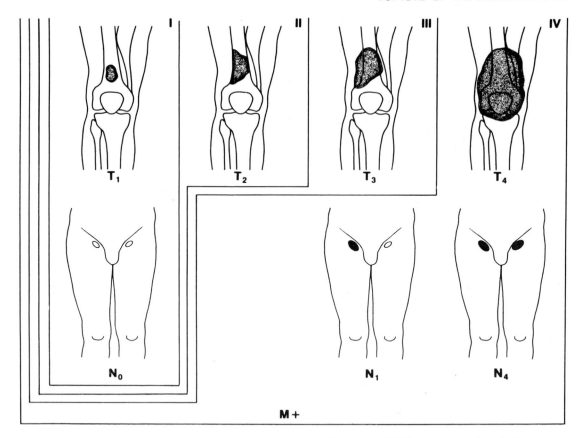

FIG. 22-28. Anatomic staging for bone tumors. Tumor (T) categories: There is no UICC attempt to categorize bone tumors; a simple system has been proposed by the AJC. A more extensive attempt is made in this schema, using T_1 for lesions confined to bone; T_2 for tumors through the cortex with reactive periosteum; T_3 for extensive soft tissue invasion; and T_4 for involvement of joints, nerves, and vessels. Node (N) category: N_1 is regional nodes, N_4 is juxtaregional and the same as a metastatic node. (Reprinted from Rubin, P., Evarts, C. M., Boros, L.: Bone tumors. In *Clinical Oncology for Medical Students and Physicians: A Multidisciplinary Approach*, 6th ed. Rubin, P. (Ed.). New York, American Cancer Society, 1983, pp. 296–307. With permission.)

limb salvage procedures, computed tomography may be necessary for more accurate evaluation of intramedullary extension.

Chest. In individuals with primary malignant tumors of bone, the lung must be reviewed for metastatic deposits before definitive, aggressive treatment. Film tomography and CT will improve the yield of nodular lesions over routine chest X-ray films but at the expense of an increased false-positive yield of nonneoplastic, granulomanous lesions. This issue is discussed in detail in the chapter on thoracic neoplasms.

Xeroradiography. Xeroradiography primarily has been used for mammography and soft tissue tumor evaluation. Because of its edge enhancement effect, xeroradiography

Table 22-2. Tumor (T), Node (N) Classification of Bone Tumors

T_1	Localized to bone of origin; outer cortex intact.
T_{1A}	<5 cm longest dimension.
T_{1B}	>5 cm longest dimension.
T_2	Tumor destroys outer cortex; no gross invasion of soft tissue.
T_3	Gross invasion of soft tissue; recognizable, palpable mass.
T_4	Primary tumor massive; invades joint space, muscle, etc.
N_0	No palpable regional nodes.
N_1	Palpable regional nodes.

Reprinted from Rubin, P., Evarts, C. M., Boros, L.: Bone tumors. In *Clinical Oncology for Medical Students and Physicians: A Multidisciplinary Approach*, 6th ed. Rubin, P. (Ed.). New York, American Cancer Society, 1983, pp. 296–307. With permission.

Table 22-3. Stage Grouping

Stage I	IA	G_1	T_1	N_0	M_0
	IB	G_1	T_2	N_0	M_0
Stage II	IIA	G_2	T_1	N_0	M_0
Stage III	—	G_3	T_{1-3}	N_0	M_0
Stage IV	—	G_{any}	T_{any}	M_{any}	M_{any}

Reprinted from Rubin, P., Evarts, C. M., Boros, L.: Bone tumors. In *Clinical Oncology for Medical Students and Physicians: A Multidisciplinary Approach*, 6th ed. Rubin, P. (Ed.). New York, American Cancer Society, 1983, pp. 296–307. With permission.

Table 22-4. Imaging Modalities for Evaluating Bone Cancers

MODALITY	STAGING CAPABILITY	COST/ BENEFIT RATIO	RECOMMENDED AS A STAGING PROCEDURE	COMMENTS
Primary Tumor (T)				
Conventional roentgenograms	High sensitivity and specificity for primary bone tumors; lower sensitivity and specificity for metastatic lesions in bone	High	Yes	Metastases tend to involve medullary canal and must be >1 cm to be detected
Film tomography	Occasionally useful to evaluate tumor for calcium/bone matrix, soft tissue extension, periosteal changes, and medullary extension	Low	No	Only to answer specific plain film questions
Xeroradiography	Occasionally useful to assess soft tissue component and marginal tumor characteristics	Low	Occasionally	Virtually replaced by CT
Angiography	Seldom useful except to serve as a vascular road map for surgery	Low	No (Yes, if considering limb salvage and clear margin from tumor not demonstrated by CT)	Essential if embolic or infusion therapy contemplated
Computed tomography	Useful to stage tumor locally for medullary and soft tissue extension as well as presence of matrix or cortical disruption	High	Yes	Essential in planning limb conservation surgery
MRI	Applications at present are speculative. Main use with soft tissue rather than bone tumors	Unknown	No	
Metastatic Evaluation (M)				
Chest roentgenograms	Essential for all tumor types	High	Yes	
Film tomography	Useful to characterize questionable plain film findings	Medium	No	If questions or concerns regarding metastases to the chest will alter the primary treatment approach, CT of the lungs should be undertaken
Computed tomography of lungs	Use in high risk patient group where treatment decisions hinge upon presence or absence of lung metastases	Medium (high in proper setting)	Yes	Highest sensitivity but lower specificity (than film tomography). Cannot usually distinguish metastatic from benign nodules in lung. Biopsy must validate CT lung nodules
Radionuclide bone scan	Essential to determine if bone lesion is monostotic or polyostotic	High	Yes	Critical to diagnosis because metastatic lesions are more common and may masquerade as primary bone tumors; many primary bone tumors metastasize to other bones or may appear initially with polyostotic disease; and may be useful in evaluation of extent of lesion in primary tumor
Lymphangiography	Limited usefulness	Low	No	Not found routinely useful in staging

allows a better analysis of the fascial planes and boundaries of a tumor in soft tissues. This technique will image bone tumors as well, but there is no advantage in using xeroradiography over conventional films. It may show the degree of extension of a bone tumor into soft tissue, but this is usually better shown with more sophisticated imaging techniques.

Radionuclide Bone Scanning. The value of radionuclide-labeled bone-seeking agents in evaluating tumors of bone has been appreciated for many decades. It is only recently, however, that advances in instrumentation and the development of newer radiopharmaceutical agents have resulted in high quality scans with radiation doses low enough to allow its use in children. ^{99m}Tc-labeled phosphate derivatives are the most common agents in use today in bone scanning. These include labeled polyphosphates, pyrophosphates, and diphosphonates. Gallium 67 is a valuable agent in that it tends to concentrate in tumors and abscesses and may give a more accurate picture of the size of a tumor. It is not, however, a specific bone-seeking agent.

Although a primary tumor of bone is usually clearly detected on plain films, its extent within the skeleton may be shown to better advantage with a radionuclide bone scan. To distinguish a metastatic from a primary bone tumor, the radionuclide bone scan will most easily determine the other sites of skeletal involvement. Admittedly, these may be metastases from a primary bone tumor, but more often the suspected primary bone tumor may prove to be a metastatic lesion. A radionuclide skeletal survey therefore is an essential component of the staging process for patients suspected of having primary bone tumors.

In the follow-up of patients with primary sarcomas of bone, the decrease in uptake as chemotherapeutic treatment proceeds may be a valuable variable for the chemotherapist to follow, suggesting that tumor necrosis is proceeding well. Unfortunately, the reactive bone resulting from extensive necrosis may complicate the interpretation of scans which may not become completely negative (cold). In most cases of good response to chemotherapy, the radionuclide scans demonstrate decreasing activity as treatment proceeds. It is important to note that multiple myeloma may not be evident on the bone scan, since the lesions of myeloma in general do not stimulate new bone formation. It is estimated that 25% to 30% of radionuclide bone scans in patients with myeloma are normal. The more reliable method of evaluating myeloma is a radiographic skeletal survey. However, some of the lesions of myeloma occasionally do show increased uptake of radionuclide, but in the routine evaluation of myeloma, plain films of the skeleton are usually more accurate in defining the extent of disease. Eosinophilic granuloma may also be relatively "cold" on a bone scan and therefore skeletal films are to be preferred in this condition, as well as in myeloma. In the long-term follow-up of patients with a variety of bone tumors, bone scans are invaluable, for they will demonstrate abnormalities many months before the roentgenograms are abnormal. In a study of 55 patients with primary tumors of the extremities, bone scans were unreliable in separating benign from malignant lesions or in reliably defining the degree of local spread.[50] Gallium scans were more accurate in delineating the local extent of malignant disease. Gallium scans have also proved valuable in the evaluation of Paget's sarcoma, as discussed previously. Widely disseminated metastatic disease, as in breast cancer or prostatic cancer, may lead to symmetrical uptake and may be misinterpreted as a negative scan. The clue to correct interpretation in these instances of the so-called "superscan" is the absence of isotope in the kidneys.

Lymphangiography. There has been a considerable drop in the number of lymphangiograms performed at Memorial Sloan-Kettering Hospital because CT imaging is frequently able to demonstrate the extent of nodal disease. Nodal metastases from primary sarcomas of bone are uncommon. In two tumors, however, malignant fibrous histocytoma and primary lymphoma of bone, nodal disease is relatively common. Lymph node metastases are seen with primary lymphoma of bone, and in the evaluation of this tumor it is important to determine whether other portions of the lymphatic system are involved. Thus, generalized involvement of the nodes in a patient suspected of having a primary malignant lymphoma of bone probably indicates that this is a generalized lymphoma with localized bone involvement. In a primary lymphoma of bone, generalized dissemination to the lymphatic system occurs late.

Angiography. Since the development of sophisticated noninvasive imaging techniques, there has been a marked decrease in the number of conventional angiographic studies performed. Digital subtraction angiography is now in general use and has reduced the number of conventional angiographic studies further. However, conventional angiography still has an occasional place in the evaluation of bone tumors. It is an invasive technique, although serious complications in experienced hands are uncommon. The common indication in the past has been to assess the vascular pattern and therefore the nature of a suspected tumor. However, hypervascularity, arteriovenous shunting, encasement of vessels, and neovascularity may be found in inflammatory lesions and also in benign tumors. Plain films are more reliable in predicting the nature of a tumor of bone than is an angiogram. However, if a primary tumor of vascular origin, such as an hemangioendothelioma, is suspected, angiography is indicated. Computed tomographic angiography has proved valuable and has largely taken the place of routine angiography. Computed tomographic studies with and without contrast in tumors of bone will give more valuable information than simple conventional angiograms. Angiography allows the surgeon to evaluate the exact relationship of the vessel to the tumor and to determine whether en bloc resection can be performed. In many cases, CT angiograms provide this information, but surgeons in general require more detailed demonstration of the anatomy of the vessel. Embolization of some tumors may be considered desirable before surgery. Transcatheter chemotherapy has been favored in the treatment of a variety of primary tumors of bone and also of soft tissue tumors. Since the intravenous route provides adequate blood levels of chemotherapeutic drugs and good results, we feel that administering the drug via the arterial route is probably unnecessary.

Ultrasonography. Ultrasonography is an extremely useful noninvasive method in the investigation of soft tissue tumors, neoplasms of liver, spleen, and kidney. It has no place in the evaluation of primary tumors of bone because bone cannot be imaged with this technique. It shows the extent of spread of a primary tumor of bone into soft tissue, and before staging the tumor, evaluation by this simple technique may be useful; however, CT demonstrates this variable more effectively.

Biopsy. Open biopsy is still the favored technique of most orthopedic surgeons for confirming a suspected primary tumor of bone.[11,35] Many will insist on performing these biopsies for probable metastatic lesions as well. The radiologist is ideally placed to indicate the optimal site of the biopsy, since frequently there is necrotic tissue present as indicated by either a CT study or an angiogram. Close cooperation between a surgeon and radiologist will reduce the number of repeat biopsies because of necrotic tissue. Percutaneous bone biopsy techniques are now in general usage throughout the United States and elsewhere, and they have become the province of the diagnostic radiologist. They are usually easily performed with no significant morbidity, frequently on an outpatient basis. Most commonly, the indication is for evaluation of the nature of a probable metastasis or the confirmation of metastases. Primary bone tumors also lend themselves to these closed biopsies and radiologists are increasingly being requested to perform these studies. In addition to an aspirate of the material, a trephine instrument should be used so that an adequate amount of tissue is obtained for histologic evaluation. The Craig biopsy instrument and modifications of it are extremely useful in evaluating lesions of the spine, since in many cases a tumor of the spine is so extensive that an open biopsy may be dangerous. Percutaneous techniques are preferred in these circumstances. With a little experi-

ence, these biopsies are easily performed without any significant morbidity. The studies are frequently done under CT control and this makes the examination much simpler. The reader interested in learning more about percutaneous skeletal biopsy techniques is referred to de Santos et al.[11] and Murphy et al.[35]

IMAGING STRATEGIES AND DECISIONS

In the selection of the sequence of imaging procedures to evaluate a suspected primary tumor of the skeleton, the approach should be chosen based upon whether or not the appendicular or axial skeleton is involved (Figure 22-29).

Appendicular Skeleton

Plain films in two planes of both bone and soft tissue are obtained. If a bony tumor is clearly present and has aggressive features, a bone scan should be performed as a baseline and also to exclude the presence of other lesions. If a second lesion is found at a distance from the involved bone, it is probably a metastasis from the primary tumor-skip lesion or possibly an incidental lesion such as a benign nonossifying fibroma, or it may suggest that both lesions are metastases from an undiscovered primary site. If a second lesion is found at a distance from the primary tumor, it represents a bony metastasis. If a primary sarcoma is found, its relationship to the vascular bundle should be evaluated with CT angiography, which should demonstrate the extent of the disease and also the possible involvement of the neurovascular bundle. Most of the patients who are referred to large bone tumor centers have already had an open biopsy and simple confirmation of the diagnosis by the pathologist is all that is necessary before treatment can begin.

Axial Skeleton

Primary sarcomas of the axial skeleton are relatively uncommon except for multiple myeloma and chondrosarcoma in the older age group and Ewing's sarcoma in younger individuals. Metastatic lesions are by far the most common tumors of the spine and pelvis. Evaluation with plain films may be inadequate, and conventional tomography is often necessary for identification of the area of destruction. The radionuclide bone scan is useful, but frequently the lack of specificity in the spine, where there frequently are associated degenerative or osteoarthritic changes, may result in false positives. A CT scan will demonstrate the extent of the lesion and also its spread into the soft tissues except in the case of multiple myeloma, when the bone scan usually appears normal despite widespread lesions.[45] If myeloma is suspected, then the diagnosis is made based on a

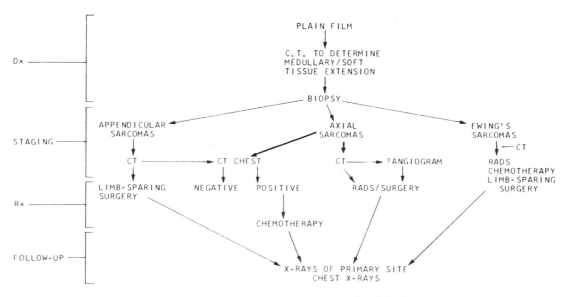

FIG. 22-29. Decision tree of imaging strategies for skeletal tumors.

serum protein profile by immunoelectrophoresis and urinalysis for Bence Jones proteins, which will usually reveal the nature of the tumor. A monoclonal increase in immunoglobulin G1(IgG1), immunoglobulin A (IgA) or immunoglobulin E (IgE) occurs in 54%, 22%, and 1%, respectively, of each[45] (Figure 22-30).

TREATMENT DECISIONS

In view of the wide variety of bone tumors that exist, the considerations here will be limited to the most common problems that arise. The management of malignant bone tumors has become multidisciplinary, not only in diagnosis but in treatment. Each of the standard modalities—surgery, radiation therapy, and chemotherapy—plays an important role in the management of these neoplasms (Table 22-5). Success has been improving, particularly in the pediatric population, and for the first time long-term survivors are beginning to appear in substantial numbers. The main challenge has been the optimization of treatment, particularly with regard to appendicular tumors, where limb preservation has been the major emphasis of modern treatment, with a gradual shift to more conservative surgical procedures, radiation therapy, and multiagent chemotherapy for controlling metastatic disease as well as the primary tumor.

Multiple Myeloma

Because the vast majority of myelomas are multiple and relentless as a result of their progressive nature, systemic chemotherapy is the most important approach to this disease. There are two exceptions. Asymptomatic patients with stable monoclonal hyperglobulinemia should be observed untreated until evidence of infections, altered blood profile, or bone pain appears. The second circumstance is solitary plasmacytomas, which simulate other bone tumors but are readily controlled with doses of 4,000 to 5,000 cGy, which can produce sterilization. If these lesions remain solitary, long-term control and cure is possible.[39,46] Alkylating agents coupled with prednisone are the treatment of choice in multiple myeloma. Melphalan and cytoxan are commonly used with corticosteroids, and usually produce an objective response in approximately 50% of patients.[1,2,45] Although the addition of more aggressive chemotherapy such as vincristine and BCNU promises to yield objective responses of 60% to 70%, it only provides for longer suppression of the disease, which eventually resurges. Palliative radiation therapy to symptomatic areas is very effective for control of pain and doses as modest as 2,000 to 3,000 cGy are most generally used for this purpose. An inverted T arrangement to treat the lower lumbar spine and sacroiliac region is the most common field shape used to produce pain relief.

Osteogenic Sarcomas

Osteogenic sarcoma, which was once refractory to most measures and overwhelmed patients with an aggressive course, has changed its natural history. The experience at the Mayo Clinic[16] has confounded the evaluation of aggressive chemotherapy because of the change in the aggressive nature of this disease. Any results must be interpreted in light of the Mayo Clinic report in 1980 by Edmondon et al.[16] Whether surgery alone, without adjuvant therapy, can provide a high degree of local control is currently undergoing trials. Nevertheless, the con-

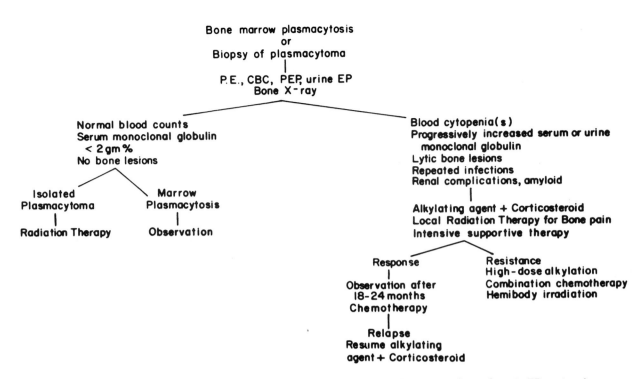

FIG. 22-30. Decision tree for multiple myeloma. PE = physical examination; PEP = protein electrophoresis; EP = urine electrophoresis. (Reprinted from Bakemeier, R. M., Zagars, G., Cooper, R. G., Rubin, P.: The malignant lymphomas: Hodgkin's disease and non-Hodgkin's lymphoma, multiple myeloma, and macroglobulinemia. In *Clinical Oncology for Medical Students and Physicians: A Multidisciplinary Approach*, 6th ed. Rubin, P. (Ed.), New York, American Cancer Society, 1983, pp. 346–369. With permission.)

Table 22-5. Treatment Decisions: Bone Tumors

STAGE	SURGERY	RADIATION THERAPY	CHEMOTHERAPY
Multiple myeloma	NR	Palliative RT 2,000–3,000 cGy	Cytoxan and prednisone
Solitary myeloma	NR	Definitive RT 5,000 cGy	NR
Osteogenic sarcoma	Conservation surgery or amputation	NR	MAC*
Ewing's sarcoma	Biopsy of soft tissue component	Definitive RT 5,000–6,000 cGy	MAC as VACA
Chondrosarcoma	Resection of tumor if possible or amputation	If residuum postoperatively RT: 5,000–7,000 cGy	NR
Histologic cell or Lymphoma	Biopsy	Definitive RT and	MAC as CHOP
Giant cell tumor (Malignant)	Resection if possible	For central axial 5,000–6,000 cGy	NR
Parosteal osteosarcoma	Conservative resection	NR	NR

RT = radiation therapy
NR = not recommended
MAC = multiagent chemotherapy
VACA = Vincristine, actinomycin D, cyclophosphamide, doxorubicin (Adriamycin)
CHOP = Cyclophosphamide, hydroxydaunomycin (Adriamycin), vincristine (Oncovin), and prednisone
*With high dose methotrexate, adriamycin, bleomycin, cyclophosphamide, actinomycin D

tribution of multiagent chemotherapy has been impressive in a variety of studies by cooperative groups.[14,19,26] Most important has been the new approach of adjuvant multiagent chemotherapy advocated by Rosen et al.[40] Primary osteogenic sarcomas are treated with high dose methotrexate and leucovorin rescue, Adriamycin, and a combination of bleomycin, cyclophosphamide, and actinomycin D four weeks before definitive surgery (Figure 22-31). If the resection specimen shows 90% necrosis, the patient is continued on the same chemotherapy. Success rates of 98% have been reported with a median of 31 months of follow-up.[40] If there is less than 90% necrosis, the program is changed to cisplatin with mannitol diuresis. A survival rate of 93% has been reported with this approach, with a median of 18 months follow-up. Limb preservation is difficult because of the radioresistant nature of osteogenic sarcoma, but more conservative subamputative surgery is being attempted to reduce the functional and psychologic morbidity of amputation.[38] To date, the disease-free survival of those patients who have had limb-sparing surgery does not appear to be different from those who have had amputation,[30] but long-term outcome needs to be assessed. The excellent results achieved by Rosen have not been reproduced by other investigators, and a recent review by a National Center Institute task force on osteogenic sar-

comas suggests that with effective chemotherapy, 60% of patients will have long-term disease-free survival.[25]

Ewing's Sarcoma

This highly malignant and widely metastasizing tumor has been brought under dramatic control with the use of all of the standard modes of therapy. Surgery has been more conservative, being limited mainly to biopsy except in the case of pelvic tumors, where resection may be attempted. The emphasis is on biopsy of the soft tissue component rather than bone, since a diagnosis can be made readily without increasing the risk of pathologic fracture. Computed tomography is particularly effective in demonstrating the large soft tissue component associated with most of these lesions. Chemotherapy has proved very effective, with cyclophosphamide, actinomycin D, Adriamycin, and vincristine offering response rates ranging from 60%[29] to 90%.[24] The actuarial survival ranges from the neighborhood of 56% in some of the cooperative group studies[32,33] to Rosen's report of 75%.[41] Limb preservation is a major part of this program, with radiation offering excellent control at doses in the neighborhood of 5,000 to 6,000 cGy. The entire bone needs to be treated, therefore doses of 4,000 to 5,000 cGy are used with a smaller boost field, which can be directed by CT or occasionally by peripheral arteri-

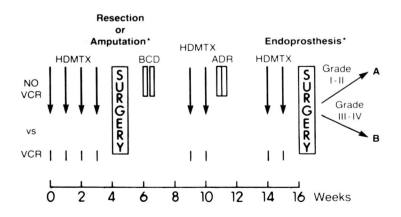

(T-10)

HDMTX - 8 - 12 gm / M^2
(delete after 12
or 16 doses)

LEUCOVORIN - 10 - 15 mg p.o.
q6h · 10 doses
start 20 hours post HDMTX

BCD - Bleomycin
15 mg / M^2 / day
Cyclophosphamide
600 mg / M^2 / day
Dactinomycin
600 mcg / M^2 / day

ADRIAMYCIN (ADR)
30 mg / M^2 / day

*Patients who are to undergo resection or amputation will have surgery at approximately four weeks.
patients who are to undergo endoprosthetic replacement will have surgery at approximately 16 weeks.

FIG. 22-31. Induction chemotherapy for osteogenic sarcoma.

ography, to deliver the maximum dose of 5,500 to 6,000 cGy and ensure coverage of the involved bone and adjacent soft tissue areas.[27]

For those interested in a more detailed management of other bone tumors, see Bakemeier,[5,6] Rosen et al.,[42] Rosenberg et al.,[43] and Rubin et al.[45]

REFERENCES

1. Alexanian, R., Bonnet, J., Gehan, E., Haut, A., Hewlett, J., Montague, L., Monto, R., Wilson, H.: Combination chemotherapy for multiple myeloma. *Cancer* 30:382–389, 1972.
2. Alexanian, R., Salmon, S., Bonnet, J., Gehan, E., Haut, A., Weick, J.: Combination therapy for multiple myeloma. *Cancer* 40:2765–2771, 1977.
3. Axtell, L. M., Myers, M. H.: Contrasts in survival of black and white cancer patients, 1960–1973. *J. Nat. Cancer Inst.* 60:1209–1215, 1978.
4. Bakemeier, R. F.: Hodgkin's disease. In *Practical Cancer Chemotherapy*. Rosenthal, S. N., Bennett, J. M. (Eds.). Garden City, Medical Examiner's Publishing Co., 1981, pp. 104–121.
5. Bakemeier, R. F., Zagars, G., Cooper, R. G., Rubin, P.: The malignant lymphomas: Hodgkin's disease and non-Hodgkin's lymphoma, multiple myeloma, and macroglobulinemia. In *Clinical Oncology for Medical Students and Physicians*, 6th ed. Rubin. P. (Ed.). New York American Cancer Society, 1983, pp. 346–369.
6. Cutler, S. J., Young, J. L.: The third national cancer survey: Incidence data. *Natl. Cancer Inst. Monogr.* 41, 1975.
7. Dahlin, D. C.: *Bone Tumors*, 3rd ed. General aspects and data on 6,221 cases. Springfield, Ill., Charles C. Thomas.
8. Dahlin, D. C., Henderson, E. D.: Chondrosarcoma, a surgical and pathological problem. Review of 212 cases. *J. Bone Joint Surg.* 38A:1025–1038, 1956.
9. Dahlin, D. C., Unni, K. K., Matsuno, K.: Malignant (fibrous histiocytoma of bone—fact or fancy. *Cancer* 39:1508–1516, 1977.
10. del Regato, J. A., Spjut, H. J., (Eds.): *Ackerman and del Regato's Cancer: Diagnosis, Treatment and Prognosis*, 5th ed. Chicago, C. V. Mosby, 1977.
11. de Santos, L. A., Lukeman, J. M., Wallace, S., Murray, J. A., Ayala, A. G.: Percutaneous needle biopsy of bone in the cancer patient. *A.J.R.* 130:641–649, 1978.
12. Durie, B. G., Salmon, S. E.: A clinical staging system for multiple myeloma. *Cancer* 36:842–854, 1975.
13. Falk, S., Alpert, M.: The clinical and roentgen aspects of Ewing's sarcoma. *Am. J. Med. Sci.* 250:492–508, 1965.
14. Fuller, L. M., Macoc-Jones, H., Hagemeister, F. B., Jr., Rodgers, R. W., North, L. B., Butler, J. J., Martin, R. G., Gamble, J. F., Schullenberger, C. C.: Further follow-up of results of treatment in 90 laparotomy-negative stage I and II Hodgkin's disease patients: Significance of mediastinal and nonmediastinal presentations. *Int. J. Radiat. Oncol. Biol. Phys.* 6:499–508, 1980.
15. Glass, A. G., Fraumeni, J. F., Jr.: Epidemiology of bone cancer in children. *J. Nat. Cancer Inst.* 44:187–199, 1970.
16. Gupta, S.: Immunodeficiencies in Hodgkin's disease. Part I: Cell-mediated immunity. *Clin. Bull.* 11:58–65, 1981; Part II: B cell immunity, complement systems, and phagocytic cell systems. *Clin. Bull.* 11:110–119, 1981.
17. Hardy, D. C., Murphy, W. A., Gilula, L. A.: Computed tomography in planning percutaneous bone biopsy. *Radiology* 134:447–450, 1980.
18. Heelan, R. T., Watson, R. C., Smith, J.: Computed tomography of lower extremity tumors. *A.J.R.* 132:933–938, 1979.
19. Hoppe, R. T.: Radiation therapy in the treatment of Hodgkin's disease. *Semin. Oncol.* 7:144–154, 1980.
20. Husband, J. E., Hobday, P. E. (Eds.): *Computerized Axial Tomog-*

21. Huvos, A. G. (Ed.): *Bone tumors: Diagnosis, Treatment and Prognosis*. Philadelphia, W. B. Saunders, 1979.
22. Huvos, A. G., Rosen, G., Bretsky, S. S., Butler, A.: Telangiectatic osteogenic sarcoma: A clinicopathologic study of 124 patients. *Cancer* 49:1679–1689, 1982.
23. Jaffe, H. L.: *Tumors and Tumorous Conditions of the Bone and Joints*. Philadelphia, Lea & Febiger, 1958.
24. Johnson, R. E., Zimbler, H., Berard, C. W., Herdt, J., Brereton, H. D.: Radiotherapy results for nodular sclerosing Hodgkin's disease after clinical staging. *Cancer* 39:1439–1444, 1977.
25. Jones, S. E., Rosenberg, S. A., Kaplan, H. S.: Non-Hodgkin's lymphoma. I. Bone marrow involvement. *Cancer* 29:954–960, 1972.
26. Keller, A. R., Kaplan, H. S., Lukes, R. J., Rappaport, H.: Correlation of histopathology with other prognostic indicators in Hodgkin's disease. *Cancer* 22:487–492, 1968.
27. Kyle, R. A.: Multiple myeloma. Review of 869 cases. *Mayo Clin. Proc.* 50:29–40, 1975.
28. Linden, G., Dunn, J. E.: Ewing's sarcoma in Negroes. *Lancet* 1:1171, 1980.
29. Long, J. C.: The immunopathology of Hodgkin's disease. *Clin. Haematol.* 8:531–566, 1979.
30. Lutzner, M., Edelson, R., Schein, P., Green, I., Kirkpatrick, C., Ahmed, A.: Cutaneous T-cell lymphomas: The Sézary syndrome, mycosis fungioides, and related disorders. *Ann. Intern. Med.* 83:534–552, 1975.
31. Marcove, R. C.: Chondrosarcoma: diagnosis and treatment. *Orthop. Clin. North. Am.* 8:811–820, 1977.
32. Mauch, P., Goodman, R., Hellman, S.: The significance of mediastinal involvement in early stage Hodgkin's disease. *Cancer* 42:1039–1045, 1978.
33. Mauch, P., Hellman, S.: Supradiaphragmatic Hodgkin's disease: Is there a place for MOPP chemotherapy in patients with bulky mediastinal disease? *Int. J. Radiat. Oncol. Biol. Phys.* 6:947–950, 1980.
34. McLeod, R. A., Stephens, D. H., Beaulont, J. W., Sheedy, P. F., II, Hattery, R.: *Semin. Roetgenol.* 13:000–000, 1978.
35. Murphy, W. A., Destouet, J. M., Gilula, L. A.: Percutaneous skeletal biopsy, 1981: A procedure for radiologists—results, review and recommendations. *Radiology* 139:545–549, 1981.
36. Murray, R. O., Jacobson, H. G.: *The Radiology of Skeletal Disorders*, 2nd ed. New York, Churchill Livingstone, 1977, pp. 772–779.
37. Otis, J., Hutter, R. V. P., Foote, F. W., Jr., Marcone, R. C., Stewart, F. W.: Hemangioendothelioma of bone. *Surg. Gynecol. Obstet.* 127:295–305, 1968.
38. Paladuga, R. R., Bearman, R. M., Rappaport, H.: Malignant lymphoma with primary manifestation in the gonad. A clinicopathologic study of 38 patients. *Cancer* 45:561–571, 1980.
39. Petrovich, Z., Fishkin, B., Hittle, R. E., Acquarelli, M., Barton, R.: Extramedullary plasmacytoma of the upper respiratory passages. *Int. J. Radiat. Oncol. Biol. Phys.* 2:723–730, 1977.
40. Rosen, G., Caparros, B., Huvos, A. G., Kosloff, C., Nirenberg, A., Cacavio, A., Marcove, R. C., Lane, J. M., Mehta, B., Urban, C.: Preoperative chemotherapy for osteogenic sarcoma: Selection of postoperative adjuvant chemotherapy based on the response of the primary tumor to preoperative chemotherapy. *Cancer* 49:1221–1230, 1982.
41. Rosen, G., Caparros, B., Nirenberg, A., Marcove, R. C., Huvos, A. G., Kosloff, C., Lane, J., Murphy, M. L.: Ewing's sarcoma: Ten-year experience with adjuvant chemotherapy. *Cancer* 47:2204–2213, 1981.
42. Rosen, G., Marcove, R. C., Caparros, B., Nirenberg, A., Kosloff, C., Huvos, A. G.: Primary osteogenic sarcoma. The rationale for preoperative chemotherapy and delayed surgery. *Cancer* 43:2163–2177, 1979.
43. Rosenberg, S. A., Suit, H., Baker, L. H., Rosen, G.: Sarcomas of the soft tissue and bone. In *Cancer—Principles and Practice of On-*

cology. DeVita, V. T., Jr., Hellman, S., Rosenberg, S. A. (Eds.). Philadelphia, J. B. Lippincott, 1982, pp. 1036-1093.

44. Rosseau, J. J., Franck, G., Grisar, I., Reznik, M., Heynen, G., Salmon, J.: Osteosclerotic myeloma with polyneuropathy and ectopic secretion of calcium. *Eur. Cancer* 14:133-140, 1977.

45. Rubin, P., Evarts, C. M., Boros, L.: Bone tumors. In *Clinical Oncology for Medical Students and Physicians: A Multidisciplinary Approach*, 6th ed. Rubin, P. (Ed.). New York, American Cancer Society, 1983, pp. 296-307.

46. Salmon, S. E. (Ed.): Myeloma and related disorders. *Clin. Haematol.* 11:1, 1982.

47. Schajowicz, J.: Juxtacortical chondrosarcoma. *J. Bone Joint Surg.* 59B:473-480, 1977.

48. Schottenfeld, D., Fraumeni, J. F., Jr.: *Cancer Epidemiology and Prevention.* Philadelphia, W. B. Saunders, 1982.

49. Sherman, R. S., Soong, K. Y.: Ewing's sarcoma. Its roentgen classification diagnosis. *Radiology* 66:529-539, 1956.

50. Simon, M. A., Kirchner, P. T.: Scintigraphic evaluation of primary bone tumors, comparison of technetium-99M phosphonate and gallium citrate imaging. *J. Bone Joint Surg.* 62A:758-764, 1980.

51. Smith, J., Botet, J. T., Yeh, S.: Bone sarcomas in Paget's Disease — A study of 85 patients. *Radiology* 152:583-590, 1984.

52. Smith, J., Ahuja, S. C., Huvos, A. G., Bullough, P. G.: Parosteal (juxtaarterial) osteogenic sarcoma. A roentgenological study of 30 patients. *J. Can. Soc. Radiol.* 29:167-174, 1978.

53. Smith, J., O'Connell, R. S., Huvos, A. G., Woodard, H. Q.: Hodgkin's disease complicated by radiation sarcoma in bone. *Br. J. Radiol.* 53:314-321, 1979.

54. Spjut, H. J., Dorfman, H. D., Fechner, R. E., Ackerman, L. V.: Tumors of bone and cartilage. *Atlas of Tumor Pathology*, Second Series, Bethesda, MD, 1971.

55. Stevens, G. M., Pugh, D. G., Dahlin, D. C.: Roentgenographic recognition and differentiation of parosteal osteogenic sarcoma. *A.J.R.* 78:1-12, 1957.

56. Taylor, W. F., Ivins, J. C., Dahlin, D. C., Edmunson, J. H., Pritchard, D. J.: Trends and variability in survival from osteosarcoma. *Mayo Clin. Proc.* 53:695-700, 1978.

57. Unni, K. K., Dahlin, D. C., Beaubout, J. W.: Periosteal osteogenic sarcoma. *Cancer* 37:2476-2485, 1976.

58. Unni, K. K., Ivins, J. C., Beaubout, J. W., Dahlin, D. C.: Hemangioma, hemangiopericytoma, and mangioendothelioma (angiosarcoma) of bone. *Cancer* 27:1403-1414, 1971.

59. Young, J. L., Asire, A. J., Pollack, E. S.: *SEER program: Cancer incidence and mortality in the United States, 1973-1976.* DHEW Publication No. (NIH)78-1837, 1978.

23 SOFT TISSUE TUMORS OF THE APPENDICULAR SKELETON

Marvin M. Lindell, Jr.
Sidney Wallace

The radiologic diagnostic procedures used for evaluating and staging appendicular soft tissue sarcomas are designed to ascertain the nature, location, and extent of disease. This information forms the basis for the selection of the appropriate therapies used to attempt complete eradication of the tumor while maintaining maximum function.[55,75,80] The more common appendicular soft tissue sarcomas are malignant fibrous histiocytoma (MFH), clear cell sarcoma, liposarcoma, and epithelioid sarcoma. Any soft tissue sarcoma may appear in an extremity: Ewing's sarcoma, fibrosarcoma, osteosarcoma, chondrosarcoma, rhabdomyosarcoma, alveolar soft part sarcoma, and others.

The value of early detection cannot be overly stressed, inasmuch as most of these tumors are aggressive and in most instances tend to metastasize, particularly as they reach large size.

The advent of computed tomography (CT) and ultrasonography (US) has provided the means to diagnose these lesions as well as diagnose them when they are still too small to be detected by conventional radiography. Computed tomography and US also provide the means for staging the primary lesion earlier and for detecting metastases.

Survival rates for soft tissue sarcomas are quite variable, depending upon tumor type, location, size, therapy, and whether and where metastases occur. Soule reported a 64% five-year survival rate for 33 patients with MFH.[77] Twenty-one cases of clear-cell sarcomas of tendons and aponeuroses were reported by Enzinger.[25] The survival rates are not well given to percentages because of many variables; delay of treatment after onset of disease, recurrent tumor, metastases, and types of therapy. Death occurred at variable periods of time, ranging from 1 to 36 years. At the time these data were published, 14 patients had died, 5 were living, and the remainder were lost to follow-up. Three additional cases were submitted by Dutra, but no survival figures are available.[19]

Of 107 patients suffering synovial sarcoma and followed five years or more, Cadman reported 11% living 10 years or more.[9] Of these, six had late recurrences after tumor-free periods of 6, 7, 8, and 11 years, and five died of metastases. Ariel and Pack reported 25 patients with synovial sarcoma, of whom 13 died within five years of diagnosis of their disease, six were living and free of disease for over five years, four were treated too recently for evaluation, and two were lost to follow-up.[4]

Edland reviewed 15 cases of liposarcoma, of which six involved the extremities.[20] Five survived just less than six years following therapy, one dying but two days after commencement of cobalt therapy.[20] Enterline reviewed 53 cases of liposarcoma, 22 occurring in the extremities. Forty of the 53 patients were followed for five years and 25 for 10 years. Nine having extremity tumors survived an average of 4.6 years, and one was lost to follow-up.[24]

Epithelioid sarcoma occurs most frequently in the extremities. Of 62 cases reported by Enzinger in 1970, 60 involved the extremities; there were 11 deaths.[27] Peimer et al. added 37 cases from a review of the literature and presented 6 additional cases.[65] Following treatment, none have succumbed, but follow-up periods range from but 6 to 36 months.

TUMOR BEHAVIOR
AND PATHOLOGY

Histopathology

Malignant Fibrous Histiocytoma. Among the first to describe malignant fibrous histiocytoma were O'Brien and Stout in 1964.[61] It is now recognized as a specific entity and is probably the most common soft tissue sarcoma of older patients, the highest incidence occurring in patients between 50 and 70 years of age. In young patients, the tumor is characterized by a lesser degree of cellular pleomorphism.[49] The thigh and shoulder regions are most commonly affected. The tumors are nodular and measure 5 to 10 cm in greatest diameter. More than other sarcomas, MFH exhibits a wide range of cellular composition and patterns, both from tumor to tumor and in different areas of the same tumor.[18] The least pleomorphic pattern is a distinct storiform or whorled pattern. As the pleomorphism increases, the storiform pattern becomes less pronounced and MFH can often be confused with adult type rhabdomyosarcoma or pleomorphic carcinoma. Malignant fibrous histiocytoma is locally invasive, at times eroding bone. Nodal metastases are common and hematogenous metastases to the lungs are not unusual.

Epithelioid Sarcoma. This is not a rare tumor, but it has been confused with several benign and malignant lesions. Superficial forms of these neoplasms have often been mistaken for necrotizing granulomatous processes or ulcerating squamous cell carcinomas. When located in deeper tissues, the tumor was often mistaken for fibrosarcoma or synovial sarcoma. At present, it is recognized as a specific entity.

Epithelioid sarcoma is a slowly progressive, firm scarlike mass arising from the fascia or deep subcutaneous layer, or less commonly, from the tendon or tendon sheath. It affects patients at any age, but most frequently those in the 20-to-40-year age group. Enzinger initially reported 62 cases and later an additional 95. Of the total 157 cases, 57% were located in the hand and forearm regions, with males being affected 70% of the time.[27] Other reports substantiate these findings.[8,31,73]

The tumor characteristically consists of large, mononuclear, polygonal, epithelium-like cells having vesicular nuclei and deeply eosinophilic cytoplasm arranged in an irregular multinodular pattern. Cellular degeneration or necrosis is not unusual. There are cellular findings that permit differentiation from synovial sarcoma.

Recurrence usually occurs before metastases are evident, the recurrence rate being reported as high as 85%; the metastasis rate is about 30%.[27] Metastases have been most commonly reported in the lungs, lymph nodes, and

scalp. The incidence of metastasis becomes even higher as follow-up periods increase. Early and aggressive surgery is necessary to combat both recurrences and metastases.

Clear Cell Sarcoma of the Tendon Sheath and Aponeurosis. This sarcoma was first described by Enzinger in 1965.[25] These are rare tumors that had earlier been classified as synovial sarcomas or fibrosarcomas in most instances. The clear cell neoplasm has been reported in both young and old patients, but most were observed in patients about 24 years of age, with women probably affected more frequently than men.

A firm, slightly movable painless mass was usually the first sign noted by these patients. When pain was present, it was not severe. A small number of these tumors showed sudden and rapid growth. The feet are most commonly involved, and the lower extremity more frequently than the upper. Most tumors were well delineated grossly and were smooth to moderately nodular. Microscopically, the neoplasms consisted of compact nests and fascicles of pale, fusiform cells of epithelioid appearance.[19,25] The cellular elements were enclosed by delicate septae of fibrous tissue, which merged with the tendinous or aponeurotic tissues. The cells were usually pale staining with indistinct borders, round nuclei, and prominent nucleoli. Mitotic figures were usually scarce, especially in the primary lesions, and the overall vasculature was sparse.[25]

Clinically, growth of this tumor is slow but relentless, with recurrences and metastases commonly observed. The more common sites of metastasis are the regional lymph nodes and the lungs; the heart, liver, and brain follow in frequency.

Liposarcoma. A common neoplasm of the soft tissue sarcoma series, liposarcoma, constitutes about 25% of the total.[26,57] All ages may be affected, but liposarcoma is unusual before the third decade and is most common during the fourth. The average age is about 52 years. The tumor is virtually nonexistent during childhood.[48] Liposarcomas of higher grade are more common in older patients. Both sexes are about equally involved, but men predominate when the tumor is of the well-differentiated type.

These neoplasms can attain very large size, but become apparent earlier in the smaller regions of the appendages. Liposarcomas have a definite predilection for the intermuscular fat planes of the thigh.

The incidence of metastasis is probably about 30% to 40%. Both hematogenous and lymphatic routes exist as well as progressive local invasion and recurrence.

Stout divided the liposarcomas into four groups: (1) well-differentiated myxoid, (2) poorly differentiated myxoid, (3) round cell, and (4) mixed.[79] Enterline has presented a modification of this classification:[24]

1. The well-differentiated type has, as the predominant finding, myxoid cells that are nonpleomorphic in nature. These lie loosely in a mucoid background stroma, rich in capillaries, particularly near the margins of the mass. There may be fibrous bands and a vague lobular pattern.

2. The poorly differentiated type is similar, but the nuclei of the cells are either occasionally or predominately larger and often lobulated and hyperchromatic. Giant cells occur with moderate frequency. Mitoses are noted occasionally but are scanty.

3. This tumor is "lipoma-like," and can easily be mistaken for lipoma or normal fat. These are not encapsulated and the tumor cells are usually mature in appearance, but variable in size, containing scattered, abnormal, often bizarre nuclei. Mitoses are usually absent, but giant cells may be present.

4. This type is myxoid mixed. These tumors are predominantly myxoid, but contain a mixture of other cells, including round cells in most instances. Giant cells, mitoses, and nuclear pleomorphism and cellularity are frequently present, as well as blood vessel invasion.

5. The last type is the nonmyxoid. Adult fat cells are rare. The round cell is predominant, having a moderately large nucleus in vacuolated cytoplasm. Giant cells and mitoses are again frequent as well as blood vessel invasion and marked nuclear pleomorphism. Osteoid at times may be noted, but is probably incidental.

Synovial Sarcoma. This highly malignant tumor is relatively rare, comprising approximately 8% of all soft tissue sarcomas, occurring about equally in men and women, with an average age of 35 years. Ariel and Pack reported over 60% of their patients were under 40 years.[4] Synovial sarcoma is the fourth most common soft tissue sarcoma of the extremities and the most common primary malignant neoplasm of the hands and feet.[9,10] The lower extremity is more frequently involved, especially about the knee. These tumors usually arise beyond the confines of the joint capsule and occasionally from a bursa or tendon sheath.

The tumor frequently recurs locally and distant metastatic disease has been reported to be as high as 65%, with the lungs the most common site. The presence of a painless mass is the usual finding when the patient first appears for treatment.

Synovial sarcomas are unencapsulated, often contain calcifications, and are mostly located near rather than in a joint. Histologically, there are two clear cut patterns: a fibrosarcomatous stroma exhibiting spindle-shaped cells with reticulum fiber and collagen; and a glandular synovial-like component, usually containing mucin. These may be elongated and plump, appearing in compact sheet cords or nests. Foci of calcification are frequently present microscopically and are discernible radiographically in approximately 30% of primary tumors.[9,10,30,62,69,72] There has been a report of calcification and ossification within pulmonary metastases.[15]

CLASSIFICATION AND STAGING

A staging system has been put forth by the American Joint Committee (Figure 23-1). The TNM system was augmented to include the grade of malignancy of the tumor as (G). The fundamental variables are type of tumor, size, and grade of malignancy. The histologists of this committee put forth the soft tissue sarcoma staging system, GTNM.

The definitions of this system are G—pathologic grade of malignancy (G_1 low, G_2 moderate, G_3 high); T—primary tumor (T_1 less than 5 cm, T_2 tumor greater than 5 cm, T_3 tumor that grossly invades bone, major vessel, or major nerve); N—regional lymph nodes (N_0, no histologic verification of metastases to nodes, N_1, histologically verified lymph node metastases); M—distant metastases (M_0, no distant metastases. M_1, distant metastases).

Inasmuch as there was difficulty in obtaining histologic verification of distant metastases in parenchymatous viscera, such verification was not required. However, radiographic evidence as well as positive nuclear scans, lymphangiograms, and angiograms were accepted as evidence of disseminated disease.[73]

Classifications of soft tissue sarcomas are many, but earlier ones include the classification by A. P. Stout in the Soft Tissue Fascicle of the *Atlas of Tumor Pathology* (1957),[78] and revised by Stout and Lattes (1967).[79] A second was presented by the World Health Organization (WHO) in 1969, compiled by an international panel of pathologists (Enzinger, Lattes, and Torloni, 1969).[29] A more current classification used at the Armed Forces Institute of Pathology is an update of the WHO version (Table 23-1).[28] M. D. Anderson Hospital has prepared a new classification of the soft tissue sarcomas, but this is not yet finalized (Table 23-2).

Using the definition for G, T, N, and M, four stages were identified, based upon 702 cases in which complete data for staging was available, including 423 cases histologically reviewed and graded by four pathologists on the Soft Tissue Task Force (Table 23-3, Figure 23-1).[5,73] Conclusions regarding prognosis were based upon the personal experiences of the Task Force, because these data were not collected in the retrospective study.

The determination of stages and substages was made from information obtained from the retrospective study of 1,215 cases, with 702 having complete staging information. Data for stages I through IV were plotted for the 702 cases with complete computer staging information.

This staging system depends upon information ana-

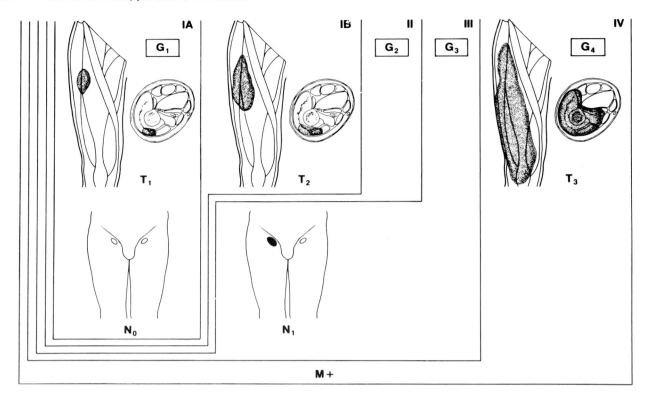

FIG. 23-1. Anatomic staging for soft tissue sarcoma. Tumor (T) categories: Size and extension to bone, major vessels, or nerves determine category. Less or more than 5 cm determines T_1 v T_2, and T_3 extension to other structures. Node (N) categories: This applies to the establishment of histologically positive nodes (N_1). Stage Grouping: This is determined by tumor grade and is a departure from cancer anatomic extent and represents a contradiction in terms. A and B distinguish the size < 5 cm or > 5 cm in diameter. Stage IV is the most advanced, with primary infiltrating surrounding structures and regional nodal and distant metastases. AJC v UICC classifications: There is accord on the classification systems recommended. Modified from AJC. (Reprinted from Pories, W. J., Murinson, D. S., Rubin, P.: Soft tissue sarcoma. In *Clinical Oncology for Medical Students and Physicians: A Multidisciplinary Approach*, 6th ed. Rubin, P. (Ed). New York, American Cancer Society, 1983, pp. 308–325. With permission.)

Table 23-1. Classification of Primary Soft Tissue Sarcomas

Tumors of Known Histogenesis
Fibrosarcoma	Synovial sarcoma
Malignant fibrous histiocy-toma	Malignant mesothelioma
Liposarcoma	Malignant schwannoma
Leiomyosarcoma	Malignant neuroepithelioma
Rhabdomyosarcoma	Extraskeletal myxoid chondro-sarcoma
Hemangiosarcoma	
Lymphangiosarcoma	Extraskeletal mesenchymal chondrosarcoma
Malignant hemangiopericy-toma	Extraskeletal osteosarcoma
	Malignant mesenchymoma

Tumors of Specific Type but Uncertain Histogenesis
Alveolar soft part sarcoma	Epithelioid sarcoma
Malignant granular cell tumor	Extraskeletal neoplasm resembling Ewing's sarcoma
Clear cell sarcoma	

Tumors, Type Undetermined
Sarcoma, type undetermined

Reprinted from Enzinger, F. M. Recent developments in the classification of soft tissue sarcomas. In *Management of Primary Bone and Soft Tissue Sarcomas*, Proceedings of the Annual Clinical Conference on Cancer sponsored by The University of Texas System Cancer Center, M. D. Anderson Hospital and Tumor Institute. Chicago, Year Book Medical Publishers, 1977, p. 220. With permission.

lyzed by the pathologist. Soft tissue lesions are notorious for extreme variations in growth patterns from one part of the tumor to another. A liposarcoma may have a pure fibroblastic growth pattern in one area and may be confused with fibrosarcoma, MFH, or even rhabdomyosarcoma.

The larger the size of the specimen, the better the reliability of the histologic analysis. A needle biopsy has the lowest reliability, whereas incisional biopsy is better. The best material would result from excisional biopsy. The histologic grade of soft tissue sarcomas is a reliable index of survival and prognosis for patients with these tumors.[73] Survival rates by stage for the 702 cases are shown in Table 23-4.[73]

IMAGING PROCEDURES AND ASSESSMENT

The diagnostic procedures presently available are conventional radiography and xeroradiography, ultrasonography, computed tomography, angiography, lymphangiography, and percutaneous needle biopsy.[80] The

Table 23-2. Classification of Soft Tissue Sarcomas—
M. D. Anderson Hospital*

Tumors of Known Histogenesis
Rhabdomyosarcoma
Most malignant fibrous histiocytomas (other than myxoid)
Liposarcoma—pleomorphic and dedifferentiated
Extraskeletal osteogenic sarcoma
Extraskeletal Ewing's sarcoma
Angiosarcoma
Most "unclassified" sarcomas
Synovial sarcoma
Leiomyosarcoma
Neurosarcoma
Alveolar soft part sarcoma

Tumors of Specific Type but Uncertain Histogenesis
Myxoid liposarcoma
Myxoid MFH
Hemangiosarcoma
Mesenchymal chondrosarcoma
Epithelioid and clear cell sarcoma
Myxoid extraskeletal chondrosarcoma
Angiomatoid MFH

Tumors, Type Undetermined
Desmoid fibromatoses
Atypical intramuscular lipomas and well differentiated liposarcoma
Dermatofibrosarcoma protuberans
Hemangioendothelioma?

---

*Temporary draft; to be finalized.
A. Actual 1–3 of grading fibrosarcoma and chondrosarcoma.
B. Synovial sarcomas are to be divided into mono- and biphasic (class III).
C. If information is provided, state "superficial" or "deep" depending upon relationship to fascia to aponeurosis.

---

investigative process should begin with the noninvasive modalities, proceeding next to the invasive, depending upon the clinical problems and the availability of equipment and technical and diagnostic expertise. The studies employed depend upon the morality and morbidity, radiation dosage, expense, and physician and patient convenience. When the therapeutic needs have been met, the search process is concluded.

Conventional Radiography

Chest Radiography and Tomography. Chest radiography (CXR), including whole lung tomography (WLT), is a routine procedure in the evaluation of all patients suspected of having a soft tissue sarcoma. At the present time, computed tomography (CT) is preferably employed in the search for pulmonary metastases.

Chest tomography is most efficacious when the higher kilovoltages are employed; 125 to 150 kVp. Whole lung tomography is most accurate when performed with the patient erect. The thinner the cuts, the higher the accuracy, but 1.0-cm tomographic cuts made from the posterior to the anterior ribs suffice for the primary examination; additional 0.3-to-0.5-cm cuts are obtained as required.[52] Computed tomography is done at 1-cm intervals through the thorax and, when applicable, closer

cuts are obtained. In comparing these three noninvasive modalities, sensitivity and specificity assume great importance. Sensitivity is defined as the proportion of patients shown to have metastases by the examination employed. Specificity pertains to those who do not exhibit metastases. False-positive results are those inter-

Table 23-3. Staging

Stage I*	
Stage IA	
$G_1T_1N_0M_0$	A grade 1 tumor less than 5 cm in diameter with no regional lymph nodes or distant metastases.
Stage IB	
$G_1T_2N_0M_0$	A grade 1 tumor 5 cm or greater in diameter with no regional lymph nodes or distant metastases.
Stage II†	
Stage IIA	
$G_2T_1N_0M_0$	A grade 2 tumor less than 5 cm in diameter with no regional lymph nodes or distant metastases.
Stage IIB	
$G_2T_2N_0M_0$	A grade 2 tumor 5 cm or greater in diameter with no regional lymph nodes or distant metastases.
Stage III‡	
Stage IIIA	
$G_3T_1N_0M_0$	A grade 3 tumor less than 5 cm in diameter with no regional lymph nodes or distant metastases.
Stage IIIB	
$G_3T_2N_0M_0$	A grade 3 tumor greater than 5 cm in diameter with no regional lymph nodes or distant metastases.
Stage IIIC	
G_{any} or $T_{1-2}N_{0-1}M_0$	A tumor of any malignancy grade or size (no invasion) with regional lymph node metastases but no distant metastases.
Stage IV	
Stage IVA	
$G_{any}T_3N_{any}M_0$	A tumor of any differentiation or malignancy demonstrating clear radiographic evidence of destruction of cortical bone (with invasion) and histopathologic confirmation of invasion of major artery or nerve with or without regional lymph node metastases but without distant metastases.
Stage IVB	
$G_{any}T_{any}N_{any}M_1$	A tumor with distant metastases.

With these definitions for G, T, N, and M, four stages were identified based on 702 cases of the series for which complete information for staging was available and including 423 cases histologically reviewed and graded by four pathologists on the Soft Tissue Task Force.
*The distinction between the stage designations of IA and IB is based solely on the 5-cm size factor.
†As in stage I, the distinction between IIA and IIB is based solely on the 5-cm size factor of the primary tumor, the G_2 being the sole qualification.
‡It was necessary to spread the gradation into three subgroups for stage III. The G_3 classification is the largest single determinant and is the common factor for stages IIIA and IIIB; the N_1 classification functions as a sole determinant for stage IIIC.
Adapted from Beahrs, O. H., Myers, M. H.: In *Manual for Staging of Cancer*, 2nd ed. 1983; and Russell, W. O., Cohen, J., Enzinger, F., Hajdu, S. I., Heise, H., Martin, R. G., Meissner, W., Miller, W. T., Schmitz, R. L., Suit, H. D.: In *Management of Primary Bone and Soft Tissue Tumors*. Chicago, Year Book Medical Publishers, 1977, pp. 271–279.

Table 23-4. Survival Rates by Stage

STAGE	NUMBER OF CASES	% SURVIVAL	YEARS AFTER DIAGNOSIS
I	177	80%	10
II	86	55%	5*
III	329	30%	10
IV	110	7%	10

*The curve of stage II was not plotted beyond five years, since at that point the standard error was 5% or higher.

preted as positive for metastases, but are proved to be negative. Sensitivity rises as one progresses from routine chest radiography to whole lung tomography to computed tomography, which is the most sensitive, producing approximately 20% more information. The degree of specificity is not yet clear.[52]

There is considerable variation in the frequency of pulmonary metastases, depending upon the size and nature of the primary tumor and the tendency of the sarcoma to metastasize, ranging from less than 0.5% for the desmoplastic sarcomas to about 50% for the alveolar soft parts sarcomas, and to over 60% for the synovial sarcomas.

Soft Tissue Radiography and Xeroradiography. Soft tissue sarcomas that contain tumor calcification and fat or that distort the fascial fat planes, may be demonstrated on soft tissue radiographs or xeroradiographs (Figure 23-2).[1] Synovial sarcomas are fourth in incidence and are most frequently adjacent to large joints, most often the knee (Figures 23-3, 23-4). The presence of fat within a tumor suggests the possibility of liposarcoma. Approximately 15% of these tumors exhibit low-density areas radiographically. Calcifications are usually nonspecific and may be seen in synovial sarcomas (30%), liposarcomas (15%), and malignant fibrous histiocytomas (10% to 15%). Some sarcomas exhibit relatively specific calcifications; amorphous calcifications in soft tissue osteosarcomas and ringlet calcifications in soft tissue chondrosarcomas (Figure 23-5). The majority of soft tissue sarcomas have similar radiographic features regardless of histology, and distinguishing between malignant and benign tumors is usually impossible.

Xeroradiography (XR) shows the fascial planes and borders of the tumor to better advantage because of the inherent property of edge enhancement. Benign or slow growing neoplasms usually have a sharp, well-defined outline, while malignant or more rapidly progressive tumors are poorly defined because of loss of the fascial fat planes, suggesting invasion (Figures 23-6, 23-7). This is best demonstrated by the xeroradiographic negative mode. Tumor calcifications and fat are better demonstrated by xeroradiography, and the presence of peri-

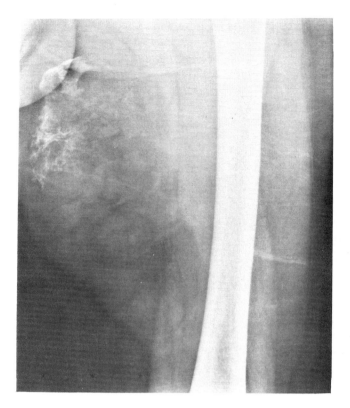

FIG. 23-2. An AP roentgenogram of the thigh showing fat density soft tissue tumor with irregular calcifications and contours: liposarcoma. (Reprinted from Lindell, M. M., Jr., Wallace, S., deSantos, L. A., Bernardino, M. E.: Diagnostic technique for the evaluation of the soft tissue sarcoma. *Semin. Oncol.* 8:160–171, 1981. With permission.)

osteal reaction and bone destruction may indicate the nature and extent of disease (Figure 23-8).

Ultrasonography. Ultrasonography (US) has become a very useful and accurate method for the evaluation of the appendicular soft tissue sarcomas.[97] The differentiation of cystic, solid, and complex masses can usually be made. One has the advantage of imaging in multiple planes, which provides better definition of the acoustical interfaces. When this interface is undetectable, it usually indicates invasion of the adjacent fascial planes. Examinations can be completed in about 5 minutes with demonstration of the exact size and shape of the neoplasm. This is a very important consideration for those patients who are to be followed after radiation or chemotherapy. At the time of the ultrasonographic scan, radiation fields can be quickly and accurately mapped on the patient's skin.

Ultrasonographic patterns of soft tissue sarcomas are frequently nonspecific, inasmuch as these may be echo-free or complex, but benign tumors may have the same findings.[32,42] Ultrasound is of value in follow-up examinations of patients with appendicular sarcomas being treated by surgical and nonsurgical means (Figure 23-9).

In a recent study comparing xeroradiography, ultrasonography, and computed tomography, the size of the lesion was most accurately defined by ultrasound in 23 of 25 cases. The internal consistency of these tumors was noted to vary widely and, in 20 cases, was nonspecific and no histologic diagnosis could be made. In 22 of the 25 patients, the anatomic relationship of the lesion to adjacent bone was determined by ultrasonography.[6] Appendicular sarcomas can be studied by static B scanning, using 3.5 to 10.0 MHz internally focused transducers. Examination consists of scans made in multiple sections through the lesion at intervals of 0.5 to 1 cm. Utilizing the electronic calipers of the digital unit, exact measurements of the length, width, and depth of the neoplasm can be made (Figure 23-10). It is quite easy to place skin markers delineating the mass at this time as an aid to the surgeon and radiotherapist.

Computed Tomography. Computed tomography (CT), while noninvasive, is a very useful radiographic procedure for the evaluation of appendicular soft tissue sarcomas. The ability to differentiate small differences in density allows the anatomic structures as well as alterations of their intrinsic architecture to be recognized. The use of contrast material serves to enhance the demonstration of the soft tissue tumor as well as its relationship to the opacified vessels. It should be borne in mind that intravenous contrast may render the neoplasm isodense, thereby obscuring the process. Contrast material is administered by drip infusion or bolus injection into a vein distal to the lesion for identification of the vascular anatomy or enhancement of the tumor. Both extremities should be visualized for comparative purposes whenever possible and scanning sections through the sarcoma are obtained at 8-mm to 10-mm levels using a 10-mm or 8-mm collimator.[6] Appropriate multiple window widths and levels are selected in recording the images for optimal display.

Soft tissue masses exhibit densities ranging from about 20 to 100 Hounsfield units. The presence of fat or calcium within the tumor may suggest the histologic diagnosis.[44] Liposarcomas have well to poorly defined margins of varying attenuation depending upon tissue contents, whereas a lipoma is usually a well-circumscribed mass of low attenuation (Figures 23-11, 23-12).[14,21] When sufficient fat is present, this is registered as negative (− 60 to − 100) Hounsfield units and is easily detectable, but the differentiation of a fatty tumor from tissue necrosis may not be possible.[7]

The size and configuration of soft tissue neoplasms can usually be accurately estimated. Whenever a sarcoma is identified on a CT scan, the tumor–bone relationship can be seen, thus showing whether or not osseous involvement is present. Computed tomography is most accurate for determination of tumor extension into the vascular bundle.[33,34] However, when all considerations are taken into account, ultrasound scanning remains the best single modality for the evaluation and diagnosis of appendicular soft tissue sarcomas and other soft tissue masses.[76]

Lesions as small as 1 to 3 mm may be detected when thinner cuts are obtained and through use of greater col-

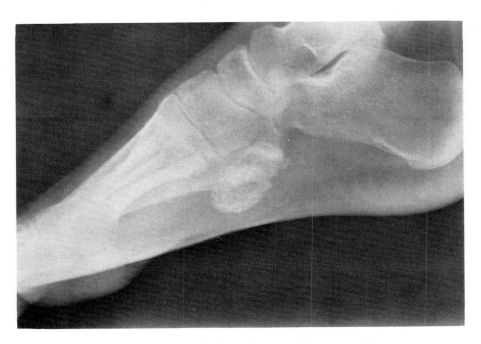

FIG. 23-3. Lateral roentgenogram of the foot showing calcifications within synovial sarcoma.

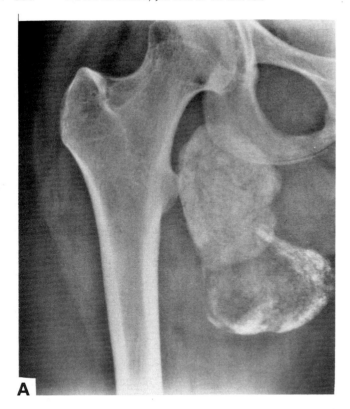

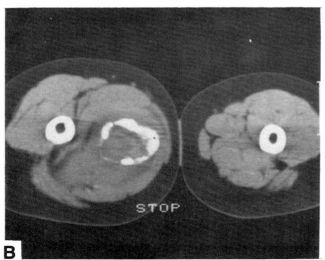

FIG. 23-4. (A) AP roentgenogram of the thigh showing a large synovial sarcoma containing calcifications. (B) A CT scan showing calcifications within the tumor.

limation. The use of overlapping cuts will provide even greater resolution.

Angiography. Angiography (arteriography and venography) was previously the primary method for diagnosing the extent and nature of soft tissue tumors, but at present it is used primarily for the solution of those problems still existing after the use of less invasive procedures.[22] Short-term hospitalization and closer supervision may be required, thus adding to patient expense. However, angiography continues to play a role in the diagnostic and therapeutic management of patients having appendicular soft tissue sarcomas.[23,41,46,70,89] Indications include (1) diagnosis of the nature of the sarcoma by analysis of neoplastic vascularity; (2) determination of the extent of the disease and its relationship to major vessels and septal and tissue planes; and (3) transcatheter therapy by infusion of chemotherapeutic agents and tumor embolization and occlusion.[2,3,11,23,41,46,47,70,74,85,86,87,88,89,92,93]

It should be stressed there are no absolute pathognomic criteria for the diagnosis of malignant neoplasia.[13,60,83] When the neovascularity is a bizarre conglomerate of vessels with pooling of contrast material, and there is vascular encasement where the vessels exhibit an abrupt and irregular change in caliber, these constitute the most consistent and reliable findings in malignancy.[8] Angiomatous lesions and myositis ossificans may be confused angiographically with malignant neoplasms based on the wildly distorted vasculature (Figure 23-13).[37,45] The extent of the tumor can be better demonstrated by angiography if the neoplasm is hypervascular, with lesions as small as 5 mm being detectable. Hypovascular lesions of about 2 cm in diameter may be defined when there is distortion and displacement of adjacent major vessels.[43,51,54,56]

Arteriography of an appendicular soft tissue sarcoma is designed primarily to demonstrate the vascular nature and extent of the neoplasm, to demonstrate encroachment on septal or fascial planes, and to determine operability.[64] When there is invasion of major vessels, local resection is negated, necessitating amputation.

When residual or recurrent tumor is suspected, angiography provides an accurate procedure for demonstrating the extent of disease. The vascularity is usually similar to that of the primary sarcoma.[36] At least two to three months should elapse before postoperative angiography inasmuch as tumor stain and vascularity may be the result of surgery. Angiography readily demonstrates the presence of intravascular extension of the sarcoma.

The lower limits of resolution of computed tomography, ultrasonography, and scintigraphy are about 0.5 to 2 cm. When the lesions are hypervascular, angiographic resolution is such that lesions as small as 5 mm may be detected, but hypovascular metastases must be of the order of 2 cm to be seen.

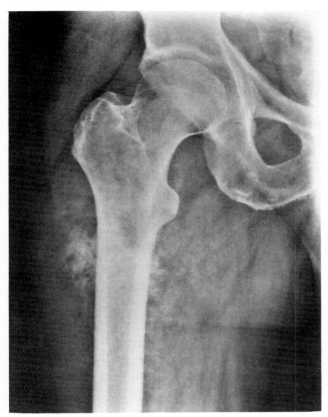

FIG. 23-5. An AP roentgenogram of the upper thigh showing a soft tissue osteosarcoma containing amorphous calcifications.

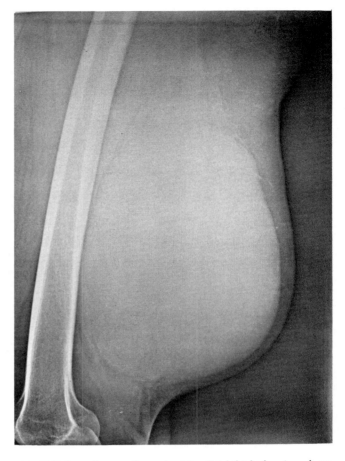

FIG. 23-7. Lateral xeroradiograph of the distal thigh showing a large, dense, soft tissue mass exhibiting a sharp peripheral contour but vague superior and interior borders: unusual dense liposarcoma.

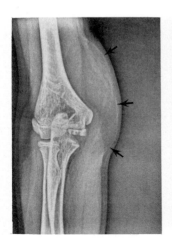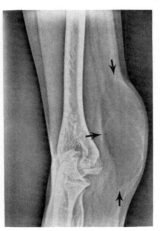

FIG. 23-6. Oblique xeroroentgenograms of the elbow showing a sharply demarcated soft tissue mass of decreased density: lipoma (arrows).

A more recent and extremely promising procedure in the treatment of soft tissue sarcomas is intraarterial chemotherapy. This is followed by surgical resection whenever possible in an attempt to control local disease without unacceptable deformity as well as treat undetected metastases. Cis-platinum (cis-diamminedichloroplatinum) and CYADIC (cytoxan, adriamycin, dimethyltriazeno imidazole carboxamide-DTIC) have proven very efficacious in the treatment of soft tissue sarcomas[74] (Fig. 23-14).

Lymphangiography. Lymphangiography (LAG) can be very useful in the staging of soft tissue sarcomas of the appendicular skeleton, providing additional information on the extent of disease.[84,90,91]

Rigid criteria are absolutely essential if the diagnosis of metastases is to be associated with a high degree of

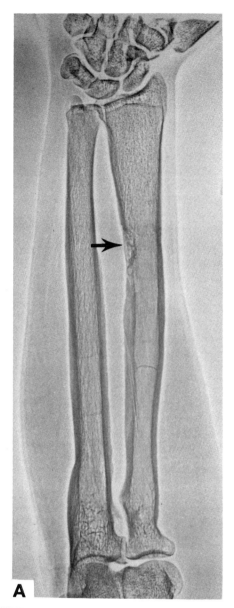

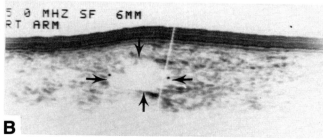

FIG. 23-8. (A) Xeroradiograph of forearm showing cortical erosion and periosteal reaction of bone secondary to recurrent desmoid fibrosarcoma (arrow). No soft tissue mass is evident. (B) Longitudinal sonogram showing soft tissue recurrence but no osseous information (arrows). (Reprinted from Bernardino, M. E., Jing, B. S., Thomas, J. L., Lindell, M. M. Jr., Zornoza, J.: The extremity soft-tissue lesion: A comparative study of ultrasound, computed tomography, and xeroradiography. *Radiology* **139**:53–59, 1981. With permission.)

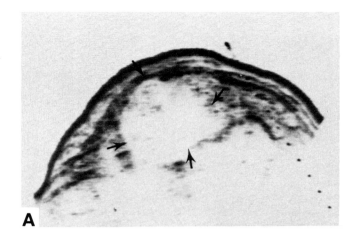

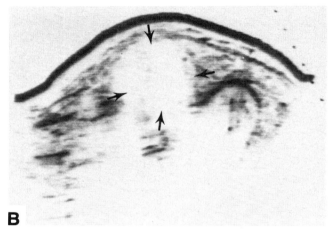

FIG. 23-9. (A) US scan showing large mass (arrows). Undifferentiated soft tissue sarcoma. (B) US scan made 2 months after radiation therapy. The mass (arrows) slightly smaller.

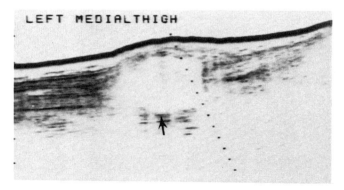

FIG. 23-10. Longitudinal sonogram of thigh showing synovial sarcoma (arrow) and black dots placed by electronic caliper for tumor measurements.

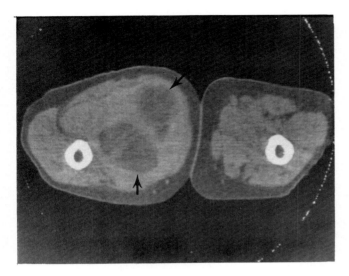

FIG. 23-11. A CT scan of the thigh showing areas of decreased attenuation: malignant fibrous histiocytoma (arrows).

accuracy of pathologic correlation. The primary criterion most commonly associated with metastatic carcinoma is a filling defect in a node not traversed by lymphatic channels (Figure 23-15). Rhabdomyosarcomas may have a pattern similar to that seen in lymphomas, whereas other soft tissue sarcomas may have patterns also seen in carcinomas. Obstruction of the lymphatic channels may occur when the nodes are partially replaced by tumor. This will often lead to opacification of collateral channels; lymphatic to prelymphatic, lymphatic to lymphatic, and lymphatic to venous. In the event of total nodal replacement, disruption of the lymphatic pathways is secondary evidence of nodal disease. Appropriate

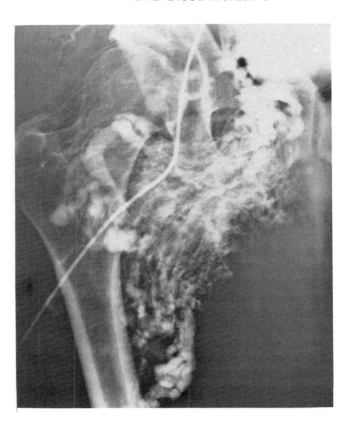

FIG. 23-13. Angiogram of the thigh showing hypervascular tumor with bizarre vessels and pooling and shunting: angiomyolipoma.

confirmatory studies should be performed next; pyelography, angiography, ultrasonography, computed tomography, and needle biopsy. The most common soft tissue sarcomas to metastasize include malignant fibrous histiocytomas, synovial sarcomas, rhabdomyosarcomas, and clear cell sarcomas of the tendon sheath and aponeurosis.[4,19,39,63,77] The fibrosarcomas and liposarcomas manifest metastases only occasionally.

Tallroth, in 1976, presented lymphangiographic findings in 71 cases of soft tissue sarcoma, 24 of which involved nodal metastases (33.8%).[82] This incidence is significantly greater than previous reports.[20,24,25,38,95] M. D. Anderson Hospital reported 16 of 81 patients who exhibited nodal metastases from all types of sarcomas (20%)[100] and unpublished data of 108 cases of soft tissue sarcoma revealed positive lymphangiograms in 23 (21%).

Percutaneous Needle Biopsy. The most important consideration in the case of a soft tissue tumor is the precise identification of its histologic nature. When this variable has been ascertained, one can proceed with therapeutic planning; surgery, radiation therapy, chemotherapy, or any combination thereof. While recurrent sarcoma can often be confirmed by percutaneous aspiration biop-

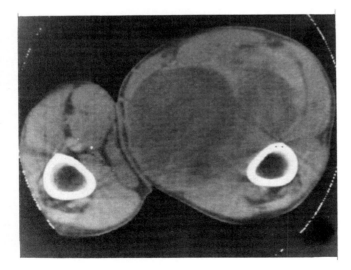

FIG. 23-12. A CT scan of the thigh showing a large tumor of fat density: liposarcoma.

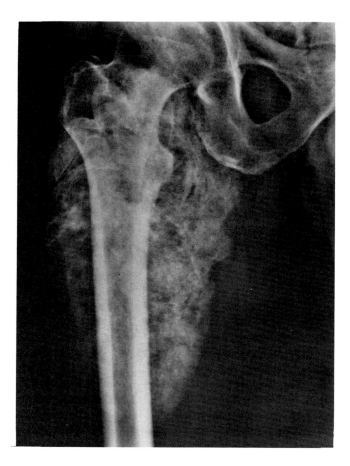

FIG. 23-14. An AP roentgenogram of the upper thigh showing dense calcification and ossification of a soft tissue osteosarcoma 6 months after intra-arterial chemotherapy and balloon occlusion. This is the same patient as shown in Figure 23-5.

sy, the diagnosis of the initial neoplasm is best made by means of core biopsy with a cutting needle. The position and contours of the mass are obtained by radiographic means, followed by needle biopsy of the most invasive area, which is rarely the center of the tumor. This region of the mass may be necrotic and should be avoided because tissue specimens are often devoid of recognizable tumor cells.

The appendicular soft tissue sarcoma lends itself to easy biopsy by the Tru-Cut needle (Travenol Laboratories, Inc., Deerfield, Ill), which obtains a 2 × 20-mm core of tissue. This core is usually quite adequate in obtaining specimen material for histopathologic and electron microscopic analyses. Percutaneous needle aspiration (18–23 gauge) is not an optimal procedure, even though frequently performed, because the cytologic specimen may be of insufficient volume and therefore inadequate for precise identification of the histologic type of sarcoma. It is, however, useful in the evaluation of possible recurrent sarcoma inasmuch as a sufficient amount of

tumor usually is obtained for demonstration of malignant sarcomatous cells that can be compared with the initial diagnostic material.

There is usually a feeling of resistance as the needle enters the neoplastic tissue, at which time the needle is firmly advanced into the tumor. One to four needle aspirations are usually sufficient to ensure adequate material for cytologic diagnosis.

The evaluation of lymph nodes suspected of containing metastatic deposits is easily resolved by means of percutaneous needle biopsy, with a 23-gauge needle under fluoroscopic guidance.[16,17,35,98,99] This procedure has the added advantage that patients usually do not require any special medication or orders and may be examined as outpatients. It is considered prudent not to use percutaneous needle biopsy on patients having abnormal bleeding variables. The complication of seeding the tumor cells along the needle track is uncommon and a minimal risk compared with the diagnostic reward.

IMAGING STRATEGIES AND DECISIONS

Imaging plays a very important role in the diagnosis of soft tissue sarcomas. This section will deal with soft tissue sarcomas in general, but mainly in the appendicular presentations. There is a partial chapter devoted to

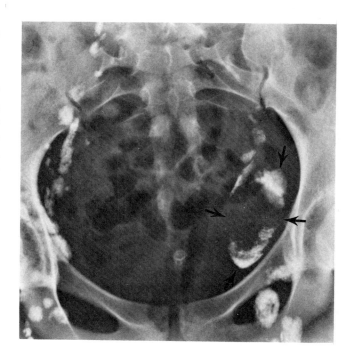

FIG. 23-15. Nodal phase of a lymphangiogram showing metastasis in pelvic node from a liposarcoma (arrows). The lymphatic phase showed that the feeding channel did not traverse the node.

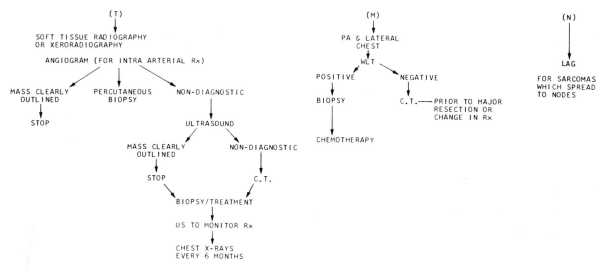

FIG. 23-16. Staging decision tree for soft tissue sarcomas.

retroperitoneal sarcomas (Chapter 15), which is considered in the differential diagnosis of adrenal tumors.

A mass in the soft tissues of the body is usually identified clinically or because it causes compression symptoms or it has invaded the underlying bone or neighboring neurovascular bundle. The first imaging modality is soft tissue radiography or xeroradiography. A percutaneous biopsy may be obtained if the mass is clearly outlined. Ultrasound and CT examinations are commonly done before a more definitive invasive biopsy is attempted. Computed tomographic examination, as noted, is the more accurate procedure in axial skeletal tumors, but ultrasound can be very effective, particularly in appendicular masses or masses in the retroperitoneal area to monitor them during treatment. As previously noted, a multimodal approach is usually used, consisting of conservation surgery, radiation therapy, and chemotherapy depending upon the histopathologic grade of the sarcoma in addition to its size.

One of the important determinants in the management of the patient once the histopathologic diagnosis is made is to determine whether there is metastatic disease. Since hematogenous spread is much more common than lymph node spread, a chest film is usually obtained. If a solitary lesion is found or if none is identified and the tumor is poorly differentiated and likely to metastasize, a CT scan of the chest is indicated. If multiple metastases are found, this is an essential step before major resection or aggressive local regional radiation therapy. If metastatic disease is identified, the patient is a candidate for chemotherapy. If liver enzyme levels are abnormal, a CT scan of the liver would be ordered. Computed tomography rather than lymphangiography would be used for evaluation of the nodal compartment de-

pending upon the origin of the tumor. Unusual bone pain or the proximity of the lesion to bone would warrant a bone scan and, if positive, targeted radiography of the area. Although brain scans would not be done as part of a routine workup once metastatic disease was identified or there was any suspicion of neurologic findings, this diagnostic study would be in order.

TREATMENT DECISIONS[29,53,67]

The histologic grade more than the pathologic type and stage determines the management of soft tissue sarcomas. Oncologic imaging, particularly CT scanning, plays a very important role in defining the muscle compartments that are involved and that need to be resected. As with bone tumors, the tendency has been toward limb preservation in soft tissue sarcomas, and resections tend to be conservative whenever possible. This has led to the use of preoperative or post-operative radiation therapy and chemotherapy, the latter therapy particularly in areas where intra-arterial infusions may be conducted (Table 23-5).

Surgery

Resection of the primary tumor usually encompasses the local extension along tissue planes and the entire muscle compartment and aponeuronic structures. Contiguous neurovascular tissues should be spared if possible, but may be included along with a regional node resection if such a step is not debilitating. If skin and subcutaneous tissues are involved they also are resected widely and skin grafts can be used for coverage. Amputation is only done when the mass cannot be encompassed by a wide excision with a 2 to 3 cm margin on all sides or a useless extremity will result because of an inadequate vascular or neurologic supply.

Radiation Therapy

The role of radiation therapy has proven to be an important one, particularly with the accomplishments of Suit,[71,81] who has firmly established preoperative or postoperative irradiation with conservative surgical resections as the preferred approach. Although randomized studies have not been done, the results in the literature indicated this approach yields excellent survival rates with fewer complications than in the past. Megavoltage techniques are required with coned-down fields as higher doses are given. Usually a large volume with generous margins receives a dose of 5,000 to 6,000 cGy with the smaller tumor receiving a boosted dose of 6,000 to 7,000 cGy. Occasionally with implantations and smaller electron fields, boost doses as high as 8,000 cGy can be delivered, but these need to be given in a protracted period of time. An alternate technique is intraoperative irradiation, where a dose of 1,500 to 2,000 cGy is applied to the area of residuum through the operative wound. This is particularly useful in axial (retroperitoneal) rather than appendicular neoplasms. The use of preoperative irradiation has reduced the size of the radiation field, and doses are usually limited to 5,000 cGy to avoid problems with healing.[81]

Chemotherapy

Previously, excellent results were being noted for multidrug regimens such as CYVADIC, which includes cyclophosphamide (Cytoxin), vincristine, Adriamycin, and DTIC. Reports indicated this to be a very active combination, with a 50% response rate, complete remissions in 17% of patients, and median survivals of 16 months.[66,96] However, this has not been substantiated and Adriamycin alone or in combination with DTIC may be yielding comparable results.[96] This has led to some questions about the efficacy of chemotherapy as an adjuvant. Instead, neoadjuvant or presurgical chemotherapy is being studied in clinical trials, which has led to wider use of agents in the form of intra-arterial infusions,[59] isolation infusions,[58] and hyperthermic infusions.[50] These latter approaches have been combined with limb sparing surgery and often with irradiation as well in an attempt to avoid amputation. To date, randomized studies have not substantiated the role of these neoadjuvant infusions.[58,68] Such drugs as phenylalanine mustard, nitrogen mustard, actinomycin D, and doxorubicin have been given intra-arterially. There are some series with impressive results using preoperative arterial Adriamycin and radiation therapy in conservative doses of 3,500 cGy in 10 fractions with surgery 7 to 10 days afterward with a radical en bloc resection of the tumor including 10 cm margins. If postoperative chemotherapy has also been given, it usually consists of vincristine, high dose methotrexate, and citrovorum rescue.[94]

The results overall of local regional control remain excellent. The five-year local control rate with postoperative irradiation is 84% at the Massachusetts General Hospital and it was 83% at the National Cancer Institute. Disease-free survival with conservation of limb in a UCLA study by Weisenberger is reported to be at a 60% level.[94]

IMPACT OF NEW TECHNOLOGY

Magnetic resonance imaging (MRI) is a rapidly emerging technique that produces high quality tomographic images similar to CT.[40] Magnetic resonance imaging is conceptually quite different from conventional imaging modalities and offers a unique set of variables for tissue characterization. Early research on pathologic tissue indicated a significant variation in the MRI variables of several soft tissue tumors compared with normal tissue.[12] Further research in this area is underway to determine the potential tissue specificity of MRI imaging measurements (Harms, S. E.: personal communication). Magnetic resonance imaging provides several other ad-

Table 23-5. Treatment Decisions: Soft Tissue Sarcoma

STAGE	SURGERY	RADIATION THERAPY		CHEMOTHERAPY
IA,B (T_1,T_2G_1)	Conservative resection	If microresiduum, postoperative RT		NR
IIA,B (T_1,T_2G_2)	Conservative resection	Pre- or postoperative RT	and/or	SAC/MAC
IIIA,B ($T_1,T_2,N_0,G_3N_1,G_{any}$)	Conservative resection	Pre- or postoperative RT	and/or	SAC/MAC
IVA ($T_3,N_{0,1},G_{any}$)	Amputation	Pre- or postoperative RT	and	SAC/MAC
B ($T_{any},N_{any},M_+,G_{any}$)	NR	Palliative RT	and	MAC

NR = not recommended
RT = radiation therapy (It consists of 5000–6000 cGY plus small field boost to 7000 cGy.)
SAC = single agent chemotherapy, as Adriamycin
MAC = multiagent chemotherapy (investigational)

vantages including (1) imaging planes are not limited to the axial section as in CT; any desirable plane can be imaged and individual planes extracted from the computer memory without repeating the scanning process; (2) the entire three-dimensional volume may be imaged and individual planes extracted from the computer memory without repeating the scanning process; (3) MRI uses no ionizing radiation, and (4) MRI data may be obtained from several nuclei to provide more specific metabolic information. The future role of MRI imaging in the evaluation of soft tissue sarcomas will be the subject of an increasing amount of clinical research.

REFERENCES

1. Abramowitz, D., Zornoza, J., Ayala, A. G., Romsdahl, M. M.: Soft-tissue desmoid tumors: Radiographic bone changes. *Radiology* **146**: 11–13, 1983.
2. Anderson, J. H., Gianturco, C., Wallace, S.: Experimental transcatheter intra-arterial infusion-occlusion chemotherapy. *Invest. Radiol.* **16**:496–500, 1981.
3. Anderson, J. H., Wallace, S., Gianturco, C., Gerson, L. P.: "Mini" Gianturco stainless steel coils for transcatheter vascular occlusion. *Radiology* **132**:301–303, 1979.
4. Ariel, I. M., Pack, G. T.: Synovial sarcoma: Review of 25 cases. *N. Engl. J. Med.* **268**:1272–1275, 1963.
5. Beahrs, O. H., Myers, M. H.: In *Manual for Staging of Cancer*, 2nd ed., p. 113. New York, American Cancer Society, 1983.
6. Bernardino, M. E., Jing, B. S., Thomas, J. L., Lindell, M. M. Jr., Zornoza, J.: The extremity soft-tissue lesion: A comparative study of ultrasound, computed tomography, and xeroradiography. *Radiology* **139**:53–59, 1981.
7. Brasch, R. C., Kim, O. H., Kushner, J. H., Rosenau, W.: Ossification in a soft tissue embryonal rhabdomyosarcoma. *Pediatr. Radiol.* **11**:99–101, 1981.
8. Bryan, R., Soule, E., Dobyns, J., Pritchard, E., Lincheid, R.: Primary epithelioid sarcoma of the hand and forearm. A review of thirteen cases. *J. Bone Joint Surg.* **56A**:458–465, 1974.
9. Cadman, N. L., Soule, E. H., Kelly, P. J.: Synovial sarcoma: An analysis of 134 tumors. *Cancer* **18**:613–627, 1965.
10. Cavanagh, R. C.: Tumors of the soft tissues of the extremities. *Semin. Roentgenol.* **3**:73–89, 1973.
11. Chuang, V. P., Wallace, S.: Arterial infusion and occlusion in cancer patients. *Semin. Roentgenol.* **16**:13–25, 1981.
12. Damadian, R., Zaner, K., Hor, D., Di Maio, T.: Human tumors detected by nuclear magnetic resonance. *Proc. Natl. Acad. Sci. USA* **71**:1471–1473, 1974.
13. Denny, M. B. M.: Vascular patterns in tumors of the extremities. *S. Afr. Med. J.* **30**:27–30, 1956.
14. deSantos, L. A., Ginaldi, S., Wallace, S.: Computed tomography in liposarcoma. *Cancer* **47**:46–54, 1981.
15. deSantos, L. A., Lindell, M. M. Jr., Goldman, A. M., Luna, M. A., Murray, J. A.: Calcification within metastatic pulmonary nodules from synovial sarcoma. *Orthopedics* **1**:141–144, 1978.
16. deSantos, L. A., Wallace, S.: Intravascular treatment of liver and bone neoplasms. In *Percutaneous Biopsy and Therapeutic Vascular Occlusion.* Anacker, H., Gullotta, U., Rupp, N. (Eds.). New York, Georg Thieme Verlag, 1980, pp. 113–116.
17. Dodd, G. D., Wallace, S., Jing, B. S., Paulus, D. D., Jr., Goldstein, H. M., Handel, S. F., Zornoza, J.: Diagnostic radiologic techniques in the detection, staging, and treatment of neoplastic disease. In *Cancer Patient Care at M. D. Anderson Hospital and Tumor Insti-*
tute. Clark, R. L., Howe, C. D. (Eds.). Chicago, Year Book Medical Publishers, 1976, pp. 769–823.
18. Dorfman, H. D., Bhagavan, B. S.: Malignant fibrous histiocytoma of soft tissue with metaplastic bone and cartilage formation: A new radiologic sign. *Skeletal Radiol.* **8**:145–150, 1982.
19. Dutra, F. R.: Clear-cell sarcoma of tendons and aponeuroses. Three additional cases. *Cancer* **25**:942–946, 1970.
20. Edland, R. W.: Liposarcoma. A retrospective study of fifteen cases. A review of the literature and a discussion of radiosensitivity. *Am. J. Roentgenol. Radium Ther. Nucl. Med.* **103**:778–791, 1968.
21. Egund, N., Ekelund, L., Sako, M., Persson, B.: CT of soft tissue tumors. *A.J.R.* **137**:725–729, 1981.
22. Ekelund, L., Herrlin, K., Rydholm, A.: Comparison of computed tomography and angiography in the evaluation of soft tissue tumors of the extremities. *Acta Radiol. [Diagn]* **23**:15–28, 1982.
23. Ekelund, L., Lunderquist, A.: Pharmacoangiography with angiotensin. *Radiology* **110**:533–540, 1979.
24. Enterline, H. T., Culberson, J. D., Rochlin, D. B., Brady, L. W.: Liposarcoma. A clinical and pathological study of 53 cases. *Cancer* **13**:932–950, 1960.
25. Enzinger, F. M.: Clear-cell sarcoma of tendons and aponeuroses. An analysis of 21 cases. *Cancer* **18**:1163–1174, 1965.
26. Enzinger, F. M.: Recent trends in soft tissue pathology. In *Tumors of Bone and Soft Tissue.* Chicago, Year Book Medical Publishers, 1965, pp. 315–332.
27. Enzinger, F. M.: Epithelioid sarcoma. A sarcoma simulating a granuloma or carcinoma. *Cancer* **26**:1029–1041, 1970.
28. Enzinger, F. M.: Recent developments in the classification of soft tissue sarcomas. In *Management of Primary Bone and Soft Tissue Tumors,* 21st Clinical Conference on Cancer 1976, at the University of Texas System Cancer Center, M. D. Anderson Hospital and Tumor Institute. Chicago, Year Book Medical Publishers, 1977, pp. 219–234.
29. Enzinger, F., Lattes, R., Torloni, H.: In *Management of Primary Bone and Soft Tissue Tumors.* Chicago, Year Book Medical Publishers, 1977, p. 220.
30. Felson, B.: *Chest Roentgenography.* Philadelphia, W. B. Saunders, 1973, pp. 465–493.
31. Gabbiani, G., Fu, Y.-S., Kaye, G. I., Lattes, R., Majno, G.: Epithelioid sarcoma. A light and electron microscopic study suggesting a synovial sarcoma origin. *Cancer* **30**:486–499, 1972.
32. Goldberg, B. B.: Ultrasonic evaluation of superficial masses. *J. Clin. Ultrasound* **3**:91–94, 1975.
33. Golding, S. J., Husband, J. E.: Radiology of soft tissue sarcoma. *J. Roy. Soc. Med.* **75**:729–735, 1982.
34. Golding, S. J., Husband, J. E.: The role of computed tomography in the management of soft tissue sarcomas. *Br. J. Radiol.* **55**:740–747, 1982.
35. Gothlin, J. H.: Post-lymphangiographic percutaneous fine needle biopsy of lymph node guided by fluoroscopy. *Radiology* **120**:205–207, 1976.
36. Granmayeh, M., Jonsson, K., McFarland, W., Wallace, S.: Angiography of abdominal leiomyosarcoma. *A.J.R.* **130**:725–730, 1978.
37. Gronner, A. T.: Muscle necrosis simulating a malignant tumor angiographically. Case report. *Radiology* **103**:309–310, 1972.
38. Guccion, J. G., Enzinger, F. M.: Malignant giant cell tumor of soft parts: An analysis of 52 cases. *Cancer* **29**:1518–1529, 1972.
39. Haagensen, C. D., Stout, D. P.: Synovial sarcoma. *Ann. Surg.* **118**:1032–1051, 1943.
40. Harms, S. E.: Current status of nuclear magnetic resonance imaging. In *Medical Diagnostic Imaging Systems: Technology and Applications.* New York, Frost and Sullivan Press, 1982.
41. Hawkins, I. F. Jr., Hudson, T.: Priscoline in bone and soft tissue angiography. *Radiology* **110**:541–546, 1974.
42. Hayama, I., Fukuma, H., Masuda, S., Kobayashi, T.: Ultrasonic tomography of tumors in the soft tissue and bone (Meeting Ab-

stract). *J. Jpn. Orthop. Assoc. (Special)*:67, 1977.

43. Hudson, T. M., Hass, G., Enneking, W. F., Hawkins, I. F.: Angiography in the management of musculoskeletal tumors. *Surg. Gynecol. Obstet.* 141:11–21, 1975.

44. Hunter, J. C., Johnston, W. H., Genant, H. K.: Computed tomography evaluation of fatty tumors of the somatic soft tissues: Clinical utility and radiographic-pathologic correlation. *Skeletal Radiol.* 4:79–91, 1979.

45. Hutcheson, J., Klatte, E. C., Kremp, R.: The angiographic appearance of myositis ossificans circumscripta. A case report. *Radiology* 102:57–58, 1972.

46. Jacobs, J. B., Hanafe, W. N.: The use of priscoline in peripheral arteriography. *Radiology* 88:957–960, 1967.

47. Bledin, A. G., Kantarjian, H. M., Kim, E. E., Wallace, S., Chuang, V. P., Patt, Y. Z., Haynie, T. P.: ^{99m}Tc-labeled macroaggregated albumin in intrahepatic arterial chemotherapy. *A.J.R.* 139:711–715, 1982.

48. Kauffman, S. L., Stout, A. P.: Lipoblastic tumors of children. *Cancer* 12:912–925, 1959.

49. Kauffman, S. L., Stout, A. P.: Histiocytic tumors (fibrous xanthoma and histiocytoma) in children. *Cancer* 29:961–976, 1972.

50. Krementz, E. T., Carter, R. D., Sutherland, C. M., Hutton, I.: Chemotherapy of sarcomas of the limbs by regional perfusion. *Ann. Surg.* 185:555–564, 1977.

51. Levin, D. C., Gordon, D. H., McSweeney, I.: Arteriography of peripheral hemangiomas. *Radiology* 121:625–630, 1976.

52. Libshitz, H. I., North, L. B.: Pulmonary metastases. *Radiol. Clin. North Am.* 20:437–451, 1982.

53. Lindberg, R. D.: Soft tissue sarcoma. In *Textbook of Radiotherapy*, 3rd ed. Fletcher, G. H. (Ed.). Philadelphia, Lea & Febiger, 1980, pp. 922–942.

54. Lindberg, R. D., Murphy, W. K., Benjamin, R. S., et al.: Adjuvant chemotherapy in the treatment of primary soft tissue sarcomas: A preliminary report. In *Management of Primary Bone and Soft Tissue Tumors*, 21st Clinical Conference on Cancer 1976, at the University of Texas System Cancer Center, M. D. Anderson Hospital and Tumor Institute. Chicago, Year Book Medical Publishers, 1977, pp. 343–352.

55. Lindell, M. M., Jr., Wallace, S., deSantos, L. A., Bernardino, M. E.: Diagnostic technique for the evaluation of the soft tissue sarcoma. *Semin. Oncol.* 8:160–171, 1981.

56. Martel, W., Abell, M. R.: Radiologic evaluation of soft tissue tumors. A retrospective study. *Cancer* 32:352–366, 1973.

57. Martin, R. G., Butler, J. J., Albores-Saavedra, J.: Soft tissue tumors: Surgical treatment and results. In *Tumors of Bone and Soft Tissue*. Chicago, Year Book Medical Publishers, 1965, pp. 333–347.

58. McBorde, C. M.: Regional chemotherapy for soft tissue sarcomas. In *Management of Primary Bone and Soft Tissue Tumors*, 21st Clinical Conference on Cancer 1976, at the University of Texas System Cancer Center, M. D. Anderson Hospital and Tumor Institute. Chicago, Year Book Medical Publishers, 1977, pp. 353–360.

59. Morton, D. L., Eilber, F. R., Townsend, C. M., Grant, T. T., Mirra, J., Wekenburgers, T. H.: Limb salvage from a multidisciplinary treatment approach for skeletal and soft tissue sarcomas of the extremity. *Ann. Surg.* 184:268–278, 1976.

60. Ney, F. G., Feist, J. H., Altemus, L., Ordinario, V. R.: The characteristic angiographic criteria of malignancy. *Radiology* 104:567–570, 1972.

61. O'Brien, J. E., Stout, A. P.: Malignant fibrous xanthomas. *Cancer* 17:1445–1455, 1964.

62. O'Keefe, M. E., Good, C. A., McDonald, J. R.: Calcification in solitary nodules of the lung. *A.J.R.* 77:1023–1033, 1957.

63. Patton, R. B., Horn, R. C. Jr.: Rhabdomyosarcoma: Clinical and pathological features and comparison with human fetal and embryonal skeletal muscle. *Surgery* 52:572–584, 1962.

64. Paushter, D. M., Borkowski, G. P., Buonocore, E., Belhobek, G.

H., Marks, K. E.: Digital subtraction angiography for preoperative evaluation of extremity tumors. *A.J.R.* 141:129–133, 1983.

65. Peimer, C. A., Smith, R. J., Sirota, R. L., Cohen, B. E.: Epithelioid sarcoma of the hand and wrist: Patterns of extension. *J. Hand. Surg.* 2:275–282, 1977.

66. Pinedo, H. M., Kenis, Y.: Chemotherapy of advanced soft tissue sarcomas in adults. *Cancer Treat. Rev.* 4:67–86, 1976.

67. Pories, W. J., Murinson, D. S., Rubin, P.: Soft tissue sarcoma. In *Clinical Oncology for Medical Students and Physicians: A Multidisciplinary Approach*, 6th ed. Rubin, P. (Ed.). New York, American Cancer Society, 1983, pp. 308–325.

68. Rantakokko, V., Ekfors, T. O.: Sarcomas of the soft tissue in the extremities and limb girdles. *Acta Chir. Scand.* 125:385–394, 1979.

69. Robbins, S. L.: Pathologic Basis of Disease. Philadelphia, W. B. Saunders, 1974, pp. 1472–1474.

70. Rockoff, S. D., Doppman, J., Block, J. B., Ketcham, A.: Variable response of tumor vessels to intra-arterial epinephrine: An angiographic study in man. *Invest. Radiol.* 1:205–213, 1966.

71. Rosenberg, S. A., Suit, H. D., Baker, L. H., Rosen, G.: Sarcomas of the soft tissue and bone. In *Cancer—Principles and Practice of Oncology*. DeVita, V. T. Jr., Hellman, S., Rosenberg, S. A. (Eds.). Philadelphia, J. B. Lippincott 1982, pp. 1036–1093.

72. Rubin, P., Green, J.: *Solitary Metastasis*. Springfield, IL, Charles C Thomas, 1968, pp. 7–51.

73. Russell, W. O., Cohen, J., Enzinger, F. M., Hajdu, S. I., Heise, H., Martin, R. G., Meissner, W., Miller, W. T., Schmitz, R. L., Suit, H. D.: In *Management of Primary Bone and Soft Tissue Tumors*. Chicago, Year Book Medical Publishers, 1977, pp. 271–279.

74. Shuman, L. S., Chuang, V. P., Wallace, S., Benjamin, R. S., Murray, J.: Intra-arterial chemotherapy of malignant fibrous histiocytoma of the pelvis. *Radiology* 142:343–346, 1982.

75. Simon, M. A., Enneking, W. F.: The management of soft tissue tumors of the extremities. *J. Bone Joint Surg.* 58A:317–327, 1976.

76. Slasky, B. S., Lenkey, J. L., Skolnick, M. L., Campbell, W. L., Cover, K. L.: Sonography of soft tissues of extremities and trunk. *Semin. Ultrasound* 3:288–330, 1982.

77. Soule, E. H., Enriquez, P.: A typical fibrous histiocytoma, malignant fibrous histiocytoma, malignant histiocytoma, and epithelioid sarcoma. *Cancer* 30:128–143, 1972.

78. Stout, A. P.: Tumors of the soft tissues. In *Atlas of Tumor Pathology*, Section 2, Fascicle 5. Washington, D.C., Armed Forces Institute of Pathology, 1953.

79. Stout, A. P., Lattes, R.: Tumors of the soft tissues. In *Atlas of Tumor Pathology*. Second Series, Fascicle 1. Washington, D.C., Armed Forces Institute of Pathology, 1967, p. 196.

80. Suit, H. D., Russell, W. O., Martin, R. G.: Management of patients with sarcoma of soft tissue in an extremity. *Cancer* 31:1247–1255, 1973.

81. Suit, H. D., Russell, W. O.: Radiation therapy of soft tissue sarcomas. *Cancer* 36:759–764, 1975.

82. Tallroth, K.: *Lymphatic Dissemination of Bone and Soft Tissue Sarcomas*. Paperi, J. A., Painotuote, K. (Eds.). Helsinki, Finland, 1976.

83. Viamonte, M. Jr., Roen, J., LaPage, J.: Nonspecificity of abnormal vascularity in the angiographic diagnosis of malignant neoplasms. *Radiology* 106:59–63, 1973.

84. Wallace, S.: Dynamics of normal and abnormal lymphatic systems as studied with contrast media. *Cancer Chemother. Rep.* 52:31–58, 1968.

85. Wallace, S.: Interventional radiology in the cancer patient. *Cancer* 37:517–531, 1976.

86. Wallace, S.: The evolution of interventional radiology. (Published as Proceedings of the First International Symposium on Intervention Radiology, Algarve, Portugal, May 29–June 2, 1979). Amsterdam, Excerpta Medica, 1981.

87. Wallace, S., Chuang, V. P.: Transcatheter management of the cancer patient. In *Cancer—Principles and Practice of Oncology*.

DeVita, V. T., Jr., Hellman, S., Rosenberg, S. A. (Eds.). Philadelphia, J. B. Lippincott, 1982, pp. 1862–1877.

88. Wallace, S., Chuang, V. P.: Transcatheter management of musculoskeletal neoplasms. In *Interventional Radiology*. Wilkins, R. A., Viamonte, M. Jr. (Eds.). Oxford, Blackwell Scientific Publications, 1982, pp. 225–240.

89. Wallace, S., Chuang, V. P., Carrasco, C. H., Charnsangavej, C., Bechtel, W., Wright, K. C., Gianturco, C.: Physioanatomic concepts and radiologic techniques for intra-arterial delivery of therapeutic agents. *The Cancer Bulletin of the University of Texas M. D. Anderson Hospital and Tumor Institute at Houston* 36: 6–14, 1984.

90. Wallace, S., Jackson, L.: Lymphangiography. *Encycl. Med.* 3:307–323, 1964.

91. Wallace, S., Jackson, L., Dodd, G. D., Greening, R. R.: Lymphangiographic interpretation. *Radiol. Clin. North Am.* 3:467–485, 1965.

92. Wallace, S., Jing, B. S.: Lymphangiography in carcinoma. In *Golden Diagnostic Radiology*. Clouse, M. (Ed.). Baltimore, Williams & Wilkins, 1977, pp. 185–273.

93. Wallace, S., Medellin, H., De Jongh, D. S., De Jongh, D., Gianturco, C.: Systemic heparinization for angiography. *Am. J. Roentgenol. Radium Ther. Nucl. Med.* 116:204–209, 1972.

94. Weisenberger, T. H., Eilber, F. R., Grant, T. T., Morton, D. L.,

Murra, J. J., Steinberg, M., Rickles, D.: Multidisciplinary "limb salvage" treatment of soft tissue and skeletal sarcomas. *Int. J. Radiat. Oncol. Biol. Phys.* 7:1495–1499, 1981.

95. Willis, R. A.: *The Spread of Tumors in the Human Body*, 3rd ed. London, Butterworths, 1973, p. 417.

96. Yap, B.-S., Baker, L. H., Sincovic, J. G., Rivkin, S. E., Bottomley, R., Thigpen, T., Burgess, M. A., Benjamin, R. S., Bodey, G. P.: Cyclophosphamide, vincristine, Adriamycin, and DTIC (CYVADIC) combination chemotherapy for the treatment of advanced sarcomas. *Cancer Treat. Rep.* 64:93–98, 1980.

97. Yiu-Chiu, V., Chiu, L. C.: Complementary values of ultrasound and computed tomography in the evaluation of musculoskeletal masses. *RG (Radiographics)* 3:46–82, 1983.

98. Zornoza, J.: *Percutaneous needle biopsy*. Baltimore, Williams & Wilkins, 1980.

99. Zornoza, J., Bernardino, M. E., Ordonez, N. E., Thomas, J. L., Cohen, M. A.: Percutaneous needle biopsy of soft tissue tumors guided by ultrasound and computed tomography. *Skeletal Radiol.* 9:33–36, 1982.

100. Zornoza, J., Wallace, S., Goldstein, H. M., Lukeman, J. M., Jing, B.: Transperitoneal percutaneous retroperitoneal lymph node aspiration biopsy. *Radiology* 122:111–115, 1977.

24 PEDIATRIC ONCOLOGY

Herman Grossman
Donald R. Kirks

In most parts of the developed world, malignant neoplasms, although rare, are second only to trauma as a cause of death in childhood. Fewer types of tumors occur in the pediatric age group than in the adult population; many of these tumors are unique to children. The behavior of many of these tumors, including response to treatment, is often unique as well. For example, the epithelioid form of Wilms' tumor, the most common renal malignancy of childhood, responds to a combination of surgery, chemotherapy, and radiation in more than 90% of cases;[91] the outcome for renal cell carcinoma, the most common adult renal malignancy, is less favorable. Similarly, the five-year survival rate for pediatric acute lymphoblastic leukemia with combined chemotherapy is greater than that for adult leukemia.[22] Among the solid tumors seen in childhood, rhabdomyosarcoma[63] and Ewing's sarcoma[70] may respond to combined therapy regimens, while neuroblastoma, a common solid tumor of childhood, has a very poor response to all therapies.[80] The one exception is neuroblastoma in children under 1 to 2 years of age, in whom the prognosis is good because of spontaneous regression of the tumor. Non-Hodgkin lymphoma in childhood responds less well to therapy than do these malignancies in adults.[62]

The pediatric neoplasms to be discussed in this chapter are Wilms' tumor, nephroblastomatosis, and neuroblastoma. The histopathology, natural history, pathways of dissemination, and therapeutic responses of childhood malignancies have been thoroughly described. An area of pediatric oncology that has not been evaluated is the efficacy of various imaging modalities in diagnosis for each type of patient. In general, the following areas need to be more closely defined: (1) evaluation of type of imaging procedures best suited for initial detection of pediatric neoplastic processes; (2) evaluation of appropriate imaging studies required to stage disease; (3) recommendation of procedures best suited for detection of distant metastatic disease; and (4) selection of procedures appropriate for assessment of complications of treatment.

In the assessment of pediatric patients there are advantages and disadvantages of the various imaging modalities. Ultrasonography has several advantages: it is cheaper than computed tomography; generally no sedation is required for an ultrasonographic examination; imaging can be performed in multiple planes; its use does not involve exposure to ionizing radiation; and ultrasonography does not require physiologic function for anatomic visualization as is necessary with excretory urography or some aspects of computed tomography. Ultrasonography is adversely affected by bone and gas artifacts. A second disadvantage is its dependence on the skill of the operator.

Computed tomography (CT) provides anatomic detail that is superior to other imaging modalities.[45,56] Enhancement with contrast medium facilitates measurement of blood flow to an organ, visualization of vascular structures, and may define pathologic abnormalities. The drawbacks to the use of CT are that sedation is generally required for children, and the paucity of fat in children makes delineation of anatomic margins in the retroperitoneum difficult.[76]

Chest CT in children warrants special mention. Although primary parenchymal malignant tumors are rare in this age group, it is frequently necessary to search for metastatic lesions in the lungs.[46] The propensity for pulmonary metastases in children is attributed to systemic venous extension of the primary tumor and embolic seeding of the rich vascular supply of the lungs.[44] The most common metastatic lung lesions of childhood are associated with Wilms' tumor, osteogenic sarcoma, and rhabdomyosarcoma. Determining the presence or absence of metastatic disease is, therefore, the most common indication for pediatric chest CT scans.[50] Since metastatic nodules are often subpleural and peripheral in location, these lesions are not apparent on chest roentgenograms or tomograms but are particularly well defined with CT evaluation. The possibility of detecting a benign nodule by chest CT has not been as thoroughly investigated in children as it has in adults. As many as 60% of nodules detected by CT in adults are benign at resection.[74] Experience indicates that pleural-based normal lymph nodes or benign granulomas are not present on chest CT scans of children; however, the radiologic-pathologic studies needed to confirm this clinical impression have not been performed. A finding of peripheral nodules in the lungs of a child with a primary malignancy is considered to represent metastatic disease and usually alters the course of radiation, surgical, or chemotherapeutic treatment chosen for the patient. The important exception is children undergoing chemotherapy. Several pediatric patients we have followed developed nodules in the lungs several months after a primary malignancy had been removed and while the patient was on chemotherapy. Because these nodules persisted while on chemotherapy, they were surgically removed. Histologic examination showed fibrous tissue only, without evidence of residual malignancy. This probably represents a nonspecific reaction to chemotherapy-induced necrosis of metastatic tumor tissue.[33]

The best method for detection of bone metastasis in patients with neuroblastoma and rhabdomyosarcoma is still under discussion. There is some dispute over whether scintigraphy or a roentgenographic skeletal survey is more sensitive for detecting early, small, metastatic lesions. Either imaging modality is satisfactory but neither is consistently accurate for detecting metastases.[40] We have examples in which one method detected a metastatic lesion while the images from the other modality appeared normal. A greater problem in this area is the use of radionuclide bone scintigraphy in growing children. It is difficult to determine the uptake in the normal growing metaphysis from some activity related to metastasis.

WILMS' TUMOR

Wilms' tumor (nephroblastoma) is the most common renal malignancy of childhood. The disease ranks third, behind leukemia and brain tumors, as a childhood malignancy. It occurs with approximately the same frequency as neuroblastoma and is slightly more common in boys than in girls. Although the lesion is seen in older children and occasionally in adults, approximately 90% of Wilms' tumors occur in patients who are less than eight years of age. The average age of diagnosis is three years. Wilms' tumors account for approximately 10% of all childhood malignancies.[24] In the United States, the annual incidence of Wilms' tumor is 7.8 per million children under 15 years of age.[12]

Wilms' tumors most frequently appear as asymptomatic abdominal masses. Less commonly, the child has specific complaints of bloody urine, malaise, poor appetite, or constipation. Hypertension is noted in more than half of patients with Wilms' tumor.[11] Wilms' tumor is bilateral in 5% to 10% of reported cases.[11]

Tumor Behavior and Pathology

Wilms' tumor is usually bulky and replaces most of the involved kidney. The tumor may originate in any portion of the kidney, except the renal pelvis, and usually expands within the renal parenchyma to displace and distort the pelvocalyceal system. The renal capsule is usually intact; it is uncommon for the tumor to break through this capsule and extend into the extrarenal space. Central hemorrhage and necrosis frequently occur. These pathologic processes account for the lucency seen during total body opacification on exretory urograms, as well as the areas of decreased echogenicity detected by ultrasonography. The tumor may extend into the ipsilateral renal vein, the inferior vena cava, and occasionally into the right atrium.

Renal blastema, which are aggregates of primitive metanephric epithelial cells with occasional tubular differentiation, are felt to be the precursors of Wilms' tumor and may be considered analogous to the existence of neuroblastoma in situ in neonates. In most patients, this renal blastema will involute. Occasionally, the patient's defense mechanisms are inadequate and a Wilms' tumor develops.[25] Nodules of renal blastema are found in approximately 15% of kidneys resected for Wilms' tumor and are particularly common if the tumor is bilateral.[12] Histologically, Wilms' tumor consists of undifferentiated renal tissues with embryonic or abortive glomeruli and tubule formation surrounded by spindle cell stroma. Tumors with these microscopic features are considered favorable histologically, with an approximate survival rate of 90%. Approximately 10% of all Wilms' tumors have unfavorable histology (UH). Four subtypes of disease are included in this category: focal anaplasia, diffuse anaplasia, "rhabdoid" sarcoma, and clear-cell sarcoma. The rhabdoid and clear-cell neoplasms have certain clinical features that are unlike Wilms' tumors. The rhabdoid tumor tends to be associated with intracerebral disease that manifests itself as deposits or as a second independent small-cell brain tumor.[66] Wilms' clear-cell sarcoma, on the other hand, is associated with its tendency to metastasize to bone.[2] Only 40% of children with the unfavorable histology of Wilms' tumor survive. In addition to the type of Wilms' histology, another factor of prognostic importance is the presence of metastases in lymph nodes or in distant structures. The actual size of the tumor and operative spillage of tumor have a minor impact on outcome.[9]

Wilms' tumors metastasize by direct invasion of adjacent tissues, lymphatic spread to retroperitoneal lymph nodes, hematogenous seeding or, rarely, ureteral spread to the distal urinary tract.[11] Renal vein invasion accounts for the hematogenous lung metastases noted in Wilms' tumor. The incidence of pulmonary metastases is 8% to 15% at the time of diagnosis.[25] As stated earlier, chest CT scans are particularly valuable in diagnosing the presence of metastatic tumor in the lung.[50] Pneumothorax occasionally occurs in patients with the sarcomatous type of Wilms' tumor secondary to pulmonary metastatic disease. Liver metastases are rare at the time of initial diagnosis of Wilms' tumor; however, during the course of the disease 8% to 10% of all patients with Wilms' tumor will develop liver metastases. The majority of those liver metastases occur in the terminal stage of the disease or are discovered at autopsy.[25]

Appropriate effective therapy for Wilms' tumor depends on the extent of involvement as determined by imaging modalities, surgery, and pathologic examination.[11,24]

Classification and Staging

A system of staging has been established by the National Wilm's Study Group III. It is outlined in Table 24-1 and Figure 24-1.[3]

Imaging Procedures, Assessment, and Strategies

One approach to rational assessment of all abdominal and pelvic masses in children is to start with ultrasonography. This study would determine whether the mass was extrarenal or intrarenal and whether it was cystic or solid. These findings, coupled with the age of the patient, lead to a diagnosis in most children. After 1 year of age, solid renal masses are usually Wilms' tumors; from infancy to 5 years of age, solid adrenal and paravertebral

Table 24-1. National Wilms' Tumor Study Group III Staging System and a Comparison to the American Joint Committee's Staging System

AJC	NWTS	ANATOMIC DESCRIPTION
T_1,N_0,M_0	Stage 1	Tumor limited to kidney and completely excised. The surface of the renal capsule is intact. Tumor was not ruptured before or during removal. There is no residual tumor apparent beyond the margins of resection.
T_2,N_0,M_0 T_1,N_{1a},M_0	Stage II	Tumor extends beyond the kidney, but is completely excised. There is regional extension of the tumor, i.e. penetration through the outer surface of the renal capsule into perirenal soft tissues. Vessels outside the kidney substance are infiltrated or contain tumor thrombus. The tumor may have been biopsied or there has been local spillage of tumor confined to the flank. There is no residual tumor apparent at or beyond the margins of excision.
	Stage III	Residual nonhematogenous tumor confined to abdomen. Any 1 or more of the following may occur.
$T_{1 \text{ or } 2},N_{1b},M_0$		a. Lymph nodes on biopsy are found to be involved in the hilus, the periaortic chains or beyond. b. There has been diffuse peritoneal contamination by tumor such as by spillage of tumor beyond the flank before or during surgery, or by tumor growth that has penetrated through the peritoneal surface.
$T_{3a},$ any N,M_0		c. Implants are found on the peritoneal surfaces.
$T_{3b},$ any N,M_0		d. The tumor extends beyond the surgical margins either microscopically or grossly.
$T_{3c},$ any N,M_0		e. The tumor is not completely resectable because of local infiltration into vital structures.
Any T, except $T_4,$ any N,M_1	Stage IV	Hematogenous metastases. Deposits beyond stage III, i.e., lung, liver, bone and brain.
$T_4,$ any $N,$ any M	Stage V	Bilateral renal involvement at diagnosis. An attempt should be made to stage each side according to the above criteria on the basis of extent of disease prior to biopsy.

Modified from Putnam, T. C., Cohen, H. J., Constine, L. S.: Pediatric Solid Tumors. In *Clinical Oncology for Medical Students and Physicians*, 6th ed. Rubin, P. (Ed.) American Cancer Society, 1983, p. 399.

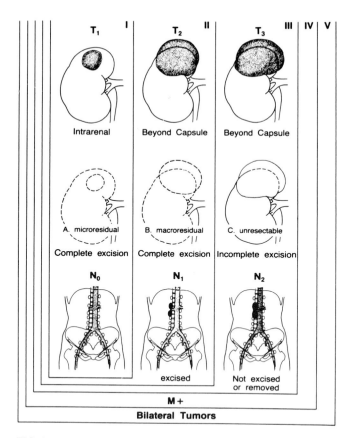

FIG. 24-1. Anatomic staging for Wilms' tumor. Tumor (T) categories: The entire thrust of pediatric tumor classification is postsurgical—whether or not the tumor is resectable. The T_1 and T_2 categories are simply tumor within the kidney capsule or beyond and T_2 v T_3 is its resectability. The division of T_3 into microresidual, macroresidual, and unresectable is the A,B,C substage. Node (N) categories: The regional nodes are involved and resectable (N_1) or incompletely resected (N_2). Stage grouping: The favorable staging is I and II, where disease is totally resected. Stage III is similar to T_3 with the addition of unresectable nodes. Stage IV is distant metastases. A special feature of Wilms' tumor is stage V, bilateral renal involvement. N_1 or T_2 are included in stage II; and N_2 or T_3 are included in stage III. AJC/UICC classification: There is no UICC staging system and the NWTS system has been adopted by the International Society of Pediatric Oncology (SIOP). (Modified from Putnam, T. C., Cohen, H. J., Constine, L. S., III: Pediatric solid tumors. In *Clinical Oncology for Medical Students and Physicians: A Multidisciplinary Approach*, 6th ed. Rubin, P. (Ed.). New York, American Cancer Society, 1983, pp. 392–427. With permission.)

masses are usually neuroblastomas. These two tumors constitute the majority of abdominal solid tumors in childhood. If a renal mass is solid on an ultrasound examination, computed tomography without and with enhancement is recommended.[4,7] Computed tomography delineates the extent of the renal mass as well as any abnormality of the liver, renal veins, or inferior vena cava.[43]

If ultrasound examination reveals the renal mass to be cystic, it is almost always benign.[27] Excretory urograms or renal nuclear scintigraphy are recommended before surgery to define any areas of renal function. Newborns

may require nuclear scintigraphy because of their poor renal function in and distortion of the pelvocalyceal system (Figure 24-2). Wilms' tumor may also compress the renal pelvis to produce obstructive hydronephrosis. In 10% of all Wilms' tumors, there is renal nonfunction. This is due to occlusion and invasion of the renal pelvis, ureter, or renal vein.[25]

If a foot vein is injected with large amounts of contrast material while a tourniquet is in place around the opposite thigh, good opacification of the inferior vena cava is obtained. The renal vein and inferior vena cava may contain intraluminal tumor thrombus or be obstructed, displaced, or distorted by the Wilms' tumor. It is often difficult to distinguish between obstruction of the vessel by tumor and extrinsic compression.[11] The appearance of occlusion may be accentuated by the normal physiologic mechanism of increased intra-abdominal pressure with crying.

Ultrasonography. There is a spectrum of ultrasonographic abnormalities in Wilms' tumor, but the hallmark is a

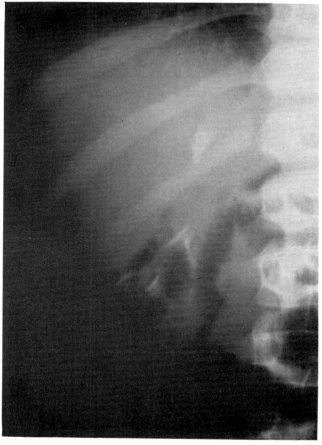

FIG. 24-2. A six-year-old boy with an asymptomatic flank mass. This excretory urogram shows splaying of the upper and middle calyces of the right kidney as a result of an intrarenal mass that proved to be a Wilms' tumor.

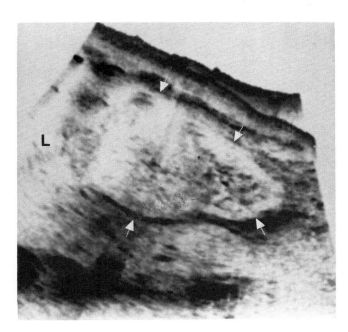

FIG. 24-3. A longitudinal ultrasonogram of the right kidney and liver (L) of the same patient as shown in Figure 24-2, shows bulging of the middle portion of the kidney as a result of an echogenic mass. The arrows outline most of the kidney and show the change in the contour of the kidney by the mass.

mixed echogenic pattern caused by the solid tumor elements (Figure 24-3). The margins of the tumor are usually well defined. Echolucent areas may be present as a result of necrosis and hemorrhage. A solid renal mass on an ultrasonogram in an older infant or child is most often a Wilms' tumor.[26,35,52]

Examination of vascular structures by ultrasound is important to search for tumor extension into the venous structures or for displacement of major vessels by the tumor. This usually requires longitudinal, transverse, and oblique imaging with real-time ultrasonography. Venous extension is diagnosed when echogenic filling defects are identified within a renal vein, the inferior vena cava (Figure 24-4A), or the right heart. Ultrasonography is most accurate for evaluating the more cephalad portion of the inferior vena cava. Since Wilms' tumors are usually large and expansile, the inferior vena cava is frequently displaced by tumor mass (Figure 24-4B). This may prevent adequate visualization of intraluminal venous structures, particularly in uncooperative children. Computed tomography with bolus contrast injection or inferior venacavography by catheter provides better visualization of the caudal portion of the vena cava and renal veins.

Computed Tomography. In patients with Wilms' tumor, excretory urography usually indicates only that a mass is within the kidney. The hallmark of ultrasonography in Wilms' tumor is the echogenic pattern. The presence of echolucent areas caused by necrosis and hemorrhage

may be misleading, but increased echogenicity should suggest the correct diagnosis. Computed tomography (CT) offers a means to specify the nature of the lesion, including its morphologic characteristics, extent of tumor, and presence of local metastases.[75] Computed tomography visualizes vascular structures, identifies nodal involvement, evaluates the liver for the presence or absence of metastases, and is the most accurate method for imaging the opposite kidney.[52] Evaluation by CT of renal veins and the infrahepatic inferior vena cava may be performed during bolus injection of contrast medium (3 mL/kg of Renografin-60) (Figure 24-5). Upper extremity vein injection is preferred for optimal visualization of the renal arteries and veins.[52] If contrast medium is injected into a foot vein, the inferior vena cava may become so densely opacified that a high-density artifact is produced.

As stated, the contralateral kidney is usually better evaluated by CT than ultrasonography (Figure 24-6A). If tumor is initially nonresectable or bilateral, CT is extremely helpful in following response to chemotherapy[8] (Figure 24-6B). Chest CT may also be performed at initial evaluation to identify pulmonary metastases, which are present in approximately 10% of children at initial diagnosis.[50] Chest roentgenograms may appear normal when CT demonstrates metastatic disease (Figure 24-7A and B).

Computed tomography is an excellent method for following patients after resection of a Wilms' tumor. The tumor bed may be extremely difficult to assess by ultrasonography since it frequently contains loops of bowel. Computed tomography provides precise anatomic delineation of the tumor bed after the use of oral and intravenous contrast medium. It may detect ipsilateral recurrence or contralateral development of Wilms' tumor. Moreover, the lungs and liver may be evaluated for metastases by CT.

Nuclear Scintigraphy. Nuclear scintigraphy has a limited role in the evaluation of Wilms' tumor. It may be used as a screening method for detection of hepatic metastases. However, marked extrinsic liver compression by a primary intrarenal tumor frequently mimics direct hepatic extension. Moreover, as experience with CT for the initial evaluation of Wilms' tumor has grown, its value in assessing hepatic involvement has become clear.[52] Bone scintigraphy may be helpful in diagnosing metastases from the sarcomatous type of Wilms' tumor (Figure 24-8) before the patient becomes symptomatic.

Angiography. Previously, aortography, bilateral selective renal arteriography, and inferior venacavography were routinely performed in the initial evaluation of Wilms' tumor. The development of less invasive imaging modalities has essentially eliminated the need for renal angiog-

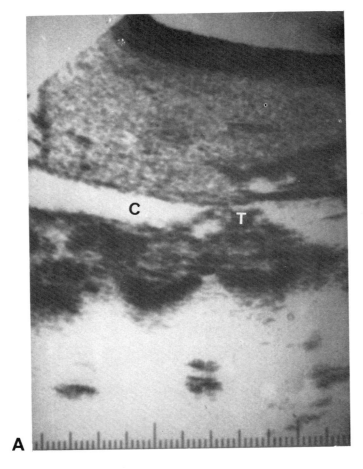

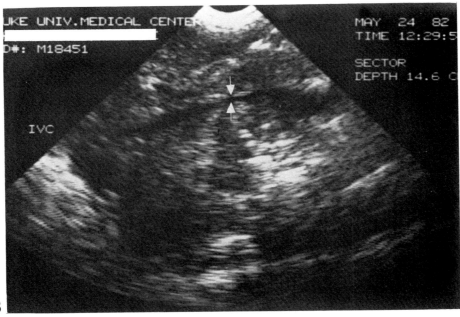

FIG. 24-4. (A) Longitudinal ultrasonogram of a five-year-old boy with an asymptomatic Wilms' tumor that was found to have tumor thrombus (T) in the inferior vena cava (C) during ultrasonographic evaluation of a right renal mass. (B) Longitudinal ultrasonogram of the inferior vena cava of the same patient as shown in Figure 24-2, shows narrowing (arrows) of the vena cava by pressure from the enlarged kidney.

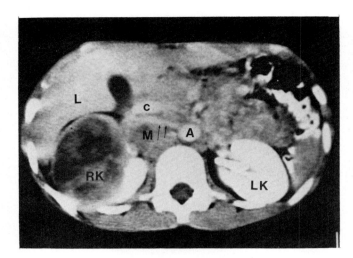

FIG. 24-5. Same patient as shown in Figure 24-2. An enhanced computed tomogram through the right renal mass demonstrates an enlarged kidney with areas of low density from hemorrhage and necrosis (RK). Tumor mass (M) extends beyond the kidney, which displaces the right renal artery (two arrows) and the inferior vena cava (C). The right renal artery is seen joining the aorta (A). The left kidney (LK) is normal. The liver (L) shows no evidence of metastatic disease.

raphy in these patients.[42] The hypervascular nature of the lesion can be detected by the newer modalities. Inferior venacavography may be required if the vessel cannot be adequately imaged by ultrasonography, excretory urography, or CT.

Figure 24-9 shows the imaging choices for the evaluation of Wilms' tumor.

Treatment Decisions

Wilms' tumor exemplifies the ten milestones in successful treatment of solid tumors in children that are the basis for the multimodal approach in modern-day cancer management. According to Hammond these are:[28]

1. Extirpative surgery.
2. Postoperative radiation therapy.
3. Activity of single chemotherapeutic agents.
4. Effective combinations of active agents.
5. Combined modality therapy.
6. Development of multidisciplinary therapy teams.
7. Identification and refinement of new prognostic variables.
8. Development and refinement of systems of staging.
9. Differential therapy approaches based on prognosis.
   a. Less aggressive therapy for patients with good prognosis.
   b. More aggressive therapy for patients with poor prognosis.
10. Widespread application of new techniques.

With this as the perspective, the management begins with surgery and progresses to chemotherapy and radiation therapy.

Surgery. Surgery consists of a transabdominal approach with exploration and complete tumor removal, with care being taken to avoid rupture and to achieve early ligation of the vascular trunk. To avoid tumor spillage, contiguous structures are usually taken in continuity with the tumor such as Gerota's fascia and the perinephric fat; the renal vein and vena cava are carefully evaluated for tumor involvement. Silver clips are used to outline the renal tumor bed to aid the radiotherapist in planning therapy.[71]

Chemotherapy. The second major line of treatment is chemotherapy and consists of actinomycin D and vincristine, with recent National Wilms' Tumor Study (NWTS) results suggesting that adriamycin added to this combination may be superior to the two-drug combination.[55] The VACA program, which also includes the addition of an alkylating agent such as cyclophosphamide, is used for more aggressive tumors.

Radiation Therapy. The role of radiation therapy has been decreasing in light of the success of chemotherapy for this disease and because it avoids later complications. In stage I patients with completely localized disease, postoperative radiation treatment is not recommended. For stage II patients with localized disease, radiation therapy is confined to the tumor bed and includes regional nodes. In stage III patients with massive tumor spillage or diffuse peritoneal seeding, whole abdominal irradiation is given with coned-down fields to the renal tumor bed.[71]

Optimization of treatment is decreasing the intensity and use of all modalities for all stages of the malignancy. The use of less aggressive treatment is exemplified by tailoring radiation prescriptions, i.e., reducing fields or doses or both, with different prognostic groups and to best interdigitate such treatment with chemotherapy programs. The third generation of protocols in the National Wilms' Tumor Study (NWTSIII) illustrate this effort with reduction in the number and length of chemotherapy cycles.

The cure rates in this disease have steadily increased from 5% in 1920 to 90% in 1980. Currently stages I, II, and III yield better than 90% two-year disease-free survival with more than 50% for metastatic stage IV indicating the value of the combined modality approach.

Nephroblastomatosis

Nephroblastomatosis is a rare dysontogenic lesion of the infantile kidney that is probably intermediate between malformation and neoplasm.[42] It is part of a complex characterized by bilateral, subcapsular aggregates of primitive metanephric epithelium that vary from mi-

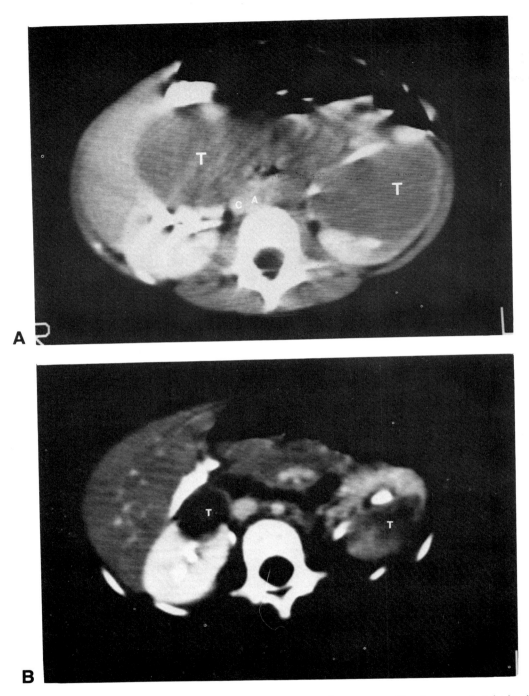

A

B

FIG. 24-6. (A) A five-year-old girl with bilateral flank masses. A computed tomogram with enhancement at the level of both kidneys demonstrates a large tumor (T) in the upper half of the right kidney and another tumor (t) in the middle portion of the left kidney. The aorta (**A**) is displaced to the right by the tumor mass from the left kidney, and the inferior vena cava is displaced downward by the tumor mass from the right kidney. (B) Six weeks later, after vincristine and actinomycin therapy, a repeat CT scan shows that the tumor masses (T) in both kidneys have decreased in size and the aorta and inferior vena cava have returned to their normal position.

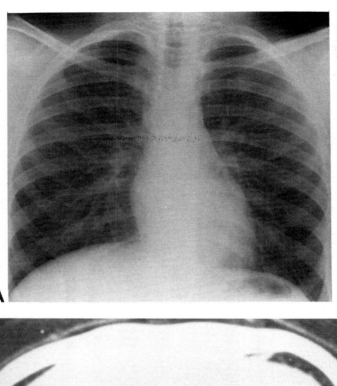

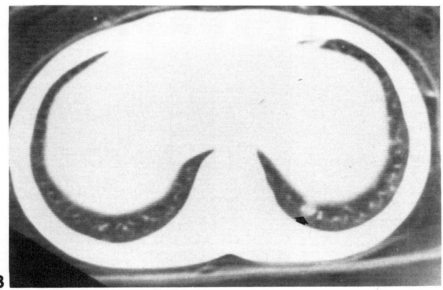

FIG. 24-7. (A) A seven-year-old boy with a Wilms' tumor on his right side who had a normal chest roentgenogram at the time of initial diagnosis. (B) A chest CT scan at the time of the initial diagnosis of Wilms' tumor shows a mass lesion (arrow) in the left lower lung field. This mass was assumed to be a metastatic Wilms' tumor. This lesion disappeared after chemotherapy, and the patient has been disease-free for two years after termination of chemotherapy.

croscopic foci to massive confluent aggregates.[57] The foci are referred to as nodular renal blastema and may be found in normal kidneys of neonates who die of other causes or in association with known Wilms' tumor. The massive confluent forms are termed nephroblastomatosis. Progression from nephroblastomatosis to Wilms' tumor may occur. Although related to Wilms' tumor and a precursor of it, nephroblastomatosis should be differentiated as a separate entity. The gross location of tumor, early in the disease, aids in differentiation from other entities.

Nephroblastomatosis is usually discovered as bilateral flank masses when the child is less than two years of age. The process is diffuse and involves the entire subcapsular portion of the kidneys. There is no definite tumor and there is an absence of necrosis or hemorrhage. Microscopically, confluent masses of nephrogenic epithelial cells are located beneath the renal capsule; these cells form immature tubules and glomeruli. Excretory urography demonstrates bilateral nephromegaly and calyceal distortion; the latter may be minimal early in the disease.

The prognosis of patients with nephroblastomatosis is

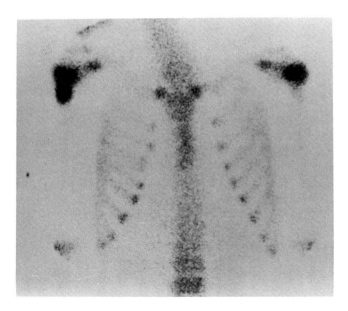

FIG. 24-8. A six-year-old boy with an asymptomatic Wilms' tumor of his right kidney with the unfavorable sarcomatous histologic type. Because this form of Wilms' tumor goes to bone, a radionuclide bone scan was performed that showed increased photon activity in the proximal right humerus. A roentgenogram of this area showed minimal demineralization and periosteal irregularity.

still uncertain,[20] although it appears to be good.[13] There is a risk of developing a Wilms' tumor with the favorable type of histologic structure. Children with bilateral Wilms' tumors may have had nephroblastomatosis initially. This is a particularly attractive consideration when no extension of tumor is detected from one kidney to the other. The good prognosis for patients with bilateral Wilms' tumors supports this thesis. The development of multidrug adjuvant chemotherapy has significantly im-

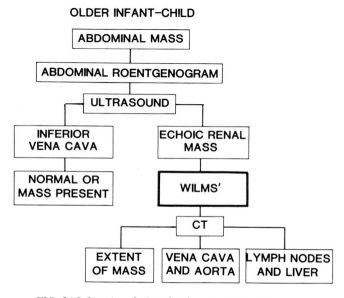

FIG. 24-9. Imaging choices for detecting Wilms' tumors.

proved the prognosis for patients with bilateral renal involvement.

Therapy has not been established for nephroblastomatosis, but it may consist of chemotherapy alone or combined with surgery, and, under some circumstances, radiotherapy. The nephroblastomatosis may return to normal spontaneously.[53] However, even with regression of the nephroblastomatosis, Wilms' tumor may develop.[69,72]

Nephroblastomatosis has been confused with adult polycystic kidney disease on excretory urograms. Ultrasonograms of nephroblastomatosis shows subcortical and parenchymal masses that have been described as demonstrating both hypoechoic and hyperechoic areas.[20,69] It is assumed that with high resolution CT scanners, subcapsular low attenuation areas would be identified.

NEUROBLASTOMA

Neuroblastoma is the second most common abdominal malignancy in older infants and children, accounting for approximately 10% of all childhood malignancies. This incidence is approximately the same frequency as Wilms' tumor. Together, Wilms' tumor and neuroblastoma comprise approximately 20% of all childhood malignant tumors.[51] Neuroblastoma is a malignant tumor of primitive neuroblasts that may arise within the adrenal medulla and sympathetic neural system. This tumor occurs primarily in the abdomen and posterior mediastinum. It has a tendency for direct spread as well as metastasis to distant sites.[10]

Approximately half of patients with neuroblastoma are 2 years of age or less at diagnosis, while 85% of patients are less than 4 years of age.[21,51] The two-year survival is 60% for patients less than 1 year old, 20% for patients aged 1 to 2 years, and 10% for patients 2 to 7 years old.[21] Thus survival is particularly good when the neoplasm is discovered in early infancy, even if it is stage IVS. The age of the patient is the most critical factor in determining prognosis.

Tumor Behavior and Pathology

Neuroblastoma usually remains clinically silent until it invades or compresses adjacent structures, metastasizes, or produces large amounts of catecholamines, which may cause diarrhea or hypertension. Approximately one fourth of all tumors are detected clinically while they are confined to their primary site of origin. More than half of all neuroblastomas arise within the abdomen, and the majority of these originate in the adrenal gland. A small number of neuroblastomas arise in the pelvis.[21,51] Extra-abdominal sites are the thorax, neck, and skull-olfactory bulb. The location of the primary lesion in some cases is never discovered.[21] Abdominal neuroblastomas may have local symptoms and signs as a result of ureteral obstruction, compression of the rectum or bladder, or extradural spinal cord compression. Occasionally, the child, parent, or pediatrician incidentally notes an abdominal mass.

Approximately 95% of patients with neuroblastoma excrete an excess of catecholamine metabolites (vanillylmandelic acid [VMA], hemovanillic acid [HVA], norepinephrine [NA], and dopamine) in their urine.[21] Therefore, chemical determination of the level of these metabolites is useful for diagnosing neuroblastoma initially and for follow-up when recurrence is suspected. Although urine spot WMA tests may be positive in neuroblastoma cases, there is a high false-positive and false-negative rate, so that 24-hour urine collections for catecholamine metabolites should be performed. An increased excretion of these metabolites indicates the presence of a neural crest neoplasm.

Histologically, neuroblastoma consists of small, round tumor cells, which may be arranged in rosettes. The presence of neurofibrils confirms the diagnosis of neuroblastoma. The additional presence of ganglion cells is diagnostic of ganglioneuroblastoma, an indication that the lesion may be converting to a benign tumor. Other tumors containing small, round cells include rhabdomyosarcomas, Ewing's sarcomas, and lymphomas. Tissue culture and electron microscopy may be helpful in distinguishing neuroblastomas from these other neoplasms.

Classification and Staging

As stated previously, the age of the patient and the site of origin primarily affect the prognosis (i.e., under 1 year of age and extra-abdominal origin have the best prognosis). The anatomic stage of the disease has some influence on prognosis but is more useful for determining treatment regimen and for planning time intervals and the type of imaging modalities to be used for following the progress of the disease. In addition to surgery and pathologic examination, the newer imaging modalities, particularly computed tomography, have influenced the process of diagnosis and staging of neuroblastoma.

Anatomic stages are outlined in Table 24-2 and Figure 24-10.[16]

Stage I neuroblastomas should have an excellent prognosis, but unfortunately 75% of patients already have metastases at the time of diagnosis. Metastatic spread may be either lymphatic or blood borne, and secondary lesions may appear in a variety of locations. Distant metastases occur rather early and widely invade bone marrow, the skeleton, brain, and the orbits. At the time that a neuroblastoma is diagnosed, metastases are noted to be in the skeleton of approximately 70% of the patients, in the regional lymph nodes of approximately 50%, in the liver of approximately 35%, and in the skull or brain of 25%.[21] They are not prone to appear initially in the lungs, as is the finding with Wilms' tumor. In babies, the liver may be massively infiltrated and replaced by tumor

and yet no metastases can be identified outside of the abdomen; such a distribution is seldom encountered in children beyond the first year of life. Distant and widespread metastases can occur from any growth, but the tendency to metastasize is lower from a primary tumor in the thorax and neck than from those in the abdomen.

Neuroblastoma has the highest recognized spontaneous cure rate (5% to 7%) of any childhood neoplasm. It may also occasionally mature to benign ganglioneuroma.[64] This spontaneous regression is most common in young infants[64] but has been reported occasionally in patients receiving irradiation to the primary tumor or associated with only biopsy of the tumor.

Imaging Procedures, Assessment, and Strategies

Abdominal Roentgenography. On roentgenograms of the abdomen in a child with a neuroblastoma, there is usually evidence of a soft tissue mass that displaces gas-filled loops of bowel. Approximately two thirds of all abdominal neuroblastomas contain calcification that is visible on plain roentgenograms. This calcification may be diffuse, finely stippled, or less frequently, coalescent.[21]

One should carefully look for erosion of the vertebral bodies and pedicles; in addition, the paravertebral soft tissues should be carefully inspected for direct extension or metastases and the liver for hematogenous metastases.

Excretory Urography with Total Body Opacification. If an excretory urogram is performed, a neuroblastoma usually appears as a dense mass during the total body opacification phase because of the increased vascularity of the neoplasm. Occasionally, lucent areas caused by hemorrhage or necrosis can be noted.[26,52]

Neuroblastoma most frequently originates in the adrenal gland, and this location tends to displace the kidney downward and laterally without intrinsic distortion of the calyces or renal pelvis (Figure 24-11). Kinking of the ureteropelvic junction may occur as the kidney is displaced inferiorly. Occasionally, a suprarenal neuroblastoma will distort the upper pole calyces and mimic an intrarenal mass. Lateral films may help in confirming the presence of downward displacement of the kidney by neuroblastoma in contrast to the intrarenal distortion of the calyces by Wilms' tumor. Neuroblastoma frequently crosses the midline and may cause extrinsic displacement of the contralateral kidney or ureter. The left adrenal gland normally overlaps the ventral portion of the upper pole of the left kidney so that a neuroblastoma of the left adrenal may directly overlie the kidney but not displace it.

Ultrasonography. A neuroblastoma is a solid tumor; therefore ultrasonography should demonstrate an echo-

Table 24-2. Postsurgical Anatomic Staging for Neuroblastoma

STAGE	AJC	ANATOMIC DESCRIPTION
I	T_1,N_0,M_0	Tumor confined to organ or structure of origin.
II	T_1 or T_{3a}, N_0 or N_{1a}, M_0	Tumor extends in continuity beyond the organ or structure of origin, but does not cross the midline. Homolateral regional lymph nodes may be involved. Tumors arising in the midline structure (such as the organ of Zuckerkandl) penetrating beyond the capsule and involving the lymph nodes on the same side should be considered stage II. Bilateral extension should be considered stage III.
III	T_{3b} or T_{3c}, N_{1a} or N_{1b}, M_0	Tumor extends in continuity beyond the midline. Bilateral regional lymph nodes may be involved.
IV	Any T, except T_4, any N, M_1	Remote disease involving skeleton, parenchymatous organs, soft tissues or distant lymph node groups.
IVS		A special category. Stage I or II with remote disease confined to 1 or more of the following sites: liver, skin or bone marrow without radiologic evidence of bone metastases on skeletal survey.
V	T_4, any N, any M	Multicentric tumor.

Modified from Putnam, T. C., Cohen, H. J., Constine, L. S.: Pediatric Solid Tumors. In *Clinical Oncology for Medical Students and Physicians*, 6th ed. Rubin, P. (Ed.) American Cancer Society, 1983, p. 401.

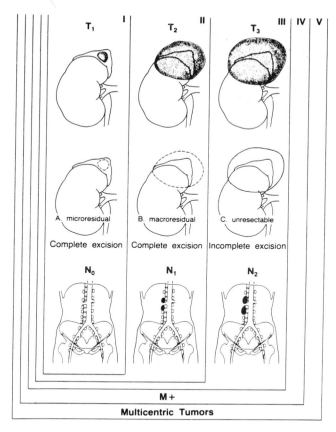

FIG. 24-10. Anatomic staging for neuroblastoma. Tumor (T) category: Extension rather than size is stressed. The major feature is a postsurgical classification—whether or not the tumor is unresectable. (Modified from Putnam, T. C., Cohen, H. J., Constine, L. S., III: Pediatric solid tumors. In *Clinical Oncology for Medical Students and Physicians: A Multidisciplinary Approach*, 6th ed. Rubin, P. (Ed.). New York, American Cancer Society, 1983, pp. 392–427. With permission.)

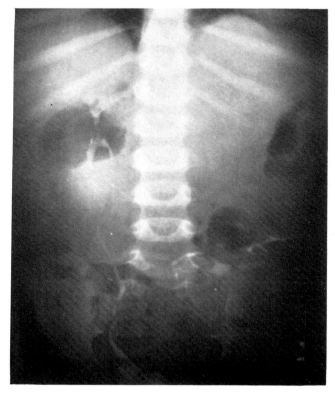

FIG. 24-11. An 18-month-old boy with a large left flank mass. This excretory urogram shows downward displacement of the left kidney. Fine punctate calcifications can be seen in the suprarenal area.

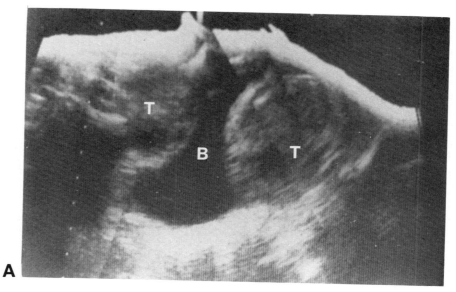

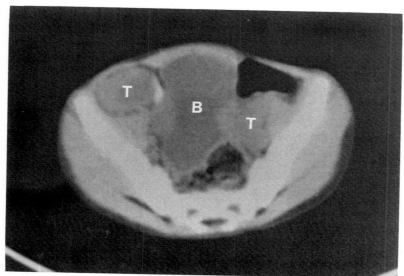

FIG. 24-12. (A) A two-year-old boy with bilateral inguinal masses noted on routine physical examination. Pelvic ultrasonography shows pelvic masses (T) indenting the bladder (**B**) bilaterally. (B) A CT scan of the same patient shows the pelvic masses (T) pressing on the bladder (**B**). The extent of the tumor masses was clearly demonstrated by multiple CT cuts. This modality was useful for following the response to therapy.

genic mass (Figure 24-12A). However, because neuroblastoma tissue may be homogeneous, the ultrasonogram may produce an anechoic pattern similar to a cystic mass; the picture can be distinguished from a cyst by the absence of transmission of sounds through the mass. Large calcium deposits may produce acoustic shadowing. Ultrasonography may identify metastases of the liver as well as extension into the kidney. The mass is imaged directly with ultrasonography rather than indirectly through renal displacement as on an excretory urogram. For this reason, ultrasonography may be particularly helpful if the mass is located ventral to the left kidney and does not displace it.[48] Ultrasonography does have

limitations in accurately determining tumor margins and local extension.[51] For this reason, CT is considered the modality of choice for imaging neuroblastomas.

Computed Tomography. Computed tomography (CT) is superior to ultrasonography for defining the morphologic details of a neuroblastoma and for documenting the extent of tumor through direct spread or lymphatic metastases.[75] The CT characteristics of neuroblastoma include irregular shape and margins, the lack of a well-defined capsule, a mixed low-density center as a result of hemorrhage and necrosis and calcification in at least 75% of patients.[52,78] The imaging capabilities of CT are particularly helpful in pelvic neuroblastoma (Figure 24-12B).[77] Computed tomography without and with contrast enhancement precisely demonstrates anatomy as well as renal function and organ vascularity. Particular attention should be paid to the prevertebral region since neuroblastoma has a propensity for surrounding the celiac axis and superior mesenteric artery. Computed tomography is usually performed with isotonic metrizamide or a comparable water-soluble contrast material injected into the subarachnoid space to determine the presence or absence of extradural tumor extension (Figure 24-13).[1,47] Computed tomography is the most accurate imaging modality for monitoring recurrences or metastases from neuroblastomas.

Nuclear Scintigraphy. Bone scintigraphy is less sensitive, particularly in the metaphyseal regions, than radiographic skeletal survey for bone metastases from neuroblastomas.[40] If a skeletal survey is negative, then bone scintigraphy may be performed if there is a strong suspicion of skeletal metastases. Since CT is indicated in all patients with neuroblastoma, liver scintigraphy is rarely performed.

Angiography. Computed tomography has virtually eliminated the need for angiography in neuroblastoma.

A decision tree outlining the imaging choices for neuroblastoma is presented in Figure 24-14.

Treatment Decisions

The success in the management of neuroblastoma is not comparable to that for Wilms' tumor and embryonal rhabdomyosarcoma. Metastatic disease occurs very frequently, and chemotherapy has affected long-term survival only slightly. Although it is producing excellent remissions, relapses are frequent. Again, the management of this malignancy is approached in the multimodal fashion, with all of the standard treatment methods being used.

Surgery. Curative surgery is possible if total resection of the tumor is achieved. Even in the presence of widespread disease, surgical removal of the primary tumor is indicated in the hopes of producing regression of metastatic disease. The usefulness of cytoreductive surgery for primary tumors in patients with metastases continues to be evaluated but is difficult to determine without a clinical trial.[71]

Radiation Therapy. Microresiduum as well as macroresiduum following surgery are managed most often with local regional postoperative irradiation. Doses are more moderate than with other childhood tumors and usually range from 2,000 to 4,000 cGy, depending upon the bulk of the disease being treated and the age of the patient.

Extra-adrenal neuroblastomas, which often are not resectable because of their anatomic location and extensions, can be treated quite successfully with high-dose definitive radiation therapy, with the majority of such patients being long-term survivors.[91] Generally, complete regressions and cure are more likely in children under 2 years of age. Since these are usually large tumors, the doses that are often delivered are limited by normal tissue tolerance and, again, are determined by the age of the patient.

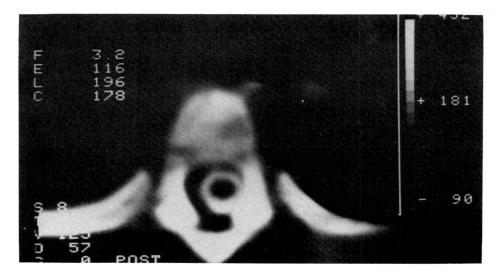

FIG. 24-13. A CT scan of the spine with metrizamide injected into the subarachnoid space demonstrates displacement of the cord by extradural tumor extension. Roentgenograms of the spine were normal.

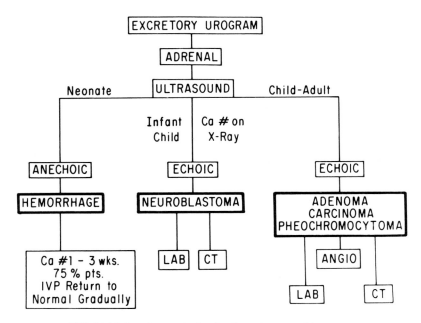

FIG. 24-14. Imaging strategies for detecting neuroblastomas.

Chemotherapy. The management of metastatic disease in adjuvant programs is by a combination of such agents as cyclophosphamide, vincristine, and DTIC (dimethyl triazeno imidazole carboxamide), with the observation that responders do survive longer than nonresponders.[71] More aggressive multidrug programs are promising better regression rates but are still in the trial design phase.

For stage I disease, treatment of infants under 2 years of age with limited disease can best be done by complete surgical resection with an outcome and survival of greater than 90%.[71] No other treatment such as radiation or chemotherapy is indicated in an adjuvant fashion for stage I patients.

For stage II patients with microresiduum, postoperative irradiation is recommended, but chemotherapy is usually withheld except for older patients and patients who have a poor prognosis in terms of histopathology.

For stage III and IV disease (advanced neuroblastoma patients), the treatment is more aggressive and surgery is used for diagnosis and staging, and for cytoreductive resection if there is no major risk in tumor removal.[19,71] Generally, radiation treatment is part of the plan and is administered in definitive doses. If the patient has metastatic disease, chemotherapy may be used first, followed by a consolidation course of radiation therapy. This is particularly true of stage IVS patients, where even hemibody irradiation in modest doses has been used, covering the extensive spread of this stage of disease. Prognosis with stage IVS patients is between that of stage I and II. A major problem in delivering large doses of radiation therapy to such wide fields is that it may interfere with the administration of chemotherapy.

RHABDOMYOSARCOMA

Rhabdomyosarcoma is the most common soft tissue sarcoma in infants and children. It represents between 10% and 15% of all childhood solid tumors and is exceeded in frequency only by brain tumors, neuroblastomas, and Wilms' tumors. Rhabdomyosarcoma is extremely malignant and invades contiguous structures, recurs early if incompletely treated, and metastasizes rapidly through blood and lymph channels. If untreated, over 90% of the patients will die within a year.[17] Both sexes are equally affected; no racial predilection has been established.

Tumor site is a factor in the incidence of rhabdomyosarcoma in different age groups. Tumors of pelvic origin and the head and neck are more prevalent in infancy and early childhood, while paratesticular rhabdomyosarcomas are largely a disease of adolescents and adults.[83] The occurrence rate for rhabdomyosarcoma of the extremities is the same at all ages in childhood through age 21 years. Orbital and trunk tumors make up a small group and are apparently unrelated to age.

Tumor Behavior and Pathology

Although rhabdomyosarcoma has been classically described as occurring in striated muscle, this tumor can occur in mesenchymal tissue at almost any site in the body. There has been a diversity of histologic types of rhabdomyosarcoma; these have been united as a single entity with pleomorphic, embryonal (including botryoid), and alveolar subtypes recognized as variants of a single tumor system. Rhabdomyoblasts are identified by light microscopy or electron microscopy in each of the varieties.

The embryonal type is seen in infants and small children. This form is found in more than two thirds of the tumors of the head and neck and in approximately one half of those in all other sites except the trunk, where it is less common than the alveolar form. The botryoid subtype of the embryonal form ordinarily extends into body cavities, such as the bladder, nasopharynx, vagina, or bile duct.

The alveolar cell type, named for a superficial resemblance to the pulmonary alveoli, is the most common form found in the muscle masses of the trunk and extremities and is seen more frequently as age advances.

The pleomorphic type presents the most bizarre histologic appearance but is only seen in a very small number of children.

The Intergroup Rhabdomyosarcoma Study (IRS)[61] described two additional types, termed *soft tissue Ewing's sarcoma* and *small cell mesenchymal sarcomas, type undetermined.*

Classification and Staging

Anatomic staging for rhabdomyosarcoma is outlined in Table 24-3 and Figure 24-15.[39]

Imaging Procedures, Assessment, and Strategies

A mass lesion in different parts of the anatomy often is an indication of a soft tissue sarcoma. Since carcinomas are so rare in children, sarcomas are immediately suspect. The most common soft tissue sarcoma is rhab-

domyosarcoma, and this applies to most anatomic sites other than the retroperitoneum. Since these tumors many times arise in different geographic sites such as the head and neck or the pelvis, where they involve the genitourinary system as well as the extremities, a roentgenographic survey followed by biopsy establishes the diagnosis, particularly if there are no signs of metastatic disease. Once the diagnosis is established, a diagnostic workup is done to determine the presence of metastases before wide surgical resection and other treatments are added to the program. This consists of routine laboratory work such as CBC and liver enzyme studies. A bone scan and bone marrow biopsy as well as ultrasonography or CT liver scan if metastases are suspected, usually follow. Where metastatic disease is the initial symptom, a biopsy of one of the accessible lesions is attempted to establish a diagnosis, and then a complete metastatic workup is done as previously described. The workup of the primary tumor would not be as rigorous, since it would not be approached surgically in this instance.

Figure 24-16 summarizes the imaging choices for rhabdomyosarcoma.

Treatment Decisions

Major gains have been made in the multimodal management of rhabdomyosarcoma compared with more than a decade ago when surgery and radiation therapy cured less than 25% of all patients, with the exception of those with tumors arising in either the orbit or the genitourinary primary sites.[14,36,37,85] With the success of combination chemotherapy, the gain both from the point

Table 24-3. Surgical Resection Staging System, Intergroup Rhabdomyosarcoma Study and American Joint Committee Comparison

IRS	AJC	ANATOMIC DESCRIPTION
Group I		Localized disease, completely resected. Regional nodes not involved.
	T_1,N_0,M_0	a. Confined to muscle or organ of origin.
	T_2,N_0,M_0	b. Contiguous involvement—infiltration outside the muscle or organ of origin, as through fascial planes; totally resected.
Group II		Regional disease
	T_{3a},N_0,M_0	a. Grossly resected tumor with microscopic residual disease. No evidence of gross residual tumor. No clinical or microscopic evidence of regional node involvement.
	T_2,N_{1a},M_0	b. Regional disease, completely resected (regional nodes involved completely resected with no microscopic residual).
	T_{3a},N_{1a},M_0	c. Regional disease with involved nodes, grossly resected, but with evidence of microscopic residual.
Group III	$T_{3b,c},N_{1a,b},M_0$	Incomplete resection or biopsy with gross residual disease.
Group IV	Any T, any N, M_1	Metastatic disease present at onset.

Modified from Putnam, T. C., Cohen, H. J., Constine, L. S.: Pediatric Solid Tumors. In *Clinical Oncology for Medical Students and Physicians,* 6th ed. Rubin, P. (Ed.) American Cancer Society, 1983, p. 407.

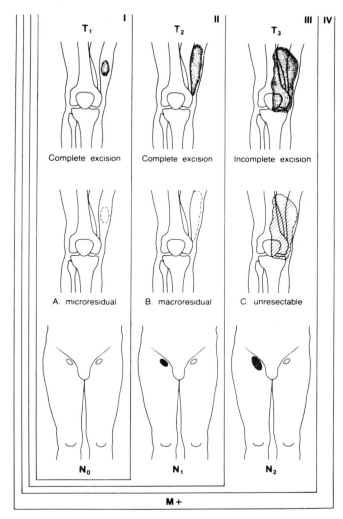

FIG. 24-15. Anatomic staging for rhabdomyosarcoma. Tumor (T) category: Extension is important for tumor staging. The major feature is postsurgical classification—whether or not the tumor is unresectable. (Modified from Putnam, T. C., Cohen, H. J., Constine, L. S., III: Pediatric solid tumors. In *Clinical Oncology for Medical Students and Physicians: A Multidisciplinary Approach*, 6th ed. Rubin, P. (Ed.). New York, American Cancer Society, 1983, pp. 392–427. With permission.)

of view of cosmesis and function has been increased considerably. The optimal sequencing of surgery, radiation therapy, and chemotherapy is evolving in intergroup protocol designs.

Surgery. Curative resection of the primary tumor including the surrounding normal tissues gives a good chance of local control, but the wide local excision need not be mutilating since it will be coupled with radiation therapy and chemotherapy. Therefore, conservation surgery is advocated, particularly in sites where the deformity would be large if such an aggressive surgical approach was used, since in most instances there will be some residual disease that will require further treatment by other modes.

Radiation Therapy. Radiation therapy has provided excellent local and regional control of residual microscopic disease in 90% of patients, particularly when it is combined with chemotherapy.[14,15,86] As surgery becomes more conservative, radiation therapy fields will need to encompass a volume well beyond the margins of the tumor to be sure that the malignancy is eradicated in its extensions. Since the radiation oncologist attempts to encompass the muscle compartment in which the tumor arose, fields can be among the most extensive of those currently used. The optimal doses usually range from 4,000 to 5,000 cGy for microscopic disease, with 5,000 to 6,000 cGy being reserved for gross macroresiduum.

The Intergroup Rhabdomyosarcoma Study group recommended the following radiation dosage: 5,000 cGy in five weeks for patients with microscopic residual disease and 6,000 cGy in six weeks for bulk disease (Clinical Groups III and IV). Dosage was graduated downward for younger patients and for some specific sites.

The effects of radiation therapy in local disease control were more difficult to evaluate. It appears, however, that patients 6 years of age and older who received less than 4,000 cGy had a rate of local recurrence that was higher than those who received more than 4,000 cGy. Among younger patients, this difference was not apparent.

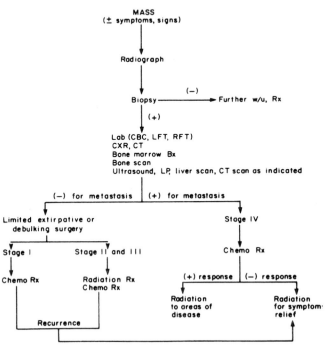

FIG. 24-16. Imaging choices for detecting rhabdomyosarcoma. (Reprinted from Putnam, T. C., Cohen, H. J., Constine, L. S., III: Pediatric solid tumors. In *Clinical Oncology for Medical Students and Physicians: A Multidisciplinary Approach*, 6th ed. Rubin, P. (Ed.). New York, American Cancer Society, 1983, pp. 392–427. With permission.)

Chemotherapy. Chemotherapy consists of the VACA program, which includes vincristine, actinomycin D, cyclophosphamide, and doxorubicin (Adriamycin). This has proved successful both in the adjuvant setting and in the treatment of metastatic disease.[23] Orbital rhabdomyosarcomas are challenging in that treatment attempts to preserve vision, relying on radiation with chemotherapeutic programs to avoid enucleation.[41,88] In other head and neck sites, the results have not been as good, with 40% of patients failing to achieve cure despite high dose radiation and combination chemotherapy.[6,84] Craniospinal irradiation should be administered when the disease involves the meninges. Prophylactic programs of high dose cranial irradiation (4,000 to 4,500 cGy) and intrathecal chemotherapy are being investigated in attempts to spare bone marrow. In the attempt to avoid the deformity caused by pelvic exenteration, which was commonly used in the era before the introduction of effective combined irradiation and chemotherapy regimens, multiagent cyclic chemotherapy is being tested with periodic reassessment and includes biopsy and second-look procedures. In the extremities, conservation surgery is being used with careful definition by tumor imaging for setting up radiation fields.

Multimodal programs have increased the effectiveness of therapy. Only with the alveolar histologic type of lesions has there been a higher recurrence and mortality rate. Botryoid tumors have the same, or even greater, sensitivity to chemotherapeutic agents than other embryonal rhabdomyosarcomas.

During the past two decades the survival rates among children with rhabdomyosarcomas has improved from approximately 20% to over 70%. This improvement can be attributed to combined therapy regimens using intense radiotherapy (5,000 to 6,000 cGy in 5 to 6 weeks), the development of more intense chemotherapy in an attempt to increase the rate of resectability or provide long-term control, and improved surgical techniques.[68,82,89]

The Intergroup Rhabdomyosarcoma Study (IRS) groups joined to carry out a prospective clinical trial to determine the role of chemotherapy in the management of rhabdomyosarcoma.[29]

In the Clinical Group I patients, those with localized and completely resected tumors, all patients received two years of vincristine, dactinomycin, and cyclophosphamide, (VAC), and randomized patients received local radiation. Local tumor recurrence rate was 3.7% in the radiation group and 5.5% in the nonradiation group. Thus, radiotherapy had no beneficial effect in Clinical Group I patients.

Patients in Group II had positive lymph nodes, microscopic residual tumor, or local extension of tumor into adjacent organs. The clinical trial concerned the evaluation of VAC for two years or intensive therapy with vincristine and dactinomycin for one year. All patients received local radiotherapy. There was no significant difference between the results of these two regimens after two years.

The Clinical Group III patients had incomplete local surgical resection, and those patients in Clinical Group IV had metastasis at the time of diagnosis. These patients had surgical procedures as indicated and received radiotherapy six weeks after the initiation of therapy. These patients were randomized between two chemotherapy regimens of vincristine, actinomycin, and cyclophosphamide (VAC) and VAC plus Adriamycin. There was no significant difference between the two regimens. Regression of tumor occurred in over 72% of the patients in Group III and over 65% in Group IV. In approximately 25%, no demonstrable tumor change was achieved.

Different Anatomic Locations

Genitourinary System Rhabdomyosarcoma. Urinary tract. Rhabdomyosarcomas may arise anywhere in the urinary tract. The urinary bladder is the most common site of involvement, with boys being affected twice as frequently as girls. The tumor usually appears during the first three years of life as either a solid, infiltrating lesion or as polypoid masses extending into the bladder. This tumor most often originates at the trigone or bladder base.[18]

On voiding cystourethrograms, ultrasound scans or computed tomography (CT), a polypoid mass at the base of the urinary bladder should suggest the diagnosis (Figure 24-17). There may be associated partial obstruction of the distal ureters with ureteropyelocaliectasis. Occasionally, the tumor prolapses into the urethra. A CT scan is often able to clearly demonstrate thickening and infiltration in determining if the tumor arises in the bladder, prostate gland, or vagina.

Prostate gland. Rhabdomyosarcoma of the prostate gland frequently manifests itself as prostatism in older children. There is early invasion of the base of the bladder and posterior urethra and there may be associated partial obstruction of the rectum or distal ureters.[32]

A voiding cystourethrogram, ultrasound scan or CT scan may reveal extrinsic deformity of the base of the bladder and posterior urethra with elevation of the bladder floor. Computed tomography has the ability to define invasion into the bladder, urethral lumen, or adjacent tissues.

Paratesticular rhabdomyosarcoma. Paratesticular rhabdomyosarcoma is a nongerminal neoplasm of the scrotal contents that is frequently encountered in children and young adults. The average age of patients with this lesion in the IRS series is nine years. Clinically it appears as a painless, movable mass within the scrotum or inguinal canal. Spread is via the lymphatics to the periaortic and renal hilar lymph nodes. Combined therapy produced major improvement in the survival of these patients.[59]

By 1975,[29] in a small series of patients in the IRS series, there had been an 89% disease-free survival rate. From this and other experiences the following recommended therapy regimen had developed: (1) total orchiectomy with high ligation of the cord structures; (2) retroperitoneal lymphadenectomy; (3) radiotherapy to the abdomen if the nodes are positive and to the scrotum for skin involvement or prior transcrotal surgical approaches, and (4) long-range chemotherapy.

Vagina. Rhabdomyosarcoma is the most common primary tumor of the vagina and external genitalia in young girls. It is usually of the sarcoma botryoides type. Clinical symptoms include vaginal discharge or bleeding, vaginal mass, or protrusion of polypoid tissue from the vaginal orifice. This tumor usually arises from the upper third of the anterior vaginal wall with growth into the lumen and infiltration of the vesicovaginal septum as well as the posterior bladder wall and urethra. The extent of the intravaginal mass and any extension to the bladder, rectum, and uterus are usually demonstrable by CT.

Before the development of effective chemotherapy–radiotherapy regimens, patients with tumors of the bladder and vagina were treated by wide local excision or exenteration and had survival rates of approximately

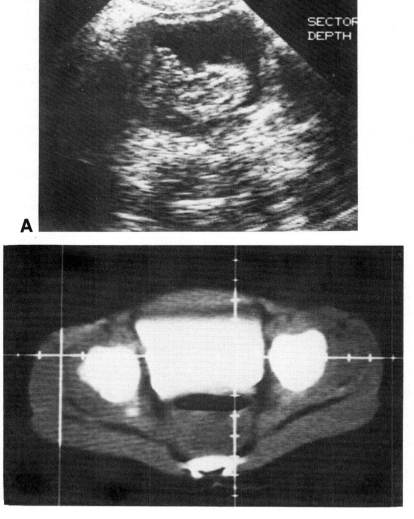

FIG. 24-17. A three-year-old girl with hematuria and white cells in the urine. (A) This ultrasound scan of the pelvis shows an echogenic mass in the bladder with attachment (origin) to the wall of the bladder. (B) A computed tomogram of the bladder shows thickening of the bladder wall as a result of an infiltrative process. The biopsy specimen proved to be embryonal cell type of rhabdomyosarcoma.

20%, while those with primary prostatic lesions rarely lived.[31]

Primary tumors of the pelvis were found to be among the most sensitive to multiple-agent chemotherapy regimens. Supplemental radiotherapy frequently is used. This combined mode of therapy has reduced the size of the local tumor to make extirpative surgical procedures feasible. There is a group of long-range, tumor-free surviving patients who have been treated in this way.

Head and Neck Rhabdomyosarcoma. Rhabdomyosarcomas of the structures of the head and neck constitute approximately one third of all rhabdomyosarcomas. Except for orbital lesions, rhabdomyosarcomas of the head and neck have a poor prognosis. Rhabdomyosarcomas of the head and neck arise primarily in the nasal pharynx, nasal sinuses, and auditory canals. Although the local lymph nodes become involved, the usually lethal spread is hematogenous or directly into the central nervous system.

Over half of the patients are male and greater than 70% of the lesions are of the embryonal cell type. More than 50% of the children were in IRS Clinical Group III. The survival rate has improved from slightly over 10% to over 50% with multimodal therapy. Recurrence of head and neck rhabdomyosarcoma in the IRS series has been predominantly local or regional initially, but ultimately has been distant. The predominant regional spread was into the central nervous system via the meningeal route adjacent to the primary tumor, and this form of extension has been uniformly lethal. Thus, the IRS now believes that patients with rhabdomyosarcoma in the parameningeal sites or those with osseous erosion at the base of the skull should have prophylactic central nervous system radiotherapy.[81]

Orbital rhabdomyosarcoma is the most frequently occurring primary malignant tumor of the orbit. The tumor histologically is predominantly embryonal and most patients are classified as IRS Clinical Group III (Figure 24-18). The prognosis for children with orbital rhabdomyosarcomas is more favorable than for children with tumors of any other site, irrespective of the form of therapy. Before effective radiotherapy or chemotherapy, these tumors were treated by orbital exenteration, with a survival rate of aproximately 50%.[38] Radiotherapy was found effective and multiple or single agent chemotherapy has improved the survival rate. Orbital exenteration is carried out only for recurrence. With this general type of therapy, the survival rates are greater than 80%.[29]

Rhabdomyosarcoma of the Extremities. Patients with rhabdomyosarcomas of the extremities have a poorer prognosis than patients with this tumor in any other location of the body. The poor outcome in these patients is probably related to the predominance of the malignant

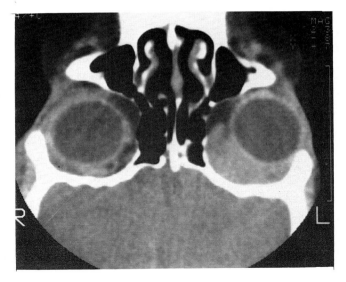

FIG. 24-18. A CT scan of a child with decreasing vision and proptosis of the left eye demonstrates a solid orbital mass that proved to be rhabdomyosarcoma of the embryonal cell type.

nature of the histologic alveolar type. Before the 1970s, radiotherapy and primary amputation were associated with a low rate of survival.[82] Survival rates varied among different institutions, from as low as 13% for all extremity sites to as high as 50% for patients with upper extremity tumors.[65] Surgery was the predominant mode of therapy and in some cases the sole mode of therapy, with chemotherapy and radiation usually employed only after recurrence.

Because of the poor results until 1970, some changes were made in the management of extremity rhabdomyosarcoma. Radiotherapy doses were increased to 6,000 to 7,000 cGy in 6 to 7 weeks, which resulted in local control of extremity lesions[58] but the effects of such therapy on the skeletal growth of the extremities in childhood were deforming.[80] This somatic effect prompted a trial of the efficacy of radiotherapy in a reduced dosage range combined with multiple-agent chemotherapy and a change in surgical extirpation.

In the IRS series, extremity lesions comprised 23% of the rhabdomyosarcomas, a higher incidence of these sites than found in most recent series.[29] Alveolar-type lesions were only slightly more common than embryonal-type tumors and this group contained most of the soft tissue Ewing's sarcoma variants. With a minimum of two years of surveillance, there has been a marked difference in survival related to IRS Clinical Groups. Of 21 patients in IRS Clinical Group I (complete local excision), the relapse rate has been 14% and the mortality rate 10% two years after diagnosis. In Clinical Group II (gross excised tumor, with microscopic residual tumor, positive nodes, or local extension), the relapse rate has been 19% and the mortality rate 9% among 32 patients two years after diagnosis. However, among the 14 patients in Clinical Group III, nine have relapsed and four have died.

The recommended approach to extremity lesions has been excision of the tumor, followed by postoperative radiation therapy and chemotherapy.

Among the patients subjected to amputation in the IRS series, 50% have relapsed, which correlates with prior studies and reflects the advanced stage of disease in these patients. The IRS data do not indicate that primary lesions of the upper extremities have as dire a prognosis as previously reported.

Rhabdomyosarcoma Arising in Less Sites. Biliary tree.

Twenty-seven cases of rhabdomyosarcoma of the biliary tree were reported before 1976,[60] and Ruymann et al.[73] have recently extracted the cases from the IRS, which brings the total to 37 patients. The histologic type is predominantly embryonal botryoides.

Most of the patients had extension of tumor from the bile ducts to liver, lymph nodes, or surrounding structures. This situation is contrary to the traditional criteria of resectability of biliary cancer. Therefore, survival of this tumor in the biliary tract has been extremely rare. It is hoped, however, that a more aggressive surgical approach, increased radiation therapy (up to 6,000 cGy to the tumor bed), and extensive chemotherapy will produce longer survival time and possibly more cures.

Ultrasonography and computed tomography should show the extent of the tumor and its effect on the biliary tree.

Retroperitoneum.[29] The dominant histologic type of rhabdomyosarcoma of the retroperitoneum has been embryonal in over 50%. Resectability of tumor in this location was about 25%. Recurrence and distant metastases were common.

Perineal (including perianal) rhabdomyosarcomas have a very poor prognosis.[79] The mean duration of survival has been 1½ years. Over 55% of the lesions are of the alveolar cell type.

Imaging Modalities for Evaluating Rhabdomyosarcomas

The key to evaluating the extent of a rhabdomyosarcoma in any part of the body is computed tomography. Ultrasonography is useful for liver and pelvic diseases. Lymphangiography may be of help with pelvic rhabdomyosarcomas and those in the lower extremities.[5]

From multiple reports,[30,54,87] several observations were noted: (1) multiple and "pulses" of chemotherapy produced dramatic responses in tumor reduction and tumor control in more than 50% of children for an indefinite period of time; tumors were not sensitive to single

chemotherapeutic agents; (2) vaginal-uterine lesions are most amenable to combined chemotherapy; prostatic and bladder tumors respond with equal effectiveness to primary chemotherapy regimens; (3) the combination of intensive chemotherapy (particularly Cytoxan) and radiotherapy may result in fibrosis and contracture of the bladder, destroying its useful function.

REFERENCES

1. Armstrong, E. A., Harwood-Nash, D. C. F., Ritz, C. R., Chuang, S. H., Pettersson, H., Martin, D. J.: CT of neuroblastomas and ganglioneuromas in children. A.J.R. 139:571, 1982.
2. Beckwith, J. B., Norkool, P. A.: Incidence and clinicopathological features of Wilms' tumor patients with bone metastases. A report of the National Wilms' Tumor Study (NWTS) Committee, (abstracted). Proceedings of the American Association for Cancer Research 20:125, 1979.
3. Belasco, J., D'Angio, G. J.: Wilms' tumor. CA 35:262, 1981.
4. Berger, P. E., Munschauer, R. W., Kuhn, J. P.: Computed tomography and ultrasound of renal and perirenal diseases in infants and children. Relationship to excretory urography in renal cystic disease, trauma and neoplasm. Pediatr. Radiol. 9:91, 1980.
5. Bergiron, C., Markovits, P., Benjaafar, M., Piekarski, J. D., Garel, L.: Lymphography in childhood rhabdomyosarcomas. Radiology 133:627, 1979.
6. Berry, M. P., Jenkin, R. D. T.: Parameningeal rhabdomyosarcoma in the young. Cancer 48:281–288, 1981.
7. Brasch, R. C., Abols, I. B., Gooding, C. A., Filly, R. A.: Abdominal disease in children: A comparison of computed tomography and ultrasound. A.J.R. 134:153, 1980.
8. Brasch, R. C., Cann, C. E.: Computed tomographic scanning in children. II. An updated comparison of radiation dose and resolving power of commercial scanners. A.J.R. 138:127, 1982.
9. Breslow, N. E., Palmer, N. F., Hill, L. R.: Wilms' tumor: Prognostic factors for patients without metastases at diagnosis: Results of the National Wilms' Tumor Study. Cancer 41:1577, 1978.
10. Chrispin, A. R., Gordon, I., Hall, C., Metreweli, C.: Diagnostic Imaging of the Kidney and Urinary Tract in Children. Berlin, Springer International, 1980.
11. Clark, R. E.: Roentgen evaluation of Wilms' tumor. CRC Crit. Rev. Radiol. Sci. 3:551–576, 1972.
12. D'Angio, G. J., Beckwith, J. B., Breslow, N. E., Bishop, H. C., Evans, A. E., Farewell, V., Fernbach, D., Goodwin, W. E., Jones, B., Leape, L. L., Palmer, N. F., Tefft, M., Wolff, J. A.: Wilms' tumor: An update. Cancer 45 (suppl 7):1791, 1980.
13. deChadarevian, J. P., Fletcher, B. D., Chatten, J., Rabinowitz, H. H.: Massive infantile nephroblastomatosis. Cancer 39:2294, 1977.
14. Donaldson, S. S.: Rhabdomyosarcoma. In Principles of Cancer Treatment. Carter, S. K., Glatstein, E., Livingston, R. B. (Eds.). New York, McGraw-Hill, 1982, pp. 852–862.
15. Dritschilo, A., Weichselbaum, R., Cassady, J. R., Jaffe, N., Green, D., Filler, R. M.: The role of radiation therapy in the treatment of soft tissue sarcomas of childhood. Cancer 42:1192–1203, 1978.
16. Evans, A. E., D'Angio, G. J., Randolph, J.: A proposed staging for children with neuroblastoma. Cancer 27:374, 1971.
17. Exelby, P. R.: Management of embryonal rhabdomyosarcomas in children. Surg. Clin. North Am. 54:849, 1974.
18. Exelby, P. R., Ghavimi, F., Jereb, B.: Genitourinary rhabdomyosarcoma in children. J. Pediatr. Surg. 13:746, 1978.
19. Finklestein, J. F.: Multiagent chemotherapy for children with metastatic neuroblastoma. Med. Pediatr. Oncol. 6:179, 1979.
20. Franken, E. A., Yiu-Chiu, V., Smith, W. L., Chiu, L. C.: Nephro-

blastomatosis: Clinicopathologic significance and imaging characteristics. *A.J.R.* **138**:952, 1982.

21. Friedland, G. W., Crowe, J. E.: Neuroblastoma and other adrenal neoplasms. In *Pediatric Oncologic Radiology.* Parker, B. R., Castellino, R. A. (Eds.). St. Louis, C. V. Mosby, 1977, pp. 267–300.

22. George, S. L., Fernbach, D. J., Vietti, T. J., Sullivan, M. P., Lane, D. M., Haggard, M. E., Berry, D. H., Lonsdale, D., Komp, D.: Factors influencing survival in pediatric acute leukemia: The SWCCSG experience, 1958–1970. *Cancer* **32**:1542, 1973.

23. Green, D. M., Jaffe, N.: Progress and controversy in the treatment of childhood rhabdomyosarcoma. *Cancer Treat. Rev.* **5**:7–27, 1978.

24. Grossman, H.: Evaluating common intra-abdominal masses in children—a systematic roentgenographic approach. *CA* **26**:219, 1976.

25. Grossman, H.: Wilms' tumor. In *Pediatric Oncologic Radiology.* Parker, B. R., Castellino, R. A. (Eds.). St. Louis: C. V. Mosby, 1977.

26. Grossman, H.: Integrated imaging for the evaluation of the urologic diseases of childhood. *Urol. Clin. North Am.* **7**:177–199, 1980.

27. Haller, J. O., Schneider, M., Kassner, E. G., Slovis, T. L., Perl, L. J.: Sonographic evaluation of mesenteric and omental masses in children. *A.J.R.* **130**:269, 1978.

28. Hammond, D.: Progress in the study, treatment, and cure of the cancers of children. In *Cancer—Achievements, Challenges, and Prospects for the 1980s,* Vol. 2. Burchenal, J. H., Oettgen, H. R. (Eds.). New York, Grune & Stratton, 1981, pp. 171–190.

29. Hayes, D. M.: The management of rhabdomyosarcoma in children and young adults. *World J. Surg.* **4**:15, 1980.

30. Hayes, D. M., Ortega, J.: Primary chemotherapy in the management of pelvic rhabdomyosarcoma in infancy and early childhood. In *Adjuvant Therapy of Cancer.* Salmon, S. E., Jones, S. E., (Eds.). Amsterdam, Elsevier/North Holland Biomedical Press, 1977, pp. 381–387.

31. Hayes, D. M., Raney, R. B., Lawrence, W., Gehan, E. A., Soule, E. H., Tefft, M., Maurer, H. M.: Rhabdomyosarcoma of the female urogenital tract. *J. Pediatr. Surg.* **16**:828, 1981.

32. Hayes, D. M., Raney, R. B.: Primary chemotherapy in the treatment of children with bladder-prostate tumors in the intergroup rhabdomyosarcoma study (IRS-II). *J. Pediatr. Surg.* **17**:812, 1982.

33. Hidalgo, H., Korobkin, M., Kinney, T. R., Lawrence, W., Tefft, M., Soule, E. H., Crist, W. F., Foulkes, M., Maurer, H. M.: The problem of benign pulmonary nodules in children receiving cytotoxic chemotherapy. *A.J.R.* **140**:21, 1983.

34. Hornbach, N. B., Homayoon, S.: Rhabdomyosarcoma in the pediatric age group. *A.J.R.* **126**:542, 1976.

35. Jaffe, M. H., White, S. J., Silver, T. M., Heidelberger, K. P.: Wilms' tumor: Ultrasonic features, pathologic correlation, and diagnostic pitfalls. *Radiology* **140**:147, 1981.

36. Johnson, D. G.: Trends in surgery for childhood rhabdomyosarcoma. *Cancer* **35**:916–920, 1975.

37. Jones, I. S., Reese, A. B., Kraut, J.: Orbital rhabdomyosarcoma: An analysis of 65 cases. *Trans. Am. Ophthalmol. Soc.* **63**:223–255, 1965.

38. Jones, I. S., Reese, A. M., Kraut, J.: Orbital rhabdomyosarcoma. *Am. J. Ophthalmol.* **61**:721, 1966.

39. Kaufman, R. A.: Practical techniques for liver–spleen computed tomography. *J. Comput. Tomogr.* **7**:42, 1983.

40. Kaufman, R. A., Thrall, J. H., Keyes, J. W., Jr., Brown, M. L., Zakem, J. F.: False negative bone scans in neuroblastoma metastatic to ends of long bones. *A.J.R.* **130**:131, 1978.

41. Kilman, J. W., Clatworthy, H. W., Newton, W. A., Grosfeld, J. L.: Reasonable surgery for rhabdomyosarcoma: A study of 69 cases. *Ann. Surg.* **178**:346–351, 1973.

42. Kirks, D. R.: Pediatric renal angiography. *Appl. Radiol.* **11**:83, 1978.

43. Kirks, D. R.: Computed tomography of pediatric urinary tract disease. *Urol. Radiol.* **5**:199, 1983.

44. Kirks, D. R.: Practical techniques for pediatric chest computed tomography. *J. Comput. Tomogr.* **7**:31, 1983.

45. Kirks, D. R.: Practical techniques for pediatric computed tomography. *Pediatr. Radiol.* **13**:48, 1983.

46. Kirks, D. R.: *Practical Pediatric Imaging: Diagnostic Radiology of Infants and Children.* Boston, Little, Brown and Co., 1984.

47. Kirks, D. R., Berger, P. E., Fitz, C. R., Harwood-Nash, D. C.: Myelography in the evaluation of paravertebral mass lesions in infants and children. *Radiology* **119**:603, 1976.

48. Kirks, D. R., Conrad, M. R., Damert, W.: Left adrenal neuroblastoma with normal conventional radiologic studies: Value of gray scale ultrasonography. *South Med. J.* **73**:389, 1980.

49. Kirks, D. R., Fram, E. K., Vock, P., Effmann, E. L.: Tracheal compression by mediastinal masses in children: CT evaluation. *A.J.R.* **141**:647, 1983.

50. Kirks, D. R., Korobkin, M.: Computed tomography of the chest wall, pleura and pulmonary parenchyma in infants and children. *Radiol. Clin. North Am.* **19**:421, 1981.

51. Kirks, D. R., Merten, D. F., Grossman, H., Bowie, J. D.: Diagnostic imaging of pediatric abdominal masses: An overview. *Radiol. Clin. North Am.* **19**:527, 1981.

52. Kuhn, J. P., Berger, P. E.: Computed tomography of the kidney in infancy and childhood. *Radiol. Clin. North Am.* **19**:445, 1981.

53. Kulkarni, R., Bailie, M. D., Bernstein, J., Newton, B.: Progression of nephroblastomatosis to Wilms' tumor. Letter to the Editor, *J. Pediatr.* **96**:178, 1980.

54. Kumar, A. P. M., Wrenn, E. L., Fleming, I. D., Hustu, H. O., Pratt, C. B.: Combined therapy to prevent complete pelvic exenteration for rhabdomyosarcoma of the vagina and uterus. *Cancer* **37**:118, 1976.

55. Leape, L. L., Breslow, N. E., Bishop, H. C.: The surgical treatment of Wilm's tumor: Results of the National Wilm's Tumor Study. *Ann. Surg.* **187**:351–356, 1978.

56. Ling, D., Grossman, H., Kirks, D. R.: Use of computed tomography in pediatric oncology. *Am. J. Pediatr. Hematol. Oncol.* **6**(3):293–311, 1984.

57. Machin, G. A.: Nephroblastomatosis and multiple nephroblastoma: Histologic, therapeutic, and theoretical aspects. *Arch. Pathol. Lab. Med.* **102**:639, 1978.

58. Mahour, G. H., Soule, E. H., Mills, S. D., Lynn, H. B.: Rhabdomyosarcoma in infants and children: A clinicopathologic study of 75 cases. *J. Pediatr. Surg.* **2**:402, 1967.

59. Malek, R. S., Kelalis, P. P.: Paratesticular rhabdomyosarcoma in childhood. *J. Urol.* **118**:450, 1977.

60. Martinez, L. A., Haase, G. M., Koep, L. J., Akers, D. R.: Rhabdomyosarcoma of the biliary tree: The case for aggressive surgery. *J. Pediatr. Surg.* **17**:508, 1982.

61. Maurer, H. M., Moon, T., Donaldson, M., Fernandez, C., Hays, D. M., Ragab, A., Sutow, W. W.: The Intergroup Rhabdomyosarcoma Study: A preliminary report. *Cancer* **40**:2015, 1977.

62. Murphy, S. B., Frizzeva, G., Evans, A. E.: A study of childhood non-Hodgkin's lymphomas. *Cancer* **36**:2121, 1975.

63. Ortega, J. A., Rivard, G. E., Issacs, H., Hittle, R. E., Hays, D. M., Pike, M. D., Karon, M. R.: The influence of chemotherapy on the prognosis of rhabdomyosarcoma. *Med. Pediatr. Oncol.* **1**:227, 1975.

64. Oterman, K., Schueller, E. F.: Maturation of neuroblastoma to ganglioneuroma. *Am. J. Dis. Child.* **120**:217, 1970.

65. Pack, G. T., Eberhart, W. F.: Rhabdomyosarcoma of skeletal muscle—report of 100 cases. *Surgery* **32**:1032, 1952.

66. Palmer, N. F., Beckwith, J. B.: Multiple primary tumor syndrome in children with rhabdoid tumor of the kidney. *Proc. Am. Soc. Clin. Oncol.* **22**:406, 1981 (abstr.).

67. Pilepich, M. V., Rene, J. B., Munzenrider, J. E., Carter, B. L.: Contribution of computed tomography in the treatment of lymphomas. *A.J.R.* **131**:69, 1978.

68. Pratt, C. B.: Response of childhood rhabdomyosarcoma to combination chemotherapy. *J. Pediatr.* **74**:791, 1969.

69. Previtt, L.: Nephroblastomatosis: A brief survey based on two case reports. Presented at the Annual Meeting of the Society for Pediatric Radiology, San Francisco, California, March, 1981.

70. Pritchard, D. J., Dahlin, D. C., Dauphine, R. T., Taylor, W. F., Beabout, J. W.: Ewing's sarcoma—a clinico-pathological and statistical analysis of patients surviving five years or longer. *J. Bone Joint Surg.* 57A:10, 1975.

71. Putnam, T. C., Cohen, H. J., Constine, L. S. III: Pediatric solid tumors. In *Clinical Oncology for Medical Students and Physicians: A Multidisciplinary Approach*, 6th ed. Rubin, P. (Ed.). New York, American Cancer Society, 1983, pp. 392–427.

72. Rosenfield, N. S., Shimkin, P., Berdon, W., Barwick, K., Glassman, M., Siegel, N. J.: Wilms' tumor arising from spontaneously regressing nephroblastomatosis. *A.J.R.* 135:381, 1980.

73. Ruymann, F. B., Donaldson, M., Lawrence, W., Tefft, M., Crist, W. M.: Extrahepatic biliary rhabdomyosarcoma. *Proc. Am. Assoc. Can. Res.* 21:388, 1980 (abstr.).

74. Schaner, E. G., Chang, A. E., Doppman, J. L., Coukle, D. M., Flye, M. W., Rosenberg, S. A.: Comparison of computed and conventional whole lung tomography in detecting pulmonary nodules: A prospective radiologic-pathologic study. *A.J.R.* 131:51–54, 1978.

75. Siegel, M. J.: Pediatric applications. In *Computed Body Tomography*. Lee, J. K. T., Sagel, S. S., Stanley, R. J. (Eds.). New York, Raven Press, 1983.

76. Siegel, M. J., Balfe, D. M., McClennan, B. L., Levitt, R. G.: Clinical utility of CT in pediatric retroperitoneal disease: 5 years experience. *A.J.R.* 138:1011, 1982.

77. Siegel, M. J., Glasier, C. M., Sagel, S. S.: CT of pelvic disorders in children. *A.J.R.* 37:1139, 1981.

78. Siegel, M. J., Sagel, S. S.: Computed tomography as a supplement to urography in the evaluation of suspected neuroblastoma. *Radiology* 142:435, 1982.

79. Srouji, M. N., Donaldson, M. H., Chatten, J., Koblenzer, C. S.: Perianal rhabdomyosarcoma in childhood. *Cancer* 38:1008, 1976.

80. Sutow, W. W., Gehan, E. A., Heyn, R. M., Kung, F. H., Miller, R. W., Murphy, M. L., Traggis, D. F.: Comparison of survival curves 1956 vs 1962 in children with Wilms' tumor and neuroblastoma.

Pediatrics 45:800, 1970.

81. Sutow, W. W., Lindberg, R. D., Gehan, E. A., Ragab, A. H., Raney, R. B., Ruymann, F., Soule, E. H.: Three year relapse-free survival rates in childhood rhabdomyosarcoma of the head and neck. *Cancer* 49:2217, 1982.

82. Sutow, W. W., Sullivan, M. P., Ried, H. L., Taylor, H. G., Griffith, K. M.: Prognosis in childhood rhabdomyosarcoma. *Cancer* 25:1384, 1970.

83. Stout, A. P.: Rhabdomyosarcoma of the skeletal muscles. *Ann. Surg.* 123:447, 1946.

84. Tefft, M., Fernandez, C., Donaldson, M. H., Newton, W., Moon, T. E.: Incidence of meningeal involvement by rhabdomyosarcoma of the head and neck in children: A report by the Intergroup Rhabdomyosarcoma Study (IRS). *Cancer* 42:253–258, 1978.

85. Tefft, M., Jaffe, N.: Sarcoma of the bladder and prostate in children: Rationale for the role of radiation therapy based on a review of the literature and a report of 14 additional patients. *Cancer* 32:1161–1177, 1973.

86. Tefft, M., Lindberg, R. D., Gehan, E. A.: Radiation therapy combined with systemic chemotherapy of rhabdomyosarcoma in children: Local control in patients enrolled in the intergroup rhabdomyosarcoma study. *Natl. Cancer Inst. Monogr.* 56:75–81, 1981.

87. Voute, P. A., Vos, A.: Combination chemotherapy as primary treatment in children with rhabdomyosarcoma to avoid mutilating surgery or radiotherapy. *Proc. Am. Assoc. Can. Res. Am. Soc. Clin. Oncol.* 327, 1977.

88. Weichselbaum, R. R., Cassady, J. R., Albert, D. M., Gonder, J. R.: Multimodality management of orbital rhabdomyosarcoma. *Int. Ophthalmol. Clin.* 20:247–259, 1980.

89. Wilbur, J. R.: Combination chemotherapy for embryonal rhabdomyosarcoma. *Cancer Chemother. Rpt.* 58:281, 1974.

90. Wolff, J. A.: Advances in the treatment of Wilms' tumor. *Cancer* 35:901, 1975.

91. Young, L., Rubin, P., Hanson, R.: The extra-adrenal neuroblastoma: High radiocurability and diagnostic accuracy. *A.J.R.* 108:75–91, 1970.

25 COMPUTED TOMOGRAPHY AND RADIATION THERAPY TREATMENT PLANNING

Robert W. Kline
W. Dennis Foley
Michael T. Gillin

Radiation therapy is a primary cancer treatment modality and, depending upon the type and stage of tumor, is delivered with the intent of either cure or palliation. The most important factors affecting the results of radiation therapy are the tumor type, its local and regional extent, the anatomic area of involvement, and the geometric accuracy with which a calculated radiation dose is delivered to a target defined in three dimensions.

Computed tomography (CT) has had a marked impact on radiation therapy. Its value for radiotherapy planning has been addressed, and efficacy studies have been reported by a number of authors.[1-3,6,7,10-12,16,19,24,26-28,30,31,33-36,39-41] Radiologists can confirm the large number of CT studies directed at oncology patients. Many can also confirm the nuisance of radiation therapists, physicists, or dosimetrists in pursuit of "treatment planning scans." Computed tomography makes very important contributions to tumor localization and diagnosis. At times CT is complimentary with barium contrast studies, angiography, lymphography, and other studies; in many cases CT is much better than conventional imaging procedures. This has been emphasized in the foregoing chapters.

In only the narrowest sense, treatment planning consists of generating isodose distributions for a set of fields that simulate a potential patient treatment. The treatment planning process is considerably broader in scope. Basic decisions relative to treatment strategies are based on the results of diagnostic studies, clinical evaluation, and the radiotherapist's knowledge of the natural course of the particular disease, his or her experience, and the treatment armamentarium. It is impossible to separate the treatment planning activities of CT from its purely diagnostic contributions. This chapter takes for granted the diagnostic capabilities of CT in tumor localization and emphasizes the technical aspects of CT-assisted radiotherapy planning. The use of CT for radiotherapy planning requires attention to a variety of details that are generally of little or no consequence to the diagnostician, generally disruptive for CT personnel, and altogether necessary.

Failure to control tumor growth is the most important cause of an adverse outcome in the management of malignant disease. Local failure occurs in a significant percentage of patients treated with radiotherapy depending upon tumor site and stage.[32] Computed tomography, with its ability to define internal anatomy, permits treatment to be given with more confidence through better definition of the treatment fields. Goitein has suggested, based upon an average dose-response relationship for tumors, that for one series of patients CT could improve the probability of local tumor control by an average of 6% and improve the chance of five-year survival by an average of 3.5%.[11] The literature contains many articles indicating changes in radiation techniques directly resulting from the use of CT. The ability of any institution to take advantage of CT-assisted radiotherapy planning depends upon a number of variables, but especially the willingness of radiotherapists to incorporate this information in a systematic way into an already complex process.

OBJECTIVES AND LIMITATIONS OF CT-ASSISTED RADIATION THERAPY PLANNING

Fundamentally, the aim of radiation therapy is to deliver a tumoricidal dose of radiation to a target volume and to limit the dose received by normal tissues to levels that avoid unacceptable morbidity. The prescribed dose for a particular patient is dependent on the type of tumor and can range from less than 30 Gy to more than 70 Gy. Because tumor control probability and adverse effects to normal tissue are strongly dose dependent, desired accuracy with which the prescribed dose should be delivered is ±5%.[23,29,37] There are numerous variables for the various tolerances associated with radiotherapy treatment that make that level of accuracy a challenging goal. These include basic treatment unit variables such as calibration, beam descriptors, and mechanical specifications. Also included are computer algorithms and patient-specific variables such as external contour and relative internal structure. The basic contributions of CT to radiotherapy planning, in the context of mapping the dose within a patient, are the display of individual patient anatomy and the unique ability of CT to determine quantitatively the X-ray attenuation properties of the tissues.

The accuracy of dose delivery is dependent upon patient positioning. Radiation treatments are often fractionated, commonly delivered five times per week for 5 to 7 weeks. This demands strict attention to reproducible patient positioning. Computed tomographic scans conducted for radiotherapy planning must use the identical patient position as that used for treatment. Most radiotherapy departments are stocked with an assortment of positioning aids and immobilization devices, many of which are used when CT scans are performed.

The accuracy required in terms of simply defining the external contour of a patient is very important. For cobalt 60 treatment, an error of 1 cm in defining the depth of a dose prescription translates into a 5% error in dose (less at higher X-ray energies). If we consider using CT images from a multiformat camera for defining external contours, a distortion of less than 0.1% per centimeter between the horizontal and vertical magnifications (minifications) of the image is required to achieve 1-cm accuracy for a patient diameter of 30 cm. Such relative distortions of the multiformat camera image are of little or no interest to the diagnostician but are of great importance for radiotherapy planning.[22]

Computed tomography can define tumor volume and the position of adjacent organs in a cross-sectional anatomic format in a manner that was impossible with previous techniques (Figure 25-1). However, there are two primary limitations to optimizing the geometric accuracy of CT-assisted radiotherapy. First, there is inaccuracy in macroscopic tumor staging by CT. This is due to the observers' inability to distinguish between contiguity of tumor to adjacent normal structures and tumor invasion.

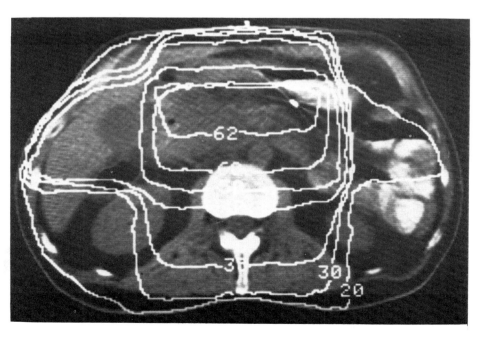

FIG. 25-1. Dose distribution representing a treatment of carcinoma of the pancreas. This plan is for a three-field treatment with 18 MV X rays: an anterior field and wedged, bilateral fields. Isodose lines are in gray. Computed tomography is of particular value in imaging the upper abdomen. Of importance in this case is definition of the target volume and the relative location of critical normal tissues of known radiation tolerance; the kidneys, liver, and spinal cord.

In addition, microscopic spread cannot be detected on CT scans. Second, there can be variation between patient positioning in the CT scanner and positioning in treatment and variation in patient positioning between individual treatments. The potential benefit of achieving a higher and more accurate radiation dose to the tumor by more accurately defining target volume can be offset by inattention to strict repositioning specifications.

In addition to displaying individual patient anatomy, CT can also provide quantitative information regarding the X-ray attenuation properties of the tissues. Computed tomographic numbers represent attenuation caused by photoelectric absorption and Compton scattering, which are dependent on atomic number and electron density, respectively. Megavoltage X-ray therapy beams are attenuated primarily by Compton interactions, and thus the distribution of dose is dependent on the electron density of the tissues. Dose computation schemes that presume the body to be of uniform water attenuation values do not provide an accurate description of dose because of the varying electron densities in different tissues of the body. This can result in a significant difference between calculated and actual radiation dose, particularly in the thorax when the lower electron density of lung tissue is not included in the calculations. With CT, it is possible to convert the image data to either the average electron density in an outlined region or to determine electron density on a pixel by pixel basis. A correction for average electron density may be sufficient to provide an estimated radiation dose that is within several percent of the actual figure, and significantly different from that obtained without a correction.

CT TECHNIQUE

The approach to a therapy planning scan is different from that for a diagnostic CT study for tumor staging. In staging examinations, a series of contiguous or closely spaced CT sections are performed. A curved tabletop is used, and for thorax scanning the arms are elevated. Intravenous contrast material is used for most staging procedures. For most therapy planning CT studies, a limited series of sections are performed, encompassing the center and the margins of the proposed treatment volume. The patient is placed on a flat tabletop insert so that the external contour will closely match that on the radiotherapy treatment couch. For lesions in the cranium, the sections of interest are transverse rather than the typical diagnostic sections, which parallel the orbital-meatal line. In many cases of treatments in the thorax, the arms are placed at the patients' sides. For tangential chest wall fields for breast tumors, only the ipsilateral arm is elevated (Figure 25-2).

The treatment positioning devices used in radiotherapy rooms, such as bilateral and ceiling lasers, should be

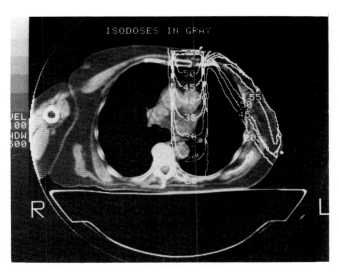

FIG. 25-2. Dose distribution representing treatment of a post-mastectomy patient with breast carcinoma. The treatment includes three 6 MV X-ray fields: an anterior field encompassing the ipsilateral internal mammary lymph nodes, and opposed tangential fields treating the chest wall. Computed tomography is useful for such patients for determination of the chest wall thickness and the amount of lung encompassed in the high dose region. However, the technical setup of this treatment conflicts with the usefulness of CT. For this setup, the ipsilateral arm must be extended out of the tangential fields. In most cases this cannot be exactly reproduced for the CT study because of the limited aperture of the CT gantry. For such a study, one attempts to minimize the discrepancy between the treatment and scan positions, and recognizes the probable inaccuracies generated by such a situation.

available. In treatment positioning for tumors of the head and neck, thoracic inlet, and upper chest, it is important to provide head and neck immobilization. Devices for this purpose often must be modified for use in CT, for example, by replacing metal components with acrylic in order to minimize reconstruction artifacts. Contrast material is not always employed for therapy planning scans. However, to obtain anatomic definition it is considered necessary to administer oral contrast for scans of the abdomen and intravenous contrast for scans of the cranium and pelvis (Figure 25-3).

Based on information from prior CT scans or other imaging tests, the location of the central ray and the margins of the proposed fields may be outlined on the patient's skin with radiopaque catheter tubing. A longitudinal localization digital radiograph is then obtained with the patient in the treatment position. The CT digital radiographs are produced by a collimated fan beam, which is pulsed as the patient is translated longitudinally through the scanning circle. This results in an image that has no geometric distortion in the cephalocaudad dimension. Thus, the location of a series of axial scans performed at anatomic levels selected from the digital radiograph corresponds exactly to the location annotated on

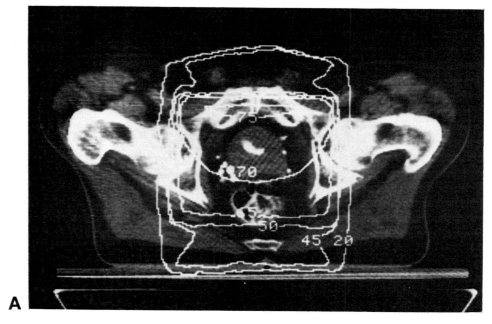

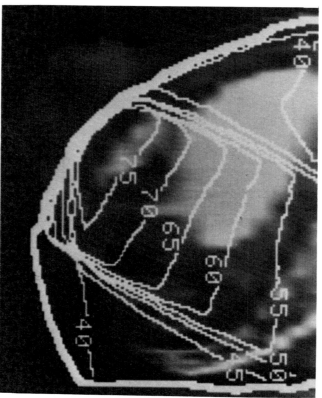

FIG. 25-3. Dose distribution for a treatment of prostate carcinoma. This plan employs opposed anterior/posterior fields and a perineal field treated with cobalt 60 radiation. Isodose lines are in gray. Two representations of the dose distribution are presented: (A) A transverse section at the level of the mid-prostate, and (B) the corresponding distribution in the midsagittal plane. The image in B has been generated as a reformatted image from a set of contiguous (1 cm) axial sections. The potential of CT to contribute to multiplane, multiview, and three-dimensional dose calculation and display is as yet untapped. Such treatment planning will certainly increase the scope of treatment planning CT scans.

the electronic image. This is of fundamental importance in that the lateral extent of a macroscopic tumor and critical organs at each selected level can be determined from the corresponding axial CT image.[17] The digital radiograph has proved invaluable in defining the locations for scans and in correlating the axial images with simulator and port films taken in radiotherapy (Figure 25-4).[8] In our practice it is usual to locate the zero level for the study at the central ray of the therapy beam. A limited series of axial sections above and below this level are performed.

For practical patient setup and study definition, a person from the radiotherapy department must attend the CT planning session. This may be a radiotherapist, a dosimetrist, a physicist, or a technologist. Optimally, both a radiotherapist and a technical person should be available. It is in the interest of both the radiotherapy staff and the CT staff that each facility develop and use a therapy planning CT request form that outlines the scope and objectives of the study and defines the technical setup to be employed. We have found that identifying a scheduled time for radiotherapy scans is greatly

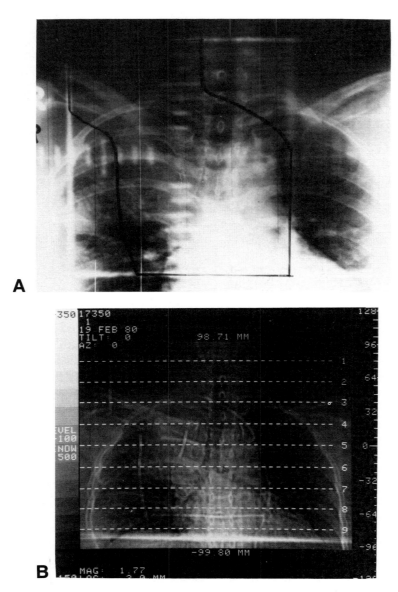

FIG. 25-4. A simulator film (A) and digital radiograph (B) for a patient with lung cancer. The proposed treatment field has been drawn on the simulator film (A). For the treatment planning CT study, the central ray and outline of this field were defined with radiopaque catheter tubing taped on the patient's skin. The zero level of the digital radiograph (B) corresponds to the central ray of the treatment field. Axial sections were taken at 2-cm intervals to cover the extent of the planned field. The lateral extent of abnormal tissue was then determined on each image and compared with the target defined in the conventional manner. For this patient, the volume of abnormal tissue as defined by CT extended beyond the target volume at levels from the central ray to the caudad border. The target volume was then expanded.

desirable. This ensures time on the CT unit for radiotherapy, eases the scheduling burden, and minimizes the disruption caused by the special demands of the procedure.

The specifications for CT scanner performance that are suggested as adequate for a therapy planning study are similar to those required for specialized diagnostic studies.[10,20] Image quality should be sufficient to define tumor extent. Images should be obtained with short scan times to reduce motion artifacts. When scans of the chest and upper abdomen are performed during breath holding, only slight inspiration is used in order to simulate as closely as possible the internal anatomy during treatment. An important feature of scanner performance is accuracy in table repositioning so that a scan that is programmed 4 cm above the central ray is, in fact, anatomically 4 cm above the central ray. The current CT scanners have tight table repositioning specifications that meet the needs of radiotherapy planning. The gantry aperture and field of view should be wide enough to allow the body contour at the level of the shoulders and hips to be included within the reconstruction circle. Tabletop inserts that accurately reproduce the flat radiotherapy couches should be available. In general, the quality of the image needed for a planning study is quite similar to that needed for a diagnostic study.

The requirements of radiotherapy relative to the filmed CT images from a multiformat camera are somewhat different from those of diagnosis. If these images are to be used for defining external contour and internal anatomy for entry into a treatment planning computer, then, as mentioned earlier, minimal geometric distortion in the filmed images is mandatory. We have found it useful to employ the largest image format available. The window and level settings for filming should preserve diagnostic information but must allow determination of the external contour. Generally, we also require overlaying a calibrated square grid (software generated on the display) on each filmed image, which facilitates viewing the series of images of the study from a geometric perspective and allows optical magnification.

Quality assurance procedures on the CT unit should be expanded to address the requirements of radiotherapy. These considerations include table repositioning specifications, multiformat camera distortion, laser alignment, calibration of CT number versus electron density.

The time of the planning CT study relative to simulation poses some interesting challenges. In conventional planning, the treatment setup is simulated before treatment; that is, the patient position is established with or without the help of immobilization devices, the central ray and the borders of the treatment field are defined and plain films are taken. If the planning CT scan is performed before simulation, the technical details of the treatment setup are not available. In many cases this is not significant, since many setups follow well-defined guidelines. However, if the subsequent simulation modifies the patient position, then a repeat planning scan may be necessary. When the planning scan is performed after simulation, the results of the study may necessitate resimulation. In most settings the time demands on the CT unit are far greater than on the simulator. Such is the case in our clinic, where, as a consequence, we will do a minor simulation or localization procedure on the simulator for many patients, then a planning CT scan, and then a normal simulation. We have found this to be particularly helpful for patients with low grade brain tumors, tumors of the oral cavity and oropharynx, maxillary antrum tumors, neuroblastomas, and tumors in the abdomen and retroperitoneum. For several years we were doing combination diagnostic/therapy studies, in which the patient was repositioned to the requirements of radiotherapy immediately after the diagnostic study, and a limited number of additional sections were taken through the region of interest. Unfortunately, we have had to abandon this technique because problems arose as a result of two studies performed on the same day.

CT-BASED TREATMENT PLANNING

Computer-based treatment planning systems were developed in the 1960s and through the 1970s became an almost necessary adjunct to radiotherapy centers. Before this development radiotherapists (usually residents), physicists, dosimetrists, or technologists spent many hours compounding isodose distributions by hand. These were generated using patient contours obtained with solder wire, plaster strips, or in some cases, relatively sophisticated contouring devices. Internal anatomy was added employing information from palpation, plain roentgenograms, or atlases of cross-sectional anatomy. The implementation of computer treatment planning systems decreased the work load associated with individual treatment plans and provided the advantages of potentially more accurate dose calculations and more sophisticated treatment planning. However, the patient-specific input data relied on existing techniques. The use of CT images for radiotherapy planning commenced as the availability of individual patient cross-sectional anatomy was recognized as a significant advance.

Commercial computer treatment planning systems use a variety of calculational approaches to model the dose distribution in a two-dimensional patient section. One can consider the dose calculation as a sequential modification of the dose distribution for a radiation beam incident at a right angle on a flat-surfaced patient of homogeneous water density. Most planning systems use measured data for such a situation as the basis of data representing a particular beam. The dose distribution in this case is simple although dependent on variables such as beam energy, field flattening, collimation, field size, and others. Using a digitized contour for the patient of interest, the computer modifies the dose distribution appropriately. The dose may be modified further to account for devices such as wedge filters or to account for tissue heterogeneity.

In most cases, more than one field is employed for a particular treatment. The computer system generates individual dose distributions for each field, which may then be combined with specified relative weights for each field. The resultant dose distribution is generally produced on a plotter as a line drawing with operator-selected isodose lines superimposed on outlines of the external contour and any entered internal structures. Several alternate distributions may be generated for different beams (energy, placement, wedge filter, etc.) or for different relative doses. Evaluation of the resultant distribution includes determination of the adequacy of the dose delivered to the target region and consideration of that received by normal tissues.

The role of CT in this process is rather obvious. It is the generation of patient-specific diagnostic and anatomic information for treatment planning. The availability of multiple transverse images is a great advantage. Target volumes and normal structures are three-dimensional and may change dramatically in the cephalocaudad direction. External patient contours can change rapidly, particularly in the head and neck and upper thorax and can significantly modify the dose distribution relative to other locations in the treated region. Multiplane treatment planning is clearly facilitated by CT.

The ability to reformat axial CT images to create an image in a sagittal or a coronal plane offers the treatment planner an opportunity to view the plan from a different perspective. In our experience, such reformatting has proved to be useful in treating upper thorax tumors and in treating perineal fields (Figure 25-3). It may prove to be valuable for treating brain tumors as we begin to think in three-dimensions more consistently.

In addition to providing valuable information for the planning of external beam radiotherapy, CT has also been shown to be of use for treatments involving intracavitary and interstitial radioactive sources.[4,5,18,25]

Beyond the diagnostic and relative anatomic information, CT also provides a quantitative description of the X-ray attenuation properties of the tissues imaged. For both megavoltage X-ray beams and electron beams, attenuation is primarily dependent on the electron density of the attenuating material. Although CT images are obtained at diagnostic energies where photoelectric attenuation is important, a relatively simple and acceptably accurate correspondence can be made between CT number and electron density. Thus, CT data can be employed to correct the dose distribution for tissue heterogeneity. Such correction is of some importance when considering radiation treatments in the thorax because of the large volume of low density lung tissue (Figure 25-5). Heterogeneity corrections are also important for planning the use of charged particle beams (electrons, protons, pi mesons).[9,21,38] A pitfall in the employment of CT data for heterogeneity corrections is the presence of contrast material in the images. (Using such corrections for an image with a constrast-opacified bladder, for example, would be ludicrous.)

The relative importance of heterogeneity corrections does depend on the treatment modality (X-ray or electron energy), the field arrangement and weighting, and the relative heterogeneity. The same treatment protocol applied to two different patients with lung tumors may result in significantly different dose distributions, because of the anatomic differences between the patients. Attention to tissue heterogeneity thus is important, not only from the standpoint of accurate dose specification, but also to achieve precision in a particular treatment protocol. These considerations have been known for years in the radiotherapy community. However, the incorporation of such corrections into routine dosimetry has yet to become the norm. The reasons for this include some justifiable inertia against modifying treatment protocols that are based on clinical experience, a previous lack of quantitative data on tissue heterogeneity, and inadequacies in the methods employed to calculate this effect. Computed tomography can now provide the required quantitative information. Commercial treatment planning computer systems are able, with various limitations in accuracy and general application, to model the effect of heterogeneities. It will be prudent of individual clinics, however, to integrate this capability into practice gradually.

The earliest and perhaps still the most common use of CT images in a treatment planning computer is indirect. For example, films from a multiformat camera may be optically projected to life size. The external contour and interesting internal structures can then be traced and digitized for entry into the computer. Alternatively, systems are now available that interface directly with the CT images. This may be done by a direct link to the CT unit or through portable media such as magnetic tape or floppy discs. Systems are available that allow generation of dose distributions on the CT computer, at the operator's console, or at an independent viewing console. Because time-sharing of the CT system with the diagnostic section generally has proved difficult, the common arrangement is an independent, dedicated treatment planning computer system that is capable of using CT images. Such systems are capable of storing and displaying archived CT images and generating and superimposing dose distributions on the images.

As mentioned earlier, treatment planning is broader

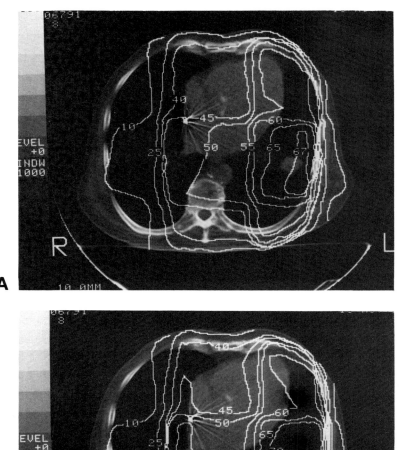

FIG. 25-5. Dose distributions for a treatment of lung carcinoma. Six fields using 18 MV X rays are employed: anterior/posterior, reduced anterior/posterior, and left/right lateral. Isodose lines are in gray. (A) The dose calculated assuming uniform (water) density. (B) The dose distribution corrected for tissue heterogeneity based on a linear relationship between CT number and electron density. In general, the lower density of lung tissue results in a higher dose than that calculated assuming unit density. This effect depends on X-ray energy and is more important at lower energies. Comparison of the two dose distributions shows significant differences. In the region of the primary lesion in the left lung the maximum dose is approximately 67 Gy (A). After correcting for heterogeneity, a somewhat larger volume of lung is shown to receive a dose in excess of 70 Gy (B). In the contralateral medial lung, a region appears to receive between 45 Gy and 50 Gy, when ignoring heterogeneity (A). With correction, this region is shown to receive 55 Gy (B).

in scope than the consideration of plotted dose distributions. Much use can be made of CT-derived information independent of computer dosimetry. With the aid of the calibrated grid on the CT images, it is possible to determine field orientations and borders. It is a common and useful practice to view simultaneously the CT images and "beam's eye" plain roentgenograms on which to draw the margins of an irregularly shaped field. In many cases, in fact, the computer-generated dose distribution serves the purpose of treatment verification rather than treatment planning.

For some patients, follow-up CT scans are useful for examining the effect of treatment. Figure 25-6 is a particularly striking example of fibrotic changes in a patient with lung cancer corresponding to the radiation fields employed for treatment. Reflection upon such studies may lead to modification of particular treatment approaches. With the internal anatomy defined so precisely, it is possible to analyze various treatment approaches in terms of the volume of a lung or other organ receiving a certain percentage of the target dose. It may even be possible to correlate changes in the CT numbers with the dose distributions.

Computed tomography has certainly increased the work load for treatment planners, both in the time associated with the examination and in incorporating the information derived from the study into the planning process. It is likely that the latter effort will expand significantly. The state of CT-assisted radiotherapy is that CT provides more information than can be used by current treatment planning systems. The available systems are essentially limited to two-dimensional planning. Further development is underway in better modeling of heterogeneity corrections, irregular fields and three-dimensional planning. Goitein has addressed the limitations of current planning systems.[13] Subsequently, Goitein et al.[14,15] have discussed the potential and implementation of three-dimensional display systems for treatment planning. These authors describe the synthesis of diagnostic information and integration of anatomic and tumor images into three-dimensional simulations that are interactive with the treatment planner. They also present multidimension planning from a beam's eye view, back projection, and projection through CT sections. The implementation of interactive three-dimensional computer

graphics in radiotherapy has lagged behind that in other fields. These techniques will become available in commercial planning systems and should permit treatment planners to take full advantage of the information available in CT imaging.

EXPERIENCE WITH CT-ASSISTED TREATMENT PLANNING

This chapter has focused on the technical aspects of the use of computed tomography for radiotherapy planning. Inclusion of CT in the treatment planning process certainly increases the time and cost associated with patient management. Justification for CT-assisted treatment planning has been demonstrated by a number of studies. Again, one cannot easily separate the diagnostic impact of CT from its contributions to the technical aspects of treatment planning.

A common approach has been to plan treatments conventionally and then to replan the treatments to include information provided by CT examinations. Using this methodology, Munzenrider et al.[28] considered 75 patients in terms of the volume treated without CT data and that at the volume treated using CT. The treatment volume including the CT data would have been unchanged in 41 (55%) patients, larger in 16 (21%), and smaller in 18 (24%). Coverage of the tumor as determined from all other studies except CT was considered clearly inadequate in 15 (20%) patients, marginal in 20 (27%), and adequate in 40 (53%). The authors judged CT scans as essential for treatment planning if their availability

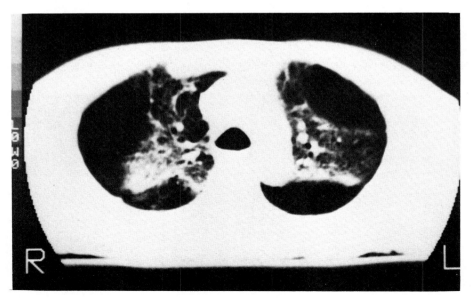

FIG. 25-6. Follow-up CT scan performed 7 weeks after completion of radiation therapy for lung cancer. The patient received 41.4 Gy through opposed anterior/posterior fields and 21.6 Gy through opposed lateral fields (heterogeneity corrections have not been incorporated in the dose calculation). The margins of the radiation changes in the lungs closely follow the borders of the treatment fields.

resulted in the volume irradiated being larger or smaller or if tumor coverage would have been inadequate or marginal without them. The CT scan was judged helpful if field placement and other treatment variables were more easily determined than with other methods. With these criteria, CT was judged essential in 41 (55%) patients, helpful in 23 (31%) patients, and not necessary in 11 (14%) patients.

The relative value of CT was noted to be dependent on the anatomic region of interest; thus, it is less important in the pelvis. The study of Munzenrider et al.[28] and a selection of similar studies have been condensed and are presented in Table 25-1. There is a significant percentage of patients for whom the CT information modified the treatment plan in all of these studies. Criticism may be directed at these studies because some patient selection was possible and attention to the conventional planning may be questioned. Nevertheless, these reports are supported by numerous other reports and are coupled with general agreement among radiotherapists and treatment planners that CT represents a significant advance for radiotherapy. It is certainly true that when a CT study is present during the discussion of a particular patient, communication is improved among all parties and there is more attention to detail.

The contribution of CT to the treatment planning process can be summarized in two major capabilities. One is the ability of CT to define the tumor volume within the patient, basically in the axial perspective. The other is the ability of CT to define internal anatomy (including X-ray attenuation properties) and external contours. Computed tomography can do this not only at a single level but at multiple levels, which can be correlated with each other. The relative importance of these two contributions depends on the site involved as well as the individual patient and the treatment philosophy and techniques of the institution. We have reflected on our six-year experience with CT-assisted treatment planning and summarized in Table 25-2 the perceived value of CT. This table is a subjective appraisal of the relative value of CT by anatomic site for tumor definition, normal tissue definition, boost field design, and heterogeneity corrections.

In treating brain tumors it is equally important to define the target volume precisely and to spare as much normal tissue as possible. This will permit the use of high doses while minimizing potential side effects. In our clinic the treatment field is defined on the simulator film by studying the axial and reformatted images and the computed radiograph. It is possible to define the initial fields and reduced fields on a centimeter-to-centimeter grid in the cephalocaudad direction. It is particularly helpful to have the center of the simulator film correspond to the zero level of the computed radiograph and the axial images.

The treatment of head and neck tumors involves a region of the body where the external contours change rapidly and where there is great variation in the internal anatomy. The spinal cord is generally the dose-limiting organ in the treatment field, but there are many other critical structures. The definition of normal anatomy by CT at various levels in the treatment field is a major contribution. Computed tomography is very helpful in determining the depth of lymph nodes or other structures from the surface and thus the electron energy appropriate for treating such structures.

Tumors located in the upper thoracic region, such as tumors of the thyroid and middle to upper esophagus, must be treated aggressively but with great care. In this region there are substantial changes in body contour as well as in the location of internal anatomy, as evidenced by the relative change in the location of the spinal cord. The definition of internal anatomy via CT is very useful. The sagittal reformatted image is of particular use here. Electron beams may be employed for treating this region, and depths to critical structures such as the spinal cord are important. The placement of the oblique fields is facilitated greatly by CT images. Again, multilevel dosimetry is very important, especially when planning field reductions.

Lung tumors may be imaged with CT; in some cases, areas of involvement can be identified that would be im-

Table 25-1. Effect of CT in Defining Tumor Volume and Modifying Treatment Plan

STUDY	SITE	NUMBER OF PATIENTS	INADEQUATE TUMOR VOLUME WITHOUT CT (%)	TREATMENT PLAN ALTERED WITH CT (%)
Brizel et al.[3]	Pelvis	72	40	61
Emami et al.[6]	Lung	32	28	53
Goitein et al.[16]	All	77	31	52
Hobday et al.[19]	All	123	26	38
Munzenrider et al.[28]	All	75	20	55
Seydel et al.[36]	Lung	23	17	26

Table 25-2. Value of CT for Treatment Planning by Site

SITE	TUMOR DEFINITION	NORMAL TISSUE DEFINITION	BOOST FIELD DESIGN	HETEROGENEITY CORRECTIONS
Cranium	Excellent	Limited	Excellent	No
Head and Neck	Moderate	Excellent	Moderate	Limited
Upper Thorax	Moderate	Excellent	Moderate	Limited
Breast	Limited	Moderate	Limited	Moderate
Lung	Excellent	Excellent	Excellent	Excellent
Abdomen	Moderate	Excellent	Moderate	No
Pelvis	Moderate	Moderate	Moderate	No
Extremities	Moderate	Moderate	Moderate	No

possible to detect with conventional radiographic studies. Normal anatomy is precisely defined. Of greatest importance beyond the diagnostic information is the availability of quantitative data for correcting doses for lung density. Heterogeneity corrections for treatment of the thorax at single levels or at composite multiple levels will certainly be required in the future and will become a standard practice (Figure 25-5). The choice of the most appropriate X-ray beam energy is facilitated through the use of CT.

Many organs in the upper abdomen, such as the liver, kidneys, stomach, and spinal cord, have critical dose-limiting tolerances. The definition of these structures is necessary when treating pancreatic carcinomas or other tumors in this region. The determination of field placement, shaping, and relative weights with the goal of limiting the dose to specific vital structures can be done with greatly increased confidence using CT (Figure 25-1).

Many types of pelvic tumors are treated with radiotherapy. Again, CT is helpful in defining normal anatomy. This is valuable when treating patients with fields other than anteroposterior parallel opposed fields. Treatment plans can be defined to limit the dose to sensitive structures such as the rectum and small bowel. Planning using reformatted sagittal images may be helpful, especially if perineal or other nonstandard fields are used (Figure 25-3).

At times CT is extremely useful for examining patients in whom an intracavitary or interstitial implant has been done. Typical gynecologic applicators cause considerable artifacts on certain axial images. The artifact problem is not nearly so severe in the case of radioactive wires and seeds. In these cases the radioactive sources can be identified relative to anatomy and the resultant dose distributions superimposed over the CT anatomy. This can be very useful for both documentation and instructional purposes.

The use of planning CT scans for tumors in the extremities can be very helpful in specific patients. External contours may change significantly in the extremities, so multilevel treatment plans are important. Field design,

mixed X-ray/electron beam treatments, and adequate doses to the target volume can be challenging problems with tumors in the extremities.

It needs be emphasized that the relative value of CT for specific sites and specific patients is perceived as and is truly different for individual clinics and clinicians. The "tumor volume" reported by the diagnostician is rarely the "target volume" to be treated. The clinical acumen of the radiation oncologist dictates determination of the target volume, and his or her training and available equipment determine treatment approaches. Certainly the use and perceived value of CT for radiotherapy planning will continue to evolve. This evolution will include enhanced capabilities of treatment planning computer systems that use the information provided by CT more fully, and also will include new imaging modalities such as nuclear magnetic resonance.

CONCLUSION

The ultimate criteria for the success of radiotherapy treatment are analysis of tumor control, duration of disease-free survival, and complications associated with treatment. Assessment of the benefit of CT to radiotherapy has been related temporally to the planning and management of treatment. There is much subjective value placed on the benefit of CT to these aspects of treatment. There is certainly a belief and a hope that CT will positively influence the results of treatment. As cited earlier, Goitein has developed a model to project the benefit of CT to the end points of radiotherapy.[11] He concludes that CT scans could improve the probability of local control by 6% and improve five-year survival by 3.5%. Retrospective studies may contribute important information about the benefit of CT scans. However, given the perceived efficacy of CT for treatment planning and its widespread and evolving implementation, randomized prospective studies to assess the long-term results of radiotherapy not assisted with CT versus CT-assisted radiotherapy may be unethical.

The CT study performed as a diagnostic procedure

provides valuable information for the radiation oncologist but usually gives inadequate quantitative anatomic information for detailed dosimetry and optimal treatment planning. Because of the precise positioning demands of radiotherapy, there frequently is a conflict between treatment position and the position that is optimum for diagnostic yield from the CT study. Also, the contrast employed for a diagnostic examination may obviate the correction of dose for tissue heterogeneity. Thus, there exists a distinct class of "treatment planning scans," with special technical demands that are required by radiotherapy.

Beyond technical considerations, the most important requisites for successful integration of CT into radiotherapy planning are dialogue and cooperation between CT personnel and radiotherapy personnel, both the professional and the technical staff members. The needs of radiotherapy and the importance of details should be communicated and appreciated. Radiotherapy personnel must be sensitive to the limitations presented by scanner capabilities and scheduling, and they must identify reasonable objectives for each study. Clearly, the benefit of CT for an individual patient's treatment should not be diminished either by an inadequately performed treatment planning scan or by its inadequate employment in treatment planning.

ACKNOWLEDGEMENTS

The computed tomography images presented in this chapter were obtained on the General Electric Model 8800 scanner at Milwaukee County General Hospital. The computer-generated dose distributions were obtained using the software of the Atomic Energy of Canada, Ltd. TP-11/THERAPLAN.

REFERENCES

1. Barrett, A., Dobbs, H. J., Husband, J. E.: The value of computed tomography in radiation therapy. CT 5:217-218, 1981.
2. Battista, J. J., Rider, W. D., Van Dyk, J.: Computed tomography for radiotherapy planning. Int. J. Radiat. Oncol. Biol. Phys. 6:99-107, 1980.
3. Brizel, H., Livingstone, P., Grayson, E.: Radiotherapeutic applications of pelvic computed tomography. J. Comput. Assist. Tomogr. 3:453-466, 1979.
4. Elkon, D., Kim, J. A., Constable, W. C.: Anatomic localization of radioactive gold seeds of the prostate by computer-aided tomography. Comput. Tomogr. 5:89-93, 1981.
5. Elkon, D., Kim, J. A., Constable, W. C.: CT scanning and interstitial therapy. CT 5:268-272, 1981.
6. Emami, B., Melo, A., Carter, B. L., Munzenrider, J. E., Piro, A. J.: Value of computed tomography in radiotherapy of lung cancer. A.J.R. 131:63-67, 1978.
7. Fullerton, G. D., Sewchand, W., Payne, J. T., Levitt, S. H.: CT determination of parameters for inhomogeneity corrections in radiation therapy of the esophagus. Radiology 126:167-171, 1978.
8. Gillin, M. T., Foley, W. D., Kline, R. W., Kun, L. E.: The computed

radiograph: a method of correlating axial tomographic images with simulation and port films. Int. J. Radiat. Oncol. Biol. Phys. 7:1603-1606, 1981.
9. Goitein, M.: The measurement of tissue heterodensity to guide charged particle radiotherapy. Int. J. Radiat. Oncol. Biol. Phys. 3:27-33, 1977.
10. Goitein, M.: Computed tomography in planning radiation therapy. Int. J. Radiat. Oncol. Biol. Phys. 5:445-447, 1979.
11. Goitein, M.: The utility of computed tomography in radiation therapy: An estimate of outcome. Int. J. Radiat. Oncol. Biol. Phys. 5:1799-1807, 1979.
12. Goitein, M.: Benefits and cost of computerized tomography in radiation therapy. J.A.M.A. 244:1347-1350, 1980.
13. Goitein, M.: Limitations of two-dimensional treatment planning programs. Med. Phys. 9:580-587, 1982.
14. Goitein, M., Abrams, M.: Multi-dimensional treatment planning: I. Delineation of anatomy. Int. J. Radiat. Oncol. Biol. Phys. 9: 777-787, 1983.
15. Goitein, M., Abrams, M., Rowell, D., Pollari, H., Wiles, J.: Multi-dimensional treatment planning: II. Beam's eye view, back projection and projections through CT sections. Int. J. Radiat. Oncol. Biol. Phys. 9:789-797, 1983.
16. Goitein, M., Wittenberg, J., Mendiondo, M., Doucette, J., Friedberg, C., Ferrucci, J., Gunderson, L., Linggood, R., Shipley, W. U., Fineberg, H. V.: The value of CT scanning in radiation therapy treatment planning: A prospective study. Int. J. Radiat. Oncol. Biol. Phys. 5:1787-1798, 1979.
17. Griffin, B. R., Shuman, W. P., Luk, K. H., Tong, D.: Locate: An application of computed tomography in radiation therapy treatment planning with emphasis on tumor localiation. Int. J. Radiat. Oncol. Biol. Phys. 10:555, 1984.
18. Herskovic, A., Padikal, T. N., Lee, S. N.: Localization in interstitial dosimetry utilizing the CT scanner. Comput. Tomogr. 3:101-103, 1979.
19. Hobday, P., Hodson, N. J., Husband, J., Parker, R. P., Macdonald, J. S.: Computed tomography applied to radiotherapy treatment planning: Techniques and results. Radiology 133:447-482, 1979.
20. Hogstrom, K. R.: Computer tomography: Interface with the treatment planning process. ICRU Report 24. Washington, DC, 1976, pp. 46.
21. Hogstrom, K. R., Smith, A. R., Simon, S. L., Somers, J. W., Lane, R. G., Rosen I. I., Kelsey, C. A., von Essen, C. F., Kligerman, M. M., Berardo, P. A., Zink, S. M.: Static pion beam treatment planning of deep-seated tumors using computerized tomographic scans. Int. J. Radiat. Oncol. Biol. Phys. 5:875-876, 1979.
22. Ibbot, G. S.: Radiation therapy treatment planning and the distortion of CT images. Med. Phys. 7:261, 1980.
23. ICRU Report 24, Determination of absorbed dose in a patient irradiated by beams for radiation therapy. Washington, DC, 1981, pp. 1.
24. Isherwood, I., Pullan, B. R., Rutherford, R. A., Strang, F. A.: Electron density and atomic number determination by computed tomography. Part I: Methods and limitations. Part II: A study of colloid cysts. Br. J. Radiol. 50:613-619, 1977.
25. Lee, K. R., Mansfield, C. M., Dwyer, S. J., Cox, H. L., III, Levine, E., Templeton, A. W.: CT for intracavitary radiotherapy planning. A.J.R. 135:809-813, 1980.
26. Male, R. S., Rideout, D. F., Bronskill, M. J.: Evaluation of computerized tomography in oncology. J. Can. Assoc. Radiol. 31:246-250, 1980.
27. Mohan, R., Chui, C., Miller, D., Laughlin, J. S.: Use of computed tomography dose calculations for radiation therapy treatment planning. CT 5:273-282, 1981.
28. Munzenrider, J. E., Pilepich, M., Rene-Ferrero, J. B., Tchakarova, I., Carter, B. L.: Use of body scanner in radiotherapy treatment plan-

ning. *Cancer* 40:170–179, 1977.

29. *NCRP Report No. 69*, Dosimetry of X-ray and Gamma-ray beams for radiation therapy in the energy range 10 keV to 50 MeV. Washington, DC, 1981, pp. 1.

30. Pilepich, M. V., Rene, J. B., Munzenrider, J. E., Piro, A. J.: Value of computed tomography in radiotherapy of lung cancer. *A.J.R.* 131:63–73, 1978.

31. Prased, S. C., Pilepich, M. V., Perez, C. A.: Contribution of CT to quantitative radiation therapy planning. *A.J.R.* 136:123–128, 1981.

32. Proceedings of the Workshop on Patterns of Failure After Cancer Treatment. *Cancer Treatment Symposia* 2, NIH Publication No. 83-2488, Washington, DC, U.S. Government Printing Office, 1983.

33. Ragan, D. P., Perez, C. A.: Efficacy of CT-assisted two-dimensional treatment plannings: Analysis of 45 patients. *A.J.R.* 131:75–79, 1978.

34. Rockoff, S. D.: The evolving role of computerized tomography radiation oncology. *Cancer* 39(2 suppl.):694–696, 1977.

35. Schlager, B., Asbell, S. O., Baker, A. S., Sklaroff, D. M., Seydel, H. G., Ostrum, B. J.: The use of computerized tomography scanning in treatment planning for bladder carcinoma. *Int. J. Radiat. Oncol. Biol. Phys.* 5:99–103, 1979.

36. Seydel, H. G., Kutcher, G. J., Steiner, R. M., Mohiuddin, M., Goldberg, B.: Computed tomography in planning radiation therapy for bronchogenic carcinoma. *Int. J. Radiat. Oncol. Biol. Phys.* 6:601–606, 1980.

37. Sternick, E. S.: Treatment aim and degree of accuracy required. In *Advances in Radiation Therapy Treatment Planning*. Wright, A. E., Rager, A. L. (Eds.), Med. Physics Monograph 9:11–15. New York, American Institute of Physics, Inc., 1983.

38. Tsuji, H., Bagshaw, M. A., Smith, A. R., von Essen, C. F., Mettler, F. A., Kligerman, M. M.: Localization of structures for pion radiotherapy by computerized tomography and orthodiagraphic projection. *Int. J. Radiat. Oncol. Biol. Phys.* 6:319–325, 1980.

39. Van Dyk, J., Battista, J. J., Cunningham, J. R., Rider, W. D., Sontag, M. R.: On the impact of CT scanning on radiotherapy planning. *Comput. Tomogr.* 1:55–65, 1980.

40. Van Houtte, P., Piron, A., Lustman-Marécahl, J., Osteaux, M., Henry, J.: Computed axial tomography (CAT) contribution for dosimetry and treatment evaluation in lung cancer. *Int. J. Radiat. Oncol. Biol. Phys.* 6:995–1000, 1980.

41. Yu, W. S., Sagerman, R. H., King, G. A., Chung, C. T., Yu, Y. W.: The value of computed tomography in the management of bladder cancer. *Int. J. Radiat. Oncol. Biol. Phys.* 5:135–142, 1979.

Additional Suggested Readings

Husband, J. E., Hobday, P. A. (Eds.): *Computerized Axial Tomography in Oncology*. London, Churchill Livingstone, 1981.

Ling, C. C., Rogers, C. C., Morton, R. J. (Eds.): *Computed Tomography in Radiation Therapy*. New York, Raven Press, 1983.

26 CONTRIBUTIONS OF INTERVENTIONAL RADIOLOGY TO DIAGNOSIS AND MANAGEMENT OF THE CANCER PATIENT

Sidney Wallace
C. Humberto Carrasco
Chusilp Charnsangavej
Jesus Zornoza
Vincent P. Chuang

Interventional radiology incorporates techniques already employed by diagnostic radiologists into a more aggressive and invasive approach to diagnosis and patient management. Percutaneous biopsies and drainage procedures became the province of the radiologist when the equipment (fluoroscopic image intensification, ultrasonography, and computed tomography) allowed precise localization and ready access to the disease process. This dramatically increased the radiologist's ability to establish the nature and extent of disease while decreasing risk and expense to the patient. Vascular occlusions, infusions, and dilatations are now percutaneous techniques adapted from established surgical procedures. These interventional radiologic techniques are particularly applicable to the diagnosis and management of cancer patients.[147]

To increase the yield of such investigation it is necessary to be familiar with the natural history of the specific disease in order to localize the most likely sites of involvement. A knowledge of the therapeutic alternatives may aid in selecting the method and depth of the search to determine the extent of disease.

In the performance of these invasive procedures, the radiologist must be aware of possible complications and must be prepared to handle acute problems. Consultative support must be available to manage other complications and side effects. This support is as essential to the radiologist as it is to all other physicians who require assistance with problems outside their immediate realm.

Our medical and surgical colleagues must realize that these interventional procedures are capable not only of great rewards but also of risks and complications. Once the radiologist participates in these procedures, he or she immediately shares responsibility with other clinicians in the medical, moral, and legal aspects. The radiologist must assess the costs to the patient as well as to himself or herself. Many intravascular and biopsy techniques increase radiation exposure, which is always an important consideration in exploring patients with overwhelming disease. The hoped-for remission, perhaps of only a few weeks' duration, should be weighed against the risk of accumulated radiation exposure.[148]

Essential to interventional radiology is the availability of research facilities to ensure that these techniques have sound experimental basis. Our laboratory was established for problem solving and as a place where difficulties in the clinical setting are defined, interpreted, and investigated. The solutions found are then translated into patient care.

The interventional radiologic techniques used in the diagnosis and management of patients with cancer are listed in Table 26-1.

PERCUTANEOUS BIOPSY TECHNIQUES

Over 750 percutaneous biopsies are performed each year by the radiologists at The University of Texas M. D. Anderson Hospital and Tumor Institute.[160] In most of these procedures, the primary objective is to establish a diagnosis and to initiate therapy, thereby obviating the need for surgical intervention. An interested cytologist

Table 26-1. Interventional Radiology in Cancer Patients

Percutaneous Biopsy
  Chest
    Lung
    Cardiac, transvascular
    Pleura
    Mediastinum
  Abdomen
    Intra-abdominal masses
    Liver: Transabdominal, transjugular
    Retroperitoneal masses
    Pancreas
    Lymph Nodes
    Kidney
    Adrenal
  Musculoskeletal
    Appendicular skeleton
    Axial skeleton
    Soft tissue masses
  Miscellaneous
    Thyroid
    Breast
    Orbital
    Cranial
Aspiration and Drainage Procedures
  Abscesses
    Lung
    Liver
    Abdominal—Subdiaphragmatic, subhepatic, pelvic
    Retroperitoneal
  Cysts
    Renal
    Hepatic
    Pancreatic pseudocyst
    Breast
    Thyroid
  Biliary Tract Drainage
  Nephrostomy
Others
  Stone Extraction
    Urinary
    Biliary
  Foreign body extraction
    Intravascular
    Urinary
    Biliary
Intracavitary Therapy
  Cysts
    Renal
    Hepatic
    Bone, steroids
  Sclerosing agents—Pantopaque blood, alcohol, or sotradecol
  Eosinophilic granuloma of bone, steroids
  Abscesses, antibiotics
  Neoplasms, chemotherapy
Transcatheter Intra-Arterial Infusions and Occlusion
  Hepatic, primary and secondary neoplasms
  Kidney and adrenals
  Bladder
  Uterine cervix and corpus
  Ovary
  Colon
  Lymph nodes
  Lung
  Bones, Primary and Secondary Neoplasms
    a. Giant cell tumor and aneurysmal bone cyst
    b. Malignant neoplasms of bone
  Soft Tissue Sarcomas

is essential to a successful biopsy procedure. Percutaneous biopsies should be performed only if the results will influence management. If a patient is to be treated without regard for the biopsy results, the rewards do not justify the risks.

Employing radiographic, fluoroscopic, ultrasonic, and computed tomographic guidance, percutaneous biopsy procedures have obtained adequate tissue specimens for histologic and cytologic evaluation of lesions of the lungs, heart, mediastinum, thyroid, breast, liver, pancreas, kidneys, adrenals, lymph nodes, intra-abdominal and retroperitoneal masses, and bones. Percutaneous biopsies of the orbit and brain monitored by computed tomography have also been reported.[160]

Equipment

At our institution the majority of biopsies are performed under fluoroscopic guidance. Most contemporary fluoroscopic suites are equipped with image-intensifier television fluoroscopy, a spot film device, and a tilting table; these are adequate to perform almost every needle biopsy. Single-plane fluoroscopy is satisfactory for most procedures and is the preferred approach. However, simultaneous fluoroscopy in two planes at right angles, when available, may be more accurate in localizing the needle point.

Ultrasonography has been widely used to demonstrate space-occupying lesions and has proved very useful in guiding percutaneous biopsies.[74] To perform the biopsy while actually visualizing the target requires a transducer with a central canal through which to introduce the needle. This procedure can be performed with any commercially available ultrasonic unit. In cystic lesions, simultaneous real-time display of the puncture target and the needle can be achieved using a multielement transducer. Sterile lubricant and a sterile transducer are needed for the procedure.

The success of computed tomography is its ability to display clearly the exact location of the needle within the lesion.[64] At M. D. Anderson Hospital, a Siemens DR3 computed tomographic scanner is most often chosen for percutaneous biopsy procedures because of the larger aperture of the gantry and instantaneous reconstruction of the image. A skin grid marker system facilitates the localization within millimeters of the needle puncture site relative to the tumor to be biopsied.[67] A control scan with a skin grid marker system in place determines the puncture site on the X axis. For accurate needle placement, the image correction factor for the computed tomographic unit can be applied. The disadvantages of computed tomographic guided biopsies are high unit cost, relatively high radiation dose, and the length of time needed to perform the procedure.

Simpler techniques such as fluoroscopy and ultrasonography are preferred when feasible; however, computed tomography provides more precise guidance for localization of small lesions and those deeply located in the liver or retroperitoneal space. With computed tomography, larger needles can be used because of the increased accuracy of CT in localizing a needle within a lesion.

Needles

The types of needles available for percutaneous biopsies include aspiration, cutting, screw type, and trephine drill needles (Figure 26-1); all are designed to provide optimal diagnostic results with minimal patient risk. The development of reliable cytologic techniques has permitted aspiration biopsy by a fine-caliber spinal-type flexible steel needle. The most frequently used needles are 18 to 23 gauge, 10 to 20 cm long with a 20° to 30° sharp-edged bevel (Cook, Inc., Bloomington, Ind.; Johannah Medical Services, Inc., Minneapolis, Minn.). Finer gauge (i.e., 22 and 23) needles are at times difficult to control because of their flexibility and may not be the best choice for biopsy. More frequently, 18 to 21 gauge needles are used.

The combination of aspiration and cutting actions in a single needle (Unique Industries, Memphis, Tenn.) is effective in collecting specimens for both cytologic and histologic examinations. Tissue cores and fragments for histologic study can be obtained with a modified Franseen cutting and aspiration needle (Cook, Inc., Bloomington, Ind.), which is an 18-gauge needle with a saw-toothed tip.[65] The Rotex biopsy instrument (Ursus Konsult AB, Stockholm, Sweden) described by Nordenström[106] is a screw-tip needle inserted through a 0.8 mm steel cannula. The Tru-Cut needle (Travenol Laboratories, Inc., Deerfield, Ill.) is available in 6-inch or 8-inch lengths, 14 gauge, with a bayonet tip and sliding shaft for the cutting edge. Trephine drill needles have also been used to advantage.[103] A Teflon sheath, through which an aspiration or cutting needle is introduced, permits multiple biopsies while the sheath remains in place and the use, at times, of a plug (Gelfoam) to occlude the tract on removal.

Needles can be fitted to different types of syringes for aspiration. Routinely, a disposable 12-mL plastic syringe is employed. Several other instruments, such as the Franzen syringe (KIFA, Solna, Sweden) or the Cameco holder (Cameco, Enebyberg, Sweden), have special handles for a one-handed grip during biopsy.

Medication

Biopsies are performed on outpatients as well as inpatients, and no fasting is usually required. Premedication and anesthesia are rarely required, except for pediatric patients. In anxious adult patients, diazepam (Valium) is given intramuscularly or, preferably, intravenously (5 to 10 mg). Meperidine hydrochloride (Demerol) is added intravenously in 25-mg increments before and during the procedure, not to exceed a total dose of 150 mg.

General Technique

The biopsy site is prepared and draped. The skin and subcutaneous tissues are anesthetized with 1% to 2% Xylocaine. A small incision is made in the skin and subcutaneous tissue with a No. 11 scalpel blade to facilitate the needle advancement by reducing skin friction. The incision also permits transmission of variations in tissue consistency to the operator's fingers without interference from adjacent skin.

Once the lesion has been impaled, accurate placement can be verified under fluoroscopic control by small movements of the needle; these should be accompanied by synchronous movements of the lesion. Biplane fluoroscopy can be helpful. It may be necessary to rotate the patient into an oblique or lateral position to confirm the depth of the needle tip relative to the lesion. A cross-table roentgenogram of the biopsy site can further localize the needle tip.

In biopsy of a large tumor, the sample should be obtained from the periphery; samples from the center often yield debris and necrotic material. Cavitary lesions should be biopsied at the outer and inner margins. If the lesion is malignant, then the specimen obtained from the interior wall usually will contain necrotic material. Tissue from the outer margin is more likely to provide reliable diagnostic material. The reverse prevails in biopsy of an inflammatory lesion. Inflammatory cavities can be injected with sterile saline solution without preservative, which is then immediately aspirated for bacteriologic examination.

When the needle tip has reached the desired location, imaging is discontinued. The needle is rotated several times in both directions on its longitudinal axis to detach cellular elements. While the patient holds his or her breath, the stylet is removed and a disposable 12-mL plastic syringe is attached to the hub. Constant suction is applied to the syringe with one hand, while the needle is advanced with a to-and-fro motion. The needle and syringe are rotated again and the negative pressure is allowed to equalize slowly to prevent ejection of aspiration material from the lumen. The patient then suspends respiration while the syringe and needle are removed as a unit.

The specimen is blown out of the needle onto a ground glass slide or into a preservative. The slide is immediately stained and evaluated by an experienced cytologist. Once a diagnosis is established, no further attempts are made. The procedure can be repeated several (two to three) times until a good specimen is obtained. After the pro-

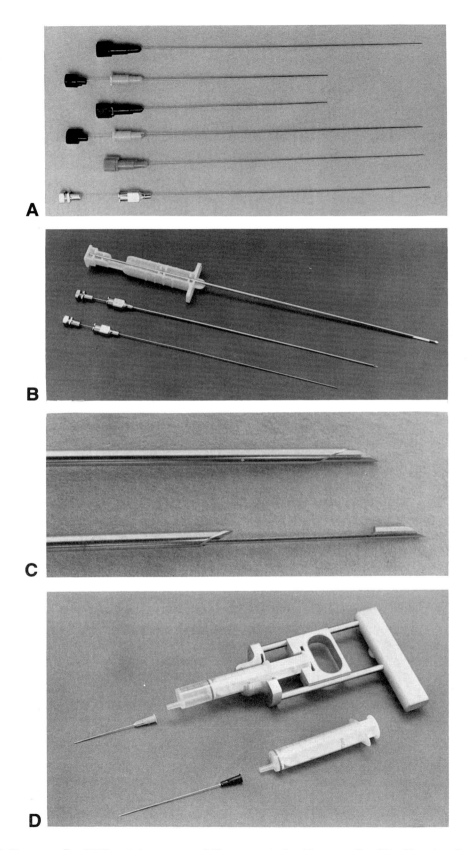

FIG. 26-1. Biopsy needles. (A) Twenty-two-gauge and 23-gauge aspiration biopsy needles, 15-to-20-cm lengths. (B) Eighteen-gauge and 20-gauge aspiration biopsy needles compared with a 14-gauge Vim Tru Cut cutting needle. (C) The cutting mechanism of a Vim Tru Cut cutting needle in the open and closed positions. (D) The handle used for needle aspiration biopsy.

cedure a sterile dressing (Band-Aid) is applied over the puncture site.

Lung. Percutaneous needle biopsy of the lungs and endobronchial brush biopsies are established radiologic procedures.[46,160,162] The success and complications depend on the nature, size, and location of the process, the status of the patient and the lungs, and the experience, competence, and confidence of both the radiologist and the cytologist (Figure 26-2).

Technique. Available chest roentgenograms locate the lesion and aid in determining the approach. A comparison

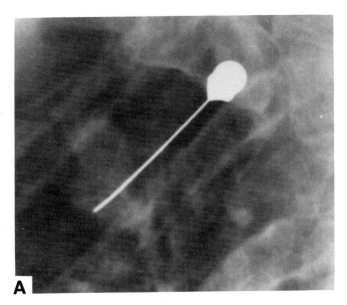

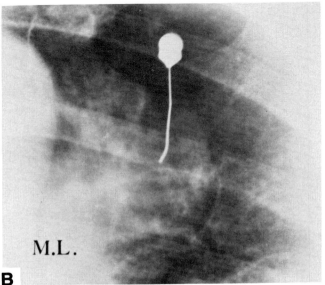

FIG. 26-2. Lung and mediastinal aspiration biopsy. (A) Biopsy of a squamous cell carcinoma of the lung. (B) Percutaneous needle biopsy of a left anterior mediastinal mass revealed a thyroma.

of the relative magnification of the chest roentgenogram to the actual chest measurements indicates the depth at the center of the lesion. The patient is placed horizontally on the fluoroscopic table and the lesion is localized. The chest wall closest to the lesion is selected for insertion of the needle, and the patient is positioned supine for an anterior approach and prone for a posterior approach. If multiple pulmonary lesions are present, the most peripheral and accessible is biopsied. Under fluoroscopic monitoring, a metallic pointer or a hemostat tip is used to localize the lesion and mark the entry site on the chest wall. The patient is allowed to breathe normally during localization. The biopsy needle should be introduced close to the upper edge of the rib to avoid intercostal vessels.

The biopsy needle is inserted into the chest wall, the parietal and visceral pleura, and the lung parenchyma. The patient is allowed to breathe normally during introduction of the needle. Holding the needle with a hemostat under fluoroscopy permits verification of position and avoids irradiation of the hand. Under intermittent fluoroscopy the needle is advanced toward the periphery of the lesion. The patient is asked to suspend respiration during attempted entry into the lesion to avoid movement of the lesion.

Often, when the needle reaches the pulmonary lesion, an increased resistance is felt. Solid neoplastic lesions offer a gritty sensation upon penetration. Benign lesions such as tuberculosis and other granulomas are difficult to impale and may slide to one side when the needle reaches the surface. On such occasions, a sharp thrust of the needle may achieve penetration. Movement of the needle accompanied by synchronous movements of the lesion establish needle position within the lesion. Lesions at the hilum and apex are generally fixed and cannot be checked in this fashion. Lesions at the lateral chest wall near the diaphragm usually are difficult to view in profile and may defy verification of accurate needle placement. Diffuse, tiny nodular lesions and lymphangitic carcinomas have been blindly biopsied when a definite nodular lesion could not be identified fluoroscopically.

Indications. Percutaneous needle biopsy should be performed only in those cases in which simpler tests have failed to provide a diagnosis.[160,162] These include the following: (1) a lung mass, most likely a primary malignancy, that is not suitable for thoracotomy as primary therapy (if a thoracotomy is to be performed anyway, a percutaneous biopsy is needless); (2) obvious metastatic disease of unknown origin; (3) multiple primary tumors; (4) a new lung lesion in a patient in remission with a known treated primary neoplasm; (5) culture and chemotherapy sensitivity testing requiring specimens of viable tumor cells; (6) Pancoast's tumors; (7) an indeterminate solitary pulmonary nodule; (8) patients with diminished immunologic competence related to both disease and drug therapy; and (9) diffuse interstitial pulmonary disease.

Contraindications. Only relative contraindications to transthoracic needle biopsy exist if histologic proof is necessary for proper treatment. Patient cooperation is essential for a safe procedure. Dyspnea, abnormal coagulation studies, pulmonary hypertension, emphysema, and contralateral pneumonectomy must be weighed against the potential benefit from the procedure. No biopsy is performed when the platelet count is below 20,000. If biopsy is essential for patient management, platelet transfusions are given immediately before biopsy to increase the platelet count to at least 50,000 to 100,000 and the transfusion is continued throughout the procedure.

Location seldom poses a serious problem with fine-gauge needles. Transthoracic needle biopsy is fraught with great risk in patients with an uncontrollable cough. Aspiration biopsy for diagnosis of centrally located lesions risks trauma to vascular structures. The inadvertent placement of a needle into the aorta, a pulmonary vein or artery, the heart, or the mediastinum has not been a significant problem. If blood is aspirated, the needle is withdrawn and redirected. Cutting or drill biopsy needles increase the hazard of vascular laceration. Cutting needle biopsies are now usually reserved for chest wall lesions (Figure 26-3).

Results. At M. D. Anderson Hospital, 425 aspiration lung biopsies[160] were performed during a three-year period (1976 to 1979). A single puncture yielded sufficient cytologic material in 73% of patients. Two passes were required in 25% of the patients and three or more in the remainder. The material obtained was diagnostic in 85% of aspiration lung biopsies. In 3.5%, subsequent open biopsies demonstrated neoplastic tumor; failure to obtain diagnostic material occurred in 11.4%.

An overall success rate of 80% with aspiration lung biopsy has been reported.[160] Of 400 biopsies performed on discrete lung lesions, 88.5% yielded a correct diagnosis.[160] A cytologic diagnosis was established in only 7 of 25 biopsies (28%) in diffuse pulmonary disease.

Complications. Pneumothorax, the principal complication of transthoracic needle biopsy, occurred in 115 (27%) of 425 patients.[160,162] A small pneumothorax resolved spontaneously in 94 patients (22%). Only 5% were symptomatic and required closed intercostal drainage. The incidence of pneumothorax was greater in patients with diffuse pulmonary lesions (35%) than in those with discrete lesions. The incidence was dependent upon the status of the patient's lungs, the patient's ability to cooperate, the site of the lesion, the number of punctures, the expertise of the operator, and the cytologist. Our incidence compares well with other series, 6% to 57%.[160]

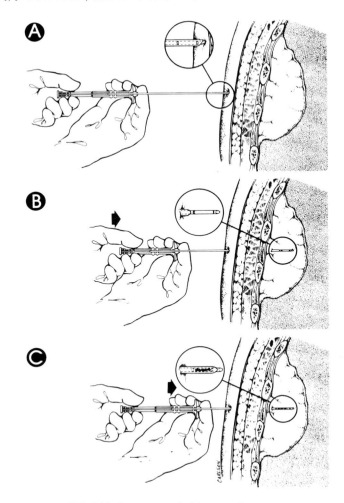

FIG. 26-3. Cutting needle biopsy technique.

In our institution, the patient remains hospitalized for 24 hours and chest roentgenograms are taken during expiration immediately after the procedure and just before discharge.

A simple catheter technique is used to treat any pneumothorax requiring prompt relief. A 14-inch, 9F Teflon catheter (Cook, Inc., Bloomington, Ind.) with multiple side holes near the tip and a No. 18 needle cannula are inserted into the second anterior intercostal space at the midclavicular line. Once in the pleural cavity, the catheter is advanced over the cannula and the catheter tip is positioned near the lung apex. A three-way stopcock is attached to the catheter hub and manual aspiration of pleural air is performed. A Heimlich valve[10] allowing one-way air flow or an Emerson pump is attached to the stopcock. The catheter is withdrawn 24 to 48 hours after complete lung re-expansion.

Hemoptysis occurred in 3% of patients in our series and was mild, requiring no treatment. Occasionally, bleeding was noted as a haziness around the lesion. Only two cases of fatal intrathoracic hemorrhage after aspiration biopsy have been documented.[72,96,117,125,129,130,154] The incidence of severe hemorrhage increases with the use of cutting and trephine needles, and several cases of fatal pulmonary bleeding have been reported.[96,117]

The incidence of inflammatory complications, i.e., emphysema, abscess, etc., is low, and the danger is more theoretical than actual.[125] The implantation of tumor cells in the needle track is also very rare; Sinner and Zajicek reported one episode in 2,700 aspiration biopsies.[130] No instance of cancer dissemination was encountered in our series. The reported fatal complications have occurred almost exclusively with cutting and trephine needles. Nearly all fatalities with cutting needles were associated with sudden massive pulmonary hemorrhage. Herman and Hessel[72] reported a 0.1% death rate in 1,562 patients undergoing aspiration lung biopsy. Of the five documented cases of death related to aspiration, two resulted from massive pulmonary hemorrhage, one from embolism, one from tension pneumothorax, and one from an unknown cause, probably air embolism.[154] The mortality rate in our lung aspiration biopsy series is zero.

Heart. The technique of transvascular endomyocardial biopsy was pioneered in Japan in the 1960s by Sakakibara and Konno,[126] and modified by the Stanford group in California. It has been extensively used to detect rejection in cardiac transplant patients.[93] Virtually all of the 1,000 cardiac biopsies performed at M. D. Anderson Hospital and Tumor Institute have been done to detect and evaluate Adriamycin cardiotoxicity.[87,91] This approach allows closer monitoring and increased use of this very effective chemotherapeutic agent. Consequently, more individualization has occurred, and it has been possible to increase total dosage to as much as three to four times that ordinarily prescribed.[45]

Technique. Conventional fluoroscopic equipment is adequate for the performance of a cardiac biopsy. A "C"-arm or biplane fluoroscope might be preferable to develop the skill necessary for positioning the bioptome.

A physiologic monitor capable of displaying and recording electrocardiographic patterns and intracardiac pressures is needed. A pericardiocentesis tray and apparatus for cardioversion and cardiopulmonary resuscitation should be available.

Cardiac biopsy specimens are obtained from the right ventricular septum at the apex usually via the right internal jugular vein but occasionally via the femoral vein. On occasion, the left ventricular septum is subjected to a biopsy via a femoral artery puncture.[93]

The internal jugular vein may be entered at the angle of the triangle formed by the two heads of the sternocleidomastoid muscle. It may also be approached higher in the neck along the medial aspect of the sternocleidomastoid muscle just below the angle of the mandible.

An intravenous infusion of 5% glucose in water is started, and most patients are premedicated with 5 mg of diazepam (Valium) administered intravenously. After the patient is prepared and draped, the bioptome insertion site is anesthetized with 1% lidocaine and a 22-gauge needle is advanced as a guide into the jugular vein. The Trendelenberg position or the Valsalva's maneuver may facilitate venous entry. Once the depth and direction of the guide needle are determined, a small skin incision with a scalpel is made adjacent to the needle. An 18-gauge thin-walled needle is then inserted into the vein and a guide wire, vessel dilator, and sheath are inserted in the usual manner. The 9F sheath remains in the vessel after removal of the guide wire and dilator.

The bioptomes are 50 cm long and are considerably stiffer than the usual cardiac catheter (Figure 26-4A). The biting jaw just fits through the 9F sheath modified by a rubber seal over the connector to prevent air from entering the venous system and to reduce bleeding in patients with elevated venous pressure.[93] The biting jaw of the bioptome can be directed from the handle, and the instrument is so designed that the finger holes in the handle always point in the direction of the jaw. The bioptome is passed through the sheath under fluoroscopic guidance with the jaw closed and pointing toward the right side. As the jaw passes into the right atrium, the handle is rotated anteriorly so that the jaw traverses the tricuspid valve more laterally. The bioptome is then turned posteriorly toward the septum and advanced to the apex of the right ventricle. The instrument actually makes an arc of 270° as it passes from the right atrium to the apex of the heart. As the jaw enters the right ventricle, frequent premature ventricular contractions are often noted, and short runs of ventricular tachycardia are not uncommon. These ectopic beats are an important part of the procedure because they confirm that the bioptome is in the right ventricle (Figure 26-4B–D). The instrument is pulled back slightly, the jaws opened, the bioptome advanced, and the jaws briskly closed. The bioptome is then removed through the sheath and the specimen is carefully removed from the opened jaws and immediately placed in 5% buffered glutaraldehyde solution for fixation. Three specimens, 2 to 3 mm in maximum dimension, are usually taken. Right heart pressures can be measured by a catheter introduced through the same sheath.

Patients undergoing cardiac biopsy describe very little discomfort or no unusual sensation at the moment of tissue removal. Cardiac biopsy procedures require 15 to 45 minutes and are usually performed on an outpatient basis. The patients are then observed in a holding area for two hours and the vital signs are monitored.

Complications. Cardiac tamponade is the primary complication associated with transjugular endomyocardial biopsy. Of over 1,000 cardiac biopsies performed in our unit, there were 10 (1%) instances of tamponade com-

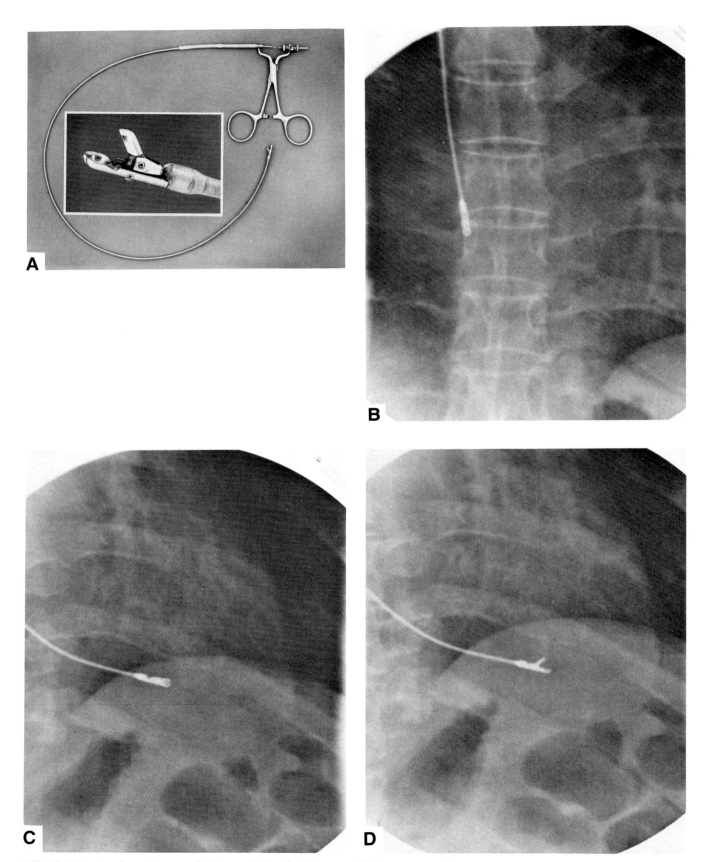

FIG. 26-4. Transjugular endomyocardial biopsy. (A) Stanford bioptome; (B) Bioptome in right atrium; (C) Bioptome in right ventricle; (D) Biopsy of the right ventricle at septum.

pared with 0.05% reported by Mason et al.[93] Minor problems related either to local anesthesia, needle puncture, or cannulation of the internal jugular vein have included local hematomas, temporary hoarseness from transient paralysis of the right recurrent laryngeal nerve, pneumothorax, and right arm pain. Rarer complications as a result of mechanical irritation or tissue removal include atrial or ventricular arrhythmia and pericarditis, which has responded to an anti-inflammatory agent, indomethacin (Indocin). No deaths have occurred from the procedure in either our series or the larger Stanford study.

Abdomen. Once the appropriate radiologic examination (conventional radiography, fluoroscopy, ultrasonography, computed tomography, angiography, etc.) has been performed to localize the lesion to be biopsied, the patient is placed on the examining table for the procedure. A transabdominal approach is used for most abdominal biopsies and only in those cases in which paravertebral, adrenal, and renal masses or the spine are to be biopsied is the posterior approach used. An anterior approach is more suitable for lesions of the pancreas and lymph nodes, which are organs that are closer to the anterior abdominal wall and can be reached without bony interference.

The patient is prepared, draped, and anesthetized locally. A small incision is made and the entry site is dilated with a hemostat. The needle is introduced perpendicular to the lesion through the anterior abdominal wall. Minimal deviation from the desired vertical course ultimately will misplace the needle, which cannot be realigned by bending the hub portion of the needle. In an obese patient or a patient with a muscular anterior abdominal wall, a thin-walled 18-gauge needle can be used to stabilize the inner 23-gauge needle, although a 20-gauge or 21-gauge needle allows better control. The position of the needle should be checked fluoroscopically after each advancement in small increments. If a 15-cm or 20-cm needle is used, it is recommended that one hand advance the needle while the other stabilizes it at the skin. Manual control of the needle is preferable to use of rubber-tipped hemostats for stability.

When the abdominal cavity has been entered, no resistance will be met until the needle tip reaches the posterior parietal peritoneum. At this time, the patient may experience pain, which can be alleviated by the injection of a small amount of Xylocaine. Small-gauge needles tend to bend at this point if they are advanced with a quick motion. Slight continuous pressure allows easier passage of the needle through the anterior retroperitoneal fascia. Because it is difficult for a patient to achieve a consistent degree of respiration and any abrupt movement is undesirable while the needle is in the abdominal cavity, the patient is allowed to breathe normally during the procedure.

Often, increased resistance to the needle indicates that the mass has been reached. The desired point to be biopsied is verified by oblique projections when fluoroscopy is used. Precise localization under CT guidance can be facilitated by injecting a small amount of contrast material during the biopsy procedure.[64,135] When biopsy of a solid lesion is performed under ultrasonographic control with a small-gauge needle, it may not be possible to verify position.[74] At the time the specimen is collected, the needle is rotated clockwise and counterclockwise along the longitudinal axis to detach cellular material. Suction is applied with a 12-mL plastic syringe attached to the hub, while the needle is gently moved up and down several times with an approximate 1-cm excursion. When the aspiration is complete, suction is relieved and the pressure is allowed to equalize before the needle is withdrawn from the lesion. This maneuver retains the tissue in the needle, from which it can be ejected onto glass slides or into a container of preservative. The procedure is repeated, if necessary, two to three times to obtain sufficient cytologic material as determined immediately after each aspiration by the cytologist present in the operating room. After biopsy, patients are observed for two to three hours in the radiology department.

Pancreas

Technique. The same radiologic examinations used to identify pancreatic masses can also be used to localize the biopsy site and the approach through the anterior abdominal wall. In biopsies performed under fluoroscopic control, barium in the duodenal loop or contrast medium in the common duct from a transhepatic cholangiogram or in the pancreatic duct after endoscopic cannulation is very useful in locating the lesion.

When angiography is used for localization, the biopsy can be performed with the catheter still in place. The catheter is advanced as close to the lesion as possible and thus marks the pancreas.[60] The pancreatic lesion can be identified with small injections of contrast material through the catheter. On other occasions, the spine can be used as a landmark. If fluoroscopy is used for guidance and biplane fluoroscopy is not available, ultrasonography can provide additional information regarding the depth of the lesion. Most often, however, the tumor is localized by the resistance offered to the needle as it penetrates the mass.

Ultrasonography[74] and computed tomography[64] are most often used to biopsy the pancreas. Abdominal ultrasound scanning can outline the mass, and its depth can be measured from the A mode display.[69,131] The puncture is performed with a special ultrasonic transducer that has a central canal through and directed along the path of the sound beam (Figure 26-5).

Computed tomography provides very precise biopsy localization, especially in small pancreatic lesions.[48,64]

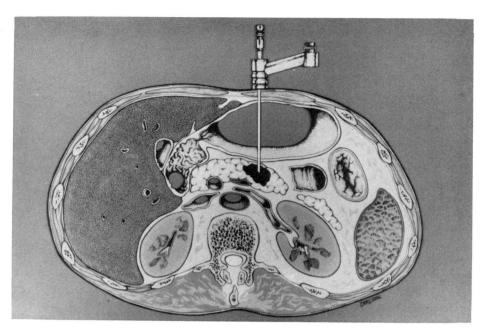

FIG. 26-5. Pancreatic biopsy—percutaneous transabdominal approach. The ultrasonic transducer was used for localization and biopsy. Note that the stomach is traversed.

Despite their excellent image resolution and three-dimensional visualization, CT biopsies are time consuming and expensive. However, CT is still preferred for small lesions and for those patients in whom other methods have failed.

In scirrhous pancreatic carcinomas, a hard gritty sensation can be felt as the needle enters the mass. Because these tumors have a large connective tissue component, it is sometimes difficult to retrieve enough material. In such cases, a larger needle (18 or 20 gauge) can obtain an adequate specimen.

Indications. Percutaneous biopsy is indicated for patients with neoplasms of the body and tail of the pancreas with clinical or radiologic evidence of unresectability, such as involvement of the liver, major extra-pancreatic vessels, or the mesenteric root. In patients who have undergone a bypass procedure in which operative biopsy was either not performed or inadequate, percutaneous biopsy prevents a second laparotomy and permits treatment by chemotherapy or irradiation. In patients with biliary obstruction, although preoperative diagnosis is not essential, it shortens operating time by avoiding frozen sections and obviates the risk of intraoperative biopsy. Bypass surgery can be avoided by permanent percutaneous biliary drainage to relieve obstruction.

Results. The combined results of percutaneous biopsies reported for 227 patients with proven malignant disease was 71%.[160] In 80 biopsies performed at our institution an overall success rate of 74% was obtained. Failure sometimes occurred in biopsy of large tumors because of associated inflammation or necrosis or both. No complications related to the procedure were encountered.

Liver

Technique. Localization of liver masses can be performed using angiography, ultrasonography, scintigraphy, and computed tomography. Fluoroscopic guidance can be used when localization is established by angiography.

With a cystic lesion, ultrasonography is the most useful method for guidance because the needle can be visualized entering the mass.[74] With small lesions or with lesions in the posterior segment of the right lobe, computed tomography provides more precise guidance[64] (Figure 26-6).

The needle should be introduced at the shortest distance from the mass perpendicularly, as long as precautions are taken to avoid other vital organs.

Conventional transabdominal liver biopsy, usually performed with a Menghini or Vim Silverman needle, is a well-established diagnostic procedure best suited for investigation of diffuse parenchymal liver disease. In focal malignant disease, the accuracy of "blind" liver biopsy decreases. Results from different studies show a diagnostic yield of 50% to 71%; this procedure is usually performed without radiologic localization.[160] Haaga and Vanek[66] using computed tomography, reported a yield of 86%. Suspicion of hemangioma or hydatid cyst and the presence of obstructive jaundice contraindicate its use. Needle biopsy of the liver by the Menghini method carries a very low mortality but a somewhat higher rate of major complications. In a review of more than 20,000 cases, Zamcheck and Klausenstock[159] found an overall mortality of 0.194%; however, in their own series, there was a 17% incidence of significant complications (hypotension, hemorrhage, bile peritonitis, and gallbladder perforation). An 11% complication rate was reported using the Vim Silverman needle.

Indications. Fine-needle (22-gauge or 23-gauge) aspiration liver biopsy is a valuable tool in diagnosis of malignant hepatic disease, especially in patients in whom metastases are suspected and who, with radiologic localization, can be spared the risk of exploratory laparotomy plus the increased cost and delay of treatment.[164] Small-gauge needle aspiration liver biopsy is not intended to replace standard needle liver biopsy. Rather, this technique represents a further adjunct to liver biopsy that may obviate exploratory surgery. Basically, small-gauge needle aspiration should be performed in patients with: (1) lesions of the left lobe of the liver or in areas of the right lobe inaccessible to the Menghini needle; (2) ascites or cholestasis in whom standard needle biopsy is contraindicated because of the relative frequency of bile peritonitis; and (3) highly vascularized lesions. Other indications include acute hepatitis, cirrhosis, and metabolic abnormalities. However, such lesions are generally diffuse and do not require radiologic localization.

Results. Our overall success rate in 88 needle aspiration biopsies of hepatic masses under radiologic guidance was 77%.[160,164] False-positive results undoubtedly occur, but only a few have been reported. Little morbidity has been reported in several hundred aspiration liver biopsies.[164]

Transjugular liver biopsy. The transjugular liver biopsy approach has been suggested for special circumstances.[68,123] This technique is usually used for patients with hepatic masses and associated cirrhosis or jaundice. The biopsy of a hypervascular neoplasm, such an angiosarcoma, is performed with probably less morbidity and mortality through the transjugular approach. Although this technique is more elaborate, it is safer because of the reduced risk of hemoperitoneum and peritonitis. The transjugular approach is similar to that described for cardiac biopsy.

Lymph Nodes. The percutaneous approach to the para-aortic and pelvic lymph node using a fine-caliber needle (22 or 23 gauge) represents a simple technique to establish or confirm the presence of metastases.[61,160,163] The histologic verification of inoperability or recurrent retroperitoneal disease also can be established readily by this technique. In view of the position of the para-aortic and pelvic lymph nodes in relation to the great vessels and in consideration of the patient's comfort, an anterior transperitoneal approach is usually more suitable. Lymphangiographic opacification of lymph nodes allows fluoroscopic guidance for biopsy (Figure 26-7); otherwise, computed tomography is necessary (Figure 26-8).

The biopsy site of a previously opacified lymph node will differ depending upon the histologic type of neoplastic disease. The most common lymphangiographic finding seen in metastatic carcinoma is a defect in a node that is not traversed by lymphatics. The remaining normally functioning portion of the node frequently appears as a crescentic configuration representing a node partially replaced by a neoplasm. Consequently, the greatest yield would result from a biopsy of that part of the node adjacent to the crescent (Figure 26-7).

Once the needle reaches the lymph node, the patient is rotated slightly to both sides to determine the relative depth of the needle. When the node is punctured it will move in concert with the needle tip, indicating an accurate placement. Because the defects biopsied are usually between 1 and 2 cm, the needle should be moved very gently to detach material. The presence of oil droplets in the aspirate demonstrates that the node, previously opacified during lymphangiography, has been punctured.

Aspiration biopsy of a lymph node containing metastatic carcinoma is more successful (72%) than of those containing lymphomas (54%). Epithelial metastases, especially those originating in the pelvic viscera, are frequently highly cellular, poorly vascularized, and readily distinguishable from the normal cells of a lymph node.[160,161,163]

Percutaneous transperitoneal lymph node biopsy involves the passage of a needle into the peritoneal cavity, at times through solid and hollow viscera. The potential complications such as intra-abdominal bleeding, pancreatitis, and bowel perforation with peritonitis, were not encountered in this study. The possibility of disseminating a neoplasm by aspiration biopsy does not seem to present a significant problem.

Kidney. Percutaneous biopsy of the kidney has been used in the diagnosis of both benign and malignant disease[142] (Figure 26-8). Percutaneous puncture is especially advantageous in the diagnosis and management of patients with simple cysts of the kidney. Once a cystic lesion is established by nephrotomography, ultrasonography, computed tomography, or angiography, cyst puncture can be performed for verification or identification. Carbon dioxide and water-soluble contrast material are exchanged for the cyst fluid, which is then examined for cytologic and biochemical content. Thus, the nature of the cystic lesion is established. Our present policy is to obtain two diagnostic studies to confirm the diagnosis

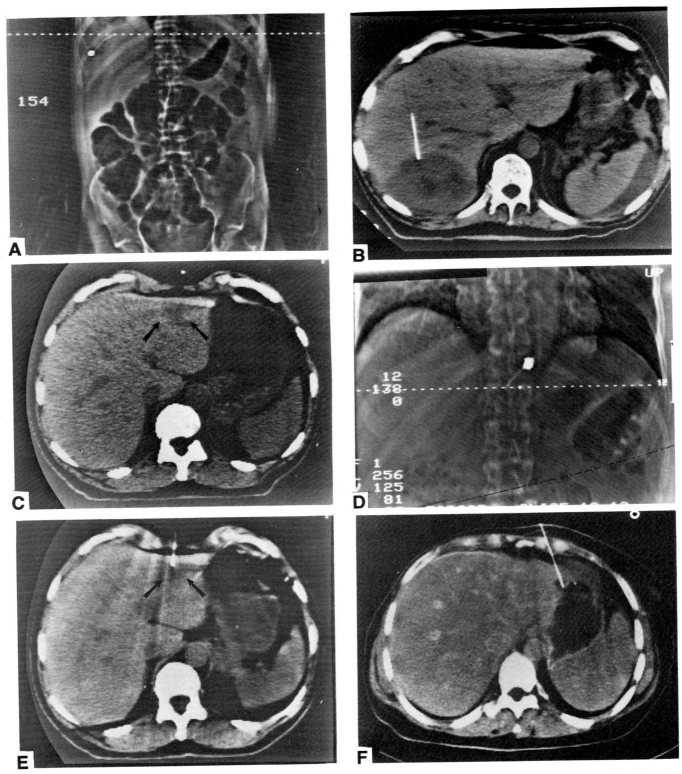

FIG. 26-6. Liver biopsy—percutaneous transabdominal approach. (A) Localization with CT. **(B)** The same patient as in A—needle biopsy of a metastatic colon carcinoma. **(C)** This patient with a carcinoma of the colon was found to have an area of low attenuation in the left lateral segment of the liver. **(D)** The same patient as in C—a topogram localized the lesion and the needle. **(E)** The same patient as in C— metastatic colonic carcinoma was diagnosed by aspiration biopsy. **(F)** Another patient with a known breast carcinoma had a single lesion of the left lateral segment of the liver and an attenuation coefficient of 20 Hounsfield units. **(G)** The same patient as in F—aspiration biopsy revealed a simple cyst.

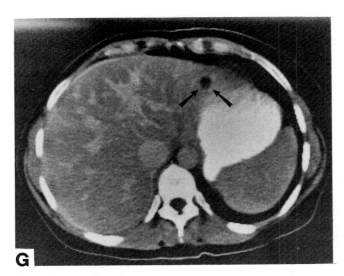

Figure 26-6, continued.

of a cyst. Puncture is reserved for those situations in which there is confusion over diagnosis.

Adrenal Glands. Percutaneous needle aspiration biopsy was performed on 22 patients at M. D. Anderson Hospital for cytologic evaluation of adrenal masses that were symptomatic at initial examination or were discovered incidentally during routine radiologic surveys for metastatic disease.[80] Needle aspiration of adrenal masses was via a posterior or anterior approach guided by fluoroscopy, ultrasonography, and, especially, computed tomography, using 18-gauge to 22-gauge spinal-type needles. In 10 cases, biopsy specimens for histologic examination were also obtained using cutting-type needles. Electron microscopy was performed on specimens obtained with either percutaneous needle aspiration or cutting needles.

Of the 22 patients with adrenal lesions, nine were demonstrated to have benign lesions, which included five benign adrenal cysts, one adrenal myelolipoma, one nodular hyperplasia, and two adenomas (Figure 26-9). Thirteen of the adrenal masses proved to be malignant. There were six primary tumors of the adrenal gland, which included four adrenocortical carcinomas and two neuroblastomas. Three patients had metastatic tumors secondary to bronchogenic carcinomas. There were in

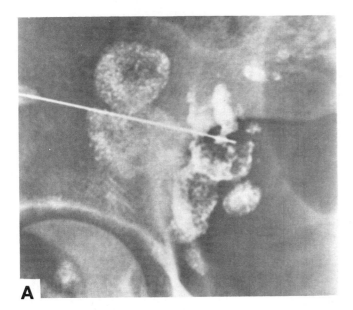

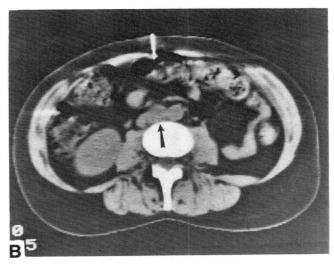

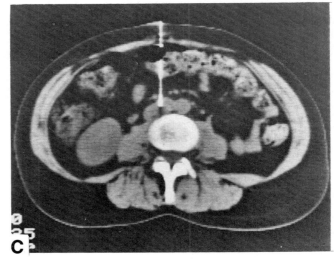

FIG. 26-7. Lymph node biopsy—percutaneous transabdominal approach. (A) Lymphangiographic opacification of a lymph node containing a metastasis from a carcinoma of the cervix. Needle aspiration was accomplished with fluoroscopic guidance. (B) Computed tomographic demonstration of an enlarged lymph node between the aorta and the inferior vena cava in a patient with an ovarian carcinoma. (C) Same patient as in B—biopsy was accomplished with CT guidance. Cytologic examination confirmed the presence of metastasis.

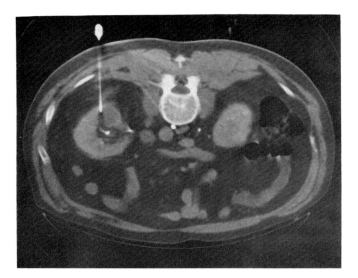

FIG. 26-8. CT-guided percutaneous renal biopsy in a patient with metastatic breast carcinoma.

addition four patients who had tumors of unknown origin who had metastatic disease to the adrenals.

The overall sensitivity of needle biopsy of the adrenal gland in detecting the presence of malignancy was 85%, while the number of patients correctly classified for all adrenal masses was 90%.

Other Abdominal and Paravertebral Masses. The technique employed is the same as that used for the pancreas and lymph nodes.[48,60,64,69,74,80,131,160,163] Abdominal masses usually are approached anteriorly, with the posterior approach preferred for paravertebral masses, renal, and adrenal masses. Localization has been performed using any or all of the radiographic methods available, with fluoroscopy and computed tomography the most frequently employed. Ultrasonography and, especially, computed tomography, are used primarily to localize small masses. The overall accuracy in 300 patients was 90%. No significant complications were encountered (Figure 26-10).

Bone. Direct visualization of the osseous lesion by fluoroscopy has made bone biopsy a safe and relatively simple procedure. Although this technique has been available for at least 50 years, only recently has the radiologist become involved.[33,37,160] The primary indications for bone biopsy in cancer patients are to establish the existence of widespread metastases, multiple myeloma, and lymphoma. With the advent of transcatheter intra-arterial infusion of osteosarcomas and arterial embolization for giant cell tumors, percutaneous biopsy of primary neoplasms has found considerable application.[5,38]

Equipment. A variety of needles is available for bone biopsy. The specific needle used depends upon the nature, consistency (osteoblastic, osteolytic, or mixed), and the site of the lesion (Figure 26-11). The Ackerman needle (Cook, Inc., Bloomington, Ind.) is a 12-gauge needle with a 13-gauge saw-toothed trocar to bore through an osteoblastic lesion or cortical bone. The Craig needle (Becton Dickinson) essentially is of the same construction except that it is of larger caliber (10 gauge). The saw-toothed trocar has a metallic handle that facilitates rotation necessary for the introduction of the needle. Because of its size it is seldom employed. The Vim Tru Cut needle (Travenol Laboratories, Deerfield, Ill.) is a 14-gauge needle with a bayonet configuration of the distal portion, which allows the sleeve to cut a 20 × 1 mm core of tissue. This needle is best suited for the biopsy of osteolytic or

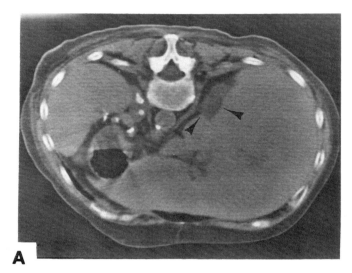

A

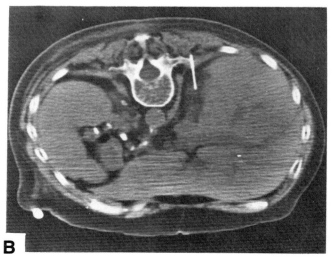

B

FIG. 26-9. (A) A right adrenal biopsy using CT guidance demonstrated an adrenal adenoma in this patient with breast carcinoma.

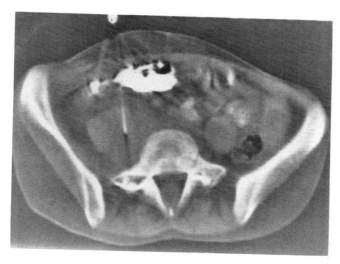

FIG. 26-10. CT-guided biopsy in a patient with recurrent uterine carcinoma.

mixed lesions or whenever the biopsy of a soft tissue component is also indicated. An orthopedic drill (5/64–3/32 inch) is at times employed to bore through the thick cortex to allow the Vim Tru Cut to sample the tumor in the medullary cavity. The Jamshidi needle (Kormed Co., Minneapolis, Minn.) is most frequently used for bone marrow biopsy but can be effective in obtaining a core biopsy of a flat bone or a relatively lytic lesion. Pediatric and adult sizes are available (11 and 12 gauge). Chiba or spinal type needles (Cook, Inc., Bloomington, Ind.) are 18 to 23 gauge thin-walled needles that can be used effectively in the biopsy of soft lesions or for obtaining cytologic material after the cortex has been perforated with any of the larger cutting needles or a drill.

Technique. With the exception of vertebral body biopsy, which is performed under general anesthesia or heavy sedation, the biopsies are usually performed as outpatient procedures. After location of the optimal point for biopsy, the patient is turned to the most advantageous position to obtain the shortest possible needle path and to prevent damage to underlying structures. The lesions of the anterior portions of the pelvis are biopsied with the patient supine, but lesions involving the ischia and posterior iliac crests are biopsied with the patient prone.

After positioning of the patient and localization of the lesion fluoroscopically, the overlying skin is prepared and the point of entry in the skin and subcutaneous tissues to the periosteum area is anesthetized with 2% Xylocaine. A small incision is made to facilitate passage of the needle. The needle is generally introduced in a trajectory perpendicular to the cortex of the bone to be biopsied while major vessels and structures are avoided. In the case of flat bones such as the scapula or ribs, an oblique approach is favored in order to obtain the maximum amount of bone and to avoid damage to the underlying structures.

When the lesion is dense radiographically or within the marrow cavity with an intact cortex, an Ackerman or Craig needle is used to obtain a core of bone. An orthopedic drill also facilitates passage of a spinal type needle or a Vim Tru Cut needle through the cortical defect into the marrow for aspiration. The biopsy of a lytic lesion or a soft tissue component is preferably performed with a Vim Tru Cut needle (Figures 26-12, 26-13). Thin needle aspiration with an 18 to 23 gauge needle is routinely performed for cytologic examination as well as culture and Gram stain studies when indicated.

The technique for percutaneous biopsy of a vertebral body varies depending on the particular anatomical location of the vertebra (Figure 26-14). For the purpose of biopsy, the cervical spine should be considered in two parts, the first three vertebral bodies and the last four bodies. For biopsy of the first three bodies, the anterior or "pharyngeal" approach is preferred (Figure 26-14A). The patient's mouth is kept open by means of a mouth opener and the nasal anesthesia tube is kept retracted to one side. A spinal needle (16 to 22 gauge) is introduced through the mouth and advanced into the vertebral body under careful fluoroscopic control. For biopsy of the lower cervical spine, either a lateral or an anterior approach may be used. To avoid damage to the carotid, thyroid, or vertebral arteries, the jugular veins, and the recurrent laryngeal nerves, the lateral approach is probably the best choice (Figure 26-14B). The needle should be kept behind the posterior margin of the sternocleidomastoid muscle perpendicular to the horizontal plane of the vertebra to be biopsied. Gentle pressure and rotation are used to insert the needle into the area of abnormality. Although a small caliber Ackerman needle has been used in this biopsy, we recommend that a 16-gauge spinal needle be used.

Biopsy of thoracic and lumbar vertebral bodies is performed via an oblique posterior approach with the patient prone. The needle is introduced approximately 7 to 8 cm from the spinous process and directed obliquely to the body (Figure 26-14C). The position is controlled by fluoroscopy and cross-table lateral films for biplane guidance. In the thoracic region, a more acute angle of the needle is required to avoid the pleura (Figures 26-14D and E, Figure 26-15).

No complications have been encountered thus far, but the potential problem of trauma to nerves, vessels, and viscera does exist. The benefits include rapid and accurate establishment of a cytologic, histologic, and electron microscopic diagnosis and avoidance of a surgical procedure with its associated risks and costs.

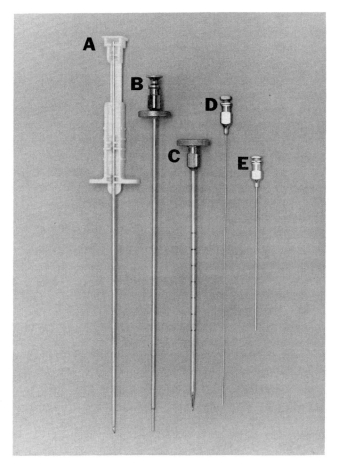

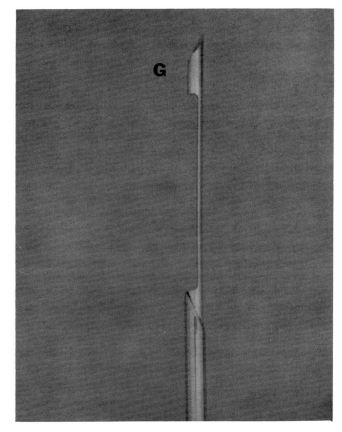

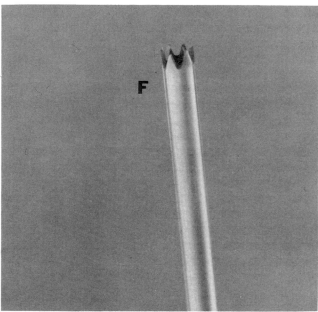

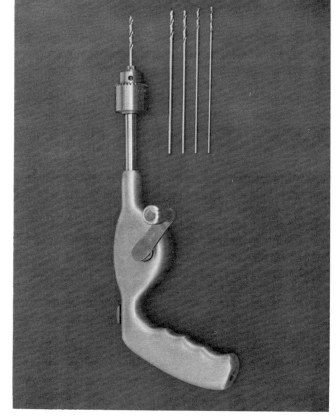

FIG. 26-11. Bone biopsy needles. (A) Vim Tru Cut; (B, C) Ackerman trephine needle set; (D, E) Aspiration needle or spinal type needle; (F) Cutting tip — detail of saw-toothed tip; (G) Cutting tip — detail of bayonet and shaft; (H) Orthopedic drill with bits.

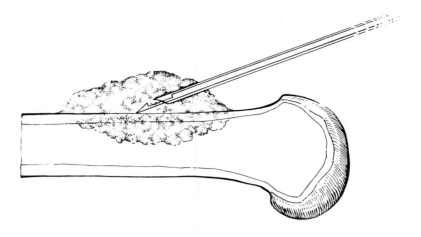

FIG. 26-12. Diagram of biopsy of an extraosseous soft tissue mass with a Vim Tru-Cut needle.

THERAPEUTIC DRAINAGE AND INJECTION PROCEDURES

Percutaneous drainage techniques using radiographic localization are available for the management of cysts and abscesses in (and about) the liver, kidneys, abdomen, retroperitoneum, and lungs. The treatment of a cyst, abscess, or neoplasm is also possible by the aspiration of the liquid content, when present, followed by the injection of chemotherapeutic agents, steroids, antibiotics, or sclerosing agents.

Renal cysts may decrease in size after puncture. With the injection of Pantopaque (acting as a sclerosing agent) into the cyst, reduction in size can be accomplished in 85% of cases.[146] Cyst puncture is still employed as a therapeutic measure if the cyst is symptomatic, i.e., if pain or discomfort is present because of size and location, or if the cyst is encroaching on the collecting system.

Liver cysts may be punctured and opacified for diagnostic and therapeutic purposes. Pantopaque instillation sometimes is effective in sclerosing a symptomatic liver cyst (Figure 26-16).[57] Adrenal cysts are approached the same way for diagnosis and management.[80]

Puncture and drainage of abscess cavities, regardless of location, may be managed by the percutaneous approach.[55,108] Once the abscess is localized radiologically, puncture and drainage are accomplished with a guide

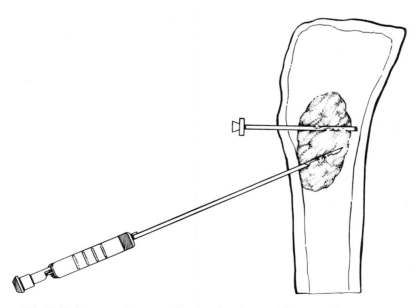

FIG. 26-13. Diagram of a biopsy of an osteolytic lesion of the proximal tibia with a trephine needle and a Vim Tru-Cut needle.

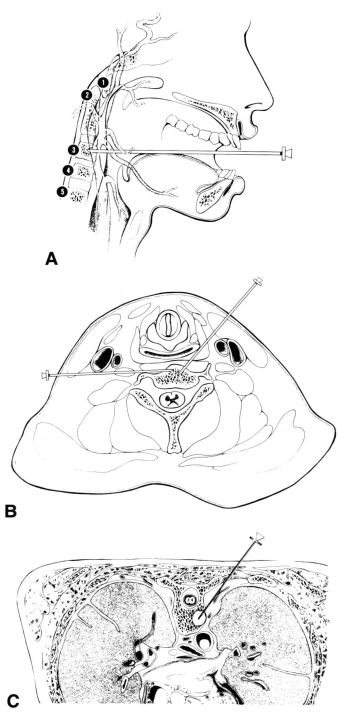

A

B

C

FIG. 26-14. Spine and pelvis biopsies. (A) Biopsy of upper cervical spine; (B) Lower cervical spine; (C) Thoracic spine; (D) Lumbar spine; (E) Pelvis.

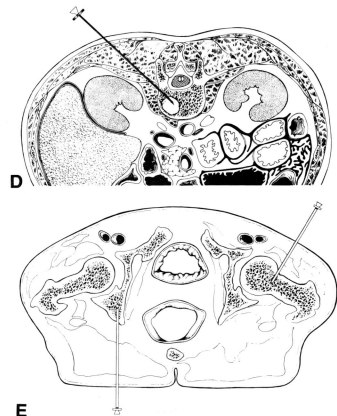

D

E

wire and a variety of catheters, preferably sump drains or pigtail catheters with multiple side-holes (Figure 26-17). These catheters allow adequate drainage and irrigation. Antibiotics may be injected to facilitate management. Multiple loculated abscesses may require surgery for adequate drainage.

Biliary Drainage

Percutaneous biliary drainage is an effective nonsurgical method of decompressing an obstructed biliary tree. This procedure is indicated in cases of extrahepatic biliary obstruction caused by locally advanced neoplasms, metastatic lymphadenopathy, failed biliary-enteric bypass, and cholangitis. This approach is also used to relieve obstructive jaundice caused by benign strictures and choledocholithiasis. For patients who are candidates for surgical biliary bypass procedures, preoperative percutaneous biliary drainage may reduce operative and postoperative percutaneous morbidity and mortality.[16,36,39,47,63,70,97,99,102,107,112,120] However, there have been studies that indicated little, if any, significant benefit from preoperative drainage.[36,102] Percutaneous drainage is generally performed in patients who are not surgical candidates in order to relieve the symptoms associated with jaundice and to improve hepatic function for subsequent administration of antineoplastic agents metabolized by the liver. The contraindications to percutaneous biliary drainage include uncorrectable hemostatic disorders and multiple areas of intrahepatic bile duct obstruction, usually secondary to hepatic metastases.

Technique. A few similar techniques for percutaneous biliary drainage have been described.[16,36,39,47,63,70,97,99,102,107,112,120] Routine predrainage measures should include (1) a check

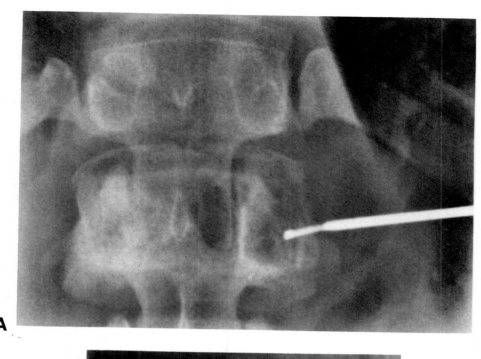

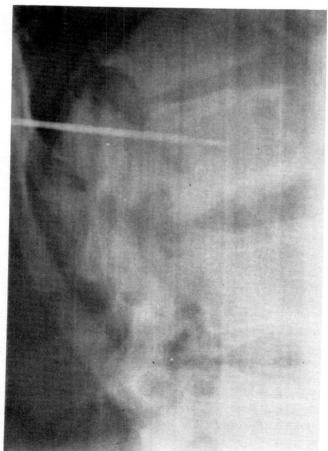

FIG. 26-15. Lumbar spine biopsy. A Tru Cut needle biopsy of a solitary lytic bone lesion in a 30-year-old man revealed a solitary plasmacytoma. (A) AP projection; (B) lateral projection.

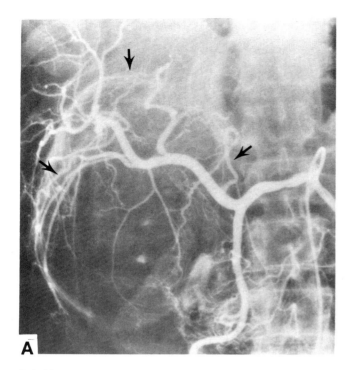

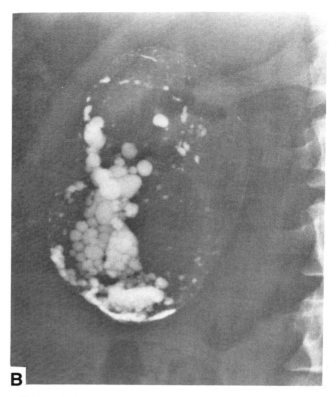

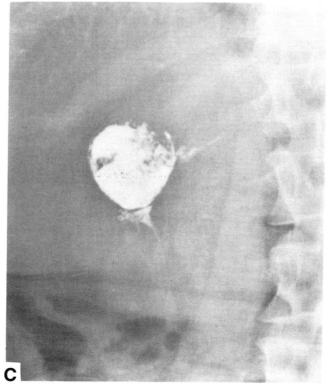

FIG. 26-16. Hepatic cyst management for pain. (A) A symptomatic hepatic cyst is demonstrated by angiography to be immediately beneath the gallbladder and cystic artery. (B) Pantopaque (10 mL) is injected into the cyst. (C) Eighteen months later there is marked decrease in the size of the liver cyst with the relief of pain.

of coagulation variables and their correction if indicated; (2) broad spectrum antibiotic coverage if cholangitis is suspected; (3) analgesic and sedative premedication; and (4) informed consent. The right upper quadrant of the abdomen is studied fluoroscopically in order to localize the lowermost extension of the pleural reflection during deep inspiration and the hepatic contour, which is outlined by gas-containing structures such as the lungs superiorly and the bowel inferiorly. We prefer to use a two-stage method for biliary drainage; a fine-needle percutaneous transhepatic cholangiogram is performed initially, followed by puncture of an intrahepatic biliary radicle with a larger sheathed needle.

The skin puncture site is marked in the anterior axillary line at a level immediately below the pleural reflection and overlying the right lobe of the liver. This area is then prepared and draped using standard sterile technique. Following infiltration of the skin and the subcutaneous tissues with a local anesthetic, a 22- or 23-gauge Chiba needle is introduced into the hepatic parenchyma. The needle should be parallel to the tabletop and should be directed toward an area just cephalad to the region of the porta hepatis, usually to the right of the 11th or 12th vertebral body. Small amounts of contrast medium are then injected while the needle is withdrawn slowly

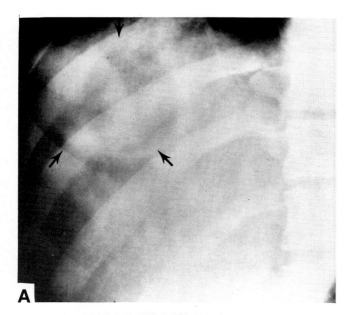

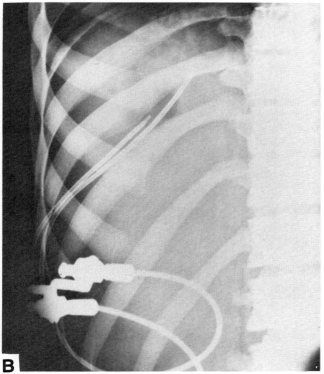

FIG. 26-17. Hepatic abscess drainage. (A) Hepatic angiogram of a patient with acute leukemia demonstrates a lesion in the right lobe of the liver with a hypervascular margin. (B) The liver abscess is drained with two catheters.

until a bile duct is opacified. Several punctures may be required before a duct is opacified depending on the degree of dilatation of the intrahepatic bile ducts. The needle should not be retracted from the hepatic parenchyma completely to avoid making several punctures through the liver capsule. Each subsequent pass should be made at a slightly different angle than the previous one. Once a bile duct is entered, the necessary amount of contrast material should be injected to opacify an intrahepatic bile duct adequately for the subsequent puncture with the sheathed needle. Care should be taken not to over-distend the biliary tree with contrast material, since this may lead to bacteremia.

Once a bile duct adequate for puncture is identified (usually a horizontal branch of the right hepatic bile duct), a small skin incision is made in the lateral abdominal wall overlying the right lobe of the liver at the anterior axillary line. An 18-gauge cannula-sheathed needle is then introduced into the hepatic parenchyma toward the intrahepatic bile duct chosen for puncture (Figure 26-18), while the Chiba needle used to opacify the bile ducts is left in place should the need arise for additional opacification of the biliary tree. As the sheathed needle traverses the duct wall, a small indentation of the duct will be observed on the fluoroscope. A tactile sensation of lesser resistance will also be noted once the needle enters the bile duct. The sheath is left in place while the inner cannula is withdrawn. Free flow of bile through the sheath indicates satisfactory duct puncture and a 0.038-inch guide wire is then threaded through the sheath into the bile duct. The length of the guide wire within the biliary tree will determine its stability, and therefore it should be advanced as far as possible. The sheath is then removed over the guide wire, and the tract is dilated using a 7F and subsequently an 8F dilator. An 8.3F polyethylene pigtail catheter with several side-holes near its tip is then introduced over the guide wire for external biliary drainage. The catheter is secured to a Molnar disc, which is taped or sutured to the skin. The catheter is then connected to a biliary drainage bag.

The catheter should be exchanged for a 10F or a 12F catheter two or three days after the initial procedure to provide adequate drainage. The catheter can also be internalized for a more physiologic drainage of bile into the duodenum (Figures 26-19, 26-20). This is performed by negotiating a guide wire through the obstructed segment into the duodenum and then passing an 8.3F to 12F catheter over it. The catheter for internal drainage should have side-holes above and below the site of the obstruction to ensure bile drainage. Hydrostatic pressures through the internal drainage catheter should measure below 20 cm of water; higher pressures represent inadequate internal biliary drainage and the catheter should be exchanged for one with external drainage only.

Catheters may remain patent for variable periods of time and should be exchanged for new ones whenever they become kinked or occluded. Patients should be instructed on how to irrigate their drainage catheters using 10 mL of saline solution daily to prevent inspissation of bile.

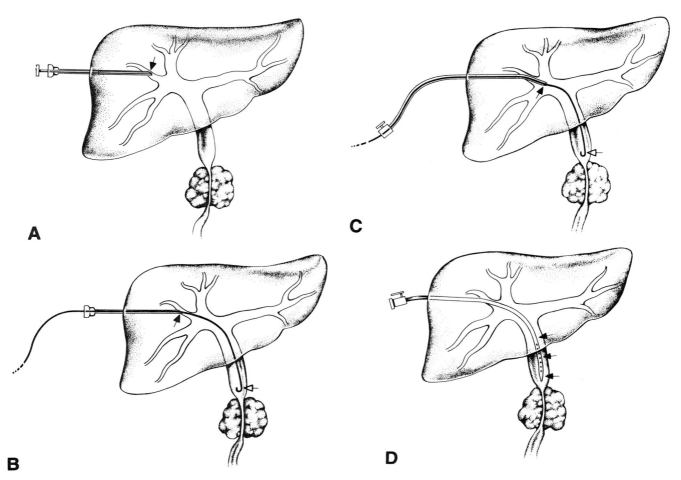

FIG. 26-18. Biliary drainage: External. (A) After opacification of a dilated biliary tract, a duct is punctured with a sheathed needle. (B) A J wire is threaded into the common bile duct. (C) A catheter is exchanged over the J wire. (D) The catheter is left in the dilated common bile duct for external drainage.

Complications. Although percutaneous biliary drainage is an effective method of decompressing an obstructed biliary system and will usually palliate the symptoms associated with jaundice, it is not without the potential for a multiplicity of problems. In a series of 161 patients with malignant biliary obstruction who underwent percutaneous biliary drainage at M. D. Anderson Hospital and Tumor Institute, we observed a high incidence of cholangitis (47%). The frequency of cholangitis in patients with internal drainage catheters was higher (67%) than in those with external drainage catheters only (36%). Partial or complete dislodgement of the catheter occurred in 18% of our cases. Partial dislodgement of the catheter may predispose the patient to cholangitis because of inadequate drainage, or to bleeding, when the side-holes abut a vessel; however, the catheter can be repositioned easily when this problem is identified. On the other hand, complete dislodgement of the drainage catheter carries a high risk of significant complications, including death.

Unless a well-formed biliocutaneous tract is present, it may be very difficult to reinsert a new drainage catheter into a nondilated biliary tree that is being decompressed into the peritoneal cavity by the track of the dislodged catheter. Surgery may not be an alternative in some of these very ill, and, at times, myelosuppressed patients.

Leakage of fluid around the catheter may be secondary to ascites, which cannot usually be corrected. Leakage of bile, however, usually signifies inadequate transcatheter drainage caused by a catheter that is either clogged or of insufficient caliber to ensure adequate drainage and warrants a catheter exchange. High volume bile output is an infrequent complication of unknown etiology and temporary in nature. Fluid and electrolyte losses may be pronounced and at times reach 7 L per day, leading to hypotension and symptomatic hyponatremia.

Other potential complications include biliopleural fistulas, pneumothorax, and intraperitoneal hemorrhage, which can be avoided by careful attention to technique.

A catheter prosthesis of preferably 12F or greater will alleviate many of the problems associated with either external or external-internal drainage.[16] The prosthesis can be introduced percutaneously through the liver, through a combined transhepatic and oral approach, or endoscopically.

The overall median survival of our patients undergoing percutaneous biliary drainage is 57 days (range, 1 to 921 days). However, depending on the aggressiveness of the neoplasm responsible for the obstruction and the effectiveness of the therapy available for that neoplasm, some patients will survive for prolonged periods of time.

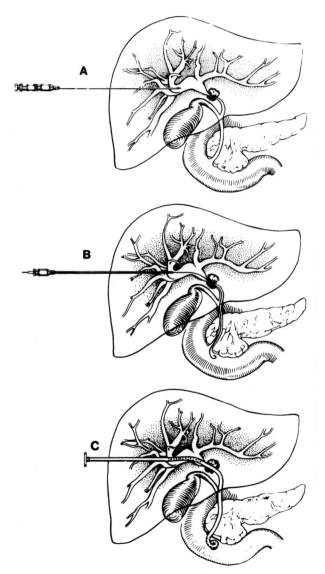

FIG. 26-19. Biliary drainage: External-internal. (A) After a transhepatic cholangiogram with a 22- to 23-gauge needle, an 18-gauge sheathed needle is used to puncture the dilated bile duct. (B) An 0.038-inch guide wire is threaded through the obstruction into the duodenum. (C) An 8.3F pigtail catheter is exchanged over the wire. The pigtail is placed in the duodenum allowing for external-internal drainage.

The interventional radiologist must assume the responsibility for care of patients in all respects related to percutaneous biliary drainage.

Nephrostomy

Percutaneous nephrostomy provides a nonsurgical approach to the urinary tract, and the indications for this procedure include relief of ureteral obstructions secondary to calculi, sloughed papillae, malignancies, and benign strictures; percutaneous removal of calculi; dilatation of benign strictures; insertion of brush biopsy instruments, nephroscopes, and ureteral stents; and instillation of antibiotics, stone dissolving solutions, and chemotherapeutic agents.[6,7,12,41,51,73,94,118,119,133,134]

In cases of bilateral urinary tract obstruction and secondary azotemia, the need for a means of relieving the obstruction is obvious, and percutaneous nephrostomy is the procedure of choice because of the high surgical risk in these patients. Unilateral ureteral obstruction without azotemia is a frequent occurrence in cancer patients, and percutaneous nephrostomy is performed in order to improve renal function before the administration of nephrotoxic antineoplastic agents.

Technique. The technique used in the insertion of a percutaneous nephrostomy is derived from the Seldinger approach to the intravascular space.[6,7,12,41,51,73,94,118,119,133,134] We prefer to use a two-step method; the pelvocalyceal system is initially opacified with contrast material through a fine needle, and subsequently it is punctured with a larger sheathed needle for the insertion of a guide wire and the drainage catheter.

Antibiotics should be administered if a urinary tract infection is suspected, and adequate analgesia and sedation should be achieved before the procedure. Intravenous contrast medium administered before the procedure may be useful in the subsequent fluoroscopic visualization of the renal collecting system depending on the renal function; however, it may be several hours before any appreciable contrast material is excreted into an obstructed pelvocalyceal system. In most patients, the renal outline can be adequately visualized under fluoroscopy without the aid of prior intravenous contrast material. Ultrasonography is frequently employed while computed tomography is rarely used for localization.

The patient is positioned in the prone oblique position with the side of interest away from the tabletop. The choice of the prone oblique position is mandated by the entrance site of the nephrostomy catheter, which should be posterolateral to decrease the likelihood of catheter kinking and provide for greater patient comfort. The patient is instructed to maintain quiet breathing and to avoid deep inspiration or expiration, particularly during the introduction of the puncture needles. The skin directly overlying the renal shadow is marked, prepared, and draped in the standard sterile manner, and

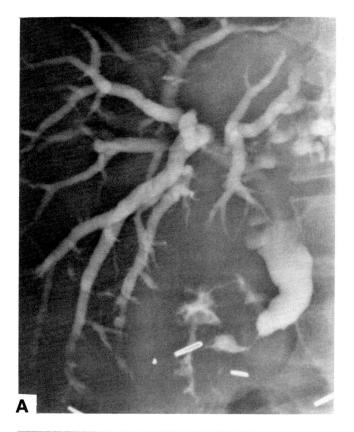

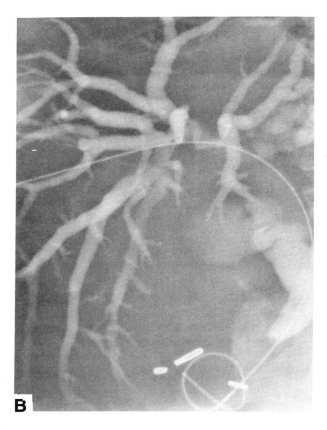

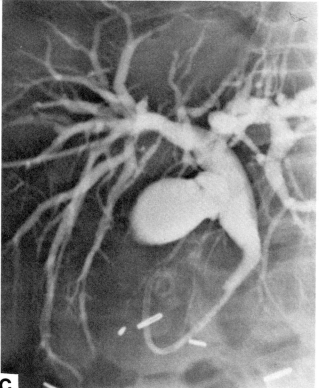

FIG. 26-20. Biliary drainage: External-internal. (A) A distal obstruction of the common bile duct is visible on this transhepatic cholangiogram of a 62-year-old patient with carcinoma of the stomach and obstructive jaundice. (B) A guide wire is passed through the obstruction into the duodenum. (C) A pigtail catheter in place in the duodenum bypassing the obstruction.

then superficial and deep infiltration of the puncture site with a local anesthetic is performed. The puncture site should be low enough to avoid violation of the pleural space. A 23-gauge Chiba needle is introduced toward the renal outline in the general region of the pelvocalyceal system. Puncture of the collecting system will be noted by a tactile sensation of diminished resistance at which time the stylet is removed and free-flow of urine is obtained. Contrast material is then injected through the Chiba needle until adequate opacification of the pelvocalyceal system is achieved. Partial drainage of the collecting system via the Chiba needle may be required to prevent excessive distention of the urinary tract, which may lead to bacteremia. The fluoroscopic table may have to be tilted temporarily to maintain the patient's head in a more dependent position and thus prevent the contrast material from flowing down the ureter.

Once adequate opacification of the pelvocalyceal system is obtained, a calyx is chosen for insertion of the nephrostomy catheter, and the skin and subcutaneous tissues overlying it are generously infiltrated with a local anesthetic. With the patient in a neutral suspended respiration and under fluoroscopic visualization, an 18-gauge sheathed needle is introduced and the chosen calyx punctured. Puncture of the renal collecting system will be identified by a tactile snap. Care should be taken not to introduce the sheathed needle beyond the collecting system, since it will then reach the renal hilum where puncture of major vessels and subsequent hemorrhage is more likely. The presence of larger vessels about the renal hilum also makes the renal pelvis an undesirable site for puncture of the collecting system. Once a calyx has been punctured, the needle is removed and the sheath is left in place. When free-flow of urine is obtained, a 0.038-inch guide wire is introduced through the sheath into the renal collecting system as far as possible, preferably into the distal ureter. The sheath is then removed and the track is progressively dilated up to a 10F size. A 10F pigtail catheter is then introduced into the renal pelvis. The guide wire is removed and the pigtail is formed within the renal pelvis where it will tend to exert less pressure on the walls of the renal collecting system. The catheter tip can be left in the bladder for external-internal drainage (Figure 26-21). The catheter is secured to a Molnar disk, which is taped or sutured to the skin and then connected to a bag for drainage by gravity.

Complications. Hematuria will almost always be present following the procedure, but it will usually clear within a few minutes. Depending on the degree of trauma inflicted on the kidney, the hematuria may last a few days, particularly in azotemic patients whose bleeding time is prolonged as a result of platelet dysfunction. In cases of severe hematuria, the catheter needs to be irrigated frequently with 10 mL of saline solution to prevent clots from obstructing it. At times streptokinase or urokinase injected through the catheter might lyse clots.

Urinary tract infections are more likely to occur in those patients undergoing prolonged nephrostomy drainage during episodes of myelosuppression. The nephrostomy catheter should be inspected every three months for kinks and for accumulation of concretions within its lumen and should be exchanged for a new one should this occur. Catheter exchanges are performed by inserting a guide wire through the nephrostomy catheter, which is then removed, leaving the wire within the renal collecting system; the new catheter is then inserted over the guide wire. When the catheter is obstructed, the hub is cut off and a sheath is placed over the catheter into the pelvocalyceal system. The catheter is withdrawn and a new one inserted.

Dislodgement of the catheter occurs rarely and if a well-formed urocutaneous tract is present a new catheter can be reinserted without difficulty. This is performed by first introducing a guide wire through the track and threading the catheter over it. When dislodgement of the catheter occurs soon after its replacement and the uro-

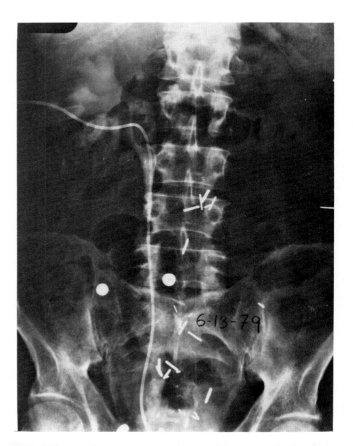

FIG. 26-21. Nephrostomy: External-internal drainage. The distal part of a catheter is coiled in the bladder, allowing for internal drainage in this patient with carcinoma of the colon with pelvic recurrence.

cutaneous tract is not yet well formed, it may not be possible to reinsert the catheter through the tract of the dislodged nephrostomy, and a new puncture will need to be performed.

Bone Cysts and Eosinophilic Granuloma of Bone

Stimulated by the success of direct injections of corticosteroids into simple bone cysts, a similar approach was employed in the management of localized eosinophilic granulomas of bone. The results of direct puncture and instillation of corticoids in cases of eosinophilic granuloma of bone have been encouraging. Ten of twelve children treated in this manner have had significant improvement in three to six months after a single injection of 150 mg of methylprednisolone.[32] Two injections were required to produce significant improvement in the other two children.

TRANSCATHETER INTRA-ARTERIAL THERAPY

The treatment of patients with neoplastic disease by intra-arterial infusion and devascularization has been employed for two to three decades with less than dramatic results.[11,34,35,92,138] Many interventional procedures were initially performed out of desperation but were soon incorporated into primary therapeutic management. The percutaneous approach to the vascular system routinely used for angiography provides the avenue for intravascular occlusion and infusion therapy primarily via selective catheterization of the arterial supply of the neoplasm.[149]

Technique

The standard angiographic techniques for catheterization are employed. Selective catheterization of the specific vessel supplying the neoplasm is preferable for optimal infusion and essential for embolization and occlusion. Most frequently 5F or 6.5F polyethylene catheters are introduced through the femoral artery. The brachial artery is the alternate avenue for prolonged infusions of five days or more and for those vessels difficult to cannulate from the femoral route. Smaller catheters (3.7F and 4F) are employed in children. Bilateral femoral artery puncture with internal iliac artery catheterization is frequently necessary for pelvic infusions.

Infusion

The rationale of intra-arterial infusion is to expose the neoplasm to a higher local concentration of chemotherapeutic agents than that obtained with intravenous administration. Most cytotoxic agents have a steep dose-response curve, i.e., the higher the concentration of the drugs, the higher the antitumor effect.[52] The systemic

concentration, and therefore systemic toxicity, will usually remain the same whether the agent is delivered intravenously or intra-arterially. However, a neoplasm that is refractory to systemic chemotherapy may respond to arterial infusion of the same agent at the same dose.

The catheter is positioned in the artery as close to the neoplasm as possible so that the infusion bathes the bulk of the tumor, but spares the maximum amount of normal tissue. The catheter is fixed in position by taping it to the skin with plastic adhesive (OP-Site, Smith and Nephew, Ind., Lachine, Quebec, Canada), covered with soft surgical tape (Microfoam, 3M Company, St. Paul, Minn.) and connected to a continuous infusion pump.

Aqueous heparin, 10,000 to 25,000 units, is given each day during the infusion to maintain a 1.5-fold prolongation of the clotting parameters to minimize thrombotic complications. If incompatible with the drug infused, i.e., Adriamycin, the heparin is given intravenously. Otherwise, it is mixed with the chemotherapeutic agents and infused intra-arterially.

For infusions longer than 24 hours, a conventional roentgenogram of the area of interest is obtained daily in order to check catheter position. Occasionally, the catheter position must be assessed fluoroscopically with test injections of contrast material. In the event of catheter displacement, which occurs in approximately 10% of cases, the external portion of the catheter is cleansed with an antiseptic solution and repositioned. The catheter is exchanged on rare occasions. The patient is then treated with wide spectrum antibiotics prophylactically until the catheter is removed. During the period of infusion the patient is usually in bed, but may be allowed limited ambulation. Ambulation is necessary, especially in prolonged infusions of longer than five days and in elderly patients.

The cytotoxic agents delivered by the intra-arterial route include 5-fluorouracil (5-FU), floxuridine (FUDR), doxorubicin hydrochloride (Adriamycin), methotrexate (MTX), cis-diamminedichloroplatinum (CDDP), vincristine sulfate, vinblastine sulfate (Velban), vindesine, 5-(3,3-dimethyl-1-triazeno)-imidazole-4-carboxamide (dacarbazine; DTIC), mitomycin-C (MTC), epipodophyllotoxin (VP-16), dactinomycin, nitrosourea (BCNU), AZQ, and AMSA. Before the use of a new agent intra-arterially, laboratory experimentation is necessary to determine the tolerable dose to the patient, the organ, and the artery used for the infusion.[3]

Occlusion

The materials available for embolization include: autologous clot and tissue; clot modified by thrombin; epsilon aminocaproic acid (Amicar); absorbable gelatin sponge (Gelfoam); Oxcel; polyvinyl alcohol foam (Ivalon); cyanoacrylates; Silastic and metallic spheres; silicone and silicone rubber; Ethibloc; microfibrillar collagen hemostat (Avitene); sodium tetradecyl sulfate (Sotradecol);

lyophilized porcine dura mater; balloon catheters and detachable balloons; ethyl alcohol; and metallic devices such as brushes and stainless steel coils. The combination of particulate emboli for the peripheral vascular bed of the neoplasm and central occlusion of the major supplying vessel is superior to either component alone. In general, in our institution, peripheral embolization is accomplished with Gelfoam particles (3-mm cubes) or Ivalon (150 to 500 μm) frequently accompanied by 2 to 5 mL of alcohol and central occlusion with Gelfoam segments ($3 \times 3 \times 30$ mm) and stainless steel coils. Stainless steel coils (Cook, Inc., Bloomington, Ind.) are available in 3 mm, 5 mm, and 8 mm helix diameters and can be introduced through 5F and 6.5F angiographic catheters, which will accept a 1-mm (0.038-inch) wire.[24,27,56,82,150]

The indications for transcatheter embolization of neoplasms are (1) to control hemorrhage; (2) to facilitate resection preoperatively by decreasing blood loss and operating time; (3) to inhibit tumor growth; (4) to relieve pain by decreasing tumor bulk; and (5) to perhaps stimulate an immune response to the ischemic neoplasm.

CONTROL OF HEMORRHAGE

The control of hemorrhage in patients with neoplastic disease is often lifesaving and may create an opportunity for more specific antitumor therapy by surgery, radiation, or chemotherapy.[8,30,58,83,122,128]

The intravenous infusion of vasopressin is at times effective in the management of diffuse gastrointestinal hemorrhage as seen in patients with leukemia. Intra-arterial vasopressin is usually ineffective in the control of gastrointestinal bleeding from malignant neoplasms but is used in the treatment of hemorrhage of benign etiology in cancer patients. Gastrointestinal bleeding from neoplasms of the liver, stomach, duodenum and rectosigmoid, as well as bleeding from radiation injury to the bowel are more readily controlled by embolization of the bleeding vessel.[30,58,122,128]

Hemorrhage from neoplasms of the genitourinary tract has been successfully treated by intra-arterial embolization. This has been accomplished in patients with neoplasms of the bladder, uterine cervix, and corpus.[128] Bleeding caused by radiation cystitis may be controlled by bilateral internal iliac artery embolization.[83]

Renal Carcinoma

The treatment for primary renal cell carcinoma confined to the renal capsule (stage I) is radical nephrectomy.[78,98] Renal artery embolization as a therapeutic modality was first suggested by Lalli et al.[84] and Lang[85] and it is now used before surgery in cases of large neoplasms in order to facilitate resection and decrease operative blood loss (Figure 26-22). It has been reported that over 50% of patients with stage I neoplasms measuring 6.5 cm in diameter or more were found to have lymph node me-

tastases.[75] Therefore, patients with stage I disease may benefit from a possible immunologic response against the neoplasm after preoperative renal infarction.

Patients with metastatic disease at the time of initial diagnosis pose a therapeutic dilemma. Chemotherapy, radiation therapy, and hormonal manipulation have generally been of no value in prolonging survival nor in causing regression of metastases in patients with renal cell carcinomas. Based on the initial work of Almgard et al.,[2] who reported stabilization of metastases in several of their patients with renal adenocarcinoma following renal artery embolization, a protocol involving renal infarction, a delay, nephrectomy, and hormonal therapy was established at M. D. Anderson Hospital and Tumor Institute[152] (Figure 26-22). Evaluation of the first 100 cases with long-term follow-up demonstrated an overall response rate (including those patients showing a complete response, a partial response, or prolonged stabilization) of 28%.[141] The median survival time for the responding patients was over 30 months, with one third surviving for five years. The overall survival rates for this group of patients do not represent a statistically significant improvement as yet when compared with historical controls treated at our institution by nephrectomy and hormonal-chemotherapeutic protocols without renal embolization. In patients with pulmonary metastases alone, however, a significant increase in the survival rates was observed in comparison with nephrectomy alone (Figure 26-23). This improvement in the survival rates was confined to that group of patients with only pulmonary parenchymal metastases. The median survival time of patients with metastases confined to the lung parenchyma was twice as high (18 months versus 9 months) as that of patients with hilar or mediastinal lymphadenopathy or pleural effusion (with or without parenchymal metastases).

The apparent clinical benefit of renal embolization and nephrectomy derived by some patients with pulmonary parenchymal metastases from renal carcinoma continues to be an empiric observation. It has been suggested that immunologic factors play a role based on the assumption that infarction of the neoplasm may release or uncover tumor antigens, thereby triggering an antineoplastic response.[140]

Our current management of patients who have pulmonary parenchymal metastases includes transcatheter embolization of the primary tumor with Gelfoam and stainless steel coils followed by radical nephrectomy approximately one week later. Following nephrectomy, these patients are treated with medroxyprogesterone acetate (DepoProvera), 400 mg intramuscularly twice weekly as long as there is no progression of their disease. Patients with metastases to sites other than the pulmonary parenchyma do not appear to benefit from infarction and nephrectomy and have therefore been offered experimental protocols including daily injections of human leukocyte interferon.[121]

Hepatic Metastases. Liver metastases from renal carcinomas occur in 14% of cases and are ominous, with a median survival of three months.[78] Two approaches have been pursued: (1) sequential hepatic embolization as well as renal embolization and nephrectomy; and (2) renal embolization and hepatic artery infusion with FAMP, (FUDR, Adriamycin, mitomycin-C and cisplatin). Thus far, the survival time in six patients treated in this manner is one year.

Skeletal Metastases. Osseous metastases occur in 30% to 45% of patients with renal carcinoma and are most frequently hypervascular. Embolization was not undertaken until at least six weeks after radiotherapy, the preferred treatment, had been completed. Arterial occlusion effectively controlled pain in 21 patients who failed to obtain relief from conventional radiation therapy.[29,132]

Preoperative arterial embolization of bone metastases from renal carcinoma can reduce the potential for major operative blood loss from internal fixation or instillation of a prosthesis.[13] The average blood loss during surgery, following embolization, was 500 mL, as compared with 3,800 mL and 7,000 mL blood loss in two patients in whom adequate occlusion could not be accomplished.

Solitary Renal Carcinoma or Metastases. Metastases to the residual kidney or second primary carcinoma in the solitary kidney create unique problems. When the patient is a good operative risk, surgical resection of a localized lesion is the preferred approach. Transcatheter occlusion might be considered if the neoplasm is localized and is supplied by a single branch of the renal artery. Three such patients have been treated for either the neoplasm or complications caused by the neoplasm, such as hemorrhage and hypercalcemia.

Absolute ethanol has been used with increasing frequency to infarct renal neoplasms.[43] Two milliliters of absolute alcohol, at a time, are injected into the renal ar-

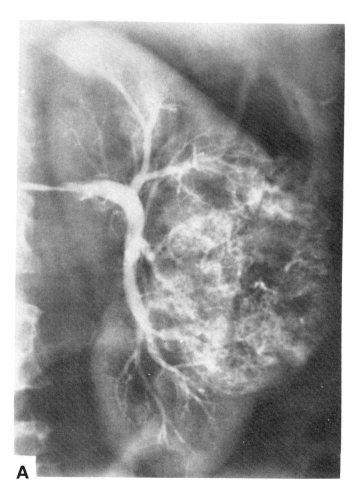

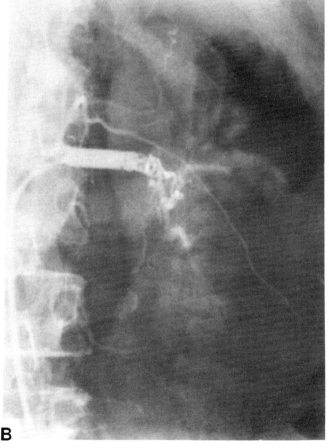

FIG. 26-22. Renal carcinoma embolization. (A) Hypervascular carcinoma in the middle portion of the left kidney. (B) The left renal artery was first embolized peripherally with Gelfoam cubes and then proximally with coils. A postembolization arteriogram shows complete occlusion of the renal artery.

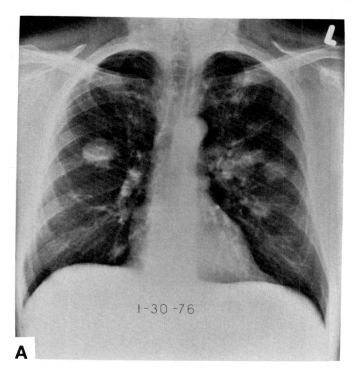

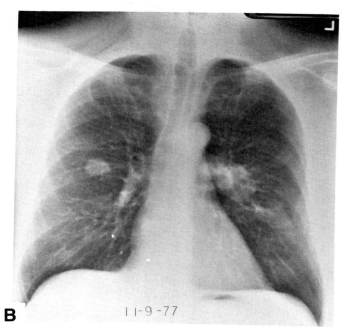

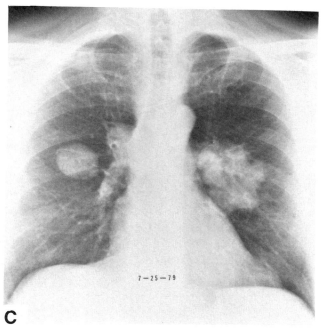

FIG. 26-23. Improvement in lung metastasis following primary renal carcinoma infarction. (A) Multiple metastatic lung tumors from a renal carcinoma. (B) Twenty-two months after renal infarction and radical nephrectomy, there is significant decrease in size and number of metastatic lung tumors. (C) Three and one-half years after initial treatment, there is gradual progression of the lung metastases.

tery, until flow slows, to a maximum of 50 mL. A more effective approach which requires less alcohol utilizes balloon occlusion of the renal artery. Two to five milliliters of ethanol are injected at a time. This allows greater contact time and more rapid occlusion. The patient experiences severe but transient pain with each injection of alcohol, which is controlled with intravenous analgesics or epidural anesthesia.

In order to stimulate a nonspecific immune response in those patients who agree, BCG, 1×10^8 organisms, is added to the Gelfoam emboli and to stainless steel coils to occlude the renal artery.[155] After a two-week interval, a nephrectomy is performed. Because of the possible negative effect of DepoProvera on the immune mechanism, this agent is deleted from the protocol. Our experience with this approach is as yet too limited to evaluate results.

Hepatic Carcinoma

Hepatic resection is still the preferred form of management when a hepatic neoplasm is located in a resectable segment of the liver. Otherwise, the management of hepatic neoplasms, whether primary or secondary, includes transcatheter hepatic arterial infusion (HAI) and occlu-

sion (HAE).[4,31,50,86,105,109] Both primary and secondary neoplasms of the liver receive their blood supply almost exclusively from the hepatic artery (90%), while the normal parenchyma has a dual supply, the hepatic artery (25%) and the portal vein (75%); 50% of the oxygen comes from each source.[15,54,71] Both infusion and occlusion therapy depend upon this concept; the treatment delivered to the hepatic artery almost selectively effects the neoplasm.

The classical distribution of the hepatic artery originating from the celiac axis occurs in approximately 55% of patients; an aberrant artery becomes a significant obstacle to HAI.[23,62,95] Transcatheter occlusion of the aberrant hepatic artery is performed to redistribute the hepatic arterial flow to a single vessel.[23] This is accomplished by the placement of stainless steel coils at the origin of the replaced hepatic artery (Figure 26-24).

Hepatic Arterial Infusion (HAI). Administration of mito-mycin-C, 15 mg/m[2], over a 2- to 24-hour period, and floxuridine (FUDR), 100 mg/m[2] per day for a five-day continuous infusion is the present protocol for treating hepatic metastases from colorectal carcinoma.[44,113-116] Adriamycin, 60 to 75 mg/m[2] given over the course of five days in three pulses of 20 to 25 mg/m[2] each, is added to the above for primary hepatocellular neoplasms or metastases from an unknown primary neoplasm. For metastases from breast carcinoma, cisplatin or vinblastine are infused; for soft tissue sarcomas, Adriamycin and DTIC are used; and for melanomas, CDDP and DTIC are used. The treatment course is repeated every four to six weeks, depending upon the patient's tolerance. Complications include gastritis, gastric and duodenal ulcers, cholecystitis, pancreatitis, hepatitis, vascular injuries such as arteritis, occlusions, and aneurysms, as well as local infection and sepsis.[4,22,28,31,59,109]

At MDAH, 20% of patients with metastatic colon carcinoma to the liver will respond to intravenous 5-FU alone or in combination.[116] Of the patients who fail to respond to the intravenous agents, 45% will show improvement when the same chemotherapy is delivered

intra-arterially.[113-116] There is also significant prolongation of life, 14 months compared with 7 months. Breast carcinoma metastases to the liver show a 30% response rate with CDDP alone and a 65% response rate with vinblastine and CDDP.

Hepatic Occlusion (HAE). Devascularization of an hepatic neoplasm can be achieved percutaneously by sequential embolization at monthly intervals with 100 to 200 mg of Ivalon granules (150 to 590 μm) alone or Ivalon with ethanol (1 to 2 mL at a time)[19,20,21,22,28,59,88,158] This method is used (1) in patients with unresectable primary hepatic neoplasms; (2) preoperatively, to facilitate resection of a hypervascular neoplasm; (3) in metastatic neoplasms that fail to respond to chemotherapy; (4) as the initial form of management of certain metastases that are usually refractory to chemotherapy; and (5) to control pain or hemorrhage from an hepatic neoplasm.

For example, 18 patients with various apudomas (hormone-producing tumors) metastatic to the liver underwent hepatic artery embolization with a 65% response rate (Figure 26-25). Of eight patients with carcinoid metastases to the liver, six have responded well with excellent control of the carcinoid syndrome, i.e., predominantly diarrhea and flushing. Embolization is now the treatment of choice to reduce tumor bulk and thus decrease the production of pharmacologically active substances in those patients with functioning tumors.[19]

The median survival for the first 100 patients from the

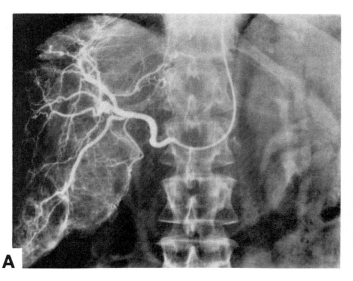
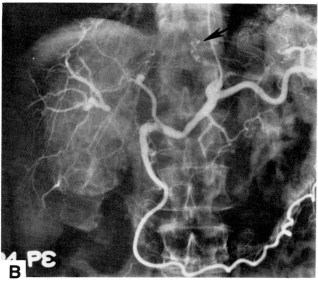

FIG. 26-24. Hepatic flow redistribution. The patient had Michel's type IV anatomy, i.e., the midhepatic artery from the common hepatic artery, the left hepatic artery from the left gastric artery, and the right hepatic artery from the superior mesenteric artery. (A) Selective right hepatic artery opacification with a catheter through superior mesenteric artery shows metastatic tumors in right lobe. The artery was embolized proximally with coils. (B) The left hepatic artery was also embolized with two coils (arrow) distal to the left gastric branches. The catheter was placed in the common hepatic artery for infusion chemotherapy. Intrahepatic interlobular collaterals developed to the right lobe of the liver. Collaterals to the lateral segment were less prominent.

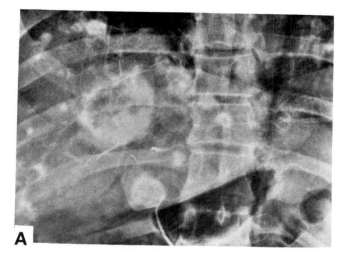

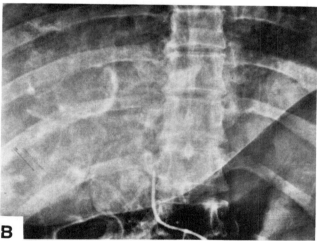

FIG. 26-25. A 45-year-old patient with ileal carcinoid metastatic to the liver and with carcinoid syndrome. Parenchymal phase of a left hepatic arteriogram before (A) and after (B) two Ivalon embolizations.

time of the HAE, usually performed after failure of all other treatment, was 11.5 months.[22,28] To date, over 400 patients have been treated by hepatic artery embolization.

A posthepatic embolization syndrome is the expected side effect and consists of pain, nausea, vomiting, and fever. Liver function studies are usually abnormal from the start and become more abnormal for one to three weeks. Of the first 100 patients treated by 150 embolizations, there were seven deaths, which occurred within one month of the procedure. Three deaths were most probably the result of hepatic failure or the hepatorenal syndrome, while four patients probably died of extensive metastases. The "hepatorenal" syndrome was observed in four patients, one of whom failed to respond to therapy consisting of hydration, electrolytes, and corticosteroids.

Primary Carcinoma of the Liver. Twenty-four patients with hepatocellular carcinoma or cholangiocarcinoma were treated with hepatic artery infusion of chemotherapeutic agents (FUDR, Adriamycin, mitomycin-C ± CDDP) in 14 patients, and hepatic artery embolization in 11 patients; one patient had a combination of two treatments. Ten of the 14 (72%) who underwent infusion demonstrated partial remissions. The median survival time was 12.3 months. Six of the nine patients (67%) who underwent embolization and for whom follow-up was available, responded to treatment. The median survival time for those patients was 17.4 months.[21]

In Japan, 120 patients with primary hepatocellular carcinoma were treated by embolization of the hepatic artery with Gelfoam. The one-, two-, and three-year cumulative survival rates were 44%, 29%, and 15%, respectively.[158] A significant decrease in α-fetoprotein levels was observed in 90% of these patients.

Portal Vein Infusion After Hepatic Artery Occlusion. The hepatic artery has been shown to be the principal nutrient supply to primary and secondary neoplasms of the liver; the portal vein is a minor nutrient supply.[15,54,71] Lin et al. reported that the contribution made by the portal vein to metastases may be substantial.[88] Ekelund et al. demonstrated in animals that the supply from the portal vein increases considerably after peripheral hepatic artery occlusion.[42] Taylor et al. described a significant increase in portal vein perfusion to metastases after hepatic artery ligation in humans.[145]

At MDAH, nine patients have been treated by portal vein infusion after hepatic artery occlusion. Four had central occlusion of the celiac or common hepatic arteries as a result of HAI in whom the infusion catheter was surgically placed in a branch of the middle colic vein. In another five patients, percutaneous transhepatic placement and infusion into the portal vein was accomplished after peripheral embolization of the hepatic arteries. The latter group thus far seems to be responding better, but it is still to early to objectively evaluate this approach.

Neoplasms of Bone

Transcatheter management of primary and secondary bone tumors includes both arterial infusion and occlusion.[1,9,16,17,25,26,40,53,76,77,101,124,139,143,153] Intra-arterial infusion of chemotherapeutic agents has been used primarily in the treatment of bone tumors, osteosarcomas, while arterial occlusion has been effective in giant cell tumors and aneurysmal bone cysts. The palliative control of bone pain secondary to metastatic renal carcinoma has already been described.

Osteosarcoma. For many years, radical surgery has been the principal mode of therapy for primary osteosarcomas. The overall three-year survival rate for patients with osteosarcomas was approximately 20%.[139] Radiologic evidence of pulmonary metastases occurred at a median of 8.5 months after potentially curative surgery and patients usually died within six months after detection of pulmonary metastases.[139]

The fatal outcome for most osteosarcoma patients after surgery led to the use of radiation therapy for local control in an effort to spare patients who were likely to develop pulmonary metastases from unnecessary mutilation. It was also believed that irradiation might change tumor cell viability and prevent implantation of cells dislodged during surgery. However, this approach yielded survival rates comparable with those achieved by surgery alone, and radiation therapy was discarded as a primary treatment modality.

Chemotherapeutic agents were also used in an attempt to improve the dismal results obtained by surgery alone. Initially, the agents used yielded far from ideal results. However, more recently, response rates of 35% to 40% have been obtained using methotrexate, Adriamycin, CDDP, and Cytoxan. Their administration alone or in combination has led to eradication of established metastases, destruction of primary tumors, and escalation of disease-free survival. The belief that osteosarcoma is microscopically disseminated at the time of diagnosis, as evidenced by the rapid onset of clinically evident pulmonary metastases soon after amputation, has led to the administration of adjuvant chemotherapy after surgery.

Advances achieved with chemotherapy led to the search for alternative methods to treat the primary tumor short of amputation, the most significant of which has been limb salvage.[1,9,17,26,40,53,76,101,124,143] Preoperative chemotherapy was also used initially in an attempt to contain the primary tumor while awaiting the production of a customized endoprosthesis for limb salvage surgery. Subsequently, preoperative chemotherapy and delayed surgery were employed with the intent of treating the primary tumor and identifying an effective chemotherapeutic agent for adjuvant therapy based on the degree of tumor necrosis. Rosen et al.,[124] using methotrexate, Adriamycin, bleomycin, Cytoxan, and dactinomycin achieved an overall disease-free rate of 72%.

Intra-arterial infusion chemotherapy was performed in order to increase the exposure of the primary osteosarcoma to the antineoplastic agents and thus attempt to improve on the results obtained by their systemic administration. Akahoshi et al.[1] used mitomycin-C, 5-fluorouracil, and methotrexate by continuous intra-arterial infusion for 8 to 48 days followed by surgery and bronchial artery infusion in 14 patients with osteosarcoma. Metastases occurred in 60% of patients during the first year. The projected five-year survival rate was 44% in those patients in whom the infusion lasted longer than three weeks compared with 26% for those who received shorter infusions. Eilber et al.[40] using intra-arterial infusions

of Adriamycin followed by radiation therapy in 36 patients, observed tumor cell necrosis in over 80% of the resected specimens. In more than half of the specimens, 90% to 100% destruction of the neoplasm was noted. Jaffe et al.[77] observed between 90% and 100% tumor destruction in three of five patients who underwent intra-arterial infusion of Adriamycin and systemic methotrexate. In another report, Jaffe et al.[76] noted one partial and three complete responses among nine patients who underwent intra-arterial infusion of methotrexate as part of a randomized study. No responses occurred in the six patients who received intravenous methotrexate.

Preoperative intra-arterial CDDP is currently being administered to patients with localized osteosarcomas at M. D. Anderson Hospital (Figure 26-26). A response rate of 66% was achieved in 18 patients treated with intra-arterial CDDP; there were nine complete and three partial responses.[26] The results were determined by clinical, angiographic, and histologic variables (needle biopsy, amputation, and local resection). Increased tumor destruction was found to be a function of the number of infusions (three or more), high CDDP concentration within the neoplasm, and tumor subtype (osteoblastic). In contrast, decreased tumor destruction was associated with less than four infusions, smaller concentrations, and the telangiectatic subtype. In another report from this institution, Benjamin et al.[9] noted 10 responses in 18 patients treated with intra-arterial CDDP and systemic Adriamycin.

Other primary bone tumors, such as malignant fibrous histiocytomas, and giant cell tumors have been treated in a similar fashion.

The complications in this group of patients included nausea and vomiting in all patients, skin reaction with edema, pain and discoloration in two patients, and transient diastolic hypertension in four pediatric patients as a result of the renal toxicity of CDDP. Although CDDP is known to produce auditory and neurologic toxicity, none of the patients in this group were so affected.[9,17,26,76]

Giant Cell Tumors. Embolization has been performed in the management of 12 patients with unresectable giant cell tumors and aneurysmal bone cysts after failure of other modes of therapy or as a primary treatment modality.[14,25,153] The tumors were located in the sacrum in four patients, the sacrum and ilium in one patient, the ilium only in two patients, and in the lumbar spine (L-4), thoracic spine (T-10), and the humerus in one patient each. All patients had some degree of pain as the initial symptom. Five of the 12 patients had failed to respond to both chemotherapy and irradiation. Two additional patients had chemotherapy alone and all had some form of surgery. Two of the 12 patients had some improvement after intra-arterial chemotherapy. Seven of the 12 patients experienced significant pain relief, but radio-

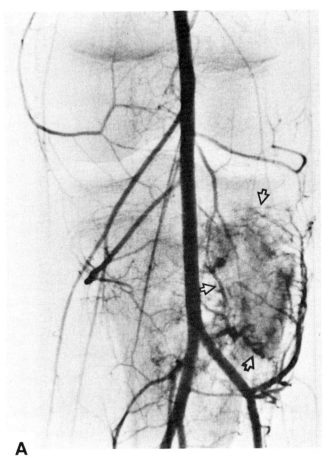

A

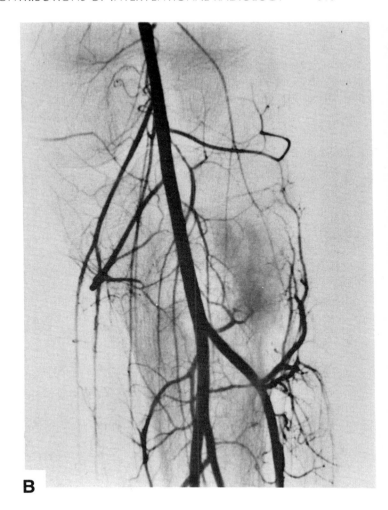

B

FIG. 26-26. Osteosarcoma of the tibia. (A) A selective popliteal arteriogram reveals marked tumor vascularity and stain in the medial aspect of the proximal metaphysis of the tibia (arrows). (B) After intra-arterial infusion of cisplatin, the tumor vascularity and stain completely clears.

graphic features of healing (calcification within the tumor and a decrease in size of the soft tissue mass) were observed in six patients. These seven patients had excellent clinical responses with a duration of 14 months to 7 years (Figure 26-27).

Bladder Carcinoma

Intra-arterial chemotherapy has been employed by Nevins and Hoffman, who surgically implanted the catheters into each internal iliac artery.[104] 5-Fluorouracil was infused for 10 days and then every other week for three months. This was combined with radiation therapy. Regression of local disease was seen in 6 of 10 patients. A mean survival of 25 months was noted in the complete responders. Intra-arterial mitomycin-c was effective in 33 patients reported by Ogata et al. in 1973.[110] None of 16 patients with T_1, and 5 of 12 patients with T_{2-3} bladder carcinomas, responded, but the myelosuppression and local irritation were significant.

With the introduction of new agents and the percutaneous approach for catheter placement, three groups of patients with D_2 carcinoma of the bladder, i.e., disease beyond the pelvis, were treated at MDAH by intra-arterial infusion.[89,90,127,136,151,156] In group I, 18 patients were given intra-arterial cis-diamminedichloroplatinum (CDDP); in group II, 29 patients received 5-fluorouracil intra-arterially during the intravenous administration of Adriamycin (doxorubicin) and mitomycin-C;[89,90,151] while in group III, 28 patients were treated with intra-arterial cis-diamminedichloroplatinum (CDDP), Cytoxan (cyclophosphamide) and Adriamycin delivered intravenously.[89,91,151]

The responses to intra-arterial CDDP of the 18 patients in group I were as follows: three of the 18 patients treated after surgery or radiation therapy had all measurable traces of the disease removed and were considered as adjuvant treatment. Of the remaining 15 patients, there were six complete responses; three partial responses;

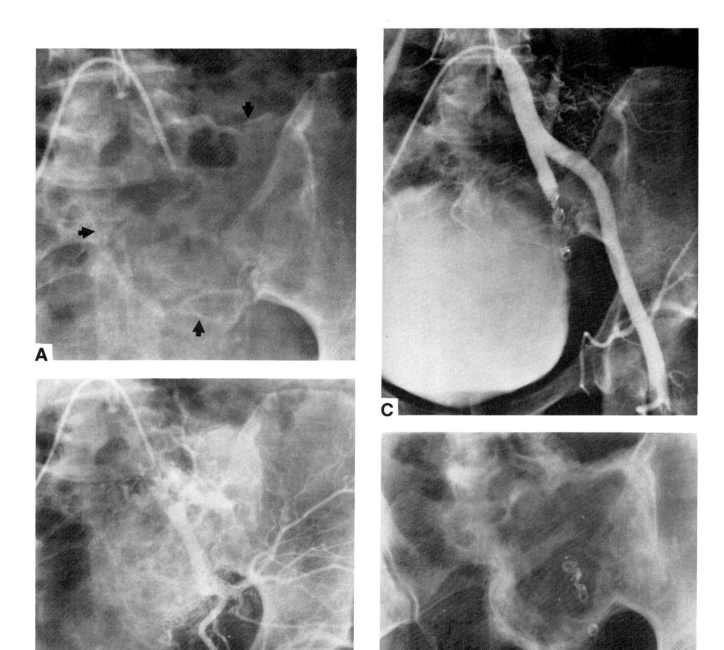

FIG. 26-27. Giant cell bone tumor. (A) Pretreatment plain roentgenogram shows large lytic lesions (arrows) in sacrum. (B) A left internal iliac arteriogram shows the tumor to be markedly hypervascular. The artery was embolized with Gelfoam cubes and coils. (C) A postembolization angiogram reveals complete occlusion of internal iliac artery. (D) A two-year follow-up study shows a solid rim of calcification of the tumor indicative of healing. The patient has been asymptomatic for seven years.

and six failures, a response rate of 9 of 15 (60%), with a median survival of 75 weeks (Figure 26-28). The pelvic pain in 12 of 15 patients and the hematuria in 8 of 15 patients were adequately controlled with intra-arterial CDDP.[151]

Seventeen (58%) of the patients in group II achieved an objective response. Twelve of 20 patients with transitional cell carcinoma responded. All four patients with adenocarcinoma responded, whereas the three patients with squamous transformation of transitional cell carcinoma failed to respond. The single patient with a spindle cell variant failed to respond while the patient with adenocarcinomatous transformation responded. The median survival time of the responding patients was 52 weeks, while the nonresponding patients had a survival time of 28 weeks.[89,90,151]

The third group of 28 patients was managed with intravenous and intra-arterial CISCA (cisplatin, Cytoxan and Adriamycin). For intra-arterial CISCA, only CDDP

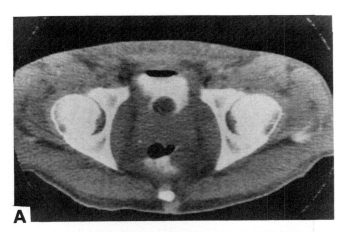

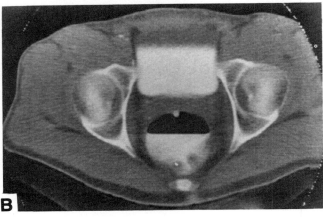

FIG. 26-28. Bladder carcinoma. (A) A pretreatment CT scan reveals a thickened and irregular bladder wall. The patient was treated with three courses of bilateral internal iliac artery infusion. (B) A posttreatment CT scan shows a normal bladder.

was administered intra-arterially; Cytoxan and Adriamycin were infused via the intravenous route. All patients either had unresectable tumor (26 patients) or had failed initial therapy consisting of cystectomy or irradiation (two patients). The tumors were of bladder origin in 26 patients and of ureteral origin in two patients. All but two patients received a combination of intra-arterial and intravenous CISCA chemotherapy. Those patients with only locally advanced disease received three courses of intra-arterial CISCA spaced one month apart. Patients with nodal metastases received their initial chemotherapy intravenously followed by intra-arterial CISCA if an objective response was achieved. The doses for CISCA consisted of Cytoxan, 650 mg/m^2, and Adriamycin, 50 to 60 mg/m^2, delivered intravenously, while cisplatin, 100 mg/m^2, was administered intra-arterially. Complete remission occurred in 11 patients (39%) with a median duration of remission, thus far, of 49 weeks (range, 25 to 108 weeks). In seven (25%) additional patients, an objective regression of tumor occurred. Ten patients (36%) failed to respond. A significant improvement in the survival rate was documented for the complete responders, but there was no difference in the survival rates between those patients achieving an objective response and the nonresponders.[89]

The complications of CDDP in group I included high output acute tubular necrosis in two patients; an embolus to the lower extremity in one patient; and transient peripheral neuropathy in seven patients.[89,151] The combination of 5-FU, Adriamycin and mitomycin-C in group II caused fatal respiratory failure from mitomycin-C interstitial pneumonia in one patient; transient pneumonia in another; and status asthmaticus and death in a third patient.[90] Inflammatory skin changes in the distribution of the gluteal vessels caused by 5-FU was seen in all patients; this lasted two to four weeks with no permanent skin ulcerations. Leukopenic fever was experienced in 59% of group II patients. 5-Fluorouracil induced transient motor neuropathy in four patients; all had complete recovery.

Pelvic occurrences of malignant urothelial tumors are among the most difficult and most poorly tolerated. These symptoms are usually the result of invasion of the sacral plexus, the external genitalia, or the urinary bladder, resulting in pain and hematuria. Our experience with this select population of carcinoma of the bladder, stage D$_2$, demonstrated the effectiveness of intra-arterial chemotherapy. Cisplatin is the most active agent available in the treatment of transitional cell carcinoma and squamous cell carcinoma of the bladder. Because of the success of the intravenous combination of CISCA (CDDP, Adriamycin and Cytoxan), the CDDP is now given intra-arterially and the other agents are administered intravenously. For those patients with adenocarcinoma of the bladder, the combination of 5-FU is delivered intra-arterially, while Adriamycin and mitomycin-C are added intravenously. The FAM regimen is also indicated when the CISCA regimen is not tolerated or when it fails. For those patients who are initially seen with hydronephrosis, percutaneous nephrostomies are performed to preserve renal function before chemotherapy, especially if CDDP is to be administered.

Carcinoma of the Uterine Cervix

Utilizing bilateral internal iliac artery infusion of bleomycin alone or in combination with mitomycin-C and vincristine in the treatment of recurrent cervical carcinoma, Morrow et al.[100] observed 2 of 15 objective remissions, while Swenerton et al. reported 3 of 20.[144] Ohta and other Japanese investigators suggested employing intra-arterial infusion before definitive radiation therapy.[111]

At MDAH, nine patients with squamous cell carcinoma of the uterine cervix were treated by bilateral internal iliac artery infusion of CDDP.[18] Six of these patients had unresectable pelvic recurrences following radiation therapy, and three patients had previously untreated large-volume primary tumors. Three patients (33%) experienced partial responses, including two patients with pelvic recurrences and one with a previously untreated tumor. The duration of the responses was six, six, and three months. The previously untreated patient demonstrated a marked reduction in tumor volume and, after three infusions of CDDP, at intervals of one month, began radiation therapy. She remained free of disease 7 months after the initiation of therapy (Figure 26-29).

In an attempt to lower local recurrence rates and improve the response rates to chemotherapy of stage III and IV patients, a study consisting of the intravenous administration of vincristine (2 mg) with intra-arterial infusion of mitomycin-C (10 mg/m²) over 24 hours every other course, bleomycin (20 to 40 mg/m²) over 24 hours, and CDDP (100 to 110 mg/m²) over 24 hours is being performed.[81] Three cycles spaced three weeks apart are given via percutaneously placed catheters into each internal iliac artery. The proportion of chemotherapy delivered with each catheter was determined by the location of the tumor on pelvic examination and the vascular pattern of the pelvis on radionuclide flow studies.[79] The initial results of this study are encouraging: seven of nine evaluable patients were considered responders and five of the responders have completed radiation therapy. The impact of this therapeutic modality on survival and local recurrence is as yet unknown. An identical drug regimen was employed in 17 patients with recurrent disease following primary irradiation, with an overall response rate of 41%. Partial responses (29%) were of short duration, however, and did not lead to a significant prolongation of the patient's survival.[81]

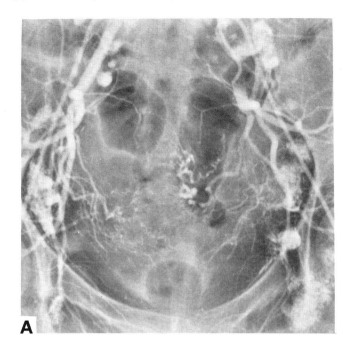

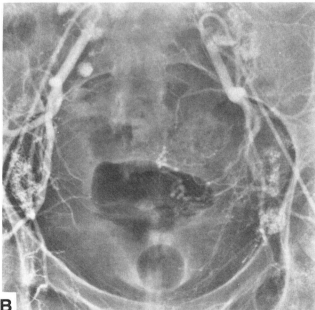

FIG. 26-29. Carcinoma of the uterine cervix. (A) A bilateral internal iliac arteriogram reveals diffuse tumor vessels involving the pelvis. (B) After infusion chemotherapy, there is a marked decrease of tumor vascularity.

Brain Tumors

Both glioblastomas multiforme and brain metastases continue to present a very poor prognosis. Intracarotid infusion has been attempted with various antineoplastic agents including methotrexate, 5-FU, Cytoxan, thiotepa, vincristine, vinblastine, and nitrogen mustard. A recent study of intracarotid bis-chlorethylnitrosourea (BCNU) reported substantial activity against intracerebral metastases from carcinoma of the lung.[157] Both primary and secondary brain tumors have responded to intravenous CDDP. In an attempt to enhance the response rate of intracerebral tumors to this drug, CDDP was delivered by the intracarotid approach at a dose of 60 to 100 mg/m² over a one-hour period following adequate hydration, intravenous mannitol, and dexamethasone.[49,137]

Thirty-five patients with progressive brain tumors have now been treated with intracarotid CDDP; 30 patients were evaluable for response (Figure 29-30).[49,137] All evaluable patients had received cranial irradiation and developed progressive disease documented by computed tomography (CT) and neurologic examination. The vast majority had also failed prior systemic chemotherapy. The life expectancy for these patients was only one to two months. Twenty-three patients with primary malignant intracerebral tumors were treated with intra-arterial CDDP. The majority (78%) had glioblastoma multiforme, which is the most aggressive and also associated with the poorest prognosis. Of 20 evaluable patients, 6 (30%) had definite improvement in neurologic function and on CT scans. Five (25%) patients had stable disease and 9 (45%) failed to respond. The median time to tumor progression for responding patients was 33 weeks and for patients with stable disease, 16 weeks.

Ten of 12 patients with metastatic brain tumors were evaluable for response to CDDP. Seven (70%) had improvement and two had stable disease. In two cases, the patients expired due to extracranial disease while the brain tumors were still responding to CDDP. One patient with a trophoblastic tumor had disappearance of her brain metastases on CT scans. Another patient with undifferentiated carcinoma required bilateral carotid infusions. He had a reduction in the size of his brain tumors that was greater than 50%. The estimated median time to progression for responders is 30 + weeks and 12 + weeks for patients with stable disease. The vast majority tolerated the procedure well.

The toxicity of intracarotid CDDP in 104 evaluable cycles included seizure (5%), transient motor weakness (7%), encephalopathy (1%), and ocular toxicity (5%).

At present, the agents delivered via the internal carotid artery include CDDP, BCNU, VP-16, CDDP and BCNU in combination, and AZQ. Once an effective treatment is formulated, attempts will be made to consistently place the catheter tip beyond the ophthalmic artery for infusions of one hour to minimize retinal damage.

CONCLUSION

The treatment procedures discussed constitute but a portion of the interventional activity now pursued. This approach is limited by the availability of effective chemo-

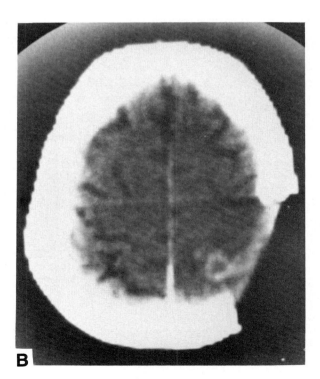

A

B

FIG. 26-30. Glioma. (A) A pretreatment CT scan shows a glioma in the left parietal area that was surgically unresectable. (B) Posttreatment with intra-arterial infusion of cisplatin shows almost complete regression of the tumor. The patient has remained stable for two years.

therapeutic agents for intra-arterial infusion and the creative initiative of radiologists as active members of the therapeutic team.

REFERENCES

1. Akahoshi, Y., Takeuchi, S., Chen, S., Nishimoto, T., Kikuike, A., Yonezawa, H., Yamamoro, T.: The results of surgical treatment combined with intra-arterial infusion of anticancer agents in osteosarcoma. *Clin. Orthop.* **120**:103–109, 1976.
2. Almgard, L. E., Fernstrom, I., Haverling, M., Ljungqvist, A.: Treatment of renal adenocarcinoma by embolic occlusion of the renal circulation. *Br. J. Urol.* **45**:474–479, 1973.
3. Anderson, J. H., Gianturco, C., Wallace, S.: Experimental transcatheter intraarterial infusion-occlusion chemotherapy. *Invest. Radiol.* **16**:496–500, 1981.
4. Ansfield, F. J., Ramariz, G., Skibba, J. L., Bryan, G. T., Davis, H. L., Jr., Wirtanen, G. W.: Intra-hepatic arterial infusion with 5-Fluorouracil. *Cancer* **28**:1147–1151, 1971.
5. Ayala, A. G., Zornoza, J.: Primary bone tumors: Percutaneous needle biopsy. *Radiology* **149**:675–679, 1983.
6. Barbaric, Z. L.: Interventional uroradiology. *Radiol. Clin. North Am.* **17**:413–433, 1979.
7. Barbaric, Z. L., Wood, B. P.: Emergency percutaneous nephropyelostomy: Experience with 34 patients and review of the literature. *A.J.R.* **128**:453–433, 1977.
8. Baum, S., Nusbaum, M.: The control of gastrointestinal hemorrhage by selective mesenteric arterial infusion of vasopressin. *Radiology* **98**:497–505, 1971.
9. Benjamin, R. S., Lindberg, R. D., Martin, R. G., Murray, J., Wallace, S. R., Chuang, V. P., Ayala, A., Romsdahl, M. M.: Limb salvage for patients with sarcomas of soft tissue and bone. *Cancer Bull.* **35**:11–15, 1983.
10. Bernstein, A., Waqaruddin, M., Shah, M.: Management of spontaneous pneumothorax using a Heimlich flutter valve. *Thorax* **28**:386–389, 1973.
11. Bierman, H. R., Byron, R. L., Miller, E. R., Shimkin, M. B.: Effects of intraarterial administration of nitrogen mustard. *Am. J. Med.* **8**:535, 1950.
12. Bigongiari, L. R.: An angiographic approach to percutaneous nephrostomy and ureteral stent placement. *Urol. Radiol.* **2**:141–145, 1981.
13. Bowers, T. A., Murray, J. A., Charnsangavej, C., Soo, C., Chuang, V. P., Wallace, S.: Bone metastases from renal carcinoma. *J. Bone Joint Surg.* **64A**:749–754, 1982.
14. Bree, R. L., Goldstein, H. M., Wallace, S.: Transcatheter embolization of the internal iliac artery in the management of neoplasms of the pelvis. *Surg. Gynecol. Obstet.* **143**:597–601, 1976.
15. Breedis, C., Young, G.: The blood supply of neoplasms of the liver. *Am. J. Pathol.* **30**:969–985, 1954.
16. Burcharth, F.: Nonsurgical drainage of the biliary tract. *Semin. Liver Dis.* **2**:75–86, 1982.
17. Calvo, D. B., Patt, Y. Z., Wallace, S., Chuang, V. P., Benjamin, R. S., Pritchard, J. D., Hersh, E. M., Bodey, G. P., Mauligit, G. M.: Phase I–II trial of percutaneous intra-arterial cis-diamminedichloroplatinum (II) for regionally confined malignancy. *Cancer* **45**:1278–1283, 1980.
18. Carlson, J. A., Jr., Freedman, R. S., Wallace, S., Chuang, V. P., Wharton, J. T., Rutledge, F. N.: Intra-arterial cisplatinum in the management of squamous cell carcinoma of the uterine cervix. *Gynecol. Oncol.* **12**:92–98, 1981.
19. Carrasco, C. H., Chuang, V. P., Wallace, S.: Apudomas metastatic to the liver: Treatment by hepatic artery embolization. *Radiology* **149**:79–83, 1983.
20. Charnsangavej, C., Chuang, V. P., Wallace, S., Soo, C. S., Bowers,
T.: Angiographic classification of hepatic arterial collaterals. *Radiology* **144**:485–494, 1982.
21. Charnsangavej, C., Chuang, V. P., Wallace, S.: Transcatheter management of primary carcinoma of the liver. *Radiology* **147**:51–55, 1983.
22. Chuang, V. P., Wallace, S.: Current status of transcatheter management of neoplasms. *Cardiovasc. Intervent. Radiol.* **3**:256–267, 1980.
23. Chuang, V. P., Wallace, S.: Hepatic arterial redistribution for intraarterial infusion of hepatic neoplasms. *Radiology* **135**:295–299, 1980.
24. Chuang, V. P., Soo, C. S., Wallace, S.: Ivalon embolization in abdominal neoplasms. *A.J.R.* **136**:723–733, 1981.
25. Chuang, V. P., Soo, C. S., Wallace, S., Benjamin, R. S.: Arterial occlusion: Management of giant cell tumor and aneurysmal bone cyst. *A.J.R.* **136**:1127–1130, 1981.
26. Chuang, V. P., Wallace, S., Benjamin, R. S., Jaffe, N., Ayala, A., Murray, J., Zornoza, J., Patt, Y., Mavligit, G., Charnsangavej, C., Soo, C. S.: The therapy of osteosarcoma by intraarterial cis-platinum and limb preservation. *Cardiovasc. Intervent. Radiol.* **4**:229–235, 1981.
27. Chuang, V. P., Wallace, S., Gianturco, C., Soo, C. S.: Complications of coil embolization: Prevention and management. *A.J.R.* **137**:809–813, 1981.
28. Chuang, V. P., Wallace, S., Soo, C. S., Charnsangavej, C., Bowers, T.: Therapeutic Ivalon embolization of hepatic tumors. *A.J.R.* **138**:289–294, 1982.
29. Chuang, V. P., Wallace, S., Swanson, D., Zornoza, J., Handel, S. F., Schwarten, D. A., Murray, J.: Arterial occlusion in the management of pain from metastatic renal carcinoma. *Radiology* **133**:611–614, 1979.
30. Chuang, V. P., Wallace, S., Zornoza, J., Davis, L. J.: Transcatheter arterial occlusion in the management of rectosigmoidal bleeding. *Radiology* **133**:605–609, 1979.
31. Clouse, M. E., Ahmed, R., Ryan, R. B., Oberfield, R. A., McCaffrey, J. A.: Complications of long term transbrachial hepatic arterial chemotherapy. *A.J.R.* **129**:799–803, 1977.
32. Cohen, M., Zornoza, J., Cangir, A., Murray, J. A., Wallace, S.: Direct injection of methylprednisolone sodium succinate in the treatment of solitary eosinophilic granuloma of bone. *Radiology* **136**:289–293, 1980.
33. Coley, B. L., Sharp, G. S., Ellis, E. B.: Diagnosis of bone tumors by aspiration. *Am. J. Surg.* **13**:215–224, 1931.
34. Creech, O., Jr., Krementz, E. T., Ryan, R. F., Winblad, J. N.: Chemotherapy of cancer: Regional perfusion utilizing an extracorporeal circuit. *Ann. Surg.* **148**:616–632, 1958.
35. Cromer, J. K., Bateman, J. C., Berry, G. N., Kennelly, J. M., Klopp, C. T., Platt, L. I.: Use of intra-arterial nitrogen mustard in the treatment of cervical and vaginal cancer. *Am. J. Obstet. Gynecol.* **63**:538–548, 1952.
36. Denning, D. A., Ellison, E. C., Carey, L. C.: Preoperative percutaneous transhepatic biliary decompression lowers operative morbidity in patients with obstructive jaundice. *Am. J. Surg.* **141**:61–65, 1981.
37. deSantos, L. A., Lukeman, J. M., Wallace, S., Murray, J. A., Ayala, A. G.: Percutaneous needle biopsy of bone in the cancer patient. *Am. J. R.* **130**:641–649, 1978.
38. deSantos, L. A., Murray, J. A., Ayala, A. G.: The value of percutaneous biopsy in the management of primary bone tumors. *Cancer* **43**:735–744, 1979.
39. Dodd, G. D., Greening, R. R., Wallace, S.: The radiologic diagnosis of cancer. In *Management of the Patient with Cancer*. Nealon, T. F., Jr. (Ed.). Philadelphia, W. B. Saunders, 1965, pp. 72–113.
40. Eilber, F. R., Grant, T., Morton, D. L.: Adjuvant therapy for osteosarcoma: Preoperative treatment. *Cancer Treat. Rep.* **62**:213–216, 1978.

41. Ekelund, L., Karp, W., Klefsgard, O., Lindstedt, E., Lindquist, S. B.: Percutaneous nephrostomy: Indicational and technical considerations. *Urol. Radiol.* 1:227–231, 1980.

42. Ekelund, L., Lin, G., Bengmark, S.: The blood supply of experimental liver tumors following intra-arterial embolization with Gelfoam powder and absolute ethanol. *Cardiovasc. Intervent. Radiol.* 7:234–239, 1984.

43. Ellman, B. A., Green, C. E., Eigenbrodt, E., Garriott, J. C., Curry, T. S.: Renal infarction with absolute ethanol. *Invest. Radiol.* 15:318–322, 1980.

44. Ensminger, W. D., Rosovsky, A., Raso, V., Levin, D. C., Glode, M., Come, S., Steele, G., Frei, E., III: A clinical-pharmacological evaluation of hepatic arterial infusions of 5-Fluoro-2-Deoxyuridine and 5-Fluorouracil. *Cancer Res.* 38:3784–3792, 1978.

45. Ewer, M. S., Ali, M. K.: Cardiac biopsy: A review of the procedure, complications, and indications. *Prac. Cardiol.* 7:7, 1981.

46. Fennessy, J. J.: Bronchographic criteria of inflammatory disease and radiologic lung biopsy techniques. *Radiol. Clin. North Am.* 11:371–392, 1973.

47. Ferrucci, J. T., Mueller, P. R., Harbin, W. P.: Percutaneous transhepatic biliary drainage: Technique, results and applications. *Radiology* 135:1–13, 1980.

48. Ferrucci, J. T., Wittenberg, J.: CT biopsy of abdominal tumors: Aids for lesion localization. *Radiology* 129:739–744, 1978.

49. Feun, L. G.: Intra-arterial chemotherapy for primary and metastatic brain cancer. *Cancer Bull.* 36:57–60, 1984.

50. Fortner, J. G., Mulcar, R. J., Solis, A., Watson, R. C., Golbey, R. B.: Treatment of primary and secondary liver cancer by hepatic artery ligation and infusion chemotherapy. *Am. Surg.* 178:162–172, 1973.

51. Fowler, J. E., Meares, E. M., Goldin, A. R.: Percutaneous nephrostomy: Techniques, indications and results. *Urology* 6:428–434, 1975.

52. Frei, E., III: Effect of dose and schedule on response. In *Cancer Medicine*, Holland, J. F., Frei, E., III (Eds.). Philadelphia, Lea & Febiger, 1973.

53. Friedman, M. A., Carter, S. K.: The therapy of osteogenic sarcoma: Current status and thoughts for the future. *J. Surg. Oncol.* 4:482–510, 1972.

54. Gelin, L. E., Lewis, D. H., Nilsson, L.: Liver blood flow in man during abdominal surgery. *Acta Hepatosplenol.* 15:21–24, 1968.

55. Gerzof, S. G., Robbins, A. H., Birkett, D. H., Johnsen, W. C., Pugatch, R. D., Vincent, M. E.: Percutaneous catheter drainage of abdominal abscesses guided by ultrasound and computed tomography. *A.J.R.* 133:1–8, 1979.

56. Gianturco, C., Anderson, J. H., Wallace, S.: Mechanical devices for arterial occlusion. *A.J.R.* 124:428–435, 1975.

57. Goldstein, H. M., Carlyle, D. R., Nelson, R. S.: Treatment of symptomatic hepatic cyst by percutaneous instillation of pantopaque. *A.J.R.* 127:850–853, 1976.

58. Goldstein, H. M., Medellin, H., Ben-Menachem, Y., Wallace, S.: Transcatheter arterial embolization in the management of bleeding in the cancer patient. *Radiology* 115:603–608, 1975.

59. Goldstein, H. M., Wallace, S., Anderson, J. H., Bree, R. L., Gianturco, C.: Transcatheter occlusion of abdominal tumors. *Radiology* 120:539–545, 1976.

60. Goldstein, H. M., Zornoza, J., Wallace, S., Anderson, J. H., Bree, R. L., Samuels, B. I., Lukeman, J.: Percutaneous fine needle aspiration biopsy of pancreatic and other abdominal masses. *Radiology* 123:319–322, 1977.

61. Gothlin, J. H.: Post-lymphangiographic percutaneous fine needle biopsy of lymph nodes guided by fluoroscopy. *Radiology* 120:205–207, 1976.

62. Granmayeh, M., Wallace, S., Schwarten, D.: Transcatheter occlusion of the gastroduodenal artery. *Radiology* 131:59–64, 1979.

63. Greenfield, A. J.: Percutaneous biliary drainage. In *Interventional Radiology*, Athanasoulis, C. A., Pfister, R. C., Greene, R. E., Roberson, G. H. (Eds.). Philadelphia, W. B. Saunders, 1982, pp. 535–556.

64. Haaga, J. R., Alfidi, R. J.: Precise biopsy localization by computed tomography. *Radiology* 118:603–607, 1976.

65. Haaga, J. R., LiPuma, J. P., Bryan, P. J.: Clinical comparison of small- and large-caliber cutting needles for biopsy. *Radiology* 146:665–667, 1983.

66. Haaga, J. R., Vanek, J.: Computed tomographic guided liver biopsy using the Menghini needle. *Radiology* 133:405–408, 1979.

67. Hammerschlag, S. B., Wolpert, S. M., Carter, B. L.: Computed tomography of the spinal canal. *Radiology* 121:361–367, 1976.

68. Hanafee, W. N., Weiner, M.: Transjugular percutaneous cholangiography. *Radiology* 88:35–39, 1967.

69. Hancke, S., Holm, H. H., Koch, F.: Ultrasonically guided percutaneous fine needle biopsy of the pancreas. *Surg. Gynecol. Obstet.* 140:361–364, 1975.

70. Hatfield, A. R. W., Tobias, R., Terblanche, J., Girdwood, H. H., Fataar, S., Harries-Jones, R., Kernoff, L., Marks, I. N.: Preoperative external biliary drainage in obstructive jaundice. A prospective controlled clinical trial. *Lancet* 2:896–899, 1982.

71. Healey, J. E., Sheena, K. S.: Vascular patterns in metastatic liver tumors. *Surg. Forum* 14:121–122, 1963.

72. Herman, P. G., Hessel, S. J.: The diagnostic accuracy and complications of closed lung biopsies. *Radiology* 125:11–14, 1977.

73. Ho, P. C., Talner, L. B., Parsons, C. L., Schmidt, J. D.: Percutaneous nephrostomy: Experience in 107 kidneys. *Urology* 16:532–535, 1980.

74. Holm, H. H., Pedersen, J. F., Kristensen, J. K., Rasmussen, S. N., Hancke, S., Jensen, F.: Ultrasonically guided percutaneous puncture. *Radiol. Clin. North Am.* 13:493–503, 1975.

75. Hulten, L., Rosencrantz, M., Seeman, T., Wahlqvist, L., Åhrén, C.: Occurrence and localization of lymph node metastases in renal carcinoma. *Scand. J. Urol. Nephrol.* 3:129–133, 1969.

76. Jaffe, N., Knapp, J., Chuang, V. P., Wallace, S., Ayala, A., Murray, J., Cangir, A., Wang, A., Benjamin, R. S.: Osteosarcoma: Intra-arterial treatment of the primary tumor with cis-diammine-dichloroplatinum II (CDP). *Cancer* 51:402–407, 1983.

77. Jaffe, N., Watts, H., Fellow, K. E., Vawter, G.: Local en bloc resection for limb preservation. *Cancer Treat. Rep.* 62:217–223, 1978.

78. Johnson, D. E., Samuels, M. L.: Chemotherapy for metastatic renal carcinoma. In *Cancer Chemotherapy—Fundamental Concepts and Recent Advances*, Proceedings University of Texas System Cancer Center, M. D. Anderson Hospital and Tumor Institute 19th Annual Clinical Conference on Cancer. Chicago, Year Book, 1975, pp. 493–503.

79. Kaplan, W. D., D'Orsi, C. J., Ensminger, W. D., Smith, E. H., Levin, D. C.: Intra-arterial radionuclide infusion: A new technique to assess chemotherapy perfusion patterns. *Cancer Treat. Rep.* 62:699–703, 1978.

80. Katz, R., Patel, S., Mackay, B., Zornoza, J.: Fine needle aspiration cytology of adrenal gland. *Acta Cytologica* 28:269–282, 1984.

81. Kavanagh, J. J.: Regional chemotherapeutic approaches to the management of pelvic malignancies. *Cancer Bull.* 36:52–55, 1984.

82. Kerber, C. W., Bank, W. O., Horton, J. A.: Polyvinyl alcohol foam: Prepackaged emboli for therapeutic embolization. *A.J.R.* 130:1193–1194, 1978.

83. Kobayashi, I., Kusano, S., Matsubayashi, T., Uchida, T.: Selective embolization of the vesical artery in the management of massive bladder hemorrhage. *Radiology* 136:345–348, 1980.

84. Lalli, A. F., Perterson, N., Bookstein, J. J.: Roentgen guided infarction of kidney and lung—A potential therapeutic technique. *Radiology* 93:434–435, 1969.

85. Lang, E. K.: Superselective arterial catheterization as vehicle for delivering radioactive infarct particles to tumors. *Radiology* 93:391–399, 1971.

86. Lee, Y. T. N.: Nonsystemic treatment of metastatic tumors of the

liver—A review. *Med. Pediatr. Oncol.* 4:185–203, 1978.

87. Legha, S. S., Benjamin, R. S., MacKay, B., Ewer, M., Wallace, S., Valdivieso, M., Rasmussen, S. L., Blumenschein, G. R., Freireich, E. J.: Reduction of doxorubicin cardiotoxicity by prolonged continuous intravenous infusion. *Ann. Intern. Med.* 96:133–139, 1982.

88. Lin, G., Hagerstrand, L., Lunderquist, A.: Portal blood supply of liver metastases. *A.J.R.* 143:53–55, 1984.

89. Logothetis, C. J., Samuels, M. L.: Intra-arterial chemotherapy for malignant urothelial tumors. *Cancer Bull.* 36:47–52, 1984.

90. Logothetis, C. J., Samuels, M. L., Wallace, S., Chuang, V., Trindade, A., Grant, C., Haynie, T. P., III, Johnson, D. E.: Management of pelvic complications of malignant urothelial tumors with combined intraarterial and IV chemotherapy. *Cancer Treat. Rep.* 66:1501–1507, 1982.

91. MacKay, B., Keyes, L. M., Benjamin, R. S., Ewer, M. S., Legha, S. S., Wallace, S.: Cardiac biopsy. *Texas Society. Electron Microscopy* 11:10–15, 1981.

92. Markowitz, J.: The hepatic artery. *Surg. Gynecol. Obstet.* 95:644–646, 1952.

93. Mason, J. W., Bristow, M. R., Billingham, M. E., Daniels, J. R.: Invasive and non-invasive methods of assessing Adriamycin cardiotoxic effects in man: Superiority of histopathologic assessment using endomyocardial biopsy. *Cancer Treat. Rep.* 62:857–864, 1978.

94. McLean, G. K., Gordon, R. D., Ring, E. J.: Interventional uroradiology. In *Interventional Radiology Principles and Techniques*, Ring, E. J., McLean, G. K. (Eds.). Boston, Little, Brown and Co., 1981, pp. 379–410.

95. Michels, N. A.: *Blood Supply and Anatomy of the Upper Abdominal Organs.* Philadelphia, J. B. Lippincott, 1965.

96. Milner, L. B., Ryan, K., Gullo, J.: Fatal intrathoracic hemorrhage after percutaneous aspiration lung biopsy. *A.J.R.* 132:280–281, 1979.

97. Molnar, W., Stockum, A. E.: Relief of obstructive jaundice through percutaneous transhepatic catheter—A new method. *A.J.R.* 122:356–367, 1974.

98. Montie, J. E., Stewart, B. H., Straffon, R. A., Barowsky, L. H. W., Hewitt, C. B., Montague, D. K.: The role of adjunctive nephrectomy in patients with metastatic renal cell carcinoma. *J. Urol.* 117:272–275, 1977.

99. Mori, K, Misumi, A., Sugiyama, M., Okabe, M., Matsuoka, T., Ishii, J., Akagi, M.: Percutaneous transhepatic bile drainage. *Ann. Surg.* 185:111–115, 1977.

100. Morrow, C. P., DiSaia, P. J., Mangan, C. F., Lagasse, L. D.: Continuous pelvic arterial infusion with bleomycin for squamous carcinoma of the cervix recurrent after irradiation therapy. *Cancer Treat. Rep.* 61:1403–1405, 1977.

101. Morton, D. L., Eilber, F. R., Townsend, C. N., Jr., Grant, T. T., Mirra, J., Weisenburger, T. H.: Limb salvage from a multidisciplinary treatment approach for skeletal and soft tissue sarcomas of the extremity. *Ann. Surg.* 184:268–278, 1976.

102. Nakayama, T., Ikeda, A., Okuda, K.: Percutaneous transhepatic drainage of the biliary tract; techniques and results in 104 patients. *Gastroenterology* 74:554–559, 1978.

103. Neff, T. A.: Percutaneous trephine biopsy of the lung. *Chest* 61:18–23, 1972.

104. Nevins, J. E., Hoffman, A. A.: Use of arterial infusion of 5-Fluorouracil either alone or in combination with supervoltage radiation as a treatment for carcinoma of the prostate and bladder. *Am. J. Surg.* 130:544–549, 1975.

105. Nilsson, L. A.: Therapeutic hepatic artery ligation in patients with secondary liver tumors. *Rev. Surg.* 23:374–376, 1966.

106. Nordenström, B.: New instruments for biopsy. *Radiology* 117:474–475, 1975.

107. Norlander, A., Kalin, B., Sunblad, R.: Effect of percutaneous transhepatic drainage upon liver function and postoperative mortality. *Surg. Gynecol. Obstet.* 155:161–166, 1982.

108. Novy, S., Wallace, S., Goldman, A. M., Ben-Menachem, Y.: Pyogenic liver abscess: Angiographic diagnosis and treatment by closed aspiration. *A.J.R.* 121:388–395, 1974.

109. Oberfield, R. A., McCaffrey, J. A., Polio, J., Clouse, M. E., Hamilton, T.: Prolonged and continuous percutaneous intra-arterial hepatic infusion chemotherapy in advanced metastatic liver adenocarcinoma from colorectal primary. *Cancer* 44:414–423, 1979.

110. Ogata, J., Migita, N., Makamura, T.: Treatment of carcinoma of the bladder by infusion of the anticancer agent (Mitomycin C) via the internal iliac artery. *J. Urol.* 110:667–670, 1973.

111. Ohta, A.: Basic and clinical studies on the simultaneous combination treatment of cervical cancer with a carcinostatic agent and radiation. *J. Tokyo Med. Coll.* 36:529–543, 1978.

112. Oleaga, J. A., McLean, G. K., Freiman, D. B., Ring, E. J.: Interventional biliary radiology. In *Interventional Radiology Principles and Techniques*, Ring, E. J., McLean, G. K. (Eds.). Boston, Little, Brown and Co., 1981, pp. 245–376.

113. Patt, Y. Z., Bedikian, A. Y., Chuang, V. P., Wallace, S., Fuqua, R., Mavligit, G. M.: New approaches to the treatment of Dukes' Colorectal carcinoma and metastatic colorectal carcinoma confined to the liver. In *Gastrointestinal Cancer*, Stroehlein, J. R., Romsdahl, M. M., (Eds.). New York, Raven Press, 1981, pp. 391–403.

114. Patt, Y. Z., Mavligit, G. M., Chuang, V. P., Wallace, S., Johnston, S., Benjamin, R. S., Valdivieso, M., Hersh, E. M.: Percutaneous hepatic arterial infusion (HAI) of Mitomycin C and Floxuridine (FUDR)—An effective treatment for metastatic colorectal carcinoma in the liver. *Cancer* 46:261–265, 1980.

115. Patt, Y. Z., Peters, R. E., Chuang, V. P., Wallace, S., Mavligit, G.: Effective retreatment of patients with colorectal cancer and liver metastases. *Am. J. Med.* 75:237–240, 1983.

116. Patt, Y. Z., Wallace, S., Freireich, E. J., Chuang, V. P., Hersh, E. M., Mavligit, G.: The palliative role of hepatic arterial infusion and arterial occlusion in colorectal carcinoma metastatic to the liver. *Lancet* 1:349–353, 1981.

117. Pearce, J. G., Patt, N. L.: Fatal pulmonary hemorrhage after percutaneous aspiration lung biopsy. *Am. Rev. Respir. Dis.* 117:346–349, 1974.

118. Pfister, R. C., Newhouse, J. H.: Percutaneous nephrostomy: Types of catheters for drainage, occlusion, dilatation and fiberoptics for endoscopy. In *Interventional Radiology*, Athanasoulis, C. A., Greene, R. E., Pfister, R. C., Roberson, G. H. (Eds.). Philadelphia, W. B. Sauders, 1982, pp. 467–496.

119. Pollack, H. M., Banner, M. P.: Percutaneous nephrostomy and related pyeloureteral manipulative techniques. *Urol. Radiol.* 2:147–154, 1981.

120. Pollock, T. W., Ring, E. R., Oleaga, J. A., Freiman, D. B. , Mullen, J. L., Rosato, E. F.: Percutaneous decompression of benign and malignant biliary obstruction. *Arch. Surg.* 114:148–151, 1979.

121. Quesada, J. R., Trindade, A., Swanson, D. A., Trindade, A., Gutterman, J. U.: Renal cell carcinoma: Antitumor effects of leukocyte interferon. *Cancer Res.* 43:940–947, 1983.

122. Rosch, J., Dotter, C. T., Brown, M. J.: Selective arterial embolization—A new method for control of acute gastrointestinal bleeding. *Radiology* 120:303–306, 1972.

123. Rosch, J., Lakin, P. C., Antonovic, R., Dotter, C. T.: Transjugular approach to liver biopsy and transhepatic cholangiography. *N. Engl. J. Med.* 289:227–231, 1973.

124. Rosen, G., Caparros, B., Huvos, A. G., Kosloff, C., Nirenberg, A., Cacavio, A., Marcove, R. C., Lane, J. M., Mehta, B., Urban, C.: Preoperative chemotherapy for osteogenic osteosarcoma: Selection of postoperative adjuvant chemotherapy based on the response of the primary tumor to preoperative chemotherapy. *Cancer* 49:1221–1230, 1982.

125. Sagel, S. S., Forrest, J. V.: Fluoroscopically assisted lung biopsy techniques. In *Special Procedures in Chest Radiology*, Sagel, S. S.

(Ed.). Philadelphia, W. B. Saunders, 1976.

126. Sakakibara, S., Konno, S.: Endomyocardial biopsy. *Jpn. Heart J.* **3**:537–543, 1962.

127. Samuels, M. L., Moran, M. E., Johnson, D. E., Bracken, R. B.: CISCA combination chemotherapy for metastatic carcinoma of the bladder. In *Cancer of the Genitourinary Tract*, Johnson, D. E., Samuels, M. L. (Eds.). New York, Raven Press, 1979, pp. 101–106.

128. Schwartz, P. E., Goldstein, H. M., Wallace, S., Rutledge, F. N.: Control of arterial hemorrhage using percutaneous arterial catheter technique in patients with gynecologic malignancies. *Gynecol. Oncol.* **3**:276–278, 1975.

129. Sinner, W. N.: Complications of percutaneous transthoracic needle aspiration biopsy. *Acta Radiol. (Diagn.)* **17**:813–826, 1976.

130. Sinner, W. N., Zajicek, J.: Implantation metastasis after percutaneous transthoracic needle aspiration biopsy. *Acta Radiol. (Diagn.)* **17**:473–480, 1976.

131. Smith, E. H., Bartrum, R. J., Jr., Chang, Y. C., D'Orsi, C. J., Lokich, J., Abbruzzese, A., Dantono, J.: Percutaneous aspiration biopsy of the pancreas under ultrasonic guidance. *N. Engl. J. Med.* **292**:825–828, 1975.

132. Soo, C. S., Chuang, V. P., Wallace, S., Charnsangavej, C.: Interventional angiography in the treatment of metastases. *Radiol. Clin. North Am.* **20**:591–600, 1982.

133. Stables, D. P.: Percutaneous nephrostomy: Techniques, indications and results. *Urol. Clin. North Am.* **9**:15–29, 1982.

134. Stables, D. P., Ginsberg, N. J., Johnson, M. L.: Percutaneous nephrostomy: A series and review of the literature. *A.J.R.* **130**:75–82, 1978.

135. Stephenson, T. F., Mehnert, P. J., Marx, A. J., Boger, J. N., Roth-Mayo, L., Balaji, M. R., Nadaraja, N.: Evaluation of contrast markers for CT aspiration biopsy. *A.J.R.* **133**:1097–1100, 1979.

136. Sternberg, J. R., Bracken, R. B., Handel, P. B., Johnson, D. E.: Combination chemotherapy (CISCA) for advanced urinary tract carcinoma. *J.A.M.A.* **238**:2282–2287, 1977.

137. Stewart, D. J., Wallace, S., Feun, L. G., Leavens, M., Young, S. E., Handel, S., Mavligit, G., Benjamin, R. S.: A phase I study of intracarotid artery infusion of cis-diamminedichloroplatinum. *Cancer Res.* **42**:2059–2062, 1982.

138. Sullivan, R. D., Norcross, J. W., Watkins, J. E.: Chemotherapy of metastatic liver cancer by prolonged hepatic artery infusion. *N. Engl. J. Med.* **270**:321–327, 1964.

139. Sutow, W. W., Sullivan, M. P., Wilbur, J. R., Cangir, A.: A study of adjuvant chemotherapy in osteogenic sarcoma. *J. Clin. Pharmacol.* **7**:530–533, 1975.

140. Swanson, D. A.: The current immunologic status of renal carcinoma. *Cancer Bull.* **31**:36–39, 1979.

141. Swanson, D. A., Johnson, D. E., von Eschenbach, A. C., Chuang, V. P., Wallace, S.: Angioinfarction plus nephrectomy for metastatic renal cell carcinoma—An update. *J. Urol.* **130**:449–452, 1983.

142. Swartz, R. D., Cho, K. J., Adams, D. F.: Percutaneous renal biopsy in the assessment of renal parenchymal disease. In *Abrams Angiography: Vascular and Interventional Radiology*, 3rd ed. Abrams, H. L. (Ed.). Boston, Little, Brown and Co., 1983, pp. 2319–2332.

143. Sweetnam, R., Knowelden, J., Seddon, H.: Bone sarcoma: treatment of irradiation, amputation or a combination of the two. *Br. Med. J.* **2**:363–367, 1971.

144. Swenerton, K. D., Evers, J. A., White, G. W., Bayes, D. A.: Intermittent pelvic infusion with vincristine, bleomycin, and mitomycin C for advanced recurrent carcinoma of the cervix. *Cancer Treat. Rep.* **63**:1379–1381, 1979.

145. Taylor, I., Bennett, R., Sherriff, S.: The blood supply of colorectal liver metastasis. *Br. J. Cancer* **38**:749–756, 1979.

146. Vestby, G. W.: Percutaneous needle-puncture of renal cysts: New method in therapeutic management. *Invest. Radiol.* **2**:449–462, 1967.

147. Wallace, S.: Interventional radiology in the cancer patient. *Cancer* **37**:517–531, 1976.

148. Wallace, S.: The evolution of interventional radiology. In *First International Symposium on Intervention Radiology, Algarve, Portugal, 1979*. Amsterdam, Excerpta Medica, 1981.

149. Wallace, S., Chuang, V. P.: Transcatheter management of the cancer patient. In *Cancer—Principles and Practice of Oncology*, DeVita, V. T. Jr., Hellman, S., Rosenberg, S. A. (Eds.). Philadelphia, J. B. Lippincott, 1982, pp. 1862–1887.

150. Wallace, S., Chuang, V. P., Anderson, J. H., Gianturco, C.: Steel coil embolus and its therapeutic applications. In *Abrams Angiography: Vascular and Interventional Radiology*, 3rd ed., Abrams, H. L. (Ed.). Boston, Little, Brown and Co., 1983, pp. 2151–2173.

151. Wallace, S., Chuang, V. P., Samuels, M., Johnson, D.: Transcatheter intra-arterial infusion of chemotherapy in advanced bladder cancer. *Cancer* **49**:640–645, 1982.

152. Wallace, S., Chuang, V. P., Swanson, D. A., Bracken, B., Hersh, E. M., Ayala, A., Johnson, D.: Embolization of renal carcinoma—Experience with 100 patients. *Radiology* **138**:563–570, 1981.

153. Wallace, S., Granmayeh, M., deSantos, L. A., Murray, J. A., Romsdahl, M. M., Bracken, R. B., Jonsson, K.: Arterial occlusion of pelvic bone tumors. *Cancer* **43**:322–328, 1979.

154. Westcott, J. L.: Air embolism complicating percutaneous needle biopsy of the lung. *Chest* **63**:108–110, 1973.

155. Wright, K. C., Soo, C. S., Wallace, S., McDonald, M. W., Ayala, A.: Experimental percutaneous renal embolization using BCG-saturated Gelfoam. *Cardiovasc. Intervent. Radiol.* **5**:260–263, 1982.

156. Yagoda, A.: Phase II trials in bladder cancer at Memorial Sloan-Kettering Cancer Center, 1975–1978. In *Cancer of the Genitourinary Tract*. Johnson, D. E., Samuels, M. L. (Eds.). New York, Raven Press, 1979, pp. 107–119.

157. Yamada, K., Bremer, A. M., West, C. R., Ghoorah, J., Park, H. C., Takita, H.: Intra-arterial BCNU therapy in the treatment of metastatic lung carcinoma. *Cancer* **44**:2000–2007, 1979.

158. Yamada, R., Sato, M., Kawabata, M., Nakatsuka, H., Nakamura, K., Takashima, S.: Hepatic artery embolization in 120 patients with unresectable hepatoma. *Radiology* **148**:397–401, 1983.

159. Zamcheck, N., Klausenstock, O.: Liver biopsy (concluded). II. The risk of needle biopsy. *N. Engl. J. Med.* **249**:1062–1069, 1953.

160. Zornoza, J.: *Percutaneous Needle Biopsy*. Baltimore, Williams & Wilkins, 1980.

161. Zornoza, J., Jonsson, K., Wallace, S., Lukeman, J. M.: Fine needle aspiration biopsy of retroperitoneal lymph nodes and abdominal masses: An updated report. *Radiology* **125**:87–88, 1977.

162. Zornoza, J., Snow, J., Lukeman, J. M., Libshitz, H. I.: Aspiration biopsy of discrete pulmonary lesions using a new thin needle. *Radiology* **123**:519–520, 1977.

163. Zornoza, J., Wallace, S., Goldstein, H. M., Lukeman, J. M., Jing, B.: Transperitoneal percutaneous retroperitoneal lymph node aspiration biopsy. *Radiology* **122**:111–115, 1977.

164. Zornoza, J., Wallace, S., Ordonez, N., Lukeman, J. M.: Fine-needle biopsy of the liver. *A.J.R.* **134**:331–334, 1980.

27 THE IMPACT OF FUTURE TECHNOLOGY ON ONCOLOGIC DIAGNOSIS

William R. Hendee

The detection of suspected cancer by methods of radiologic imaging followed by histologic analysis of a biopsy sample of suspected tissue is almost an exact science, limited only by the capability of the imaging system to reveal the presence of cancer in the first place. This limitation, however, should not be taken lightly, because dissemination of the cancer by metastasis or invasion of the primary cancer into critical tissues often has occurred by the time the cancer is detected radiologically. Improved methods of radiologic detection are required to identify the presence of cancer in an earlier state of development where it is more amenable to treatment. These methods depend on future technologic developments in radiologic imaging, the course of which can only be speculated upon at this time. In any field, speculations on the future are subject to substantial misjudgments, especially if the field is experiencing rapid technologic evolution. Such an evolution is occurring today in radiologic imaging, and speculations on the future are educated guesses at best. Still, such speculations are necessary so that individuals specializing in the field, and especially students of the discipline, can prepare themselves educationally and technically to exploit new developments when they become available. Furthermore, a speculative approach is required to address the title of this chapter; not only is the course of new technology to be predicted, but also the impact of this technology on oncologic diagnosis is to be estimated.

For any radiologic imaging system, the quality of the images and their value in cancer detection can be characterized in terms of four fundamental properties. These properties are spatial resolution, contrast discrimination, image noise, and the presence of distortion or artifacts (Table 27-1). Of these four properties, contrast discrimination probably is the variable in greatest need of improvement if major advances are to be realized in the early detection and diagnosis of cancer. A growing awareness of the importance of improvements in this imaging characteristic is the principal reason for the current interest in new imaging technologies such as digital radiography and magnetic resonance imaging (MRI) as well as for the sustained interest in developing improved contrast agents for various imaging modalities and in identifying quantitative techniques for differentiation of pathologic from normal tissues. Because of the adverse influence of image noise on contrast discrimination, considerable effort also is being directed toward the reduction of noise in different imaging modalities. Improvements in spatial resolution also are important if tumors are to be detected in an earlier state of development. However, the significance of this image property pales alongside the importance of contrast discrimination to earlier radiologic detection of the majority of cancers. Finally, image distortion and the presence of artifacts invariably interfere with the visualization of tumors that are marginally detectable under the best of circumstances. Selected images from various imaging modalities are compared in Figures 27-1, 27-2, and 27-3.

There can be little argument with the observation that radiologic imaging is in the midst of a technologic revolution, with many exciting developments implemented over the past ten years and many more just a few months

Table 27-1. Imaging Characteristics of Selected Diagnostic Systems

MODALITY	SPATIAL RESOLU-TION	CONTRAST RESOLU-TION	TEMPORAL RESOLU-TION	SIGNAL-TO-NOISE RATIO	DISTORTION AND ARTIFACTS	WIDE-SPREAD APPLI-CATION	COST
Roentgenography	E	P	E	E	F	E	E
Fluoroscopy	F	P	E	F	F	F	F
Digital Subtraction Angiography	P	E	E	P	F	P	F
X-ray Computed Tomography	F	E	F	P	F	F	P
Ultrasonography	F	P	E	F	F	F	E
Positron Tomography	P	F	P	F	F	P	P
Nuclear Medicine	P	P	P	P	F	F	E
Magnetic Resonance	P	E	P	P	F	F	P

E = excellent; F = fair; P = poor. Reprinted from *Diagnostic Imaging,* May, 1983. With permission.

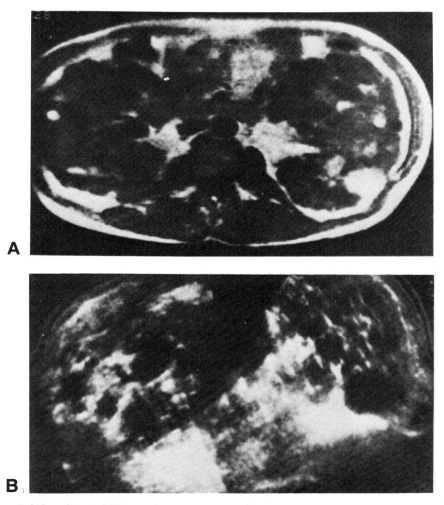

FIG. 27-1. Polycystic kidney disease. (A) Magnetic resonance image shows both kidneys to be markedly enlarged. The renal parenchyma is replaced by cysts of various size. There are different signal intensities in the cysts ranging from low values for simple cysts to a high-intensity cyst with T_1 and T_2 relaxation times suggestive of hemorrhagic cysts. The largest hemorrhagic cyst is seen at the posterior lateral aspect of the left kidney. (B) A transverse supine sonogram at a similar anatomic level shows both kidneys to be large. The renal parenchyma is replaced by cysts of various sizes. All of the cysts have similar echo characteristics, and differentiation between simple and hemorrhagic cysts is not possible. (Reprinted from Hricak, H., Crooks, L., Sheldon, P., Kaufman, L.: Nuclear magnetic resonance imaging of the kidney. *Radiology* 146:425–432, 1983. With permission.)

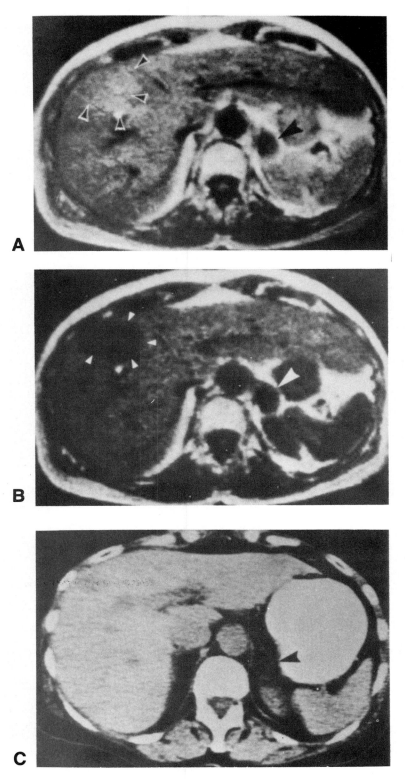

FIG. 27-2. Carcinoid tumor metastatic to the left adrenal (large arrow-head) and liver (small arrowheads). (A) The metastatic focus appears as a low-intensity mass with a slight heterogeneous interior on this spin-echo MR image. The round structure adjacent to the metastasis is the stomach. (B) This IR 1000/420 image exhibits greater tissue contrast, with tissues having a relatively long T_1 appearing darker. The hepatic metastasis is seen best on this view. (C) The metastasis has low attenuation and a homogeneous center (arrowhead) on this CT scan. (Reprinted from Moon, K. L., Jr., Hricak, H., Crookes, L. E., Gooding, C. A., Moss, A. A., Engelstad, B. L., Kaufman, L.: Nuclear magnetic resonance imaging of the adrenal gland: A Preliminary Report. *Radiology* **147**: 155–160, 1983. With permission.)

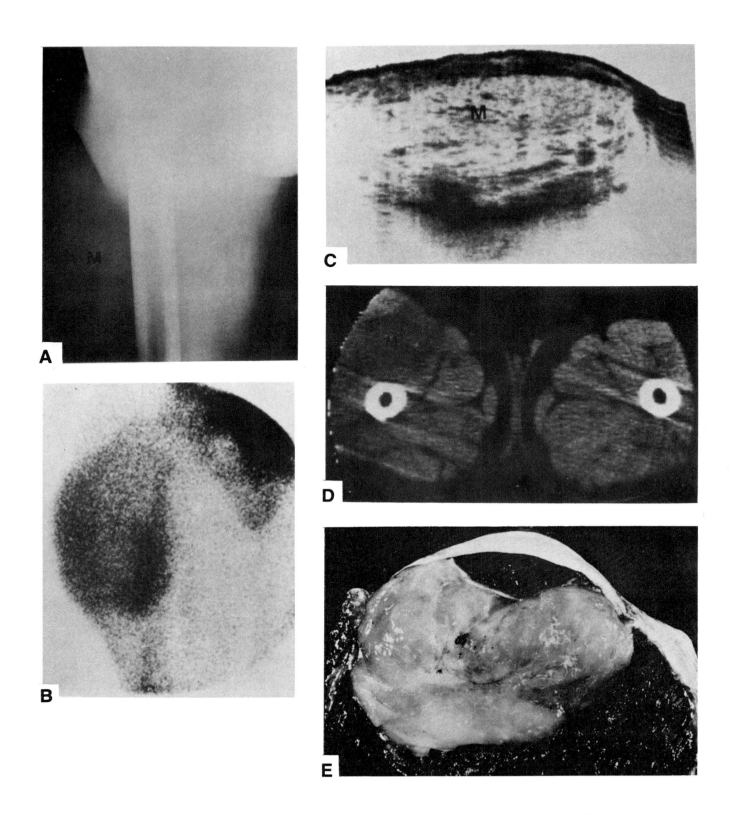

FIG. 27-3. (A) A conventional roentgenogram shows a large soft tissue mass (M) involving the lateral aspect of the right thigh. (B) An anterior radionuclide bone scan shows an area of increased activity in the soft tissue corresponding to the position of the mass seen on the roentgenogram. (C) A longitudinal ultrasonogram demonstrates a well-defined echogenic mass (M). (D) A CT scan shows a low attenuation mass (M) involving the anterior compartment. (E) The resected specimen confirms a diagnosis of a malignant fibrous histiocytoma. (Reprinted from Yiu-Chiu, V. S., Chiu, L. C.: Complementary values of ultrasound and computed tomography in the evaluation of musculoskeletal masses. *Radiographics* 3:46–82, 1983. With permission.)

or years away (Table 27-2). With identification of the improvements needed to enhance the contribution of radiologic imaging to the earlier detection of cancer, these developments can be channeled in part to attain this objective. It is towards attainment of this objective that this chapter is dedicated.

MAGNETIC RESONANCE

Since the 1940s, nuclear magnetic resonance (NMR)* has been used in physics and chemistry to study the structure of organic and biochemical molecules and other complex chemical configurations. The importance of NMR was acknowledged in 1952 when Bloch and Purcell received the Nobel Prize for development of this analytical tool.[9,96] More recently, applications of NMR have been extended to investigations of the biochemistry of living tissues. For example, NMR analysis of the concentration of different chemical forms of phosphorus in tissue can reveal the metabolic state of the tissue and the presence of various disease processes.[19,79,103] Even the biochemistry of internal organs can be studied in vivo by NMR.[1,32,89,98]

In 1971, Damadian proposed that certain properties characteristic of cancerous tissue may be detectable by NMR.[25] This proposal stimulated several investigations of the utility of NMR as a tool for cancer detection and diagnosis. Some of the investigations revealed differences between normal and cancerous tissue,[10,13,31,110] primarily in the values of relaxation times associated with the NMR signal. In general, however, these differences have been identified in extracted tissue samples where the NMR signals from cancerous and surrounding normal tissue can be compared without the perturbing influence of the remainder of the body. Extension of these results to in vivo detection of cancer by quantitative measure-

Table 27.2. Emerging Imaging Technologies
Important to Oncologic Diagnosis

Very Important
    Magnetic resonance
    Digital radiography
    Monoclonal antibody imaging
Probably Important
    Emission computed tomography
    Quantitative methods in imaging
        Transmission computed tomography
        Ultrasound
Possibly Important
    Diaphonography (transillumination)
    Microwave thermography

---

*In laboratory applications, the expression nuclear magnetic resonance (NMR) is used to connote analytic techniques utilizing the magnetic properties of nuclei. In the imaging applications of these techniques, the expression magnetic resonance (MR) or magnetic resonance imaging (MRI) is preferred.

ment of relaxation times of the NMR signal has been relatively unproductive, at least up to the present time. One application of NMR to the detection of cancer may be its usefulness in distinguishing differences in blood perfusion or extracellular fluid space between tumors and adjacent normal tissues.[24]

Damadian's original proposal concerning the detection of cancer by NMR included the hypothesis that the spin-lattice relaxation time T_1 of hydrogen is longer in tumors than in normal tissues.[25] Since the relaxation time of hydrogen is related in part to the freedom of motion of water molecules, this hypothesis led to speculation that the concentration of structurally bound water is different in cancerous and noncancerous tissues. A difference in bound water has even been postulated to extend to noncancerous organs and sera of tumor-bearing animals and patients. Termed a *systemic effect*,[7] this whole-body response to cancer might lead to longer relaxation times for the sera of cancer patients and, thereby, a sensitive mechanism for detection of the presence of cancer anywhere in the body. However, investigations of the systemic effect have led to the conclusion that elevated NMR measurements of hydrogen relaxation times in sera can reflect a variety of disease states and are not a specific indication of cancer.[58]

At the present time, the most promising application of NMR for the detection and diagnosis of cancer, as well as for the variety of other disease processes, is as a clinical imaging instrument. Magnetic resonance imaging (MRI) probably is the most exciting development in medical imaging since the advent of X-ray transmission computed tomography in the early 1970s. This development was proposed originally by Lauterbur in 1973[70] and offers at least five fundamental characteristics of tissues as imaging variables. The characteristics are (1) the concentration of a particular element in the tissues; (2) the spin-lattice relaxation time T_1 of the element in the tissues; (3) the spin-spin relaxation time T_2 of the element in the tissues; (4) frequency shifts associated with the chemical compounds into which the element is incorporated; and (5) motion caused, for example, by flowing blood in the tissues. The spin-lattice relaxation time T_1 (also termed the thermal or longitudinal relaxation time) reflects the exchange of energy between an excited nucleus and other atoms in the surrounding molecular lattice. The relaxation time T_1 describes the time required for decay of the magnetic resonance signal as a result of realignment after application of a radio frequency energy pulse. The spin-spin relaxation time T_2 (also termed the transverse relaxation time) reflects the exchange of energy between an excited nucleus and other precessing nuclei in a magnetic field. The relaxation time T_2 describes the time required for decay of the magnetic resonance signal as a result of dephasing after application of a radio-frequency energy pulse.

The physical properties of flow and spectral shift can be evaluated by magnetic resonance techniques. The first property can be measured as a result of the alteration in an MR signal resulting from the flow of blood into the sample region; measurement of the change in signal strength provides an indirect measure of the flow rate of blood into the region. The second property is an indication of the molecular configuration of the element of interest. To date, most spectral shift measurements in clinical medicine have been confined to hydrogen; however, other elements, especially phosphorus, are receiving increasing attention.

In vivo images of MRI variables have been confined to the element hydrogen, primarily because of the generous signal-to-noise ratio of this element compared with other elements and because of its relatively high concentration in biologic tissues. In the body, hydrogen occurs primarily in body water and secondarily in fat; therefore, MRI images of hydrogen depict primarily the distribution of body water and, to a somewhat lesser degree, the lipid content of various tissues. Other elements in the body that may be amenable to MRI include phosphorus, sodium, and, possibly, fluorine as a contrast agent; however, the resolution attainable with these elements will be far inferior to that achievable with hydrogen. Although other elements, including nitrogen, oxygen, carbon, potassium, and chlorine, yield an MRI signal, their low concentrations and poor signal-to-noise ratios probably preclude their serious consideration as elements for imaging.[23,54,68] On the other hand, quantitative MRI measurements of these elements in localized regions of tissue may reveal the presence of selected disease processes, including cancer.

As mentioned earlier, MRI offers the possibility for obtaining images with excellent contrast resolution for the element hydrogen and with spatial resolution that is competitive with that in computed tomographic images. Spatial resolution as fine as 1 mm or so has been attained for MRI, and multi-slice scanning techniques have been developed that yield 15–20 contiguous cross-sectional images in times as short as a few minutes.[12,58]

Although the contrast resolution of MR images is excellent, it may be enhanced in specific regions by administration of one of several potential contrast agents. These agents, known as paramagnetic substances, possess unpaired electrons that introduce nonuniformities in their immediate magnetic environment. The nonuniformities influence the spin-lattice relaxation times of nearby hydrogen nuclei to produce a stronger MR signal, thereby yielding an enhancement of the region in the MR image. Paramagnetic elements that may serve as useful contrast agents include the lanthanides, transition series metals, and nitroxide stable-free radicals.

The rate of advancement in the clarity of information in MR images has been little short of spectacular over the past few years. Of similar spectacular proportions has been the commitment of the medical imaging industry to the commercialization of MRI. A number of imaging instruments have been developed that use permanent, resistive, and superconducting magnets. It now appears that image clarity is improved at higher magnetic field strengths. For this reason, superconducting systems operating between 0.3 and 2 tesla may have some advantages over magnetic resonance units using magnets of lower field strengths.

Magnetic resonance imaging represents the most recent application of advanced technology to medical imaging[51,52] and promises to provide significant advances not only in clinical imaging but also in the acquisition of data related to a variety of physiologic and metabolic processes and their disturbance by pathologic conditions. In particular, MR imaging promises to yield significant improvements in the detection and diagnosis of cancer because of its exquisite rendition of low contrast information[108] and because of its ability to reveal information in bony regions (e.g., the posterior fossa and the pelvis) that are not readily accessible by techniques employing ionizing radiation (Figures 27-1–27-3). Although these potential advances are viewed with considerable enthusiasm by medical imagers, their expense is not insignificant in terms of both the initial investment and operating costs. In addition, extensive training of physicians and operating personnel will be required if this new technology is to be exploited to its fullest. These promises and problems make MRI one of the more stimulating and challenging areas for both basic and clinical research associated with the adoption of advanced technology to medical problems, including cancer detection and diagnosis.

RADIOACTIVELY TAGGED ANTIBODIES

For almost a century, antibodies have been used clinically for a variety of purposes, including tissue and blood typing, identification of micro-organisms, and passive immunization.[105] With the development of radiolabeled and enzyme-linked immunoassay procedures over the past three decades, the usefulness of antibodies has been extended to the detection and quantification of a wide spectrum of substances, including hormones, drugs, and enzymes. Today, antibodies are a major diagnostic tool in virtually every clinical laboratory.

Even though antibody techniques are used widely in medicine, they have been handicapped considerably by the unavailability of methods for making specific antibodies in a dependable and reproducible manner. In many ways, the production of specific antibodies has been more of an art than a science.[113] In the past few years, however, a method has evolved to produce almost unlimited quantities of homogeneous antibodies. These monoclonal antibodies promise to open new arenas for immunoassay procedures, possibly including the detection and diagnosis of cancer.

The body is capable of producing millions of different antibodies, with each antibody designed to react with one of the seemingly endless variety of antigens present in nature. By their electrophoretic behavior, these antibodies, also termed immunoglobulins, can be categorized within the class of serum proteins known as gamma globulins. The basic structure of any antibody molecule is four polypeptide chains, with two identical chains possessing a molecular weight of 55,000 to 75,000 and two other identical chains exhibiting a molecular weight of about 25,000. The chains are attached to each other by disulfide bonds. One end of the antibody molecule, termed the constant (or carboxy terminal) region, is restricted in the number of amino acid sequences available to each chain. This restriction determines the class of the antibody as well as the class of the heavy and light chains, with two classes of light chains and eight or nine classes of heavy chains available. In general, different classes of antibodies exhibit different biologic activities.

The chains at the opposite (amino terminal) end of the antibody molecule have much greater variability in the sequence of amino acids. It is this variable end of the antibody molecule that determines the antigenic specificity of the antibody. It is also this end of the antibody that makes contact with an antigen. The structural heterogeneity of the variable end of the antibody molecule provides a wide assortment of three-dimensional binding sites, with complementarity between antigen and antibody at only one site required for an antibody to attach to an antigen.

If an antigen is introduced into the body, it ultimately is presented to cells (B lymphocytes or their progeny, plasma cells) that contain a surface antibody that reacts with the antigen. Following this reaction, the cells are stimulated to generate clones of plasma cells that secrete antibodies to the antigen. That is, each of the many antigenic determinants in a macromolecular antigen stimulates the production of antibodies that interact specifically with that determinant. For this reason, even a very pure antigen leads to a mixture of antibodies with different antigenic specificities in the serum. In the inoculation of animals with an antigen for the production of antigerm, for example, the resulting mixture of antibodies may vary from one animal to the next and even in the same animal from one inoculation to the next. It is this nonspecificity that has made the isolation of specific antibodies so difficult, at least until monoclonal antibodies become available.

In 1975, Köhler and Milstein[66] developed a method for producing large quantities of monoclonal antibodies. The method involves the fusion (hybridization) of plasma cells with myeloma cells. In the final product (hybrid-oma), the plasma cells contribute the capacity to secrete a specific antibody and the myeloma cells provide the properties of longevity in culture and tumorigenicity in animals. By selecting plasma cells for the hybridization process that produce a specific antibody of interest, relatively large quantities of a specific antibody can be produced. Details of the technique for producing hybridomas are available.[63,89,105,114]

Once a hybridoma has been created, it provides a source of specific antibody for an indefinite period of time. The antibody can be extracted from the tissue culture medium supporting the antibody or in even larger quantities by injecting the hybridoma cells into mice, where they form ascitic tumors and produce antibody in the ascitic fluid. From an inoculated mouse, 10 to 15 ml of ascitic fluid can be obtained with a concentration of antibody 100 to 1,000 times greater than that in an immunized animal.

Hybridoma technology promises to provide significant advances in a variety of fields, including the detection and diagnosis of cancer. For example, Levy et al.[72] have developed two hybridomas that produce antibody capable of distinguishing malignant from normal cells in the peripheral blood and bone marrow of children with acute lymphocytic leukemia. Ritz et al.[99] have produced a monoclonal antibody that recognizes an antigen (CALLA) present on the cells of many patients with acute lymphoblastic leukemia and some patients with chronic myelogenous leukemia. Investigators[85] in the same laboratory have developed an antibody that appears to characterize a subgroup of poorly differentiated lymphomas.

Currently, two obstacles impede the application of monoclonal antibody technology to human disease. The first is the lack of suitable human monoclonal antibodies. Antibodies produced by animal hybridomas are suitable for in vitro studies, but they could cause allergic reactions if administered repeatedly to humans. The work of Olsson and Kaplan[89] with hybridomas derived from human cells promises to provide guidance in overcoming this obstacle. The second obstacle is the derivation of hybridomas from malignant cells; conceivably, human administration of antibodies from such hybridomas could result in transmission of virus particles associated with malignancy to the recipient.

Considerable interest has evolved in the use of monoclonal antibodies as a mechanism for in vivo delivery of agents for the diagnosis and treatment of cancer. Some cancer cells may be characterized by a loss of certain antigens associated with their normal cell counterparts, as well as by the addition of certain other antigens. The added antigens often display fetal characteristics and are known as oncofetal or carcinoembryonic antigens (CEAs).[40] Ferritin is another antigen often found at elevated concentrations in tumor cells.[8,60,76,90,104] Other tumor-associated antigens have been detected by gel precipitation,[84,96] lymphocyte cytotoxicity studies,[113] and radioimmunoassay.[4] Some of these antigens may be present on the surface of selected tumor cells, where they are accessible to antibodies. This accessibility suggests that a radioactively tagged antibody specific for one or more of these surface antigens might serve as a biologic marker for the identification of cancer cells. Although a single unique antigen characteristic of all human cancer cells has not yet been identified, the presence of a spectrum of antigens associated with cancer cells of different types offers the potential for use of multiple antibody markers to identify the presence, metastasis, and recurrence of cancer in a variety of patients.

A number of investigators have explored the use of specific antibodies labeled with radioactive isotopes of iodine and technetium to identify the presence of tumor cells in experimental animals.[4,5,26,38,43,44,57,67,74,75,112] These studies have been extended to humans with less than complete success to date, principally because the antibodies do not yield an overall sensitivity and a specificity for tumor cells adequate for purposes of definitive imaging.[27,28,42,106] For example, a labeled antibody to the antigen ferritin has been compared with Ethiodol for lymphangiographic staging of breast cancer, with equivocal results.[112] In addition, some efforts have been directed towards use of radiolabeled antibodies for cancer therapy.[91,93,94] Although some success has been reported in this experimental approach to tumor therapy, repeated injections of radiolabeled antibodies have caused treatment-related mortality in animals, probably because of reactions of the antibodies with normal tissue constituents. Studies also have been reported in which labeled antibodies are used in combination with alkylating agents to enhance the therapeutic effect or to serve as a carrier for boron in neutron activation.[35,37,49,80,86,92,98] Another possible application of tumor-specific antibodies is their use as tools in targeting cytotoxic agents to tumors.[114]

The eventual role of radiolabeled antibodies in the detection and treatment of cancer is difficult to predict. Although initial efforts have revealed a number of difficulties associated with the sensitivity and specificity of the techniques employed, no intractable problems have been identified. With 10^2 to 10^5 antigenic sites per tumor cell and with 10^6 or so cells per cubic millimeter of tumor, the potential exists for tagging subclinical microscopic foci of cancer with up to 10^8 to 10^{11} radiolabeled antibodies. For an antibody labeled with a single ^{99m}Tc atom, this number of tagging sites translates to 0.09 to 90 μCi ($3.3 \times 10^3 - 3.2 \times 10^6$ 13 q) per cubic millimeter of tumor.

Continued research is needed on the isolation of antibodies with higher specificities for selected tumor cells, together with intelligent deployment of methods to circumvent present impediments associated with low target-to-nontarget ratios of the labeled antibodies. Among these methods may be tomographic imaging techniques for improved isolation of concentrations of radioactivity in tissue together with image manipulation techniques to suppress background radioactivity.[100]

QUANTITATIVE TECHNIQUES IN RADIOLOGY

Radiology is a discipline devoted to the production and interpretation of medical images. Within this discipline, however, the potential is developing for the interpretation of quantitative data for the purpose of more explicit detection and diagnosis of disease, including cancer. At the moment, this potential is most apparent in two radiologic modalities: transmission computed tomography and ultrasonography.

Transmission Computed Tomography

In transmission computed tomography, CT numbers are directly related to the linear attenuation coefficients of the corresponding tissues in a cross-sectional slice through the body. Since the linear attenuation coefficients reflect primarily the volume electron density (electrons/cm³) of the tissues, it is conceivable that analysis of a group of CT numbers could be used to characterize tissue composition. Although this potential has been discussed for years, it has not been realized to any significant degree for a variety of reasons. Included among these reasons are the problems of statistical imprecision and physical artifacts (e.g., beam hardening and volume averaging) in quantitative CT data and uncertainties in the correlation between observed CT numbers and chemical composition. Other obstacles to quantitative computed tomography include the design of CT units to display images more readily than quantitative data, the siting of CT units in image-oriented radiology departments, and the high demand for clinical CT studies, which precludes the use of most CT units for extensive research studies. In spite of these problems, quantitative computed tomography is a promising area for a selected number of applications, possibly including the detection and diagnosis of cancer.

Because of its anatomic simplicity, the brain has been the organ most studied by techniques of quantitative computed tomography. For example, Arimitsu et al. have compiled a listing of CT numbers without and with contrast medium for a number of structural components of the brain.[3] Fullerton[35] has described changes in CT numbers associated with the progression of a hematoma from early formation to eventual dissolution. Siegelman et al.[107] evaluated the CT numbers associated with pulmonary nodules in 88 patients in an effort to establish quantitative criteria for distinguishing benign from malignant lesions. For each nodule, the 32 volume elements with the highest CT values were identified and described by a single mean CT number. For malignant lesions, the highest mean CT number was 147 Hounsfield units (HU), while most of the benign lesions exhibited mean values of 164 HU and above. The higher values of the benign lesions probably was due to diffuse calcification. Other investigators have been unable to reproduce these quantitative criteria exactly, probably because of differences in CT equipment and techniques for procedure normalization. Nevertheless, qualitative agreement has been noted and offers encouragement for the increased application of quantitative computed tomography to other medical problems.

To increase the sensitivity of quantitative computed tomography to small differences in composition among similar tissues, the approach of multiple energy imaging may be useful.[51,52] In its simplest version, X-ray transmission data are collected at two distinct kilovolt peaks. Analysis of these data yields the distributions of atomic number and electron density across the tissue section of interest, within the limitations of statistical imprecision in the small differences in X-ray transmission measured at the two kilovolt peaks. Quantitative densitometry employing the dual kilovolt peak technique has been used in studies of the liver,[41] the brain,[31,77] and bone mineralization in normal and diseased patients.[11,36,47,73,103] The usefulness of multiple energy transmission measurements for tumor localization has not been resolved and presents a challenging arena for further research and development.

The evolution of quantitative computed tomography to a level where it contributes significantly to the detection and diagnosis of cancer depends upon the development of solutions to several problems. For example, specific tissues often exhibit a range of CT numbers, partly as a result of biologic variability and partly as a consequence of artifacts and imprecision in the processes of collecting transmission data and forming diagnostic images. To provide greater statistical certainty in measured CT numbers, improved software corrections for beam hardening and volume averaging are needed. In addition, techniques are required to normalize CT measurements to values near those characteristic of tissues of interest rather than to values representative of water, at least for those cases where the tissue CT values are greatly different from those for water. Also, improvements in the stability of computed tomographic equipment are needed to provide CT numbers of greater precision both temporally and spatially. As techniques are developed for improved reliability of CT values, and as more baseline data are accumulated for values of CT numbers characteristic of normal and diseased tissues, the quantitative use of CT numbers for the detection and diagnosis of cancer and other disease processes could conceivably become an important feature of transmission computed tomography.

Ultrasonography

As a pulse of ultrasound energy is propagated through or reflected in tissue, many changes occur in the pulse that are indicative of the physical characteristics of the tissue constituents and of the boundaries between these constituents. As a consequence, the ultrasound pulse emerging from the tissue is modulated extensively, and analysis of this modulation has the potential for revealing considerable information about tissue characteristics. This analysis of tissue signatures or "fingerprints" on ultrasound pulses propagated or reflected in tissue has been discussed for many years as a promising approach to definitive assessment of the characteristics of normal and diseased tissues. In 1976, for example, the statement was published that ". . . there is no question that research into quantitative tissue characterization will ultimately result in dramatic improvements in the capability of medical ultrasound. When combined with real time, high resolution imaging and implemented routinely in a clinical environment, these techniques could revolutionize medical diagnosis."[73] Unfortunately, this rather optimistic prediction of the potential role of quantitative ultrasound in medical diagnosis has not been matched by substantial progress in the analysis of tissue signatures in the eight years since its appearance.

The rather disappointing level of progress in quantitative ultrasonography is a result of at least three impediments to advances in the discipline. First, commercial instrumentation associated with diagnostic ultrasonography continues to emphasize the production of images, and this emphasis is not necessarily conducive to quantitative analysis of transmitted and reflected pulses of ultrasound. Second, the analysis of tissue signatures has proved to be more difficult than originally envisioned, primarily because the propagation of ultrasound pulses through tissue produces a variety of effects, including attenuation, reflection, diffraction, refraction, scattering, frequency dispersion, and velocity changes, and these effects are difficult to separate during analysis of the propagated pulses. Certainly the quantitative assessment of these effects is very complex compared with an analysis of the effects of tissue on transmitted X rays. A third limitation to the progress of quantitative ultrasonography may be that clinical applications of this approach have been confined primarily to analyses of normal and neoplastic breast tissue. The biologic characteristics of these analyses are especially complicated, even though breast tissues are readily accessible to study by transmitted and reflected ultrasound.

One approach to quantitative ultrasound analysis that has shown some progress is computed tomography with ultrasound. In this technique, ultrasound pulses transmitted through a particular body part are analyzed in much the same way as transmitted X-ray beams are evaluated to form transaxial images in X-ray computed tomography. To date, ultrasonic computed tomography has used pencil-like and fan-shaped ultrasound beams and a simple translate-rotate geometry for data acquisition similar to that employed in first-generation X-ray CT scanners. However, more sophisticated geometries such as purely rotational motion of transmitting and receiving transducers are certainly feasible.

A wide spectrum of ultrasonic characteristics of tissues are accessible by transmission computed tomography with ultrasound. For example, measurements of the amplitude of transmitted pulses can be analyzed by reconstruction mathematics to yield a two-dimensional matrix of attenuation coefficients similar to those obtained in transmission X-ray computed tomography.[47] These coefficients can be displayed as gray scale attenuation images or analyzed quantitatively to depict differences in attenuation from one region of tissue to another. However, the data are distorted somewhat by physical processes such as reflection and refraction. This distortion yields a relatively significant imprecision in the resulting data that can mask the small differences in attenuation that may distinguish normal from neoplastic tissue.

The speed of propagation of ultrasound through tissue is a second ultrasonic characteristic that is measurable by computed tomographic techniques. Compared with attenuation data, this characteristic promises somewhat greater return in terms of clinical usefulness. The speed of sound is determined by measuring the transmit time of the leading edge of an ultrasound pulse through the tissue. By obtaining these measurements at a variety of translational positions and angular orientations, a matrix of ultrasound speeds can be reconstructed for quantitative analysis or for display as a gray scale image. Speed of sound reconstructions have been compiled by Greenleaf and Johnson[46] at the Mayo Clinic, Glover and Sharp at the General Electric Company,[39] and Carson et al.[20,21] at the Universities of Colorado and Michigan. Each of these groups has reported that speed of sound measurements reveal distinct differences between normal and neoplastic tissue in breasts examined by ultrasound computed tomography.

In addition to attenuation and ultrasonic speed, other ultrasonic characteristics of tissues have been proposed for analysis by reconstructive techniques. Among these characteristics are variations in ultrasonic attenuation with changes in the frequency of the ultrasound pulse,[65] absorption as distinguished from attenuation of ultrasound in biologic tissues, and acoustic impedance (the product of the mass density of the tissue and the speed of ultrasound through the tissue).[53] The quantitative determination of ultrasound scattering[30] and measurement of the velocity of moving fluids in the body[53] also have been proposed as potential applications of ultrasound computed tomography.

From measurements of the speed of sound, it may be possible to construct tomographic maps of the temperature distribution in tissues, including thermal maps that facilitate the use of hyperthermia as an adjunct to radiation therapy.[59] It may also be possible to use speed of sound measurements to determine corrections for ultrasound refraction in B-mode reflection and CT attenuation images.[48,82] Development of these and other applications requires sophisticated methods for analysis of transmitted (and reflected) ultrasound signals and may not materialize until the fundamental interactions of ultrasound energy in tissue are understood more completely. Initial applications of more sophisticated techniques for signal analysis include iterative corrections for refraction of the ultrasound beam[59] and reconstruction algorithms that assume weak scattering of the beam.[82] Jones et al.[61] and Kak and Dines[62] also have attempted to characterize the ultrasonic properties of tissues by reconstruction methods.

Bone and gas interfere with the transmission of ultrasound, and quantitative ultrasonography employing transmitted beams of ultrasound energy probably is limited to regions of the body where these disturbing influences are not present. Among these regions are the female breast, the male genitals, the infant head and, possibly, certain parts of the extremities such as the wrist. Application of ultrasound computed tomography to other body parts probably requires the use of reflected rather than transmitted ultrasound, with the concomitant increase in complexity of reconstruction techniques.[30,87] Up to this time, ultrasound computed tomography has been directed primarily to the production of transmission reconstruction images of the breast. Although the clinical utility of this application is still unresolved, initial results are promising, especially in combination with B-mode reflection images.[20,45]

DIGITAL RADIOGRAPHY

Considerable interest has developed in the application of digital techniques of data acquisition, manipulation, and display to the traditional field of roentgenographic imaging. To date this application has centered primarily around the method of digital fluoroscopy, where the electronic signal from a television camera coupled optically with an image intensifier is digitized before its entry into a dedicated computer. Digital fluoroscopy has been applied almost exclusively to cardiac and visceral angiography, where it is proving to be moderately useful for real-time temporal subtraction.[56,79] At this time the technique is important to the detection and localization of cancer only to the extent that real-time subtraction techniques in angiography yield more information about the vasculature in selected regions and its perturbation because of the presence of a tumor.

A second approach to digital radiography that is under investigation is scan projection radiography.[15,71] In this method, a bank of detectors scans across the patient to measure the transmitted X-ray intensity. The method resembles X-ray transmission computed tomography and in fact evolved from a method developed in computed tomography to localize planes for transaxial tomographic imaging. The electronic signal is digitized and transmitted to a dedicated computer for processing and formatting of the final image. Although scan projection radiography is not very useful for temporal subtraction, it is very compatible with energy subtraction techniques in which images obtained at different X-ray energies are subtracted to reveal variations in tissue composition that are not detectable in the originals. The original as well as the subtraction image can be displayed on a video terminal where the density and contrast can be varied in a manner similar to that in transmission computed tomography. The potential of scan projection radiography is under evaluation at the present time; the ability of the technique to enhance image contrast by energy subtraction and image manipulation offers some promise that the method may be useful in the future for detection and diagnosis of selected types of cancer.

Digital fluoroscopy and scan projection radiography are very limited glimpses of the true potential of digital radiography. Many of the roentgenographic images captured today on film may ultimately be recorded, developed, and stored by digital methods. Before this potential can be realized, fundamental problems must be solved in the production of digital data directly from the impinging X-ray beam and in the rapid transmission and storage of these data in a digital format. Neither of these problems is close to solution today, although advances towards the solutions are being made continuously. These advances promise that true digital radiography may become a reality in another five to ten years, and that its adaptability to techniques of image enhancement and contrast modification may yield significant improvements in the detection and diagnosis of cancer.

EMISSION COMPUTED TOMOGRAPHY

The principles of computed tomography are applicable to the investigation of radionuclides within the body as well as to the study of X-ray and ultrasound transmission through the body. In this application, termed *emission computed tomography* (ECT), tomographic images are reconstructed that reveal the distribution of a radioactive nuclide in selected regions of the body. Compared with conventional nuclear medicine procedures, ECT can

yield improved image contrast and spatial resolution at depth. More importantly, functional and physiologic processes can be evaluated in ways not accessible by more conventional imaging methods. The technique has shown some potential for the evaluation of tumors in the brain, uterus, and other body sites and has been proposed as a promising method for monitoring the course of radiotherapy and chemotherapy of cancer.[16]

The subject of emission computed tomography can be separated into two topics: (1) single photon emission tomography, and (2) positron emission tomography.

Single Photon Emission Computed Tomography

In single photon emission computed tomography (SPECT), radiopharmaceuticals may be used that are identical with those employed for conventional nuclear medicine imaging. Two approaches to SPECT have been developed. In the first approach, termed longitudinal tomography, images are formed along planes parallel to the long axis of the patient's body. The second approach provides images perpendicular to the long axis. This approach is described as transaxial tomography.

Longitudinal Tomography. In the late 1960s, Anger attempted to produce analogue tomographic images with the scintillation camera.[2] These efforts led ultimately to the first commercial instrument, the "Pho-Con,"* designed to produce tomographic nuclear medicine images. In this instrument, two 9.3-inch diameter by 0.5-inch thick scintillation detectors scan in synchrony on opposite sides of the patient. During the scanning process, γ-ray emission data are accumulated and used to form the tomographic image. Data for as many as 12 tomographic planes can be obtained from one transverse scan. These data can be used to form transaxial as well as longitudinal tomographic images.[50]

Longitudinal tomographic images also can be produced by using coded apertures in place of the conventional collimators employed with stationary scintillation cameras. The use of coded apertures was pioneered by Barrett,[6] who used a Fresnel zone plate as a coded aperture. With the zone plate positioned in front of the scintillation camera, each point of radioactivity in the patient projects a unique image of the zone plate onto a film. By the illumination of the processed film with laser light, tomographic images at various depths can be formed. Compared with conventional collimators, zone plate apertures provide greater sensitivity because fewer γ-rays are absorbed in the collimating material. However, images obtained with zone plates have been rather disappointing

---

*The Pho-Con was developed by Searle Radiographics, Inc. (now Siemens Gammasonics, Inc.)

to date, primarily because of a high level of background noise, especially in images of large anatomic regions.

A somewhat different approach to zone plate apertures is the use of time-coded multiple apertures developed by Rogers et al.[101] In this approach, a lead plate with several pinholes is moved in stepwise fashion across a second plate with additional pinholes. The second plate is attached to the face of the scintillation camera. At each step, projections formed by the transmission of γ-rays through the sets of pinholes are analyzed to form longitudinal tomographic images at separations as close as 1 cm. Limitations in time-coded multiple apertures are similar to those for stationary zone plates, and the approach has not yet yielded an acceptable solution to tomographic imaging in the clinical arena.

In 1978, Vogel et al.[111] developed the stationary multiple pinhole technique for forming longitudinal tomographic images. In this approach, multiple stationary pinholes in the detector collimator project separate images of the distribution of radioactivity onto distinct regions of the scintillation crystal. From these separate projections, tomographic images can be produced through an iterative reconstruction process. With the multiple pinhole technique, all of the projection data can be obtained during a single exposure of about the same duration as that required for a conventional scintillation camera image. Lateral resolution is reasonably satisfactory, with some degradation at greater depths in the patient. Depth resolution is rather poor, and the field of view is limited to relatively small regions. Advantages of the stationary pinhole approach include relatively low cost and the ability to expand a conventional camera to tomographic imaging by addition of a multiple pinhole collimator and the appropriate software packages. Multiple pinhole collimators and appropriate software are offered commercially by several companies as attachments to conventional scintillation cameras.

A number of alternatives have been developed to the multiple pinhole approach to tomographic imaging in nuclear medicine. Among the alternatives are rotating slant-hole collimators[34,54,82] and quadrant-hole collimators.[22,109] Compared with stationary pinhole collimators, these alternatives offer a larger field of view, increased sensitivity, and improved lateral resolution at depth. Also, positioning of the patient is less critical. Disadvantages of the alternatives include their greater mechanical complexity and the need to acquire individual projections sequentially rather than simultaneously, somewhat compromising the usefulness of slant-hole and quadrant-hole collimators for dynamic imaging.

Transaxial Tomography. Single photon transaxial tomography was introduced by Kuhl and Edwards,[69] who used multiple detectors surrounding the patient to measure the emission of γ-rays from a region of interest. The approach has been pursued principally for the detection of tumors and other anomalies of the brain. Commercial units modeled after the Kuhl and Edwards scanner showed some promise clinically, but did not capture a large enough fraction of the marketplace to maintain their commercial viability.[55] One of the major disadvantages with all multicrystal transaxial tomographic scanners has been the rather lengthy times required for data collection.

An alternate approach to transaxial tomography has been developed that employs a single-crystal scintillation crystal.[66,84] Although the approach can be implemented by rotating the upright patient in front of a scintillation camera, a preferred approach is to rotate the camera with the patient remaining stationary. Over the past few years, many of the major suppliers of imaging instrumentation for nuclear medicine have introduced rotating scintillation cameras and associated computer software for transaxial tomographic imaging. Although the clinical usefulness of the technique has not been thoroughly documented, initial clinical results appear promising for a variety of studies, including those of tumor detection. One advantage of the rotating camera for transaxial tomography is its usefulness for conventional as well as tomographic imaging of the distribution of radioactivity within patients.

Comparative evaluations of multiple pinhole, rotating collimator, multicrystal, and rotating camera tomographic systems have recently begun to appear.[17,18]

Most applications of single photon tomography to date have been directed to cardiac studies, where proponents of the technique claim that tomographic sections are useful in delineating pathologic conditions not readily visible in nontomographic projections. The definitive evaluation of these claims remains to be made. Other applications of single photon tomography, including those of detection and diagnosis of various tumors, are less well developed, and the usefulness of the technique for these purposes is even less certain.

Positron Emission Tomography

For a number of years investigators have explored the feasibility of producing images by detecting the annihilation radiation released during positron decay of radionuclides distributed within the body. This approach to radionuclide imaging has two advantages.

(1) the only readily available radioisotopes of carbon, nitrogen, and oxygen (^{11}C, ^{13}N, ^{15}O) are positron emitters. These nuclides can be labeled isotopically into compounds of biologic interest, resulting in radiopharmaceuticals that are more stable and possibly more specific for selected tissue sites than are those radiopharmaceuticals tagged nonisotopically with radionuclides such as ^{99m}Tc and ^{131}I. Furthermore, these nuclides can be tagged

to compounds that are metabolically active, such as deoxyglucose, so that direct imaging studies of metabolism may be possible.

(2) The detection of annihilation radiation by coincidence counting eliminates the need for mechanical collimators, currently the major limitation to improvements in sensitivity and spatial resolution in nuclear medicine imaging. Positron imaging presents an opportunity to improve the sensitivity of nuclear medicine imaging by factors as high as five- to ten-fold with no significant deterioration in spatial resolution.[54]

In commercial positron cameras, three approaches have been taken to the design of the detector geometry. In the parallel-opposed multicrystal array pioneered by Brownell et al.,[17] opposing banks of 140 2×2-cm NaI crystals are operated to provide 2,848 possible coincidence pairs of detectors. During a single scan, the crystal banks collect data at 29 angular positions to yield 23 separate tomographic sections spaced 1 to 4 cm apart.

In their PETT I–IV scanners (PETT = Positron Emission Transaxial Tomography), Ter Pogossian et al.[110] have pursued the hexagonal array approach to the design of detector assemblies for positron tomography. In one version of this approach (PETT IV), 66 NaI crystals are distributed in a hexagonal configuration to provide six banks of 11 crystals each, with each detector operated in coincidence with all 11 detectors in the opposite bank. In this manner, 363 coincidence pairs of detectors are available. During a scan, the detector banks move linearly for a few centimeters, then rotate between 5° and 10° and repeat the translational motion. The sequence is repeated over several angular increments until the entire detector assembly has rotated through 60°.

Most recent units for positron tomography employ one or more rings of scintillation detectors completely surrounding the patient. Compared with earlier positron cameras, these units capture more of the annihilation photons and provide as many as nine tomographic sections simultaneously. The spatial resolution of the images is about 7 to 8 mm for the ring-type positron cameras and may be improved to 4 to 5 mm in the near future. Improvements in spatial resolution beyond 4 to 5 mm are limited by the finite range of positrons in tissue and the slight divergence of annihilation photons from a straight line through their origin. The latest versions of the PETT scanner (PETT V and VI) employ a ring geometry, as do the positron cameras marketed by several manufacturers.

With the use of newer scintillation detectors (e.g., bismuth germanate and cesium fluoride) with fluorescence decay times shorter than that for sodium iodide, the potential has materialized for time-of-flight positron tomography, in which differences are measured in the time of arrival of annihilation photons at opposing detectors. These difference measurements permit determination of the origin of the photons along a line between the two detectors. Time-of-flight measurements ultimately may yield further improvements in the spatial resolution of positron tomographic images.

Positron tomography is an expensive process. First, positron cameras are expensive to purchase. Their optimum use requires the availability of ^{11}C, ^{13}N, and ^{15}O, all short-lived radionuclides that require a cyclotron for their production. In addition, a sophisticated radiochemical laboratory is necessary for separation of the desired radionuclides from the highly radioactive cyclotron targets and for incorporation of these radionuclides into the pharmaceuticals of interest. The initial investment required for positron tomography is $2 million to $3 million. In addition, a substantial operating budget is required. For this reason, positron tomography is being pursued in only a few institutions at present, and the technique is at present more a research tool than a clinical modality. This status could change, however, if positron tomography were to prove useful for early detection of diseases such as senile dementia or certain types of cancer that are not accessible to other imaging modalities.

CONCLUSIONS

Advances are occurring at such a rapid rate in medical imaging that the field often is described as experiencing a technologic revolution. Many of these advances are associated with introduction of the computer into imaging systems and the concomitant enhanced flexibility for display of information useful in medical diagnosis. For example, the techniques of magnetic resonance, quantitative computed tomography, ultrasound computed tomography, digital radiography, and emission computed tomography discussed above depend on the availability of computers and rather sophisticated software packages for the handling and display of data. These techniques offer the potential for significant improvements in the detection and diagnosis of a large spectrum of disease processes, including cancer. Other new approaches to diagnostic imaging, such as real-time ultrasonography, microwave thermography, diaphonography, and heavy ion radiography, are also exciting developments, although their ultimate role in the detection and diagnosis of cancer is far from clear.[14] It is for this reason, as well as for the sake of brevity, that these exciting developments are mentioned only in passing.

With the wide spectrum of new radiologic technologies emerging into the medical arena, the outlook is optimistic for major improvements in the detection and diagnosis of cancer. Any attempt to realize these improvements, however, must be accompanied by an appreciation of the high cost of some of the new technologies and the need for careful evaluation of their diagnostic return before widespread introduction into the clinical arena. In addition, protocols must be designed for evaluation of the complementary imaging techniques and for identification of methods to triage patients through the maze of alternative imaging modalities if the improvements are to be used in an optimum manner.

REFERENCES

1. Ackerman, J. J. H., Grove, T. H., Wong, G. G., Gadian D. G., Radda, G. K.: Mapping of metabolites in whole animals by ^{31}P NMR using surface coils. *Nature* **283**:167–170, 1980.
2. Anger, H. O.: The scintillation camera for radioisotope localization. In *Radioisotope in der Lokalisations-Diagnostik.* Hoffman, G., Sheer, K. E. (Eds.). Stuttgart, F. K. Schattauer Verlag, 1967, p. 18.
3. Arimitsu, T., Di Chiro, G., Brooks, R. A., Smith, P. B.: White-gray matter differentiation in computed tomography. *J. Comput. Assist. Tomogr.* **1**:437–445, 1977.
4. Avis, F., Mosonov, I., Haughton, G.: Antigenic cross-reactivity between benign and malignant neoplasms of the human breast. *J. Natl. Cancer Inst.* **52**:1041–1049, 1974.
5. Ballou, B., Levine, G., Hakala, T., Karancheti, A., O'Dennell, W. F., Hakala, T. R., Schwentker, F. N., Steicher, F. M.: Tumor locations detected with radioactively labeled monoclonal antibody and external scintigraphy. *Science* **206**:545–548, 1979.
6. Barrett, H. H.: Fresnel zone plate imaging in nuclear medicine. *J. Nucl. Med.* **13**:382–385, 1982.
7. Beall, P. T., Medina, D., Chang, D. C., Seitz, P. K., Hazlewood, C. F.: Systematic effect of benign and malignant mammary tumors on the spin-lattice relaxation time of water protons in mouse serum. *J. Natl. Cancer Inst.* **59**:1431–1433, 1977.
8. Bieber, C. P., Bieber, M. M.: Detection of ferritin as a circulating tumor-associated antigen in Hodgkin's disease. *Natl. Cancer Inst. Monogr.* **36**:147–157, 1973.
9. Bloch, F.: The principle of nuclear induction. *Science* **118**:425–450, 1953.
10. Bottomley, P. A.: In vivo tumor discrimination in a rat by proton nuclear magnetic resonance imaging. *Cancer Res.* **39**:468–470, 1979.
11. Boyd, D. P., Gould, R. G., Quinn, J. R., Sparks, R., Stanley, J. H., Hermannsfeldt, W. B.: A proposed dynamic cardiac 3-D densitometer for early detection and evaluation of heart disease. *IEEE Trans. Nucl. Sci.* **NS-26**:2724–2727, 1979.
12. Bradley, W. G.: *NMR Tomography.* Milpitas, Calif., Diasonics, Inc., 1982.
13. Brady, T. J., Burt, C. T., Goldman, M. R., Pyrett, I. I., Buonnanno; F. S., Kistler, J. P., Newhouse, J. H., Hinshaw, W. S., Pohost, G. M.: Tumor characterization using ^{31}-P NMR spectroscopy. In *NMR Imaging—Proceedings of an International Symposium on NMR Imaging.*. Witcofski, R. L., Karstaedt, N., Partain, C. L. (Eds.). Winston-Salem, NC, Bowman-Gray School of Medicine, 1981, pp. 175–180.
14. Bragg, D. G., Hendee, W. R. (Eds.): *Tumor Imaging.* Norwalk, CT, Appleton-Century-Crofts, 1982.
15. Brody, W. R. (Ed.): *A Conference on Digital Radiography.* Proc. SPIE 314, Society of Photo-Optical Instrumentation Engineers, Bellingham, WA, 1981.
16. Brownell, G. L.: Advances in medical imaging. Presented at the annual meeting of the Society of Nuclear Medicine, Miami Beach, 1982.
17. Brownell, C. L., Burnham, C. A., Chesler, D. A., Correia, J. A., Correll, J. E., Hoop, B., Jr., Parker, J. A., Subramanyam, R.: Transverse section imaging of radionuclide distribution in heart, lung and brain. In *Reconstruction Tomography in Diagnostic Radiology and Nuclear Medicine.* TerPogossian, M. M., Phelps, M. E., Brownell, G. L., Cox, J. R. Jr., Davis, D. O., Evens, R. G. (Eds.). Baltimore, University Park Press, 1977, pp. 293–308.
18. Budinger, T. F.: Physical attributes of single-photon tomography. *J. Nucl. Med.* **21**:579–592, 1980.
19. Burt, C. T., Glonek, T., Barany, M.: Analysis of living tissue by phosphorus-31 magnetic resonance. *Science* **195**:145–149, 1977.
20. Carson, P. L., Meyer, C. R., Scherzinger, A. L., Oughton, T. V.: Breast imaging in coronal planes with simultaneous pulse echo and transmission ultrasound. *Science* **214**:1141–1143, 1981.
21. Carson, P. L., Scherzinger, A. L., Oughton, T. V., Kubitschek, J. E., Lambert, P. A., Dunne, M. G.: Progress in ultrasonic computed tomography (CT) of the breast. In *Application of Optical Instrumentation in Medicine VII,* Proc. SPIE. Bellingham, WA, 1980, pp. 618–635.
22. Chang, W., Lin, S. L., Henkin, R. E.: A rotatable quadrant slant hole collimator for tomography (QSH): A stationary scintillation camera based SPECT system. In *Single Photon Emission Computed Tomography and Other Selected Computer Topics.* Society of Nuclear Medicine, 1980, pp. 81–94.
23. Crooks, L. E., Hoenninger, J. C., Arakawa, H.: Tomography of hydrogen with NMR and the potential for imaging other body constituents. *Inserm.* **88**:19–34, 1979.
24. Crooks, L., Singer, J. R.: Some magnetic studies of normal and leukemia blood. *J. Clin. Engr.* **3**:237, 1978.
25. Damadian, R.: Tumor detection by nuclear magnetic resonance. *Science* **171**:1151–1153, 1981.
26. Day, E. D., Planinsek, J. A., Pressman, D.: Localization of radio-iodinated rat fibrinogen in transplanted rat tumors. *J. Natl. Cancer Inst.* **23**:799–812, 1959.
27. DeLand, F. H., Kim, E. E., Goldenberg, D. M.: Lymphoscintigraphy with radionuclide-labeled antibodies to carcinoembryonic antigen. *Cancer Res.* **40**:2997–3000, 1980.
28. DeLand, F. H., Kim, E. E., Simmons, G., Goldenberg, D. M.: Imaging approach in radioimmunodetection. *Cancer Res.* **40**:3046–3049, 1980.
29. Di Chiro, G., Brooks, R. A., Kessler, R. M., Chiro, G. D., Johnston, G. S., Jones, A. E., Hendt, J. R., Sheridan, W. T.: Tissue signatures with dual-energy computed tomography. *Radiology* **131**:521–523, 1979.
30. Duck, F. A., Hill, C. R.: Mapping true ultrasonic backscatter and attenuation distribution in tissue. A digital reconstruction approach. In *Ultrasonic Tissue Characterization II.* Linzer, M. (Ed.). NBS Spec. Pub. 525, Washington, D.C., U.S. Government Printing Office, 1979, pp. 247–254.
31. Eggleston, J. C., Saryan, L. A., Hollis, D. P.: Nuclear magnetic resonance investigations of human neoplastic and abnormal non-neoplastic tissues. *Cancer Res.* **35**:1326–1332, 1975.
32. Epstein, F. H. Nuclear magnetic resonance—a new tool in clinical medicine. *N. Engl. J. Med.* **304**:1360–1361, 1981.
33. Ettinger, D. S., Dragon, L. H., Klein, J., Sgagias, M., Order, S. E.: Isotopic immunoglobulin in an integrated multimodal treatment program for a primary liver cancer: A case report. *Cancer Treat. Rep.* **63**:131–134, 1979.
34. Freedman, G. S. Gamma camera tomography. Theory and preliminary clinical experience. *Radiology* **102**:365–369, 1972.
35. Fullerton, G. D.: Fundamentals in CT tissue characterization. In *Medical Physics of CT and Ultrasound: Tissue Imaging and Characterization.* Fullerton, G. D., Zagzebski, J. A. (Eds.). New York, American Institute of Physics, 1980.
36. Genant, H. K., Boyd, D. P., Rosenfeld, D., Abols, Y., Cann, C. E.: Quantitative bone mineral analysis using computed tomography in non-invasive measurements of bone mass and their clinical ap-

plications. In *Non-Invasive Measurements of Bone Mass and Their Clinical Applications.* Cohn, S. (Ed.). New York, CRC Press, 1981.

37. Ghose, T., Guclu, A., Tai, J., MacDonald, A. S., Norvell, S. T., Aquino, J.: Antibody as carrier of ^{131}I in cancer diagnosis and treatment. *Cancer* 36:1646–1657, 1975.

38. Ghose, T., Tai, J., Guclu, A., Norvell, S. T., Bodurtha, A., Aquino, J., MacDonald, A. S.: Antibodies as carriers of radionuclides and cytotoxic drugs in the treatment and diagnosis of cancer. *Ann. N. Y. Acad. Sci.* 277:671–689, 1976.

39. Glover, G. H., Sharp, J. C.: Reconstruction of ultrasound propagation speed distributions in soft tissue: Time-of-flight tomography. *IEEE Trans. Sonics Ultrasonics* 24:229–234, 1977.

40. Gold, P., Freeman, S. O.: Demonstration of tumor-specific antigens in human colonic carcinomata by immunological tolerance and absorption techniques. *J. Exp. Med.* 121:439–462, 1965.

41. Goldberg, H. L.: Differential diagnosis of diffuse liver disease with use of dual energy CT. *J. Comput. Assist. Tomogr.* 3:858–860, 1979.

42. Goldenberg, D. M. An introduction to the radioimmunodetection of cancer. *Cancer Res.* 40:2957–2959, 1980.

43. Goldenberg, D. M., Kim, E. E., DeLand, F. H., Van Nagell, J. R. Jr., Javadpour, N.: Clinical radioimmunodetection of cancer with radioactive antibodies to human chorionic gonadotropin. *Science* 208:1284–1286, 1980.

44. Goldenberg, D. M., Preston, D. F., Primus, F. J., Hansen, H. J.: Photoscan localization of GW-39 tumors in hamsters using radio-labeled anticarcinoembryonic antigen immunoglobulin G. *Cancer Res.* 34:1–9, 1974.

45. Greenleaf, J. F., Bahn, R. C.: Clinical imaging with transmissive ultrasonic computerized tomography. *IEEE Trans. Biomed. Eng.* BME-28:177–185, 1981.

46. Greenleaf, J. F., Johnson, S. A.: Algebraic reconstruction of spatial distributions of acoustic velocities in tissue from their time-of-flight profiles. *Acoustical Holography* 6:71–90, 1974.

47. Greenleaf, J. F., Johnson, S. A., Lee, S. L., Herman, G. T., Wood, E. H.: Algebraic reconstruction of spatial distributions of acoustic absorption within tissue from their two-dimensional acoustic projections. *Acoustic Holography* 5:591–603, 1975.

48. Greenleaf, J. F., Johnson, S. A., Samayoa, W. F., Hansen, C. R.: Refractive index by reconstruction: Use to improve compound B-scan resolution. *Acoustical Holography* 7:263–273, 1977.

49. Hawthorne, M. F., Wiersema, R. J., Takasugi, M.: Preparation of tumor-specific boron compounds. I. In vitro studies using boron-labeled antibodies and elemental boron as neutron targets. *J. Med. Chem.* 15:449–452, 1972.

50. Hendee, W. R.: *Medical Radiation Physics*, 2nd ed. Chicago, Year Book, 1979.

51. Hendee, W. R.: New technologies. *Radiographics* (Special Edition) RSNA [19]81 Exhibition Review, 47, 1981.

52. Hendee, W. R.: Nuclear magnetic resonance and its impact on medical imaging. In *Application of Optical Instrumentation in Medicine X*, Vol. 347. Society of Photo-Optical Instrumentation Engineers, 1982, pp. 330–333.

53. Hendee, W. R.: Advances in transmission computed tomography. In *Medical Diagnostic Imaging Systems*. New York, Frost & Sullivan, Inc. 1983, pp. 113–121.

54. Hendee, W. R.: *Physical Principles of Computed Tomography.* Boston, Little, Brown & Company, 1983.

55. Hill, T. C., Costello, P., Gramm, H. F., Lovett, R., McNeill, B. J., Treves, S.: Early clinical experience with a radionuclide emission computed tomographic brain imaging system. *Radiology* 128:803–806, 1978.

56. Hillman, B. J., Ovitt, T. W., Nudelman, S., Fisher, H. D., Frost, M. M., Capp, M. P., Roehrig, H., Seeley, G.: Digital video subtraction angiography of renal vascular abnormalities. *Radiology* 139:277–280, 1981.

57. Hoffer, P. B., Lathrop, K., Bekerman, C., Fang, V. S., Refetoff, S.: Use of ^{131}I-CEA antibody as a tumor scanning agent. *J. Nucl. Med.* 15:323–327, 1974.

58. Hoult, D. I.: *An Overview of NMR in Medicine.* National Center of Health Care Technology Monograph Series. Washington, D.C., U.S. Department of Health and Human Services, 1981.

59. Johnson, S. A., Greenleaf, J. F., Samayoa, W. F., Duck, F. A., Sjostrand, J. D.: Reconstruction of three-dimensional velocity fields and other parameters by acoustic ray tracing. *IEEE Ultrasound. Symp. Proc.* CHP 994-4SU, 46, 1975.

60. Jones, P. A. E., Miller, F. M., Worwood, M., Jacobs, A.: Ferritinaemia in leukemia and Hodgkin's disease. *Br. J. Cancer* 27:212–217, 1973.

61. Jones, S. M., Kitsen, F. L., Carson, P. L., Bayly, E. J.: Investigation of phase incoherent and other signal processing with a simulated array of ultrasonic CT. In *Proc. IEEE-EMBS Conf. Frontiers of Engineering in Health Care,* Oct., 1979.

62. Kak, A. C., Dines, K. A.: Signal processing of broadband pulsed ultrasound: Measurement of attenuation of soft biological tissues. *IEEE Trans. Biomed. Eng.* 25:321–344, 1978.

63. Kennett, R. H., McKearn, T. J., Bechtal, K. D. (Eds.): *Monoclonal Antibodies.* New York, Plenum Press, 1980.

64. Keyes, J. W., Jr., Orlandea, N., Heetderks, W. J., Leonard, P. F., Rogers, W. L.: The Humongotron—a scintillation-camera transaxial tomograph. *J. Nucl. Med.* 18:381–387, 1977.

65. Klepper, J. K., Brandenburger, G. H., Busse, L. J., Miller, J. G.: Phase cancellation, reflection and refraction effects in quantitative ultrasonic attenuation tomography. *Proc. IEEE Ultrasound Symp.* (IEEE #77, CH1264-1SU), 182–188, 1977.

66. Köhler, G., Milstein, C.: Continuous cultures of fused cells secreting antibody of predefined specificity. *Nature* 256:495–497, 1975.

67. Koji, T., Ishii, N., Munehisa, T., Kusumoto, Y., Nakamura, S., Tamenshi, A., Hara, A., Tsukada, Y., Nishi, S., Hirai, H.: Localization of radioiodinated antibody to α-fetoprotein in hepatoma transplanted in rats and a case report of a α-fetoprotein antibody treatment of a hepatoma patient. *Cancer Res.* 40:3013–3015, 1980.

68. Kramer, D. M.: Imaging of elements other than hydrogen. In *Nuclear Magnetic Resonance Imaging in Medicine.* Kaufman, L., Crooks, L. W., Margulis, A. R. (Eds.). Tokyo, Igaku-Shoin, 1981, p. 184.

69. Kuhl, D. E., Edwards, R. Q.: Image separation radioisotope scanning. *Radiology* 80:653–662, 1963.

70. Lauterbur, P. C.: Image formation by induced local interactions: Examples employing nuclear magnetic resonance. *Nature* 242:190–191, 1973.

71. Lehmann, L. A., Alvarez, R. E., Macovski, A., Brody, W. R., Pek, N. J., Riederer, S. J., Hall, A. L.: Generalized image combinations in dual kVp digital radiography. *Med. Phys.* 8:659–667, 1981.

72. Levy, R., Dilley, J., Fox, R. I., Warnke, R.: A human thymus-leukemia antigen defined by hybridoma monoclonal antibodies. *Proc. Natl. Acad. Sci. USA* 76:6552–6556, 1979.

73. Linzer, M. (Ed.): *Ultrasonic Tissue Characterization.* NBS Spec. Pub. 453, U.S. Dept. of Commerce, 1976.

74. Mach, J.-P., Carrel, S., Merenda, C., Sordat, B., Cerottini, J.-C.: In vivo localisation of radiolabelled antibodies to carcinoembryonic antigen human colon carcinoma grafted into nude mice. *Nature* 248:704–706, 1974.

75. Carrel, S., DeLisle, M. C., Mach, J. P.: Antiserums against carcinoembryonic antigen (CEA) can induce a specific lysis of colon carcinoma cells by normal lymphocytes. *Schweiz Med. Wochenschr.* 108(25):954–958, 1978.

76. Marcus, D. M., Zinberg, N.: Isolation of ferritin from human mammary and pancreatic carcinomas by means of antibody immunoadsorbents. *Arch. Biochem. Biophys.* 162:493–501, 1974.

77. Marshall, W. H., Easter, W., Zatz, L. M.: Analysis of the dense

lesion at computed tomography with dual kVp scans. *Radiology* 124:87–89, 1977.

78. Marx, J. L.: NMR research: Analysis of living cells and organisms. *Science* 202:958–960, 1978.

79. Mistretta, C. A., Crummy, A. B., Strother, C. M.: Digital angiography: A perspective. *Radiology* 139:273–276, 1981.

80. Mizusawa, E., Dahlman, H. L., Bennett, S. J., Goldenberg, D. M., Hawthorne, M. F.: Neutron-capture therapy of human cancer: In vitro results on the preparation of boron-labeled antibodies to carcinoembryonic antigen. *Proc. Natl. Acad. Sci. USA* 79:3011–3014, 1982.

81. Muehllehner, G.: A tomographic scintillation camera. *Phys. Med. Biol.* 16:87–96, 1981.

82. Mueller, R. K., Kaveh, M., Wade, G. Acoustical reconstruction tomography. *IEEE Proc.* 67:567–587, 1979.

83. Muller, M., Grossman, H.: An antigen in human breast cancer sera related to the murine mammary tumour virus. *Nature* 237:116–117, 1972.

84. Murphy, P. H., Thompson, W. L., Moore, M. L., Burdine, J. A.: Radionuclide computed tomography of the body using routine radiopharmaceuticals. I. System characterization. *J. Nucl. Med.* 20:102–107, 1979.

85. Nadler, L. M., Stashenko, P., Hardy, R., Schlossman, S. F.: A monoclonal antibody defining a lymphoma-associated antigen in man. *J. Immunol.* 125:570–577, 1980.

86. Newman, C. E., Ford, C. H. J., Davies, D. A. L., O'Neill, G. J.: Antibody–drug synergism: An assessment of specific passive immunotherapy in bronchial carcinoma. *Lancet* 2:163–166, 1977.

87. Norton, S. J., Linzer, M.: Tomographic reconstruction of reflectivity images. Presented at the 3rd International Symposium on Ultrasound Imaging and Tissue Characterization, Gaithersburg, MD, June 5–6, 1978 (abstr.).

88. Nunnally, R. L.: Localized measurements of metabolism by NMR methods: Some current and potential applications. In *NMR Imaging — Proceedings of an International Symposium on NMR Imaging.* Witcofski, R. L., Karstaedt, N., Partain, C. L., (Eds.). Winston-Salem, N.C., Bowman-Gray School of Medicine, 1981, pp. 181–184.

89. Olsson, L., Kaplan, H. S.: Human–human hybridomas producing monoclonal antibodies of predefined antigenic specificity. *Proc. Natl. Acad. Sci. USA* 77:5429–5431, 1980.

90. Order, S. E., Colgan, J., Hellman, S.: Distribution of fast- and slow-migrating Hodgkin's tumor-associated antigens. *Cancer Res.* 34:1182–1186, 1974.

91. Order, S. E., Donahue, V., Knapp, R.: Immunotherapy of ovarian carcinoma. An experimental model. *Cancer* 32:573–579, 1973.

92. Order, S. E., Kirkman, R., Knapp, R.: Serologic immuno-therapy: Results and probable mechanism of action. *Cancer* 34:175–183, 1974.

93. Order, S. E., Klein, J. L., Ettinger, D., Alderson, P., Siegelman, S., Leichner, P.: Phase I–II study of radiolabeled antibody integrated in the treatment of primary hepatic malignancies. *Int. J. Radiat. Oncol. Biol. Phys.* 6:703–710, 1980.

94. Order, S. E., Klein, J. L., Ettinger, D., Alderson, P., Siegelman, S., Leichner, P. Use of isotopic immunoglobulin in therapy. *Cancer Res.* 40:3001–3007, 1980.

95. Priori, E. S., Anderson, D. E., Williams, W. C., Dmochowski, L.: Immunological studies on human breast carcinoma and mouse mammary tumors. *J. Natl. Cancer Inst.* 48:1131–1135, 1972.

96. Purcell, E. M.: Research in nuclear magnetism. *Science* 118:431–436, 1953.

97. Radda, G. K., Chan, L., Bore, P. B.: Clinical applications of ^{31}P NMR. In *NMR Imaging — Proceedings of an International Symposium on NMR Imaging.* Witcofski, R. L., Karstaedt, N., Partain, C. L. (Eds.). Winston-Salem, NC, Bowman-Gray School of Medicine, 1981, pp. 159–170.

98. Reif, A. E., Li, R. W., Robinson, C. M.: Passive immuno-therapy for mouse leukemias with antisera of "directed" specificity: Synergism with the action of cyclophosphamide. *Cancer Treat. Rep.* 61:1499–1508, 1977.

99. Ritz, J., Pesando, J. M., Notis-McConarty, J., Lazarus, H., Schlossman, S. F.: A monoclonal antibody to human acute lymphoblastic leukemia antigen. *Nature* 283:583–585, 1980.

100. Rockoff, S. D., Goodenough, D. J., McIntire, K. R.: Theoretical limitations in the immunodiagnostic imaging of cancer with computed tomography and nuclear scanning. *Cancer Res.* 40:3054–3058, 1980.

101. Rogers, W. L., Koral, K. F., Mayans, R., Leonard, P. F., Thrall, J. H., Brady, T. J., Keyes, J. W. Jr.: Coded-aperture imaging of the heart. *J. Nucl. Med.* 21:371–378, 1980.

102. Ross, B. D., Radda, G. K., Gadian, D. G., Rocker, R., Esiri, M., Falconer-Smith, J.: Examination of a case of suspected McArdle's syndrome by ^{31}P nuclear magnetic resonance. *N. Engl. J. Med.* 304:1338–1342, 1981.

103. Rüegsegger, P., Elsasser, U., Anliker, M., Gnehm, H., Kind, H., Prader, A.: Quantification of bone mineralization using computed tomography. *Radiology* 121:93–97, 1976.

104. Sarcione, E. J., Smalley, J. R., Lema, M. J., Stutzman, L.: Increased ferritin synthesis and release by Hodgkin's disease peripheral blood lymphocytes. *Int. J. Cancer* 20:339–346, 1977.

105. Scharff, M. D., Roberts, S., Thammana, P.: Hybridomas as a source of antibodies. *Hosp. Pract.* 16:61–66, 1981.

106. Sfakianakis, G. H., DeLand, F. H.: Radioimmunodiagnosis and radioimmunotherapy. *J. Nucl. Med.* 23:840–850, 1982.

107. Siegelman, S. S., Zerhouni, E. A., Leo, F. P., Khouri, N. F., Stitik, F. P.: CT of the solitary pulmonary nodule. *A. J. R.* 135:1–13, 1980.

108. Smith, F. W., Hutchison, J. M. S., Mallard, J. R., Johnson, G., Redpath, T. W., Selbie, R. D., Reid, A., Smith, C. C.: Oesophageal carcinoma demonstrated by whole-body nuclear magnetic resonance imaging. *Br. Med. J.* 282:510–512, 1981.

109. Stokely, E. M., Tipton, D. M., Buju, L. M., Lewis, S. E., DeVous, M. D., Sr., Bonte, F. J., Parkey, R. W., Willerson, J. T.: Quantitation of experimental canine infarct size with multipinhole and rotating-slanthole tomography. *J. Nucl. Med.* 22:55–61, 1981.

110. TerPogossian, M. M., Raichle, M. E., Sobel, B. E.: Positron-emission tomography. *Sci. Am.* 243:170–181, 1980.

111. Vogel, R. A., Kirch, D., LeFree, M., Steele, P.: A new method of multiplanar emission tomography using a seven pinhole collimator and an Anger scintillation camera. *J. Nucl. Med.* 19:648–654, 1978.

112. Wright, T., Sinanan, M., Harrington, D., Klein, J. L., Order, S. Immunoglobulin: Applications to scanning and treatment. *Appl. Radiol.* 8:120–124, 1979.

113. Yelton, D. E., Scharff, M. D.: Monoclonal antibodies. *Am. Sci.* 68:510–516, 1980.

114. Yelton, D. E., Scharff, M. D.: Monoclonal antibodies: A powerful new tool in biology and medicine. *Ann. Rev. Biochem.* 50:657–680, 1981.

INDEX

Key: Letters following page numbers indicate figures (*f*) and/or tables (*t*).